Problem Solving in Radiology
Cardiovascular Imaging

Problem Solving in Radiology

Cardiovascular Imaging

Suhny Abbara, MD, FSCCT
Associate Professor of Radiology
Harvard Medical School
Director, Cardiac Imaging Fellowship
Department of Radiology
Director of Education
Cardiac MR/PET/CT Program
Massachusetts General Hospital
Boston, Massachusetts

Sanjeeva P. Kalva, MD, FSIR
Associate Division Head
Vascular Imaging and Intervention
Director, Center for Image-Guided Cancer Therapy
Massachusetts General Hospital
Assistant Professor of Radiology
Harvard Medical School
Boston, Massachusetts

ELSEVIER
SAUNDERS

SAUNDERS

1600 John F. Kennedy Blvd.
Ste 1800
Philadelphia, PA 19103-2899

PROBLEM SOLVING IN RADIOLOGY: CARDIOVASCULAR IMAGING   ISBN: 978-1-4377-2768-5
Copyright © 2013 by Saunders, an imprint of Elsevier Inc.

Notices

Knowledge and best practice in this field are constantly changing. As new research and experience broaden our understanding, changes in research methods, professional practices, or medical treatment may become necessary.

Practitioners and researchers must always rely on their own experience and knowledge in evaluating and using any information, methods, compounds, or experiments described herein. In using such information or methods, they should be mindful of their own safety and the safety of others, including parties for whom they have a professional responsibility.

With respect to any drug or pharmaceutical products identified, readers are advised to check the most current information provided (i) on procedures featured or (ii) by the manufacturer of each product to be administered to verify the recommended dose or formula, the method and duration of administration, and contraindications. It is the responsibility of practitioners, relying on their own experience and knowledge of their patients, to make diagnoses, to determine dosages and the best treatment for each individual patient, and to take all appropriate safety precautions.

To the fullest extent of the law, neither the Publisher nor the authors, contributors, or editors assume any liability for any injury and/or damage to persons or property as a matter of products liability, negligence, or otherwise, or from any use or operation of any methods, products, instructions, or ideas contained in the material herein.

Library of Congress Cataloging-in-Publication Data
Problem solving in radiology. Cardiovascular imaging / [edited by] Suhny Abbara, Sanjeeva P. Kalva.
    p. ; cm.—(Problem solving in radiology)
Cardiovascular imaging
Includes bibliographical references.
ISBN 978-1-4377-2768-5 (hardcover : alk. paper)
I. Abbara, Suhny. II. Kalva, Sanjeeva P. III. Title: Cardiovascular imaging. IV. Series: Problem solving in radiology.
[DNLM: 1. Cardiovascular Diseases—diagnosis. 2. Diagnostic Imaging—methods. 3. Diagnostic Techniques, Cardiovascular. WG 141]
    616.1'0757--dc23   2012040007

Content Strategist: Helene Caprari
Content Development Specialist: Joanie Milnes
Publishing Services Manager: Anne Altepeter
Senior Project Manager: Doug Turner
Designer: Steve Stave

Printed in China

Last digit is the print number: 9 8 7 6 5 4 3 2 1

Foreword

Early in the twentieth century, physicians recognized the power of noninvasive imaging to guide diagnosis and patient management in cardiovascular disease. By the 1980s both echocardiography and rest and stress nuclear perfusion imaging had become part of routine patient assessment, which focused primarily on the assessment of left ventricle function and perfusion. At the time, however, assessment of coronary artery disease was limited to invasive coronary angiography, and structural imaging of the myocardium was not yet possible; thus imaging remained a small and easily overlooked field within cardiovascular medicine. We have come a long way since as we have seen a revolution in cardiovascular imaging driven by the introduction and development of cardiac computed tomography (CT) and magnetic resonance imaging (MRI).

In the early 1990s, IMATRON, a small company out of San Francisco, introduced cardiac electron beam CT (EBCT) to the general public, and that changed cardiovascular medicine forever. I remember how impressed I was as a medical student examining patients on an EBCT prototype in Erlangen, Germany, as part of my medical thesis. The EBCT scanner needed a second large room to accommodate the cooling system and computer power, but it allowed for the motion-free visualization of the coronary artery tree with an assessment of stenosis on a regular basis because an image could be acquired within 50 msec (while traditional CT scanners at the time needed 1 full second). The EBCT era culminated in an article by Stephan Achenbach in 1998 published in the *New England Journal of Medicine,* but surprisingly EBCT technology was used primarily to detect and quantify coronary artery calcification in the setting of primary prevention on the West Coast of the United States. However, it triggered the development of multidetector CT (MDCT), a technology developed by Willy Kalender from Erlangen. What started in the late 1990s with four-slice MDCT has now grown into a technology with submillimeter spatial resolution and an image acquisition time of less than 1 second that reliably allows noninvasive assessment of coronary artery stenosis and atherosclerotic plaque morphology and composition. With this improvement in CT technology came the ability to assess complex cardiac morphology, heart valves, and myocardial perfusion and function. Today more than 3000 cardiac imaging–capable units can be found in the United States alone.

Although cardiac MRI has been around more than 10 years longer than CT, it has matured more slowly. Probably the most important and novel finding was published in the *New England Journal of Medicine* in 2000 by Raymond Kim and Bob Bonow from Northwestern University in which they described the phenomenon of delayed myocardial enhancement, which allowed for the prediction of functional recovery after revascularization. This triggered further development of the assessment of myocardial structure and perfusion, and today we are able to differentiate and predict infarct territory, including the core of microvascular obstruction with irreversible loss of function from myocardial edema and reversible dysfunction. In fact, in coronary disease, coronary CT angiography has developed into the primary assessment tool for patients without known coronary artery disease, whereas MRI is a very potent guide for revascularization in patients with already known coronary artery disease, a group of patients that is steadily growing. MR technology has also developed from 1.5T to 3T magnets, and today cardiac MRI is a routine diagnostic tool available at most major institutions.

Thus today's imagers are faced with an ever-increasing choice of advanced and steadily evolving imaging techniques and increasing subspecialization in all aspects of the diagnosis and management of cardiovascular disease. Given today's economic constraints in the health care sector and the increasing need for efficient patient management, it is important to provide educational materials that comprehensively cover the multiple modalities across cardiovascular imaging and decision support for ordering physicians.

Drs. Abbara and Kalva, two well-recognized experts in the field, have brought together a wide range of authors who are leaders in their respective fields. All can be congratulated for providing unique and in-depth coverage to the entire spectrum of cardiovascular disease, including anatomy, diagnosis and patient management, and technical and risk benefit aspects across modalities.

Published within the well-known Problem Solving series, this book provides a compendium that also offers complimentary online access to regularly updated web content, which will ensure that readers can keep track of ongoing breakthroughs in this exciting field.

Problem Solving in Radiology: Cardiovascular Imaging is an excellent guide and source for residents, fellows, and practitioners in both cardiology and radiology and for those who want to refresh their knowledge in the multimodality field of cardiovascular imaging.

Udo Hoffmann, MD, MPH
Associate Professor of Radiology
Harvard Medical School
Division Head, Cardiac Imaging
Department of Radiology
Director, Cardiac MR/PET/CT Program
Massachusetts General Hospital
Boston, Massachusetts

Preface

This cardiovascular imaging textbook in the Problem Solving series publishes at a remarkable time. Since the early 2000s there have been dramatic developments in the field of cardiovascular medicine and imaging. These developments include (among many others) the creation and maturation of multidetector coronary computed tomographic angiography, newer noncontrast magnetic resonance angiography (MRA) and blood pool–contrast MRA, magnetic resonance imaging (MRI)-based scar and viability imaging, particle tracking and other novel techniques, the ripening of alternatives to radionuclide imaging to demonstrate myocardial ischemia, and many novel therapies. Most notable is the development of novel image-guided minimally invasive therapies, which often rely on noninvasive preprocedure imaging for planning purposes. These procedures include, but are not limited to, endoluminal stent graft placement to treat aortic aneurysms, pulmonary vein isolation procedures to treat atrial fibrillation, transcatheter device treatment of septal and other shunts, and transcatheter aortic valve implantation/replacement (TAVI/R) to treat stenotic aortic valves, just to name a few. Hence many new applications and indications for cross-sectional cardiac and vascular imaging have surfaced since 2000. New or underrecognized disease entities have been brought to light and the incidence of some anomalies, normal variants, or conditions have had to be revised now that we have better tools to visualize their respective structures. We have called upon a cadre of more than 90 expert contributors to systematically review the many new developments and present them in a didactically meaningful way.

The text is organized to systematically review the technical nuances and acquisition methods of the various imaging modalities at our disposal, including multidetector computerized tomography, MRI, radionuclide imaging, ultrasound and echocardiography, and catheter angiography. This is followed by a review and illustration of the respective appearance of cardiac and vascular anatomy within each of the imaging modalities and a critical review of when to use which test. After this general discussion, this book is organized by disease entities that affect the cardiovascular system. Each disease entity or spectrum of entities is reviewed in-depth, with a special emphasis on the role of imaging, problem solving, and the multimodality imaging appearance of the diseases and their differential diagnostic entities.

We hope that this initiative will prove useful in the day-to-day care of patients with cardiovascular disease, serve as a stimulus for future research in basic and clinical science, and provide a utilitarian reference source for all health care professionals, trainees, scientists, and biomedical researchers active in the field of cardiovascular medicine in the twenty-first century. Hopefully, in some way, all of the effort and expertise brought together here will help advance our field. And on behalf of all the authors, we truly hope that you will find this text informative, enjoyable, and helpful, whether you are a radiologist, cardiologist, nuclear medicine specialist, resident, fellow medical student, or technologist.

Suhny Abbara, MD, FSCCT
Sanjeeva P. Kalva, MD, FSIR

Acknowledgments

I am very grateful to all the contributing authors and to my co-workers in radiology and cardiology, including our fellows, residents, students, and technologists, for their invaluable direct and indirect contributions. Their many contributions to this work, and to the field of cardiovascular imaging in general, may not always be directly apparent.

At the risk of overlooking some important contributors (if such is the case, please forgive me), special thanks go to Drs. Tom Brady, Sanjeev Francis, Brian Ghoshhajra, Udo Hoffmann, Fred Holmvang, and Jim Thrall for enabling this work, and to our outstanding technologists, Steve Bradley, Maggie Hird, Dave Brennan, Jim Hickey, Jake Calkins, and Steve Barry, to name just a few. Our students' and trainees' academic curiosity and various backgrounds challenge us to keep learning and truly enrich the academic environment—thank you. Special thanks go to Dr. Gladwin Hui for proofreading many of the chapters and to the editorial team at Elsevier for their excellent support.

Thanks also go to Dr. Sanjeeva Kalva for accepting my invitation to edit the vascular portion of this text; I know how many hours this took out of his academic and private life. His expertise was invaluable, and he did a phenomenal job seeing this through.

Last but not least, I am grateful to my wife, Dr. Amanda Fox. Juggling the clinical, on-call, and scholarly responsibilities for two professionals while maintaining a rich family life is not easy and requires extraordinary organizational talent. Thank you, Amanda, for making it all possible!

Suhny Abbara, MD, FSCCT

Sincere thanks to Dr. Suhny Abbara, who trusted me and invited me to edit the vascular section of this textbook. Thanks to all the contributors who spent their significant family and personal time to author their chapters.

No words of thanks are sufficient to express my gratitude to my mentors, teachers, colleagues, residents, and fellows who inspire me every day and contribute to my learning. Thanks to my nurses and technologists, who every day make my life easy with their excellent teamwork.

Special thanks to Kakarla Subbarao, Mathew Cherian, and Christos Athanasoulis, who have played significant roles in my life during my radiology career. Thanks to Jim Thrall, whose continued support and encouragement made this book a reality. Thanks to Dushyant Sahani, Sanjay Saini, Peter Mueller, Chieh-Min Fan, Arthur Waltman, Stuart Geller, Alan Greenfield, and Stephan Wicky for giving me the opportunity to learn, collaborate, and work together at Massachusetts General Hospital. Thanks to the editorial team at Elsevier for their support.

Thanks to my wife, Vijaya, and sons, Praneeth and Praveen, who supported my efforts with love and pride.

Sanjeeva P. Kalva, MD, FSIR

Contributors

Suhny Abbara, MD, FSCCT
Associate Professor of Radiology
Harvard Medical School
Director, Cardiac Imaging Fellowship
Department of Radiology
Director of Education
Cardiac MR/PET/CT Program
Massachusetts General Hospital
Boston, Massachusetts
Comparative Anatomy
Cardiac Valves
Cardiac Devices
Cardiac Masses
Pericardial Disease
Thoracic Aorta and Its Branches

Gerald F. Abbott, MD
Associate Professor
Harvard Medical School
Associate Radiologist
Massachusetts General Hospital
Boston, Massachusetts
Pulmonary Arteries

Stephan Achenbach, MD
Professor of Medicine
Department of Cardiology
University of Giessen
Giessen, Germany
Coronary Arteries: Coronary Atherosclerotic Disease

Chaitanya Ahuja, MD
Clinical Fellow
Dotter Interventional Institute
Oregon Health and Science University
Portland, Oregon
Lower Extremity Arteries

Tharakeswara K. Bathala, MD
Assistant Professor
Department of Diagnostic Radiology
The University of Texas MD Anderson Cancer
  Center
Houston, Texas
Vascular Ultrasound

Sanjeev Bhalla, MD
Professor of Radiology
Mallinckrodt Institute of Radiology
Washington University School of Medicine
St. Louis, Missouri
Imaging for Congenital Cardiovascular Disease

Ron Blankstein, MD, FACC
Co-Director, Noninvasive Cardiovascular Imaging
  Training Program
Cardiovascular Division and Department
  of Radiology
Brigham and Women's Hospital
Assistant Professor in Medicine and Radiology
Harvard Medical School
Boston, Massachusetts
When to Choose What Test (Cardiac)

Thorsten A. Bley, MD
Associate Professor of Radiology
Department of Radiology
University Medical Center Hamburg-Eppendorf
Hamburg, Germany
Inflammatory and Infectious Vascular Disorders

Matthew J. Budoff, MD
Professor of Medicine
David Geffen School of Medicine
University of California, Los Angeles
Los Angeles, California
Director of Cardiac CT
Los Angeles Biomedical Research Institute
Torrance, California
Atherosclerosis: Role of Calcium Scoring

Brett W. Carter, MD
Director and Section Chief, Thoracic Imaging
Baylor University Medical Center
Dallas, Texas
Cardiac Devices
Cardiac Masses
Pulmonary Arteries

Alexander Oscar Quiroz Casian, MD
Rush University Medical Center
Chicago, Illinois
Vascular Devices

Meghna Chadha, MD, DNB
Assistant Professor
Department of Radiology Wayne State University
Detroit, Michigan
Lower Extremity Arteries

Mathew P. Cherian, MD
Chief of Radiology Services
Director, Interventional Radiology
Department of Diagnostic and Interventional
  Radiology
Kovai Medical Center and Hospital
Coimbatore, India
Bronchial Arteries

Jonathan H. Chung, MD
Assistant Professor
Department of Radiology
National Jewish Health
Denver, Colorado
Thoracic Aorta and Its Branches

Kristopher W. Cummings, MD
Assistant Professor
Cardiothoracic Imaging
Mallinckrodt Institute of Radiology
Washington University School of Medicine
St Louis, Missouri
Imaging for Congenital Cardiovascular Disease
Myocardial Nonischemic Cardiomyopathies

Stephan Danik, MD
Instructor in Medicine
Cardiology Division
Massachusetts General Hospital
Boston, Massachusetts
Role of Magnetic Resonance Imaging in Cardiomyopathies

Milind Y. Desai, MD, FACC, FAHA, FESC
Associate Professor of Medicine
Department of Cardiovascular Medicine
Heart and Vascular Institute
Cleveland Clinic
Cleveland, Ohio
Pulmonary Veins, Atria, and Atrial Appendage

Jonathan D. Dodd, MD, MSc, MRCPI, FFR(RCSI)
Consultant Radiologist
St. Vincent's University Hospital
Associate Professor
University College Dublin
Dublin, Ireland
Cardiac Anatomy on Magnetic Resonance Imaging
Coronary Arteries: Anomalies, Normal Variants, Aneurysms,
  and Fistulas

Sharmila Dorbala, MD, MPH
Director, Nuclear Cardiology
The Noninvasive Cardiovascular Imaging Program
Departments of Radiology (Division of Nuclear
  Medicine and Molecular Imaging) and Medicine
  (Cardiology)
Brigham and Women's Hospital
Boston, Massachusetts
Radionuclide Imaging (Cardiac)
Myocardial Ischemic Disease: Nuclear

Daniel W. Entrikin, MD
Associate Professor
Chief, Section of Cardiothoracic Radiology
Director of Computed Tomography
Departments of Radiology and Internal Medicine
Section on Cardiology
Wake Forest University School of Medicine
Winston-Salem, North Carolina
Valves: Computed Tomography

Chieh-Min Fan, MD
Associate Director
Division of Angiography and Interventional
  Radiology
Brigham and Women's Hospital
Assistant Professor
Department of Radiology
Harvard Medical School
Boston, Massachusetts
Venous Insufficiency

Khashayar Farsad, MD, PhD
Assistant Professor
Dotter Interventional Institute and Diagnostic
  Radiology
Oregon Health and Science University
Portland, Oregon
Bronchial Arteries
Abdominal Aorta and Branches

Kathryn J. Fowler, MD
Instructor of Radiology
Director, Abdominal and Pelvic MRI
Mallinckrodt Institute of Radiology
Washington University School of Medicine
St. Louis, Missouri
Magnetic Resonance Angiography: Technique

Christopher J. François, MD
Assistant Professor
Cardiovascular and Chest Sections
Department of Radiology
University of Wisconsin School of Medicine
  and Public Health
Madison, Wisconsin
Inflammatory and Infectious Vascular Disorders

Matthias G. Friedrich, MD, FESC, FACC
Professor of Medicine
Department of Cardiology
Université de Montréal
Adjunct Professor of Medicine
Departments of Cardiac Sciences and Radiology
University of Calgary
Director, CMR Research at the Montreal Heart
  Institute
Hornstein Chair in Cardiovascular Imaging
Montreal Heart Institute
Montréal, Quebec, Canada
*Current Role of Magnetic Resonance Imaging for Suspected
  Myocarditis*

Felix M. Gonzalez, MD
Radiology Resident
Department of Diagnostic Radiology and Nuclear
  Medicine
University of Maryland
Baltimore, Maryland
*Cardiac Computed Tomography for the Evaluation of Acute
  Coronary Syndrome in the Emergency Department*

Nikhil Goyal, MD
Section Chief, Cardiac Imaging
Department of Radiology
Staten Island University Hospital
Staten Island, New York
Pericardial Disease

John D. Grizzard, MD
Associate Professor
Department of Radiology
Virginia Commonwealth University
Richmond, Virginia
Myocardial Ischemic Disease: Magnetic Resonance Imaging

Martin L. Gunn, MD
Associate Professor
Department of Radiology
University of Washington
Seattle, Washington
Thoracic Aorta and Its Branches

Jörg Hausleiter, MD
Professor of Medicine, Cardiology
Medizinische Klinik und Poliklinik I
Ludwig-Maximilians-Universität München
Munich, Germany
Radiation Issues

Sandeep S. Hedgire, MD
Clinical Research Fellow
Division of Abdominal Imaging and Intervention
Massachusetts General Hospital
Harvard Medical School
Boston, Massachusetts
Catheter Angiography (Vascular)
Upper Extremity Arteries

Travis S. Henry, MD
Assistant Professor of Radiology
Emory University School of Medicine
Atlanta, Georgia
Myocardial Nonischemic Cardiomyopathies

Laura E. Heyneman, MD
Associate Clinical Professor of Radiology
UNC Health Care
Chapel Hill, North Carolina
Imaging the Postoperative Thoracic Aorta

Gladwin Hui, MD, MPH
Clinical Fellow, Cardiac Imaging
Department of Radiology
Massachusetts General Hospital
Harvard Medical School
Boston, Massachusetts
Cardiac Devices

David T. Hunt, RVT, RDMS, RT(S)
Sonographer
Neurovascular Laboratory
Massachusetts General Hospital
Boston, Massachusetts
Carotid and Vertebral Arteries

Brian G. Hynes, MB, BCh
Fellow in Interventional Cardiology
Massachusetts General Hospital
Boston, Massachusetts
Coronary Angiography: Technique
Cardiac Anatomy on Coronary Angiography

Jill E. Jacobs, MD
Professor of Radiology
New York University Medical Center
New York, New York
Cardiac Anatomy on Computed Tomography

Carlos Jamis-Dow, MD
Associate Professor of Radiology
Penn State Milton S. Hershey Medical Center
Hershey, Pennsylvania
Cardiac Devices

Ik-Kyung Jang, MD, PhD
Professor of Medicine
Cardiology Division
Massachusetts General Hospital
Boston, Massachusetts
Coronary Angiography: Technique
Cardiac Anatomy on Coronary Angiography

Christoph J. Jensen, MD
Research Fellow
Duke Cardiovascular Magnetic Resonance Center
Duke University Medical Center
Durham, North Carolina
Myocardial Ischemic Disease: Magnetic Resonance Imaging

Philip R. John, MBChB, DCH, FRCR, FRCPC
Associate Professor
Department of Medical Imaging
University of Toronto
Director, Vascular Anomalies Clinic
Division Head, Interventional Radiology
The Hospital for Sick Children
Toronto, Ontario, Canada
Vascular Anomalies

Jason M. Johnson, MD, USAFR
Clinical Instructor in Radiology
Department of Radiology
Massachusetts General Hospital
Harvard Medical School
Boston, Massachusetts
Carotid and Vertebral Arteries

Sanjeeva P. Kalva, MD, FSIR
Associate Division Head
Vascular Imaging and Intervention
Director, Center for Image-Guided Cancer Therapy
Massachusetts General Hospital
Assistant Professor of Radiology
Harvard Medical School
Boston, Massachusetts
Catheter Angiography (Vascular)
Vascular Devices
Thoracic Aorta and Its Branches
Bronchial Arteries
Upper Extremity Arteries
Lower Extremity Arteries
Deep Venous Thrombosis

Avinash Kambadakone, MD, DNB, FRCR
Instructor of Radiology
Division of Abdominal Imaging and Intervention
Massachusetts General Hospital
Boston, Massachusetts
Computed Tomography Angiography (Vascular)
Vascular Anatomy and Variants

Niamh M. Kilcullen, MB, BCh
Clinical and Research Fellow in Medicine
Massachusetts General Hospital
Research Fellow in Medicine
Harvard Medical School
Boston, Massachusetts
Echocardiography
Valves: Echocardiography

Ronan Kileen, MB
Consultant Radiologist
Department of Radiology
Hermitage Medical Clinic
Dublin, Ireland
Cardiac Anatomy on Magnetic Resonance Imaging
*Coronary Arteries: Anomalies, Normal Variants, Aneurysms,
    and Fistulas*

Raymond J. Kim, MD
Professor of Medicine and Radiology
Director, Duke Cardiovascular Magnetic Resonance
    Center
Duke University Medical Center
Durham, North Carolina
Myocardial Ischemic Disease: Magnetic Resonance Imaging

Angela S. Koh, MBBS, MRCP(UK)
Clinical Fellow
Noninvasive Cardiovascular Imaging Program
Brigham and Women's Hospital
Harvard Medical School
Boston, Massachusetts
Consultant Cardiologist
National Heart Centre Singapore
Singapore
Radionuclide Imaging (Cardiac)
Myocardial Ischemic Disease: Nuclear

Raymond Y. Kwong, MD, MPH
Director of Cardiac Magnetic Resonance Imaging
Assistant Professor of Medicine
Brigham and Women's Hospital
Harvard Medical School
Boston, Massachusetts
Cardiac Magnetic Resonance Imaging: Techniques and Protocols

Sampson K. Kyere, MD, PhD
Resident
Department of Diagnostic Radiology
University of Maryland Medical Center
Baltimore, Maryland
*Cardiac Computed Tomography for the Evaluation of Acute
    Coronary Syndrome in the Emergency Department*

John P. Lichtenberger III, MD
Chief of Cardiothoracic Imaging
Department of Radiology
David Grant Medical Center
Travis Air Force Base, California
Assistant Professor
Department of Radiology and Radiological Sciences
Uniformed Services University of the Health
    Sciences
Bethesda, Maryland
Cardiac Devices
Cardiac Masses

Victoria L. Mango, MD
Assistant Professor of Radiology
Columbia University Medical Center
New York, New York
Cardiac Anatomy on Computed Tomography

Santiago Martínez-Jiménez, MD
Associate Professor of Radiology
Saint Luke's Hospital of Kansas City
University of Missouri, Kansas City
Kansas City, Missouri
Imaging the Postoperative Thoracic Aorta

Anna Meader, MD(c), BS
Neurovascular Sonographer
Tufts University School of Medicine
Department of Neuroradiology
Massachusetts General Hospital
Boston, Massachusetts
Carotid and Vertebral Arteries

Stephen W. Miller, MD
Thoracic Radiologist
Massachusetts General Hospital
Associate Professor of Radiology
Harvard Medical School
Boston, Massachusetts
Cardiovascular Anatomy and Pathology on Radiography

François-Pierre Mongeon, MD, SM, FRCPC
Clinical Assistant Professor of Medicine
Université de Montréal
Noninvasive Cardiology Service
Department of Medicine
Montreal Heart Institute
Montréal, Quebec, Canada
Cardiac Magnetic Resonance Imaging: Techniques and Protocols

Venkatesh L. Murthy, MD, PhD
Assistant Professor of Medicine and Radiology
Divisions of Cardiovascular Medicine, Nuclear
    Medicine, and Cardiothoracic Radiology
University of Michigan
Ann Arbor, Michigan
When to Choose What Test (Cardiac)

John W. Nance Jr., MD
House Officer
Russell H. Morgan Department of Radiology
    and Radiological Science
Johns Hopkins Hospital
Baltimore, Maryland
Myocardial Ischemic Disease: Computed Tomography

Vamsi R. Narra, MD, FRCR
Professor of Radiology
Chief, Abdominal Imaging Section
Chief of Radiology
Barnes-Jewish West County Hospital
Mallinckrodt Institute of Radiology
Washington University School of Medicine
St. Louis, Missouri
Magnetic Resonance Angiography: Technique

Smita Patel, MBBS, MRCP, FRCR
Associate Professor
Division of Cardiothoracic Radiology
Cardiovascular Center
University of Michigan Health System
Ann Arbor, Michigan
Coronary Artery Bypass Grafts

Michael H. Picard, MD
Professor
Harvard Medical School
Director, Clinical Echocardiography
Massachusetts General Hospital
Boston, Massachusetts
Echocardiography
Valves: Echocardiography

Anil Kumar Pillai, MD
Assistant Professor
Department of Diagnostic Radiology
Rush University Medical Center
Chicago, Illinois
Vascular Devices

Ferenc Czeyda-Pommersheim, MD
Assistant Professor
Department of Radiology
University of Pittsburgh
Pittsburgh, Pennsylvania
Imaging for Congenital Cardiovascular Disease

Prabhakar Rajiah, MD, MBBS, FRCR
Clinical Fellow
Cleveland Clinic Foundation
Cleveland, Ohio
Pulmonary Veins, Atria, and Atrial Appendage

Constantine A. Raptis, MD
Assistant Professor of Radiology
Director, Thoracic MRI
Mallinckrodt Institute of Radiology
Washington University School of Medicine
St. Louis, Missouri
Magnetic Resonance Angiography: Technique

Gautham P. Reddy, MD, MPH
Professor of Radiology and Vice Chair for Education
University of Washington
Seattle, Washington
Valves: Magnetic Resonance Imaging

Otávio Rizzi Coelho-Filho, MD, MPH
Cardiac MRI and CT Program
State University of Campinas—UNICAMP
Campinas, São Paulo, Brazil
Cardiac Magnetic Resonance Imaging: Techniques and Protocols

Carlos Andres Rojas, MD
Assistant Professor
Department of Radiology
University of South Florida
Tampa, Florida
Comparative Anatomy
Pericardial Disease
Septal Defects and Other Cardiovascular Shunts

Javier M. Romero, MD
Director of Ultrasound
Staff Neuroradiologist
Associate Director of Neurovascular Laboratory
Massachusetts General Hospital
Assistant Professor of Radiology
Harvard Medical School
Boston, Massachusetts
Carotid and Vertebral Arteries

Sion K. Roy, MD
Cardiology Fellow
Harbor-University of California, Los Angeles
Torrance, California
Atherosclerosis: Role of Calcium Scoring

Jeremy Ruskin, MD
Cardiac Arrhythmia Service
Massachusetts General Hospital
Boston, Massachusetts
Role of Magnetic Resonance Imaging in Cardiomyopathies

U. Joseph Schoepf, MD, FAHA, FSCBT-MR, FSCCT
Professor of Radiology, Medicine, and Pediatrics
Director of Cardiovascular Imaging
Department of Radiology and Radiological Science
Medical University of South Carolina
Charleston, South Carolina
Myocardial Ischemic Disease: Computed Tomography

Vikram Venkatesh, MD
Cardiac Radiologist
Assistant Clinical Professor
(Adjunct) Radiology
McMaster University
Department of Radiology
Grand River Hospital
Kitchener, Ontario, Canada
Cardiac Valves

Emmanuelle Vermes, MD
Research Fellow
Stephenson Cardiovascular MR Centre
Libin Cardiovascular Institute of Alberta
Departments of Cardiac Sciences and Radiology
University of Calgary
Calgary, Alberta, Canada
Current Role of Magnetic Resonance Imaging for Suspected Myocarditis

Dharshan Raj Vummidi, MBBS, MRCP, FRCR
Division of Cardiothoracic Radiology
Cardiovascular Center
University of Michigan Health System
Ann Arbor, Michigan
Coronary Artery Bypass Grafts

Christopher M. Walker, MD
Cardiothoracic Imaging Fellow
Department of Radiology
Massachusetts General Hospital
Boston, Massachusetts
Valves: Magnetic Resonance Imaging

Arthur C. Waltman, MD
Staff Radiologist
Department of Radiology
Massachusetts General Hospital
Boston, Massachusetts
Upper Extremity Arteries

William Guy Weigold, MD
Director, Cardiac CT Program
MedStar Washington Hospital Center
Washington, District of Columbia
Cardiac Gated Computed Tomography

Charles S. White, MD
Professor of Radiology
Director of Thoracic Imaging
University of Maryland
Baltimore, Maryland
Cardiac Computed Tomography for the Evaluation of Acute Coronary Syndrome in the Emergency Department

James Kin Ho Woo, MD, BSc
Radiologist
Ellesmere X-ray Associates
Toronto, Ontario, Canada
Cardiovascular Anatomy and Pathology on Radiography

Joo Heung Yoon, MD
Research Fellow
Division of Cardiology
Massachusetts General Hospital
Boston, Massachusetts
Cardiac Anatomy on Coronary Angiography

Contents

SECTION I   Imaging Technique

1. Echocardiography   3
   Niamh M. Kilcullen and Michael H. Picard

2. Coronary Angiography: Technique   37
   Brian G. Hynes and Ik-Kyung Jang

3. Cardiac Gated Computed Tomography   60
   William Guy Weigold

4. Cardiac Magnetic Resonance Imaging: Techniques and Protocols   79
   François-Pierre Mongeon, Otávio Rizzi Coelho-Filho, and Raymond Y. Kwong

5. Radionuclide Imaging (Cardiac)   91
   Sharmila Dorbala and Angela S. Kohl

6. Vascular Ultrasound   111
   Tharakeswara K. Bathala

7. Computed Tomography Angiography (Vascular)   121
   Avinash Kambadakone

8. Magnetic Resonance Angiography: Technique   131
   Constantine A. Raptis, Kathryn J. Fowler, and Vamsi R. Narra

9. Catheter Angiography (Vascular)   155
   Sandeep S. Hedgire and Sanjeeva P. Kalva

10. When to Choose What Test (Cardiac)   163
    Venkatesh L. Murthy and Ron Blankstein

SECTION II   Anatomy

11. Cardiovascular Anatomy and Pathology on Radiography   179
    Stephen W. Miller and James Kin Ho Woo

12. Cardiac Anatomy on Computed Tomography   215
    Victoria L. Mango and Jill E. Jacobs

13. Cardiac Anatomy on Magnetic Resonance Imaging   225
    Jonathan D. Dodd and Ronan Kileen

14. Cardiac Anatomy on Coronary Angiography   232
    Joo Heung Yoon, Brian G. Hynes, and Ik-Kyung Jang

15. Vascular Anatomy and Variants   248
    Avinash Kambadakone

16. Comparative Anatomy   267
    Carlos Andres Rojas and Suhny Abbara

SECTION III   Devices

17. Cardiac Valves   279
    Vikram Venkatesh and Suhny Abbara

18. Cardiac Devices   298
    John P. Lichtenberger III, Gladwin Hui, Brett W. Carter, Carlos Jamis-Dow, and Suhny Abbara

19. Vascular Devices   313
    Anil Kumar Pillai, Alexander Oscar Quiroz Casian, and Sanjeeva P. Kalva

SECTION IV   Special Situations

20. Imaging for Congenital Cardiovascular Disease   335
    Kristopher W. Cummings, Ferenc Czeyda-Pommersheim, and Sanjeev Bhalla

21. Role of Magnetic Resonance Imaging in Cardiomyopthies   357
    Stephan Danik and Jeremy Ruskin

22. Atherosclerosis: Role of Calcium Scoring   370
    Sion K. Roy and Matthew J. Budoff

23. Cardiac Computed Tomography for the Evaluation of Acute Coronary Syndrome in the Emergency Department   382
    Felix M. Gonzalez, Sampson K. Kyere, and Charles S. White

24. Imaging the Postoperative Thoracic Aorta   394
    Santiago Martínez-Jiménez and Laura E. Heyneman

25. Inflammatory and Infectious Vascular Disorders   412
    Thorsten A. Bley and Christopher J. François

26. Current Role of Magnetic Resonance Imaging for Suspected Myocarditis   423
    Emmanuelle Vermes and Matthias G. Friedrich

27. Radiation Issues   431
    Jörg Hausleiter

SECTION V   Disease Entities by Anatomic Region

28. Myocardial Ischemic Disease: Magnetic Resonance Imaging   441
    John D. Grizzard, Christoph J. Jensen, and Raymond J. Kim

29. Myocardial Ischemic Disease: Nuclear   464
    Sharmila Dorbala and Angela S. Koh

30. Myocardial Ischemic Disease: Computed Tomography   490
    John W. Nance Jr. and U. Joseph Schoepf

31. Myocardial Nonischemic Cardiomyopathies   505
    Travis S. Henry and Kristopher W. Cummings

32. Cardiac Masses   522
    John P. Lichtenberger III, Brett W. Carter, and Suhny Abbara

33. Pericardial Disease   539
     Nikhil Goyal, Carlos Andres Rojas, and Suhny Abbara

34. Valves: Echocardiography   551
     Niamh M. Kilcullen and Michael H. Picard

35. Valves: Magnetic Resonance Imaging   571
     Christopher M. Walker and Gautham P. Reddy

36. Valves: Computed Tomography   587
     Daniel W. Entrikin

37. Coronary Arteries: Anomalies, Normal Variants, Aneurysms, and Fistulas   606
     Ronan Kileen and Jonathan D. Dodd

38. Coronary Arteries: Coronary Atherosclerotic Disease   616
     Stephan Achenbach

39. Coronary Artery Bypass Grafts   632
     Dharshan Raj Vummudi and Smita Patel

40. Pulmonary Veins, Atria, and Atrial Appendage   643
     Prabhakar Rajiah and Milind Y. Desai

41. Septal Defects and Other Cardiovascular Shunts   657
     Carlos Andres Rojas

42. Pulmonary Arteries   668
     Brett W. Carter and Gerald F. Abbott

43. Carotid and Vertebral Arteries   685
     Jason M. Johnson, Anna Meader, David T. Hunt, and Javier M. Romero

44. Thoracic Aorta and Its Branches   701
     Jonathan H. Chung, Martin L. Gunn, Sanjeeva P. Kalva, and Suhny Abbara

45. Bronchial Arteries   719
     Khashayar Farsad, Mathew P. Cherian, and Sanjeeva P. Kalva

46. Abdominal Aorta and Branches   726
     Khashayar Farsad

47. Upper Extremity Arteries   758
     Sanjeeva P. Kalva, Sandeep Hedgire, and Arthur C. Waltman

48. Lower Extremity Arteries   772
     Meghna Chadha, Chaitanya Ahuja, and Sanjeeva P. Kalva

49. Deep Venous Thrombosis   786
     Sanjeeva P. Kalva

50. Venous Insufficiency   800
     Chieh-Min Fan

51. Vascular Anomalies   813
     Philip R. John

IMAGING TECHNIQUE

CHAPTER 1

Echocardiography

Niamh M. Kilcullen and Michael H. Picard

Echocardiography uses high-frequency sound waves to generate images of cardiac structures and to provide information regarding blood flow and valvular function. The introduction of two-dimensional (2-D) echocardiography into routine clinical practice in the 1970s transformed the assessment of cardiac disease. Since then, the technology has evolved with the development of multiplanar transducers, harmonic imaging, and more recently, the introduction of three-dimensional (3-D) imaging. Transthoracic echocardiography (TTE) is a noninvasive imaging modality, without radiation, that allows immediate assessment of chamber size, valves, and ventricular function. TTE is often the initial imaging test of choice in acutely ill patients. In patients presenting with myocardial infarction, echocardiography can provide immediate information regarding left ventricular systolic function, in addition to the presence or absence of regional wall motion abnormalities. Echocardiography can exclude cardiac tamponade in patients with unexplained hypotension and evaluate right ventricular size, function, and right ventricular systolic pressure in patients presenting with pulmonary embolism. TTE is often requested for suspected endocarditis, in patients with and without preexisting valve disease. Outside the acute setting, indications for requesting TTE include diagnosis and monitoring of patients with significant valve disease, left ventricular dysfunction, right-sided heart disease, congenital heart disease, ascending aortic dilatation, and aneurysms. Three-dimensional echocardiography is also developing at a rapid pace and has many useful applications in the assessment of patients with cardiac disease.

■ STANDARD VIEWS FOR A TRANSTHORACIC ECHOCARDIOGRAM

Careful positioning of the patient is important to optimize image quality. Most echocardiographers are right handed and thus scan patients in the left lateral decubitus position at approximately 45 degrees. Ideally, the patient's left arm is placed behind the head to increase the spacing between ribs. A clear electrocardiogram (ECG) trace is important to have before imaging starts, so that digital images can be captured by triggering on the R wave. If the rhythm is very irregular, however, images can be acquired according to a set time interval, rather than by ECG trigger. The standard TTE transducer

positions, or "windows," are parasternal, apical, subcostal, suprasternal, and right parasternal.

Parasternal Long-Axis View

The first view is the parasternal long-axis view, which is obtained by positioning the transducer in the third or fourth intercostal space to the left of the sternum. Depending on imaging quality, the echocardiographer may need to move the probe up or down an intercostal space to obtain clear images. In this view, the mitral (A2 and P2, the middle portion of the valve leaflets) and aortic (right and noncoronary cusps) valves are typically seen (Fig. 1-1, *A* and *B*). The left ventricle, with the exception of the apex, is also well visualized. The mitral subvalvular apparatus, comprising the papillary muscles and chordae tendineae, are assessed in this view, although they may require some medial or lateral angulation. The right ventricle is also partially seen. If the M-mode line of interrogation can be properly aligned, it can be used to measure the aortic root, left atrial and left ventricular cavity dimensions, and left ventricular wall thickness; otherwise, measurements from 2-D imaging are preferred.

The parasternal long-axis view is the optimal view for diagnosing mitral valve prolapse, which is present in approximately 2% of the population. In mitral valve prolapse, one or both leaflets are displaced at least 2 mm above the plane of the mitral annulus into the left atrium. For a diagnosis of classic mitral valve prolapse, mitral leaflet thickening (>5 mm) is also required. The color Doppler sector is placed over the aortic and mitral valves to look for evidence of stenosis or regurgitation. The smaller the sector is, the higher the color Doppler frame rate will be. Other structures that can be assessed in the parasternal long-axis view include the pericardium and the descending thoracic aorta, which lies posterior to the left atrium. The examiner can differentiate between pericardial effusion and pleural effusion in this view because pericardial effusion courses between the heart and the descending aorta, whereas pleural effusion is noted posterior to the descending aorta (see Fig. 1-1, *D*).

Right Ventricular Inflow

By angling the probe upward and medially, the right ventricular inflow comes into view, thus displaying the

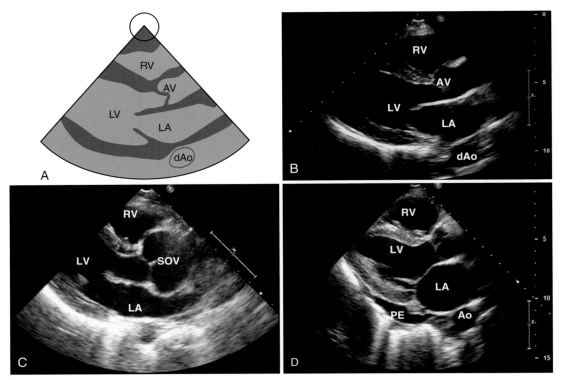

Figure 1-1 Transthoracic parasternal long-axis view. **A,** Schematic representation of normal parasternal long-axis view. **B,** Normal two-dimensional echocardiographic view. **C,** Dilated sinuses of Valsalva. **D,** Small posterior pericardial effusion. *AV,* Aortic valve; *dAo,* descending thoracic aorta; *LA,* left atrium; *LV,* left ventricle; *PE,* pericardial effusion; *RV,* right ventricle; *SOV,* sinuses of Valsalva.

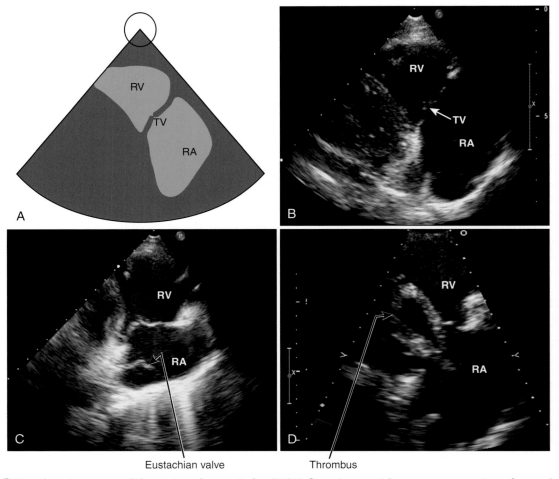

Figure 1-2 Transthoracic parasternal long-axis right ventricular (RV) inflow view. **A,** Schematic representation of normal parasternal long-axis RV inflow view. **B,** Normal two-dimensional echocardiographic view. **C,** Prominent eustachian valve, an embryonic remnant that is normal and should not be confused with a thrombus or mass. **D,** Large thrombus prolapsing across the tricuspid valve in diastole. *RA,* Right atrium; *TV,* tricuspid valve.

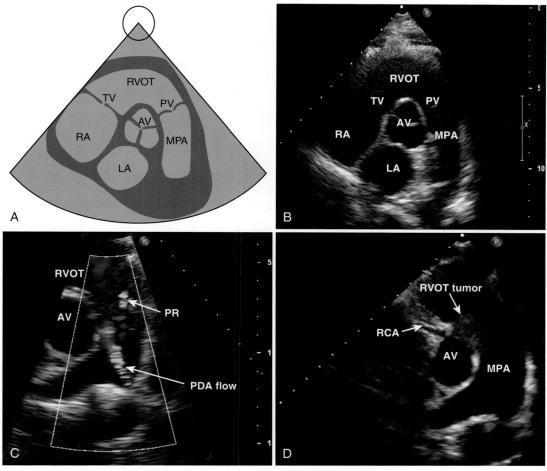

Figure 1-3 Transthoracic parasternal short-axis view, at the level of the aortic valve (AV). **A,** Schematic representation of normal parasternal short-axis view at the level of the aortic valve. **B,** Normal two-dimensional echocardiographic view. **C,** Trace pulmonary regurgitation and evidence of a patent ductus arteriosus (PDA) by color Doppler. **D,** Tumor in the right ventricular outflow tract (RVOT), in close proximity to the right coronary artery (RCA). A parasternal long-axis view of the same tumor can be seen in Figure 1-41, *A.* This tumor was confirmed as a paraglionoma following surgical resection. *LA,* Left atrium; *MPA,* main pulmonary artery; *PV,* pulmonary valve; *PR,* pulmonary regurgitation; *RA,* right atrium; *TV,* tricuspid valve.

right atrium, tricuspid valve, and right ventricle (Fig. 1-2, *A* and *B*). The inferior vena cava and coronary sinus can often be seen as they enter the right atrium. The right atrium contains several embryologic structures that can easily be mistaken for abnormalities. The crista terminalis is a muscular ridge separating the smooth portion of the right atrium from the more trabeculated portion. A prominent eustachian valve may be seen is some individuals at the junction of the inferior vena cava and the right atrium (see Fig. 1-2, *C*). This structure may be associated with a Chiari network that, in early life, was connected to the crista terminalis and the fossa ovalis and extended from the inferior vena cava to the superior vena cava. In the right ventricular view, the anterior and posterior leaflets of the tricuspid valve can be seen. The moderator band, a prominent muscular band, is usually seen traversing the right ventricle near the apex. Color flow mapping is used to look for tricuspid regurgitation, and the right ventricular inflow view is often good for evaluating the tricuspid regurgitation velocity, which can be used to estimate the right ventricular systolic pressure.

Right Ventricular Outflow View

By angling the probe upward and laterally, the right ventricular outflow tract comes into view. This view shows the right ventricular outflow tract, the pulmonary valve, and the pulmonary artery. Color flow mapping is used to look for evidence of pulmonary stenosis or regurgitation.

Parasternal Short-Axis View

The parasternal short-axis view is obtained by rotating the probe approximately 90 degrees in a clockwise direction. The optimal view shows the three cusps of the aortic valve in the center of the image (Fig. 1-3, *A* and *B*). In the case of a bicuspid valve, the right and left cusps are most commonly fused, followed by fusion of the right and noncoronary cusps. The examiner should assess the morphology and opening pattern of the aortic valve in systole because a bicuspid valve with raphe may appear tricuspid during diastole when the valve is closed. The right ventricular outflow tract lies anterior to the aortic valve, the main pulmonary artery, and its bifurcation on

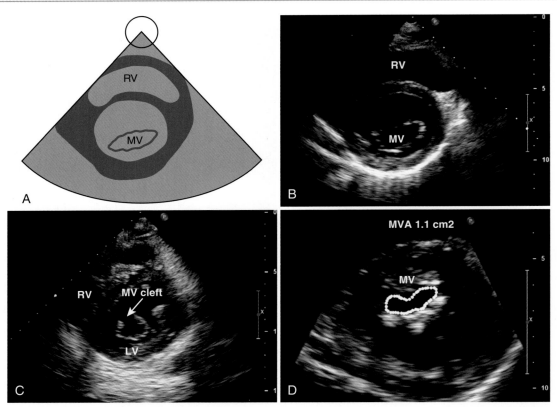

Figure 1-4 Transthoracic parasternal short-axis view at the level of the mitral valve (MV). **A,** Schematic representation of normal parasternal short-axis view at the level of the MV. **B,** Normal two-dimensional echocardiographic view showing the characteristic "fish-mouth" appearance of the leaflets when open. **C,** Cleft of the anterior MV leaflet. **D,** Direct planimetry of the MV area (MVA) in a patient with mitral stenosis. *LV,* Left ventricle; *RV,* right ventricle.

the right, the tricuspid valve and the right atrium on the left, and the left atrium posteriorly.

Color flow mapping is used to assess for evidence of tricuspid or pulmonary regurgitation. Pulsed wave and continuous wave Doppler images are used to measure the velocity across the pulmonary valve and to determine whether any stenosis or regurgitation is present. Color flow mapping can also be used to look for evidence of a left-to-right shunt across the inter-atrial septum. By angling the transducer inferiorly, the mitral valve leaflets are visualized in cross section (Fig. 1-4, *A* and *B*). This view is used in mitral stenosis to assess the mitral valve area by direct planimetry (see Fig. 1-4, *D*). Moving down the ventricle, the papillary muscles in the left ventricle come into view, and a portion of the right ventricle is also seen (Fig. 1-5. *A* and *B*). This view is used in the qualitative assessment of left ventricular systolic function and to evaluate for regional wall motion abnormalities (a sign of myocardial infarction). By angling the probe inferiorly, the left ventricular apex may be visualized (Fig. 1-6, *A* and *B*).

Apical Four-Chamber View

The apical four-chamber view is obtained by placing the probe at the left ventricular apex (Fig. 1-7, *A* and *B*). The transducer is manipulated to depict the maximal long axis of the left ventricle and both the mitral and tricuspid valve leaflets. The apex is identifiable as

the thinnest part of the myocardium, with minimal motion during the cardiac cycle. The examiner must take care not to foreshorten the ventricle because this may cause apical abnormalities such as thrombus or an aneurysm to be missed. In the apical view, both atria and ventricles are clearly seen. The superoinferior and mediolateral dimensions of the atria can be measured in this view. Color flow sector is placed across the mitral and tricuspid valves. Pulsed wave and continuous wave Doppler images allow the assessment of velocity across these valves. Pulsed wave Doppler imaging of flow in the pulmonary veins provides information regarding left atrial pressure, which can be assessed in the apical four-chamber view. The right upper pulmonary vein is usually the most easily accessible for Doppler assessment.

Apical Five-Chamber View

In the apical five chamber view, the tip of the probe is angled superiorly, and the aortic valve can be brought into view (Fig. 1-8, *A* and *B*). Color flow mapping and pulsed and continuous wave Doppler images are recorded across the aortic valve to evaluate for aortic stenosis and regurgitation. Using pulsed wave Doppler in the left ventricular outflow tract, the presence of subvalvular obstruction may be identified secondary to conditions such as hypertrophic cardiomyopathy or a subaortic membrane.

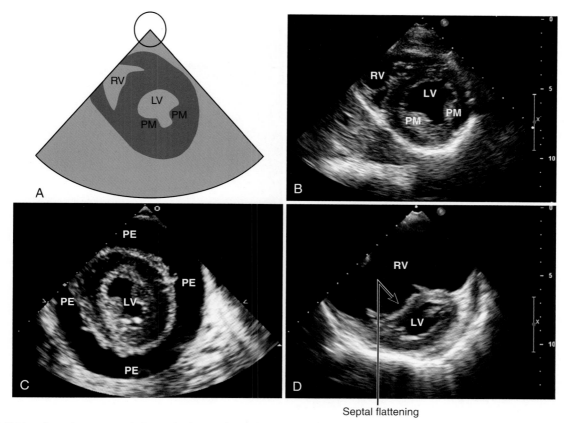

Figure 1-5 Transthoracic parasternal short-axis view at the midventricular or papillary muscle level. **A,** Schematic representation of normal parasternal short-axis view at the papillary muscle (PM) level. **B,** Normal two-dimensional echocardiographic view. **C,** Large circumferential pericardial effusion (PE). **D,** Marked dilatation of the right ventricle (RV) and flattening of the interventricular septum in a patient with RV volume and pressure overload. *LV,* Left ventricle.

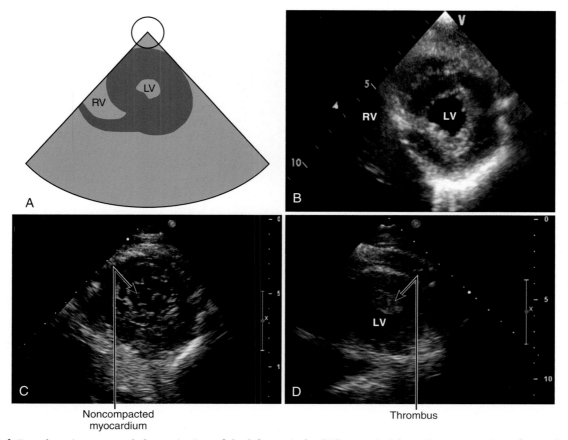

Figure 1-6 Transthoracic parasternal short-axis view of the left ventricular (LV) apex. **A,** Schematic representation of normal parasternal short-axis view of the LV apex. **B,** Normal two-dimensional echocardiographic view. **C,** Noncompaction of the left ventricular myocardium at the apex. The end-systolic ratio of noncompacted endocardial layer to the compacted myocardium is greater than 2. **D,** Large apical thrombus. *RV,* Right ventricle.

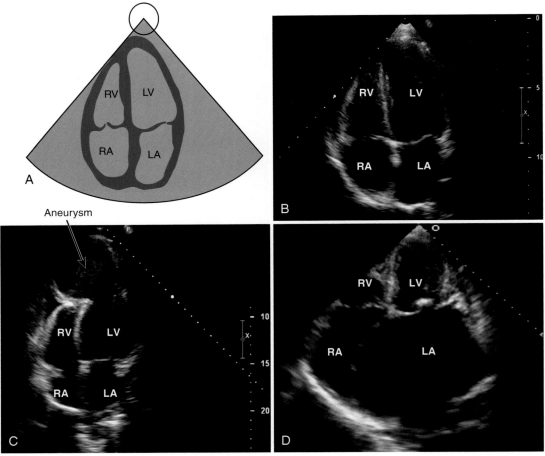

Figure 1-7 Transthoracic apical four-chamber view. **A,** Schematic representation of normal apical four-chamber view. **B,** Normal two-dimensional echocardiographic view. **C,** Large left ventricular apical aneurysm. Note the spontaneous echo contrast present in the aneurysm that represents sluggish flow. **D,** Markedly dilated left atrium (LA) in a patient with severe mitral stenosis. *LV,* Left ventricle; *RA,* right atrium; *RV,* right ventricle.

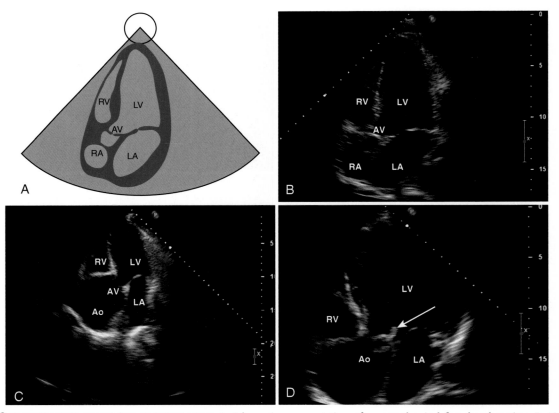

Figure 1-8 Transthoracic apical five-chamber view. **A,** Schematic representation of a normal apical five-chamber view. **B,** Normal two-dimensional echocardiographic view. **C,** Large aneurysm of the ascending aorta (Ao). The right atrium (RA) is not visualized in this image as a result of the aortic dilatation. **D,** Large vegetation on the aortic valve (AV) leaflets *(arrow).* *LA,* Left atrium; *LV,* left ventricle; *RV,* right ventricle.

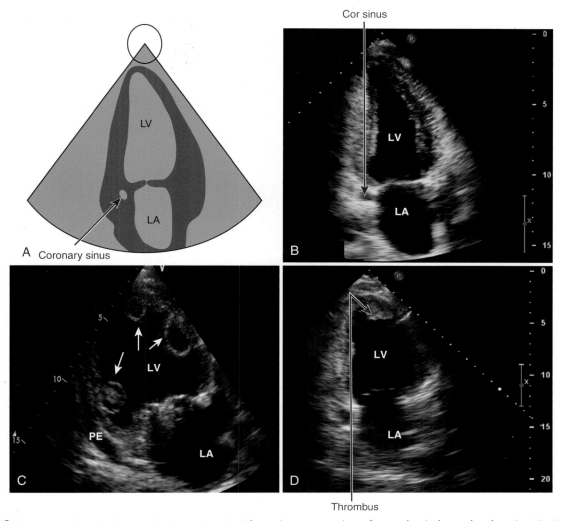

Figure 1-9 *Transthoracic apical two-chamber view.* **A,** Schematic representation of normal apical two-chamber view. **B,** Normal two-dimensional echocardiographic view. **C,** Multiple hydatid cysts *(arrows)* adherent to the left ventricular (LV) myocardium. These cysts are prone to rupture and embolization. **D,** Thrombus in the LV apex. *Cor,* Coronary; *LA,* left atrium; PE, pericardial effusion.

Apical Two-Chamber View

The apical two-chamber view is obtained by rotating the probe approximately 90 degrees in an counterclockwise direction (Fig. 1-9, *A* and *B*). In this view, the inferior and anterior walls of the left ventricle can be assessed for wall motion abnormalities. Color flow mapping and pulsed continuous wave Doppler images are recorded across the mitral valve. The coronary sinus and the descending thoracic aorta can be seen in this view.

Apical Long-Axis View

The apical long-axis view is obtained by rotating the probe further counterclockwise, so the aortic valve is brought into view (Fig. 1-10, *A* and *B*). Color flow mapping and continuous wave Doppler are used to assess for aortic regurgitation and to record velocity across the aortic valve. This view is also used to evaluate for mitral valve prolapse and the presence of systolic anterior motion of the mitral valve in patients with hypertrophic cardiomyopathy.

Subcostal View

The subcostal view is obtained by placing the probe in the subxiphoid area, with the patient lying supine. It may be helpful to ask the patient to bend the knees because this maneuver relaxes the abdominal muscles. In the subcostal view, the heart is imaged from below; therefore, the right side of the heart is on the top of the image, with the left side of the heart below it (Fig. 1-11, *A* and *B*). This view is good for examination of the inter-atrial septum when evaluating for evidence of a patent foramen ovale (PFO) or an atrial septal defect (ASD), lipomatous hypertrophy (see Fig. 1-11, *C*), or an inter-atrial septal aneurysm.

By rotating the probe counterclockwise, the inferior vena cava can be seen to enter the right atrium (Fig. 1-12, *A* and *B*). The right atrial pressure may be estimated by determining the diameter of the inferior vena cava and its respirophasic response. The diameter of the inferior vena cava should be measured at the end of expiration, just proximal to the hepatic veins that lie 0.5 to 3.0 cm proximal to the ostium of the right atrium. By

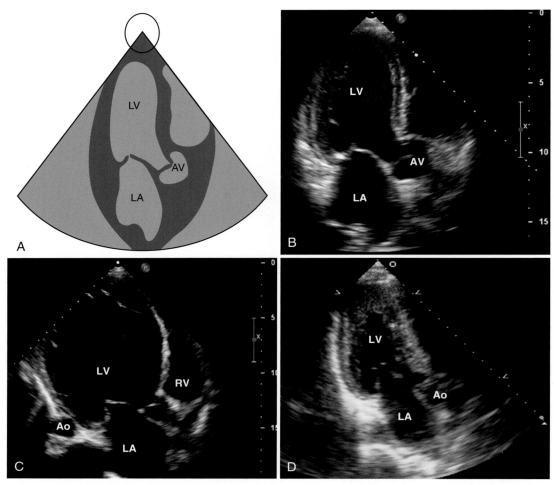

Figure 1-10 *Transthoracic apical long-axis view.* **A,** Schematic representation of normal apical long-axis view. **B,** Normal two-dimensional echocardiographic view. **C,** Markedly dilated left ventricle (LV) with thinning of the myocardium in a patient with dilated cardiomyopathy. **D,** LV hypertrophy in a patient with hypertrophic cardiomyopathy. *Ao,* Aorta; *AV,* aortic valve; *LA,* left atrium; *RV,* right ventricle.

further rotation of the probe, the abdominal aorta can be seen in long axis. The subcostal view is good when looking for evidence of diastolic flow reversal, by pulsed wave Doppler, in patients with moderate to severe aortic regurgitation. In some patients, such as supine patients ventilated in intensive care units or those with significant respiratory disease, the subcostal view may be the best view obtainable.

Suprasternal View

To obtain the suprasternal view, the probe is placed in the suprasternal notch with the patient supine and the neck extended, if possible. The suprasternal view allows the aortic arch and head and neck vessels to be visualized (Fig. 1-13, *A* and *B*). Pulsed and continuous wave Doppler imaging is used to examine flow in the descending thoracic aorta. This is the standard view used to evaluate for coarctation of the aorta (Fig. 1-14).

Right Parasternal View

To obtain the right parasternal view, the patient should be lying on the right side. This view is useful in patients

with right ventricular enlargement and when the heart is positioned more medially. The interatrial septum is often clearly visualized in this view. The ascending aorta may also be well visualized, and this view is particularly useful when assessing aortic valve gradients using the stand-alone, nonimaging continuous wave Doppler probe.

■ MEASUREMENTS

M-mode recordings are occasionally used for left ventricular, aortic root, and left atrial dimensions, although 2-D measurements are performed routinely in most laboratories (Table 1-1). Because of its superior temporal resolution, M-mode imaging of the aortic and mitral valve leaflets can provide additional information regarding valve function. M-mode measurements are made in the parasternal long-axis and parasternal short-axis views. For accurate M-mode measurements, the cursor must be perpendicular to the structure of interest; however, this may not be achievable in all patients. By convention, at the end of expiration, M-mode measurements are made from leading edge to leading edge, whereas 2-D measurements are from inner edge

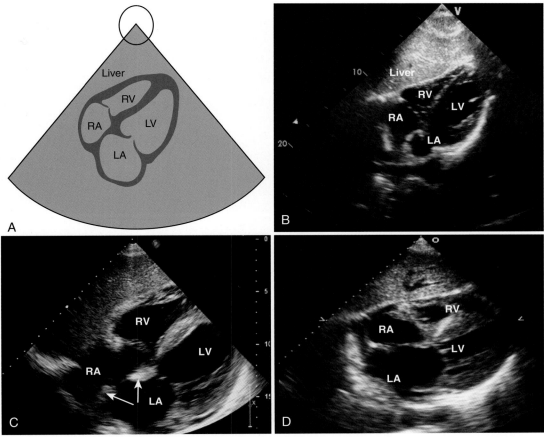

Figure 1-11 Transthoracic subcostal view. A, Schematic representation of normal subcostal view. **B,** Normal two-dimensional echocardiographic view. **C,** Subcostal view showing lipomatous hypertrophy of the interatrial septum with the characteristic "dumbbell" appearance (*arrows*). **D,** Subcostal view in a patient with cardiac amyloidosis. Note the hypertrophy of both ventricles and dilated atria in relation to the ventricular size. *LA,* Left atrium; *LV,* left ventricle; *RA,* right atrium; *RV,* right ventricle.

to inner edge. If the M-mode cannot be adequately aligned, then measurements by 2-D are preferred. These measurements should be averaged over several beats, particularly if the rhythm is irregular. Postpremature ventricular contraction beats should not be measured.

Left ventricular cavity dimensions and left ventricular wall thickness are measured at the level of the mitral valve leaflet tips at end-diastole and end-systole. The examiner should correct for body surface area by indexing left ventricular cavity dimensions. The left ventricular outflow tract diameter is measured in the parasternal long-axis view within 0.5 to 1.0 cm of the valve. Aortic root diameters include measurements at the annulus, the sinus of Valsalva, and the sinotubular junction. The aortic annulus is defined as the hinge point of the aortic leaflets. The sinotubular junction is where the sinuses of Valsalva transition to the ascending aorta.

The anteroposterior diameter of the left atrium is usually measured in the parasternal long-axis axis view at end-systole; however, although this single dimension measurement is the most reproducible, it does not always reflect true left atrial size. The left atrium may enlarge in a superoinferior or mediolateral dimension, rather than anteroposteriorly, and these measurements should be obtained in the apical four-chamber view. Left atrial volumes can be calculated with the modified

Simpson rule using apical two- and four-chamber views at end-systole. Left atrial volumes by echocardiography compare favorably with other modalities such as magnetic resonance imaging (MRI) and computed tomography (CT). The American Society of Echocardiography recommends that indexed left atrial volumes should be routinely measured in clinical practice. The reference range for indexed left atrial volumes is 22 ± 6 mL/m^2.

Right ventricular outflow tract dimensions are measured in the parasternal long-axis view (proximal portion) and parasternal short-axis view at the level of the pulmonary valve (distal portion). Right ventricular size is best measured at end-diastole, in the apical four-chamber view. Guidelines indicate that the right ventricle is dilated when the base is larger than 42 mm, the midventricle is larger than 35 mm, and the longitudinal dimension is greater than 86 mm.

Right ventricular wall thickness is measured in end-diastole in the subcostal view using either 2-D or M-mode imaging. Right atrial size can be assessed by measuring the superoinferior and mediolateral dimensions in the apical four-chamber view. Right atrial volumes can also be calculated using the modified Simpson rule. Guidelines suggest that right atrial dilatation is confirmed when the superoinferior dimension in the apical four-chamber views is greater than 53 mm and the mediolateral dimension is

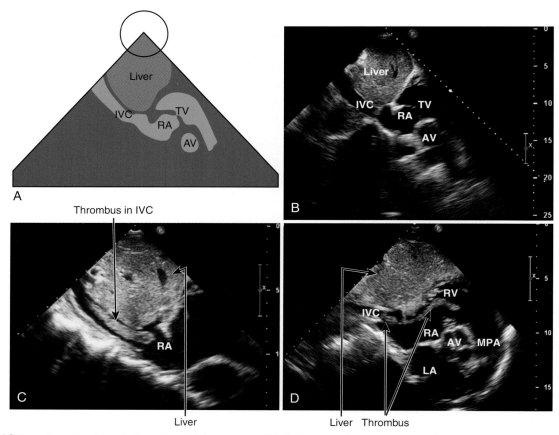

Figure 1-12 Transthoracic subcostal view of the inferior vena cava (IVC). **A,** Schematic representation of the IVC entering the right atrium (RA). **B,** Normal two-dimensional echocardiographic view. **C,** Large thrombus in the IVC that extends into the RA and **D,** prolapses across the tricuspid valve (TV) in diastole. *AV,* Aortic valve; *LA,* left atrium; *MPA,* main pulmonary artery; *RV,* right ventricle.

greater than 44 mm. A right atrial area larger than 18 cm² also suggests enlargement. The inferior vena cava dimension and inspiratory collapsibility should be assessed from the subcostal view. An inferior vena cava 2.1 cm or smaller and with more than 50% collapse on inspiration suggests normal right atrial pressure (range, 0 to 5 mm Hg). An inferior vena cava larger than 2.1 cm and with less than 50% collapse, with a sniff, suggests high atrial pressure (range, 10 to 20 mm Hg).

Assessment of Left Ventricular Function

Left ventricular function can be assessed echocardiographically both qualitatively and quantitatively. Ejection fraction can be calculated using left ventricular end-diastolic and end-systolic dimensions; however, the Simpson biplane is the recommended method for assessment of left ventricular volumes and ejection fraction. In this method, the endocardial borders are traced at end-diastole and end-systole in the apical two- and four-chamber views. The long-axis is then divided into 20 equal portions, to create 20 disks. Left ventricular volume is calculated from the summation of the volume of these disks. In patients with dilated cardiomyopathy, in whom the normal geometry is distorted, 3-D echocardiography may now be used to calculate a more accurate ejection fraction (Fig. 1-15):

$$\text{Ejection fraction (\%)} = \frac{\text{LVEDV} - \text{LVESV}}{\text{LVEDV}} \times 100$$

in which LVEDV is left ventricular end-diastolic volume and LVESV is left ventricular end-systolic volume.

Regional left ventricular function is assessed based on a 17-segment model introduced in 2002 by the American Heart Association. Each segment, except the apical cap (seventeenth segment), should be assessed for motion and systolic thickening. By convention, segments are described as normal, hypokinetic, akinetic, dyskinetic, or aneurysmal. A wall motion score or index can also be calculated if additional quantitative data are required. More sophisticated tools for the assessment of left ventricular function have emerged since 2000. Tissue Doppler imaging and strain imaging are now routinely used in the assessment of patients with left ventricular dyssynchrony and other cardiomyopathies. Circumferential, longitudinal, and radial strain can be calculated and displayed graphically. Figure 1-16 shows an example of radial strain. This technology continues to advance and has great potential for identifying patients with subclinical left ventricular dysfunction, whose ejection fraction is within the normal range. Early identification of patients with evolving cardiomyopathies may facilitate closer follow-up of patients or consideration of medical treatment, if appropriate.

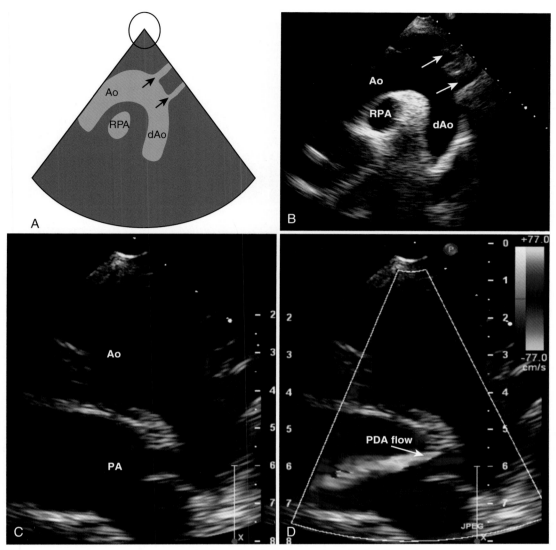

Figure 1-13 *Transthoracic suprasternal long-axis view showing the aortic arch.* **A,** Schematic representation of the suprasternal long-axis view showing the aortic arch. **B,** Normal two-dimensional echocardiographic view. The left common carotid artery and left subclavian artery are noted by the *upper* and *lower arrows*, respectively. The right brachiocephalic artery is not clearly visualized in this image. **C,** Patent ductus arteriosus (PDA) is confirmed by color flow imaging (**D**), which shows flow entering the pulmonary artery (PA) from the aorta (Ao). *dAo,* Descending aorta; *RPA,* right pulmonary artery.

■ DOPPLER ECHOCARDIOGRAPHY

Doppler echocardiography provides important hemodynamic information in real time (Table 1-2). The Doppler principle states that "the frequency of reflected ultrasound is altered by a moving target, such as red blood cells." The Doppler shift (change of frequency of a received ultrasound pulse compared with the transmitted pulse) relates to the velocity of red blood cells and the direction of blood flow. By convention, blood flowing toward the transducer is positive, and blood flowing away from the transducer is negative.

$$\text{Doppler equation}: V = \frac{\Delta F \times c}{2F_0 \times \text{Cos } \theta}$$

in which V is velocity, ΔF is the Doppler shift, F_0 is the transducer frequency, c is the velocity of sound in tissue (1540 m/second), and Cos θ is the cosine of the angle of incidence.

The three Doppler modalities used in clinical practice are pulsed wave Doppler, continuous wave Doppler, and color flow mapping. The Doppler principle can also be applied to the myocardium and is referred to as tissue Doppler. This technique has an important role in the assessment of diastolic function and left ventricular dyssynchrony. Pulsed wave Doppler measures velocity in a small sample area but is unable to measure high velocities because of aliasing. This threshold is referred to as the Nyquist limit and is determined by the pulsed repetition frequency. Pulsed wave Doppler is used to determine normal velocities across valves, measure cardiac output, and quantify intracardiac shunts. It is also used in the assessment of diastolic function and in the evaluation of cardiac tamponade and constrictive physiology.

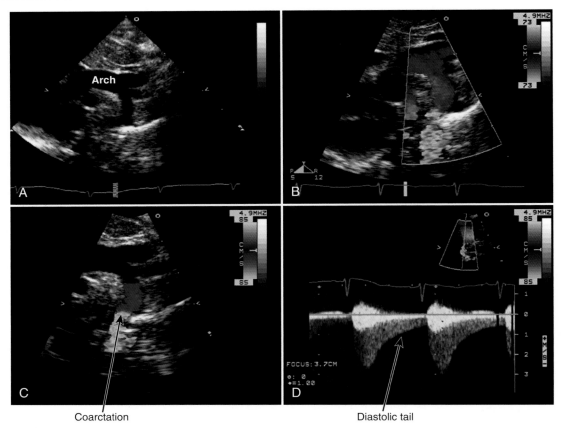

Coarctation   Diastolic tail

Figure 1-14 A, Transthoracic suprasternal view, showing coarctation of the aorta. **B,** Flow acceleration proximal to the narrowed area is demonstrated by turbulent flow on color Doppler. **C,** The area of narrowing is identified using color flow imaging. **D,** Continuous wave Doppler across the coarctation reveals a characteristic diastolic tail indicating continued flow throughout diastole.

Continuous wave Doppler can measure high velocities but is unable to determine where along the beam the maximum velocity occurs. Continuous wave Doppler is primarily used to determine the gradients across stenotic valves (e.g., aortic stenosis) or orifices (e.g., coarctation of the aorta). The peak velocity allows estimation of the peak gradient across a valve by the simplified Bernoulli equation, and the velocity time integral can be measured by tracing the Doppler waveform.

Color flow mapping uses the pulsed wave Doppler principle, but it also includes other pixels from the 2-D image. For all these regions, a flow velocity is superimposed on the 2-D images and is displayed with a color scale. By convention, flow away from the transducer is displayed as blue, and flow toward the transducer is displayed as red (BART). Because color flow mapping is based on pulsed wave Doppler, it is also affected by aliasing. To maximize the frame rate when using color flow mapping, the examiner should reduce the sector width and adjust the depth to include only the area of interest.

Doppler echocardiography has high sensitivity and specificity. It is used to determine the velocity across valves and provides information on stenosis and regurgitation. The velocity across a stenotic valve can be converted into a pressure gradient by using the simplified Bernoulli equation. The equation correlates well with invasive measurements, provided the velocity proximal to the obstruction is 1.5 m/second or less. Using the simplified Bernoulli equation, right ventricular systolic pressure may be estimated from the tricuspid regurgitation velocity profile. In the absence of pulmonary stenosis, the sum of the peak right ventricular systolic pressure and the right atrial pressure reflects pulmonary artery systolic pressure. Right atrial pressure is estimated from the assessment of inferior vena cava size and inspiratory collapse.

$$\text{Simplified Bernoulli equation}: \text{Pressure gradient} = 4V^2$$

$$\text{Flow} = \text{CSA} \times \text{Velocity}$$

$$\text{SV} = \text{CSA} \times \text{VTI}$$

in which V is velocity, CSA is cross-sectional area, SV is stroke volume, and VTI is velocity time integral.

Ideally, the cross-sectional area should not change significantly between systole and diastole. For this reason, stroke volume is best measured at the left ventricular outflow tract, given that the aortic annulus diameter does not change significantly in systole. The continuity equation is based on the principle that the flows proximal and through a valve are equal, provided no shunts

Table 1-1　Normal Dimensions

	View	Normal Values (mm)
Ascending aorta (end-diastole)	PLAX	<36
Sinus of Valsalva (end-diastole)	PLAX	24-39
Aortic annulus (end-diastole)	PLAX	<26
Left atrium (end-systole)	PLAX	≤38
Left ventricle (end-diastole)	PLAX	37-53
Interventricular septum (end-diastole)	PLAX	7-11
Posterior wall (end-diastole)	PLAX	7-11
Right ventricular outflow tract (end-diastole)	PLAX PSAX	≤33 ≤27
Main pulmonary artery (end-diastole)	PSAX	≤29
Proximal right pulmonary artery (end-diastole)	PSAX	≤17
Proximal left pulmonary artery (end-diastole)	PSAX	≤14
Right ventricle at base (end-diastole)	Apical four-chamber	≤42
Right ventricular wall thickness (end-diastole)	Subcostal	≤5
Inferior vena cava (end-diastole)	Subcostal	≤21

PLAX, Parasternal long-axis; *PSAX*, parasternal short-axis.

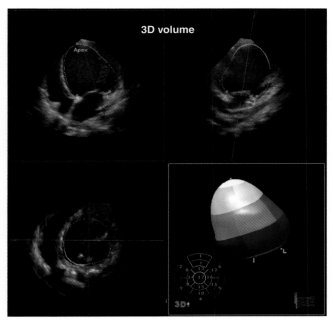

Figure 1-15 Three-dimensional left ventricular volume assessment in a patient with dilated cardiomyopathy. Multiplanar reconstruction from three cropped planes of the three-dimensional volume of ultrasound is shown. Three-dimensional data are displayed as a shell *(bottom right)*. Use of the 17-segment model allows assessment of regional wall motion. Note the marked distortion of normal anatomy of the left ventricle.

are present. The continuity equation is most commonly used in clinical practice to calculate aortic valve area in aortic stenosis.

$$\text{Continuity equation}: CSA1 \times V1 = CSA2 \times V2$$

$$CSA2 = \frac{CSA1 \times V1}{V2}$$

$$AVA = \frac{LVOT\ area \times LVOT\ VTI}{Aortic\ valve\ VTI}$$

Although the continuity equation can be used to estimate mitral valve area in the evaluation of mitral stenosis, pressure half-time is the preferred method:

$$\text{Pressure half-time}: MVA = \frac{220}{Pt\frac{1}{2}}$$

in which MVA is the mitral valve area and $Pt\frac{1}{2}$ is pressure half-time.

The assessment of regurgitation, particularly mitral regurgitation, is more challenging and is discussed in greater detail in Chapter 34. The echocardiographer can estimate the regurgitant flow and effective regurgitant orifice area by measuring the proximal isovelocity surface area, or flow convergence. This approach is based on the principle that as blood approaches a circular regurgitant orifice, concentric hemispherical shells of increasing velocity form. The regurgitant flow is then equal to the velocity of one of these shells times the area of that hemispherical shell. Because this method is based on several assumptions and has limitations, advances in 3-D imaging may help in refining the evaluation of mitral regurgitation.

$$EROA \times Regurgitant\ VTI = Regurgitant\ flow$$

$$EROA = \frac{Regurgitant\ volume}{Regurgitant\ VTI}$$

$$Regurgitant\ volume = 2\pi r^2 \times Va\ (aliasing\ velocity)$$

$$EROA = \frac{(2\pi r^2 \times Va)}{Pk\ Vreg}$$

$$Pk\ Vreg\ (peak\ regurgitant\ velocity)$$

in which EROA is the effective regurgitant orifice area, VTI is the velocity time integral, r is the PISA radius, Va is the aliasing velocity, and PkVreg is the peak regurgitant velocity.

Important Caveats Regarding Echocardiography and Doppler

■ The Doppler equation requires parallel orientation of the ultrasound beam to the blood flow. Small deviations are permissible (<20 degrees); however, larger

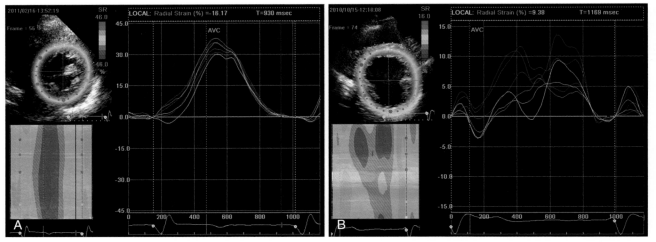

Figure 1-16 Two-dimensional radial speckle strain measured from a parasternal short-axis view at the level of the mitral annulus. The left ventricle is divided into six color-coded segments for analysis. The radial strain is displayed graphically for each segment. In systole, the myocardium thickens, and this is shown as a positive deflection. **A,** Example of normal radial strain. **B,** Radial strain in a patient with significant left ventricular dyssynchrony showing varying time to peak contraction in the six segments.

Table 1-2   Normal Doppler Measurements

	Normal Values
Mitral Valve	
Mitral E wave velocity	<1.2 m/sec
Mitral A wave velocity	<0.8 m/sec
E/A ratio*	0.75-1.5
Mitral E deceleration time†	<220 msec
Septal e′ velocity‡	6-9 cm/sec
Lateral e′ velocity‡	7-11 cm/sec
Tricuspid Valve	
Tricuspid E wave velocity	<0.6 m/sec
RVSP (estimated from peak TR velocity)§	<35 mm Hg
LVOT and Aortic Valve	
LVOT velocity	<1.5 m/sec
Aortic velocity	<2.0 m/sec
Pulmonary Valve	
Pulmonary outflow tract velocity	<0.9 m/sec

*E/A ratio decreases with age.
†Deceleration time increases with age (≤275 msec normal for individuals >60 years old).
‡Velocities decrease with age.
§RVSP is calculated from peak TR velocity using simplified Bernoulli equation. RVSP = $4V^2$ + right atrial pressure, which is estimated from inferior vena cava size and degree of collapse on inspiration.
LVOT, Left ventricular outflow tract; *RVSP,* right ventricular systolic pressure; *TR,* tricuspid regurgitation velocity.

deviations result in inaccurate velocity measurements and significant underestimation of the true pressure gradient.
■ For detection of high velocities such as in severe aortic stenosis, use of the stand-alone (nonimaging) continuous wave probe is recommended because it has a higher signal-to-noise ratio.

■ The simplified Bernoulli equation to measure peak gradient is accurate except in the following situations: (1) when velocity proximal to the stenosis is greater than 1.5 m/second, (2) in the presence of two stenotic lesions in series such as subvalvular and valvular stenosis, and (3) in the presence of long tubular stenosis. In the first situation, the proximal gradient can be subtracted from the distal gradient.
■ In aortic stenosis, examiners often note a difference between catheter measurements and Doppler findings. Doppler measures the maximum instantaneous pressure difference across the aortic valve, whereas in the catheterization laboratory, the peak-to-peak gradient (difference between peak left ventricular and peak aortic pressure) is measured. The mean gradient therefore more closely reflects the invasive mean measurement in clinical practice.
■ Underestimating eccentrically directed regurgitant jets is easy.
■ In the assessment of mitral regurgitation, one may incorrectly assume that the proximal isovelocity surface area is always hemispherical. Advances in 3-D imaging are likely to allow more accurate quantification of mitral regurgitation.
■ Assessing the degree of regurgitation in prosthetic valves is often difficult.
■ When calculating the ratio of pulmonary to systemic flow (Qp/Qs), the pulmonary annulus is difficult to visualize, and the right ventricular outflow tract contracts in systole. This results in a rate of calculation errors of up to 20%.
■ Pressure half-time for the mitral valve area is not applicable if the patient has a rapid heart rate, significant aortic regurgitation, or conditions affecting left atrial or ventricular compliance. The pressure half-time equation is not applicable *for up to 72 hours* after mitral valvuloplasty.
■ Valve gradients are dynamic and may vary significantly with changes in heart rate and blood pressure

Table 1-3 Tips and Tricks for Transthoracic Echocardiography

Problem	Solution
Poor views on transthoracic echocardiography	■ Reposition patient ■ Optimize machine settings (adjust frequency, gain, sector width, depth) ■ Use adequate gel to reduce impedance ■ Acquiring images in expiration or inspiration may be helpful ■ Subcostal views are often most useful in ventilated patients
Poor endocardial definition and inability to visualize left ventricular apex	■ Use left ventricular contrast
Poor tricuspid regurgitation signal or underestimation of RVSP	■ Use agitated saline to enhance signal
Misdiagnosis of normal structures	■ Be aware and recognize normal structures (Chiari network, eustachian valve, Lambl excrescences)
Inaccurate Doppler measurements	■ Parallel orientation to beam required
Failure to diagnose left superior vena cava	■ Insert an intravenous line in the patient's left arm for agitated saline contrast studies

RVSP, Right ventricular systolic pressure.

Table 1-4 Tips and Tricks for Transesophageal Echocardiography

Problem	Solution
Difficulty inserting the probe	■ Ensure no history of esophageal disease ■ Ensure adequate use of local anesthetic and sedation ■ Reschedule transesophageal echocardiography with anesthesia support if unsafe to proceed
Poor contact between probe and esophagus	■ Rotate probe 360 degrees or advance into stomach to dispel air
Artifacts mimicking disease such as a dissection flap or mass	■ Be aware of common artifacts ■ Know how to differentiate between actual disease and an artifact ■ Use multiple views of the same anatomy
Misdiagnosis of normal structures	■ Be aware and recognize normal structures (Chiari network, eustachian valve, Lambl excrescences)
"Blind spot" in the aorta proximal to the innominate arteries	■ Be aware of this spot and use alternative imaging (CT or MRI) if indicated
Unclear distinction between patent foramen ovale and intrapulmonary shunt	■ Perform an agitated saline contrast study and image where the right upper pulmonary vein enters the left atrium
Inaccurate sizing of atrial septal defect	■ Use three-dimensional imaging to determine the shape and size of the defect

CT, Computed tomography; *MRI,* magnetic resonance imaging.

and in the presence of inotropic drugs. The examiner must record blood pressure at the time of an echocardiogram because loading conditions can underestimate or overestimate the severity of valve disease (e.g., mitral regurgitation may appear less severe in the operating room when the blood pressure is lower than baseline).

■ Tables 1-3 and 1-4 provide troubleshooting tips.

Left Ventricular Diastolic Function

Left ventricular diastolic dysfunction is common in patients with left ventricular systolic dysfunction and is characterized by impaired myocardial relaxation and reduced compliance of cardiac chambers. The assessment of diastolic function is important in all patients with cardiac disease, particularly in patients presenting with unexplained dyspnea. Several parameters are used in echocardiography to evaluate diastolic function, including mitral inflow velocity patterns, deceleration time, tissue Doppler imaging of the mitral annulus, pulmonary vein flow, and right ventricular systolic pressure. Diastole is the period from aortic valve closure to mitral valve closure and consists of four distinct phases: isovolumetric relaxation, early filling, diastasis, and atrial contraction.

Assessment of diastolic function begins with pulsed wave Doppler across the mitral valve tips in the apical four-chamber view to evaluate the mitral inflow velocity profile. A normal profile consists of two peaks: a tall E wave and a smaller A wave. The E and A velocities

represent early passive filling and the flow during atrial contraction, respectively. In normal individuals, the E velocity is less than 1.2 m/second, the A velocity is less than 0.8 m/second, and the E/A ratio is 0.75 to 1.5 (Fig. 1-17, *A*). With increasing age, however, this ratio may be lower than 0.5 in older individuals, a finding reflecting the impaired or delayed relaxation that occurs with aging. Deceleration time is the time from the peak of the E wave to the time the E wave would reach 0 m/second; in normal individuals, it is 150 to 260 msec. Isovolumetric relaxation time is the time from aortic valve closure to mitral valve opening. To obtain this measurement, the continuous wave Doppler image is aligned to include aortic valve closure and the onset of mitral inflow. The isovolumetric relaxation time in normal individuals is 80 msec. The isovolumetric relaxation time decreases with increasing left atrial pressure.

Left atrial size and pulmonary vein flow are also helpful in the evaluation of diastolic function. Increased left atrial size is typically associated with chronic elevations in left atrial pressure. To obtain a pulmonary vein flow profile, pulsed wave Doppler imaging of the pulmonary vein is performed in the apical four-chamber view with the sample volume just inside the vein. The right upper pulmonary vein is usually the easiest vein to visualize, and it permits proper alignment for Doppler assessment. The normal pulmonary vein velocity profile consists of systolic and diastolic components, representing forward flow and a brief period of reversed flow during

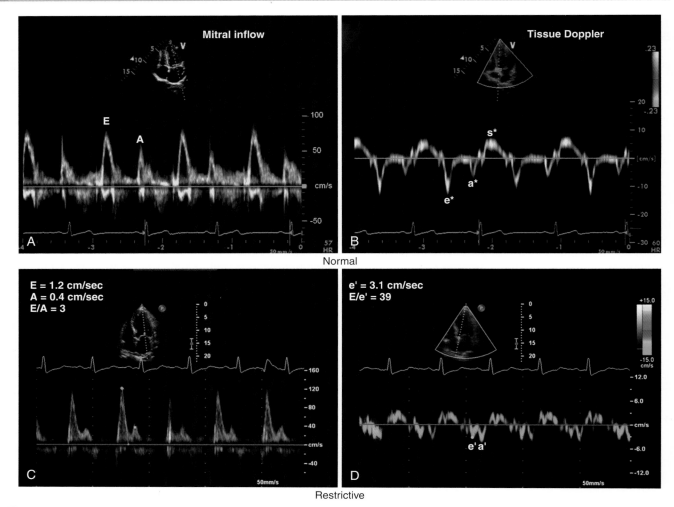

Figure 1-17 A, Pulsed wave Doppler across the mitral valve in the apical four-chamber view. The normal mitral inflow profile shows a large E wave reflecting early filling of the left ventricle and a smaller A wave, following atrial contraction. The normal E/A ratio is 0.75 to 1.5. **B,** Pulsed wave tissue Doppler imaging of the septum showing normal e′ and a′ velocities. **C,** Example of restricted filling pattern with a tall E wave and a small A wave. The E/A ratio is elevated at 3. The E wave slope is steep, and the deceleration time is reduced. **D,** Pulsed wave tissue Doppler imaging of the septum in a patient with diastolic dysfunction showing low e′ and a′ velocities. The E/e′ ratio is high at 39, suggesting elevated left atrial pressure, in the setting of left ventricular systolic dysfunction.

atrial contraction. Blunting of the systolic wave suggests elevated left atrial pressure in patients with impaired left ventricular systolic function.

Tissue Doppler imaging is now routinely used in the assessment of diastolic function in patients with cardiac disease. Pulsed wave Doppler imaging of the septal and lateral annulus of the mitral valve provides an assessment of the velocity at which the left ventricle enlarges during its filling. The diastolic annular velocities are thus lower than the baseline. The e′ and a′ peak velocities are measured (see Fig. 1-17, B). In patients with cardiac disease, the E/e′ ratio can be used to assess left ventricular filling pressures. An E/e′ ratio lower than 8 suggests normal left atrial pressure, and an E/e′ ratio greater than 15 suggests elevated left atrial pressure (see Fig. 1-17, D). Individuals with E/e′ ratios between 8 and 15 are in an indeterminate zone, and therefore other parameters of diastolic function must be closely evaluated. The E/e′ ratio is not accurate in normal individuals, in patients with marked

mitral annular calcification or mitral valve disease, or in patients with constrictive pericarditis. The assessment of diastolic function is complex, and in several clinical conditions, including atrial fibrillation, mitral stenosis, hypertrophic cardiomyopathy, and pulmonary hypertension, the foregoing parameters must be carefully interpreted in the context of the clinical history.

■ ADDITIONAL ECHOCARDIOGRAPHIC TOOLS

Agitated Saline Contrast

A contrast study (commonly referred to as a bubble study) is often requested in young patients presenting with stroke, to evaluate for evidence of a PFO (found in approximately 25% of the population). Color flow mapping may show evidence of left-to-right flow across the interatrial septum. An agitated saline contrast study

Contrast study

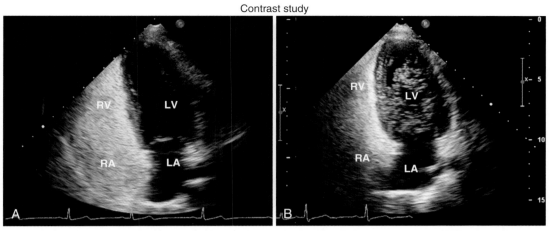

Figure 1-18 A, Transthoracic echocardiographic apical four-chamber view showing right heart opacification following the administration of agitated saline contrast material. No contrast is seen in the left side of the heart. **B,** A second injection is administered with a Valsalva maneuver, and this shows contrast in the left ventricle (LV) within three to five cycles, thus indicating right-to-left interatrial shunting consistent with a patent foramen ovale. *LA,* Left atrium; *RA,* right atrium; *RV,* right ventricle.

LV contrast

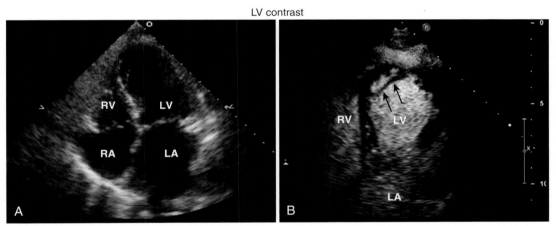

Figure 1-19 A, Transthoracic echocardiographic apical four-chamber view showing poor endocardial definition of the left ventricle (LV). **B,** Apical four-chamber view, zoomed on the LV, following the administration of LV contrast. The LV endocardium is now well visualized (prominent trabeculations indicated by *arrows*). *LA,* Left atrium; *RA,* right atrium; *RV,* right ventricle.

is performed to evaluate whether right-to-left shunting is present across the interatrial septum. To perform an agitated saline contrast study, two 10-mL syringes are connected to a three-way stopcock. In one syringe, 9 mL of saline is mixed with less than 1 mL of air (some centers substitute 1 mL of saline for 1 mL of the patient's blood). The second syringe is empty. The mixture is agitated between the two syringes.

Approximately 5 to 6 mL of agitated saline is then injected rapidly into a large antecubital vein during imaging, typically in the apical four-chamber view. The right side of the heart should opacify quickly as the agitated saline enters it. The presence of contrast material in the left ventricle three to five cycles after right-sided heart opacification suggests right-to-left interatrial shunting. Late bubbles may represent shunting at the pulmonary level. Two injections are usually administered, the first at rest and the second during a Valsalva maneuver (Fig. 1-18). On release of the Valsalva maneuver, the increase in venous return to the right atrium and the increase in right atrial pressure

may "open" a PFO. If possible, the examiner should place the intravenous catheter in the left antecubital fossa, so that a left-sided superior vena cava is not overlooked. When a patient has a left-sided superior vena cava, contrast material can be seen to enter the dilated coronary sinus before the right atrium. With a right-sided injection, this variation will not be appreciated, and consequently the diagnosis of a left-sided superior vena cava may be missed.

Contrast for Left Ventricular Opacification

In some patients, the left ventricular endocardium is poorly visualized because of body habitus or coexisting lung disease. Contrast agents have been routinely used for left ventricular opacification because these agents improve endocardial border definition (Fig. 1-19). These contrast agents consist of microbubbles containing a high-molecular weight gas, such as perfluorocarbon. These agents are administered intravenously

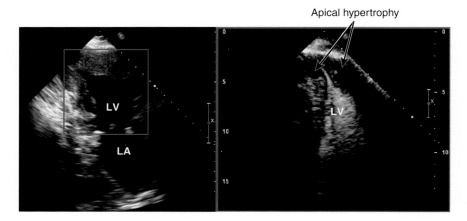

Figure 1-20 Transthoracic echocardiographic apical two-chamber view before and following the administration of left ventricular (LV) contrast. The image shows significant apical hypertrophy, which was not well appreciated on two-dimensional imaging. *LA,* Left atrium.

and are safe to use in most patients. The microbubbles are smaller than red blood cells and pass through the lungs, cardiac chambers, and myocardium without any adverse hemodynamic effects. The use of contrast for left ventricular opacification can be particularly helpful in patients in intensive care settings, where imaging is often suboptimal because of patient positioning, postoperative changes, and limited windows.

Contrast administration is contraindicated in patients with a documented right-to-left, bidirectional, or transient right-to-left cardiac shunt. Depending on the composition of the contrast agent, it is also contraindicated in patients allergic to perflutren, blood products, or albumin. Patients with significant pulmonary hypertension or unstable cardiopulmonary conditions require additional monitoring of vital signs, ECG monitoring, and cutaneous oxygen saturation determinations for up to 30 minutes after administration of contrast. An arbitrary cutoff of 55 mmHg is often used to define significant pulmonary hypertension. Adverse events have been reported for all approved agents; these events are typically mild, occur infrequently, and include symptoms such as headache, weakness, palpitations, nausea, and back or chest pain. Allergic reactions are rare (1 in 10,000). Severe anaphylactic reactions are thought to be related to nonimmunoglobulin E–mediated or anaphylactoid reactions from local complement activation. Most commercially available echocardiography machines can be set to optimize left ventricular opacification following the administration of an echocardiographic contrast agent. The examiner must lower the mechanical index to minimize premature disruption of microbubbles.

Indications for Left Ventricular Opacification

1. Quantification of left ventricular volumes and ejection fraction
2. Determination of the presence of the following abnormalities:
   - Apical hypertrophy (Fig. 1-20)
   - Noncompaction
   - Thrombus
   - Endomyocardial fibrosis
   - Left ventricular apical ballooning (Takotsubo)
   - Left ventricular aneurysm
   - Left ventricular pseudoaneurysm
   - Myocardial rupture
3. Characterization of cardiac masses
4. Optimization of Doppler signals
5. Stress echocardiography (permits more accurate assessment of ejection fraction and wall motion)

Stress Echocardiography

Stress echocardiography is a powerful, noninvasive tool for diagnosis and risk stratification in patients with known or suspected ischemic heart disease. The sensitivity and specificity both range from 80% to 85%. Exercise stress echocardiography may be performed using a treadmill, upright bicycle or supine bicycle. Dobutamine stress echocardiography is an alternative test for patients who are unable to exercise. For patients with hypertrophic cardiomyopathy, exercise stress echocardiography is helpful in determining dynamic changes in the left ventricular outflow tract gradient when the resting gradient is low. Stress echocardiography also plays an important role in the assessment of patients with valve disease, such as mitral stenosis and low-flow, low-gradient aortic stenosis.

Transesophageal Echocardiography

Transesophageal echocardiography (TEE) is routinely performed in clinical practice for both inpatients and outpatients. The proximity of the transducer to the heart, the use of higher frequencies, and the use of 2-D or 3-D imaging probes results in improved spatial resolution and image quality. The average size of the tip of the TEE probe is 13 mm in diameter. The transducer can be maneuvered in multiple dimensions. It can be moved up and down the esophagus. It can also be rotated clockwise and counterclockwise in the esophagus. The tip of the probe may be flexed or retroflexed for better visualization of specific cardiac structures. The tip of the probe may also be moved from side to side, although this is rarely required. The imaging planes are changed by adjusting the scan plane from 0 to 180 degrees. TEE is routinely used in the operating room, where it provides valuable information for both the surgeon and the anesthesiologist.

Common Indications

1. Suspected endocarditis in a patient with moderate or high test-pretest probability
2. Exclusion of a left atrial appendage thrombus before DC cardioversion
3. Exclusion of a cardiac source of emboli (including vegetation, valve tumor, PFO, left atrial appendage thrombus, aortic thrombus, or atheroma)
4. Evaluation of valve disease (mechanism of regurgitation, valve morphology)
5. Evaluation of prosthetic valve dysfunction (paravalvular leaks)
6. Evaluation of a mass
7. Evaluation of intracardiac shunts, such as total anomalous pulmonary venous drainage
8. Guiding of percutaneous interventions (PFO, ASD closure, transcatheter aortic valve implantation, left atrial appendage closure devices, mitral valvuloplasty)
9. Guiding of intraoperative procedures (valve repair or replacement, aortic graft, excision of cardiac mass)
10. Evaluation of left and right ventricular function if TTE views are limited
11. Exclusion of aortic dissection (less common now because CT is usually the first-line investigation)
12. Evaluation of patients with cardiogenic shock, especially to assess mechanical complications after acute myocardial infarction
13. Poor or limited TTE windows

TEE is a semi-invasive procedure usually performed with conscious sedation. General anesthesia is advisable for higher-risk cases, such as patients with significant pulmonary disease (e.g., obstructive sleep apnea requiring continuous positive airway pressure) or patients who would be difficult to sedate secondary to high analgesic requirements. TEE is often performed in patients who are intubated and ventilated. TEE is not without risk, and unlike esophagogastroduodenoscopy, the procedure involves blind intubation of the esophagus. Consequently, patients should have no contraindications to TEE, such as swallowing problems, esophageal disease including pharyngeal pouch, esophageal varices, or ulceration. Recent hematocrit, clotting, and renal function test results should be available. Patients are fasted for 6 to 8 hours before the procedure, and informed written consent should be obtained from all patients, their families, or the responsible physicians.

Although TEE is a routine imaging test, complications occasionally arise. Therefore, TEE should be performed only in areas where full resuscitation equipment is available. Minor complications include transient bronchospasm, hypoxia, arrhythmias, and oropharyngeal bleeding (<1 in 500 cases). Serious complications include death, sustained ventricular tachycardia, and angina and occur in less than 1 in 5000 cases. Esophageal perforation is fortunately very rare; in a study of more than 10,000 consecutive patients undergoing TEE, 1 case of hypopharyngeal perforation and 2 cases of esophageal perforation occurred.

For patients undergoing TEE with conscious sedation, local anesthetic mouthwash and throat spray facilitates probe insertion. With the patient in left lateral decubitus position, a bite block is inserted between the teeth, and midazolam and fentanyl are titrated until the patient is adequately sedated. The probe, slightly flexed, is advanced to the back of the patient's mouth, at which time the patient is asked to swallow, thus permitting advancement of the probe into the esophagus. Most imaging is done from the midesophagus, starting with the four-chamber view (Fig. 1-21, A and B). The left side of the heart is displayed on the right side of the screen; the right side of the heart appears on the left side of the screen; the atria are shown superiorly and the ventricles inferiorly. From the midesophagus, all valves, the left atrial appendage, and the interatrial septum can be visualized (Figs. 1-22 to 1-26).

By advancing the probe from the midesophagus into the stomach, transgastric views are obtained (Figs. 1-27 and 1-28). It is usually necessary for the examiner to flex the probe to visualize the heart clearly. Deep transgastric views are used to obtain gradients across the aortic valve. Transgastric views are particularly good for the assessment of left ventricular function and allow better Doppler alignment for aortic gradients. Furthermore, transgastric views often provide better visualization of the tricuspid valve and right ventricle, in addition to evaluating the presence or absence of a pericardial effusion.

The examiner must have a systematic approach when performing TEE to ensure that all structures are adequately evaluated. Figure 1-29 is a guide to performing a comprehensive study. Most operators adapt and modify their study depending on the specific clinical question.

The development of 3-D TEE probes has allowed more detailed assessment of cardiac structures, thereby providing additional information. Three-dimensional imaging plays an important role in the assessment of ASDs. Increasing evidence indicates that many ASDs are not circular as they often appear on 2-D imaging. Furthermore, 3-D imaging is now used in the assessment of mitral valve disease and facilitates preoperative planning for surgical repair. Three-dimensional imaging is especially superior to 2-D imaging in the assessment of prosthetic mitral valve paravalvular leaks and in the identification of mitral valve clefts in patients with myxomatous mitral valve prolapse.

■ COMMON ARTIFACTS

Artifacts are common in TTE and TEE. The operator must be aware of these and know how to differentiate them from true abnormalities. To minimize artifacts, echocardiographers should lower the gain when imaging highly reflective surfaces, examine structures in multiple views, and have a good understanding of normal

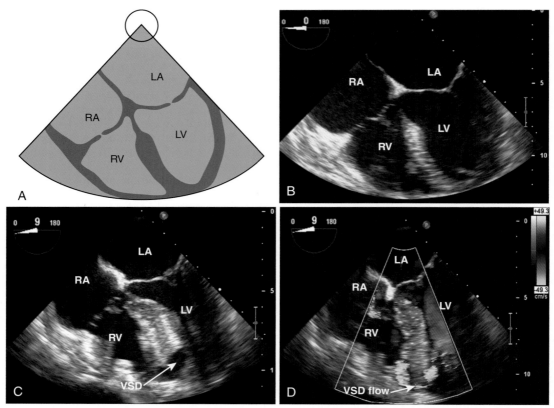

Figure 1-21 Transesophageal echocardiographic midesophageal four-chamber view. **A,** Schematic representation of normal midesophageal four-chamber view. **B,** Normal two-dimensional echocardiographic view. **C,** Large ventricular septal defect (VSD) in a patient after acute myocardial infarction. **D,** Continuous flow Doppler shows evidence of left-to-right flow across the VSD. *LA,* Left atrium; *LV,* left ventricle; *RA,* right atrium; *RV,* right ventricle.

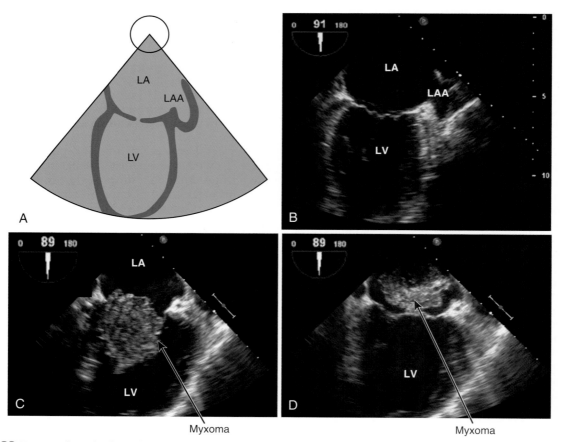

Figure 1-22 Transesophageal echocardiographic midesophageal two-chamber view. **A,** Schematic representation of normal midesophageal two-chamber view. **B,** Normal two-dimensional echocardiographic view. **C,** A large left atrial myxoma prolapsing across the mitral valve in diastole. **D,** Large left atrial myxoma that was attached to the interatrial septum. *LA,* Left atrium; *LAA,* left atrial appendage; *LV,* left ventricle.

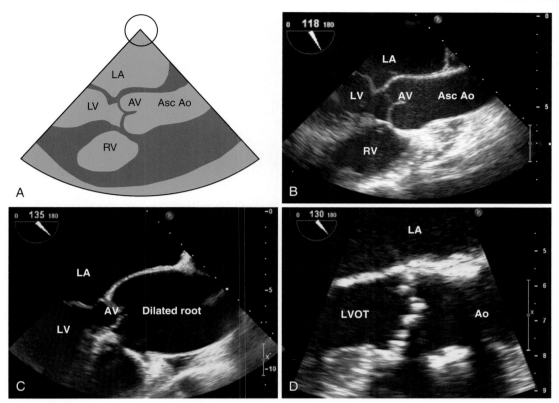

Figure 1-23 Transesophageal echocardiographic midesophageal long-axis aortic valve (AV) view. **A,** Schematic representation of normal midesophageal long-axis AV view. **B,** Normal two-dimensional echocardiographic view. **C,** Markedly dilated aortic root with effacement of the sinotubular junction. Incomplete closure of the AV leaflets secondary to annular dilatation (annuloaortic ectasia) is noted. **D,** Heavily calcified AV in a patient with severe aortic stenosis. *Asc Ao,* Ascending aorta; *LA,* left atrium, *LV,* left ventricle; *LVOT,* left ventricular outflow tract; *RV,* right ventricle.

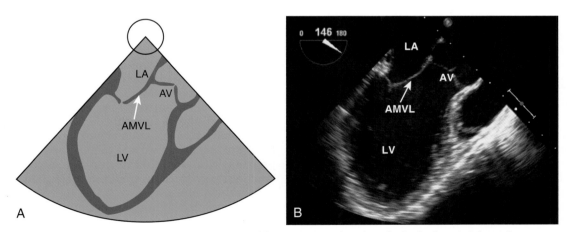

Figure 1-24 Transesophageal echocardiographic midesophageal long-axis view of aortic and mitral valves. **A,** Schematic representation of normal midesophageal long-axis view of aortic and mitral valves. **B,** Normal two-dimensional echocardiographic view. *AMVL,* Anterior mitral valve leaflet; *AV,* aortic valve; *LA,* left atrium; *LV,* left ventricle.

anatomy. Some of the most common artifacts encountered are as follows:

■ Reverberation artifacts (TTE and TEE) arise from a strong reflector, such as calcium, pacing wires, or a prosthetic metallic valve.

■ Side lobe artifacts (TTE) are caused by low-energy side lobes of the main ultrasound beam. When strong reflectors are present, they are displayed as if they originated from the central beam. Structures that may

often result in side lobe artifacts include the atrioventricular groove and the fibrous skeleton of the heart.

■ Mirror-image artifacts (TEE) in the transverse and descending thoracic aorta give the appearance of a double-barrel aorta. This appearance is caused by the aorta-lung interface, which acts as a reflector.

■ Linear artifacts (TEE) may mimic an intimal flap in the ascending aorta, particularly when the aortic diameter exceeds the left atrial diameter.

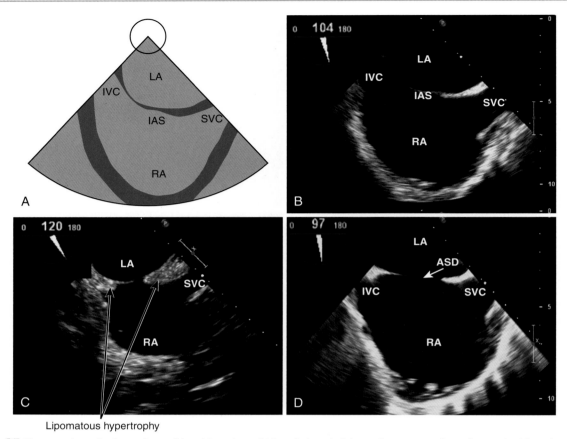

Lipomatous hypertrophy

Figure 1-25 Transesophageal echocardiographic midesophageal bicaval view. **A,** Schematic representation of normal midesophageal bicaval view. **B,** Normal two-dimensional echocardiographic view. **C,** Lipomatous hypertrophy of the interatrial septum (IAS). This is often described as having a "dumbbell" appearance and should not be mistaken for a mass. **D,** Secundum atrial septal defect (ASD). *IVC,* Inferior vena cava; *LA,* left atrium; *RA,* right atrium; *SVC,* superior vena cava.

■ Acoustic shadowing (TTE and TEE) is commonly seen with prosthetic metallic valves.

■ SPECIFIC STRUCTURES AND DISORDERS

Aorta

TTE and TEE are both excellent noninvasive modalities for the diagnosis and follow-up of patients with aortic aneurysms and dissection. In patients with a newly diagnosed aortic aneurysm on echocardiography, many physicians obtain a CT or MRI scan to delineate the exact location and size of the aneurysm. If the aneurysm is fully visualized on TTE and if the measurements correlate well with CT or MRI, then it is reasonable to follow up with serial TTEs to minimize radiation exposure (see Figs. 1-1, *C,* 1-8, *C,* and 1-23, *C*).

A patent ductus arteriosus is best visualized in a parasternal short-axis view, at the level of the main pulmonary artery and its bifurcation, or alternatively in the suprasternal view (see Figs. 1-3, *C,* and 1-13, *C* and *D*). TTE aortic arch views are also helpful in the diagnosis and follow-up of patients with coarctation of the proximal descending thoracic aorta. In most patients, the coarctation is located just distal to the left subclavian artery. Color flow mapping identifies turbulent flow and flow acceleration proximal to the narrowed area,

and continuous flow Doppler is used to assess the gradient across the coarctation. The gradient typically persists in diastole resulting in the characteristic "diastolic tail" seen on the Doppler profile (see Fig. 1-14, *D*). The gradient obtained may differ (overestimate) from the gradient obtained at the time of catheterization, and this may in part be a result of pressure recovery. The conversion of potential energy to kinetic energy across the narrowed area results in high velocity and a drop in pressure. Distal to the narrowing, flow decelerates. Some kinetic energy is reconverted into potential energy with a recovery in pressure.

The presence of aortic atheroma and thrombus is usually well visualized with TEE imaging (Fig. 1-30). The sensitivity and specificity of TEE in aortic dissection are high, at 97% to 99% and 97% to 100%, respectively (Fig. 1-31). The advantage of TEE is that it is quick, can be performed at the bedside, and does not require contrast which may be a consideration in patients with renal impairment. TEE also provides information regarding the aortic valve, the degree of aortic regurgitation if present, and involvement of the coronary ostia. TEE has, however, a slightly lower sensitivity and specificity when compared with CT and MRI; one potential disadvantage of TEE is a 2-cm blind spot proximal to the innominate arteries, where a discrete dissection flap may not be appreciated. CT and MRI

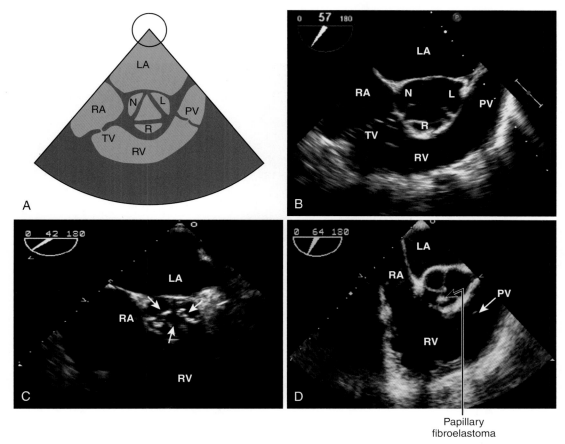

Figure 1-26 Transesophageal echocardiographic midesophageal short-axis view showing the aortic valve and right ventricular (RV) inflow and outflow tracts. **A,** Schematic representation of normal midesophageal short-axis view showing the aortic valve and RV inflow and outflow tracts. **B,** Two-dimensional echocardiographic view. **C,** Severe calcific aortic stenosis. **D,** Papillary fibroelastoma attached to the right coronary cusp. *L,* Left coronary cusp; *LA,* left atrium; *N,* noncoronary cusp; *PV,* pulmonary valve; *R,* right coronary cusp; *RA,* right atrium; *TV,* tricuspid valve.

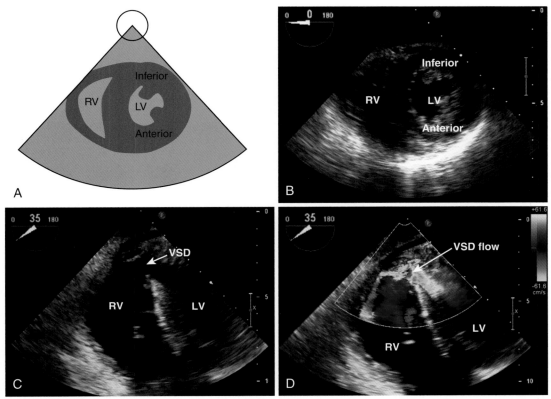

Figure 1-27 Transesophageal echocardiographic transgastric view short-axis view showing the right ventricle (RV) and left ventricle (LV). **A,** Schematic representation of normal transgastric short-axis view of the ventricles. **B,** Normal two-dimensional echocardiographic view. **C,** Large ventricular septal defect (VSD). **D,** Evidence of left-to-right (L-R) flow is shown by color Doppler. The VSD was best visualized with the probe flexed at 35 degrees.

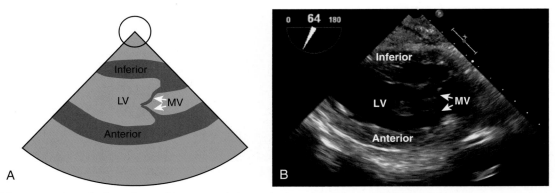

Figure 1-28 Transesophageal echocardiographic transgastric long-axis view of the left ventricle (LV). **A,** Schematic representation of the normal transgastric long-axis view of the LV. **B,** Normal two-dimensional echocardiographic view of the LV. *MV,* Mitral valve.

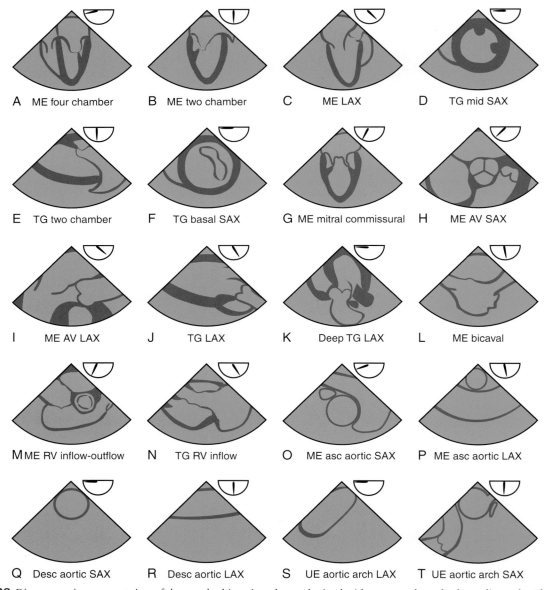

Figure 1-29 Diagrammatic representation of the standard imaging planes obtained with transesophageal echocardiography. The multiplane angle for each view is shown. *AV,* Aortic valve; *LAX;* long-axis; *ME,* midesophageal; *RV,* right ventricle; *SAX,* short-axis; *TG,* transgastric; *UE,* upper esophageal. (Reprinted with permission from the *Journal of the American Society of Echocardiography* from Shanewise JS, Cheung AT, Aronson S, et al. ASE/SCA guidelines for performing a comprehensive intra-operative transesophageal examination: recommendations of the American Society of Echocardiography and the Society of Cardiovascular Anesthesiologists Task Force for Certification in Perioperative Transesophageal Echocardiography. *J Am Soc Echocardiogr.* 1999;12:887.)

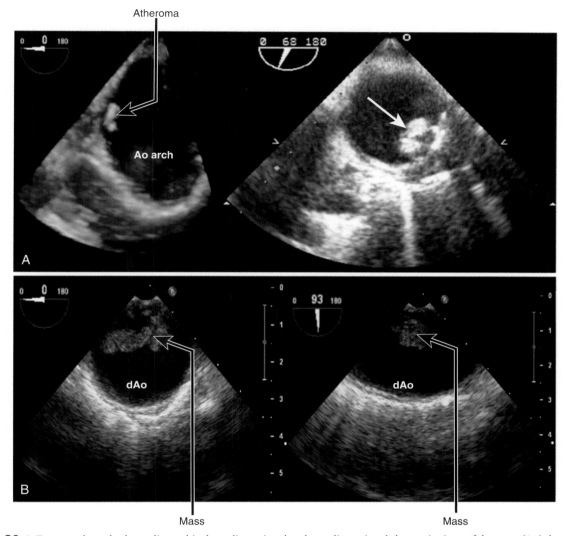

Figure 1-30 **A,** Transesophageal echocardiographic three-dimensional and two-dimensional short-axis views of the aorta (Ao) that show varying degrees of atheroma *(arrow).* **B,** Short-axis and long-axis views of the descending aorta (dAo) that show a large mobile mass with the appearance of thrombus.

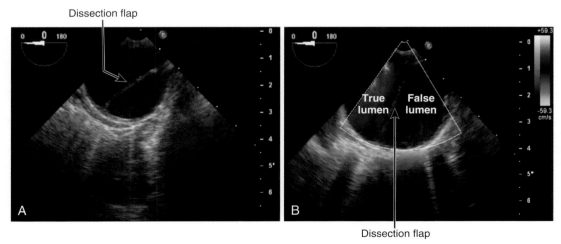

Figure 1-31 Chronic aortic dissection. **A,** Transesophageal echocardiographic two-dimensional short-axis view showing a dissection flap in the descending aorta. **B,** Color flow Doppler shows flow in the true lumen only because the false lumen is thrombosed.

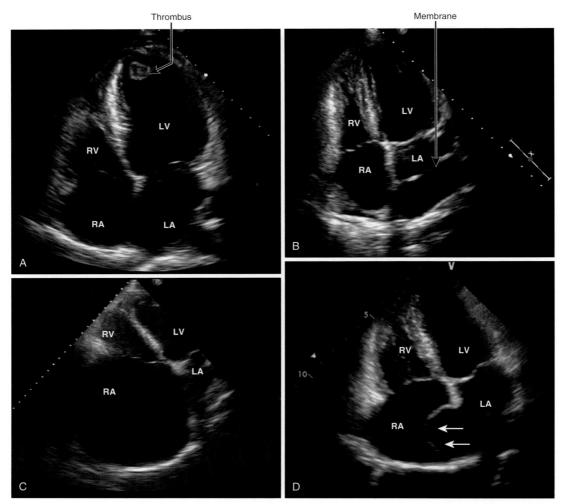

Figure 1-32 **A,** Transthoracic echocardiographic apical four-chamber view showing a thrombus in the left ventricular (LV) apex. **B,** Apical four-chamber view showing a membrane in the left atrium (LA) consistent with cor triatriatum. **C,** Apical four-chamber view, showing a markedly dilated right atrium. **D,** Apical four-chamber view, showing an aneurysm of the interatrial septum *(arrows)*. This is defined as mobile, redundant tissue in the region of the fossa ovalis that demonstrates phasic excursion of 10 to 15 mm during the cardiac cycle. *RA,* Right atrium; *RV,* right ventricle.

are superior to TEE for assessment of the aortic arch vessels, which are often involved in patients with type A aortic dissection.

Atria

Atrial abnormalities such as dilatation, cor triatriatum, and interatrial septal aneurysms can be assessed by TTE (see Figs. 1-7, *D,* and 1-36, *D*; Fig. 1-32, *B* to *D*). An interatrial septal aneurysm is defined as mobile, redundant tissue in the region of the fossa ovalis that demonstrates phasic excursion of 10 to 15 mm during the cardiac cycle. It may be seen in up to 2% of patients referred for a TTE. Patients often have an associated PFO or ASD.

PFO and ASDs are often evaluated using TTE and TEE imaging (see Fig. 1-25, *D*; Fig. 1-33). If percutaneous device closure is being considered, TEE is important to confirm the location and type of ASD and to ensure that there is no evidence of a sinus venosus defect, which may not be appreciated by TTE, if present.

Moreover, the examiner must ensure that a sufficient rim of septal tissue surrounds the defect for anchoring the device. A careful assessment of all four pulmonary veins is also helpful to exclude partial anomalous pulmonary venous return. The maximum diameter of the ASD is measured in the anteroposterior (approximately 45-degree view where the aortic valve is seen) and inferosuperior (bicaval view) orientations. An ASD suitable for percutaneous closure measures less than 30 mm with a rim of tissue (≥5 mm) around the defect, to prevent obstruction to surrounding structures following deployment of the device.

The left atrial appendage varies in size and shape and is well visualized by TEE (Fig. 1-34, *A* and *B*). Examiners may see more than one lobe (see Fig. 1-34, *C*). For that reason, the appendage should be imaged in multiple planes to avoid missing thrombus in an accessory lobe. Pectinate muscles may be prominent and should not be mistaken for thrombus. Color flow mapping can be helpful in differentiating thrombus from pectinate muscles. In patients with atrial fibrillation, the emptying

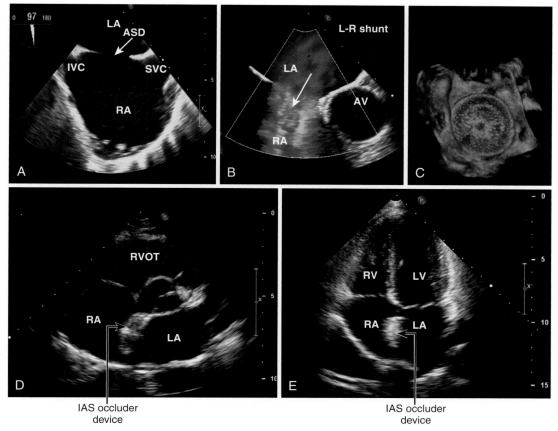

Figure 1-33 **A,** Transesophageal echocardiographic midesophageal bicaval view, showing a large secundum atrial septal defect. **B,** Color flow mapping shows laminar flow with left to right shunting. **C,** Midesophageal three-dimensional view of the interatrial septum, showing an atrial septal closure device following deployment. **D,** Transthoracic echocardiographic parasternal short-axis view at the level of the aortic valve showing the appearance of an atrial septal closure device. **E,** Transthoracic echocardiographic apical four-chamber view showing an atrial septal closure device. AV, Aortic valve; ASD, atrial septal defect; IAS, interatrial septal; IVC, inferior vena cava; L-R, left to right; LA, left atrium; LV, left ventricle; RA, right atrium; RV, right ventricle; SVC, superior vena cava.

velocities obtained using pulsed wave Doppler are often low (<40 cm/second), thus reflecting mechanical dysfunction (Fig. 1-35, *B*).

Cardiomyopathies

Echocardiography plays an important role in the assessment of cardiomyopathies. TTE facilitates classification and diagnosis of various cardiomyopathies including ischemic, dilated, hypertrophic, infiltrative, arrhythmogenic right ventricular cardiomyopathy or dysplasia (ARVC/D), as well as isolated ventricular noncompaction (IVNC).

Ischemic cardiomyopathy is common in patients with ischemic heart disease and is characterized by impaired left ventricular systolic function and the presence of regional wall motion abnormalities. TTE is often one of the first imaging tests requested for patients presenting with acute chest pain, especially when the ECG findings are confusing. The detection of a new wall motion abnormality by echocardiography may identify patients with acute ischemia and facilitate early invasive intervention, if appropriate. Furthermore, echocardiography is the imaging test of choice in evaluating complications of acute myocardial infarction. These patients tend

to be clinically unstable, and TTE can quickly identify many abnormalities including papillary muscle rupture, ventricular septal rupture, right ventricular infarction, cardiac tamponade, and pseudoaneurysm, thereby facilitating appropriate therapy (see Figs. 1-21, *C* and *D*, and 1-27, *C* and *D*).

In dilated cardiomyopathy, patients have dilation of one or both ventricles, with global impairment of systolic function (see Fig. 1-10, *C*; Fig. 1-36, *C*). Occasionally, left ventricular function may be globally impaired with regional variation, as a result of preserved basal function, or abnormal septal motion resulting from left bundle branch block. "Functional" mitral or tricuspid valvular regurgitation may result from annular dilatation and incomplete valve closure. Dilated cardiomyopathy has several causes, and determining the exact etiology is often difficult. The most common causes seen in clinical practice are idiopathic and secondary to viral infections. Other less common but important causes includes peripartum stress (Takotsubo), and tachycardia-mediated cardiomyopathy.

Restrictive cardiomyopathies can be challenging to diagnose and may be difficult to differentiate clinically from constrictive pericarditis. The most common

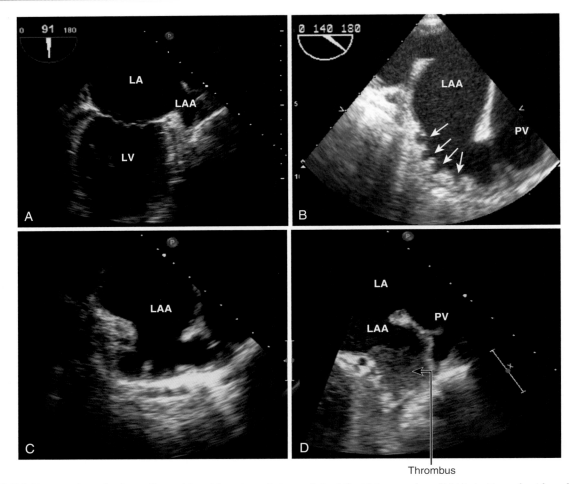

Figure 1-34 Transesophageal echocardiographic midesophageal views of the left atrial appendage (LAA). **A,** Normal midesophageal two-chamber view. **B,** Normal appearance of LAA pectinate muscles *(arrows)*. **C,** LAA showing two separate lobes. The LAA should be evaluated in different planes and transducer angles because a thrombus may be present in only one lobe. **D,** LAA thrombus. *LA,* Left atrium; *LV,* left ventricle; *PV,* pulmonary vein.

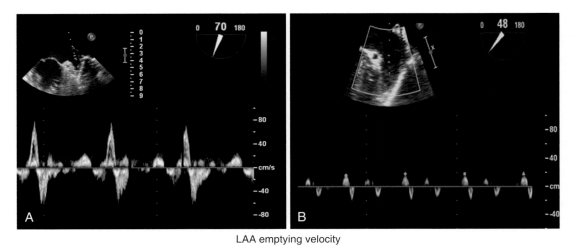

LAA emptying velocity

Figure 1-35 Pulsed wave Doppler of the left atrial appendage on a transesophageal echocardiogram. The normal left atrial appendage emptying velocity is greater than 40 cm/second. The risk of developing a thrombus is higher if the left atrial appendage velocity is less than 40 cm/second. **A,** Normal left atrial appendage normal emptying velocities. **B,** Abnormal left atrial emptying velocities at 20 cm/second.

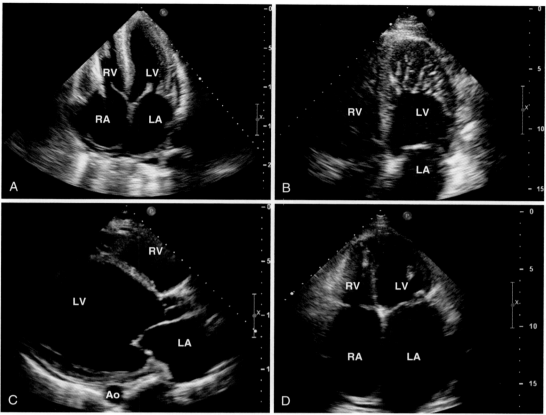

Figure 1-36 **A,** Transthoracic echocardiographic apical four-chamber view from a patient with amyloid heart disease that shows the characteristic speckled appearance of the myocardium. Note also the dilated atria and hypertrophied ventricles. A pacing wire is noted in the right ventricle (RV). **B,** Apical four-chamber view, zoomed on the left ventricle (LV), showing noncompaction of the LV myocardium. The end-systolic ratio of the noncompacted endocardial layer to the compacted myocardium is greater than 2. **C,** Parasternal long-axis view showing a markedly dilated LV in a patient with dilated cardiomyopathy. **D,** Apical four-chamber view in a patient with restrictive cardiomyopathy. Note the massively dilated atria and small ventricles. *Ao,* Aorta; *LA,* left atrium; *RA,* right atrium.

infiltrative cardiomyopathy seen on echocardiography is amyloid, which is associated with a characteristic highly reflective granular speckled appearance of the myocardium. In this restrictive cardiomyopathy, the classic appearance is that of dilated atria and small hypertrophied ventricles with evidence of diastolic dysfunction. Examiners not uncommonly see a small associated pericardial effusion (see Figs. 1-11, *D,* and 1-36, *A*).

Hypertrophic cardiomyopathy is an inherited disorder characterized by otherwise unexplained left ventricular hypertrophy, with left ventricular walls 15 mm or thicker in a nondilated left ventricle. The hypertrophy may be asymmetric, concentric, or predominantly apical. Asymmetric septal hypertrophy with a septal-to-posterior wall ratio of 1.3 to 1.0 is the most common pattern seen on TTE (Fig. 1-37, *A*). Systolic anterior motion of the anterior mitral valve leaflet is often associated with asymmetric septal hypertrophy (see Fig. 1-37, *B*). With these findings, Doppler imaging may reveal a resting late systolic gradient across the left ventricular outflow tract (see Fig. 1-37, *C*). This gradient may be significantly higher with reduced preload (a Valsalva maneuver) and decreased with reduced afterload (hand grip). Although the mitral valve is structurally normal, mitral regurgitation often results from the systolic anterior motion of the mitral valve leaflet.

Therefore, the examiner must distinguish between the Doppler velocity profile of the mitral regurgitation jet and the left ventricular outflow tract gradient jet. In symptomatic patients, if the resting left ventricular outflow tract gradient is low, a stress echocardiogram is often requested to evaluate for dynamic obstruction with increased contractility.

ARVC/D is a genetic condition in which the right ventricular myocardium is replaced by fibrofatty tissue. The exact incidence of the condition is unknown; however, the prevalence is thought to be 1 in 1000. TTE findings include dilated right ventricle or right ventricular outflow tract, right ventricular free wall sacculations or aneurysm formation, trabecular derangement, hyperreflective moderator band, and impaired right ventricular function. The diagnosis of ARVC/D is based on the collective findings from clinical history and routine investigations, which include signal averaged ECG, TTE, MRI, endomyocardial biopsy, and genetic testing. In 2010, updated guidelines for the diagnosis of ARVC/D were published, and these include revised criteria regarding right ventricular measurements by echocardiography. ARVC/D is a progressive disorder, and it is not exclusive to the right ventricle. Left ventricular involvement typically affecting the posterior lateral wall is not uncommon.

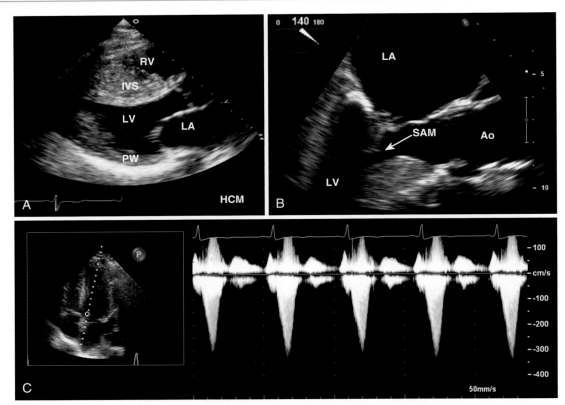

Figure 1-37 Hypertrophic cardiomyopathy (HCM). A, Transthoracic echocardiographic two-dimensional parasternal long-axis view showing asymmetric septal hypertrophy. **B,** Transesophageal echocardiographic midesophageal long-axis view of the aortic and mitral valves showing systolic anterior motion (SAM) of the anterior mitral valve leaflet. **C,** Continuous wave Doppler in the left ventricular outflow tract, showing a late peaking systolic gradient. This acceleration of flow in mid- to late systole may be seen in patients with HCM at rest or with a Valsalva maneuver. If the resting gradient is low, evidence of dynamic obstruction can be assessed during an exercise stress echocardiogram. *IVS,* Interventricular septum; *LA,* left atrium; *LV,* left ventricle; *PW,* posterior wall; *RV,* right ventricle.

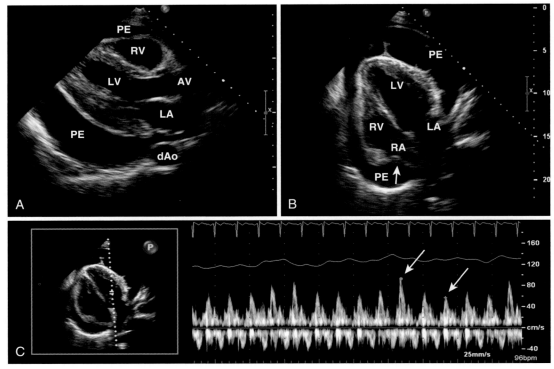

Figure 1-38 A, Transthoracic echocardiographic parasternal long-axis view showing a large circumferential pericardial effusion (PE). **B,** Apical four-chamber view with evidence of fibrinous strands around the left ventricular (LV) apex and lateral wall. Inversion of the right atrial (RA) wall *(arrow)* is evident. **C,** Continuous wave Doppler across the mitral valve that shows respiratory variation in the transmitral flow consistent with elevated intrapericardial pressure *(arrows). AV,* Aortic valve; *dAo,* descending aorta; *LA,* left atrium; *RV,* right ventricle.

IVNC, another genetic disorder, results from intrauterine arrest of the normal process of compaction of the myocardium (see Figs. 1-6, *C*, and 1-36, *B*). The diagnostic echocardiographic criteria for IVNC include (1) absence of coexisting cardiac abnormalities, (2) a maximum end-systolic ratio of noncompacted endocardial layer to the compacted myocardium of more than 2, (3) noncompacted myocardium in more than 80% of cases in apical and midventricular areas of the inferior and lateral wall, and (4) evidence of deeply perfused intertrabecular recesses by color Doppler imaging or contrast. The examiner must be aware that the echocardiographic and MRI criteria for IVNC are different because MRI uses a maximum ratio in diastole of noncompacted to compacted myocardial thickness of more than 2.3, as assessed in the long-axis view.

Pericardium

TTE is an excellent imaging modality for the detection and evaluation of pericardial effusions. Important information regarding the size and location of the effusion can help determine whether percutaneous pericardiocentesis is safe and feasible. Pericardial effusions smaller than 0.5 cm are regarded as small, and those greater than 2 cm are large (see Figs. 1-1, *D*, and 1-5, *C*). Cardiac tamponade is a clinical diagnosis; however, TTE provides additional information regarding the hemodynamic significance of a pericardial effusion. As the intrapericardial pressure rises, right atrial inversion during ventricular systole and right ventricular free wall inversion in early-diastole are seen. The inferior vena cava is often dilated and demonstrates less than 50% collapse with inspiration. In cardiac tamponade, the normal respiratory variation in mitral and tricuspid inflow velocities is exaggerated, reflecting ventricular interdependence. With inspiration, the tricuspid flow velocity increases, the mitral flow velocity decreases, and, as a consequence, left ventricular stroke volume is reduced (Fig. 1-38).

The diagnosis of pericardial constriction is difficult and often requires several imaging studies, both invasive and noninvasive. Pericardial thickening and or calcification is best evaluated by MRI and CT, respectively; however, TTE is often the initial imaging test requested. TTE may show evidence of restricted left ventricular filling, respiratory variation in transmitral flow, and other evidence of ventricular interdependence, such as abnormal motion of the interventricular septum with respiration.

Cardiac Masses

Echocardiography is an excellent imaging modality for the assessment and evaluation of cardiac masses. Normal variants may occasionally be mistaken for primary cardiac masses, however, and may lead to inappropriate interventions. Therefore, echocardiographers must have a thorough knowledge of normal anatomic structures. Differentiating between a thrombus and a tumor is often difficult; however, the location, appearance, and mobility often favor one diagnosis over the other. Left ventricular thrombi are typically seen in the apex in the setting of wall motion abnormality secondary to an apical infarct (see Figs. 1-6, *D*, 1-9, *D*, and 1-32, *A*). Patients with atrial fibrillation are at risk of left atrial appendage thrombi, as seen in Figure 1-34, *D*. Thrombus in right heart chambers may also be seen, particularly in patients with right heart catheters or pacing leads (see Figs. 1-2, *D*, and 1-12, *C* and *D*; Fig. 1-39).

Benign pericardial cysts are occasionally seen on TTE or TEE and do not require treatment unless they are causing local compression of cardiac chambers. A more unusual cardiac mass that may occasionally be encountered is a hydatid cyst (see Fig. 1-9, *C*). Several reports have noted cardiac hydatid cysts resulting from infection with the *Echinococcus* parasite. These cysts are usually seen in the left or right ventricles or pericardium.

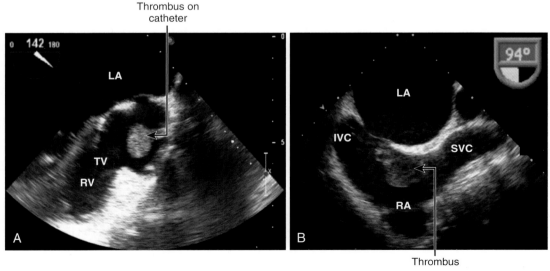

Figure 1-39 **A,** Transesophageal echocardiographic midesophageal modified bicaval view showing a large thrombus attached to the tip of a catheter entering the right atrium (RA) from the superior vena cava (SVC). **B,** Midesophageal bicaval view showing a thrombus in the RA attached to the interatrial septum. *IVC,* Inferior vena cava; *LA,* left atrium; *RV,* right ventricle; *TV,* tricuspid valve.

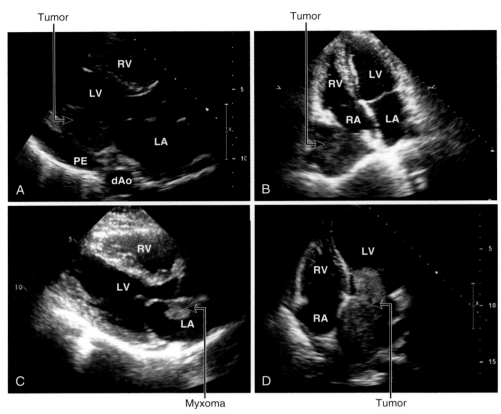

Figure 1-40 A, Transthoracic echocardiographic parasternal long-axis view showing a large tumor in the left ventricle (LV), adjacent to the posterior wall. This tumor was confirmed as a sarcoma. Note the small posterior pericardial effusion (PE). **B,** Apical four-chamber view showing a large angiosarcoma impinging on the right atrium (RA). **C,** Parasternal long-axis view showing a left atrial myxoma attached to the interatrial septum. **D,** Apical four-chamber view showing a large tumor filling the left atrium (LA) and prolapsing across the mitral valve in diastole. This was a metastatic lung tumor with direct invasion through the pulmonary veins. *dAo,* Descending aorta; *RA,* right artery; *RV,* right ventricle.

Patients often have multiple cysts, which may embolize or rupture. Surgical intervention is advised in addition to medical treatment; however, the prognosis often remains poor despite aggressive management.

Primary cardiac tumors are exceptionally rare, with an incidence of 0.002% to 0.3%, and most (estimated at 75%) of these are benign. Cardiac metastases are 20 to 40 times more common than primary cardiac tumors. The most common benign tumors are myxoma in adults and rhabdomyoma in children. Although myxomas are histologically benign, they can embolize or obstruct. Myxomas classically are pedunculated tumors found in the left atrium (75%), attached to the interatrial septum in the region of the fossa ovalis, and they often prolapse across the mitral valve in diastole (see Fig. 1-22, C and D; Fig. 1-40, C). Myxomas are usually globular and irregular and appear heterogenous on echocardiography. Doppler imaging is useful to assess the degree of obstruction across the mitral valve. Myxomas are often multiple, so it is imperative to exclude additional tumors. In most cases, surgical excision of the myxoma is performed. Patients must have follow-up imaging after excision because myxomas are known to recur.

Primary malignant tumors are fortunately rare in children. Sarcomas are the most common malignant primary cardiac tumors seen in adults and include angiosarcoma, rhabdomyosarcoma, and fibrosarcoma. These tumors are usually found in a right heart chamber, are extremely aggressive, and are associated with a poor prognosis (see Fig. 1-40, A and B; Fig. 1-41, B). Metastatic cardiac tumors are relatively common in patients with certain malignant diseases, especially when widespread metastatic disease is present. Tumors can invade the heart directly or by hematogenous spread. For example, metastatic renal cell carcinoma may invade the right atrium through the inferior vena cava; whereas metastatic bronchogenic carcinoma may invade the left heart through a pulmonary vein (see Figs. 1-40, D, and 1-41, C). Pericardial metastases are usually associated with pericardial effusion.

■ ECHOCARDIOGRAPHY TO GUIDE INTERVENTION

TTE and TEE are now routinely used to guide percutaneous interventional procedures in the catheterization and electrophysiology laboratories. TTE may be used in addition to fluoroscopy, to guide pericardiocentesis. Echocardiography is helpful in determining the size of the effusion and in identifying the most suitable approach (subcostal or apical) for aspiration. TTE allows direct visualization of the needle as it enters the pericardial space.

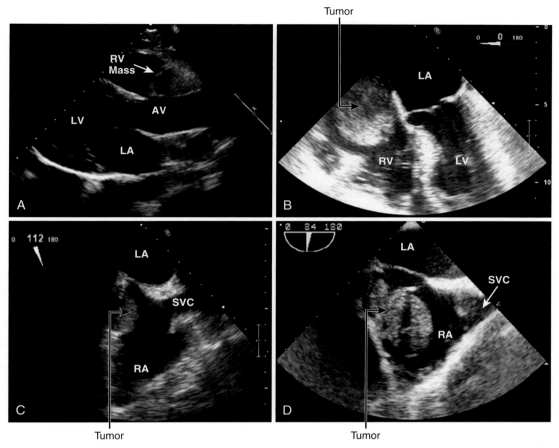

Figure 1-41 **A,** Transthoracic echocardiographic parasternal long-axis view showing a large mass in the right ventricle (RV). A parasternal short-axis view of the same mass is shown in Figure 1-3, *D*. This tumor was confirmed as a paraganglionoma following surgical resection. **B,** Transesophageal echocardiographic midesophageal four-chamber view showing a large tumor in the right atrium (RA) that prolapses across the tricuspid valve in diastole. This tumor was confirmed as a low-grade sarcoma. **C,** Transesophageal echocardiographic midesophageal bicaval view showing a large tumor invading the RA from the inferior vena cava in a patient with metastatic renal cell carcinoma. **D,** Transesophageal echocardiographic midesophageal bicaval view showing a large tumor in the RA that originated from the inferior vena cava. This tumor was confirmed as a fibroma. *AV,* Aortic valve; *LA,* left atrium; *LV,* left ventricle; *SVC,* superior vena cava.

Furthermore, agitated saline contrast can be injected to confirm that the introducer needle is in the pericardial space, before insertion of a dilator and pigtail drain.

TTE provides assessment of mitral valve function and the degree of mitral regurgitation immediately after percutaneous mitral valvuloplasty. TTE is also used to guide alcohol septal ablation treatment of hypertrophic cardiomyopathy. TEE or intracardiac ultrasound is used to facilitate percutaneous PFO or ASD closure in the catheterization laboratory. TEE allows assessment of the size, shape, and location of the defect. Furthermore, TEE can detect discrete fenestrations that may be relevant when the size of the closure device is being selected. Following deployment of the device, the examiner must ensure that the device is well seated and that it is not interfering with aortic or mitral valve function. Patients should have

no evidence of obstruction to systemic venous flow or pulmonary venous obstruction (see Fig. 1-33).

TEE is also used to guide procedures such as percutaneous closure of paravalvular leaks, ventricular septal defects, and implantation of left atrial appendage closure devices (Fig. 1-42). TEE plays a pivotal role in guiding percutaneous implantation of aortic valves, a procedure currently undergoing evaluation in clinical trials. TEE allows accurate measurements of the aortic valve annulus and root that dictate the size of the stent mounted valve selected for implantation. Under TEE and fluoroscopic guidance, the stent mounted prosthesis is carefully positioned before deployment. The positioning of the stent-mounted prosthesis is crucial because it determines the successful or failure of the procedure, and little room for error exists.

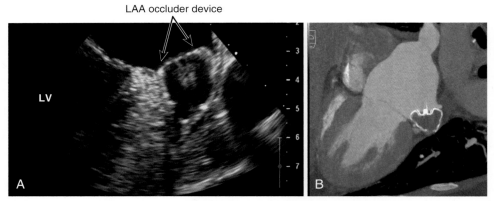

LAA occluder device

Figure 1-42 A, Transesophageal echocardiographic midesophageal view of the left atrial appendage (LAA) that shows an LAA occluder device. These occluder devices are deployed with transesophageal guidance to ensure that they are well seated with no residual flow into the LAA. **B,** Computed tomography appearance of an LAA occluder device. *LV,* Left ventricle.

Bibliography

Appelbe AF, Walker PG, Yeoh JK, et al. Clinical significance and origin of artifacts in transesophageal echocardiography of the thoracic aorta. *J Am Coll Cardiol.* 1993;21:754-760.

Armstrong WF, Ryan T. *Feigenbaum's Echocardiography.* 7th ed. Philadelphia: Lippincott Williams & Wilkins; 2010.

Baumgartner H, Hung J, Bermejo J, et al. Echocardiographic assessment of valve stenosis: EAE/ASE recommendations for clinical practice. *J Am Soc Echocardiogr.* 2009;22:1-23.

Bhan A, Kapetanakis S, Monaghan MJ. Three-dimensional echocardiography. *Heart.* 2010;96:153-163.

Blessberger H, Binder T. Two dimensional speckle tracking echocardiography: clinical applications. *Heart.* 2010;96:2032-2040.

Bruce CJ. Cardiac tumors: diagnosis and management. *Heart.* 2011;97:151-160.

Daniel WG, Erbel R, Kasper W, et al. Safety of transesophageal echocardiography: a multicenter survey of 10,419 examinations. *Circulation.* 1991;83: 817-821.

Douglas PS, Garcia MJ, Haines DE, et al. ACCF/ASE/AHA/ASNC/HFSA/HRS/SCAI/SCCM/SCMR 2011 appropriate use criteria for echocardiography: a report of the American College of Cardiology Foundation Appropriate Use Criteria Task Force, American Society of Echocardiography, American Heart Association, American Society of Nuclear Cardiology, Heart Failure Society of America, Heart Rhythm Society, Society for Cardiovascular Angiography and Interventions, Society of Critical Care Medicine, Society of Cardiovascular Computed Tomography, and Society for Cardiovascular Magnetic Resonance. *J Am Soc Echocardiogr.* 2011;24:229-267.

Freed LA, Levy D, Levine RA, et al. Prevalence and clinical outcome of mitral-valve prolapse. *N Engl J Med.* 1999;341:1-7.

Geyer H, Caracciolo G, Abe H, et al. Assessment of myocardial mechanics using speckle tracking echocardiography: fundamentals and clinical applications. *J Am Soc Echocardiogr.* 2010;23:351-369.

Jenni R, Oechslin EN, van der Loo B. Isolated ventricular non-compaction of the myocardium in adults. *Heart.* 2007;93:11-15.

Johri AM, Passeri JJ, Picard MH. Non-invasive imaging: three dimensional echocardiography: approaches and clinical utility. *Heart.* 2010;96:390-397.

Khandaker MH, Espinosa RE, Nishimura RA, et al. Pericardial disease: diagnosis and management. *Mayo Clin Proc.* 2010;85:572-593.

Lang RM, Bierig M, Devereux RB, et al. Recommendations for chamber quantification: a report from the American Society of Echocardiography's Guidelines and Standards Committee and the Chamber Quantification Writing Group, developed in conjunction with the European Association of Echocardiography, a branch of the European Society of Echocardiography. *J Am Soc Echocardiogr.* 2005;18:1440-1463.

Levine RA, Stathogiannis E, Newell JB, et al. Reconsideration of echocardiographic standards for mitral valve prolapse: lack of association between leaflet displacement isolated to the apical four chamber view and independent echocardiographic evidence of abnormality. *J Am Coll Cardiol.* 1998;11:1010-1019.

Leeson P, Mitchell A, Becher H. *Echocardiography.* Oxford Specialist Handbooks in Cardiology. Oxford: Oxford University Press; 2007.

Marcus FI, McKenna WJ, Sherrill D, et al. Diagnosis of arrhythmogenic right ventricular cardiomyopathy/dysplasia: proposed modification of the task force criteria. *Circulation.* 2010;121:1533-1541.

Min JK, Spencer KT, Furlong KT, et al. Clinical features of complications from transesophageal echocardiography: a single-center case series of 10,000 consecutive examinations. *J Am Soc Echocardiogr.* 2005;18:925-929.

Mulvagh SL, Rakowski H, Vannan MA, et al. American Society of Echocardiography consensus statement on the clinical applications of ultrasonic contrast agents in echocardiography. *J Am Soc Echocardiogr.* 2008;21:1179-1201.

Nagueh SF, Appleton CP, Gillebert TC, et al. Recommendations for the evaluation of left ventricular diastolic function by echocardiography. *J Am Soc Echocardiogr.* 2009;22:107-128.

Otto CM. *Textbook of Clinical Echocardiography.* 4th ed. Philadelphia: Saunders; 2009.

Peters PJ, Reinhardt S. The echocardiographic evaluation of intracardiac masses: a review. *J Am Soc Echocardiogr.* 2006;19:230-240.

Quiñones MA, Otto CM, Stoddard M, et al. Recommendations for quantification of Doppler echocardiography: a report from the Doppler Quantification Task Force of the Nomenclature and Standards Committee of the American Society of Echocardiography. *J Am Soc Echocardiogr.* 2002;15:167-184.

Reddy VY, Homes D, Doshi SK, et al. Safety of percutaneous left atrial appendage closure: results from the Watchman left atrial appendage system for embolic protection in patients with AF (PROTECT AF) clinical trial and the continued access registry. *Circulation.* 2011;123:417-424.

Rudski LG, Lai WW, Afilalo J, et al. Guidelines for the echocardiographic assessment of the right heart in adults: a report from the American Society of Echocardiography. *J Am Soc Echocardiogr.* 2010;23:685-713.

Shanewise JS, Cheung AT, Aronson S, et al. ASE/SCA Guidelines for performing a comprehensive intraoperative multiplane transesophageal echocardiography examination: recommendations of the American Society of Echocardiography and the Society of Cardiovascular Anesthesiologists Task Force for Certification in Perioperative Transesophageal Echocardiography. *J Am Soc Echocardiogr.* 1999;12:884-900.

Vignon P, Spencer KT, Rambaud G, et al. Differential transesophageal echocardiographic diagnosis between linear artifacts and intraluminal flap of aortic dissection or disruption. *Chest.* 2001;119:1778-1790.

Zoghbi WA, Enriquez-Sarano M, Foster E, et al. Recommendations for evaluation of the severity of native valvular regurgitation with two-dimensional and Doppler echocardiography. *J Am Soc Echocardiogr.* 2003;16:777-802.

Zoghbi WA, Chambers JB, Dumesnil JG, et al. Recommendations for evaluation of prosthetic valves with echocardiography and Doppler ultrasound. *J Am Soc Echocardiogr.* 2009;22:975-1014.

CHAPTER 2

Coronary Angiography: Technique

Brian G. Hynes and Ik-Kyung Jang

■ BACKGROUND

Despite major advances in other imaging modalities, invasive cardiac catheterization remains a critical component of cardiovascular care. More than 1.1 million cardiac catheterization procedures, in addition to approximately 1.3 million percutaneous coronary interventions (PCIs), were performed in the United States in 2006. Tremendous advances in digital imaging and procedural equipment have occurred since the last American College of Cardiology/American Heart Association (ACC/AHA) guidelines were published in 1999. This chapter aims to provide the reader with an overview of the practical fundamentals of performing invasive coronary angiography.

■ INDICATIONS FOR PERFORMING CORONARY ANGIOGRAPHY

Selective catheterization of the left coronary artery and the right coronary artery (RCA), combined with intra-arterial injection of radiopaque contrast media, allows radiographic imaging of the coronary arterial system. A complete assessment of coronary artery bypass grafts (arterial and venous) also entails selective cannulation and contrast media injection. Critical information concerning the presence (and burden) or absence of obstructive coronary artery disease (CAD) may be obtained from invasive coronary angiography. However, coronary angiography is a luminogram, which shows only the contrast-filled arterial lumen and densely calcified plaque. Noncalcified or lightly calcified nonobstructive atherosclerotic plaque may remain undetected in the absence of luminal narrowing. Although coronary angiography has undoubtedly had an impact on many aspects of cardiovascular care, the widespread availability of this imaging technique has perhaps influenced the management of patients with acute coronary syndrome the most. For example, primary PCI is the superior treatment modality for patients with acute ST-segment elevation myocardial infarction.

Detailed guidelines concerning indications for coronary angiography are summarized in Box 2-1. This list is not meant to be exhaustive and serves merely to highlight some of the most common clinical indications for invasive coronary angiography. The reader is directed to the ACC/AHA guidelines for coronary angiography for further information. As can be seen from these comprehensive guidelines, risk stratification plays an important role in assessing patient suitability for invasive coronary angiography. A study of patients without known CAD who underwent coronary angiography from January 2004 through April 2008 examined almost 400,000 patients enrolled in the ACC National Cardiovascular Data Registry. The investigators defined obstructive CAD as stenosis of 50% or more of the diameter of the left main coronary artery (LMCA) or stenosis of 70% or more of the diameter of a major epicardial artery. No CAD (defined as <20% stenosis in all vessels) was found in 39.2% of all patients. Among those patients with a positive result on noninvasive testing, the number was 41%. The investigators concluded that better risk stratification is required in clinical practice to ensure a higher diagnostic yield.

■ PATIENT EVALUATION BEFORE ANGIOGRAPHY

Before performing diagnostic coronary angiography, the physician should be fully aware of the patient's complete medical history and indications for proceeding to PCI if necessary. In particular, the physician must have a detailed discussion regarding the risk-to-benefit ratio of angiography with or without PCI before the patient receives sedatives. This discussion may not always be possible in the emergency setting, in which prompt revascularization with minimal delay is mandatory (e.g., ST-segment elevation myocardial infarction). Nevertheless, a focused history can elucidate key details such as allergies, risk of bleeding, and increased risk of potential adverse effects (e.g., contrast-induced nephropathy [CIN], arterial access difficulties), in addition to providing the opportunity to allay patient's concerns and obtain informed consent. The patient should also be given a brief step-by step-account of what he or she can expect to experience in the cardiac catheterization laboratory.

Physical examination should include, at a minimum, detailed vital signs (e.g., blood pressure, heart rate) and evaluation of cardiovascular, respiratory, and peripheral arterial systems. The results of these evaluations will influence arterial access choice, level of sedation, and suitability to proceed with percutaneous revascularization if deemed necessary. Results of basic

BOX 2-1 Indications for Coronary Angiography

Patients With Known or Suspected Coronary Artery Disease Who Are Symptomatic or Have Stable Angina

Class 1

CCS class III and IV angina in patients receiving medical therapy

Presence of high-risk criteria on noninvasive testing

After cardiac arrest or in patients with sustained monomorphic VT or nonsustained polymorphic VT

Class IIa

CCS class III or IV angina that improves with medical therapy

Progressive worsening abnormalities on serial noninvasive testing

Patients with angina who are unsuitable for noninvasive testing

CCS I or II unresponsive to or in patients intolerant of medical therapy

Certain occupations with abnormal but not high-risk stress tests or those deemed high risk

Class IIb

CCS class I or II angina with known ischemia in the absence of high-risk criteria on noninvasive testing

Asymptomatic man or postmenopausal woman with two or more major clinical risk factors and an abnormal stress test without high-risk criteria without known CAD

Asymptomatic patients with prior MI with normal left ventricle and ischemia in the absence of high-risk criteria

Follow-up evaluation after cardiac transplant

Non–cardiac transplantation workup in patients 40 years old or older

Class III

Angina in patients who refuse revascularization

Angina in patients unsuitable for coronary revascularization or in whom revascularization is unlikely to improve the quality or duration of life

Screening test for asymptomatic patients

Postrevascularization status without evidence of ischemia

Coronary calcification on noninvasive testing without criteria listed earlier

Indications in Patients With Nonspecific Chest Pain

Class I

High-risk findings on noninvasive testing

Class IIb

Recurrent admissions for chest pain with abnormal (but not high-risk) or equivocal noninvasive test findings

Class III

All other patients with nonspecific chest pain

Indications in Acute Coronary Syndrome

Class I

High or intermediate risk for adverse outcomes in patients with UA unresponsive to medical therapy

High risk with UA

High or intermediate risk with UA that stabilizes with medical therapy

Initially low-risk UA that has high-risk features on non-invasive testing

Suspected Prinzmetal variant angina

Class IIb

Low–short-term-risk UA without high risk on noninvasive testing

Class III

Recurrent chest discomfort suggestive of UA without objective signs of ischemia with a normal angiogram within 5 years

UA in patients not deemed suitable for revascularization for whom revascularization will not lead to improved quality or length of life

Postrevascularization Ischemia Indications

Class I

Suspected acute failure of coronary angioplasty or stenting after PCI

Recurrent angina or high-risk criteria on noninvasive testing within 9 months of percutaneous revascularization

Class IIa

Recurrent symptomatic ischemia within 12 months of CABG

High-risk criteria after CABG

Recurrent angina after revascularization refractory to medical therapy

Class IIb

Asymptomatic post-PCI patients with suspected restenosis but without noninvasive high-risk test features

Recurrent angina in absence of high-risk features on noninvasive testing more than 1 year after CABG

Asymptomatic post-CABG patients with deterioration in noninvasive test parameters in the absence of high-risk features

Class III

Post-CABG symptoms in patients not deemed suitable for repeat revascularization

Routine angiography in asymptomatic patients after PCI or surgery

Acute ST-Segment Elevation Myocardial infarction

Class I

ST-elevation MI in patients who are eligible for primary or rescue PCI

Patients with cardiogenic shock who are suitable for revascularization

Patients for surgical repair of ventricular septal rupture or severe mitral regurgitation

Ongoing hemodynamic or electrical instability

Class III

Coronary angiography not indicated in patients deemed unsuitable for revascularization (e.g., because of severe comorbidities)

BOX 2-1 Indications for Coronary Angiography—cont'd

Acute Coronary Syndrome Unstable Angina and Acute Non–ST-Segment Elevation Myocardial Infarction

Class I

Diagnostic angiography with intent to perform revascularization in UA and non–ST-segment elevation MI with refractory angina or hemodynamic or electrical instability

Patients directed toward an early invasive strategy

Class IIb

As part of an invasive strategy for patients with chronic kidney disease

Class III

Diagnostic angiography as part of an invasive strategy not indicated in patients deemed unsuitable for revascularization (e.g., because of severe comorbidities)

Patients with acute chest pain and a low likelihood of acute coronary syndrome

Patients who refuse an invasive strategy

Perioperative Evaluation for Noncardiac Surgery

Class I

Patients with known or suspected CAD

High-risk features on noninvasive testing

Angina refractory to medical therapy

UA

Equivocal noninvasive test results in high–clinical risk patients undergoing high-risk surgery

Class IIa

Multiple intermediate–clinical risk features and planned vascular surgery

Ischemia on noninvasive testing without high-risk features

Equivocal noninvasive test result in intermediate– clinical risk patient with planned high-risk noncardiac surgery

Urgent noncardiac surgery after recent acute MI

Class IIb

Perioperative MI

Stable CCS III or IV angina and planned low-risk surgery

Class III

Low-risk noncardiac surgery, in patients with known CAD without high-risk features on noninvasive testing

Asymptomatic patients after coronary revascularization and excellent exercise capacity (≥7 METS)

Patients deemed unsuitable for revascularization (e.g., because of severe comorbidities)

Patients With Valvular Heart Disease

Class I

Before valve surgery or balloon valvotomy in patients with chest discomfort or noninvasive ischemia, or both

Before valve surgery in patients with multiple risk factors for CAD

Infective endocarditis with evidence of coronary embolization

Class IIb

During LHC before atrioventricular valve or mitral valve surgery in patients without symptoms or noninvasive features of CAD

Class III

Before surgery for infective endocarditis in patients with no evidence of coronary embolization or risk factors for CAD

Asymptomatic patients without planned surgery

Before cardiac surgery when preoperative LHC is unnecessary and patients have neither risk factors for nor evidence of CAD

CABG, Coronary artery bypass grafting; *CAD,* coronary artery disease; *CCS,* Canadian Cardiovascular Society; *LHC,* left heart catheterization; *MET,* metabolic equivalent; *MI,* myocardial infarction; *PCI,* percutaneous coronary intervention; *UA,* unstable angina; *VT,* ventricular tachycardia.

BOX 2-2 Contraindications to Cardiac Catheterization

Coagulopathy

Anemia

Electrolyte abnormalities

Contrast allergy

Worsening renal dysfunction

Decompensated heart failure

Infection around planned arteriotomy site

Uncontrolled severe hypertension

laboratory tests such as renal function, complete blood count, coagulation profile, and liver function parameters should be available and reviewed. Abnormalities may require case deferral, depending on the clinical setting. Box 2-2 shows contraindications to cardiac catheterization.

■ CARDIAC CATHETERIZATION

Coronary angiography is performed in a fully equipped specially designed catheterization laboratory (see Fig. 2-3, *A*). For minimally invasive cardiac procedures to be performed in a safe and efficient manner, a dedicated, fully trained multidisciplinary team including cardiac nurses, technicians, and an interventional cardiologist is required. Common femoral arterial sheath placement using the modified Seldinger technique remains the most frequently employed access route for coronary angiography in the United States. Despite a surge of interest in using radial artery access, ACC National Cardiovascular Data Registry data suggest that less than 2% of all cardiac catheterization procedures are performed using the radial approach. Safe arterial access before any cardiac catheterization procedure is of critical importance to the success of the entire diagnostic or subsequent PCI procedure. A thorough knowledge of this procedure and its potential complications (Table 2-1)

Table 2-1   Femoral Arterial Access Complications

Diagnostic Cardiac Catheterization: Vascular Complications	0.40% Overall Complication Rate
PCI	
Femoral access hematoma (>6 cm)	5-23%
Retroperitoneal hematoma	0.15-44%
Pseudoaneurysm	0.5-6.3%
Atriovenous fistula	0.2-2.1%
Infection	<0.1%

Data from Antman EM, Anbe DT, Armstrong PW, et al. ACC/AHA guidelines for the management of patients with ST-elevation myocardial infarction—executive summary: a report of the American College of Cardiology/American Heart Association Task Force on Practice Guidelines (Writing Committee to Revise the 1999 Guidelines for the Management of Patients with Acute Myocardial Infarction). *J Am Coll Cardiol.* 2004;44:671-719; Tobis JM, Mallery JA, Gessert J, et al. Intravascular ultrasound cross-sectional arterial imaging before and after balloon angioplasty in vitro. *Circulation.* 1989;80:873-882; and Uren NG, Melin JA, De Bruyne B, Wijns W, Baudhuin T, Camici PG. Relation between myocardial blood flow and the severity of coronary-artery stenosis. *N Engl J Med.* 1994;330:1782-1788.

BOX 2-3   Risk for Vascular Complications During Percutaneous Coronary Intervention

Advanced age
Female sex
Smaller body surface area
Congestive heart failure, coagulopathy, chronic
    obstructive pulmonary disease, renal impairment,
    liver dysfunction, immunosuppression, prior
    coronary artery bypass grafting
Urgent or emergency procedure
Multivessel coronary artery disease
Intraaortic balloon pump counterpulsation use
Antiplatelet therapy (e.g., antiglycoprotein IIb/IIIa
    agents)
Increased lesion complexity

Data from Antman EM, Anbe DT, Armstrong PW, et al. ACC/AHA guidelines for the management of patients with ST-elevation myocardial infarction—executive summary: a report of the American College of Cardiology/American Heart Association Task Force on Practice Guidelines (Writing Committee to Revise the 1999 Guidelines for the Management of Patients with Acute Myocardial Infarction). *J Am Coll Cardiol.* 2004;44:671-719; and Arzamendi D, Ly HQ, Tanguay JF, et al. Effect on bleeding, time to revascularization, and one-year clinical outcomes of the radial approach during primary percutaneous coronary intervention in patients with ST-segment elevation myocardial infarction. *Am J Cardiol.* 2010;106:148-154.

is mandatory for all operators. Femoral arterial access complications may lead to limb viability compromise and even death in severe cases.

What Is the Risk Associated With Arterial Access in My Patient?

Several patient- and procedure-specific features may be used to estimate an increased risk of vascular access complications in patients who subsequently require PCI (Box 2-3). Patients undergoing vascular access for diagnostic angiography alone are deemed at low risk for complications (<1% complication rate). These procedures usually entail the use of smaller arterial sheaths, often with no systemic anticoagulation. Other

characteristics of low risk include elective procedures, male sex, normal renal function, and short procedure duration. Patients at moderate risk (1% to 3%) of vascular access complications include those undergoing routine PCI. In addition, increasing age, female sex, renal impairment, use of larger arterial sheaths (6 to 7 Fr), anticoagulation, and antithrombotic treatments are associated with greater risk. High-risk (>3%) features are coexisting peripheral arterial disease (PAD), renal and coagulation abnormalities, increasing age and sheath size (≥8 Fr), and female sex. Furthermore, emergency and challenging procedures such as primary or multivessel PCI and complex prolonged procedures increases the vascular access complication profile. Procedures that require even larger arterial sheaths, such as balloon aortic valvuloplasty (≥10 Fr), may carry an access complication rate of 11% to 17%.

Guide to Obtaining Arterial Access

The anatomic landmarks necessary for safe common femoral arterial access are illustrated in Figure 2-1, *A*, and should be identified before puncture. The inguinal ligament usually lies inferior to the inguinal skin crease and is crossed by the femoral artery at the one third medial–two thirds lateral point. The relation of the inguinal skin crease to the midfemoral head is routinely assessed radiographically with artery forceps (see Fig. 2-1, *B*). This assessment is particularly important because considerable variation in distance may exist between the inguinal skin crease and the inferior border of the femoral head, especially in obese patients.

An example of equipment commonly used is shown in Figure 2-3, *B*. After informing the patient of what to expect, the clinician administers 10 to 12 mL of 2% lidocaine subcutaneously, initially with a 25-gauge needle and then with a 22-gauge needle over the chosen skin puncture site. Care must be taken always to aspirate before injection, to avoid intraarterial or venous lidocaine administration. Once sufficient local anesthetic has been given, all remaining agent is discarded, to avoid mistaken intravascular administration at a later stage during the procedure. A small superficial nick using the tip of a number 11 scalpel is made; this nick can then be enlarged with blunt dissection using mosquito forceps. Care must be taken to avoid trauma to the femoral artery, especially in very thin patients.

Remembering the relation of the skin entry site to the inferior femoral head, the operator holds an 18-gauge needle to the skin, usually at a 30- to 45-degree angle, while the left index and middle fingers palpate the chosen arteriotomy site. The femoral pulse is usually approximately 2 cm inferior to the inguinal ligament. The needle is then advanced slowly toward the chosen arteriotomy site until resistance is met and the needle is felt to puncture the anterior wall. Brisk arterial flow should then be encountered. Care must be taken not to puncture the posterior wall of the artery because this may potentially lead to serious complications such as hematoma or retroperitoneal hemorrhage, especially

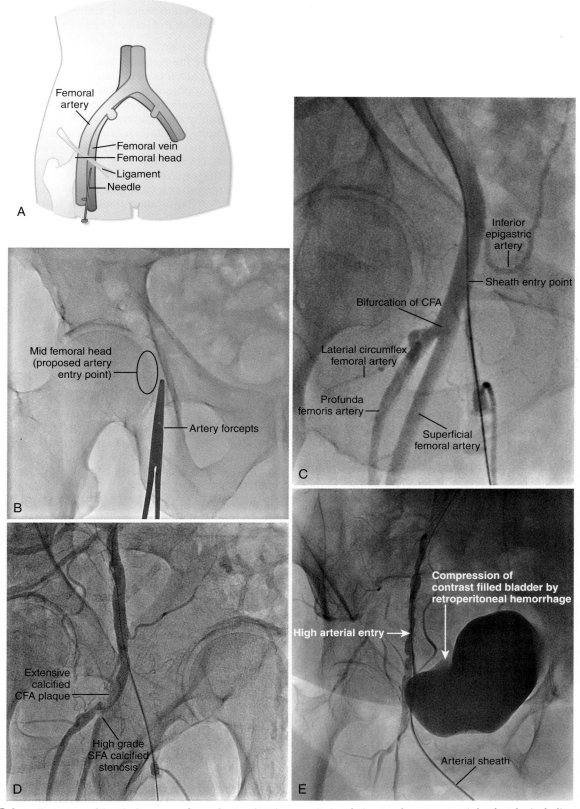

Figure 2-1 **A,** Illustration of the ideal common femoral artery (CFA) access site in relation to relevant anatomic landmarks, including the femoral head and inguinal ligament. **B,** Anteroposterior fluoroscopic image illustrating the forceps landmarks (midfemoral head) for the appropriate access site. **C,** Postaccess arteriogram in the right anterior oblique (RAO) projection demonstrates ideal CFA access. **D,** RAO projection in a different patient demonstrates calcified atherosclerotic CFA plaque. SFA, superficial femoral artery. **E,** RAO projection in a different patient demonstrates high artery entry leading to a retroperitoneal hematoma with resultant compression of the bladder filled with contrast.

if a subsequent PCI necessitating full anticoagulation is performed. Furthermore, bleeding from a back wall puncture may initially be unrecognized until hemodynamic compromise occurs.

Using his or her right hand, the operator advances a long 0.035-inch J-tipped wire through the needle while the left hand carefully fixes the needle in position within the artery. Use of a long 0.035-inch guidewire with a soft atraumatic tip, such as the Hi-Torque Versacore guidewire (Abbott Vascular, Abbott Park, Ill), is advisable, especially in patients with known or likely PAD. The wire should advance smoothly, without resistance. If any resistance is encountered, the wire should be withdrawn and spun while it is advanced slowly under fluoroscopic guidance, thus ensuring that the wire tip moves freely and is not subintimal. If this maneuver is not possible, the wire should be withdrawn, and pulsatile needle blood flow should be confirmed. If the needle blood flow is poor or absent, the operator may try carefully repositioning the needle by changing the angle of entry. If satisfactory blood flow cannot be achieved, the best approach is to withdraw the needle completely and maintain thorough hemostasis with firm manual compression for 5 to 6 minutes or until oozing ceases.

Once the first 5 to 10 cm of the guidewire is advanced, then the operator continues to advance the wire under fluoroscopic guidance to the descending thoracic aorta. The needle is removed, and pressure is applied with the left hand to maintain hemostasis over the arteriotomy site, while the guidewire is cleaned with a sterile, nonfibrous swab and loaded with the chosen sheath. The sheath is then advanced into the artery smoothly, with gentle rotation to reduce resistance if necessary. When any extra resistance is encountered, the sheath should not be advanced without examining its position and that of the guidewire under fluoroscopy. This is also the case if any undue discomfort is experienced by the patient. After allowing the sheath to bleed back, the operator should consider performing check femoral angiography in the right anterior oblique (RAO) projection with the guidewire in situ (see Fig. 2-1, C). The guidewire may be directed medially by using a towel to aid identification of the arteriotomy site under fluoroscopy. When a long sheath is used, it is advanced approximately 10 cm before femoral angiography and then readvanced over the reinserted dilator and indwelling guidewire.

Checking femoral angiography at the outset of the procedure serves many uses. It identifies femoral artery anatomy and the presence of significant PAD (Box 2-4; see Fig. 2-1, D [e.g., calcification, tortuosity]), and it may prove vital in minimizing vascular complications if the patient requires PCI, in which larger sheaths may be needed. It also aids identification of possible complications, such as pseudoaneurysm formation in the case of low arterial puncture, and likely difficulty with manual compression and risk of hematoma or retroperitoneal hemorrhage in the case of high arterial puncture. For example, Figure 2-1, E, demonstrates a high puncture with bladder compression from an extensive retroperitoneal hemorrhage. Femoral angiography is advised to assess for suitability before arterial closure device use.

BOX 2-4   Problem Solving: Common Femoral Artery Access in Presence of Peripheral Arterial Disease

1. Aim to use the common femoral artery on the side with less PAD, if possible (stronger pulse, lesser claudication or objective evidence of lower PAD burden on the basis of arterial noninvasive testing, computed tomography angiography, or prior angiography).
2. Identify key anatomic landmarks carefully as in item 1.
3. Perform arterial entry under fluoroscopic guidance.
4. Use a 0.035 steerable long guidewire with an atraumatic tip (e.g., Versacore wire, Abbott Vascular).
5. Use a long sheath (23 cm at a minimum).
6. Perform femoral angiography on successful sheath placement.
7. Always exchange catheters over the guidewire by using the desheathing technique.
8. When significant atherosclerotic disease is present at the arteriotomy site, avoid all active arteriotomy closure devices.

PAD, Peripheral arterial disease.

Radial Access

The radial approach for coronary angiography was initially described in 1989 by Campeau. Three years later, elective PCI through this approach was detailed by Kiemeneij and associates. Radial access as the default strategy has been embraced widely in many centers because of perceived benefits regarding patient comfort, early mobilization, and discharge, together with a significant reduction in morbidity and mortality after PCI in some series. Jolly and colleagues demonstrated a greater than 70% reduction in major bleeding rates with radial versus femoral access for diagnostic angiography or PCI. Significant bleeding as a consequence of femoral access vascular complications has been shown to have a negative impact on long-term survival mainly because of increasing 30-day mortality. Doyle and associates reviewed outcomes in more than 17,900 patients and found that greatest risk was seen with patients requiring transfusion of 3 or more units of blood. The most effective method of reducing the rate of major hemorrhage appears to be to employ the transradial approach. By virtue of its anatomy, the radial artery is very superficial and is not surrounded by any large veins or nerves, thus facilitating easy puncture and hemostasis. In addition, when the palmar arch is patent, the radial is not functionally an end artery, and so the hand should not be susceptible to ischemic complications should occlusion occur (Fig. 2-2, A and B). Given these data, the obvious question is this: Why is the radial approach for arterial access so infrequently used?

Diagnostic angiography and subsequent PCI may be more technically challenging and may thereby lead to longer procedure duration, greater radiation exposure, and higher failure rates requiring crossover to femoral access. Other perceived difficulties include upper extremity arterial anomalies, radial artery spasm, and occlusion. However, one study of low- to medium-volume operators who performed transradial PCI was

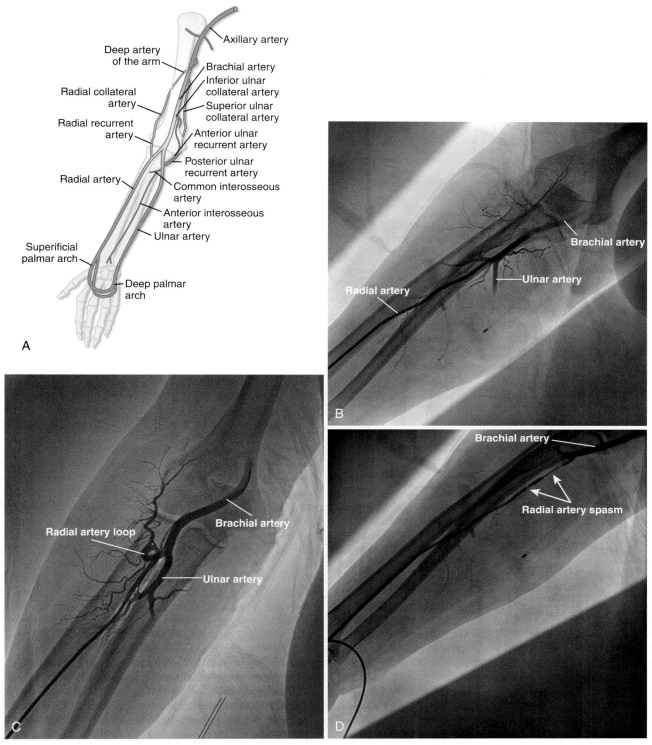

Figure 2-2 **A,** Illustration of upper extremity arteries. **B,** Radial-brachial angiogram in the anteroposterior projection shows normal anatomy. **C,** Radial-brachial angiogram in a different patient shows a proximal radial artery loop. **D,** Radial-brachial angiogram in a different patient shows significant catheter- or wire-induced radial artery spasm.

encouraging. The investigators reported a failure rate of less than 5%. Predictors of transradial failure included age older than 75 years, prior coronary artery bypass grafting, and short stature. Initial failure rates approaching 10% appear to decline rapidly to less than 2% as initial experience is gained with radial catheterization.

TECHNIQUE
A good understanding of upper extremity arterial anatomy is a prerequisite to safe radial cardiac catheterization. This anatomy is detailed in Figure 2-2, *A.* Use of the radial access site generally involves the same skill set of that of the transfemoral approach, with several additional

unique features. These features stem primarily from working with a smaller-caliber artery and negotiating the upper extremity arterial system en route to the ascending aorta. The major contraindication to radial access is the absence of collateral circulation between the ulnar and radial arteries because radial artery occlusion rates as high as 10% have been reported in some series.

Following sterile preparation and draping of the chosen wrist, 1 to 2 mL of 2% lidocaine is administered subcutaneously 1 to 2 cm proximal to the styloid process, again with aspiration before injection, to avoid intravascular administration. The operator's left-hand middle two to three fingers are used to define the location and path of the radial artery. Two methods are commonly used for sheath placement: the modified Seldinger technique and the Seldinger technique. The former consists of front wall arterial puncture, whereas the latter involves the through-and-through technique. The Seldinger method commonly involves using a cannula premounted on a needle.

The anterior wall of the artery is punctured, usually at an angle of approximately 30 degrees to the wrist. This results in brisk blood return, and the operator continues advancing the needle and cannula until blood flow ceases. The needle is withdrawn, and the cannula is then retracted very slowly (1 mm at a time) while the operator carefully assesses for arterial blood flow return. When brisk blood flow returns, the operator's left hand immobilizes the cannula, and the operator then advances the 0.018-inch hydrophilic guidewire, which should advance without resistance. Fluoroscopy may aid confirmation of correct wire placement.

Force should never be employed if resistance is encountered. This is particularly important where radial loops (see Fig. 2-2, C) may be found because excessive force may result in arterial dissection or even perforation. These forearm loops can be traversed under fluoroscopic guidance, often with a hydrophilic or 0.014-inch coronary wire. After sheath aspiration and flushing with heparinized saline, an intraarterial spasmolytic cocktail of verapamil (2.5 to 5 mg) and nitroglycerin (200 to 300 mcg) is injected. In addition, intravenous heparin (45 to 50 units/kg) may be administered. Refinement of radial catheterization has resulted in routine administration of antispasm and anticoagulation medications in addition to hydrophilic sheath use.

Despite these maneuvers, severe spasm may still occur, especially if the sheath needs to be enlarged, before PCI (see Fig. 2-2, before and after changing to a 6-Fr sheath, which induced severe spasm). Administration of intraarterial nitroglycerin, combined with intravenous delivery of sedation and anxiolytics, usually results in resolution of spasm. Furthermore, the technique of maintaining intraradial artery flow with concomitant hemostasis after sheath removal appears to reduce radial artery occlusion. Relative contraindications to this approach include the presence of severe innominate-subclavian artery disease, patients likely to require an arteriovenous fistula, and the presence of Raynaud syndrome. A list of common difficulties encountered among angiographers transitioning from

Table 2-2 Problem Solving: Overcoming Transradial Difficulties in Arterial Sheath Insertion

Arterial puncture	Identify artery using extensive palpation Puncture more proximally
Failure of wire advancement	If brisk arterial flow, advance wire while spinning under fluoroscopic guidance to ensure free movement of wire tip If poor flow, remove wire and needle and repuncture
Difficult sheath advancement	Ensure satisfactory wire placement with fluoroscopy Use hydrophilic sheaths, and advance with wet swap Make small skin incision
Radial artery spasm	Inject verapamil and nitroglycerin intra-arterially Use a smaller sheath
Failure of wire to advance in forearm	Manipulate under fluoroscopic guidance Use hydrophilic wire Perform angiogram to assess for loops
Failure to reach ascending aorta	Instruct patient to inspire deeply Direct guidewire (e.g., Hi-torque Versacore) with Judkins right catheter

Adapted from Hamon M, Baron JC, Viader F. Periprocedural stroke and cardiac catheterization. *Circulation.* 2008;118:678-683.

the transfemoral to the transradial approach is provided in Table 2-2.

Transbrachial Approach

Percutaneous transbrachial catheterization may also be used as an alternative approach. Similar to the transradial approach, it overcomes difficulties relating to severe lower extremity PAD. Advantages over the radial approach include the ability to employ larger sheath sizes. Indeed, numerous reports have noted intraaortic balloon pump insertion by this approach. Performing transbrachial angiography also involves many of the steps outlined in the transfemoral approach. A micro-puncture kit (Cook, Inc, Bloomington, Ind) is used routinely, and the artery is punctured approximately 1 cm above the antecubital crease. This site is readily identifiable under fluoroscopy because it projects over the olecranon process. At this site, the brachial artery is usually readily palpable, and hemostasis may be achieved after sheath withdrawal by compression against the distal humerus. Routine anticoagulation is administered to prevent thrombosis.

The brachial approach has fallen from favor because of the higher rate of complications compared with the transradial route. Major vascular access site complications were significantly higher in the brachial compared with the radial group (2.3% versus 0%; P = .035) in a randomized comparison composed of 279 patients. Complications secondary to percutaneous brachial access for endovascular procedures most commonly manifest as pseudoaneurysm formation or brachial artery thrombosis. In a retrospective study from the Cleveland Clinic in Ohio of almost 290 patients undergoing brachial access for endovascular procedures, pseudoaneurysms occurred in 11 patients, and brachial

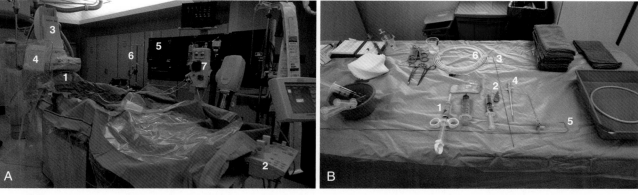

Figure 2-3 **A,** Photograph of the general cardiac catheterization laboratory setup: *1,* patient draped; *2,* C-arm and table controls; *3,* C-arm image intensifier; *4,* mobile radiation shield; *5,* monitor stack incorporating fluoroscopy live and review monitors, hemodynamic and electrocardiographic monitors, and intravascular ultrasound and echocardiographic image monitors; *6,* defibrillator cart; and *7,* automated contrast injector. **B,** Prepared table equipment: *1,* lidocaine syringe; *2,* arterial needle with cannula and radial access scalpel; *3,* 0.018-inch hydrophilic radial wire; *4,* 5-Fr radial artery sheath; *5,* 5-Fr Jacky radial catheter; *6,* 0.035-inch 260-cm guidewire.

artery thrombosis in 7 patients. Female patients in particular had a higher complication rate of 11.5% compared with 2.7% (*P* = .003) in men.

Angiography of the Left Coronary System

Information on detailed coronary anatomy, in addition to commonly encountered normal variants and pathology, is provided in Chapter 14. A basic catheterization laboratory setup for routine coronary angiography is shown in Figure 2-3, *A* and *B.* Fundamentals of coronary angiography include comprehensive assessment of all coronary artery anatomy and disease. Lesions should be outlined in at least two orthogonal views to facilitate accurate morphologic assessment. Specific risks include stroke, air embolism, artery thrombosis, and dissection. A key concept involves transitioning wires and catheters to avoid trauma to the aorta and thereby minimize the risk of catheter- or wire-induced atheroembolism.

Before every wire or catheter insertion, the sheath should be back bled and flushed with heparinized saline solution unless a contraindication to heparin exists. Thrombus may form quickly within the sheath and may then be propagated all the way to the coronary ostia, with potentially devastating consequences. The Judkins Left number 4 (JL4) catheter is loaded with the 0.035-inch guidewire, and the catheter tip is inserted into the sheath. The wire is then advanced smoothly under fluoroscopic guidance in the anteroposterior (AP) projection into the abdominal aorta. Then with the wire leading, both are advanced toward the ascending aorta. When the wire reaches the proximal portion of the ascending aorta, it is fixed, and the catheter is advanced until it reached the last couple of inches of the wire and is seen to configure to its predetermined shape. The wire is then carefully withdrawn under fluoroscopic guidance (moved to the 30-degree left anterior oblique [LAO] position) while the catheter is fixed with the operator's left hand to prevent

inadvertent engagement of the LMCA. The wire is wiped, wrapped, and placed in the heparinized saline bowl.

The catheter is connected to the manifold, and 4 to 6 mL of blood is aspirated and discarded through the waste valve. If the operator cannot freely aspirate blood at this stage, the catheter should be withdrawn under fluoroscopic guidance until the tip is free and aspiration is possible. Before contrast injection, the arterial pressure is checked to ensure that a satisfactory waveform is present.

Once the catheter is aspirated, a small injection of contrast agent can be made to opacify the catheter. Gentle manipulation of the catheter is usually all that is required to engage the LMCA successfully. This manipulation consists of gentle advancement, occasionally requiring concomitant minimal clockwise rotation. The configuration of the catheter in the aortic arch is important to appreciate, and it aids engagement of the left coronary sinus (Fig. 2-4, *A*). If the catheter tip appears below the left coronary sinus, gentle retraction with counterclockwise rotation is done. If these maneuvers fail, a change in catheter size is usually necessary to avoid unnecessary manipulation within the aortic root. Larger roots seen typically with aortic regurgitation may require a JL5 or JL6 or indeed an Amplatz Left (AL) 1-3 catheter.

Extreme aortic root dilatation may make selective angiography extremely challenging. In Figure 2-5, *D*, in which the patient had a massive aortic root pseudoaneurysm secondary to bioprosthetic aortic valve regurgitation, an alternative strategy was necessary. A 7-Fr Sones catheter was needed to engage the RCA, and a 125-cm Davis catheter was required for left coronary angiography. In general, selective angiography with the Sones catheter requires greater manipulation than does standard Judkins catheterization because the catheter must be advanced toward the left coronary cusp, again in the LAO projection. With further advancement against the valve, the relatively straight catheter tip is deflected upward toward the LMCA. Minimal counterclockwise

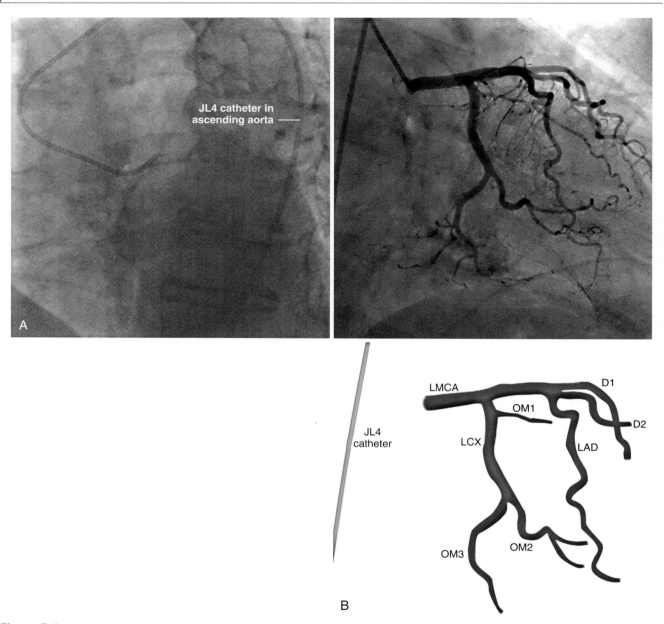

Figure 2-4 **A,** Anteroposterior (AP) projection of the aorta with a Judkins catheter (JL4) in the ascending aorta. **B,** Injection of the left main coronary artery (LMCA) in the right anterior oblique caudal projection using a JL4 catheter. *D1* and *D2,* First diagonal and second diagonal; *LAD,* left anterior descending coronary artery; *LCX,* left circumflex coronary artery; *OM1* to *OM3,* obtuse margin 1 to 3.

rotation usually facilitates LMCA engagement. A similar method is employed for the RCA, with initial advancement and rotation toward the right coronary cusp (see Fig. 2-5, *D*).

During catheter removal or exchange, the catheter should be retracted under fluoroscopic guidance to disengage the coronary ostium atraumatically. The catheter is disconnected from the manifold, and the cleaned guidewire is advanced until it is just proximal to the catheter tip. The wire is then fixed while the catheter is retracted fully. Again, these maneuvers are done to minimize the release of atheroemboli. For active catheters such as the Amplatz or Extra Back-up guide catheters (Medtronic Vascular, Galway, Ireland),

counterclockwise rotation during pullback is required to prevent deeper engagement of the artery that potentially could cause artery trauma. These catheters require careful manipulation to reduce the risk of iatrogenic arterial dissection.

When engaged, the arterial tracing should demonstrate a sharp waveform, as opposed to that seen where the catheter may be occluding arterial flow. Catheter-related arterial occlusion may be identified by blunting or ventricularization of the pressure waveform. Contrast injection should not be performed because catheter occlusion may induce ischemia and malignant arrhythmia or possible coronary dissection if the tip is embedded in the artery wall.

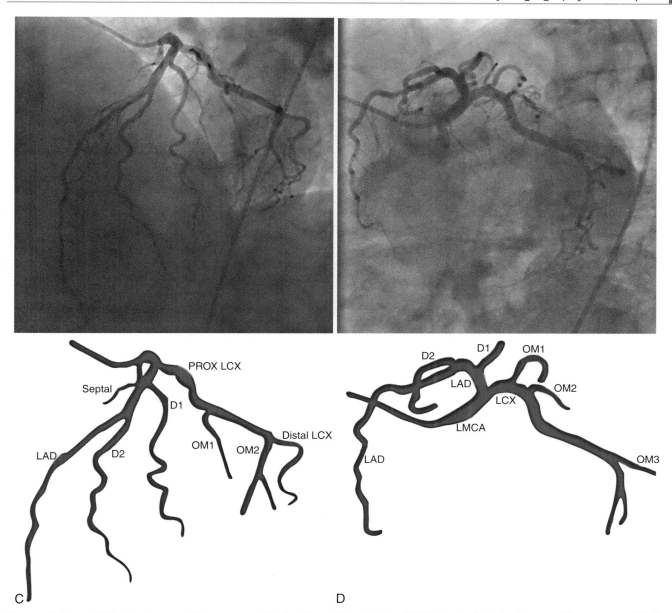

Figure 2-4, cont'd C, Angiogram of the same vessel in the AP cranial projection. *PROX,* Proximal. **D,** Angiogram of the same vessel in the spider view.

Prevention of Iatrogenic Complications

Ventricularization of Pressure Waveform

If no blood can be aspirated at this stage even though the catheter tip is free, the safest option is to withdraw the catheter externally and completely under continuous negative suction and reflush and clean it outside the body to ensure that it is clot free.

Contrast injection should not be performed when damping or ventricularization (loss of diastolic pressure waveform component) is evident. Damping may result from catheter tip occlusion secondary to clot or from being embedded in the arterial wall. Forceful injection may lead to potentially devastating com-

plications such as coronary occlusion or dissection. Ventricularization of the arterial waveform may occur when the coronary artery is occluded by the catheter, a condition that may induce ischemia and provoke arrhythmia. The syringe and manifold must also be thoroughly checked for air or any thrombus before injection.

Coronary Air Embolism

Air embolism, a rare but potentially devastating complication of coronary angiography, has an incidence of 0.1% to 0.3%. It usually arises from poor operator technique and inadequate catheter aspiration and flushing. Entrainment of air may also result from overzealous advancement or removal of equipment (e.g.,

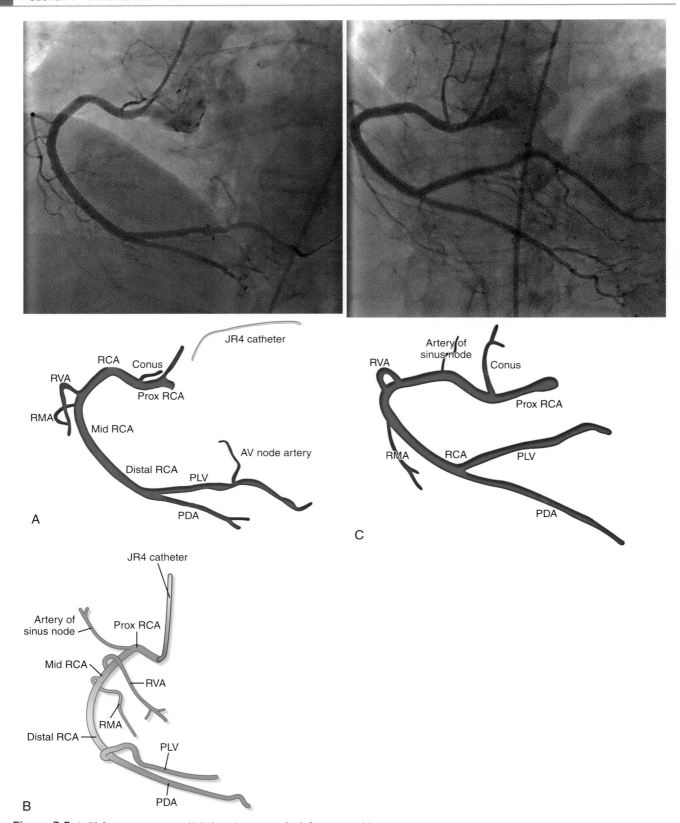

Figure 2-5 A, Right coronary artery (RCA) angiogram in the left anterior oblique (LAO) projection. *PDA,* Posterior descending coronary artery; *PLV,* posterior left ventricular; *RMA,* right marginal artery; *RVA,* right ventricular apical. **B,** Right anterior oblique (RAO) projection of the same vessel. **C,** Anteroposterior cranial angiogram of the same vessel.

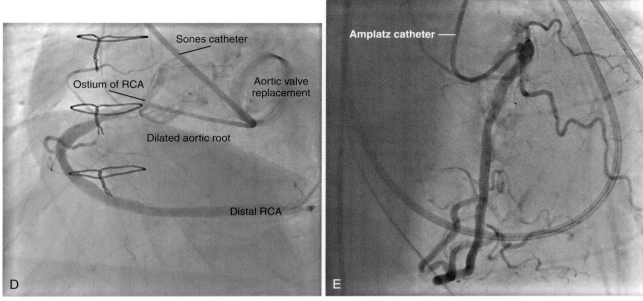

Figure 2-5, cont'd D, A different patient's RCA angiogram in the LAO projection using a Sones catheter. E, Another patient's RCA angiogram in the RAO projection using an Amplatz (AL1) catheter.

guidewires, angioplasty balloon or stent catheters). This is particularly relevant in the case of smaller-French catheter systems. Injection of air may cause chest pain, hypotension, electrocardiographic changes indicative of ischemia, and arrhythmias including bradycardia, heart block, asystole, and ventricular fibrillation. Careful review of the angiogram may reveal passage of air bubbles down the coronary system and associated arterial spasm and slow flow.

Prevention of air embolism with meticulous technique is a crucial part of safe angiography. Before all injections are administered, the syringe must be checked for air, and it should also be held as vertically as possible to reduce the chance of air delivery during injection. Symptoms related to microbubble injection are usually mild and transient. Nevertheless, expert help should always be sought immediately. Management options include delivery of 100% oxygen; in some cases, hemodynamic supportive measures such as inotropes and intraaortic balloon pump counterpulsation may be needed. Intravenous analgesia may also be necessary. Other techniques described include forceful coronary injection of saline solution to help break up air pockets, in addition to antispasm medications such as adenosine. The use of thrombus aspiration catheters to suck the air out has also been reported.

Angiographic Views

Some of the most common standard views are detailed in the following subsections (see Fig. 2-4, *B* to *D*). Several standard views of the left system are obtained to unmask overlapped coronary segments. Variations of these views are often necessary to delineate specific coronary lesions, depending on individual body position and habitus. All views are generally obtained during the patient's held inspiration when possible, with the exception of the RAO caudal projection. This is not always convenient if the patient is unable to cooperate or when thoracic motion during inspiration reduces catheter stability. The anatomic configurations in each of the standard views are outlined here. A few general principles may aid vessel recognition for the novice angiographer. The left circumflex (LCx) artery moves in the general direction of the image intensifier (i.e., the fluoroscopy tube), and the left anterior descending (LAD) artery moves in the opposite direction. Cranial angulation moves the LCx artery toward the top of the screen, with the LAD artery moving in the opposite direction. In general, caudal projections (RAO, LAO, and AP) enhance visualization of the LCx artery, whereas LAO views aid assessment of the middle and distal LAD artery.

The LMCA may be defined as the coronary artery segment that runs from the ostium of the left coronary artery to the bifurcation into the LAD and LCx arteries. Occasionally, the LMCA may be very short, or the LAD and LCx arteries may have separate ostia. A study of 1000 angiograms reported a mean LMCA length of 11.6 ± 5.0 mm and a mean diameter of 4.9 ± 1.0 mm. Although this segment of the coronary artery tree is usually less than 15 mm, disease within this portion of the left coronary system carries the worst prognosis because of the large area of myocardium it supplies. Mortality rates approaching 40% at 3 years for untreated LMCA stenosis have been described. Careful visualization of the LMCA is vital during angiography. Furthermore, major adverse events may arise during diagnostic angiography in patients with significant LMCA disease, particularly those with ostial disease. LMCA atherosclerotic disease, when present, more often affects the bifurcation (>60%), but it may also be confined to the middle or ostial segments. Aggressive or uncontrolled catheter engagement may lead to dissection plaque embolism or vessel occlusion. When ostial LMCA disease is suspected, a nonselective angiogram is useful. In addition to the standard left coronary views, a magnified angiogram of the LMCA in the straight AP or shallow RAO view may be informative.

Left Anterior Descending Coronary Artery

The LAD artery arises at the bifurcation of the LMCA and runs over the anterior interventricular sulcus toward the apex (see Fig. 2-4). Its length is subject to considerable variability because it may terminate proximal to, distal to, or at the apex. When it extends beyond the apex, the LMCA tracks along the posterior interventricular groove. Along its course, it gives rise to diagonal branches (supplying the anterolateral left ventricle [LV]) and the septal arteries (usually four to six), which course close to the endocardium on the right side of the interventricular septum. The ostium and proximal LAD artery may be assessed in the LAO caudal views. Considerable foreshortening of the LAD artery occurs in the caudal views. In general, the entire LAD artery (with the exception of the proximal portion) is usually better seen in the cranial views. The LAO cranial view, in particular during deep inspiration, aids full visualization of the LAD artery and its diagonal branches. Often, RAO projection has LCx artery overlap across the proximal LAD artery. Sometimes, a left lateral projection may aid detection of disease of the LAD artery or diagonal bifurcation.

Left Circumflex Coronary Artery

The LCx artery originates at a steep angle from the LMCA and courses along the left atrioventricular sulcus. It gives rise to marginal and left atrial branches, and it ends before the obtuse margin of the LV (see Fig. 2-4). The LCx artery may also continue proximal to or distal to the crux cordis. In 40% of cases, the sinus node artery arises from the LCx artery, as opposed to the RCA. The posterior descending artery originates from the LCx artery (i.e., left dominant system) in approximately 10% of patients. Standard views of the left coronary system are outlined in Figure 2-4.

Right Coronary Artery

The RCA arises from the right coronary sinus and courses along the right atrioventricular sulcus, again frequently exhibiting a variable termination point from person to person. In the case of nondominance, the RCA may end between the acute margin of the right ventricle and the crux cordis. When the RCA is dominant, it may continue farther, to provide arterial supply to the posterolateral LV wall through variable numbers of posterolateral branches. At the crux cordis, the posterior descending artery arises from the RCA bifurcation to supply the inferior interventricular septum through variable septal branches. Other important RCA branches are the conus artery and the acute marginal artery, which supplies the right ventricular anterior wall. Standard RCA views are shown with diagrams in Figure 2-5.

Technique

For the novice angiographer, RCA imaging often proves more challenging because greater catheter manipulation may be required, compared with left coronary artery engagement. From the transfemoral approach, the JR4 catheter is the default catheter in most catheterization laboratories. The catheter is advanced to the aortic root in the same manner as described for left coronary angiography. After catheter preparation as detailed earlier, the catheter is retracted approximately 2 cm from the aortic valve, and in the LAO projection, it is torqued in a clockwise fashion approximately 180 degrees so that it faces anteriorly. Gentle retraction should then enable engagement of the RCA. Depending on the site and angulation of the RCA ostium, this technique may need to be repeated at different levels above and below the initial starting point. Other catheters, such as a 3-DR or no-torque right, may be necessary if repeated attempts with the JR4 fail. For RCAs with anterior or posterior takeoffs, catheters with a longer reach, such as the Amplatz Right (AR) or AL 0.75-1, may prove useful. Nonselective angiography or an aortic root shot in the LAO view with a pigtail catheter and a power injector may also facilitate localization of the RCA ostium and configuration. The operator must monitor the arterial pressure waveform at all times to ensure that dampening does not result from deep intubation, ostial spasm, or selective conus artery engagement. Injection of contrast in this setting is ill advised because it may precipitate coronary dissection, ischemia, or ventricular fibrillation. In general, less force and smaller volume are needed during RCA angiography, again bearing in mind that ventricular fibrillation may result from excess vigor during injection. Although deep inspiration may aid visualization of the RCA, it may also precipitate catheter disengagement because catheter stability is less than that of the JL4. Standard views are outlined in Figure 2-5.

Left Ventriculography

Standard left ventriculography is performed using a multiholed pigtail catheter, which is advanced over a 0.035-inch guidewire to the aortic root in a similar fashion as described earlier. The catheter is then unsheathed by wire withdrawal, thus allowing it to assume its pigtail configuration. The guidewire is left a few centimeters proximal to the tip, to impart extra torque, which facilitates crossing of the aortic valve. An angled pigtail catheter is commonly used for the groin approach, whereas a straight pigtail catheter may be preferable going from the upper extremity. Under fluoroscopic guidance, usually in the AP or RAO projection, the pigtail catheter is advanced to the aortic valve and then is simultaneously withdrawn and moved counterclockwise; this maneuver usually results in successful valve crossing. The wire is then withdrawn, and the catheter is aspirated and carefully flushed with heparinized flush before the LV end-diastolic pressure is recorded. When this method fails, the valve may be crossed initially with the J-tipped 0.035-inch guidewire, which is then fixed while the pigtail is advanced across the valve. In patients with severe aortic stenosis, a straight 0.035-inch wire is often required in conjunction with an AL1 catheter.

Once the AL1 catheter is positioned in the aortic root in standard fashion, the J wire is exchanged for the 0.035-inch straight wire. Both catheter and wire (with the wire leading by 2 to 3 cm) are advanced toward the aortic valve and are rotated clockwise or counterclockwise until they are in the jet emanating from the LV. Both are then advanced across the aortic valve in a smooth fashion. Care must be taken not to induce trauma to the aorta, LMCA, or LV with this method.

Once across the valve, the straight wire is exchanged for a long (260-cm) J-tipped guidewire that enables the AL1 to be exchanged out over the wire for the pigtail catheter. When any delay is encountered with this maneuver, the risk of atheroembolic events increases substantially. Meticulous detail to flushing of catheters (performed at a minimum of 3-minute intervals during attempted valve crossing) and sheaths, in addition to thorough wire cleaning, is vital. In the case of known aortic stenosis, anticoagulation is routinely administered before proceeding. The necessity of crossing the aortic valve must always be examined before the procedure because one study detailed the occurrence of new cerebral ischemic lesions detected by diffusion-weighted magnetic resonance imaging in more than 20% of patients with severe aortic stenosis who underwent retrograde catheterization of the valve. The correct orientation of the pigtail catheter is shown in Figure 2-6. The operator must ensure that it is free within the mid-LV cavity and not entangled in the mitral valve apparatus. Furthermore, repositioning is required when excessive ventricular ectopy is experienced because this will impair accurate LV systolic function and mitral regurgitation assessment.

The left ventriculogram is generally contraindicated in the presence of elevated LV end-diastolic pressure (>25 mm Hg), severe aortic stenosis, and significant LV dysfunction and in patients with critical LMCA stenosis. Standard views for left ventriculography are depicted with the relevant anatomy below in Figure 2-6. For satisfactory opacification, a mechanical power injector is used to deliver 10 to 15 cc/second for a total volume of 30 to 40 mL, with a rate rise of 0.4 at a pressure of 600 psi. Standard LV views shown with diagrams are illustrated in Figure 2-6. Aortography performed with the pigtail catheter just above the aortic valve in the LAO position may be used to assess for aortic regurgitation.

Graft Angiography

When available, the patient's operative report from coronary artery bypass grafting surgery should be reviewed because this provides invaluable information. A few caveats are worth entertaining (Box 2-5). Unless a specific contraindication exists, anticoagulation should be administered after arterial access has been obtained. Following native coronary angiography, the grafts are then selectively engaged. After RCA catheterization, the JR4 is moved in counterclockwise fashion and is retracted under fluoroscopic guidance in the LAO view. The

saphenous venous graft (SVG) to the RCA system usually originates in the anterior aortic wall just superior to the native RCA ostium (Fig. 2-7, A). Those RCA grafts with a steep inferior angulation may require use of the right bypass graft catheter or multipurpose 1 catheter. In addition to straight RAO and LAO views, the LAO view with cranial projection or the AP cranial view may prove useful in visualization of the distal vessel. A free radial graft to the RCA also usually arises in the same location (see Fig. 2-7, B).

The next graft that arises superior and posterolateral to the RCA graft is usually the SVG to the LAD or diagonal system (see Fig. 2-7, C). This may be engaged in the LAO or RAO projections with the JR4 or left coronary bypass graft catheter. On withdrawal from the RCA graft ostium, the catheter requires 30- to 45-degree clockwise rotation as it is withdrawn gently superiorly. In the LAO projection, this causes the catheter tip to appear foreshortened. Commonly, a catheter with more reach, such as an AL1 or AL2, may be necessary. The SVG to the LCx system (see Fig. 2-7, D) commonly arises superior to the SVG to the LAD and diagonal system and can be engaged with the same catheters. Some operators prefer to add cranial angulation in the case of the LAD grafts and caudal angulation for SVG-LCx angiography. Again, gentle catheter manipulation under fluoroscopic guidance is vital during selective engagement and disengagement, to avoid SVG trauma.

Left Internal Mammary Artery

When the aortic arch is tortuous, an aortogram in the LAO 40-degree projection provides valuable information on the origin of the left subclavian artery (see Fig. 2-7, E). Excessive catheter manipulation and scraping must be avoided because embolization to the carotid or vertebral arteries may result in significant morbidity and mortality. Visualizing the ostium and the proximal left subclavian artery proximal to the left internal mammary artery (LIMA) takeoff is important, to rule out potentially hemodynamically important stenosis. The patient should be notified that he or she will experience flushing or warm sensations in the left upper extremity and head during contrast injection. Use of dilute contrast agent is preferred until the IMA is selectively engaged. The JR4 catheter may be used in the AP projection to engage the left subclavian artery selectively. First, the catheter is advanced around the aortic arch with the 0.035-inch guidewire leading. Then the wire is withdrawn, and the catheter is retracted and torqued in a counterclockwise direction so that it is oriented superiorly. As it is gently withdrawn, the catheter is seen to pass by the ostia of the brachiocephalic and left common carotid artery before engaging the left subclavian artery. The catheter is then rotated and advanced slightly to ensure that it is coaxial with the left subclavian artery. This may be further verified by a satisfactory artery tracing confirming that the catheter is not embedded in the sidewall.

Angiography is usually performed in the RAO projection to evaluate the ostium. An exchange-length Versacore wire is then advanced with continuous spinning out the subclavian artery and care taken not

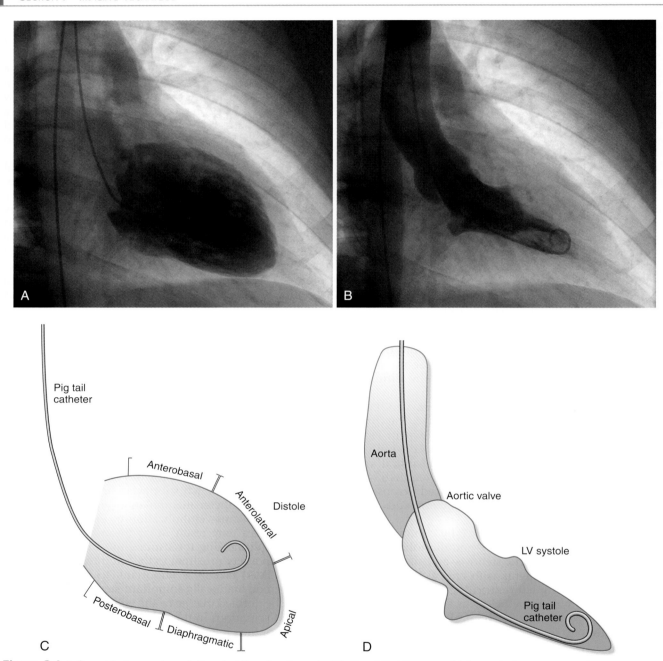

Figure 2-6 Left ventriculogram in end-diastole (**A**) and end-systole (**B**). **C** and **D**, Diagrams of left ventriculogram in end-diastole and end-systole. *LV,* Left ventricle.

to traumatize the vertebral artery or IMA. In the case of more complex aortic arch configurations, dedicated carotid catheters such as the Davis, Simmons, or Vitek (Cook, Inc, Bloomington, Ind) catheters may be necessary. The Vitek catheter in particular has some unique features and requires experience to form it safely in the descending aorta and advance it facing upward to engage the subclavian artery actively in a nontraumatic manner. An IMA catheter is advanced over the wire beyond the LIMA origin and is withdrawn following wire removal. Gentle contrast injection aids selective LIMA engagement. Care must be taken at all times to avoid excessive

or rapid catheter manipulation, which may result in LIMA dissection. Angiography of the LIMA is performed in the AP projection, followed by RAO and LAO views (see Fig. 2-7, *F* and *G*). Panning is necessary to view the entirety of the graft and bypassed artery. Additional helpful views concentrating on the anastomosis site include the left lateral and AP caudal projections.

Transradial Angiography Issues

Although most of the fundamentals of coronary angiography from the radial approach are shared with access

BOX 2-5   Problem Solving: Finding Grafts

Review coronary artery bypass grafting operative notes before the procedure.

Review earlier graft studies when available, to reference graft ostia to sterna wires and clips and duplicate angle of projection.

When multiple grafts are in close proximity, taking angiograms straight RAO and LAO projections is often helpful.

Aortography in the 30-degree LAO view may aid identification and serve as reference image.

LAO, Left anterior oblique; RAO, right anterior oblique.

from the radial artery, radial access has some unique features of practical importance to the angiographer (see Table 2-2). The learning curve is steeper, and often greater catheter manipulation may be required with the transradial approach. For beginners, a more comfortable approach may be to obtain radial access with the patient's arm abducted and the wrist hyperextended. Following sheath insertion, placement of adhesive tape or a suture is helpful to prevent inadvertent sheath removal, especially when left radial access is used. Once the sheath is in place, the patient's arm should be positioned alongside the patient's thigh, to allow the operator to work with a setup similar to that of the femoral

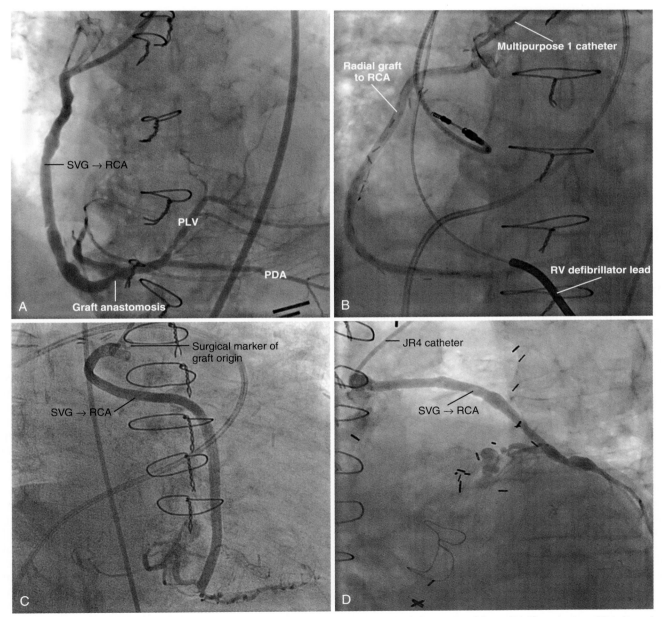

Figure 2-7 A, Saphenous vein graft (SVG) of the right coronary artery (RCA) in the left anterior oblique (LAO) projection. *PDA,* Posterior descending coronary artery; *PLV,* posterior left ventricular. **B,** Radial graft to the right posterior descending artery in the LAO cranial projection. *RV,* Right ventricular. **C,** SVG of the diagonal system. **D,** SVG of the left circumflex coronary artery.

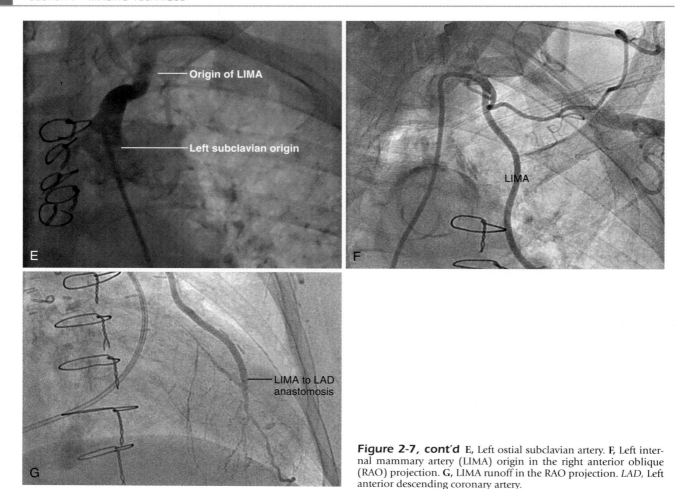

Figure 2-7, cont'd **E,** Left ostial subclavian artery. **F,** Left internal mammary artery (LIMA) origin in the right anterior oblique (RAO) projection. **G,** LIMA runoff in the RAO projection. *LAD,* Left anterior descending coronary artery.

approach. In the case of left radial access, the left arm can be slightly flexed and adducted, thus bringing it close to the left groin. This position can be supported with folded sheets to stabilize the upper extremity. Initially, the right coronary catheter is advanced over a 0.035-inch Versacore wire, which facilitates the traversing of any tortuous upper limb arteries. Deep inspiration may aid direction of the wire from the subclavian into the ascending aorta. For the left system, a JL catheter a 0.5 size smaller than for the femoral approach is commonly used. The guidewire should be withdrawn 1 to 2 cm and left in place during torquing of the catheter to aid successful coronary engagement. From the left radial artery, an AR catheter may be more suitable than the JR4. For left ventriculography, a straight pigtail catheter is used. Several dedicated radial catheters have been developed, such as the Jacky and Tiger (Terumo Corporation, Somerset, NJ). These catheters are designed to be used to engage both coronary ostia and the LV, thereby reducing the risk of radial artery spasm by minimizing exchanges. Exchange-length (260-cm) guidewires are very useful for catheter exchanges by reducing radiation exposure and procedure times. Graft studies may also be more technically challenging to begin with and require familiarity with many different diagnostic catheters. Engagement of the LIMA is easier from the left radial artery, but newer dedicated catheters such as the right IMA catheter are now available.

Complications of Cardiac Catheterization

The operator must remain mindful at all times of the risk of precipitating complications relating to invasive catheterization. Although the rate of cerebrovascular accident (CVA) arising as a consequence of angiography is low, the resultant sequelae can have a devastating effect on the patient. Stroke occurring in the setting of left heart catheterization or PCI has been reported to occur in 0.2% to 0.38% of cases. Patient characteristics linked with an increased risk include diabetes mellitus, renal failure, and prior CVA. Procedure-related factors include longer and urgent cardiac catheterization procedures, the use of larger volumes of contrast agent, and intraaortic balloon counterpulsation. As described earlier, the operator must remain vigilant to the risk of atheroembolic disease at every step of the procedure. He or she must studiously avoid catheter scraping of the aorta as much as possible by employing transitioning techniques. Keely and Grines reported that scraping of the aorta may occur in more than half of all PCIs and is more common with larger catheters. Other mechanisms of iatrogenic CVA include air embolus and thrombus formation and propagation from the catheter tip. Methods to reduce the risk of CVA include careful transitioning of catheters over wires and wire desheathing, frequent catheter and sheath flushing with heparinized saline solution, and anticoagulation use in high-risk settings. Use of an access site (i.e., radial) that may avoid traversing an abdominal aorta with a high plaque burden may also be considered. The procedure should be performed efficiently by avoiding prolonged periods of intraarterial catheter or wire placement.

Renal function may also be adversely affected during cardiac catheterization as a consequence of atheroembolic disease. Atheroembolic renal disease or cholesterol embolization to the renal parenchymal vasculature results in significant morbidity and mortality. One series described that almost 25% of patients with atheroembolic renal disease progressed to end-stage renal failure; the 5-year mortality rate was almost 40%, and most of these deaths were attributable to cardiovascular causes.

Another mechanism of procedure-related renal dysfunction is CIN, which may be defined as a rise in serum creatinine of more than 0.5 mg/dL (44 micromol/L) or 25% higher than baseline within 48 hours of contrast delivery. Creatinine usually peaks 5 to 7 days after the procedure. Although the overall incidence is thought to be less than 2%, CIN may be seen in as many as 50% of high-risk patients such as those with chronic renal impairment, diabetes mellitus, and anemia, as well as in older patients. A diagnosis of CIN carries serious consequences, with an almost 40% in-hospital mortality and 20% 2-year mortality in patients needing dialysis. When possible, every effort should be undertaken to reduce the risks of CIN by employing appropriate prehydration, withdrawal of potentially nephrotoxic drugs, and minimizing the dose of the contrast agent. The efficacy of other drug treatment regimens for CIN prevention, such as N-acetyl-L-cysteine, remains unclear. Uncontrolled or deep catheter engagement may induce iatrogenic coronary artery or aortic dissection. Dissection limited to the aortic sinus of Valsalva may often be managed conservatively. Infrequently, retrograde extension of the dissection plain into the ascending aorta may occur. Usually, the entry point of the dissection may be sealed with stent deployment; however, extensive open surgical repair may be warranted in some cases when the dissection extends more than 40 mm beyond the coronary os. A study of more than 50,000 coronary angiography and PCI procedures showed iatrogenic LMCA dissection in 38 (0.07%) patients, with the incidence during PCI almost twice that of diagnostic catheterization alone. In this study, 1 death occurred as a consequence. Most patients (82%) underwent subsequent revascularization (PCI or coronary artery bypass grafting), whereas 16% were treated conservatively.

Arterial Sheath Removal

In the case of diagnostic transfemoral angiography, when no anticoagulation has been administered, the sheath may be pulled and manual compression to achieve hemostasis applied for 12 to 15 minutes or until complete hemostasis is achieved. Bed rest for a minimum of 4 hours is recommended. For larger sheaths and anticoagulation, different protocols are necessary, such as prolonged bed rest and deferral of sheath removal until coagulation has normalized. Various active and passive closure devices are readily available, and details pertaining to their safe use are outlined in an AHA guideline document to which the reader is directed. Dedicated passive closure wrist bands (e.g., Terumo TR band, Terumo Corporation, Somerset, NJ) exist for managing hemostasis after radial sheath removal. These devices are attached around the wrist, and the compression balloon is gently inflated to achieve hemostasis as the sheath is withdrawn. The balloon is deflated (0.5 to 1 mL at a time) just to the point where blood flow returns and then is reinflated with an extra 2 cc of air. In addition, a wrist splint prevents unnecessary wrist movement. Both are usually left in place for 2 or 4 hours following diagnostic angiography or PCI, respectively.

■ LIMITATIONS OF CORONARY ANGIOGRAPHY

Conventional coronary angiography does have some fundamental limitations when it comes to assessing atherosclerotic CAD. In particular, angiographic stenoses may correlate poorly with hemodynamic significance, especially in the case of stenoses of intermediate severity (40% to 70%). Although this may be improved with quantitative coronary angiography, the functional impact of a stenosis remains challenging to ascertain especially in the setting of collateral circulation and downstream myocardial viability. Severe vessel tortuosity, multiple overlapping segments, contrast underfilling, and failure to obtain perpendicular x-ray angulation are some of the reasons for inaccuracies reported with conventional coronary angiography.

■ ADDITIONAL LESION EVALUATION TECHNIQUES IN THE CATHETERIZATION LABORATORY

To overcome the limitations of luminography, particularly in the assessment of indeterminate lesions, certain additional structural imaging and physiologic techniques have been introduced. Fractional flow reserve (FFR) is performed using a 0.014-inch angioplasty guidewire equipped with a pressure sensor (Fig. 2-8, A). FFR may be defined as the ratio of flow in the poststenotic artery to that of the theoretically normal artery. Pressure in a normal artery is equal to that of the aorta. After inducing hyperemia, usually with intracoronary or intravenous adenosine, the FFR across the lesion is calculated. FFR has been demonstrated to be a reproducible measurement of lesion severity independent of changes in heart rate, blood pressure, or the presence of downstream infracted myocardium. The clinical utility of FFR in managing indeterminate lesions was demonstrated in several studies showing that an FFR recording of less than

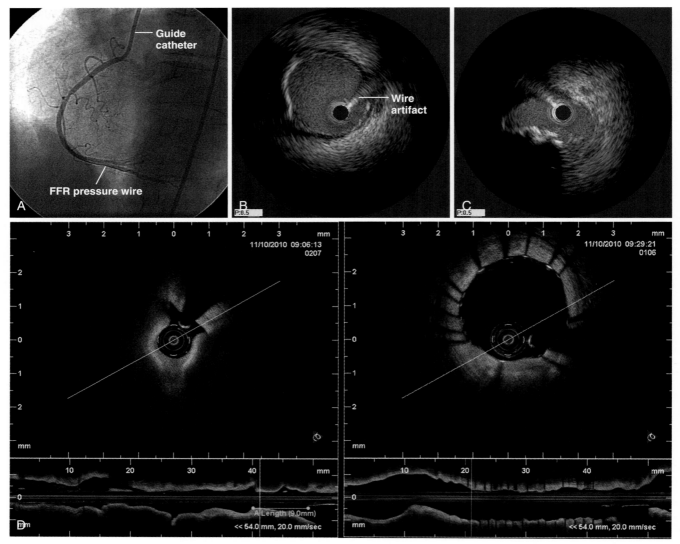

Figure 2-8 A, Fractional flow reserve (FFR) pressure wire placed across a midright coronary artery stenosis. **B,** Intravascular ultrasound (IVUS) distal to a lesion in the left anterior descending coronary artery. **C,** IVUS of the left main coronary artery illustrating significant eccentric arterial stenosis. **D,** Optical coherence tomography before and after successful stent deployment.

0.75 correlates with demonstrable ischemia, whereas lesions with values greater than 0.75 may be safely managed medically.

Structural Intravascular Imaging

Intravascular ultrasound (IVUS) is performed by advancing an ultrasound imaging catheter over a 0.014-inch coronary guidewire and thus enabling the generation of cross-sectional images of the coronary vessel (see Fig. 2-8, *B*). IVUS provides the operator with detailed information concerning the minimum luminal diameter and area of a stenotic lesion. Furthermore, characterization of atherosclerotic plaque, such as the degree of calcification and fibrous content, and PCI guidance (e.g., stent size selection, expansion) are facilitated by IVUS. IVUS has also proved useful in the assessment of atherosclerotic LMCA disease and in transplant vasculopathy.

Structural Optical Coherence Tomography

Optical coherence tomography (OCT) is an infrared light emission–based intravascular imaging system with higher resolution than IVUS (see Fig. 2-8, *C*). It may be used to assess the severity of lesions with higher accuracy than conventional angiography by detailing the minimal luminal area; an area smaller than 4 mm^2 is frequently cited as significant in vessels larger than 3 mm. OCT has also been used to characterize atherosclerotic plaques and to image inflammatory cell composition. Limitations of OCT include the necessity of imaging in a bloodless field and difficulty assessing large-caliber vessels and atherosclerotic plaques that are more than 1.3 to 1.5 mm thick. However, the introduction of second-generation frequency domain OCT has helped this exciting imaging modality gain increasing use in the clinical field. The hope is that future OCT studies will significantly aid

BOX 2-6   **Indications for Use of Swan-Ganz Catheter**

Cardiogenic shock
Discordant right- and left-sided heart failure
Severe chronic heart failure during supportive therapy
Hemodynamic diagnosis and assessment of pulmonary hypertension
Transplantation workup
Differentiation of septic from cardiogenic shock
Not indicated as routine pulmonary artery catheterization in high-risk cardiac and noncardiac patients

Adapted from Webb JG, Pate GE, Humphries KH, et al. A randomized controlled trial of intravenous N-acetylcysteine for the prevention of contrast-induced nephropathy after cardiac catheterization: lack of effect. *Am Heart J.* 2004;148:422-429.

BOX 2-7   **Potential Risks Associated With Pulmonary Artery Catheterization**

Pneumothorax
Carotid artery cannulation
Internal jugular thrombosis
Pulmonary infarction
Right atrial, right ventricular, or pulmonary artery rupture
Arrhythmia
Pacemaker or defibrillator lead dislodgment
Tricuspid regurgitation

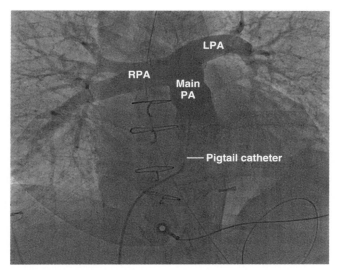

Figure 2-9 Pulmonary angiogram in the anteroposterior projection shows normal anatomy. *LPA,* Left pulmonary artery; *Main PA,* main pulmonary artery; *RPA,* right pulmonary artery.

the ability to identify vulnerable atherosclerotic coronary plaques.

Right Heart Catheterization

Central Venous Access

Uses of right heart catheterization include determining the cause of hypotension and shock, managing optimal hemodynamic status in terms of fluid status, and administering inotropic therapy (Box 2-6). This technique also has a useful role in hemodynamic monitoring during cardiac and noncardiac surgery. However, its utility in certain clinical situations has been questioned. The clinical indication for right heart catheterization often influences the chosen venous access site. To minimize infection in patients with indwelling pulmonary artery (PA) catheters, the internal jugular (IJ) site is most commonly used unless a specific contraindication (e.g., local infection, jugular venous thrombosis) exists. Femoral venous access during coronary angiography is also routinely performed. Intravascular wire placement and sheath placement are similar to those outlined for arterial access. IJ venous cannulation is routinely performed under ultrasound and fluoroscopic guidance to minimize complications, as outlined in Box 2-7. Briefly, after identification of the anatomic landmarks, a micropuncture (Cook Micropuncture Introducer set, Cook, Inc, Bloomington, Ind) needle attached to a syringe is used to gain IJ access. The 0.018-inch guidewire is then advanced gently and smoothly under fluoroscopic guidance, which is used to confirm satisfactory placement. The needle is withdrawn, and the 5-Fr sheath is advanced into the vein and is then exchanged over a 0.035-inch guidewire. Finally, the 7- or 8-Fr introducer sheath is placed. A small skin nick may be necessary before final sheath insertion. Care must be taken to avoid carotid artery cannulation or trauma. If the carotid artery is inadvertently accessed with the sheath, a vascular surgical consultation is warranted immediately.

Pulmonary Artery Catheter Insertion

Insertion of an inflatable balloon-tipped PA catheter is usually straightforward from the right IJ approach. Greater manipulation may be required from the femoral approach, which sometimes necessitates the use of a 0.018- or 0.021-inch guidewire. From the IJ approach, the right atrium (RA) is reached with approximately 15 to 20 cm of catheter advancement. Further advancement from the IJ approach usually results in easy passage across the tricuspid valve into the right ventricular outflow tract (RVOT) forming a U shape and on to the PA. The corresponding RA distance from the common femoral vein is 65 to 70 cm. From the common femoral vein approach, counterclockwise torque and simultaneous advancement are needed to negotiate the RVOT into the PA. Alternatively, the tricuspid valve may be traversed by looping the catheter using the RA wall; this results in a configuration that facilitates traversal of the RVOT into the PA. Any catheter loops should be undone before pressure recording. The PA catheter enables right-sided pressures and waveforms, in addition to blood saturation and cardiac output measurement. Potential complications include arrhythmia, valve trauma, thrombosis, and cardiac or PA rupture. Several designated catheters are also available for right heart catheterization including the balloon wedge and the Cournand catheters. A pigtail catheter may be used to perform right ventriculography and PA angiography (Fig. 2-9, *A,* which shows a PA angiogram in the AP projection).

Bibliography

Agostoni P, Biondi-Zoccai GG, de Benedictis ML, et al. Radial versus femoral approach for percutaneous coronary diagnostic and interventional procedures: systematic overview and meta-analysis of randomized trials. *J Am Coll Cardiol.* 2004;44:349-356.

Alvarez-Tostado JA, Moise MA, Bena JF, et al. The brachial artery: a critical access for endovascular procedures. *J Vasc Surg.* 2009;49:378-385:discussion 385.

Amoroso G, Kiemeneij F. Transradial access for primary percutaneous coronary intervention: the next standard of care? *Heart.* 2010;96:1341-1344.

Anderson JL, Adams CD, Antman EM, et al. ACC/AHA 2007 guidelines for the management of patients with unstable angina/non–ST-elevation myocardial infarction: a report of the American College of Cardiology/American Heart Association Task Force on Practice Guidelines (Writing Committee to Revise the 2002 Guidelines for the Management of Patients With Unstable Angina/Non–ST-Elevation Myocardial Infarction) developed in collaboration with the American College of Emergency Physicians, the Society for Cardiovascular Angiography and Interventions, and the Society of Thoracic Surgeons endorsed by the American Association of Cardiovascular and Pulmonary Rehabilitation and the Society for Academic Emergency Medicine. *J Am Coll Cardiol.* 2007;50:e1-e157.

Antman EM, Anbe DT, Armstrong PW, et al. ACC/AHA guidelines for the management of patients with ST-elevation myocardial infarction: a report of the American College of Cardiology/American Heart Association Task Force on Practice Guidelines (Committee to Revise the 1999 Guidelines for the Management of Patients With Acute Myocardial Infarction). *J Am Coll Cardiol.* 2004;44:e1-e211.

Antman EM, Anbe DT, Armstrong PW, et al. ACC/AHA guidelines for the management of patients with ST-elevation myocardial infarction—executive summary: a report of the American College of Cardiology/American Heart Association Task Force on Practice Guidelines (Writing Committee to Revise the 1999 Guidelines for the Management of Patients With Acute Myocardial Infarction). *J Am Coll Cardiol.* 2004;44:671-719.

Arzamendi D, Ly HQ, Tanguay JF, et al. Effect on bleeding, time to revascularization, and one-year clinical outcomes of the radial approach during primary percutaneous coronary intervention in patients with ST-segment elevation myocardial infarction. *Am J Cardiol.* 2010;106:148-154.

Baim DS. *Grossman's Cardiac Catheterization: Angiography and Intervention.* 7th ed. Baltimore: Lippincott Williams & Wilkins; 2006.

Bech GJ, De Bruyne B, Bonnier HJ, et al. Long-term follow-up after deferral of percutaneous transluminal coronary angioplasty of intermediate stenosis on the basis of coronary pressure measurement. *J Am Coll Cardiol.* 1998;31:841-847.

Brasselet C, Blanpain T, Tassan-Mangina S, et al. Comparison of operator radiation exposure with optimized radiation protection devices during coronary angiograms and ad hoc percutaneous coronary interventions by radial and femoral routes. *Eur Heart J.* 2008;29:63-70.

Brueck M, Bandorski D, Kramer W, Wieczorek M, Holtgen R, Tillmanns H. A randomized comparison of transradial versus transfemoral approach for coronary angiography and angioplasty. *JACC Cardiovasc Interv.* 2009;2:1047-1054.

Caixeta A, Mehran R. Evidence-based management of patients undergoing PCI: contrast-induced acute kidney injury. *Catheter Cardiovasc Interv.* 2010;75(suppl 1):S15-S20.

Campeau L. Percutaneous radial artery approach for coronary angiography. *Cathet Cardiovasc Diagn.* 1989;16:3-7.

Capodanno D, Di Salvo ME, Seminara D, et al. Epidemiology and clinical impact of different anatomical phenotypes of the left main coronary artery. *Heart Vessels.* 2011;26:138-144.

Chase AJ, Fretz EB, Warburton WP, et al. Association of the arterial access site at angioplasty with transfusion and mortality: the M.O.R.T.A.L. study (Mortality benefit Of Reduced Transfusion after percutaneous coronary intervention via the Arm or Leg). *Heart.* 2008;94:1019-1025.

Chatterjee K. The Swan-Ganz catheters: past, present, and future: a viewpoint. *Circulation.* 2009;119:147-152.

de Bruyne B, Bartunek J, Sys SU, Pijls NH, Heyndrickx GR, Wijns W. Simultaneous coronary pressure and flow velocity measurements in humans: feasibility, reproducibility, and hemodynamic dependence of coronary flow velocity reserve, hyperemic flow versus pressure slope index, and fractional flow reserve. *Circulation.* 1996;94:1842-1849.

Dehghani P, Mohammad A, Bajaj R, et al. Mechanism and predictors of failed transradial approach for percutaneous coronary interventions. *JACC Cardiovasc Interv.* 2009;2:1057-1064.

Doyle BJ, Ting HH, Bell MR, et al. Major femoral bleeding complications after percutaneous coronary intervention: incidence, predictors, and impact on long-term survival among 17,901 patients treated at the Mayo Clinic from 1994 to 2005. *JACC Cardiovasc Interv.* 2008;1:202-209.

Dunning DW, Kahn JK, Hawkins ET, O'Neill WW. Iatrogenic coronary artery dissections extending into and involving the aortic root. *Catheter Cardiovasc Interv.* 2000;51:387-393.

Eshtehardi P, Adorjan P, Togni M, et al. Iatrogenic left main coronary artery dissection: incidence, classification, management, and long-term follow-up. *Am Heart J.* 2010;159:1147-1153.

Fergusson DJ, Kamada RO. Percutaneous entry of the brachial artery for left heart catheterization using a sheath: further experience. *Cathet Cardiovasc Diagn.* 1986;12:209-211.

Fitzgerald PJ, Oshima A, Hayase M, et al. Final results of the Can Routine Ultrasound Influence Stent Expansion (CRUISE) study. *Circulation.* 2000;102:523-530.

Fuchs S, Stabile E, Kinnaird TD, et al. Stroke complicating percutaneous coronary interventions: incidence, predictors, and prognostic implications. *Circulation.* 2002;106:86-91.

Garg S, Stone GW, Kappetein AP, Sabik 3rd JF, Simonton C, Serruys PW. Clinical and angiographic risk assessment in patients with left main stem lesions. *JACC Cardiovasc Interv.* 2010;3:891-901.

Gruberg L, Mehran R, Dangas G, et al. Acute renal failure requiring dialysis after percutaneous coronary interventions. *Catheter Cardiovasc Interv.* 2001;52:409-416.

Hamon M, Baron JC, Viader F. Periprocedural stroke and cardiac catheterization. *Circulation.* 2008;118:678-683.

Hayes MA, Timmins AC, Yau EH, Palazzo M, Hinds CJ, Watson D. Elevation of systemic oxygen delivery in the treatment of critically ill patients. *N Engl J Med.* 1994;330:1717-1722.

Huang D, Swanson EA, Lin CP, et al. Optical coherence tomography. *Science.* 1991;254:1178-1181.

Hutchins GM, Nazarian IH, Bulkley BH. Association of left dominant coronary arterial system with congenital bicuspid aortic valve. *Am J Cardiol.* 1978;42:57-59.

Jang IK, Bouma BE, Kang DH, et al. Visualization of coronary atherosclerotic plaques in patients using optical coherence tomography: comparison with intravascular ultrasound. *J Am Coll Cardiol.* 2002;39:604-609.

Jolly SS, Amlani S, Hamon M, Yusuf S, Mehta SR. Radial versus femoral access for coronary angiography or intervention and the impact on major bleeding and ischemic events: a systematic review and meta-analysis of randomized trials. *Am Heart J.* 2009;157:132-140.

Kandzari DE, Colombo A, Park SJ, et al. Revascularization for unprotected left main disease: evolution of the evidence basis to redefine treatment standards. *J Am Coll Cardiol.* 2009;54:1576-1588.

Keeley EC, Grines CL. Scraping of aortic debris by coronary guiding catheters: a prospective evaluation of 1,000 cases. *J Am Coll Cardiol.* 1998;32:1861-1865.

Kelly AM, Dwamena B, Cronin P, Bernstein SJ, Carlos RC. Meta-analysis: effectiveness of drugs for preventing contrast-induced nephropathy. *Ann Intern Med.* 2008;148:284-294.

Kern MJ. Cardiac catheterization on the road less traveled: navigating the radial versus femoral debate. *JACC Cardiovasc Interv.* 2009;2:1055-1056.

Kern MJ. *The Cardiac Catheterization Handbook.* 4th ed. St. Louis: Mosby; 2003.

Kern MJ, de Bruyne B, Pijls NH. From research to clinical practice: current role of intracoronary physiologically based decision making in the cardiac catheterization laboratory. *J Am Coll Cardiol.* 1997;30:613-620.

Kern MJ, Lerman A, Bech JW, et al. Physiological assessment of coronary artery disease in the cardiac catheterization laboratory: a scientific statement from the American Heart Association Committee on Diagnostic and Interventional Cardiac Catheterization, Council on Clinical Cardiology. *Circulation.* 2006;114:1321-1341.

Khan M, Schmidt DH, Bajwa T, Shalev Y. Coronary air embolism: incidence, severity, and suggested approaches to treatment. *Cathet Cardiovasc Diagn.* 1995;36:313-318.

Kiemeneij F, Laarman GJ. Percutaneous transradial artery approach for coronary stent implantation. *Cathet Cardiovasc Diagn.* 1993;30:173-178.

Kiemeneij F, Laarman GJ, Odekerken D, Slagboom T, van der Wieken R. A randomized comparison of percutaneous transluminal coronary angioplasty by the radial, brachial and femoral approaches: the access study. *J Am Coll Cardiol.* 1997;29:1269-1275.

Lazar JM, Uretsky BF, Denys BG, Reddy PS, Counihan PJ, Ragosta M. Predisposing risk factors and natural history of acute neurologic complications of left-sided cardiac catheterization. *Am J Cardiol.* 1995;75:1056-1060.

Leesar MA, Abdul-Baki T, Akkus NI, Sharma A, Kannan T, Bolli R. Use of fractional flow reserve versus stress perfusion scintigraphy after unstable angina: effect on duration of hospitalization, cost, procedural characteristics, and clinical outcome. *J Am Coll Cardiol.* 2003;41:1115-1121.

Lloyd-Jones D, Adams R, Carnethon M, et al. Heart disease and stroke statistics—2009 update: a report from the American Heart Association Statistics Committee and Stroke Statistics Subcommittee. *Circulation.* 2009;119:480-486.

Louvard Y, Lefevre T, Morice MC. Radial approach: what about the learning curve? *Cathet Cardiovasc Diagn.* 1997;42:467-468.

Maiello L, La Marchesina U, Presbitero P, Faletra F. Iatrogenic aortic dissection during coronary intervention. *Ital Heart J.* 2003;4:419-422.

Manske CL, Sprafka JM, Strony JT, Wang Y. Contrast nephropathy in azotemic diabetic patients undergoing coronary angiography. *Am J Med.* 1990;89:615-620.

McCullough PA, Wolyn R, Rocher LL, Levin RN, O'Neill WW. Acute renal failure after coronary intervention: incidence, risk factors, and relationship to mortality. *Am J Med.* 1997;103:368-375.

McKay RG. The Mansfield Scientific Aortic Valvuloplasty Registry: overview of acute hemodynamic results and procedural complications. *J Am Coll Cardiol.* 1991;17:485-491.

Mehra MR, Ventura HO, Stapleton DD, Smart FW, Collins TC, Ramee SR. Presence of severe intimal thickening by intravascular ultrasonography predicts cardiac events in cardiac allograft vasculopathy. *J Heart Lung Transplant.* 1995;14:632-639.

Nasser TK, Mohler 3rd ER, Wilensky RL, Hathaway DR. Peripheral vascular complications following coronary interventional procedures. *Clin Cardiol.* 1995;18:609-614.

Nikolsky E, Aymong ED, Halkin A, et al. Impact of anemia in patients with acute myocardial infarction undergoing primary percutaneous coronary intervention: analysis from the Controlled Abciximab and Device Investigation to Lower Late Angioplasty Complications (CADILLAC) Trial. *J Am Coll Cardiol.* 2004;44:547-553.

Nissen SE, Yock P. Intravascular ultrasound: novel pathophysiological insights and current clinical applications. *Circulation.* 2001;103:604-616.

Noel BM, Gleeton O, Barbeau GR. Transbrachial insertion of an intra-aortic balloon pump for complex coronary angioplasty. *Catheter Cardiovasc Interv.* 2003;60:36-39:discussion 40.

Omran H, Schmidt H, Hackenbroch M, et al. Silent and apparent cerebral embolism after retrograde catheterisation of the aortic valve in valvular stenosis: a prospective, randomised study. *Lancet.* 2003;361:1241-1246.

Onorati F, Impiombato B, Ferraro A, et al. Transbrachial intraaortic balloon pumping in severe peripheral atherosclerosis. *Ann Thorac Surg.* 2007;84: 264-266.

Pancholy S, Coppola J, Patel T, Roke-Thomas M. Prevention of Radial artery Occlusion-Patent Hemostasis Evaluation Trial (PROPHET study): a randomized comparison of traditional versus patency documented hemostasis after transradial catheterization. *Catheter Cardiovasc Interv.* 2008;72:335-340.

Patel MR, Jneid H, Derdeyn CP, et al. Arteriotomy closure devices for cardiovascular procedures: a scientific statement from the American Heart Association. *Circulation.*122:1882-1893.

Patel MR, Peterson ED, Dai D, et al. Low diagnostic yield of elective coronary angiography. *N Engl J Med.* 2010;362:886-895.

Pepine CJ, Allen HD, Bashore TM, et al. ACC/AHA guidelines for cardiac catheterization and cardiac catheterization laboratories: American College of Cardiology/American Heart Association ad hoc Task Force on Cardiac Catheterization. *Circulation.* 1991;84:2213-2247.

Pijls NH, De Bruyne B, Peels K, et al. Measurement of fractional flow reserve to assess the functional severity of coronary-artery stenoses. *N Engl J Med.* 1996;334:1703-1708.

Piper WD, Malenka DJ, Ryan Jr TJ, et al. Predicting vascular complications in percutaneous coronary interventions. *Am Heart J.* 2003;145:1022-1029.

Prati F, Regar E, Mintz GS, et al. Expert review document on methodology, terminology, and clinical applications of optical coherence tomography: physical principles, methodology of image acquisition, and clinical application for assessment of coronary arteries and atherosclerosis. *Eur Heart J.* 2010;31:401-415.

Raffel OC, Tearney GJ, Gauthier DD, Halpern EF, Bouma BE, Jang IK. Relationship between a systemic inflammatory marker, plaque inflammation, and plaque characteristics determined by intravascular optical coherence tomography. *Arterioscler Thromb Vasc Biol.* 2007;27:1820-1827.

Rao SV, Ou FS, Wang TY, et al. Trends in the prevalence and outcomes of radial and femoral approaches to percutaneous coronary intervention: a report from the National Cardiovascular Data Registry. *JACC Cardiovasc Interv.* 2008;1:379-386.

Rathore S, Stables RH, Pauriah M, et al. Impact of length and hydrophilic coating of the introducer sheath on radial artery spasm during transradial coronary intervention: a randomized study. *JACC Cardiovasc Interv.* 2010;3:475-483.

Ron W. Comparison of closure strategies after balloon aortic valvuloplasty: suture mediated vs. collagen based vs. manual. *Catheter Cardiovasc Interv.* 2011 Jan 13:[Epub ahead of print].

Sanmartin M, Gomez M, Rumoroso JR, et al. Interruption of blood flow during compression and radial artery occlusion after transradial catheterization. *Catheter Cardiovasc Interv.* 2007;70:185-189.

Scanlon PJ, Faxon DP, Audet AM, et al. ACC/AHA guidelines for coronary angiography: a report of the American College of Cardiology/American Heart Association Task Force on Practice Guidelines (Committee on Coronary Angiography). Developed in collaboration with the Society for Cardiac Angiography and Interventions. *J Am Coll Cardiol.* 1999;33:1756-1824.

Sciahbasi A, Pristipino C, Ambrosio G, et al. Arterial access-site-related outcomes of patients undergoing invasive coronary procedures for acute coronary syndromes (from the ComPaRison of Early Invasive and Conservative Treatment in Patients With Non–ST-ElevatiOn Acute Coronary Syndromes [PRESTO-ACS] Vascular Substudy). *Am J Cardiol.* 2009;103:796-800.

Scolari F, Ravani P, Pola A, et al. Predictors of renal and patient outcomes in atheroembolic renal disease: a prospective study. *J Am Soc Nephrol.* 2003;14:1584-1590.

Solodky A, Birnbaum Y, Assali A, Ben Gal T, Strasberg B, Herz I. Coronary air embolism treated by bubble aspiration. *Catheter Cardiovasc Interv.* 2000;49:452-454.

Stone GW, Marsalese D, Brodie BR, et al. A prospective, randomized evaluation of prophylactic intraaortic balloon counterpulsation in high risk patients with acute myocardial infarction treated with primary angioplasty: Second Primary Angioplasty in Myocardial Infarction (PAMI-II) Trial Investigators. *J Am Coll Cardiol.* 1997;29:1459-1467.

Taggart DP, Kaul S, Boden WE, et al. Revascularization for unprotected left main stem coronary artery stenosis stenting or surgery. *J Am Coll Cardiol.* 2008;51:885-892.

Tepel M, Aspelin P, Lameire N. Contrast-induced nephropathy: a clinical and evidence-based approach. *Circulation.* 2006;113:1799-1806.

Tobis J, Azarbal B, Slavin L. Assessment of intermediate severity coronary lesions in the catheterization laboratory. *J Am Coll Cardiol.* 2007;49:839-848.

Tobis JM, Mallery JA, Gessert J, et al. Intravascular ultrasound cross-sectional arterial imaging before and after balloon angioplasty in vitro. *Circulation.* 1989;80:873-882.

Uren NG, Melin JA, De Bruyne B, Wijns W, Baudhuin T, Camici PG. Relation between myocardial blood flow and the severity of coronary-artery stenosis. *N Engl J Med.* 1994;330:1782-1788.

Webb JG, Pate GE, Humphries KH, et al. A randomized controlled trial of intravenous *N*-acetylcysteine for the prevention of contrast-induced nephropathy after cardiac catheterization: lack of effect. *Am Heart J.* 2004;148:422-429.

CHAPTER 3

Cardiac Gated Computed Tomography

William Guy Weigold

■ GENERAL PRINCIPLES

Cardiac computed tomography (CT) is a specialized form of chest CT. All the technical principles that govern the acquisition and reconstruction of chest CT also apply to cardiac CT. However, the nature of cardiac anatomy and function requires that the system image small, complex structural elements in a rapidly moving organ that often contains a mixture of hard and soft densities. This requires several modifications to the standard chest CT technique. The primary modifications are the use of electrocardiogram (ECG) gating or triggering and special reconstruction algorithms required to generate motion-free images of the moving heart, as well as the use of very thin-slice, high-resolution scanning and reconstruction, which are required to image the small structures of interest and generate an isotropic data set.

ECG gating truly distinguishes cardiac CT from standard chest CT. ECG gating refers to the monitoring, collection, and use of ECG data before, during, and after the scan acquisition, all of which are needed to achieve the ultimate goal of cardiac CT: motion-free tomographic images of the heart. Gating is required for cardiac imaging because standard chest CT scan acquisition and image reconstruction parameters do not account for the motion of the heart, but are concerned only with image reconstruction in the spatial x-y plane. Standard chest CT does not take into account the timing of the reconstruction relative to any time point within the cardiac cycle. The resultant images of the heart are often blurred by motion artifact and appear in random cardiac contraction phases because although the reconstruction correctly renders *where* the anatomy is in the x-y plane, it does not take into account *when* the anatomy relative to the cardiac cycle is rendered. Cardiac reconstruction algorithms use ECG data to parse out the data and reconstruct the images at a single time point within the cardiac cycle, usually late diastole, when the heart briefly comes to rest (Fig. 3-1).

The addition of ECG gating or triggering introduces its own technical limitations and potential problems to the standard CT scan method. In a standard CT scan, the scan mode is either axial or helical. In an axial scan, the gantry, holding an x-ray tube on one side and a detector array on the opposite side (or two such pairs in case of dual source CT), spins around the patient while the table remains motionless. The x-ray tube is turned on

(triggered at a predetermined time point of the ECG) over an approximately 180- to 360-degree arc around the patient and then is turned off. As the gantry continues to spin with the x-ray tube off, the table is advanced by an increment approximately equal to the coverage of the detector array and then is stopped. The x-ray tube is again turned on, acquires another arc of attenuation data, and then is turned off, and the table is advanced again. This cycle repeats until the entire desired scan length is covered. Data acquisition occurs in slices that are in the transverse (i.e., axial) plane of the patient's body. These slices are put together to reconstruct a volume of data.

In a helical scan, the x-ray tube is turned on once at the beginning of the scan as the table begins a continuous translational sliding motion through the gantry. The x-ray tube stays on throughout the duration of the scan as the table continues to move, and once the entire desired scan length is covered, the tube is turned off, and table motion stops. Data collection occurs as one continuous helix around the patient. Transverse or axial plane images are reconstructed by interpolation of this helix of data.

In a cardiac CT scan, the collection of ECG information during the scan is added to this process. The ECG captures the time of occurrence of each QRS complex during the scan and thereby defines the beginning and end of each cardiac cycle. In all scan modes, the ECG information is used during image reconstruction to select a subset of the attenuation data for reconstruction, usually during diastasis. Diastasis is the relatively quiescent period of slow ventricular filling that occurs just before the atrial kick (atrial systole). Usually, only data collected during late diastasis are used, and late diastasis is estimated to occur approximately three fourths of the way through each cardiac cycle. In some cases, the real-time ECG events during the scan are also used to trigger data acquisition and drive the scan (i.e., to turn the x-ray tube on at the beginning of diastasis and off at the end of diastasis). In these cases, the ECG is used to predict, in a prospective fashion, when the next diastasis will occur, and hence this procedure is referred to as prospectively ECG-triggered cardiac CT. In other cases, the x-ray tube is turned on by some other event (e.g., arrival of contrast material in the ascending aorta), and the ECG information is simply collected along with the attenuation data and is used only during image reconstruction. The ECG

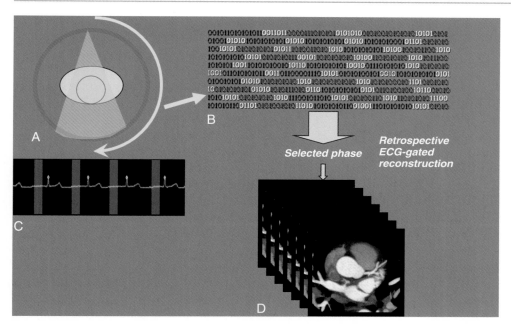

Figure 3-1 Diagram illustrating the concept of retrospective scanning. During helical data acquisition (A), a large attenuation data set is collected (all the 0s and 1s in B). After data acquisition, the software performs reconstruction using only the data acquired during the specified portion of each cardiac cycle (the reconstruction window) (*yellow bars* in C and *highlighted numbers* in B). The resultant images (D) are therefore a product of a subselection of the acquired data. This process is called retrospectively electrocardiogram (ECG)–gated reconstruction.

information is still used, but only after the scan, when it is used to gate the attenuation data (select out the data acquired during diastasis), during the process of image reconstruction. Hence, this procedure is referred to as retrospectively ECG-gated cardiac CT.

The axial scanning method in cardiac CT is always prospectively ECG triggered. The helical scanning method in cardiac CT was the original method of mechanical cardiac CT and is traditionally a retrospectively ECG-gated method. However, one scanner type (dual source CT scanner) can perform a helical scan that is prospectively triggered by the ECG. The ECG information is used to predict when diastasis will occur and then perform an extremely fast helical scan of the heart in that brief instant in time. This procedure requires high table speed and so is referred to as a high-pitch helical scan. (Pitch is a helical CT term that relates table speed to detector coverage. Higher pitch indicates higher table speed.)

Adding the element of ECG gating makes cardiac CT possible, but it also makes the technique vulnerable to gating-related problems and limitations. For ECG gating to work, certain conditions of heart rate and rhythm must be met to provide at least one window of time within each cardiac cycle during which the heart briefly ceases to move, or else the images will be blurred and distorted by motion. Generally, all cardiac CT scan types are trying to reconstruct images in diastasis, so in all cases, if diastasis is too short, or the reconstruction window is too long, then the heart will be moving during some portion of the acquisition, and the resultant images will contain motion, blurring, and artifacts. In addition, ECG-based tube current modulation, ECG-triggered axial scanning, and ECG-triggered high-pitch helical scanning all use the ECG in real time during the scan to turn the x-ray tube on and off, drive tube output, and determine the timing of the actual data acquisition on the fly and so require a regular, steady, predictable cardiac rhythm. Arrhythmia can therefore also result in

motion, blurring, and artifacts. In addition, noise and artifacts in the ECG signal itself (e.g., caused by a loose electrode or in a very obese patient) can produce misgating during the scan. Hence, for ECG gating to work ideally, the heart rate and rhythm should be slow and steady, and the scanner should receive a clean, strong ECG signal.

In addition to using ECG gating, imaging of coronary arteries also requires high-resolution thin-slice scanning and reconstruction because of the small size of the structures of interest: normal coronary arteries range in caliber from 5 mm to less than 2 mm. Thin slices are also required to generate an isotropic data set: the cardiac, and especially coronary, anatomy is complex insofar as the arteries are curvilinear and sometimes quite tortuous. Evaluation of this complex anatomy requires visualization and manipulation of the data in all three dimensions, and this is best done using an isotropic data set wherein the z-axis dimension of the voxels is as small as the dimensions in the x- and y-axes, such that each voxel is a cube. Hence, very thin slices, and very thin detector collimation, must be used (Fig. 3-2).

Again, this distinguishing modification of the standard body CT method makes the cardiac technique vulnerable to additional limitations and problems that result from thin-slice image reconstruction. By comparison with standard chest CT (2.5- to 5-mm-thick slices) or even chest CT angiography (CTA; usually 1.25- to 2.5-mm-thick slices), cardiac CT uses extremely thin slices (<1 mm thick); therefore, only small quantities of attenuation data are used for reconstruction of any given slice. At baseline, random fluctuations in the attenuation data are always present: even an image of nothing (air) contains random fluctuations and noise.

Attenuation data derived from imaging structures also contain random fluctuations in their data, or noise, which appear in the image as grain or granularity. The goal of image reconstruction is to map the real fluctuations in the attenuation data produced by

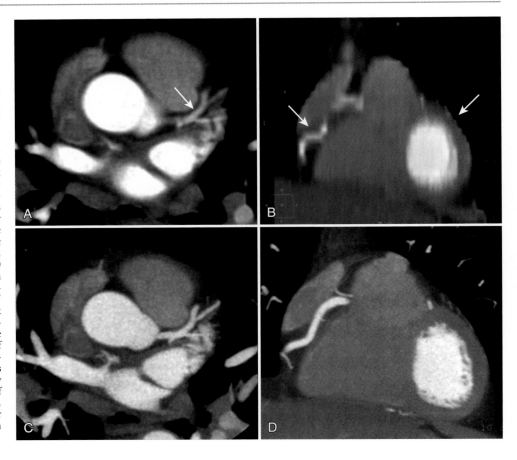

Figure 3-2 A, Axial (transverse) plane reconstruction using a standard computed tomography (CT) slice thickness (5 mm). Note blurring of edges and loss of detail, particularly of the coronary arteries *(arrow),* a result of volume averaging. **B,** Coronal reformat of the same image set, demonstrating the stair steps and blurring *(arrows)* indicative of a z-axis resolution that is insufficient for such a reformat. **C,** Axial plane image reconstructed from the same attenuation data set using 0.5-mm slice thickness and combining 10 of these thinner cuts to generate a 5-mm-thick slab (maximum intensity projection). The same "slice" of anatomy is represented, but now with improved z-axis resolution, which minimizes the volume averaging. **D,** Coronal reformat of the same, thin-cut image set, demonstrating much improved z-axis resolution. Analysis of coronary CT angiography requires the use of multiple nonaxial plane reformats, and curved plane reformats, for which high z-axis resolution is an absolute necessity.

the differential radiodensity of adjacent structures and so produce an image of these structures. Image quality depends on the ratio of the amplitude of these real fluctuations to that of random fluctuations. Given a sufficient quantity of attenuation data to feed into the reconstruction algorithm, the degree of noise can be reduced by averaging the data while preserving the real fluctuations from actual structures, thus boosting the signal-to-noise ratio. However, when reconstructing very thin slices by using only a small quantity of attenuation data, less opportunity exists for averaging data and reducing noise, and therefore the signal-to-noise ratio can be low. This relatively larger degree of noise in the image appears as a grainy, noisy image, a consequence of the requirement for very thin sections. This problem is not significant in small or average-weight individuals, but it can significantly limit interpretability in very obese patients.

Finally, the inherent nature of the heart and coronary artery disease may itself pose a problem: calcium and metal within the heart are notorious for degrading image quality in cardiac CT and can obscure visualization of the coronary arteries and reduce diagnostic accuracy. These elements are unavoidable in the cardiac patient population and in some cases may preclude the use of cardiac CT. However, some tools and tricks of the trade are available to compensate for the influence of calcium and metal on image quality, as discussed later.

Hence, the technical considerations of performing cardiac CT include those of any standard chest CT, as well as those particular to cardiac CT. Standard chest CT requires the patient to hold his or her breath during the scan and to cooperate with the scan instructions; the scan needs to be properly timed to achieve optimum opacification of the cardiovascular structures of interest; and a full evaluation of the heart requires the use of intravenous iodinated contrast medium and x-ray radiation. In addition to these requirements, for ideal image quality, a cardiac CT scan yields best results when the heart rate is slow, the rhythm is regular, and no ectopy is present, and the patient should have a reasonable body habitus and, one hopes, a minimal degree of cardiac or coronary metal and calcification.

These modifications to the standard CT technique, the nature of imaging cardiac and coronary artery disease, and the increased potential for technical challenges require special expertise, attention to detail, and the ability to troubleshoot on the part of all those involved in the preparation, performance, and interpretation of these studies. Problem solving is a daily occurrence in a high-quality laboratory striving to achieve the goal of this kind of imaging.

The goal, of course, is to perform the scan in such a way that it maximizes the diagnostic power of the study while exposing the patient to only the minimum amount of radiation necessary to achieve that diagnostic power. Three key elements interplay in every clinical scenario to balance diagnostic quality against radiation exposure: scanner factors, patient factors, and the clinical question (Box 3-1 and Fig. 3-3).

Scanner Factors

Gantry configuration (number of x-ray sources or
  detector arrays)
Gantry rotation speed
X-ray tube power
Detector configuration (number of rows; row width)
Scan modes
Radiation exposure reduction methods
Reconstruction methods

Patient Factors

Age
Sex
Weight, body mass index, body habitus
Intravenous access
Renal function
Heart rate
Heart rhythm
Blood pressure
Respiratory status (ability to hold breath)
Cognitive status (ability to follow breathing
  instructions)
Medical and surgical history

Clinical Situation

Indication
Clinical question
Expected impact on patient management
Appropriateness

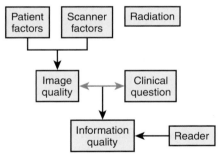

Figure 3-3 Diagram demonstrating the various factors that influence information quality. Patient and scanner factors influence image quality. Radiation exposure is also a by-product of these factors. The interplay between the image quality and the clinical question, and between the experience and ability of the reader, will then determine the quality of the information yielded by the study.

Key scanner factors include gantry hardware (e.g., number of x-ray tubes), gantry rotation speed, x-ray tube power, detector configuration (e.g., number of detector rows and detector row width), available scan modes (e.g., prospectively ECG-triggered scanning), available radiation exposure reduction methods (e.g., eclipse collimation, ECG-based tube current modulation), and available reconstruction methods (e.g., iterative reconstruction). Key patient factors include age, sex, weight, body mass index, body habitus or shape, intravenous access, renal function, heart rate, blood pressure,

respiratory status, cognitive status, and, of course, prior cardiac history.

The clinical scenario is the main indication for the scan It also determines the clinical question, what will be done with the information, and therefore how the scan will be performed.

As an example of the interplay of these elements, consider x-ray tube power. This critical technical specification has significant implications for diagnostic ability and radiation exposure. In knowing this technical specification of the scanner system and understanding its implications, the examiner will quickly realize whether a given patient fits into the technical capabilities of the scanner. For example, imaging the coronary arteries of a very obese patient may be possible if the system has a very strong x-ray tube, but if tube power is insufficient, the study will most likely be nondiagnostic. If that patient also has a high heart rate, then diagnostic imaging will need high temporal resolution, most likely involving the use of the traditional helical scan technique. If the coronary arteries turn out to be normal, the examiner may possibly determine this despite some degradation of image quality by the noise and motion artifact, but if the coronary arteries are heavily diseased and densely calcified, fully evaluating the entire coronary tree for presence and degree of coronary stenosis will be impossible. Moreover, if the clinical question in this patient is whether a 2.5-mm stent contains in-stent restenosis, a cardiac CT scan will probably be able to answer that question, given those scanner and patient factors. Even if it were feasible to image the coronary arteries of the obese patient with a high heart rate and to rule out stenosis if the coronary arteries are normal, this can be achieved today only by using a technique involving high radiation exposure (traditional helical CT). Therefore, if our example patient were a young woman with a low likelihood of obstructive coronary disease who presents with atypical chest discomfort, then it would be prudent to consider other modalities that could answer the question without exposing her to radiation.

Safe, reliable, high-quality cardiac CT will result from understanding what these three key elements (scanner factors, patient factors, clinical scenario) imply and how they interact to define the capabilities, limitations, and appropriate use of this technology. With these general concepts in mind, the next section discusses a few potentially problematic clinical scenarios that may be encountered when performing cardiac CT, the mechanisms behind the problems, and ways to avoid or ameliorate them.

■ PROBLEM SOLVING

High Heart Rate

Background

Coronary CTA is one of the most demanding tasks that can be asked of a CT scanner. Not only must the three-dimensional anatomy be imaged, but also all the image data needed for complete image reconstruction must be acquired within the brief instant in time in which the heart is not moving. Fortunately, today's scanners are exceedingly fast and efficient. However, the speed of cardiac CT is both its beauty and its vulnerability: although the best current scanners can acquire all the data needed for imaging the heart in less than one half-second, it has to be the *right* half-second. That half-second must contain perfect synchronization of arrival of contrast, settling of the heart into mechanical quiescence, the correct table position relative to the gantry, the appropriate time point within the cardiac cycle, and a good patient breath hold. Part of the trick is fitting the data acquisition within one of the two available moments of cardiac quiescence.

Cardiac Quiescence: End-Systole and Diastasis

The two temporal windows during which the heart may briefly come to rest are end-systole, which occurs during isovolumic relaxation, and late diastole, which occurs after passive filling and before atrial systole (diastasis). The end-systolic window is brief, although it is consistent across a range of heart rates and rhythms. The late-diastolic window is usually longer, although its length is more variable, increasing with lower heart rates and decreasing with higher heart rates. In addition, diastasis practically disappears at heart rates higher than 80 beats/minute, and it is the phase more commonly interrupted by ectopy. Nonetheless, because it is relatively easy to achieve a diastasis that is usually longer in duration than end-systolic isovolumic relaxation, and because of the desire to image the coronary arteries when they are elongated and lengthened, the usual goal is to image the coronary arteries in diastasis. Ideally, then, coronary CTA is performed with a heart rate of 55 to 60 beats/minute, to provide a comfortably lengthy diastasis. The goal of the scan is to acquire all the projection attenuation data needed for image reconstruction within this window of opportunity.

Acquisition Time

The acquisition time is the key scanner characteristic that determines whether the previously stated goal will be possible. It is simply the amount of time required to acquire the attenuation data needed to reconstruct the axial images. As long as the acquisition time is less than or equal to the duration of diastasis, then the heart will remain motionless during data collection, and reconstruction of the collected data will produce motion-free images. If diastasis is too short, or the acquisition time is too long, however, then the heart will be moving during data collection, and the images will be blurred by motion. Acquisition time is determined by several factors, but principal among them are scanner mechanics and scan mode.

The key scanner mechanics elements are the number of x-ray sources and the gantry rotation speed. CT works by collecting attenuation data from multiple view angles around the patient's body and then using computational algorithms to reconstruct digital representations of the patient's anatomy. Assigning grayscale values to the numbers then produces an image that the human senses can interpret. Although the earliest scanners used the full 360 degrees of projections for image reconstruction, newer algorithms make it possible to use essentially one half rotation, or approximately 180 degrees of projections, to generate images. Hence, for a standard single source scanner (one x-ray tube and one detector array), the time required to collect all the needed information for reconstruction (i.e., the acquisition time) is approximately one half the gantry rotation time. The fastest single source scanner on the market today spins at 270 msec per rotation, for a nominal acquisition time of approximately 135 msec. For a dual source scanner, the acquisition time is approximately one fourth the gantry rotation time because the two detector arrays (positioned at ~90 degrees to each other on the gantry) cover the arc in half the time. The fastest dual source scanner on the market today spins at 280 msec per rotation, for a nominal acquisition time of approximately 70 msec. The temporal resolution (shutter speed) of the scan is essentially the same as the acquisition time.

Multicycle Reconstruction

In addition to scanner mechanics, scan mode is a key determinant of acquisition time or temporal resolution. In a traditional helical, retrospectively gated cardiac CT scan, temporal resolution can be improved by double or triple acquiring the attenuation data. Today's detector arrays consist of multiple (32 to 320) rows of detectors. The thickness of each row ranges from 0.5 to 0.625 mm; hence the total z-axis width of the detector arrays ranges from 20 to 160 mm of coverage. This can be thought of as the thickness of the swath of anatomy being scanned by every pass of the gantry.

In helical mode, attenuated photons passing through any given slice level of the patient's chest strike each of the rows of the detector array in turn as the patient slides through the gantry. If the heart rate is sufficiently high and the table speed is sufficiently slow, not only may the slice be multiply exposed, but also it may be multiply exposed in diastasis. For example, in a scanner with 64 rows of detectors, at a pitch of 0.2, given a heart rate in the 70s or 80s, any given slice of the heart may be imaged in diastasis twice or thrice.

This multiple imaging of the heart can be used to advantage during reconstruction. Rather than reconstructing the images from one single 180-degree arc of attenuation data, the images can be reconstructed from two adjacent 90-degree arcs: the first 90 degrees (e.g., the 0- to 90-degree scan angle) from heart beat 1 and the second 90 degrees (e.g., the 90- to 180-degree scan angle) from heart beat 2. Alternatively, three adjacent 60-degree arcs could be used, again given a high enough heart rate and slow enough table speed.

Because the acquisition of data *within each heartbeat* is now occurring over a smaller scan angle, the time required for acquisition is shorter: whereas a 180-degree acquisition takes 135 msec, a 90-degree takes 67 msec, and a 60-degree acquisition takes 45 msec. As a result, the temporal resolution improves from 135 msec to, in theory, as fast as 45 msec. This can greatly improve visualization of fast-moving structures, such as valve leaflets and coronary arteries. However, the degree of improvement of the temporal resolution is variable and greatly depends on the exact heart rate. Often, no improvement can be achieved.

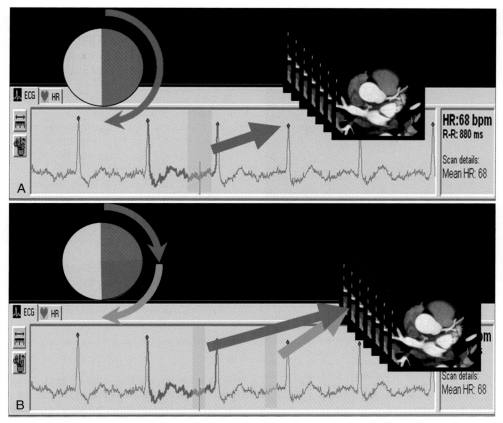

Figure 3-4 **A,** Image reconstruction using a single cardiac cycle (single cycle reconstruction). Approximately 180 degrees of data (view angles) are always required to reconstruct an axial image. In single cycle reconstruction, data acquired during one cardiac cycle are used to reconstruct a portion of the axial image set. The time required to acquire the data needed for this reconstruction is equivalent to the time required for the gantry to collect approximately 180 degrees of view angles (e.g., 135 msec for a single source scanner with a rotation time of 270 msec). This can be thought of as the "shutter speed" of the scanner: for a motion-free image, the structures imaged must remain motion free, usually in diastasis, for this amount of time. If diastasis is shorter than this time period, whether because of a high heart rate (HR) or from interruption by a premature beat, such that the structures begin moving during this acquisition time period, then that movement will be reflected in the resultant reconstructed images as blurring, streaks, and other motion artifacts. **B,** The solution is to shorten the acquisition time. This is a diagrammatic representation of image reconstruction using multiple cardiac cycles (multicycle reconstruction). Using wide, multirow detector arrays and slow-pitch helical scanning or zero-pitch whole heart scanning, any given slice level through the heart will be imaged, in diastasis, two or three times. It may be possible to gather the needed 180 degrees of data by combining acquisitions from these two or three adjacent beats. In this illustration, data from two beats are used for reconstruction. Now the time required to acquire the needed data is equivalent to the time required for the gantry to collect only 90 degrees of view angles. For the same 270-msec rotation time scanner, this is equivalent to 77 msec. The shutter speed has increased from 135 to 77 msec. This shorter acquisition time is more likely to fit within the available diastasis (barring interruption of diastasis by a premature beat), and the scanner is more likely to be able to capture motion-free data and hence to reconstruct motion-free images. In this way, multicycle reconstruction improves the temporal resolution of the scan. *bpm,* Beats per minute; *ECG,* electrocardiogram.

The process of stitching these arcs together is referred to as multicycle reconstruction, and in this case, the more beats the better. Multicycle reconstruction is more effective at higher heart rates (Fig. 3-4).

Three caveats should be mentioned. First, radiation exposure is not low. Table speed is slow; the pitch of less than 1 indicates overlapping x-ray exposure; and exposure time is relatively long compared with today's low-exposure techniques (e.g., axial scanning or high-pitch helical scanning). Second, this technique does not work when the heart and the gantry are in sync (i.e., the cardiac cycle length is a multiple of half the gantry rotation time). For example, if gantry rotation time is 420 msec, then multicycle reconstruction cannot be used for a heart rate of 95 beats/minute, because this represents a cardiac cycle length of 1.5 times the gantry rotation time (630 msec). In this situation, every time the heart returns to diastasis, the x-ray tube returns to the same angular position (or the position directly opposite the gantry); hence the requisite *adjacent* scan angles can never be collected. Third, multicycle reconstruction requires a *regular* cardiac rhythm: the heart must behave the same way, come to rest in the same position, with the same cardiac cycle length, from beat to beat, for practically every beat of the scan. If this is the case, results can be surprisingly good (Fig. 3-5). Any variation, especially in cardiac cycle length, during the scan will result in blurring.

Multicycle reconstruction is not limited strictly to helical scanning. A scanner with a wide enough detector array to cover the entire heart in one rotation, such as the 320-row scanner, can perform not just one scan, but two or potentially even three, and again combine these acquisitions to improve the "virtual" temporal resolution. The tradeoff is, of course, that each scan delivers the x-ray exposure of an entire cardiac scan. Therefore, a two-exposure scan delivers twice the exposure, and a

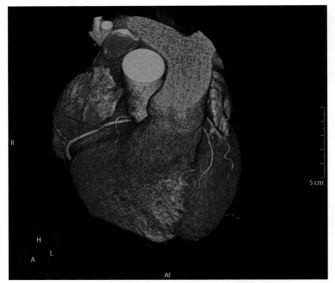

Figure 3-5 Example demonstrating the capability of multicycle reconstruction. This patient was in atrial flutter at a heart rate of 142 beats/minute during the scan. The helical computed tomography scan was performed to evaluate the left atrium and pulmonary veins before radiofrequency ablation, but it also happened to capture high-quality images of the coronary arteries, a testament to the occasional ability of multicycle reconstruction to compensate for high heart rates. Cardiac rhythm is key to the success of this strategy: the monotonous rhythm of atrial flutter makes this result possible, even at this high rate, but other conditions characterized by fluctuation in the cardiac cycle length do not elicit such clear results.

three-exposure scan delivers an exposure that reaches the levels of helical scanning, in which case one may as well perform a regular helical scan to accommodate the high heart rate.

Whatever scan mode is used, and whether or not multicycle reconstruction is used, the selected scan and reconstruction methods will result in a particular acquisition time. This acquisition time must fit within the duration of time of whichever cardiac phase (end-systole or late diastole) is selected for acquisition and reconstruction.

A low heart rate (bradycardia) results in a relatively long, motionless diastasis and therefore ample time for data collection to produce crisp, motion-free images. Although some individuals present with such a low heart rate, much more commonly the resting heart rate of the patient is between 65 and 85 beats/minute. Even in patients presenting with a low initial heart rate, anxiety about the scan and the use of sublingual nitroglycerin to increase the size and visibility of the coronary arteries may result in an increase in rate from an initially favorable bradycardia to a more problematic higher heart rate. The high heart rate can be problematic if temporal resolution is insufficient to image the moving structures because this results in motion blurring and potentially a nondiagnostic or poorly diagnostic study.

Different scanners possess differing degrees of capability to compensate for higher heart rates. Some scanners have a limited ability to compensate for high heart rate and are more vulnerable to potential motion artifacts at a heart rate that other scanners can compensate

---

Ideal heart rate for coronary computed tomography angiography: <60 beats/minute

Heart rate modulation (pharmacotherapy) for heart rates >65 beats/minute

Default scan mode (favorable heart rate <65 beats/minute)

  Prospectively ECG-triggered sequential (axial or step and shoot) scan targeting late diastole

  Prospectively ECG-triggered helical (high-pitch) scan targeting late diastole

  Retrospectively ECG-gated helical scan with ECG-based tube current modulation targeting late diastole

Mildly elevated heart rates (65 to 75 beats/minute)[*]

  Prospectively ECG-triggered sequential scan targeting end-systole

  Retrospectively ECG-gated helical scan with ECG-based tube current modulation targeting end-systole

Elevated heart rates (>75 beats/minute)

  Retrospectively ECG-gated helical scan (without tube current modulation)

[*]If low likelihood of significant coronary disease.

---

for to produce motion-free images. In general, however, virtually all experts agree that no matter which scanner is used, lower heart rates produce better image results, and for this reason pharmacologic heart rate modulation is usually the first step taken to avoid motion artifact.

Some patients may have a physiologic reason for a higher heart rate (e.g., cardiomyopathy or valvular heart disease). In these patients, lowering the heart rate may be clinically undesirable and even potentially dangerous. Of course, knowing the patient's medical history and any drug precautions or contraindications is paramount before administering medications. In some cases, the heart rate may remain unfavorable even after pharmacologic manipulation.

Approach to High Heart Rate

The best approach to a high heart rate balances patient factors, scanner factors, and the clinical scenario (Box 3-2). Patient factors may prevent reaching the target heart rate despite administration of the full dose of beta-blocker, or they may preclude using any medications at all.

Scanner factors influence the options for scan mode or scan modification that are available to compensate for a higher heart rate. The default mode should be a prospective ECG-triggered scan. Most scanners today offer this mode, which exposes the patient to a relatively low dose of radiation (~80% lower than the traditional helical method). This may be an axial step and shoot scan or a helical scan mode. Results of the step and shoot scan are usually best when the scan is performed with a wide detector system (e.g., 128 rows or higher), whereas the prospective helical scan is best (and only) performed with a high-speed dual source system. Older, basic 64-slice systems can use ECG-based tube current modulation to achieve an approximately 40% dose reduction. In either case, a relatively lengthy acquisition

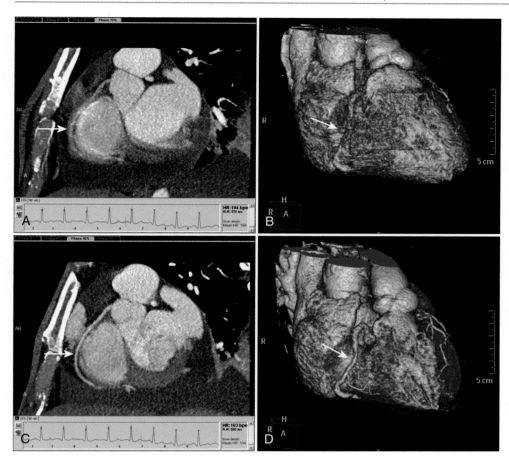

Figure 3-6 Multiplanar reformat (A) and volume-rendered image (B) of a scan during a heart rate (HR) of 104 beats/minute (bpm). Reconstruction in the diastasis phase results in severe motion artifact, especially of the right coronary artery (RCA) *(arrow)*. Diastasis essentially ceases to exist at a heart rate of more than 80 beats/minute. The RCA is uninterpretable. **C** and **D**, Reconstruction in end-systole is much improved (the distal RCA is out of plane). The RCA is virtually motion free *(arrow)*. This is another example of the ability of multicycle reconstruction to handle high heart rates effectively.

window is required for optimal quality, corresponding to a heart rate lower than 65 beats/minute, and ideally lower than 60 beats/minute. Hence, for higher heart rates, another mode must be chosen.

If gantry speed is sufficiently fast (<300 msec per rotation), the examiner may possibly in some cases target end-systole for acquisition using a prospective ECG-triggered mode. This approach usually produces sufficient image quality to exclude stenosis in patients with a low level of atherosclerotic disease burden, but image quality may not be sufficient to perform detailed analysis of heavily diseased and calcified vessels. This is also not a good option for attempting to evaluate coronary stents.

Similarly, if one is using a dual source scanner, which provides excellent temporal resolution, it is not unreasonable to consider performing an ECG-gated helical scan using dose modulation and targeting end-systole for acquisition, as well as using minimum dose tube modulation to reduce tube current outside of this end-systolic window significantly (down to 4%).

When none of the foregoing procedures are available or likely to succeed, the standard ECG-gated helical scan mode, without dose modulation, is always available as the old standby. Gantry configuration and speed still play a role in determining image quality, but the use of full helical mode permits the most flexibility in image reconstruction and manipulation and should allow the examiner eventually to reconstruct the correct image set and provide motion-free images (Fig. 3-6).

Finally, clinical scenario also plays a role here, primarily by indicating the stringency of image quality required. For example, a scan performed to evaluate the morphology of the left atrium and pulmonary veins is less likely to suffer from motion artifact, and has a lower image quality requirement, than a scan performed to evaluate the patency of a midright coronary artery stent. Similarly, a scan in a 40-year-old woman with atypical chest pain and a low likelihood of significant coronary disease may be able to performed with a low-exposure technique, even if it means risking a small amount of motion artifact, compared with a scan in an 80-year-old man with atypical chest pain and a history of prior angioplasty. In the young woman with normal coronary arteries, a small amount of motion artifact is unlikely to render the study uninterpretable, because one could still confidently exclude stenosis. However, the same motion artifact in the setting of multiple coronary plaques and calcifications in the older patient is likely to render the study inconclusive, and all efforts should be applied to maximize image quality, even at the cost of higher radiation exposure, because the higher exposure is of less clinical consequence for him.

Irregular Rhythms: Ectopy and Atrial Fibrillation

Ectopy

Ectopy manifesting as isolated premature atrial and ventricular complexes is not uncommon in cardiac patients,

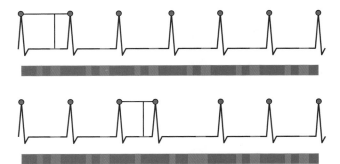

Figure 3-7 Diagram illustrating the problem of ectopy during scan acquisition. *Top*, The ideal situation, with a 1:1 correlation between electrical and mechanical events. Each QRS complex is followed by a complete isovolumic relaxation phase and a complete diastasis phase *(green bars)*. Diastasis occurs approximately 75% of the way through the cardiac cycle. Hence, reconstruction of the 75% phase *(pink bar)* uses data acquired during a motion-free interval. *Bottom*, The fourth beat is early (ectopic). This disrupts the normal electromechanical relationship of the preceding (interrupted) beat, which contains a complete isovolumic relaxation phase, but no diastasis. Hence, reconstruction as usual, attempting to use the diastasis phase, uses data acquired during a period of cardiac motion. The resultant images contain motion artifact and are likely to be uninterpretable.

but it is usually intermittent and infrequent. Atrial or ventricular bigeminy may also be present, although this is a rarer phenomenon. The scanner's ECG algorithm usually tracks these ectopic beats quite well, by tagging each premature QRS complex just as it would any normal beat. The problem with ectopy during cardiac CT is in acquisition and reconstruction of the data. Ectopy can present a problem especially if an ECG-triggered scan is performed.

The variable cycle lengths and interruption of diastasis result in an inaccurate prediction of diastasis and therefore improper triggering (too early or too late). Consequently, the acquisition is out of step with the desired late diastolic window, and so acquisition occurs during a portion of the cardiac cycle when the heart is moving, thus resulting in motion artifact (Fig. 3-7). Some scanners can detect this arrhythmia in real time during a scan and adjust for it. The scanner aborts the acquisition when it detects a premature beat, waits for next beat, and then acquires data from a normal, full-length cardiac cycle. This usually resolves the problem. However, this approach is less likely to work well in the setting of very frequent ectopy or bigeminy. In general, when performing a prospectively ECG-triggered scan, the examiner should remember that the ability to edit the ECG and fix the problem offline after the scan is limited. Therefore, the decision to proceed with a triggered scan in this setting must be made with caution.

Helical scans with dose modulation actually have a problem similar to that seen with triggered scans, in that tube current modulation is inaccurately timed. As a result, although the helical scan mode ensures that data acquisition is occurring during diastasis, that acquisition may occur when tube current is inadvertently turned down by the mistimed dose modulation. Such images have poor quality because of underexposure and are likely inadequate for coronary evaluation.

Conversely, a full helical scan without dose modulation permits editing of the ECG after the scan to fix these problems. By tagging the premature complex as an early beat, the scan alerts the system that the preceding cardiac cycle is interrupted, and shortened, and does not contain a normal diastasis. The scanner software then excludes that cardiac cycle from the reconstruction (Fig. 3-8).

Again, the extent to which the reconstruction process can be modified is limited. In incessant premature atrial or ventricular contractions, even editing the ECG has limited effectiveness because so many beats are interrupted by ectopy, but not all these beats can be excluded from reconstruction. In this case, one can attempt reconstruction using an end-systolic window.

The approach to dealing with ectopy starts with keeping eyes on the ECG during the patient setup and preparation. This is a good time to watch for arrhythmia and ectopy and its frequency and pattern. If ectopy is present and a triggered scan is considered, the examiner still may be able to perform this scan if the ectopy is infrequent and the scanner software is robust enough to detect and adjust for it in real time during the scan. Otherwise, it is safest to revert to a helical scan without dose modulation. Some examiners have reported using lidocaine to suppress ventricular ectopy. This approach may sometimes be an effective way to suppress this rhythm. Beta-blockers may have little impact on ectopy. In fact, in some cases, ectopy may become more frequent in the presence of lower heart rate or depressed sinus node activity.

Atrial Fibrillation

In general, attempting to image the coronary arteries in atrial fibrillation is not recommended. In some cases, imaging may be possible, but the results are highly dependent on available equipment, operator experience, and luck. Even in experienced hands and using the latest equipment, the results are mixed. For this reason diagnostic images of the coronaries cannot reliably be expected, so coronary imaging during atrial fibrillation is generally not recommended.

However, other indications for cardiac CT in atrial fibrillation exist, chief among these being evaluation of the left atrium and pulmonary veins before radiofrequency ablation of atrial fibrillation. Cardiac CT can be helpful in this situation to evaluate the morphology of the left atrium and pulmonary veins, identify anomalous or variant pulmonary arteries, identify anomalous or variant superior or inferior vena cava, identify abnormalities of the interatrial septum that may become important if transseptal puncture is required, and exclude left atrial appendage thrombus. Fortunately, these structures are easier imaging targets than are the coronary arteries.

Atrial fibrillation represents two problems: irregular rhythm and potentially high heart rate. Given this situation, the use of helical scans without dose modulation in all these patients is tempting. This approach ensures maximum flexibility for reconstruction, but it also results in maximum x-ray exposure.

However, the examiner should consider the imaging targets: the left atrium, the left atrial appendage, and the

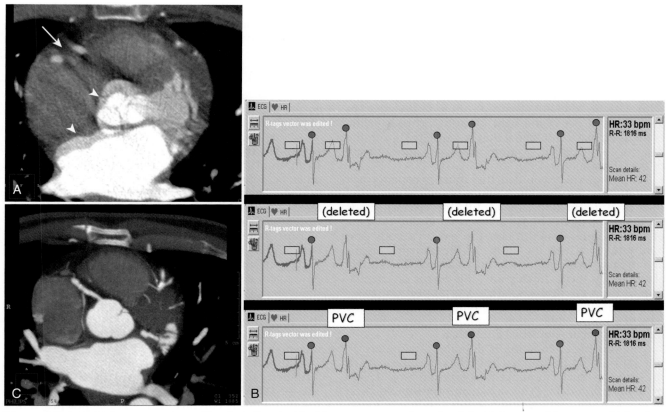

Figure 3-8 A, Multiple severe motion artifacts including double right coronary artery *(arrow)* and double borders of the aorta and left atrium *(arrowheads)*. Such artifacts should prompt a review of the electrocardiogram (ECG) for heart rate (HR) and rhythm. **B,** *Top,* The ECG reveals ventricular bigeminy. Each QRS complex has been appropriately tagged *(red dots),* but an attempt at typical reconstruction, defining diastasis as the 75% phase of each cardiac cycle, results in reconstruction of an interrupted cardiac cycle in every other beat. *Middle,* Simply deleting the tags from the premature ventricular contractions (PVCs) does prevent reconstruction from this shortened cardiac cycle, but it also shifts the reconstruction window of the full-length cycles to an earlier time point, too early for diastasis. *Bottom,* Instead, the PVCs should be marked as such, in this way allowing the software to discriminate between the normal beats and PVCs, and reconstruct only from the normal cardiac cycles, by using the correct, diastasis window. **C,** After editing the ECG in this fashion, reconstruction now reveals a good-quality, motion-free image. This ECG editing capability is available on most systems today. *bpm,* Beats per minute.

pulmonary veins. None of these are highly mobile structures. They are also relatively large and hence are easier imaging targets and are well opacified by large volumes of contrast material. Moreover, the intensity of analysis is lower than in coronary imaging because it usually consists of just a visual description of morphology and standard dimensions and volumes. Hence, helical scanning with full-dose radiation as in coronary CTA probably represents overscanning. How can one lower the dose? First, the examiner can consider lowering the tube voltage and current, depending on the patient's body habitus. Then, the scan technique can be considered: helical with dose modulation or prospective scan. The selection depends on the heart rate. Both scan types use a prospective element: the dose modulation or the data acquisition itself. The key point to remember is that in an ectopic or irregular rhythm, diastasis is interrupted; therefore, diastasis should be avoided, and the prospective element should be designed around the end-systolic window. For a helical scan, this means dose modulation around 30% to 50% of the cardiac cycle length (slightly later 35% to 55% if heart rate is >80 beats/minute), and for a prospective scan, this means using an end-systolic trigger. For maximum dose reduction (young female

patients), a reasonable choice is prospective ECG-triggered CT using an end-systolic trigger. Many sites even use nongated acquisitions to minimize dose. High-pitch spiral ("flash") acquisitions are an attractive alternative because of the very low associated radiation dose while maintaining synchronization with the cardiac cycle, but they require a dual source scanner.

The CTA in atrial fibrillation may reveal a filling defect in the left atrial appendage. However, this does not necessarily indicate the presence of a thrombus. Such a filling defect often reflects slow filling of the appendage secondary to the slow blood flow within the left atrium that accompanies atrial fibrillation. To distinguish thrombus from slow flow, one may perform a second scan immediately after the first scan and look for contrast to "fill in" the appendage, thus indicating slow flow and no thrombus.

Obese Patients

The detector array is the most expensive part of a CT scanner. Since 2000, scanner manufacturers have produced remarkable advances in detector technology that have resulted in smaller size, better scalability, and improved sensitivity. At their fundamental level, however, detectors of all generations, current and past, have done one thing: count photons.

The key ingredient of any photodetector is the small crystal that sits within its core and that, when struck by an x-ray photon, absorbs it and emits in return a photon of visible light. This emission of light allows the x-ray photon to be counted: electronic photodiodes adjacent to the crystal detect the light photon and register the event as an electronic signal that is transferred from the detector to the digital electronic hardware and software of the CT scanner system.

For photons to be counted, they must, of course, reach the detectors. Between their source (the x-ray tube) and their final destination (the scintillation crystal) stands (or lies) the patient's body (in this case, the chest). Some of the photons pass through the patient's body and hardly interact with the atoms of the patient's organs and tissues, whereas others are scattered or entirely absorbed by them. In this way, the degree of attenuation of the x-ray beam is variable; a proportion passes through relatively unaffected by passage through the patient's body, while other proportions are deflected, lose energy, or are absorbed altogether.

This variable attenuation is desirable. Examiners do not want all the photons that leave the x-ray tube to reach the detectors; such a homogenous exposure would yield no attenuation data. (This is like an overexposed chest radiograph in which the lungs appear uniformly black, without any detail.) Nor do examiners want only a few photons to make it through the patient's body; such underexposure would also yield no attenuation data; in fact, the only variation that would be present in the attenuation data would be that of random noise. (This is like an underexposed chest radiograph in which the lungs appear uniformly white or fuzzy, and structural details cannot be seen.) Ideally, some middle ground of variable attenuation of the x-ray beam is desired, such that high-density structures attenuate a large fraction of the photons, but not all of them, and low-density structures attenuate a small fraction of the photons, but not none of them.

In this ideal situation, a large difference in photon flux exists at the detector level between rays passing through high-density structures such as bone or iodine and rays passing through low-density structures such as lung or fat. Such a difference, or contrast, in photon flux is reflected in the digital signal coming from the detector array, and it leaves a similarly large digital footprint on the raw attenuation data that is further reflected in the final reconstructed image (as a large difference in the CT values) and readily perceived by the human eye (as a large difference in the grayscale).

Hence, in a small or normally sized individual, images contain little noise or granularity, and in fact in smaller patients, studies can be done with lower than usual x-ray exposure. In the obese patient, however, the enveloping layer of fat around the patient's thorax can immediately absorb a good percentage of all the photons, thus leaving fewer photons overall to do the work of trying to demonstrate some difference in variable attenuation caused by the actual intrathoracic structures

themselves. The result is a relative decrease in the difference or contrast in photon flux sensed at the detectors, not because of a decrease in x-ray density of the intrathoracic structures themselves, but because fewer photons are hitting the detectors to demonstrate the difference. The detectors register absolute (not relative) counts. Hence, for obese patients, steps must be taken to ensure that the detectors are receiving adequate counts of photons.

Approach to the Problem

To accomplish the foregoing goal, the x-ray tube settings must be adjusted. X-ray tubes have two settings that can be adjusted by the user: tube potential (kVp, often referred to as voltage) and tube current (mA) (or tube current × time product [mAs]) (Box 3-3).

Tube potential, the potential difference between the cathode and anode, determines the energy of the photon beam. This energy determines the penetrating power of the photons and their ability to pass through the patient's body; and in real numbers, it determines the proportion of photons that will pass through. Again, this proportion should be neither too great nor too small; too great an energy leads to overexposure, and too small leads to underexposure.

Within the standard tube settings of a CT scanner is a limited range of choices, currently typically 80, 100, 120, or 140 kVp, although tubes with a minimal potential of 70 kVp are entering the market. In practical terms, all these settings lead to some degree of absorption and some degree of pass-through. None of these settings will lead to an all-or-none overexposure or underexposure, but the degree is key, especially in the obese patient, in whom the tube voltage may need to be increased in some cases to ensure adequate penetration.

A tube potential of 100 kVp or lower should not be used. Such a weak x-ray beam is too highly attenuated by the patient's mass. In most cases of "typical" obesity (up to a body mass index of approximately 40 to 45 kg/m²), a tube potential of 120 kVp may deliver enough energy to provide adequate variable attenuation. Beyond this, and certainly at a body mass index of more than 50 kg/m², a tube potential of 140 kVp is required.

Maximum allowable tube current declines as a result of using the higher voltage setting, but the final results are better at the higher potential even though lower current is used, because the absolute number of photons reaching the detectors is greater, and the absolute count

---

BOX 3-3 Approach to the Obese Patient

Minimum tube voltage of 120 kVp, and 140 kVp for BMI ≥50 mg/m²
High tube current (maximum for BMI ≥50 mg/m²)
Aggressive heart rate modulation, to enable use of prospective scanning
High injection rates up to 7 mL/second
Soft reconstruction filter or kernel
Increase reconstructed slice thickness (1.25 to 1.5 mm)
Iterative reconstruction

BMI, Body mass index.

per unit time is the key metric. The other, perhaps more significant, tradeoff is a significant increase in x-ray radiation exposure.

Although x-ray exposure increases linearly with tube current, it increases exponentially with tube potential. Therefore, doubling of tube current doubles radiation exposure, but theoretical doubling to tube potential actually quadruples radiation exposure. Obese patients also require a higher tube current (mA) because more of the photons are absorbed. Consequently, to send the same number of photons to the detector as in a regular-sized person, the tube current or photon flux must be increased. In short, during cardiac CT of obese patients, tube output is generally at maximum.

That said, it does not mean that methods to otherwise limit radiation exposure cannot be used. In fact, in the obese patient, these other methods become even more important. The main method of reducing exposure (other than minimizing the scan length in z-axis) is the use of a scan mode that limits the exposure time, such as prospectively ECG-triggered axial scanning or ECG-triggered high-pitch helical scanning. For these methods to work most effectively with the least amount of artifact, a long diastasis (i.e., bradycardia) is required. Modifications can also be made to the image reconstruction parameters to offset any residual image noise that may be present despite the high tube output.

Various options are available to reduce image noise in the reconstruction, as follows:
1. Increasing slice thickness (to a maximum of 1.25 to 1.5 mm), which averages more of the attenuation data together in the z-axis; the tradeoff is a loss of z-axis resolution, which becomes quite severe at slice thicknesses greater than 1.5 mm.

2. Using a soft reconstruction kernel or filter, which reduces granularity in the x-y plane at the cost of lower sharpness.
3. Using iterative reconstruction, which is a newer method that is different from the standard filtered back projection and further reduces image noise.

Given these modifications, one can achieve diagnostic-quality coronary CTA even in the morbidly obese patient (Fig. 3-9). However, image quality is not equal to that of a normal-weight individual, and attempts to distinguish obstructive from nonobstructive disease in a coronary arterial tree riddled with diffuse atherosclerotic disease are quite difficult. Coronary CTA in the very obese patient is best done when the expectation is that coronary disease is not present, and the scan is performed to prove that. If coronary disease is present, interpretation will be extremely difficult (Fig. 3-10). Otherwise, another method should be used.

Again, best possible results are achieved by the harmonious balance of patient factors (achieving good bradycardia), scanner factors (capability for a triggered, low-exposure scan), and clinical scenario (reserving this technique for patients with low likelihood of disease).

Calcium and Other High Densities

The heart and coronary arteries are a rich source of calcium and metal. Sources include de novo calcification of atherosclerotic lesions of the native coronary arteries and metal of coronary stents. In addition, increasing numbers of devices are implanted in the heart, including pacemakers and defibrillators, closure devices of the interatrial and interventricular septum, occluders of the left atrial appendage, surgically and percutaneous

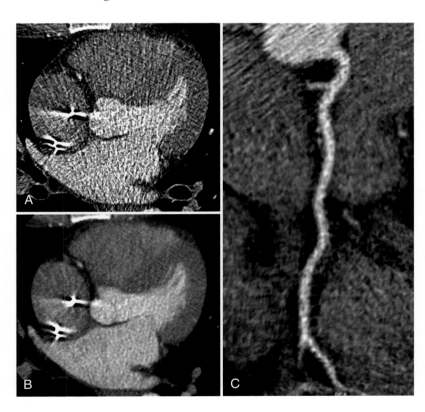

Figure 3-9 A 58-year-old woman presenting with a history of hypertension, hypercholesterolemia, and prior pacemaker implantation following atrioventricular node ablation for atrial fibrillation who now has atypical chest discomfort. She is 5 ft tall, weighs 285 lb, and has a body mass index of 55.7 kg/m². **A,** Images generated by standard reconstruction (0.75-mm slice thickness with semisharp filter) demonstrate significant granularity. **B,** Repeat reconstruction using 1.5-mm slice thickness and a soft filter significantly reduces this image noise. **C,** Curved multiplanar reformat of the right coronary artery derived from the modified reconstruction. By modifying the reconstruction in this manner, one can produce diagnostic-quality coronary images, and, in cases of minimal or no coronary disease, confidently exclude significant disease. However, these modifications cannot overcome the combination of obesity and diffuse plaque burden, in which it becomes much more difficult to exclude stenosis.

implanted prosthetic valves of various materials and designs, and ventricular assist devices (Fig. 3-11). The problem with all these lesions and devices is the high degree of attenuation they exert relative to the typical strength of x-ray beam used for body imaging, as well as the inadequacy of reconstruction algorithms meant for soft, tissue-density structures.

The high density of calcium and metal, especially in the setting of a relatively soft x-ray beam, results in scatter, beam hardening, and overattenuation of those rays passing through the dense object. As a result, the scanner has fewer data, and less accurate data, to use for image reconstruction. Cardiac reconstruction algorithms are generally not designed for these kinds of data. The result is image distortion, characterized by streak artifacts, beam hardening artifacts (dark areas), and obscure visualization of some or all of the coronary arteries. The problem is significantly compounded by any degree of motion. Calcium or metal, in motion, almost always produces serious artifacts.

Approach to the Problem

First and foremost, one must be aware of the presence of calcium and metal, usually obtained from the patient's history of coronary disease, stents, bypass, and implanted devices (Box 3-4). If a question of a potentially significant degree of coronary calcification exists, the examiner can always start with a noncontrast calcium scan and elect not to perform CTA if the coronary arteries are extremely densely calcified.

Second, the imaging target and the devices must be considered. Metal leads of a dual chamber pacemaker

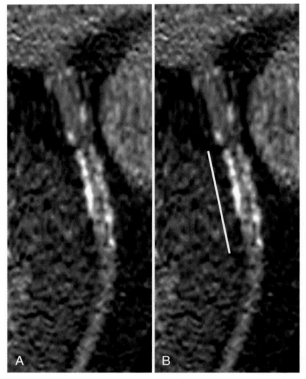

Figure 3-10 **A,** High-quality image clearly demonstrating a patent stent in the midleft anterior descending (LAD) coronary artery. **B,** Morbidly obese 48-year-old woman with prior myocardial infarction and stenting of the proximal LAD coronary artery (adjacent to the *line*) 3 months earlier who now presents with atypical chest pain. The earlier angiogram demonstrated no other significant disease, and the clinical suspicion of obstructive disease or in-stent restenosis is low, but given this image quality, one cannot declare either stent patency or restenosis.

BOX 3-4   Sources of High-Density Elements and Imaging

High-Density Elements (Calcium and Metal)
Coronary calcification (+ to +++)
Dual chamber pacemakers or defibrillators (+)
Biventricular pacemakers or defibrillators (+++)
Prosthetic valves (+)
Closure or occlusion devices (+)
Ventricular assist devices (++ to +++)

Approach to Imaging High-Density Elements
Maintain high tube voltage (120 to 140 kVp)
Maintain high tube current
Maximize heart rate lowering and coronary vasodilation
Low threshold for helical scanning
Thin-slice or small-increment slice reconstruction
Sharp kernel or filter
Iterative reconstruction

+, Minimal impact; +++, significant impact.

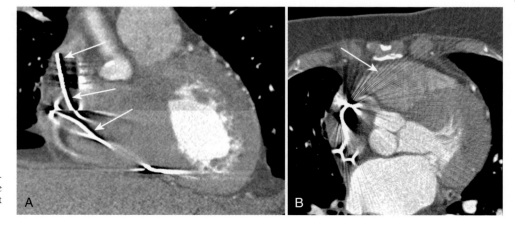

Figure 3-11 A, Beam hardening artifact (extremely hypodense areas) *(arrows)*. **B,** Streak artifact *(arrow)*.

are not usually problematic for coronary artery imaging. Many pacemakers are also defibrillators, which have a thick coil wrapped around the leads in the right atrium and ventricle; this configuration may partially obscure the right coronary artery, but often, coronary imaging can still be successfully performed. Biventricular pacemakers, conversely, can be very problematic because the left ventricular lead often obscures visualization of the circumflex artery system. Prosthetic valves and occlusion devices, perhaps surprisingly, produce little metal artifact and usually do not obscure the coronary arteries. Ventricular assist devices obscure visualization of the distal left anterior descending coronary artery and any other branches near the left ventricular apex. Of course, the coronary status of these patients is usually already known.

Finally, the scan protocol should be modified for the presence of calcium or metal. Tube voltage should be kept up (≥120 kVp), even for thin patients. In some cases, increasing the voltage to 140 kVp may be advisable. Similarly, tube current should be kept up to at least nominal current. The examiner should make the best effort possible to optimize heart rate lowering and coronary vasodilation. Especially considering that tube voltage and current must be maintained at a high level, a prospectively triggered scan mode may be the only way to reduce x-ray exposure subsequently, and this is best performed with a bradycardic heart. Motion artifact in any form must be absolutely avoided, especially in the setting of calcium or metal. If heart rate modulation cannot be achieved (with a target heart rate of <60 beats/minute), then helical scanning should be performed. The examiner should have a low threshold for performing a full helical scan. Reconstruction should be performed with thin slices and small increments, and the examiner should consider using a 33% increment instead of the usual 50% to 66% increment. Reconstruction is performed with a sharp filter or kernel (Fig. 3-12). Iterative

reconstruction (small or mild degree) is used in addition to the sharp filter to suppress excessive image noise or granularity.

Scan Timing: Low Cardiac Output and Congenital Heart Disease

In addition to optimizing temporal and spatial resolution and minimizing image granularity, another technical goal of the imaging procedure is optimal opacification of the structures of interest. A typical contrast-enhanced CT scan is performed by injecting contrast medium, waiting for some prespecified or calculated period of time called the delay or delay time, and then scanning. The delay ensures that image acquisition begins when the structures of interest are at peak opacification. Maintaining opacification of the structures of interest throughout the duration of the scan is also desirable, and this is accomplished through the design of the contrast injection protocol.

In peripheral CTA, timing is even more important because bright opacification of the arterial structures and minimal opacification of the venous structures are usually desired, even required, and the examiner has a short window of time between the peak of contrast material in the arteries and the onset of its arrival in the veins. For this reason, some form of dynamic timing is usually implemented in which the behavior of the contrast bolus is itself used to time the scan more accurately. Two methods are used to time the scan: injecting a separate timing bolus and then performing a series of timing run scans; or injecting the full bolus of contrast medium, tracking contrast density in or near the structures of interest, and then initiating the scan when the contrast density reaches a predefined threshold. The drawbacks of the timing bolus method are that it introduces an additional step in the procedure and requires the use of extra contrast medium.

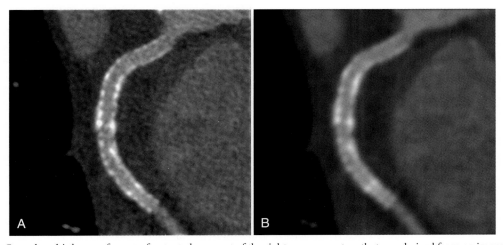

Figure 3-12 A, Curved multiplanar reformat of a stented segment of the right coronary artery that was derived from an image set reconstructed using a standard reconstruction filter or kernel. Image granularity is minimal, but the edges are blurry, and a blooming effect from the stent metal that encroaches on the stent lumen makes lumen evaluation difficult. **B,** Reconstruction using a sharper filter reduces the blurring and blooming and enhances the edge detail, although image granularity is increased and may be difficult to distinguish from intimal hyperplasia. Although the selection of a sharper filter cannot overcome tremendous metal or calcium artifacts, it can often provide enough incremental improvement to enable a more complete evaluation of what would otherwise be a potentially indeterminate result.

The bolus tracking method was devised to omit this extra step and to use the study contrast injection itself to determine the scan timing and start the scan. This is achieved by tracking contrast density in the structures of interest in real time during the contrast injection and then initiating the scan when the contrast density reaches a certain threshold. For example, in coronary CTA, one could track contrast density in the ascending aorta and start the scan sequence when contrast density reaches a predefined threshold (e.g., 120 HU), with the scan itself beginning usually after a 5-second delay after contrast density reaches this threshold. Some form of delay after threshold is required to allow time for the scanner to instruct the patient to hold his or her breath and for the patient to take in a breath and hold it. This procedure also requires extra contrast (5 seconds multiplied by the injection rate); therefore, the net amount of contrast in both the bolus tracking and timing bolus methods is equal.

However, this approach is problematic in the patient with cardiomyopathy or valvular heart disease or other forms of low–cardiac output states in that the rate of rise of contrast density at any point within the cardiovascular system, especially left-sided structures, is slower, and potentially much slower, than normal. In these cases, the threshold and delay used for patients with normal cardiac output can result in lower contrast opacification in the coronary arteries and potentially a nondiagnostic scan (Fig. 3-13).

Approach to the Problem

In patients with abnormal left or right ventricular function, or significant valvular heart disease, either valvular stenosis or regurgitation, the timing bolus method should be used. In a timing bolus, approximately 15 to 20 mL of contrast medium is injected at 4.0 to 5.0 mL/second, followed by 40 to 50 mL of saline solution at the

same rate, and a series of periodic (e.g., one per second) timing run scans are performed at the same slice level that includes the structures of interest. As the contrast bolus passes through the structures of interest, one can monitor the incremental rise and fall of contrast density in the region of interest and in this way determine the time to peak enhancement.

This time to peak enhancement is then used to time the subsequent scan, which is the actual CTA scan with a full bolus of contrast medium. Usually, approximately 2 to 5 seconds of additional time may be added to the time to peak, to take into account the slightly later time to peak that will be seen by a larger bolus of contrast.

The timing bolus method is also the optimal method for determining scan delay in patients with congenital heart disease. In addition, this method should be used when dissection is known or suspected in the ascending aorta because bolus tracking may fail if the region of interest is inadvertently placed in the false lumen.

Radiation Exposure

The advent of cardiac CT, and coronary CTA in particular, brought a tremendous wealth of invaluable information and made this information accessible to more patients and physicians. What previously required an invasive procedure can be gained noninvasively with high fidelity and exquisite detail. In particular, coronary CTA has proved extremely sensitive for the detection of the coronary atherosclerotic process in its early stage.

In the early days of cardiac CT, helical scanning using 120-kVp voltage was the only available scan mode. With meticulous attention to the scan technique, one could achieve a lower end of dose of approximately 10 mSv. This dose was still greater than that used for invasive angiography or routine chest CT, although it was on par with or even lower than that used in most single photon

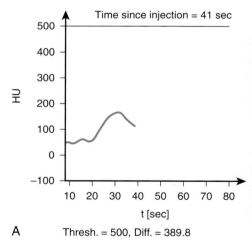
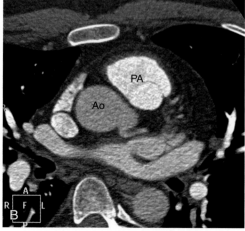

Figure 3-13 **A,** Time-attenuation curve depicting the change in attenuation (HU) over time (t) in a region of interest in the ascending aorta. The time to peak attenuation is 31 seconds, relatively long compared with most scans. This patient had moderate left ventricular dysfunction, and the associated reduced cardiac output is reflected in this prolonged time to peak. **B,** In patients with depressed cardiac output, the standard post-threshold delay used for bolus tracking may underestimate the time to peak, thus resulting in an early scan, as reflected in this image, which shows poor contrast opacification in the aorta (Ao) and left heart structures, including the coronary arteries, and bright opacification of the pulmonary artery (PA). This is the opposite of what is normally expected in a typical cardiac computed tomography scan, in which the left heart structures are preferentially opacified. In cases of known low cardiac output, the timing bolus method of scan timing should be preferred to the bolus tracking method.

emission CT scans. At the opposite end of the spectrum, one could and still can perform these scans by using a much greater x-ray exposure, up to 20 or even 30 mSv.

The primary concern regarding this issue is the theoretical risk of inducing cancer by exposing a patient to x-ray radiation. Whether medical radiation can induce oncogenic transformation is debated. No randomized trial has ever been, or ever will be, conducted to test this theory. However, because very large radiation exposures (e.g., atomic bomb detonations and nuclear reactor meltdowns) are known to be able to induce cancer, investigators have theorized that small radiation exposures may also do so. Therefore, the recommended practice is to use medical radiation in accordance with the ALARA (as low as reasonably achievable) principle: using the least amount of radiation exposure required to achieve diagnostic accuracy.

Today, the field of cardiac imaging has many technical options that allow one to obtain the same degree and quality of information but with much lower radiation exposure, as low as 1 mSv or even less (Fig. 3-14). Nonetheless, many factors determine the ultimate x-ray exposure of any one particular scan. Although obtaining the scan and answering the clinical question are possible with a low-exposure scan technique in many cases, the use of a low-exposure technique jeopardizes diagnostic accuracy in certain other cases, and a more traditional radiation dose is required. To achieve the goal of the best image quality with the least amount of required radiation exposure, one must again understand how scanner factors, patient factors, and the clinical scenario interact.

The scanner factors that determine radiation exposure include the following: tube potential (often referred to as voltage), which determines the energy spectrum of the x-ray beam and is predominantly driven by the patient's body habitus; tube current, which determines the flux of x-ray photons from the x-ray tube and is also predominantly driven by body habitus; and exposure time, which is the total duration of time that any given slice level of the patient's chest is exposed to x-ray. Exposure time is not equivalent to scan time or acquisition time. It is determined by the confluence of scanner mechanics and scan mode and some elements that are automatically programmed on the basis of the patient's heart rate. With these basic concepts in mind, the examiner must know a particular scanner's capabilities and dose-reduction options.

If one considers standard, retrospectively ECG-gated helical CT using 120 kV, 500 mA, a pitch of 0.2, and 800 mAs to be the baseline scan (and the one that delivers the highest radiation exposure), a particular scanner may have some or all of the following options to reduce the radiation exposure incrementally (Box 3-5):

1. Limit the number of scans. For example, a calcium score or a noncontrast and nongated chest scan is often unnecessary before coronary CTA.
2. Limit the scan range. If a calcium scan is performed, the images from that scan can be used to identify the table positions and scan length that will adequately cover the heart without overscanning the patient. The tendency is to overscan, so using the calcium

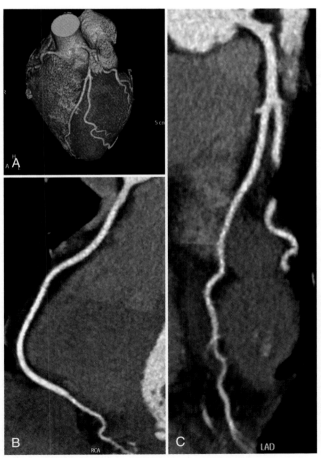

Figure 3-14 Volume-rendered image (**A**) and curved multiplanar reformats (**B** and **C**) from a scan performed using 0.8 mSv. Given the right conditions and scanner capabilities, obtaining excellent image quality does not necessarily require large radiation exposure. *LAD,* Left anterior descending coronary artery; *RCA,* right coronary artery.

BOX 3-5   Strategies to Minimize Radiation Exposure

Limit the number of scans
Limit the scan range
Decrease tube voltage (100 kV for patients <80 to 90 kg, potentially 80 kVp)
Decrease tube current
  Decrease nominal tube current (for patients <80 to 90 kg)
  Use ECG-based tube current modulation (if heart rate and rhythm permit)
Decrease exposure time
  Use prospectively ECG-triggered scanning (if heart rate and rhythm permit)
  Minimize acquisition window (to 0%)
Modify reconstruction to reduce noise (in conjunction with decreased tube current)
  Soft filter or kernel (in the absence of calcium or metal)
  Iterative reconstruction

ECG, Electrocardiogram.

scan images in this way usually results in a significant reduction in x-ray exposure.

3. Decrease the tube voltage from the standard 120 kV to 100 kV if body weight is sufficiently small and chest size and weight distribution permit. A recommended cutoff is 180 lb or 80 kg, but even if the patient's weight is 190 or 200 lb, 100 kV can be used if the weight is predominantly distributed in the lower body. In particularly thin individuals or young patients with questions of coronary anomalies (less fine detail is required), 80 kV may suffice.

4. Decrease the tube current to the minimum required. Again, this factor is predominantly driven by weight and body habitus, as described earlier, and automatic exposure control software that uses a user-predefined desired noise level may be available to help achieve this goal.

5. Decrease the average tube current using ECG-based tube current modulation. This technique requires preselection of one of the quiescent phases of the cardiac cycle (end-systole or late diastasis) for acquisition. The scanner prospectively predicts when this phase will occur for each upcoming cardiac cycle, in real time, as the scan proceeds. As the preselected phase approaches, tube current is ramped up to the programmed nominal tube current (i.e., the appropriate, required tube current for good, diagnostic coronary image quality), maintained throughout that phase, and then ramped down again to a low level throughout the rest of that cardiac cycle. This process repeats for each cardiac cycle (Fig. 3-15). Two points are important. First, data acquired while tube current is reduced are too noisy and grainy for coronary interpretation (Fig. 3-16). Only data acquired during

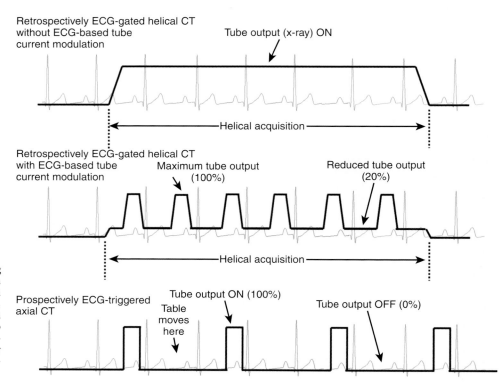

Figure 3-15 Diagram depicting the three most commonly used scan modes. The tube current remains on throughout helical scanning *(top)*, but it can be cycled up and down in time with the cardiac rhythm to spare some dose *(middle)*. Alternatively, tube current can be selectively applied only during diastasis *(bottom)* and otherwise remain off.

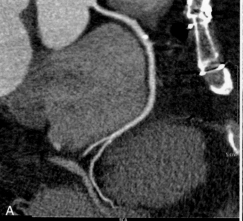
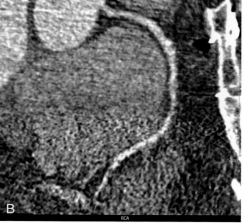

Figure 3-16 A, Curved multiplanar reformat of the right coronary artery in diastasis that demonstrates good image quality. **B,** Reconstruction of the same data set in end-systole. No motion artifact is present, but because electrocardiogram-based tube current modulation was used, and tube current was reduced during systole, the subsequent images are too grainy and noisy for accurate coronary interpretation.

the preselected phases are adequate. This data acquisition is most reliable when the heart rate is slow and diastasis is used for acquisition. Second, this prospective technique may fail if the rhythm is irregular or if the heart rate changes substantially during the scan because the scanner will not be able to predict the optimal acquisition window accurately. In fact, in patients with a mildly irregular rhythm, the use of dose modulation around a systolic window may be better because usually diastasis is interrupted by ectopy or arrhythmia. In a patient with a truly high heart rate, dose modulation should not be used in case reconstruction of both systolic and diastolic phases may be necessary. Dose modulation works best when the heart rate is slow and regular and diastasis can be well predicted. Of course, using the best current scanners, when the heart rate and rhythm are low and regular, prospective triggered CT is the scan mode of choice unless cardiac function analysis is also required.

6. Decrease the exposure time. This goal can be achieved by using one of the two currently available prospectively triggered scan modes: axial step and shoot scanning or high-pitch helical flash scanning. In the case of axial scanning, if the heart rate and rhythm are truly slow and steady, one can limit exposure even further by turning off any padding or phase tolerance (i.e., reducing the exposure window to just the absolute minimum required for reconstruction of just a single phase of the cardiac cycle).

7. Modify the reconstruction process to reduce image noise. This modification can include using a softer filter or kernel and using iterative reconstruction. This change is performed as an adjunct to using lower tube current, to reduce the image noise that would otherwise result. In this way, these techniques can restore image quality to the same level as that derived from traditional (higher) tube current.

8. Finally, the ultimate dose reduction strategy is to not scan with CT. If concerns about radiation exposure are very high, the examiner may be able to obtain guidance for patient management on the basis of a non–x-ray test such as an ultrasound, magnetic resonance imaging, or exercise ECG. Of course, the accuracy and disease detection ability of these techniques must be weighed against those of cardiac CT.

With an understanding of these scanner factors, one must then consider the patient factors relevant to radiation exposure, and these include age, sex, weight and body habitus, heart rate and rhythm, and the patient's medical and surgical history. Examiners would like to use all dose reduction strategies in younger patients and in women, but this goal is either permitted or thwarted by the patient's body weight and body habitus, as well as the heart rate and rhythm. The medical and surgical history alerts the examiner to the presence or absence of complicating factors that may also thwart or permit dose reduction strategies.

Finally, the examiner must consider the clinical scenario and question: What is the imaging target? Evaluating coronary stents for in-stent restenosis requires the highest image quality, a level of quality necessitating the use of more radiation exposure than one would use in imaging a young man in the emergency department who has a low likelihood of coronary disease.

In a young woman with a heart rate in the 80s that remains uncontrollable even after beta-blockade, the hope is to use the minimum radiation exposure. However, if the examiner is attempting to evaluate this patient for in-stent restenosis and her heart rate cannot be controlled, then a higher-exposure technique (helical scanning) will be needed, or the examiner may decide to forgo coronary CTA and try another approach.

Conversely, in an older man with a heart rate in the 50s but a rhythm that is irregular with frequent premature atrial contractions, less concern exists about minimizing radiation. If the clinical question is whether this man has obstructive coronary artery disease, based on a mildly abnormal single photon emission CT scan, and he has frequent ectopy, the examiner would most likely proceed with helical scanning and therefore higher x-ray exposure, but with the assurance of artifact-free images after manipulation of the ECG information during image reconstruction.

■ PEARLS AND PITFALLS

■ In developing scan protocols, examiners must understand how scanner factors, patient factors, and the clinical scenario interact to influence image quality and radiation exposure.

■ Protocols suited to a particular patient population should be developed after obtaining a detailed knowledge of the technical specifications, capabilities, and limitations of particular scanners.

■ The latest model scanners of all the manufacturers offer a prospectively ECG-triggered scan mode; this should be the default scan mode for cardiac CT.

■ Beta-blockers are not absolutely required for coronary CTA, but image quality is always improved when the heart rate is low.

■ In ECG-triggered axial scanning, three factors are of vital importance to image quality: gantry speed, detector coverage, and tube power.

■ In obese patients, good intravenous access (preferably 18 gauge) and the delivery of contrast medium at a higher flow rate (preferably >5.0 mL/second) and higher volume are important elements of achieving robust contrast opacification.

■ The examiner should ask about recent use of phosphodiesterase inhibitors before administering nitroglycerin.

■ Before the scan is performed, the patient should practice a breath hold for 20 seconds, and the examiner should evaluate the ability of the patient to hold his or her breath adequately.

■ Small slice increments should be used to preserve and intensify z-axis resolution, both when using thin-slice reconstruction (stents, calcifications) and when using thicker slices (obese patients). An example of reconstruction in a patient with calcium or a stent is a slice width of 0.9 mm, with an increment of 0.3 mm; an example of reconstruction in an obese patient is a slice width of 1.2 mm, with an increment of 0.4 mm.

- Increasing the matrix size and reducing the reconstructed field of view will improve image resolution in patients with calcium or stents. These techniques preserve image quality when magnifying the image, but they do not alter the actual spatial resolution of the scan.
- The average rendering mode can also be used to reduce noise or granularity of images.
- In the obese patient, heart rate lowering through pharmacotherapy is especially important for optimizing image quality and minimizing radiation exposure.

■ CONCLUSION

Ensuring best image quality results from an optimal combination of scanner factors, patient factors, and clinical scenario. By balancing these factors, in the appropriate clinical setting, diagnostic image quality can be obtained without undue or excessive x-ray exposure, to yield the information to answer the clinical question. An emerging body of literature, including appropriateness criteria and guidelines for performance and interpretation of cardiac CT, can guide clinicians and managers in this effort. The field continues to move rapidly and is still in its relatively early years. Although cardiac CT is nothing more than a highly specialized form of chest CT, it is nothing less than a revolutionary breakthrough in cardiac imaging that will continue to influence the practice of cardiovascular medicine dramatically for years to come.

Bibliography

Abbara S, Arbab-Zadeh A, Callister TQ, et al. SCCT guidelines for performance of coronary computed tomographic angiography: a report of the Society of Cardiovascular Computed Tomography Guidelines Committee. *J Cardiovasc Comput Tomogr.* 2009;3:190-204.

Abbara S, Chow BJ, Pena AJ, et al. Assessment of left ventricular function with 16- and 64-slice multi-detector computed tomography. *Eur J Radiol.* 2008;67:481-486.

Abbara S, Soni AV, Cury RC. Evaluation of cardiac function and valves by multidetector row computed tomography. *Semin Roentgenol.* 2008;43:145-153.

Bamberg F, Abbara S, Schlett CL, et al. Predictors of image quality of coronary computed tomography in the acute care setting of patients with chest pain. *Eur J Radiol.* 2010;74:182-188.

Blankstein R, Bolen MA, Pale R, et al. Use of 100 kV versus 120 kV in cardiac dual source computed tomography: effect on radiation dose and image quality. *Int J Cardiovasc Imaging.* 2011;27:579-586.

Halliburton SS, Abbara S. Practical tips and tricks in cardiovascular computed tomography: patient preparation for optimization of cardiovascular CT data acquisition. *J Cardiovasc Comput Tomogr.* 2007;1:62-65.

Kröpil P, Rojas CA, Ghoshhajra B, et al. Prospectively ECG-triggered high-pitch spiral acquisition for cardiac CT angiography in routine clinical practice: initial results. *J Thorac Imaging.* 2012;27:194-201.

Lee AM, Engel LC, Shah B, et al. Coronary computed tomography angiography during arrhythmia: radiation dose reduction with prospectively ECG-triggered axial and retrospectively ECG-gated helical 128-slice dual-source CT. *J Cardiovasc Comput Tomogr.* 2012;6:172-183.

Shapiro MD, Pena AJ, Nichols JH, et al. Efficacy of pre-scan beta-blockade and impact of heart rate on image quality in patients undergoing coronary multidetector computed tomography angiography. *Eur J Radiol.* 2008;66:37-41.

Sheth T, Dodd JD, Hoffmann U, et al. Coronary stent assessability by 64 slice multi-detector computed tomography. *Catheter Cardiovasc Interv.* 2007;69:933-938.

Taylor CM, Blum A, Abbara S. Patient preparation and scanning techniques. *Radiol Clin North Am.* 2010;48:675-686.

Techasith T, Ghoshhajra BB, Truong QA, et al. The effect of heart rhythm on patient radiation dose with dual-source cardiac computed tomography. *J Cardiovasc Comput Tomogr.* 2011;5:255-263.

Weigold WG, Abbara S, Achenbach S, et al. Standardized medical terminology for cardiac computed tomography: a report of the Society of Cardiovascular Computed Tomography. *J Cardiovasc Comput Tomogr.* 2011;5:136-144.

CHAPTER 4

Cardiac Magnetic Resonance Imaging: Techniques and Protocols

François-Pierre Mongeon, Otávio Rizzi Coelho-Filho, and Raymond Y. Kwong

Cardiac magnetic resonance imaging (MRI) sequences are numerous, and possible imaging planes are infinite. Each sequence is designed to provide specific information about function, anatomy, or tissue characteristics. Each sequence also has its set of parameters that can be modified to improve image quality. Although any imaging plane can be obtained with MRI, standard orientations that follow echocardiographic planes are suitable for most examinations. The cardiac imaging specialist is therefore faced with the following challenges:

How do cardiac MRI sequences produce images, and what key parameters can be adjusted to optimize image quality?

How should imaging planes be prescribed?

How can sequences and imaging planes be combined to form comprehensive and efficient imaging protocols designed to answer clinical questions?

This chapter reviews the commonly used MRI techniques, describes the geometry of standard imaging planes, and outlines protocols tailored to common indications for cardiac MRI.

■ TECHNIQUES

Gating

Gating refers to the timing of events of the imaging sequence according to the cardiac or respiratory cycle. Synchronization of image acquisition to the electrocardiogram (ECG) is required because of cardiac motion. The quality of the signal depends on ECG electrode placement. Rearrangement of the electrodes can improve the signal. ECG gating is either prospective or retrospective. In prospective gating (or triggering), ECG events, often the R wave, trigger the events of the imaging sequence such as radiofrequency pulses or the start of a delay to image acquisition. In retrospective gating, data are acquired throughout the cardiac cycle, and images are reconstructed subsequently, based on the relationship of acquired data with ECG events. Retrospective gating is commonly used for cine imaging. The ECG signal may be distorted by the B_0 (static) magnetic field, by the B_1 magnetic field (the radiofrequency pulse), or by the magnetohydrodynamic effect. The *magnetohydrodynamic effect* refers to amplification of the T wave by the blood flow through the vessels. The use of vectorcardiography helps distinguish true ECG waves from

artifacts. Sequences using k-space data sharing and partial k-space acquisition, as well as sequences acquired within one R-R interval (single shot sequences), are less sensitive to the quality of ECG gating. Three techniques are used to compensate for respiratory motion. Breath holding is usually used when the acquisition fits within approximately 15 seconds, because most patients cannot suspend breathing for a longer period. If the patient is breathing freely, respiratory motion averaging can be used. Navigator-based techniques allow tracking of diaphragmatic motion and therefore data acquisition at the same phase of each respiratory cycle with simultaneous synchronization to the ECG. Real-time images, like the ones produced by echocardiography, can be obtained with MRI. In that case, image quality does not depend on gating, but spatial and temporal resolution are low.

Types of Sequences and Overview of T1 and T2 Weighting

Spoiled gradient echo and spin echo sequences are most commonly used to produce MRI images. Spoiled gradient echoes are generated by the controlled application of magnetic field gradients after a single radiofrequency pulse. *Spoiling* refers to destruction of residual transverse magnetization before application of the next radiofrequency pulse. Spin echoes are produced by a 90-degree radiofrequency pulse followed by single (conventional spin echo) or multiple (turbo spin echo) 180-degree refocusing pulses. The time between each 90-degree radiofrequency pulse is called the repetition time (TR), and the time delay between the radiofrequency pulse and the generation of an echo is called the echo time (TE). When the application of a radiofrequency pulse stops, the spins of the protons begin to return to their original state. This process has two components: the recovery of longitudinal magnetization and the loss of transverse magnetization. The recovery of longitudinal magnetization, or T1 relaxation, is an exponential process with a time constant, T1. Loss of transverse magnetization occurs because protons lose phase coherence. It is also an exponential process with a time constant, T2*. Loss of phase coherence occurs because of interaction with neighboring protons (spin-spin interaction, T2 relaxation) and because of inhomogeneities in the B_0 magnetic field. MRI uses differences in T1 and T2 relaxation to produce contrast between different soft tissues.

For spin echoes, TR and TE determine the weighting of the image. T1 weighting is obtained with a short TR and a short TE. T1-weighted spin echo images are used for anatomic imaging. Fat has a bright (high) signal, and fluid has a low signal intensity. In practice, a short TR corresponds to one R-R interval. T2 weighting is obtained with a long TR and a long TE. The 180-degree refocusing pulse ensures that the effects of field inhomogeneities are canceled and that loss of phase coherence depends only on spin-spin interactions. T2-weighted spin echo images are used for edema imaging because fluid has a high T2 signal. In practice, a long TR corresponds to two or three R-R intervals. For spoiled gradient echoes, TR, TE, and the flip angle determine the T1 or T2* weighting of the images. T1-weighted spoiled gradient echoes are obtained with a short TR, a short TE, and a flip angle of approximately 30 degrees. T2*-weighted spoiled gradient echoes are obtained with a long TR and TE. These images are sensitive to magnetic susceptibility effects and are therefore well suited to detect tissue iron.

Black-Blood Sequences

Morphologic Imaging

T1-weighted black-blood turbo spin echo sequences with a double inversion recovery preparation are often used for morphologic imaging. The double inversion preparation applies a nonselective inversion pulse to the whole volume to be imaged, followed by a second slice selective inversion pulse that restores signal in the slice of interest. The 90-degree pulse of the spin echo sequence is applied after a time delay, to allow the recovering signal of the blood to cross the zero line. This delay is called the inversion time (TI), and it also allows blood that has experienced only the first inversion pulse to fill the slice. In practice, the double inversion preparation is triggered by the R wave, and the spin echoes are produced 400 to 600 milliseconds later, which correspond to diastole. Turbo spin echo sequences acquire multiple lines of k-space after a single 90-degree pulse by repeating the 180-degree refocusing numerous times, called the echo train length. An echo train length of 15 to 20 echoes usually allows the acquisition of one or two slices in a single breath hold.

A common pitfall of double inversion recovery turbo spin echo imaging is loss of signal of the myocardium as a result of cardiac motion. Structures of interest may move out of the slice, where they do not experience the second inversion pulse. This situation is remedied by increasing the thickness of the slice selective pulse. Structures with a very short T1 time (e.g., fat) recover signal very fast and appear bright on T1 weighted images. Signal from fat can be suppressed by adding a third inversion pulse immediately before the spin echo sequence or by suppressing signal with the resonance frequency of fat molecules. Figure 4-1 shows an example of morphologic assessment of anomalous right upper pulmonary vein connection to the superior vena cava by using a T1-weighted black-blood turbo spin echo sequence (see Fig. 4-1, *A*) and a post-gadolinium contrast volume interpolated gradient echo sequence (see Fig. 4-1, *B*).

Edema Imaging

Lengthening of TR and TE produces black-blood images with T2 weighting. Water-bound protons have a longer T2 time. Thus, T2-weighted imaging is sensitive to the water content of the myocardium and, consequently, to the presence of myocardial edema. Fat saturation is usually applied in addition to blood suppression to increase the contrast between normal and edematous myocardium. Double inversion recovery T2-weighted black-blood imaging has been used to delineate the area at risk after myocardial infarction and to identify myocardial edema and inflammation in myocarditis (Fig. 4-2).

Bright-Blood Sequences

Gradient Echoes

Gradient echoes produce images in which blood appears white. They are mainly used for cine imaging depicting the contraction of the heart and the flow of blood during the cardiac cycle. Gradient echo sequences feature excitation pulses separated by a constant TR. Gradients are applied along each axis for slice selection, phase, and frequency encoding. Each excitation pulse tips the longitudinal magnetization in the transverse plane of a certain flip angle. Short TRs are used for fast imaging, which means that excitation pulses are delivered at small intervals. Little time exists for recovery of longitudinal magnetization between excitation pulses. The signal of the stationary tissue in the imaged slice is reduced as it becomes saturated. Blood that flows in the imaged slice has not been excited before and generates a high signal. This phenomenon is called inflow enhancement and provides contrast between blood and myocardium, as well as the blood enhancement in time of flight magnetic resonance angiography (MRA).

Balanced Steady-State Free Precession

The most commonly used bright-blood sequence is a modification of the gradient echo sequence called balanced steady-state free precession (bSSFP). A detailed review of bSSFP is beyond the scope of this chapter and can be found in dedicated publications such as by Scheffler et al. Briefly, if the flip angle, dephasing from T1 and T2 relaxation, and TR are kept constant, a steady state of magnetization will be reached after a few TRs. bSSFP relies on application of excitation pulses with flip angles of alternating polarity on a single magnetization vector that has reached a steady state. The repeated excitation therefore leads to oscillation of magnetization around the z-axis. The magnetization vectors at the beginning and at the end of each TR are identical because all gradients applied during a TR cancel each other. Loss of phase coherence across the field of view as a result of magnetic field inhomogeneity modifies the steady state. A patient-specific process called dynamic shimming may be required to keep the magnetic field homogenous and to allow the use of bSSFP at higher magnetic fields. Contrast in bSSFP sequences is composed of T1 and T2 contributions. T2 and T1 weighting is ideal for differentiation among blood, myocardium, and fat. bSSFP offers the highest

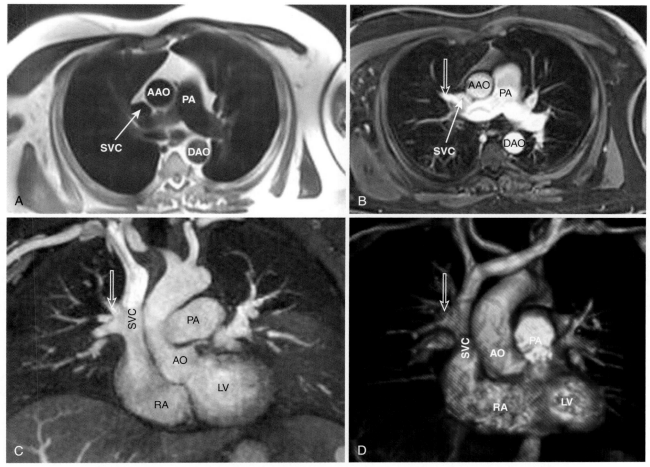

Figure 4-1 Morphologic assessment of anomalous right upper pulmonary veins connection. **A,** Abnormal shape of the superior vena cava (SVC, *white arrow*) on an axial single shot black-blood cardiovascular magnetic resonance image at the level of the pulmonary bifurcation. **B,** Immediate postgadolinium contrast volume interpolated gradient echo axial image for fast vascular anatomy assessment depicting the teardrop shape of the SVC *(white arrow)* where it is joined by a right upper pulmonary vein *(open arrow).* **C,** Reformatted maximum intensity projection magnetic resonance angiography. **D,** Three-dimensional volume rendering magnetic resonance angiography confirming the presence of multiple right upper pulmonary veins entering the SVC *(arrow).* *AAO,* Ascending aorta; *AO,* aorta; *DAO,* descending aorta; *LV,* left ventricle; *PA,* pulmonary artery; *RA,* right atrium.

signal-to-noise ratio for assessment of function and wall motion (Fig. 4-3).

Cine Imaging

Cine imaging sequences require short TR and are produced using turbo gradient echo sequences. Data are acquired at multiple time points throughout the cardiac cycle; each time point is called a (cardiac) phase. Data acquired during each phase fills a separate k-space bin corresponding to an image in a different phase. Images are then played sequentially as a movie. The more phases are acquired, the better is the temporal resolution. Turbo gradient echo sequences are repeated to acquire numerous lines of k-space per cardiac phase (a shot) during each R-R interval. These fast acquisitions are segmented. The acceleration factor is the number of lines of k-space acquired in each shot and is called the number of segments, the views per segment, or the turbo factor. Increasing the acceleration factor reduces the acquisition time, but it increases the temporal resolution.

Reducing the acceleration factor increases the scan time but also the number of phases and improves temporal resolution from a routine 45 milliseconds to 15 to 30 milliseconds. Temporal resolution is calculated as the product of TR times turbo factor (or number of views per segment). However, the apparent temporal resolution can be improved by interpolation of data between adjacent phases, a technique known as view sharing. The acceleration factor must be reduced if the heart rate increases because the number of lines of k-space that can be acquired within an R-R interval decreases. This is especially relevant during stress cardiac MRI examinations. Parallel imaging techniques can reduce the acquisition time by using information obtained from multiple channels on imaging coils. Adding parallel imaging to any imaging sequence reduces its signal-to-noise ratio. Cine gradient echo sequences are less susceptible to artifacts resulting from turbulent blood flow than is cine bSSFP. Thus, cine gradient echo sequences may be preferred for assessment of valve stenosis or regurgitation.

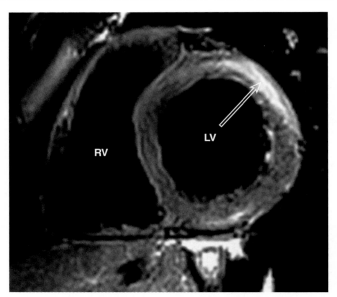

Figure 4-2 Double inversion recovery T2-weighted black-blood imaging in the midventricle short-axis view demonstrating near transmural myocardial edema in the anterolateral wall of the left ventricle (LV; *arrow*). *RV,* Right ventricle.

T2*-Weighted Imaging

T2*-weighted imaging can be obtained with gradient echo sequence and is used for measurement of myocardial iron content. Iron overload causes signal loss in affected tissues because iron deposits become magnetized in the scanner. These deposits induce local irregularities in the magnetic field that cause water protons around these deposits to lose phase coherence. This effect is concentration dependent. T2*-weighted images are obtained using a single breath-hold multi-echo technique. A single short-axis midventricular slice is acquired at eight TEs ranging between approximately 2 and 18 milliseconds with 2-millisecond increments. A region of interest (ROI) is then drawn in the interventricular septum to measure the signal intensity at each TE. Plotting the signal intensity against the TE produces an exponential decay curve. T2* is calculated from the equation $SI = Ke^{-TE/T2*}$ where SI is signal intensity and K is a constant. A myocardial T2* less than 20 milliseconds is abnormal and indicates probable iron overload, and a myocardial T2* less than 10 milliseconds indicates severe iron overload.

Phase Contrast Imaging

Phase contrast imaging allows quantification of blow flow velocities and flow rates. The phase is the angular position of a proton spin vector in relation to a frame

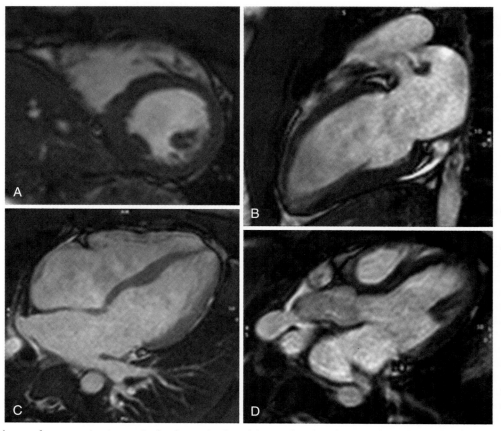

Figure 4-3 Steady-state free precession images in the short-axis plane (**A**), two-chamber plane (**B**), four-chamber plane (**C**), and three-chamber plane (**D**).

of reference. Spins moving in a magnetic field acquire a phase shift in comparison with stationary spins. The phase shift is proportional to the velocity of blood. Transverse magnetization can acquire a phase shift, and a phase contrast sequence begins with an excitation pulse to induce transverse magnetization. Then, bipolar gradients oriented in the direction of blood flow and with opposite dephasing and rephasing lobes are applied to each frame of the imaging slice. Repeating the measurement with an inverted bipolar gradient cancels the phase shifts of stationary tissues and those induced by the sequence. The phase shift, or difference, that remains after subtraction of the two measurements represents motion resulting from blood flow. Phase shift for each voxel is expressed in degrees and ranges from +180 to −180 degrees. A greater velocity results in a greater phase shift. Data from a phase contrast acquisition are displayed side by side in a magnitude image, which resembles a bright-blood image, and in a velocity image. The gray scale in the velocity image contains the velocity data for each voxel. The directions of black and white flows depend on the selected velocity encoding direction (head to foot, anterior to posterior, or left to right).

ROIs are usually drawn around the vessel of interest on the velocity images, but they should be cross-checked on magnitude images for appropriate anatomic orientation. Small ROIs are used for peak velocity measurement, and large ROIs are used for flow measurements. The instantaneous blood flow (cm^3/second) is obtained by multiplying the velocity (cm/second) of each voxel by the area (cm^2) for each phase of the cardiac cycle. Phase contrast acquisitions use a FLASH gradient echo sequence with retrospective gating. The acquisition is segmented, as for cine imaging, and can be done with breath holding or free breathing with multiple signal averages. Although breath-held acquisition are shorter, free breathing is usually preferred to avoid changes in intracardiac blood flows induced by the respiratory cycle. All measured velocities are averaged over a range of cardiac cycles. The temporal resolution can be calculated as follows: 2 × TR × views per segment. Each k-space line is sampled twice using the same TR, and the data from the two acquisitions are subtracted. The sequence can be optimized by using the shortest TR and TE possible, especially if the flow of interest is highly accelerated. Slice thickness is usually between 6 and 8 mm but can be reduced to 5 mm for small vessels. The operator must adequately set the velocity encoding (Venc) parameter, which is expressed in cm/second. The Venc should be set just above the anticipated peak velocity of the blood flow of interest. A Venc that is too high leads to a reduced signal-to-noise ratio. A Venc that is too low leads to aliasing. Aliasing is wrapping around of the velocity within a voxel. Correction for aliasing can be done manually or with specialized software, but it is usually best to repeat the acquisition with a higher Venc setting. Setting up the imaging plane is also operator dependent.

For flow measurement, the imaging plane should be perpendicular to the direction of flow (through-plane flow; Fig. 4-4). Velocity measurements can be made both in plane and through plane. An artery that appears ovoid usually indicates deviation from the optimal plane. Partial volume effect can occur if the pixel size exceeds one third of the vessel diameter. Spatial resolution must therefore be increased to image small vessels.

Contrast Enhancement

First-Pass Myocardial Perfusion

First-pass myocardial perfusion imaging follows a bolus of contrast agent as it travels through the coronary circulation. Perfusion imaging is complex, and the interested reader is referred to a detailed review by Gerber et al. With seven unpaired electrons, gadolinium is the most effective paramagnetic agent. Gadolinium chelates remain extravascular and extracellular and produce signal enhancement by shortening the T1 of adjacent protons. Thus, perfusion sequences are designed to have strong T1 contrast to allow normally perfused areas to display a high signal and hypoperfused or nonperfused areas to appear dark. T1 contrast is generated by a saturation pulse followed by an ultrafast gradient echo or bSSFP sequence. The saturation pulse eliminates any remaining magnetization from a previous pulse. Between three and five slices of the heart in views that cover most of the myocardium are acquired repeatedly every heart beat during the injection of a bolus of 0.05 to 1 mmol/kg of gadolinium chelate at 3 to 5 mL/second. Patients are asked to breath hold during the initial phase of the sequence and are allowed to take small breaths toward the end of the acquisition, which lasts 45 to 60 seconds. More slices can be acquired by using interleaved acquisitions and parallel imaging. Typical sequence parameters include a slice thickness of 5 to 10 mm and an in-plane spatial resolution of 1.5 to 3 mm. Gradient echo sequences are the most robust, especially at 3 Tesla, although SSFP sequences have a higher signal-to-noise ratio.

A common pitfall of first-pass perfusion imaging is the presence of a dark rim artifact. This artifact is a transient dark rim visible in the subendocardial layer that can mimic a hypoperfused area. Distinguishing features from a true perfusion defect are as follows: (1) the artifact normally lasts for a few heart beats, (2) it varies temporally as the contrast bolus passes through the left ventricle, and (3) signal intensity drops to less than the baseline level preceding the arrival of the contrast agent. Perfusion defects seen both under stress and at rest without infarcted areas by late gadolinium enhancement (LGE) should be interpreted as dark rim artifacts. The cause of the dark rim artifact remains unclear, but it may relate to a Gibbs ringing artifact in the phase encoding direction and to magnetic susceptibility associated with high gadolinium concentration in the bolus.

Late Gadolinium Enhancement

Gadolinium chelates are extravascular, extracellular contrast agents. Therefore, they concentrate in areas of extracellular matrix expansion. Myocardial extracellular matrix expansion can result from replacement fibrosis or from accumulation of abnormal substances, as occurs in infiltrative heart disease. Areas of fibrosis therefore have a shorter T1 because of the presence

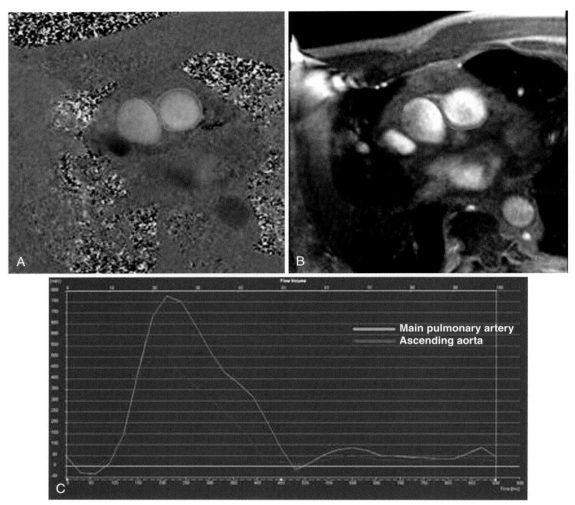

Figure 4-4 Hemodynamic assessment of a left-to-right shunt. **A,** Through-plane phase encoded cardiovascular magnetic resonance image of the ascending aorta (red contour) and the main pulmonary artery (green contour). The encoding velocity was 150 cm/second. **B,** Magnitude image corresponding to **A. C,** Graphic depiction of the systemic (aortic, red curve) cardiac output (Qs) and of the pulmonary (Qp, green curve). The Qp (159 mL/beat) is greater than the Qs (95 mL/beat) resulting from the left-to-right shunt caused by anomalous connection of the right upper pulmonary veins to the superior vena cava (Qp/Qs = 1.7).

of gadolinium (Fig. 4-5). Signal enhancement is optimal 10 to 15 minutes after the injection of 0.1 to 0.2 mmol/kg of gadolinium. LGE images are produced using a segmented fast gradient echo sequence with an inversion recovery preparation. The R wave triggers a 180-degree inversion before the pulse; then follows a user-defined delay, called the inversion time or TI, after which the image readout pulses are initiated. The image readout is aimed to happen at the time when the signal intensity time curve of the normal myocardium crosses the null point (normal myocardium is black). Because infarcted myocardium has a different (higher because of delayed washout) amount of gadolinium, its signal intensity time curve is different (faster T1 recovery) from that of normal myocardium, and the infarct will look bright. Image readout occurs in diastole to minimize cardiac motion. The k-space lines are acquired following excitation pulses with a small flip angle (20 to 30 degrees) to retain the differences in magnetization that result from the inversion pulse and TI. Because of continued washout of

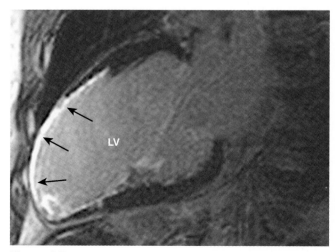

Figure 4-5 Late gadolinium enhancement sequence in a two-chamber view demonstrating a transmural infarction in the middle and distal anterior walls *(arrows)* corresponding to the proximal left anterior descending artery territory. *LV,* Left ventricle.

gadolinium, the optimal TI increases during acquisition of multiples slices and may have to be progressively increased by the operator. LGE sequences are prospectively gated with the inversion pulse applied every second R wave.

If the heart rate is greater than 100 beats/minute, the inversion pulse may need to be applied every third heart beat to allow sufficient recovery. If the heart rate is lower than 50 beats/minute, the inversion pulse can be applied every R wave. The TI can be selected based on experience and on the time since gadolinium injection. A Look-Locker (TI scout) sequence provides multiple images, each taken at a different TI to allow for fast selection of the TI that results in optimal nulling of the myocardium. The technique of phase sensitive inversion recovery produces LGE images using a nominal instead of a precise TI. This technique uses signal polarity (phase) to provide contrast between normal and fibrotic myocardium across a wide range of TI. LGE images of the whole heart are usually obtained in short-axis slices matching the position of the cine slices for ease of differentiating enhanced myocardium and blood pool. Sufficient time, usually 10 minutes, should be allowed for the blood pool signal to decrease after gadolinium injection.

Contrast-Enhanced Magnetic Resonance Angiography

MRA enhanced with gadolinium contrast is the main angiography technique used in cardiac MRI. The T1 shortening effect of gadolinium provides high signal intensity in the lumen of the vessels. Contrast depends on the data located in the center of k-space. Therefore, the center of k-space must be filled at peak vessel enhancement. Centric filling of the k-space is useful for MRA of the aorta. Contrast-enhanced MRA uses a three-dimensional (3-D) T1-weighted fast gradient echo sequence. The imaging plane of the 3-D slab must be optimized, depending on the structure to image. For example, a sagittal plane works well for the aorta, but a coronal plane is best for the pulmonary veins. MRA is usually performed using 0.2 mmol/kg of gadolinium, which is injected at a rate ranging between 2 and 3 mL/second. The injected bolus is tracked using a real-time sequence, and the MRA sequence is started when the contrast agent fills a structure of interest. This technique, called fluoroscopic triggering, must take into account the motion of the contrast agent during the acquisition as well as cardiac function. Alternatively, a timing bolus scan may be used. The patient is instructed to breath hold for the acquisition, which should be planned to be less than 20 seconds. A second phase can be acquired immediately and takes advantage of the recirculation of contrast material, especially in venous and late-enhancing structures.

A mask of background structure is acquired before MRA and can be subtracted for optimization of the vascular images. MRA images comprise a 3-D dataset that can be reconstructed and displayed in any plane using multiplanar reconstruction tools. A time resolved MRA depicts the transition of a bolus of contrast material step by step through the vascular structures. It is useful for delineation of complex vascular structures and collateral vessels. Figure 4-1, *C* and *D* provides examples of MRA images.

■ IMAGING PLANES

Conventional Planes

A cardiac MRI examination typically starts with fast localizing sequences obtained in three orthogonal planes: axial, coronal, and sagittal. These survey images allow rapid identification of thoracic structures for orientation and allow screening for extracardiac diseases. Straight axial, coronal, and sagittal images require little planning and can be of great help to delineate complex congenital heart disease, the pericardium, or masses with extracardiac extension.

Oblique Planes

Starting with a view of the heart from the axial localizer, a plane bisecting the left ventricular apex and the mitral valve produces a vertical long-axis pilot, which looks somewhat like a left ventricular two-chamber view. A plane bisecting the left ventricular apex and the mitral valve on the vertical long-axis pilot produces a horizontal long-axis pilot, which somewhat resembles a four-chamber view. A true short-axis view (see Fig. 4-3, *A*) is obtained by placing a plane perpendicular to both the vertical and horizontal long-axis pilots at the midventricular level. In the short-axis view, a plane bisecting the center of the left ventricle and the right ventricular acute margin (angle between anterior and diaphragmatic right ventricular walls) defines the four-chamber view (see Fig. 4-3, *C*). On the four-chamber view, a plane bisecting the left ventricular apex and the mitral valve center defines the left ventricular two-chamber view (see Fig. 4-3, *B*). The stack of short-axis views covering the whole ventricle that is used to measure ventricular size and function can then be planned from the four- and two-chamber views.

Care should be taken to start the coverage in the atria and to extend it beyond the apex, to avoid missing parts of the ventricles. Scrolling through a cine loop to ensure that coverage is sufficient at end-diastole, when the ventricles are the largest, is also helpful. The short-axis slices typically have a thickness of 6 to 8 mm, with or without a 2-mm interslice gap. The three-chamber or left ventricular outflow tract view is obtained by placing a plane parallel to the left ventricular outflow on the short-axis view and parallel to the interventricular septum on the four-chamber view. A coronal oblique left ventricular outflow tract view is obtained by placing a plane perpendicular to the aortic valve and parallel to the aorta on the three-chamber view. The plane of the right ventricular two-chamber view bisects the tricuspid valve and the right ventricular apex on the four-chamber view and is perpendicular to the right ventricular outflow tract on the short-axis view. Finally, the right ventricular outflow tract plane bisects the pulmonary bifurcation on an axial view and is therefore parallel to the main pulmonary artery. Trabeculations can help distinguish the right ventricle from the right atrium at the basal inflow level. Volumes are derived from tracings using the modified Simpson rule. Ejection fraction is calculated as follows: (end-diastolic volume – end-systolic volume)/end-diastolic volume × 100%.

■ PROTOCOLS

Published protocols for conducting cardiac MRI studies, such as that by Kramer et al, provide a useful framework for most clinical indications.

Ventricular Size and Function

Quantitative assessment of ventricular size and function is an integral part of every cardiac MRI study. Multiple short-axis slices parallel to the mitral valve and covering the whole heart are usually acquired. Slice thickness should be 6 to 8 mm, with a 0- to 4-mm interslice gap in an adult. Image analysis is performed using commercially available software. Epicardial and endocardial contours are traced at end-diastole and at end-systole. Watching the slice in movie format while tracing or correcting the contours can be very helpful, for example, to help differentiate the atria from the ventricles near the valve planes. Papillary muscles may or may not be included in the left ventricular cavity, as long as the same convention is used through time to allow serial comparison. The aortic valve forms the superior boundary of the left ventricle. At the base of the heart, some investigators have used the convention that slices were considered to be within the left ventricle if the blood volume was surrounded by 50% or more of ventricular myocardium. The pulmonary valve forms the superior boundary of the right ventricle. The left ventricular mass is obtained as follows: 1.05 × (epicardial volume – endocardial volume). Normal values for ventricular volumes, mass, and ejection fraction have been published. Images of the ventricles in long-axis planes are also obtained to assess valves and wall motion. Atrial volumes can be measured in a similar way.

Ischemic Heart Disease

Acute Myocardial Infarction

In addition to ventricular size and function, T2-weighted imaging is performed to assess myocardial edema (see Fig. 4-2). First-pass perfusion can be used to detect areas of microvascular obstruction. However, the main focus of the examination is delayed enhancement imaging to detect and quantify the extent of the infarct. The area of late gadolinium hyperenhancement (LGE) can overestimate the infarct size in the first 2 weeks after acute myocardial infarction because of the presence of myocardial edema. Microvascular obstruction typically appears as dark area completely surrounded by bright LGE, without any adjacent layer of normal myocardium (Fig. 4-6). Investigators have shown that within 12 hours of primary percutaneous intervention for acute myocardial infarction, the LGE volume provides the strongest association with systolic dysfunction 6 months later.

Chronic Ischemic Heart Disease and Viability

The assessment of ischemic cardiomyopathy relies on quantification of function and LGE. In dysfunctional

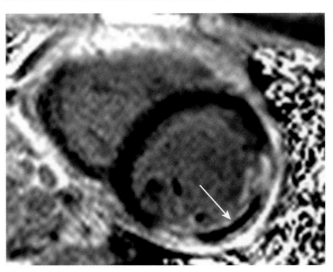

Figure 4-6 Microvascular obstruction depicted as a dark area *(arrow)* completely surrounded by late gadolinium enhancement, without any adjacent layer of normal myocardium. This late enhancement image was produced using the phase sensitive inversion recovery technique.

myocardial segments, the transmural extent of the LGE is associated with the likelihood of functional recovery after revascularization. Therefore, a viability study requires only ventricular function sequences and LGE imaging. A viability study can be combined with ischemia assessment using dobutamine or vasodilator stress.

Vasodilator Stress Perfusion Study

Vasodilator stress myocardial perfusion MRI can be used for diagnosis and for prognostic evaluation of patients with suspected coronary artery disease. Both dipyridamole and adenosine can be used for vasodilator stress myocardial perfusion MRI. Adenosine is a direct agonist of the alpha$_2$-receptor of blood vessels, whereas dipyridamole is a prodrug. Both drugs induce maximal hyperemia in the normal myocardium. When a significant coronary stenosis is present, the magnitude of perfusion increase with a vasodilator is compromised compared with the normal myocardium, which appears as a perfusion defect. Side effects of adenosine or dipyridamole are similar and include flushing, chest discomfort, headache, atrioventricular block, bronchospasm, and cerebral hypoperfusion. Contraindications to their use include severe conduction abnormalities, chronic obstructive pulmonary disease, asthma, and severe carotid stenosis. Patients must abstain from caffeinated beverages for 24 hours before the examination. MRI-compatible monitoring equipment and personnel trained in advanced cardiac life support must be available. ECGs should be recorded before and after the stress test. Because the effects of dipyridamole last for approximately 30 minutes, rest perfusion images are acquired first. Then, function images are obtained while a dose of 0.56 mg/kg of dipyridamole is injected over 4 minutes. A supplemental dose of 0.28 mg/kg of dipyridamole injected over 2 minutes can be added. Stress perfusion images are acquired 10 minutes after the beginning of the dipyridamole infusion. Aminophylline can be used as needed to reverse the effects of dipyridamole. LGE imaging is performed approximately 10 minutes after the last injection of gadolinium contrast. Adenosine is infused at 0.14 mg/kg/minutes for 3 to 6 minutes (total dose, 0.48 to 0.84 mg/kg), and stress perfusion images are acquired during the final portion of the adenosine infusion. Two intravenous lines are needed for gadolinium contrast to be infused at the same time as adenosine. Adenosine is stopped when the contrast infusion is completed. Function images are acquired followed by stress perfusion images and LGE images.

Perfusion defects persist for a very short time after injection of contrast. Therefore, temporal resolution should be maximized. The operator should also allow sufficient clearance of gadolinium between stress and rest perfusion images. In clinical practice, interpretation of perfusion images is largely qualitative. The absence of scar with uniform enhancement at stress and at rest indicates the absence of ischemia. The presence of LGE and a matching defect on stress and rest images indicate a fixed perfusion defect without ischemia. A stress-induced perfusion defect that normalizes at rest without matching LGE is positive for ischemia. Finally, an area of stress-induced perfusion defect that is greater than the matching area of LGE indicates periinfarct ischemia.

Dobutamine Stress Study

The increase in contractility provoked by dobutamine raises myocardial oxygen demand and leads to ischemia in areas supplied by stenotic coronary arteries. Severe side effects include myocardial infarction, ventricular fibrillation, and sustained ventricular tachycardia. Intravenous beta-blockers can reverse the effects of dobutamine. Monitoring requirements are the same as for a vasodilator stress study. For that reason, beta-blockers must be omitted for 24 hours before a dobutamine stress cardiac MRI. Dobutamine is administered intravenously at 3-minute stages at doses of 10, 20, 30, and 40 mcg/kg/minute and stopped at the dose when at least 85% of age-predicted maximal heart rate is reached. Supplemental atropine (0.25 mg; maximal dose, 1 mg) can be used to help reach and maintain the target heart rate. A dobutamine stress test should be stopped at the patient's request or if new wall motion abnormalities, chest discomfort, dyspnea, decrease in systolic blood pressure of more than 40 mm Hg, arterial hypertension (>240/120 mm Hg), severe arrhythmias, or other serious adverse effects occur. A set of MRI cine images in three short-axis planes (apical, middle, basal) and four-chamber, three-chamber, and two-chamber views (see Fig. 4-3) are acquired at rest and at each dose of dobutamine. Side-by-side display is helpful for image analysis. Wall motion abnormalities that appear during stress indicate ischemia. Wall motion abnormalities observed at rest that improve during low-dose stress but deteriorate during peak stress also indicate inducible myocardial ischemia. Wall motion abnormalities at rest without deterioration at peak stress are considered negative. As the heart rate increases and the R-R interval shortens, the operator must decrease the views per segment. Perfusion imaging is also performed using dobutamine. Rest first-pass perfusion is acquired before the infusion

of dobutamine, and stress perfusion is acquired at the 20 mcg/kg/minute dose of dobutamine. LGE imaging can be performed after completion of the stress study.

Diseases of the Thoracic Aorta

Cardiac MRI allows evaluation of the heart and aorta in a single study. Ventricular size and function should be measured, especially if the patient has aortic valve regurgitation. Short-axis views of the aortic valve and aortic root are also helpful. T1-weighted black-blood imaging in the axial plane through the aorta should be done to look for dissection or intramural hematoma. Cine imaging in an oblique sagittal plane parallel to the aorta is useful for visualization of the aortic arch. Contrast-enhanced MRA of the aorta is the single most important technique in the evaluation of the aorta. Measurements should be taken in true short-axis view of the lumen at each level using multiplanar reconstruction. Phase contrast acquisitions at the level of the aortic valve and at the level of the sinotubular junction in the ascending aorta allow quantification of aortic regurgitant volume and fraction. In the presence of aortic valve stenosis, phase contrast acquisition in the left ventricular outflow tract is used to measure the forward flow. Analysis of the flow profile using phase contrast imaging in the descending aorta can display holodiastolic reversal in severe aortic valve regurgitation or diastolic persistence of flow with slow upstroke in coarctation of the aorta.

Anomalous Coronary Arteries

MRI can display the course and assess patency of the proximal coronary arteries. Ventricular function should be assessed for potential wall motion abnormalities. Transaxial cine or black-blood imaging at the level of the aortic root and coronary artery ostia can show the origin of the coronary arteries and help plan the coverage of the coronary MRA. Coronary MRA is often performed using a free-breathing 3-D navigator-gated sequence. The trigger delay and acquisition window are adjusted for imaging during diastole, which is identified on a high-resolution cine loop in the four-chamber view. One should look for the phase of diastole with minimal motion of the right atrioventricular groove where the right coronary artery courses. Coronary MRA sequences are available with or without contrast enhancement. LGE imaging can be added to the examination, especially if myocardial infarction has occurred or to rule out myocardial fibrosis in a patient with syncope. In the young adult with chest pain, combining a vasodilator or dobutamine stress with an evaluation of the proximal coronary arteries allows an extensive workup of the major causes of chest pain in a single examination. In this case, one may need to replace the rest first-pass perfusion imaging with coronary artery imaging with enhanced coronary MRA.

Pulmonary Vein Evaluation

The goal of pulmonary vein evaluation is threefold: (1) to delineate anatomy before the ablation procedure, (2) to identify pulmonary stenosis after such procedure, and

(3) to identify abnormal pulmonary venous connections. All can be obtained from contrast-enhanced MRA of the pulmonary veins, which is best prescribed in the coronal plane. Assessing ventricular function and anatomy is usually advisable as well, because atrial fibrillation can be associated with structural heart disease. LGE imaging is optional. Normal variations in pulmonary veins anatomy are common and should be recognized.

Nonischemic Cardiomyopathy and Myocarditis

Ventricular size and function are essential parts of this examination. The focus of the rest of the study is tissue characterization to identify myocardial inflammation, infiltration, or fibrosis. T2-weighted black-blood imaging in the ventricular short-axis view is performed before contrast administration. Hypersignal on T2-weighted imaging indicates myocardial edema. A T2* sequence may also be helpful in the cardiomyopathy protocol to evaluate for iron overload. In the particular setting of suspected myocarditis, a T1-weighted turbo (or fast) spin echo sequence can be acquired before and immediately after contrast administration to assess early enhancement with gadolinium. Early gadolinium enhancement indicates hyperemia and capillary leak and is regarded as a sign of myocardial inflammation. The examination is completed with LGE imaging. The combination of hypersignal on T2-weighted imaging, early gadolinium enhancement, and subepicardial or midwall areas of LGE is consistent with myocarditis. Please also see Chapter 26 for more details.

The pattern of left ventricular LGE can reveal the cause of nonischemic cardiomyopathy. For example, a midwall linear area of fibrosis suggests dilated cardiomyopathy. Abnormal gadolinium kinetics and global subendocardial LGE suggest cardiac amyloidosis. If cardiac amyloidosis is suspected on the basis of thick left ventricular walls and diastolic dysfunction, LGE imaging should be started within 5 minutes of contrast administration, and difficulty in setting the appropriate TI can be expected. Stress cardiac MRI can be combined with an examination for cardiomyopathy to exclude ischemic heart disease confidently. For hypertrophic cardiomyopathy, end-diastolic wall thickness from cine bSSFP images should be reported. The peak velocity in the left ventricular outflow tract is measured with phase contrast imaging. Dephasing jets consistent with obstruction resulting from systolic anterior motion of the anterior mitral valve leaflet are seen on cine bSSFP.

Arrhythmogenic Right Ventricular Dysplasia or Cardiomyopathy

Diagnostic criteria by cardiac MRI for arrhythmogenic right ventricular dysplasia or cardiomyopathy include regional right ventricular akinesia or dyskinesia or dyssynchronous right ventricular contraction and either right ventricular dilatation or dysfunction. This information can be obtained from analysis of ventricular function and volume from a short-axis stack of cine images. Cine imaging in the axial plane to cover the right ventricle is also helpful to assess right ventricular wall motion. Wall motion abnormalities are more convincing when they are seen in orthogonal planes. Fatty infiltration of the myocardium by MRI is not among the consensus diagnostic criteria. Fibrofatty infiltration appears as areas of bright signal on T1-weighted black-blood imaging that is usually performed in the axial plane across the right ventricle. The exact same slice location is used to repeat the images with application of fat saturation. Bright signal within the myocardium that disappears after fat saturation represents fatty infiltration. The diagnostic yield of such a finding for arrhythmogenic right ventricular dysplasia is controversial. The fibrotic component of the infiltration can be recognized using LGE imaging. Performing LGE imaging of the right ventricle is more challenging, however, and the optimal TI may not be the same as for the left ventricle. The presence of LGE is not yet a diagnostic finding in arrhythmogenic right ventricular cardiomyopathy.

Congenital Heart Disease

Congenital heart defects range from simple lesions such an atrial septal defect to complex malformations such as transposition of the great arteries. In the adult population, many patients will have undergone surgical repair or palliation, and, therefore, knowledge of baseline and postsurgical anatomy is essential to plan cardiac MRI. Indications for cardiac MRI in adults with congenital heart defects have been published. Simple defects can be imaged using standard imaging planes. In complex heart defects, a useful approach is to start the examination with transaxial cine or black-blood imaging through the chest and upper abdomen. This allows anatomic orientation and helps to plan other imaging planes, including ventricular short-axis views for quantification of volumes and function. Coronal imaging is also helpful to image the outflow tracts. Gadolinium-enhanced MRA provides valuable information in congenital heart disease. LGE may or may not be part of the examination. Fibrosis is often found around patches for closure of septal defects and at the insertion of conduits. Patients with pulmonary hypertension may also have LGE at the septal insertions of the right ventricle. Flow measurements play a major role in the evaluation of congenital heart disease. At the minimum, stroke volumes are measured in the ascending aorta and in the main pulmonary artery for calculation of the Qp/Qs ratio.

Valvular Heart Disease

Indications for valve surgery include consideration of ventricular size and function. Therefore, quantification of ventricular volumes and ejection fraction by cardiac MRI will likely play an increasing role in decision making for valve repair or replacement. Patients with valvular prosthesis can safely undergo cardiac MRI at 1.5 or 3 Tesla. Valve anatomy is studied in cine imaging. Cine gradient echo may depict turbulent jets better than bSSFP (Fig. 4-7). The anatomy of the aortic valve is studied in three-chamber and left ventricular outflow

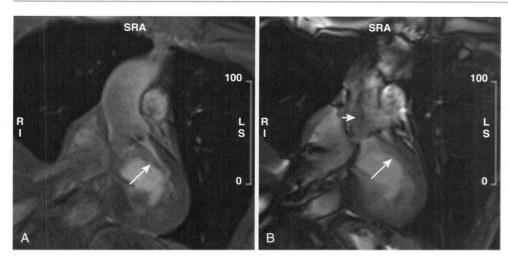

Figure 4-7 Comparison of gradient echo (**A**) and balanced steady-state free precession (bSSFP, **B**) sequences in the left ventricular outflow view for depicting the jet of aortic regurgitation (*arrow*). Note the better delineation of the jet on the gradient echo image (**A**) and the artifacts caused by turbulent flow in the ascending aorta on bSSFP (**B**, *arrowhead*).

tract views (see Fig. 4-7). A short-axis view through the aortic root may depict the anatomy of the leaflet and allow identification of a bicuspid valve. The mitral valve anatomy is demonstrated in long-axis views of the left ventricle. Potential prolapse of mitral valve leaflet scallops should be assessed only by using a stack of slices through the mitral valve in the three-chamber orientation, because other planes may lead to false-positive results. Basal short-axis four-chamber views and right ventricular two-chamber views best show the tricuspid valve. The pulmonary valve is well seen in the right ventricular outflow tract plane and sometimes in the straight sagittal orientation. High-resolution slices for the purpose of planimetry are oriented parallel to the valve plane. Such images require that the operator decrease the views per segment.

Phase contrast MRI in the plane perpendicular to the valve is used for quantification of transvalvular flows. Choosing the appropriate Venc (just above the anticipated peak velocity) in the presence of stenosis and regurgitation is of critical importance because each jet has a different velocity. The best approach is to take measurements at the level where the jet is less turbulent and to consider separate acquisitions with Venc selection targeted to a specific jet. Eccentric jets are difficult to quantify directly. Calculation of regurgitant volumes and fraction should be performed with multiple methods and compared for internal consistency. Peak velocities for valve stenosis may be underestimated by phase contrast MRI. MRA of the pulmonary arteries or of the aorta may demonstrate secondary findings associated with valve disease such as aneurysm or coarctation.

Pericardial Diseases

Ventricular volumes and function should be routinely obtained. Pericardial thickness is measured on T1-weighted black-blood imaging in the axial and short-axis planes (Fig. 4-8). Thus, stacks covering the ventricles in both planes should be obtained. Obtaining black-blood images in T2-weighted spin echo is worthwhile to detect pericardial edema, which suggests active pericarditis. T1- and T2-weighted images also

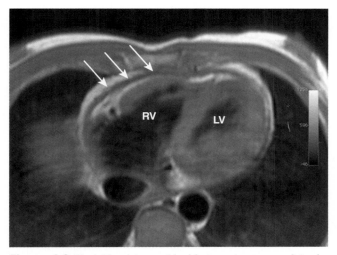

Figure 4-8 Black-blood image (double inversion recovery) in the axial plane demonstrating thickening of the anterior pericardium (*arrows*). *LV*, Left ventricle; *RV*, right ventricle.

characterize pericardial fluid. A transudate appears dark on both sequences. Pericardial adhesions may be seen in cine imaging acquired in the same orientations. The effect of adhesions can be made more conspicuous by using myocardial tagging. Tagging is produced by application of pulses that saturate the magnetization of water protons in a line or grip pattern immediately before systolic contraction. Because they are saturated, protons in these lines produce no signal when the cine sequence starts. The protons move synchronously with the deformation of the myocardium that occurs when the heart contracts. The tag lines should be applied perpendicular to the portion of pericardium that is investigated. The tag lines normally break at the interface between the epicardium and the pericardium, as the two layers of pericardium freely slide along each other. If the heart and the adjacent structures move synchronously, without any breaking and slippage of the tag lines, then pericardial adhesions are likely present (adhesions disallow free motion or sliding of the adjacent pericardial layers). Tagging is applied to selected slices in axial and short-axis planes. Free-breathing real-time imaging is used in ventricular short-axis planes to show the typical septal bounce indicating ventricular interdependence in constrictive physiology. The examination is usually completed with LGE imaging. Pericardial LGE indicates pericardial fibrosis, or inflammation if concomitant hypersignal is present on T2-weighted images.

Masses

Cardiac MRI offers an array of tools to characterize cardiac masses. The location of the mass and its plane of motion should first be identified using cine imaging. Then, the mass is imaged sequentially in T1-weighted turbo spin echo with and without fat saturation, T2-weighted turbo fast spin echo, first-pass perfusion, and LGE imaging. The behavior of the mass with each modality offers clues on its tissue composition and suggests a differential diagnosis. The definitive diagnosis can be obtained only by biopsy. Invasion of the myocardium or adjacent structures should be described because it has therapeutic implications.

■ CONCLUSION

This chapter reviews the most commonly used sequences in cardiac MRI, along with the parameters that affect image quality and the geometry of standardized imaging planes. Finally, these tools are organized in comprehensive protocols that can efficiently answer common clinical questions.

Bibliography

Aletras AH, Tilak GS, Natanzon A, et al. Retrospective determination of the area at risk for reperfused acute myocardial infarction with T2-weighted cardiac magnetic resonance imaging: histopathological and displacement encoding with stimulated echoes (dense) functional validations. *Circulation*. 2006;113:1865-1870.

Alfakih K, Plein S, Thiele H, Jones T, Ridgway JP, Sivananthan MU. Normal human left and right ventricular dimensions for MRI as assessed by turbo gradient echo and steady-state free precession imaging sequences. *J Magn Reson Imaging*. 2003;17:323-329.

Anderson LJ, Holden S, Davis B, et al. Cardiovascular T2-star (T2*) magnetic resonance for the early diagnosis of myocardial iron overload. *Eur Heart J*. 2001;22:2171-2179.

Baumgartner H, Bonhoeffer P, De Groot NM, et al. ESC guidelines for the management of grown-up congenital heart disease (new version 2010). *Eur Heart J*. 2010;31:2915-2957.

Cawley PJ, Maki JH, Otto CM. Cardiovascular magnetic resonance imaging for valvular heart disease: technique and validation. *Circulation*. 2009;119: 468-478.

Friedrich MG, Sechtem U, Schulz-Menger J, et al. Cardiovascular magnetic resonance in myocarditis: a JACC white paper. *J Am Coll Cardiol*. 2009;53:1475-1487.

Gerber BL, Raman SV, Nayak K, et al. Myocardial first-pass perfusion cardiovascular magnetic resonance: history, theory, and current state of the art. *J Cardiovasc Magn Reson*. 2008;10:18.

Karamitsos TD, Francis JM, Myerson S, Selvanayagam JB, Neubauer S. The role of cardiovascular magnetic resonance imaging in heart failure. *J Am Coll Cardiol*. 2009;54:1407-1424.

Kato R, Lickfett L, Meininger G, et al. Pulmonary vein anatomy in patients undergoing catheter ablation of atrial fibrillation: lessons learned by use of magnetic resonance imaging. *Circulation*. 2003;107:2004-2010.

Kim RJ, Shah DJ, Judd RM. How we perform delayed enhancement imaging. *J Cardiovasc Magn Reson*. 2003;5:505-514.

Kim RJ, Wu E, Rafael A, et al. The use of contrast-enhanced magnetic resonance imaging to identify reversible myocardial dysfunction. *N Engl J Med*. 2000;343:1445-1453.

Klem I, Heitner JF, Shah DJ, et al. Improved detection of coronary artery disease by stress perfusion cardiovascular magnetic resonance with the use of delayed enhancement infarction imaging. *J Am Coll Cardiol*. 2006;47:1630-1638.

Kramer CM, Barkhausen J, Flamm SD, Kim RJ, Nagel E. Standardized cardiovascular magnetic resonance imaging (CMR) protocols, Society for Cardiovascular Magnetic Resonance: Board of Trustees Task Force on Standardized Protocols. *J Cardiovasc Magn Reson*. 2008;10:35.

Larose E, Rodes-Cabau J, Pibarot P, et al. Predicting late myocardial recovery and outcomes in the early hours of ST-segment elevation myocardial infarction traditional measures compared with microvascular obstruction, salvaged myocardium, and necrosis characteristics by cardiovascular magnetic resonance. *J Am Coll Cardiol*. 2010;55:2459-2469.

Lotz J, Meier C, Leppert A, Galanski M. Cardiovascular flow measurement with phase-contrast MR imaging: basic facts and implementation. *Radiographics*. 2002;22:651-671.

Maceira AM, Joshi J, Prasad SK, et al. Cardiovascular magnetic resonance in cardiac amyloidosis. *Circulation*. 2005;111:186-193.

Marcus FI, McKenna WJ, Sherrill D, et al. Diagnosis of arrhythmogenic right ventricular cardiomyopathy/dysplasia: proposed modification of the task force criteria. *Circulation*. 2010;121:1533-1541.

McCrohan JA, Moon JC, Prasad SK, et al. Differentiation of heart failure related to dilated cardiomyopathy and coronary artery disease using gadolinium-enhanced cardiovascular magnetic resonance. *Circulation*. 2003;108:54-59.

Nagel E, Lehmkuhl HB, Bocksch W, et al. Noninvasive diagnosis of ischemia-induced wall motion abnormalities with the use of high-dose dobutamine stress MRI: comparison with dobutamine stress echocardiography. *Circulation*. 1999;99:763-770.

Ridgway JP. Cardiovascular magnetic resonance physics for clinicians: part I. *J Cardiovasc Magn Reson*. 2010;12:71.

Sakuma H, Ichikawa Y, Suzawa N, et al. Assessment of coronary arteries with total study time of less than 30 minutes by using whole-heart coronary MR angiography. *Radiology*. 2005;237:316-321.

Salton CJ, Chuang ML, O'Donnell CJ, et al. Gender differences and normal left ventricular anatomy in an adult population free of hypertension: a cardiovascular magnetic resonance study of the Framingham Heart Study offspring cohort. *J Am Coll Cardiol*. 2002;39:1055-1060.

Scheffler K, Lehnhardt S. Principles and applications of balanced SSFP techniques. *Eur Radiol*. 2003;13:2409-2418.

Steel K, Broderick R, Gandla V, et al. Complementary prognostic values of stress myocardial perfusion and late gadolinium enhancement imaging by cardiac magnetic resonance in patients with known or suspected coronary artery disease. *Circulation*. 2009;120:1390-1400.

Westwood M, Anderson LJ, Firmin DN, et al. A single breath-hold multiecho T2* cardiovascular magnetic resonance technique for diagnosis of myocardial iron overload. *J Magn Reson Imaging*. 2003;18:33-39.

CHAPTER **5**

Radionuclide Imaging (Cardiac)

Sharmila Dorbala and Angela S. Koh

▪ PRINCIPLES OF NUCLEAR CARDIAC IMAGING AND PERFORMING SINGLE-PHOTON EMISSION COMPUTED TOMOGRAPHY AND POSITRON EMISSION TOMOGRAPHY STUDIES

Cardiac imaging using nuclear techniques plays a critical role in the diagnostic and therapeutic decision-making process in management of patients with coronary artery disease (CAD). Nuclear cardiac imaging involves the administration of a radionuclide agent (radiolabeled isotope) that is that is bound to a radiopharmaceutical. The chemically unstable isotope decays and emits energy in the form of gamma radiation or charged particles that are detected by the scanner to form an image of the heart. Cardiac single-photon emission computed tomography (SPECT) imaging is widely used in clinical practice. Cardiac positron emission tomography (PET) imaging, previously used primarily in research, is gaining wider acceptance as an important clinical diagnostic tool. Inherently, PET has higher spatial, temporal, and contrast resolution than SPECT and great sensitivity for quantifying physiologic processes in the heart. One of the essential requirements for producing high-quality SPECT or PET images is understanding the basis of nuclear cardiac imaging techniques so that imaging data can be acquired with consistency and reported with accuracy. This chapter focuses on the techniques, and Chapter 29 focuses on the clinical applications of nuclear cardiac imaging.

Scanners and Advances in Technology

Four types of scanners are most commonly used in nuclear cardiac imaging:

1. Conventional SPECT scanners, based on the Anger gamma camera
2. Newer scanners with solid-state and semiconductor detectors
3. Conventional PET scanners
4. Hybrid SPECT or PET scanners combined with computed tomography (CT) scanners

A conventional SPECT system or a scintillation scanner (Anger gamma camera) consists of the following elements: a collimator, with lead septa to localize the source of the emitted gamma rays; a sodium iodide crystal, which scintillates when gamma rays interact with it and produces visible light; photomultiplier tubes, which amplify the emitted light signal and convert energy from visible light into an electric signal; pulse height analyzers and positioning circuitry to localize the signal; and an analog or digital computer designed to determine the location and energy of a photon striking the crystal. Patients are imaged in the supine or prone position by using a step and shoot acquisition mode, in which the scanner starts imaging in the right anterior oblique position, moves to the next position (3 degrees) and takes another projection image, and so on until a 180-degree rotation is completed (left posterior oblique) and tomographic images are calculated. The images obtained are processed using postprocessing filters and reconstructed into three cardiac views (short-axis, vertical long-axis, and horizontal long-axis views). The spatial resolution of the SPECT system is approximately 9 to 12 mm.

Advances in scintillation scanner technology have resulted in the development of solid-state detectors using cesium iodide coupled to photodiodes or novel semiconductor-based detectors using cadmium zinc telluride (CZT). The latest of these newer technologies is the CZT detector, which directly converts gamma radiation to an electronic pulse and thereby eliminates the need for a scintillating crystal and photomultiplier tubes. Some of the detector systems are open and L-shaped or C-shaped with an array of detector elements, as opposed to the circular gantry (Fig. 5-1). Some of the newer scanners also offer imaging with the heart at the focal point of the detector array (cardiofocal imaging), thereby improving image resolution. Because the heart volume is imaged simultaneously, rather than in a step and shoot mode, dynamic images can be acquired in a tomographic mode. With some of these systems, imaging is performed with the patient in an upright (sitting) position in a chair, rather than in the supine position in bed. In addition, high-speed imaging is possible such that acquisition of the stress and rest data takes only 4 and 2 minutes, respectively, and the entire stress-rest SPECT protocol can be completed within 30 minutes.

Myocardial count rates and image quality are higher than in conventional SPECT systems. Studies are currently under way to determine whether this improvement in image quality may translate into more accurate assessment of patients with CAD. A multicenter trial by Maddahi et al validated a half-time acquisition protocol and demonstrated that the rapid gated rest-stress upright system acquired perfusion and functional information comparable to that obtained with the conventional system. Clinical validation of the D-SPECT system (Spectrum Dynamics, Haifa, Israel) was performed by

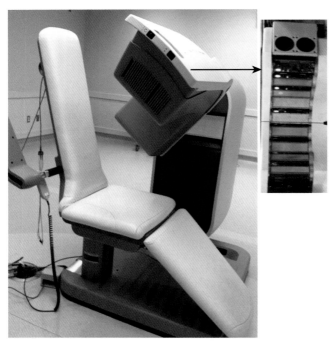

Figure 5-1 An example of a newer-generation dedicated ultrafast acquisition scanner containing multiple (cadmium zinc telluride) detector columns *(inset on the right)* arranged in an L-shape configuration *(left)* that simultaneously image the heart. Each detector column uses a tungsten parallel-hole collimator that fans back and forth and hence allows the object of interest to be viewed from hundreds to thousands of different "viewing" angles. These scanners have the potential for a five- to tenfold increase in count sensitivity with gain in resolution. The patient is also able to sit in an upright position during image acquisition.

comparing the newer camera with a conventional SPECT camera. The newer high-speed camera produced images with higher counts and excellent linear correlation between the extent of perfusion abnormality at stress and rest compared with the conventional system. Taking into account the more linear relationship between myocardial uptake and blood flow at high flow rates of thallium-201 (Tl-201) than technetium-99m (Tc-99m), a fast sequential stress Tl-201 and rest Tc-99m sestamibi dual isotope protocol was accomplished within 20 minutes with image quality and dosimetry similar to those of a rest-stress Tc-99m protocol. Furthermore, CZT detectors have higher spatial and energy resolution when compared with sodium iodide systems. This superiority in energy resolution allows discrimination of photons of different energies and hence provides the opportunity to perform simultaneous acquisition of Tl-201 and Tc-99m. A comparison of simultaneous dual tracer rest Tl-201 and stress Tc-99m sestamibi on a solid-state D-SPECT scanner with a conventional SPECT camera by Ben-Haim et al showed that fast and high-quality imaging is feasible and diagnostically comparable to conventional SPECT and separate rest Tl-201 and stress Tc-99m acquisition.

PET scanners have higher spatial (4 to 6 mm) and temporal resolution, and they detect paired photons of 511 keV energy produced by annihilation of a positron. A positron is an unstable particle with a positive charge that can travel some distance (positron range) before it interacts with an electron and is annihilated, thus releasing two 511-keV photons at 180-degrees angle from each other. Photons striking diametrically opposing detectors within a short time interval (coincidence interval of approximately 20 nsec) are considered true coincidences and are imaged by the scanner. Higher-energy positrons have a longer positron range, which can limit image resolution (Table 5-1). PET imaging is performed in a two-dimensional (2-D) mode with septa or in a three-dimensional (3-D) mode without septa. Because the 3-D mode offers higher count sensitivity, including more scatter and randoms, it requires more efficient crystals with shorter dead time and high

Table 5-1   Single-Photon Emission Computed Tomography and Positron Emission Tomography Radionuclide Characteristics

SPECT Radionuclides	Production	Decay	Emission (keV)	Half-life	Role
Thallium-201	Cyclotron	Electron capture	68–80 (x-ray); 167 (10%; gamma ray)	73 hr	Flow tracer
Iodine-123	Cyclotron	Electron capture	159 (gamma ray)	13 hr	Metabolic tracer
Technetium-99m	Generator	Internal transition	140 (gamma ray)	6 hr	Flow tracer

PET Radionuclides	Production		Positron Energy (keV)	Half-life	Role
Oxygen-15	Cyclotron		735	122 sec	Flow tracer
Nitrogen-13	Cyclotron		491	9.96 min	Flow tracer
Carbon-11	Cyclotron		385	20.3 min	Flow tracer
Fluorine-18	Cyclotron		248	110 min	Metabolic tracer
Rubidium-82	Generator		1523	1.3 min	Flow tracer

PET, Positron emission tomography; *SPECT,* single-photon emission computed tomography.

computing capabilities. PET detectors are made up of bismuth germanate (BGO), lutetium oxyorthosilicate (LSO), gadolinium oxyorthosilicate (GSO), or lutetium yttrium orthosilicate (LYSO). BGO has limited energy and timing resolution compared with LSO, LYSO, and GSO crystals. Hence, BGO is more commonly used in 2-D PET systems, which have lower count sensitivity, and LSO, LYSO, and GSO are more commonly used in 3-D PET systems.

Most PET scanners have built-in attenuation correction. Attenuation from soft tissues is estimated using a transmission scan based on a radionuclide source (germanium-68, gallium-68, or cesium-137) or a CT image. Typically, the transmission and emission scans are obtained sequentially while the patient is kept in the same position. The CT in PET-CT systems allows for a rapid transmission scan (10 seconds versus 3 to 6 minutes for a radionuclide transmission scan), that permits improved laboratory throughput and reduced patient motion. Time of flight PET technology may improve the noise quality in the images by better delineating the origin of the photons, but it is not yet widely used in cardiac applications.

Software Advances

Software techniques have evolved to improve image quality, shorten image acquisition time and thus improve patient comfort and minimize motion, and reduce radiation dose to the patient. The major advances in software and reconstruction techniques include resolution recovery, noise reduction, wide beam reconstruction, and improved scatter and attenuation correction algorithms. For example, resolution recovery methods are used to improve spatial resolution and reduce noise. By using recovery algorithms from a database of known detectors and collimator characteristics, resolution recovery mathematically corrects for resolution degradation that occurs inherently with parallel-hole collimators and increasing distance from the scintillation crystal.

Commercial manufacturers have developed different versions of resolution recovery algorithms that include not only improved resolution but also reduced image noise. For noise reduction, filters are applied either to the original projection or after reconstruction. In addition, these newer algorithms also include Compton scatter and attenuation correction techniques. Using these newer software techniques, SPECT myocardial perfusion imaging (MPI) may be performed using half the conventional scan time with preserved or even improved image quality. In several studies, half-time processing (Astonish [Philips, San Jose, Calif.]) has been associated with superior image quality and interpretative certainty compared with full-time ordered subset expectation maximization (OSEM). This has the advantage of reducing scan acquisition time and, potentially, patient radiation exposure with half-dose full-time wide beam reconstruction.

Current methods for normal limits-based quantification of myocardial perfusion on SPECT use ungated normal limits and derive perfusion information from summed images. However, image blurring caused by motion may have a significant effect on quantification. Initial evaluation of a novel motion-frozen display and quantification method for gated MPI that potentially eliminates the problem of image blurring by cardiac motion has been performed. In this proposed method, gated perfusion images are analyzed after cardiac motion tracking and 3-D motion correction. These motion-frozen images visually resemble end-diastolic frames, but they contain counts from all cardiac cycles and hence are less noisy and of higher resolution than summed images. Initial results with this method show an improvement in image quality and good diagnostic performance.

Practical Points

- The direct conversion of photons into electrical signal without the need for photomultiplier tubes and diodes results in improved efficiency and a smaller footprint of cardiac-specific scanners. The disadvantage of the newer cardiac-specific SPECT systems is that some of them do not allow for noncardiac nuclear medicine scanning, thus limiting their utility in combined practices.
- The open detector configuration in some of the newer scanners can be helpful in patients with claustrophobia.
- Upright imaging reduces attenuation from diaphragm and interference from subdiaphragmatic activity. However, imaging with the patient in the sitting position may not be feasible, particularly in hospitalized patients with comorbidities.
- Attenuation may affect different regions of the heart in the upright position compared with the supine position. For instance, in female patients, breast tissue attenuation affects the anterior or lateral walls in the supine position, and it may affect the apex and the inferior wall with upright imaging.
- Because of the high sensitivity of the newer systems, low-dose imaging with longer scan durations (8 to 10 minutes) is feasible. This imaging is still faster compared with conventional scanners with sodium iodide crystals. This approach may reduce the radiation dose to the patient significantly and decrease the risk of patient motion.
- With the newer systems, the heart volume is imaged simultaneously, rather than in a step and shoot mode. This technique permits dynamic tomographic imaging, which enables noninvasive quantification of myocardial blood flow using SPECT.
- Two photons are required for coincidence detection; hence, if one of them is attenuated or scattered, the scanner will ignore the event as a random event. Therefore, PET imaging is more susceptible to attenuation, and only attenuation-corrected PET images can be used in clinical interpretation.
- PET tracers with higher-energy positrons have a longer positron range and a somewhat lower spatial resolution.
- Advances in software reconstruction algorithms (resolution recovery, noise reduction, and scatter correction algorithms) allow for improved image quality, faster image acquisition, and lower radiation dose to

the patients. The advantage of the software advances is that they can be used with conventional scanners to reduce dose and improve image quality and may be more economical than purchasing a dedicated cardiac scanner for low-dose imaging (e.g., in practices with conventional scanners for general nuclear medicine imaging).

Radiotracers

The typical clinically radiotracers used in nuclear cardiac imaging can be characterized broadly as tracers to study myocardial blood flow (perfusion tracers) and tracers to study metabolic processes in the heart (see Table 5-1).

Single-Photon Emission Computed Tomography Radiotracers

For SPECT MPI, Tc-99m compounds are frequently used as radiotracers. Tc-99m (the m indicates that it is a metastable nuclear isomer of Tc-99) is produced from beta decay of molybdenum-99 (half-life of 66 hours), through a molybdenum-99–Tc-99m generator. Generators are devices that allow separation of a radionuclide from a long-lived parent. This allows for the continuous production of Tc-99m, the daughter radionuclide, inside the generator at a location remote from a nuclear reactor. Tc-99m emits 140-keV gamma rays and has a half-life of 6 hours. Tc-99m enters the cells passively through its lipophilic properties. Once it enters the myocyte, Tc-99m binds to the mitochondria as a free cationic complex and redistributes minimally. For Tc-99m sestamibi, as opposed to Tc-99m tetrofosmin, hepatobiliary uptake is high, with minimal redistribution.

Tl-201 is similar to potassium (K^+) and enters the myocytes through the sodium-K^+ adenosine triphosphatase pump. Tl-201 is produced by a cyclotron, emits low-energy mercury x-rays at 69 to 83 keV, and has a half-life of 73 hours. Once Tl-201 enters the cell proportional to myocardial blood flow, constant redistribution across the cell membrane reflects myocardial viability.

Iodine I-123 (I-123) beta-methyl-iodophenyl-pentadecanoic acid (BMIPP) is a tracer used to image fatty acid metabolism with SPECT. I-123 BMIPP emits 159 keV gamma rays and has a half-life of 13 hours. BMIPP is a methyl branched-chain fatty acid that does not readily undergo beta oxidation. This fatty acid tracer is trapped by normal myocardium. Thus, imaging fatty acid metabolism with BMIPP permits identification of regions of myocardial ischemia that have reduced fatty acid uptake, which manifests as a defect on these images.

Positron Emission Tomography Radiotracers

Rubidium-82 (Rb-82) and nitrogen-13 (N-13) ammonia are clinically used PET perfusion tracers, whereas oxygen-15 (O-15) water is a research perfusion tracer. Rb-82 is the most commonly used PET perfusion tracer, with a half-life of 76 seconds, and is produced by a strontium-83 generator. The strontium generator has a half-life of 23 days and is replaced every 4 to 6 weeks. Rb-82 is similar to K^+ and is taken up by the myocytes in relation to myocardial blood flow with a first-pass extraction fraction of approximately 65%. Because of kinetics similar to those of K^+ and Tl-201, delayed retention of Rb-82 may provide information about myocardial viability.

N-13 ammonia is produced by a cyclotron and has a physical half-life of 9.96 minutes. Therefore, an on-site cyclotron is necessary for its use. N-13 ammonia diffuses freely across the cell membranes and becomes incorporated into glutamine in the myocardium by the enzyme glutamine synthetase. The uptake of N-13 ammonia is related to the capillary blood flow and to the myocardial extraction characteristics. N-13 ammonia has a high extraction fraction of approximately 85%.

O-15 water is not approved by the U.S. Food and Drug Administration (FDA) and is primarily a research radiotracer. It is a freely diffusible radiotracer produced by a cyclotron and has a short half-life of 2.1 minutes. The uptake of O-15 water is linearly related to myocardial blood flow even at high flow rates.

Fluorine-18 (F-18) fluorodeoxyglucose (FDG) is a glucose analogue used to study myocardial glucose metabolism and to assess myocardial viability. F-18 FDG is a cyclotron-produced radiotracer with a half-life of 109 minutes. Uptake of F-18 FDG is through the glut-4 receptors. Once F-18 FDG enters the myocyte, it is converted by glucose-6-phosphate into FDG-6-phosphate, which is not metabolized any further and remains trapped in the myocyte. F-18 FDG uptake is exquisitely dependent on myocardial substrate use. The uptake of F-18 FDG is high when plasma glucose and insulin levels are high, and uptake is low when plasma free fatty acid levels are high.

Another F-18 PET perfusion tracer (F-18 flurpiridaz) is currently under development. This tracer is produced by a cyclotron and has a half-life of 109 minutes. It targets the mitochondria and shows rapid and high myocardial uptake with better myocardial extraction fraction than technetium compounds.

Practical Points

TECHNETIUM-99M VERSUS THALLIUM-201

The higher energy of Tc-99m gamma rays and the shorter half-life translate into higher image resolution and lower radiation dose to patients when compared with Tl-201. With Tl-201, the low-energy mercury x-rays make them more susceptible to scattering, attenuation, and limited gated images. In addition, the longer physical half-life of Tl-201 (half-life, 73-hours) limits the ability to administer higher doses and hence results in lower image quality. However, Tl-201 has a high first-pass extraction (approximately 85%) compared with Tc-99m agents (approximately 65%). Therefore, Tl-201 images can provide a better measure of hyperemic myocardial blood flow and may be more sensitive than Tc-99m images for the detection of milder degrees of stenosis. This property has been used, and newer protocols using Tl-201 for stress and Tc-99m agents for rest have been developed for some of the newer higher-sensitivity cardiac SPECT scanners. Although the first-pass extraction of Tc-99m agents is lower than that of Tl-201, the shorter half-life of Tc-99m allows for the use of a higher radiotracer dose that emits higher-energy gamma rays (less prone to attenuation) and results in better image quality compared with Tl-201.

TECHNETIUM-99M AGENTS

Because of the high hepatobiliary uptake of Tc-99m sestamibi, one must wait 45 to 60 minutes for optimal myocardial images and good clearance of hepatic uptake. The more rapid liver clearance of tetrofosmin compared with sestamibi significantly improves the ratios of cardiac to digestive activity, especially after exercise or at rest, and images can be obtained sooner after injection (10 to 15 minutes). Moreover, although tetrofosmin is reconstituted with Tc-99m, it can be allowed to stand at room temperature, unlike sestamibi, which requires boiling. This property, in addition to more rapid liver clearance and earlier image acquisition after tetrofosmin injection, is useful for performing studies in patients with acute chest pain, with higher patient throughput and image quality comparable to that with sestamibi.

POSITRON EMISSION TOMOGRAPHY RADIOTRACERS

The main advantage of Rb-82 is the ability to perform PET MPI without an on-site cyclotron. However, the necessary strontium-83 generator is very expensive, and this factor should be considered, especially if patient volumes are limited. The ultrashort half-life of Rb-82 of 76 seconds requires that the generator be directly connected to the intravenous line of the patient so that dose can be delivered directly to the patient during PET imaging. Repeat imaging is uncomplicated, and preintervention and postintervention studies are simple to perform without a time lag. The short physical half-life of N-13 ammonia of just less than 10 minutes makes an on-site cyclotron necessary for its use. N-13 ammonia produces better-quality perfusion images with high signal-to-noise ratio, low background, and low liver activity. At high flow rates (>3 mL/g/minute), N-13 ammonia may result in some underestimation of myocardial blood flow. Because O-15 water is freely diffusible and metabolically inert, it is an ideal perfusion agent and does not underestimate flow even at high flow rates. However, its freely diffusible state can lead to poor image contrast resolution and requires correction of blood pool activity or myocardial activity with a separate scan to improve signal-to-noise ratio. F-18 flurpiridaz, the investigational PET perfusion tracer, would be suitable for exercise stress imaging because of its half-life of 109 minutes. Also because of its long half-life, this radiotracer can be transported to remote (but still accessible) locations and does not need an on-site cyclotron or a generator. The lower-energy positron to F-18 compared with Rb-82 and N-13 ammonia results in sharper images related to shorter positron range. For viability imaging, myocardial F-18 FDG uptake is imaged (Fig. 5-2, *I*). Myocardial uptake of F-18 FDG highly depends on the substrate milieu. Therefore, good patient preparation is paramount to obtaining interpretable diagnostic images (Tables 5-2 and 5-3; see Fig. 5-3) and may be time-consuming and difficult to implement without protocols in place. For more details, readers are referred to the excellent review on this topic by Machac et al.

In addition, F-18 FDG PET can be used to image cardiac sarcoid (see Fig. 5-2, *J*). F-18 FDG PET is emerging as a promising diagnostic modality in identifying cardiac involvement of sarcoidosis. In these studies, localized uptake of F-18 FDG is a hallmark of active inflammatory change and potentially may also prove to be a useful indicator of response to steroid therapy (see Chapter 29 for more information).

The higher energy of PET radiotracers compared with SPECT radiotracers can result in greater penetration through the subject and can thereby lower the radiation dose to the patient. However, the radiation burden to the staff may be higher because more gamma rays are emitted from the patient and may reach the staff. The shorter the half-life of the radiotracer, the faster the protocols and lower the radiation dose to the patient will be. Extremely short half-life radiotracers such as O-15–labeled water (and sometimes Rb-82) are challenging to use for exercise stress testing because of decay of the radiotracer before the patient can be transferred from the treadmill to the scanner. Therefore, pharmacologic stress testing is preferable with short half-life radiotracers, and exercise or pharmacologic stress testing can be performed with longer half-life radiotracers. The short half-life radiotracers have a significant advantage in that rest and stress imaging can be performed using equal doses of radiotracer injection. In addition, if the dose has inadvertently infiltrated subcutaneously, rather than being injected intravenously, another scan can be obtained immediately after reinjection of another dose (rest imaging with repeat stress imaging is determined based on the half-life of the stress agent). Finally, for short half-life radiotracers produced by a cyclotron, the clinical schedule must be closely coupled with the cyclotron production schedule, thus making it less suitable for high-volume imaging. High-volume imaging using PET MPI is best performed with generator-produced radiotracers such as Rb-82 or with unit dose tracers such as the novel F-18 flurpiridaz (when it is approved by the FDA).

How to Decide Which Radioisotope to Use

This decision is based on a balance of several factors:
1. The type of stress protocol
2. The clinical question: ischemia assessment, viability assessment, assessment of ischemic memory
3. The availability for routine clinical use
4. The physical property of the radioisotope
5. Image quality

The decision to use SPECT or PET can be based on a simple algorithm (Fig. 5-3). Exercise is the preferred modality for stress imaging. Hence, any patient able to exercise is scheduled for an exercise MPI study (SPECT study for normal weight and N-13 ammonia PET when available, for obese individuals). When resources are not constrained and both SPECT and PET imaging techniques are available, PET is preferred for all pharmacologic studies. For SPECT imaging, Tc-99m agents are the most widely used; less than 10% of laboratories use Tl-201. Tc-99m sestamibi and Tc-99m tetrofosmin appear to be equally efficient, except for the differences mentioned earlier. Tl-201 has superior extraction characteristics and can be used to improve the test sensitivity for detection of ischemia, particularly with the

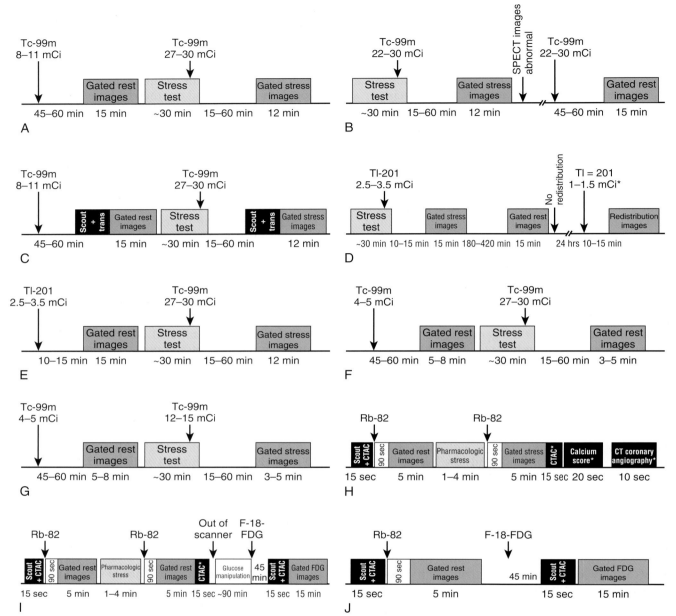

Figure 5-2 Imaging protocols for single-photon emission computed tomography (SPECT) and positron emission tomography (PET). Protocols using technetium-99m (Tc-99m) or thallium-201 (Tl-201) myocardial perfusion imaging (MPI), as well as fluorine-18 fluorodeoxyglucose (FDG) PET, are shown. **A** to **G**, various SPECT protocols. **H**, Conventional PET MPI protocol using rubidium-82 (Rb-82). Patients are imaged supine with arms raised above their shoulders. A scout scan is a simple topographic image of the body obtained to ensure appropriate patient positioning. A scout image is obtained using a low-energy computed tomography (CT) scan (10 mA, 120 keV), with the upper border defined by the tracheal bifurcation and the lower border defined by the lower margin of the heart. A transmission scan obtained by CT to provide anatomically specific density maps of the thorax is used to correct PET emission data for photon attenuation (CT attenuation correction; CTAC). The dose of radiotracer for Rb-82 is 40 to 60 mCi and 15 to 25 mCi for two-dimensional (2-D) and three-dimensional (3-D) modes, respectively. Stress testing using pharmacologic and exercise stress is followed by radiotracer injection. Image acquisition in the list mode is preferred whenever feasible. The images are acquired (as gated or static images) or reconstructed (when acquired as a list mode file) with a prescan delay of 70 to 90 seconds for Rb-82. If longer circulation time is anticipated, a higher value of pre-scan delay is used. *Optional CTAC, calcium score, or CT coronary angiography. For nitrogen-13 (N-13) ammonia studies, the dose of radiotracer is 20 to 30 mCi for 2-D imaging (15 to 25 mCi for 3-D), with a prescan delay of 180 to 240 seconds. A minimum of 50 minutes should elapse between the first and second injection of N-13 ammonia (to allow for decay of the first injection). **I**, PET viability protocol with F-18-FDG in conjunction with resting MPI or stress MPI. Following rest or stress MPI, glucose manipulation is performed (outside the gantry; see text), and F-18-FDG is injected. Hence, scout and CTAC images are obtained again, followed by gated FDG images. **J**, FDG PET protocol for cardiac sarcoid. This protocol requires special dietary preparation with a low-carbohydrate, high-fat diet (with or without intravenous heparin to promote lipolysis). This dietary preparation allows for suppression or minimization of glucose use by normal myocytes, and areas of FDG uptake are considered abnormal. Perfusion imaging is also performed in conjunction with FDG images, with PET perfusion tracers such as Rb-82 or N-13 ammonia. (Data from Yamagishi H, Shirai N, Takagi M, et al. Identification of cardiac sarcoidosis with ^{13}N-NH[3]/^{18}F-FDG PET. *J Nucl Med.* 2003;44:1030-1036.)

Table 5-2   Guidelines for Performing Fluorine-18 Fluorodeoxyglucose Cardiac Positron Emission Tomography

Procedure	Technique
Fast patient	6-12 hr
Load oral glucose	If fasting BG <~250 mg/dL (13.9 mmol/L), give 25-100 g glucose orally; then monitor BG based on Table 5-3 If fasting BG >~250 mg/dL, notify physician
Inject FDG	After monitoring BG (see Table 5-3), when BG is ~100-140 mg/dL (5.55-7.77 mmol/L), inject FDG intravenously
Begin PET imaging	Start PET imaging ~90 min after FDG injection

Adapted with permission from Machac J, Bacharach SL, Bateman TM, et al. Positron emission tomography myocardial perfusion and glucose metabolism imaging. *J Nucl Cardiol.* 2006;13:e121-e151.
BG, Blood glucose, *FDG,* fluorine-18 fluorodeoxyglucose; *PET,* positron emission tomography.

Table 5-3   Guidelines for Blood Glucose Maintenance After Oral Glucose Administration for Optimal Fluorodeoxyglucose Cardiac Uptake*

Blood Glucose 45 to 60 Min After Administration	Possible Restorative Measure (Intravenous)
130-140 mg/dL (7.22-7.78 mmol/L)	1 unit regular insulin
140-160 mg/dL (7.78-8.89 mmol/L)	2 units regular insulin
160-180 mg/dL (8.89-10 mmol/L)	3 units regular insulin
180-200 mg/dL (10-11.11 mmol/L)	5 units regular insulin
>200 mg/dL (>11.11 mmol/L)	Notify physician

Adapted with permission from Machac J, Bacharach SL, Bateman TM, et al. Positron emission tomography myocardial perfusion and glucose metabolism imaging. *J Nucl Cardiol.* 2006;13:e121-e151.
*The aim is to achieve a blood glucose concentration of approximately 100 to 140 mg/dL (5.55 to 7.77 mmol/L) at the time of fluorine-18 fluorodeoxyglucose injection.

high-sensitivity scanners and improved image quality. Moreover, Tl-201 has less hepatic uptake and can occasionally be used in patients with excessive subdiaphragmatic activity from Tc-99m tracers that cannot be resolved with delayed imaging, feeding, or prone imaging. When the clinical question involves assessment of myocardial viability when PET is not available, Tl-201 perfusion imaging with delayed imaging can be performed.

Imaging of ischemic memory is being explored with I-123 BMIPP. This technique enables identification of ischemic episodes approximately 24 hours before rest imaging with I-123 BMIPP and may play a role in imaging of patients with acute chest pain and a nondiagnostic electrocardiogram (ECG).

When to Consider Positron Emission Tomography Myocardial Perfusion Imaging

PET offers several advantages compared with SPECT (Box 5-1). PET yields higher-resolution images than

SPECT. The unique opportunity to measure peak stress left ventricular ejection fraction (LVEF) during PET is also an advantage over current SPECT protocols, which acquire poststress LVEF. LVEF reserve (peak stress minus rest LVEF) has been shown to be an important diagnostic tool for identifying multivessel disease, and a low LVEF reserve appears to have adverse prognostic implications. Images are acquired simultaneously in multiple projections that allow quantification of absolute blood flow at rest, and peak stress is a distinct advantage of PET. Because conventional SPECT and PET techniques rely on the concept of flow heterogeneity and compare relative uptake of radiotracer within the myocardium, they may potentially underdiagnose multivessel disease.

If all segments of the myocardium are ischemic to similar degrees, a situation known as balanced ischemia can result. In PET, perfusion tracers such as Rb-82, N-13 ammonia, and oxygen-15 water allow for absolute quantification of myocardial blood flow in which resting and peak stress myocardial blood flow is measured. This approach may be useful for detecting the presence of multivessel CAD. In addition, absolute quantification of PET tracer uptake permits the detection of abnormal flow reserve in preclinical states before the development of significant epicardial coronary stenoses in which abnormal microvascular or endothelial function causes vascular dysfunction. Quantitative blood flow estimation can allow the study of progression or regression of atherosclerosis and appears to add incremental prognostic value to relative perfusion imaging. The indications and clinical applications for PET MPI and quantitative PET MPI are discussed in Chapter 29.

How to Choose Among Perfusion Imaging Protocols

The choice of imaging protocol depends on the following:
1. The clinical question
2. Considerations for the appropriate radiation dose for each patient
3. The availability of radiopharmaceutical agents
4. The logistics for patients and laboratory personnel
5. The throughput of the laboratory

Single-Photon Emission Computed Tomography Myocardial Perfusion Imaging

Conventional protocols for SPECT acquisition studies using Anger camera technology and filtered back projection or OSEM (iterative) reconstruction are shown in Figure 5-2, *A* to *E*. The advantages and disadvantages of each of the protocols are listed in Table 5-4. The reader is also referred to the American Society of Nuclear Cardiology (ASNC) imaging guidelines for nuclear cardiology procedures, available in the article by Machac et al, for detailed protocols and image acquisition parameters.

The most commonly used SPECT MPI protocol is a single-day, low-dose rest study followed by a high-dose stress Tc-99m study, acquired as a gated study and reconstructed using filtered back projection or OSEM reconstruction. The images are acquired using standard parameters, as listed in the ASNC guidelines (Table 5-5).

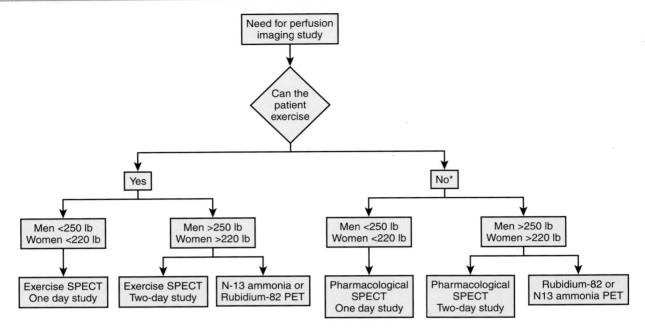

Figure 5-3 Algorithm for selection of an appropriate myocardial perfusion study (single-photon emission computed tomography [SPECT] versus positron emission tomography [PET]). Asterisk, Pharmacologic PET preferred when available; N-13, nitrogen-13.

BOX 5-1   Advantages and Disadvantages of PET over SPECT

Advantages
Higher spatial and temporal resolution
Accurate and depth-independent attenuation correction
Lower radiation dose
Faster protocols and laboratory throughput
Peak stress left ventricular ejection fraction
Quantitative myocardial blood flow assessment
Assessment of myocardial viability

Disadvantages
High cost
Lack of wide availability
Difficulty of exercise stress
Need for cyclotron or rubidium generator
Less expertise

Protocols for newer scanners are not yet well defined, but laboratories with newer CZT scanners may elect to use lower-dose imaging (see Fig. 5-2, *F*), rather than faster imaging with the usual dose of radiotracer (see Fig. 5-2, *G*).

For viability assessment, at sites using SPECT technology, a rest-redistribution Tl-201 study and a dual isotope (Tc-99m stress, Tl-201 rest) study acquired as gated images are commonly used. When PET is available, perfusion and viability imaging can be performed using FDG PET. Typical protocols for assessment of myocardial viability include myocardial perfusion assessment using gated SPECT or PET (preferred) and imaging myocardial glucose metabolism using F-18 FDG. Assessment of myocardial viability is combined with assessment of ischemia, unless stress testing is contraindicated (critical CAD or hemodynamically unstable patient) or ischemia evaluation is deemed not necessary and a decision is made to proceed with revascularization of critical coronary stenoses pending viability assessment.

Gated Myocardial Perfusion Imaging
ECG-gated SPECT is an accurate and reproducible technique used to measure LVEF, volumes, and regional wall motion. At each step of a conventional Anger scanner, several images (8 to 16 images) are acquired in relation to the surface ECG (Fig. 5-4). The newer SPECT scanners and PET scanner allow for list mode image acquisition in which image frames are acquired in relation to the ECG, as well as a time signal (see Fig. 5-4). The list mode files can be unlisted into a static or a gated image file. Gating with a higher frame rate improves temporal resolution for assessment of regional wall motion, and the overall LVEF may be comparable or slightly higher. The gated images are reconstructed using parameters similar to those used for the static images, and they are reviewed using commercial software packages for computation of LVEF and volumes. *In patients who have irregular heart rates, gated information may be inaccurate, and acceptance windows can be specified to reject cycle lengths that do not fall within the predetermined R-R interval range.*

Cardiac Positron Emission Tomography
The most commonly used PET MPI protocol is a resting study followed by a vasodilator stress Rb-82 study acquired as gated or dynamic images, in list mode when available (see Fig. 5-2, *H*), with CT- or radionuclide-based attenuation correction. Cardiac PET imaging has three main steps: a localizer scan to locate the heart position, a transmission scan for attenuation correction, and

Table 5-4   Advantages and Disadvantages of Various Single-Photon Emission Computed Tomography Acquisition Protocols*

Protocol	Advantages	Disadvantages
Technetium-Based Protocols		
Single-day rest-stress	1-day protocol	Suboptimal contrast between stress defect and rest
	Enhanced stress image quality	Long procedure time (~3-4 hr)
	Well-validated quantitative programs	
2-day stress-rest	Ideal protocol for image quality	Long procedure time (2 days)
	Improved defect and reversibility detection (no shine through of rest radiotracer activity)	
	If stress test result normal, rest test can be safely avoided, with resultant time and radiation savings	
Thallium-Based Protocols		
Single-day stress-rest with or without reinjection-rest-redistribution Tl-201	Potential to improve the assessment of myocardial ischemia and viability of patients with apparent irreversible defects	Rapid peak of myocardial concentration within 5 min of Tl-201 injection (rapid redistribution means that imaging must be done quickly and scanner must be readily available)
		Higher radiation dose to the patient
Single-Day Dual Isotope Thallium-201 and Technetium-99m		
Tl-201 at rest and Tc-99m after stress	Reduced waiting time between rest and stress image acquisition	Higher radiation dose to the patient
	Rest Tl-201 study can be reimaged after a 4-hr or 24-hr delay for viability assessment	Differences in defect resolution and photon scatter may exist when comparing two different radiotracers
	Can be used during Tc-99m shortages	Images may demonstrate apparent transient ischemic dilatation from inherent resolution differences between Tl-201 and Tc-99m

*Single-day, single-isotope, protocols with low-dose stress followed by high-dose rest are not commonly used. Images are inherently limited because of count-poor stress images.
Tc-99m, Technetium-99m; *Tl-201*, thallium-201.

an emission scan for rest and peak stress myocardial perfusion images, respectively. In certain patients, the gated CT scan can be used for quantification of coronary calcium score or a CT angiogram (CTA) immediately after myocardial perfusion, with hybrid PET-CT scanners and high–temporal resolution CT devices (at least 6-slice CT for calcium score and 64-slice CT for CTA). When both perfusion PET and CTA are required, performing the coronary CTA after the PET scan avoids interference of beta-blockers (used for heart rate control during CTA) with the chronotropic and hyperemic responses during pharmacologic stress.

Radionuclide Angiography

First-Pass Imaging
In first-pass imaging, high–temporal resolution sequential (or list mode) images of the central circulation are obtained as the radioactive tracer is administered intravenously. Conventionally, first-pass images have been acquired as planar images in either the anterior or left anterior oblique (LAO) projection. The radiotracer must be administered as a tight bolus in a small volume for an accurate first-pass study. The images depict the transit of the radioactivity through the heart's chambers with a

sufficient temporal resolution to permit measurement of right and left ventricular function. First-pass imaging had been used to assess for shunts and to evaluate for right ventricular ejection fraction and LVEF.

Multigated Acquisition
A second method of assessing ventricular performance is gated radionuclide ventriculography. This study has several names: gated equilibrium study, gated cardiac blood pool study, equilibrium radionuclide angiography, radionuclide ventriculography, and multigated acquisition study (MUGA). Gated radionuclide angiography is an imaging technique that images the intravascular blood pool. Tc-99m is the most commonly used radioisotope for MUGA scans.

PROCEDURE
The patient's blood is drawn, and red blood cells (RBCs) are labeled with Tc-99m pertechnetate, with the use of a reducing agent (stannous ion) that helps facilitate RBC binding to Tc-99m. The in vitro tagging technique involves adding 5 to 10 mL of the patient's blood to a heparinized syringe containing stannous (tin) ions in the form of stannous chloride. Approximately 20 minutes later, Tc-99m pertechnetate (20 to 25 mCi or 740

Table 5-5 *Example of a Standard Single-Photon Emission Computed Tomography Acquisition Protocol Based on a Rest-Stress Technetium-99m Protocol*

Parameter	Rest Study	Stress Study
Dose	8-12 mCi	24-36 mCi
Position	Supine	Supine
Delay time to imaging From injection to imaging From rest to stress imaging	30-60 min	15-60 min 30 min-4 hr
Acquisition protocol		
Energy window	15%-20% symmetric	15%-20% symmetric
Collimator	LEHR	LEHR
Orbit	180 degrees (45 degrees RAO to 45 degrees LPO)	180 degrees (45 degrees RAO to 45 degrees LPO)
Orbit type	Circular *or* noncircular	Circular *or* noncircular
Pixel size	6.4 ± 0.4 mm	6.4 ± 0.4 mm
Acquisition type	Step and shoot *or* continuous	Step and shoot *or* continuous
Number of projections	60-64	60-64
Matrix	64 × 64	64 × 64
Time/projection	25 sec	20 sec
ECG gating Frames/cycle R-to-R window	8 or 16 100%	8 or 16 100%

Adapted with permission from Holly TA, Abbott BG, Al-Mallah M, et al. Single photon-emission computed tomography. *J Nucl Cardiol.* 2010;17:941-973.
ECG, Electrocardiographic; *LEHR,* low-energy high-resolution; *LPO,* left posterior oblique; *RAO,* right anterior oblique.

to 925 MBq) is added. Ten minutes later (to allow for labeling of the RBCs), the labeled blood is injected into patient, and imaging is started. Other tagging techniques include the modified in vivo and in vivo techniques or the use of a commercial kit (e.g., UltraTag kit, [Mallinckrodt, St. Louis, Mo.]) for labeling. The in vivo and modified in vivo techniques have slightly lower labeling efficiency (approximately 90%) compared with the in vitro technique (approximately 95%). Care must be taken to avoid excessive agitation of the blood or use of a small intravenous needle, to avoid damage to the RBCs that can result in lysis and excessive splenic uptake (RBC sequestration) and can interfere with image analysis. In addition, the utmost care must be taken to ensure that the patient's blood is labeled appropriately and is reinjected correctly into the same patient.

The MUGA images can be acquired as planar images in the anterior or LAO projection (Fig. 5-5) or as SPECT techniques using 16- to 32-frame gating and count-based acquisition. Images are typically acquired until 5 million counts are acquired in each projection (variable time). The LAO view is typically acquired first, followed by other views. The LAO projection is the best septal view (not necessarily a 45-degree LAO view). This view provides good separation of the left and right ventricles, although a small caudal tilt (10 degrees) may be required to separate the atrial activity. A stable R-R interval is needed for gated radionuclide ventriculography. Patients with frequent ectopic beats, irregularly paced rhythms, or atrial fibrillation with uncontrolled ventricular response should be stabilized before they are referred for gated imaging.

LVEF is calculated as follows:

$$LVEF = (LVEDC - BC) - (LVESC - BC) / (LVEDC - BC)$$

In other words,

$$LVEF = (LVEDC - LVESC) / (LVEDC - BC)$$

where EDC represents end-diastolic counts, ESC represents end-systolic counts, and BC indicates background counts.

The background counts cancel out in the numerator, and the final formula incorporates background counts in the denominator. As a result, selection of the background counts is critical for accurate estimation. The background region of interest should be placed in a representative region approximately 1 cm from the heart silhouette, but ensuring that it is not overlying areas of overly low or high counts, to avoid artificially low (low background) or artificially high LVEF (high background), respectively.

Why Perform Stress Testing?

Regulation of Coronary Blood Flow

MPI is critical not only to identify coronary artery stenosis but also to identify whether lesions found on coronary angiography are hemodynamically significant. The epicardial coronary arteries supply blood to the myocardium through an array of minute arterioles and capillaries. The epicardial arteries (1 to 4 mm) are conduit vessels that provide no resistance to blood flow in health and can be affected by atherosclerosis. The myocardial blood flow is maintained primarily by vasomotion of the coronary microvasculature (coronary arteries <400 mcm), which is not affected by atherosclerosis, but highly sensitive to metabolic regulation by risk factor–mediated coronary vasodilating and vasoconstricting signals. When the epicardial arteries develop atherosclerosis, a flow gradient is noted across the coronary artery stenosis. As a consequence of the reduced perfusion pressure distal to the stenosis, the microvasculature vasodilates and maintains normal resting blood flow. Therefore, resting myocardial blood flow is maintained in both normal and diseased coronary artery segments with no angina symptoms at rest. However, in response to exercise or vasodilator stress, healthy coronary artery blood flow can increase to three to eight times normal. In contrast, the diseased segments dilate less (because of baseline vasodilation), and ischemia and angina can result (Fig. 5-6). Nuclear techniques rely on imaging the flow heterogeneity between the normal and the diseased segments during stress to identify myocardial ischemia. Therefore, for the identification of hemodynamically

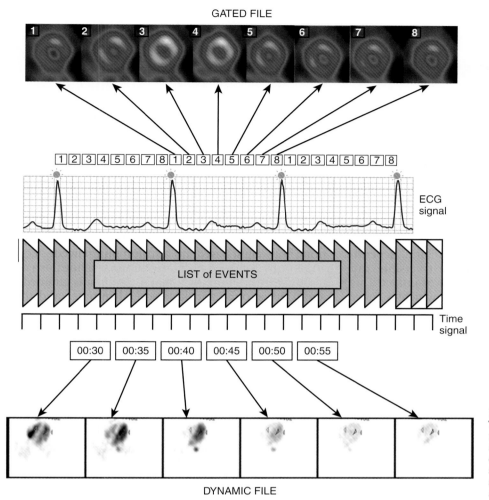

GATED FILE

ECG signal

LIST of EVENTS

Time signal

00:30 00:35 00:40 00:45 00:50 00:55

DYNAMIC FILE

Figure 5-4 List mode acquisition. This figure shows a schematic of list mode image acquisition. The data are acquired and stored with an electrocardiographic (ECG) signal and a time signal and can be reconstructed into static, gated, or dynamic image files for analysis.

significant CAD, resting MPI is insufficient, and stress testing is necessary.

Options for Stress Testing

Several options are available for stress testing. The choice between exercise stress and pharmacologic stress is determined by various factors (Table 5-6). First and foremost, all patients who can exercise should be encouraged to exercise because it provides a more comprehensive evaluation of the functional capacity of the patient compared with pharmacologic stress. Besides ECG variables, exercise capacity, heart rate recovery, heart rate reserve, chronotropic response, and ventricular ectopy all have prognostic importance during exercise. The sensitivity of ischemia testing during exercise is optimized when the patient performs exercise to a maximal tolerable safe level, which is usually accepted to be at least 85% of the patient's age-predicted maximal heart rate, defined arbitrarily as 220 minus age. Indications to terminate the exercise when it may be unsafe to continue include a significant drop in blood pressure, significant angina, sustained ventricular tachycardia, or ST-segment elevation. In such situations, if the exercise is terminated before the target heart rate is reached, the sensitivity of

the test for identifying ischemia will be reduced. Even after attaining the target rate, the patient should continue the exercise at the maximum level for at least 1 to 2 minutes after injection of the radiotracer, so that adequate circulation and uptake of the radiotracer within the heart is maintained and reflects coronary perfusion at maximal stress.

If the patient has exercise limitations or attains a submaximal heart rate with exercise (<85% age-predicted maximal heart rate), the physician should consider pharmacologic stress with vasodilator agents (adenosine, dipyridamole, or regadenoson; see the later section on novel stress agents) or dobutamine (in patients with contraindications to vasodilator stressors). In the setting of pharmacologic stress, the sensitivity approaches that of an exercise stress test at 85% of target heart rate, provided the patient has abstained from medications containing methylxanthines and foods containing caffeine, which may potentially block adenosine receptors on arterial smooth muscle cells and limit the effectiveness of these vasodilator drugs.

Practical Points

■ If the patient has left bundle branch block, vasodilator stress is recommended over exercise or dobutamine.

LAO	Anterior	Left lateral

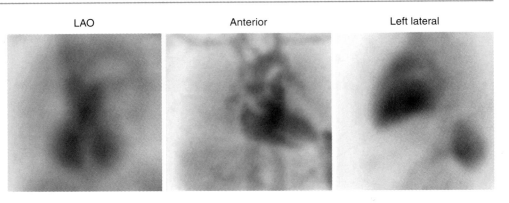

Figure 5-5 Multigated analysis. Standard left anterior oblique (LAO), anterior, and left lateral views are obtained. The LAO projection shows good separation of the left and right ventricles without overlap of atrial activity and a vertical septum. The anterior and left lateral projections show good separation from splenic activity.

Left bundle branch block is a conduction abnormality in which conduction to the left ventricle comes from the right ventricle and is delayed. This condition can result in artificial septal defects on MPI and, depending on whether the defect is fixed or reversible, can be mistakenly read as septal ischemia or infarct. This effect is accentuated by tachycardia, which is more common when exercise or dobutamine is used than with vasodilator stress.

■ If the patient has had a recent acute coronary syndrome, the safest maximal stress test to use is also a vasodilator stress test, provided the event occurred at least 48 hours before the stress test.

■ Nonspecific vasodilator stress agents can cause bronchoconstriction. Hence, in patients with bronchospastic airway disease who cannot exercise, dobutamine is preferred over vasodilator stress.

■ Combined vasodilator stress with low-level exercise (1.7 mph) can also be performed. This combination reduces side effects of vasodilators and improves image quality by improving the target-to-background ratio with a variable increase in blood pressure, heart rate, and the double product.

■ Moreover, for the evaluation of the hemodynamic significance of anatomic CAD such as myocardial muscle bridge or coronary anomalies, exercise stress with SPECT imaging is the test of choice. If that is not feasible, dobutamine stress is preferred over vasodilator stress. With dobutamine stress, the patient should attain a maximal heart rate, with additional atropine (0.25-mg increments to a maximum of 2 mg) given as needed to maintain maximal hyperemia and test sensitivity.

Novel Pharmacologic Stress Agents

Adenosine and dipyridamole (which acts by increasing endogenous adenosine levels) are nonspecific coronary vasodilators that bind to the coronary A1, A2A, A2B, and A3 receptors. Coronary A2A receptors are responsible for vasodilation, whereas A1, A2B, and A3 receptors cause the undesirable side effects of heart block, peripheral vasodilation, and bronchospasm, respectively. Therefore, newer pharmacologic stress agents that selectively bind only to the adenosine A2A receptors and cause vasodilation without the side effects have been conceived and developed. Several agents have been tested.

Regadenoson, also known as the CVT 3146 agent, has a low affinity for the adenosine A2A receptor. This agent was studied in more than 3000 patients and has been approved by the FDA for clinical use since 2008. Regadenoson is administered as a 400-mcg bolus injection (not weight based, no infusion pump needed) over 10 seconds, followed by 5 mL of normal saline flush and radiotracer injection. Maximal hyperemia is attained in about 30 seconds and lasts several minutes and then diminishes.

Other adenosine A2A receptor agonists that are being tested include Binoadenoson and Apadenoson. Binoadenoson, also known as MRE 0470 or WRC 0470, has a slightly longer duration of action and is not yet approved by the FDA. Another agent, Apadenoson, also known as BMS 068645, is currently undergoing clinical testing and is not yet FDA approved for clinical use.

Because of bolus dosing and non–weight-based injection, regadenoson is easy to use. Although it is not approved for this indication, regadenoson is well suited for use in patients with submaximal heart rate response to exercise stress. Previously, in these patients with submaximal heart rate, exercise was terminated, and an adenosine or dipyridamole infusion was prepared. Now, a novel protocol may involve the use of regadenoson at maximal treadmill exercise, followed by the injection of radiotracer to complete the study. This method allows for better tolerability of the vasodilator agent because of fewer side effects, as well as time savings. In addition, exercise treadmill information is available for clinical use. This protocol is currently under investigation by several centers.

Protocols for Stress Testing

Stress testing is performed using standard protocols. Continuous ECG monitoring is recommended during exercise and 10 minutes into recovery or until ischemic ECG changes have resolved. The blood pressure should be measured and recorded at least every 2 to 3 minutes during exercise, at peak exercise and peak hyperemia, and for 10 minutes into recovery. SPECT image acquisition can be performed within 15 to 60 minutes after exercise and 45 to 60 minutes after pharmacologic stress testing. Indications to terminate exercise and pharmacologic stress testing are shown in Box 5-2. Severe side effects, especially bronchospasm from adenosine, dipyridamole, or regadenoson, can be reversed with intravenous aminophylline, given 1 to 2 minutes after tracer injection (if possible, to ensure adequate tracer uptake) injected over 1 minute at 50 to 100 mg and repeated to a total dose of 250 to 300 mg.

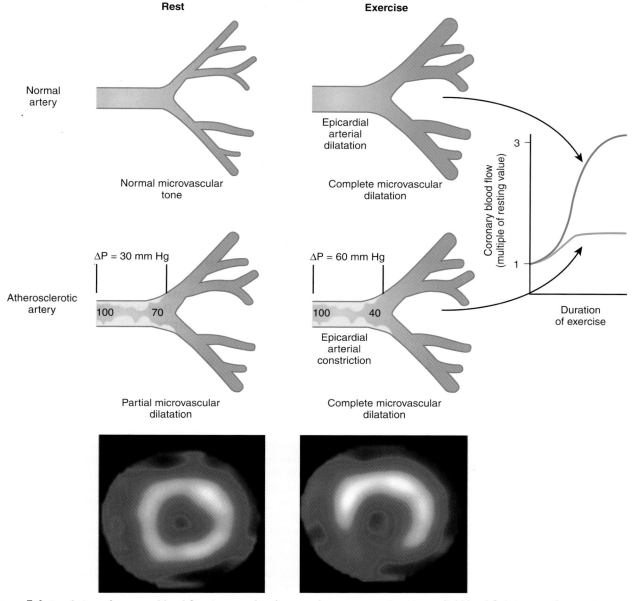

Figure 5-6 Regulation of coronary blood flow in normal and stenosed coronary arteries. Myocardial blood flow is normal at rest in a normal coronary artery. During exercise, in a normal artery, one sees dilation of the epicardial conduit vessels and the microvasculature that increases blood flow severalfold. In contrast, in the atherosclerotic artery, at rest, one sees a pressure gradient across the stenosed coronary artery and compensatory vasodilation of the microvasculature to maintain resting blood flow. During exercise, the epicardial artery constricts slightly, the pressure drop across the stenosis increases, and the microvessels have limited additional capacity to vasodilate; the result is blood flow that is inadequate to meet the demands of exercise. Consequently, the fractional flow reserve is reduced (0.4) in the stenotic artery. This difference in the flow between the normal and the stenosed coronary arteries forms the basis for myocardial perfusion imaging. In the images at the *bottom,* from a patient with 85% right coronary artery stenosis, normal rest perfusion the right coronary artery distribution (inferior wall) is seen on the *left,* whereas a perfusion defect in the inferior wall is visible on the *right.* (Reproduced with permission from Wilson RF. Assessing the severity of coronary-artery stenoses. *N Engl J Med.* 1996;334:1735-1737.)

1. Exercise stress testing: The standard Bruce protocol is a commonly used exercise treadmill protocol. A modified Bruce protocol that adds a stage 0 (1.7 mph at 0% grade) and stage ½ (1.7 mph at 5% grade) can be used in patients with impaired exercise capacity or for patients after myocardial infarction. Symptom-limited exercise stress is recommended, with exercise terminated for fatigue, rather than purely because target heart rate is reached. The radiotracer is

injected at peak heart rate, and exercise is continued for an additional minute.
2. Dipyridamole stress testing: Dipyridamole is infused as a weight-based infusion of 0.56 mg/kg over 4 minutes using an infusion pump or by hand injection. The radiotracer is injected 3 minutes after completion of the infusion. Dipyridamole is diluted in normal saline solution to minimize local discomfort at the time of injection.

Table 5-6   How to Select an Appropriate Stress Test

Patient's Profile	Stress Test of Choice
Ability to exercise to target heart rate	Exercise
Presence of left bundle branch block or pacemaker, presence of large abdominal aortic aneurysm, recent myocardial infarction (<30 days), inability to exercise adequately	Vasodilator*
Presence of bronchospastic disease with active wheezing, recent intake of caffeine (<12 hours), theophylline or oral dipyridamole use within 48 hours	Dobutamine
Reason for the test: coronary artery anomalies or myocardial muscle bridge	Exercise stress; if not feasible, dobutamine stress

From Gibbons RJ, Balady GJ, Beasley JW, et al. ACC/AHA guidelines for exercise testing: a report of the American College of Cardiology/American Heart Association Task Force on Practice Guidelines (Committee on Exercise Testing). *J Am Coll Cardiol.* 1997;30:260-311.
*Adenosine, dipyridamole, or regadenoson.

BOX 5-2   Indications to Terminate Stress Testing

Indications to Terminate Exercise Stress Testing
Decrease in systolic blood pressure by >10 mm Hg with other features of ischemia
Significant angina, dyspnea, fatigue, severe lightheadedness, or syncope
Sustained ventricular or supraventricular tachycardia
ST-segment elevation >1 mm in non–Q-wave leads
ST depression of >2 mm in the presence of angina or >3 mm in the absence of angina
Patient's desire to stop
Inability to monitor blood pressure or electrocardiogram for technical reasons

Indications to Terminate Pharmacologic Stress Testing
Sustained hypotension
Sustained ventricular or supraventricular tachycardia
Sustained heart block that does not resolve with hand exercise
Development of wheezing
Patient's desire to stop

---

3. Adenosine stress testing: Adenosine is infused as a continuous weight-based infusion of 140 mcg/kg/minute using an infusion pump over 4 to 6 minutes, with radiotracer injection at the midpoint of the infusion. Transient heart block is frequently seen at the time of radiotracer injection, and this typically resolves with hand or leg exercise in bed.
4. Regadenoson stress testing: Regadenoson is injected as a non–weight-based injection of 400 mcg over 10 seconds from a prefilled syringe, followed by 10 mL of normal saline solution. A more rapid injection (<10 seconds) can result in more side effects.
5. Dobutamine stress testing: Dobutamine is infused as a weight-based infusion starting at 10 mcg/kg/minute, increasing every 3 minutes to 20, 30, and

40 mcg/kg/minute. If the target heart rate is not reached at a dose of 40 mcg/kg/minute, atropine is used intravenously, in 0.5- to 1-mg increments to a total dose of 2 mg. Atropine is contraindicated in patients with obstructive uropathy, glaucoma, and myasthenia gravis. Tracer is administered at the target heart rate, and the infusion is continued to another 1 minute. If the heart rate remains high after completion of the study, intravenous metoprolol may be used in 5-mg increments.

■ APPROACH TO THE PATIENT AND INTERPRETING SINGLE-PHOTON EMISSION COMPUTED TOMOGRAPHY AND POSITRON EMISSION TOMOGRAPHY STUDIES

Quality Assurance and Troubleshooting Single-Photon Emission Computed Tomography and Positron Emission Tomography Imaging

After imaging is completed, several potential patient-related factors need to be looked for prior to sending the patient home. The rotating projection images should be reviewed and if there is significant patient breathing or motion artifacts, SPECT imaging should be repeated with instructions not to move during imaging and appropriate breathing instructions. In the presence of significant bowel or liver uptake that may interfere with image interpretation, SPECT imaging should be delayed until there is sufficient time for liver clearance and bowel uptake to be diverted away from region around the heart. Tables 5-7 and 5-8 outline the methods used to troubleshoot frequently encountered problems during SPECT MPI and PET MPI, respectively. The images should be reviewed to ensure that there are no high risk exercise stress or scan features that may necessitate hospitalization of the patient (see Chapter 29).

Systematic Image Interpretation

Orientation and display of data into vertical long-axis and horizontal long-axis and short-axis planes should be reviewed and should be consistent between stress and rest studies. The long axis of the left ventricle is defined on the vertical and horizontal long-axis slices to bisect the ventricle into approximately equal halves. This approach produces appropriately oriented short-axis images orthogonal to the long-axis planes. Inappropriate plane selection can cause misalignment between rest and stress images and can result in inappropriate interpretation and artifactual reversibility. The apex and base slice selection for the perfusion images should be checked and appropriately placed because this influences the computation of the transient cavity dilation ratio. A region of interest may be placed to define the myocardial contours for the polar plots, to avoid extracardiac uptake. Then, the raw data should be evaluated in a cine

Table 5-7   Troubleshooting Problems Frequently Encountered During Single-Photon Emission Computed Tomography Acquisition

Problems	Solutions
Patient motion	Properly instruct the patient. Acquire postexercise images at least 15 to 30 minutes after exercise to avoid cardiac creep. Use a multiheaded SPECT camera system for faster image acquisition. Motion correction software can help for minor motion. Consider prone imaging, which minimizes patient motion. Repeat acquisition is usually the best solution for motion-degraded images.
Gating artifacts	Check ECG lead placement and ECG tracing with the patient's arms raised above the shoulders. Check for arrhythmia. Repeat imaging, if needed. Discount gating in the presence of count loss or flashing of rotating raw projection images. Check the setting of the gating histogram width (wide histogram indicates arrhythmia).
Photon attenuation or decreased counts	Use a weight-based dosing regimen for radioisotopes. Ensure that the intravenous line is working well and that the dose is not infiltrated subcutaneously. Consider 2-day studies.
Breast or anterior attenuation	Female patients should undergo imaging without their bra, to ensure similar breast position during rest and stress imaging. Check raw data in cine format to identify breast attenuation and ensure that the attenuation pattern is similar during rest and stress. Image the patient in the exact same position during rest and stress to avoid shifting breast attenuation. Correct attenuation by CT or radionuclide transmission imaging.
Subdiaphragmatic activity	Use the optimum delay between acquisitions (45 min for sestamibi), to allow subdiaphragmatic activity to clear. Repeat imaging with a longer delay. Use prone imaging. Add low-level exercise along with pharmacologic stress to increase skeletal muscle blood flow, away from splanchnic blood flow. Rarely, repeat imaging with Tl-201 may help in patients with excessive subdiaphragmatic activity that is not cleared by any of the foregoing techniques. If filtered back projection is causing a Ramp filter artifact, consider reprocessing the images using OSEM or iterative reconstruction algorithms.
Image reconstruction artifacts	Images must be carefully reviewed for reconstruction artifacts. Camera failure or photomultiplier tube malfunction can sometimes result in geometric defects that are best seen on review of the raw projection images.

CT, Computed tomography; *ECG,* electrocardiogram; *OSEM,* ordered subset expectation maximization; *SPECT,* single-photon emission computed tomography; *Tl-201,* thallium-201.

Table 5-8   Troubleshooting Problems Encountered During Positron Emission Tomography Acquisition

Problems	Solutions
High ratio of blood pool to heart counts	Ensure optimal prescan delay: N-13 ammonia (90-180 sec), Rb-82 (70-130 sec) in healthy subjects. Consider prescan delay at the higher end of the range in selected patients (severe LV and RV systolic dysfunction, primary lung disease, or any reason for increased arm-to-heart circulation time). Obtain dynamic or list mode imaging, so that the framed images can be summed (prescan delay changed) to provide optimal separation of the blood pool and myocardial activity.
Misregistration of transmission or emission images	Review emission-transmission alignment. When misalignment is noted, use software to realign, generate new attenuation map, and correct images using the new attenuation map.
Count-poor emission images	This is typically as a result of a mismatch between patient size and the injected dose of radiotracer. With Rb-82, the end of the generator life, imaging patients larger than 300 lb, or using a 2-D mode can result in count-poor images. Attempt imaging in a 3-D mode (20-mCi Rb-82 dose) or reset the generator to deliver a rapid injection of 30-40 mCi over 30 sec.
Count-poor transmission images	This can be seen when the source used for attenuation correction is old. A transmission scan for a longer duration may help.
Patient motion	Patient motion can be challenging to detect with PET imaging. A review of the transaxial images or the multiple frames of images (if acquired as dynamic or list mode) can be helpful to identify motion. Careful instruction to patients and avoidance of motion are critical. If images are acquired in a list mode or dynamic mode, the frames with motion can be eliminated and the remaining images summed to generate a motion-free image. This may be possible for long image acquisitions such as N-13 ammonia, but it may be more difficult with Rb-82. If this is not an option, repeat imaging should be considered. Motion correction software is not typically used for PET.
Image reconstruction artifacts	Images should be carefully reviewed for reconstruction artifacts. If observed, repeat reconstruction may help. In large patients, image truncation artifacts may be seen. These artifacts can sometimes resolve with the use of a large field of view reconstruction.

2-D, Two-dimensional; *3-D,* three-dimensional; *LV,* left ventricular; *N-13,* nitrogen-13; *PET,* positron emission tomography; *Rb-82,* rubidium-82; *RV,* right ventricular.

mode to identify sources of artifacts and extracardiac findings. On the summed perfusion images (not end-diastolic or end-systolic, but summed), the size of the left ventricle and the right ventricle, radiotracer uptake in the right ventricle, and transient cavity dilation of the left ventricle are evaluated. The location, size, severity, and reversibility of perfusion defects are evaluated. Quantitative perfusion analysis is performed using commercially available software. The gated images are evaluated for global and regional ventricular function by using commercially available software. Finally, the clinical history of patient is reviewed after the images are interpreted (to avoid bias) and before the final interpretation of study.

Image Display and Quantification of Myocardial Perfusion Imaging

SPECT and PET myocardial perfusion images are interpreted based on the presence, location, extent, and severity of the perfusion defects by using a standard ASNC/American Heart Association/American College of Cardiology 17-segment model (see Fig. 14-4, A 7) and visual scoring. Serial short-axis slices are displayed from apex to base, horizontal long-axis slices are displayed from the inferior to anterior walls, and vertical long-axis slices are displayed from medial (septal) to lateral walls from left to right. By convention, stress images are displayed above the rest images. Semiquantitative criteria used to score the 17 segments and to compute the summed stress score (SSS), the summed rest score (SRS), and the summed difference score (SDS). The SSS is a measure of both fixed defects and reversible defects. The activity in each segment is scored visually, as follows: 0 is normal, 1 is a mild defect, 2 is a moderate defect, 3 is a severe defect, and 4 is absent radiotracer uptake. Similarly, the SRS is derived from the rest study, and the SDS is the difference between the two scores and is a measure of reversible defects. The score can be computed into percentage of left ventricle abnormality by dividing it by the maximum score by the numbers of segments times maximal segmental score ($17 \times 4 = 68$, for a 17-segment model and a 0 to 4 scale of scoring). Based on the SSS, the scans can be categorized as normal (0 to 4), mildly abnormal (5 to 8), moderately abnormal (9 to 13), or severely abnormal (>13). The degree or amount of defect reversibility is based on the SDS and is considered mild (1 to 3), moderate (4 to 7), or high (≥8).

Defect Interpretation

A *reversible defect* is one that is present on stress images and is not present on rest or redistribution images; this is the hallmark of stress-induced ischemia. A *fixed perfusion defect* that persists on both stress and rest or redistribution and reinjection images may reflect an attenuation artifact, myocardial scar, or myocardial hibernation. *Partially reversible defects* are stress defects that improve but do not normalize completely on rest or redistribution and reinjection images; these defects likely reflect nontransmural scar with periinfarct ischemia. A defect is said to exhibit *reverse redistribution* if it is present on rest or redistribution images and is absent on stress images. Reverse redistribution, initially described with Tl-201 imaging, has been identified in patients with multivessel

CAD and in patients with acute myocardial infarction, and it may reflect a differential wash-out of the perfusion tracer. Reverse redistribution may also indicate the technical artifact of oversubtraction of background activity on the rest and redistribution images (Table 5-9). Features of high-risk MPI scans are elaborated in Chapter 29.

Gated Single-Photon Emission Computed Tomography Interpretation

The gated SPECT images must be reviewed with and without the automatic contours generated by the computer. Global and regional wall motion is assessed visually without the contours. Calculation of LVEF is based on automatic edge detection techniques that permit the tomographic (3-D geometric) evaluation of ventricular volumes. Verification and adjustments of computer-generated endocardial contours and valve planes are essential for accurate assessment of LVEF. Volumes at end-diastole (EDV) and end-systole (ESV) are measured, and LVEF is calculated as follows:

$$LVEF\ (\%) = (EDV - ESV) / EDV \times 100$$

Regional wall motion should be analyzed visually, using standard nomenclature: normal, hypokinesis, akinesis, and dyskinesis. A semiquantitative scoring system can be used in which 0 is normal, 1 is mild hypokinesis, 2 is moderate hypokinesis, 3 is severe hypokinesis, 4 is akinesis, and 5 is dyskinesis. Dyskinesis may be difficult to evaluate using MPI. *The LVEF may be overestimated in patients with small LV cavities because the ESV may be underestimated as a result of the resolution limitations of the technique.* At present, gated SPECT imaging may also assist in differentiation of attenuation artifacts from scar.

Common Clinical Applications of Radionuclide Ventriculography

Radionuclide ventriculography is used clinically to assess the severity of regional and global right and left ventricular dysfunction. Because ejection fraction measurements obtained with this imaging technique are count based and do not depend on assumptions about the shape of the ventricle (unlike echocardiography methods), they are highly reproducible if the imaging study is performed properly. However, cardiac MRI has mostly replaced radionuclide angiography for several indications, including the following:

- Cardiomyopathy, to assess changes in ventricular function during treatment (e.g., chemotherapy regimens with cardiotoxic drugs)

Table 5-9   Defect Interpretation

Stress	Rest (or Early Redistribution)	Interpretation
Normal	Normal	Normal
Defect	Normal	Ischemia
Defect	Defect	Scar (or hibernation)
Normal	Defect	Reverse redistribution

- Regurgitant valvular diseases
- For accurate estimation of LVEF in patients with CAD (less common). This was more frequently used before the advent of cardiac MRI imaging. The advantages include ability to quantify global LVEF and regional wall motion accurately even in patients with dense scars, thus eliminating the need for software to perform edge detection in areas of dense scar because the blood pool is imaged.

■ REDUCING RADIATION RISK IN NUCLEAR CARDIAC IMAGING

Throughout this chapter and in Chapter 29, the powerful diagnostic and risk stratification data provided by SPECT and PET techniques are discussed. Nevertheless careful assessment of the risks and benefits of any imaging modality that uses ionizing radiation is imperative, so that exposure to radiation is in accordance with the ALARA principle (as low as reasonably achievable). In this context, the physician must keep in mind not only the radiation dose to the patients but also the radiation the dose to the staff and personnel involved with testing.

Strategies to Reduce Radiation Dose

Nuclear cardiac imaging involves injection of a relatively small amount of radioactive material. A detailed description of radiation physics is beyond the scope of this chapter. The amount of radioactive tracer, the duration of exposure, the type of radiation, the biologic variability (children and female patients are more sus-

ceptible than adults and male patients, respectively), and several other factors determine the radiation risk associated with a test. The effects of radiation have been extensively studied without definitive results. Most of these data come from the Life Span study of malignant diseases associated with radiation exposure in survivors of the atomic bomb explosion in Japan in 1945; this study was the principal source for the development of these risk estimates. However, whether the downward extrapolation of the effects observed from acute high-dose exposure to the low dose resulting from diagnostic testing should indeed be linear is unclear. Therefore, as with any noninvasive test, the basic principles of (uncertain) risk versus benefit must be considered.

Physicians must be educated to understand the indications for appropriate use of nuclear cardiac imaging tests. The reason for the test must be closely scrutinized, and only appropriate and indicated tests should be performed. Repeat testing should be avoided unless clearly it is indicated. Testing in asymptomatic individuals should be minimized. When the test is indicated, then a study protocol must be carefully developed to ensure that testing is performed with the lowest possible dose, while maintaining diagnostic-quality imaging. Patients should be educated, to allay unnecessary fears of radiation risk when the test is indicated. When a test is not performed because of concern about radiation dose, the physician should consider the risks of missing important diagnostic information by not performing the test. Effective patient radiation doses from various SPECT and PET studies are shown in Table 5-10. Injected amounts of radiotracer (and therefore resulting radiation doses) may differ among laboratories (see Table 5-10).

Table 5-10   Estimates of Effective Doses of Myocardial Perfusion Imaging Protocols*

| Protocol | Injected Activity (mCi) | | Effective Dose (mSv/MBq) |
	Rest	Stress	
Tc-99m sestamibi rest-stress	10.0	27.5	11.3
Tc-99m sestamibi stress only	0.0	27.5	7.9
Tc-99m sestamibi 2-day	25	25	15.7
Tl-201 stress-redistribution	0.0	3.5	22.0
Tl-201 stress-reinjection	1.5	3.0	31.4
Dual isotope Tl-201-Tc-99m sestamibi	3.5	25.0	29.2
Tc-99m–labeled erythrocytes	22.5	0.0	5.7
Rb-82[†]	50.0	50.0	~4 mSv
N-13 ammonia	15.0	15.0	2.4
O-15 water	29.7	29.7	2.5
F-18 FDG	10.0	0.0	7.0

F-18, Fluorine-18; *FDG*, fluorodeoxyglucose; *N-13*, nitrogen-13; *O-15*, oxygen-15; *Rb-82*, rubidium-82; *Tc-99m*, technetium-99m; *Tl-201*, thallium-201.
*Calculations performed with the use of International Commission on Radiological Protection publication no. 60 on tissue weighting factors and average radionuclide activities specified in current American Society of Nuclear Cardiology guidelines. Data from Hesse B, Tagil K, Cuocolo A, et al. EANM/ESC procedural guidelines for myocardial perfusion imaging in nuclear cardiology. *Eur J Nucl Med Mol Imaging*. 2005;32:855-897; and Conversion coefficients for use in radiological protection against external radiation: adopted by the ICRP and ICRU in September 1995. *Ann ICRP*. 1996;26:1-205.
†Rb-82 dose estimates data from Senthamizhchelvan S, Bravo PE, Lodge MA, Merrill J, Bengel FM, Sgouros G. Radiation dosimetry of 82Rb in humans under pharmacologic stress. *J Nucl Med*. 2011;52:485-491; and Senthamizhchelvan S, Bravo PE, Esaias C, et al. Human biodistribution and radiation dosimetry of 82Rb. *J Nucl Med*. 2010;51:1592-1599.

Specific Strategies

SINGLE-PHOTON EMISSION COMPUTED TOMOGRAPHY

Items listed in points 1 to 4 minimize the radiation dose to patients and staff.

1. Use single isotope protocols whenever feasible. If possible, use Tc-99m–labeled agents instead of Tl-201, except for specific indications, such as need for a viability assessment or in patients with increased gastrointestinal tracer uptake with Tc-99m.
2. Use newer iterative reconstruction methods, solid-state cameras, high-sensitivity crystals, and multidetector systems if available.
   a. These methods allow for a lower injected radiotracer dose.
   b. Consider obtaining newer-generation scanner and software systems when replacing systems, if feasible.
3. Consider using stress-only studies and omit the rest study if the stress study result is normal.
   a. May be considered in low to intermediate risk subjects.
   b. This approach works well with attenuation corrected SPECT and gated SPECT.
   c. This may be an option in laboratories without access to the newer scanner or software algorithms that allow low-dose imaging.
4. Use weight-based radiotracer dosing.
   a. Use lower activity in smaller patients.
5. Encourage adequate hydration after imaging and early micturition.
6. Use prospective ECG-triggering CT acquisition of the attenuation correction CT scan.
7. Minimize tube current for the attenuation correction CT scan. Diagnostic-quality chest CT scans may not be necessary.

POSITRON EMISSION TOMOGRAPHY

■ Consider the 3-D acquisition mode.
■ The 3-D mode enables use of significantly lower radiotracer dose compared with the 2-D mode.
■ The use of shorter half-life radiotracers, when available, can reduce the dose.
■ The use of stress-only techniques may work well, but it has not been thoroughly tested with PET scanning.
■ Do not perform hybrid PET and diagnostic CTA unless a specific clinical need or question exists.
■ Implement strategies to reduce the radiation dose to the staff.
■ The radiation dose from occupational exposure can be minimized by following the basic principles of time, distance, and shielding.
■ Radiation must be handled carefully, by using gloves and tongs when appropriate.
■ Staff members must maintain a distance from radioactive patients.
■ Avoid close contact with radioactive patients. Radiation decreases with the square of distance. Hence, stepping away from a radioactive patient is a simple and effective means to reduce personal exposure.
■ Minimize the time of contact with radioactive patients.

■ Local radiation safety practices must be followed.
■ Laboratories must choose imaging protocols with the most minimal possible radiation dose to patients, and this will also reduce staff exposures.

Bibliography

Al Jaroudi W, Iskandrian AE. Regadenoson: a new myocardial stress agent. *J Am Coll Cardiol.* 2009;54:1123-1130.

Anger HO. Scintillation camera with multichannel collimators. *J Nucl Med.* 1964;5:515-531.

Beller GA, Bergmann SR. Myocardial perfusion imaging agents: SPECT and PET. *J Nucl Cardiol.* 2004;11:71-86.

Beller GA, Watson DD. Physiological basis of myocardial perfusion imaging with the technetium 99m agents. *Semin Nucl Med.* 1991;21:173-181.

Ben-Haim S, Kacperski K, Hain S, et al. Simultaneous dual-radionuclide myocardial perfusion imaging with a solid-state dedicated cardiac camera. *Eur J Nucl Med Mol Imaging.* 2010;37:1710-1721.

Berman DS, Kang X, Tamarappoo B, et al. Stress thallium-201/rest technetium-99m sequential dual isotope high-speed myocardial perfusion imaging. *JACC Cardiovasc Imaging.* 2009;2:273-282.

Boger LA, Volker LL, Hertenstein GK, Bateman TM. Best patient preparation before and during radionuclide myocardial perfusion imaging studies. *J Nucl Cardiol.* 2006;13:98-110.

Bonow RO. High-speed myocardial perfusion imaging: dawn of a new era in nuclear cardiology? *JACC Cardiovasc Imaging.* 2008;1:164-166.

Borges-Neto S, Pagnanelli RA, Shaw LK, et al. Clinical results of a novel wide beam reconstruction method for shortening scan time of Tc-99m cardiac SPECT perfusion studies. *J Nucl Cardiol.* 2007;14:555-565.

Brown KA, Heller GV, Landin RS, et al. Early dipyridamole (99m)Tc-sestamibi single photon emission computed tomographic imaging 2 to 4 days after acute myocardial infarction predicts in-hospital and postdischarge cardiac events: comparison with submaximal exercise imaging. *Circulation.* 1999;100:2060-2066.

Buechel RR, Herzog BA, Husmann L, et al. Ultrafast nuclear myocardial perfusion imaging on a new gamma camera with semiconductor detector technique: first clinical validation. *Eur J Nucl Med Mol Imaging.* 2010;37:773-778.

Callahan RJ, Froelich JW, McKusick KA, Leppo J, Strauss HW. A modified method for the in vivo labeling of red blood cells with Tc-99m: concise communication. *J Nucl Med.* 1982;23:315-318.

Campisi R, Di Carli MF. Assessment of coronary flow reserve and microcirculation: a clinical perspective. *J Nucl Cardiol.* 2004;11:3-11.

Cerqueira MD. Advances in pharmacologic agents in imaging: new A2A receptor agonists. *Curr Cardiol Rep.* 2006;8:119-122.

Cerqueira MD, Allman KC, Ficaro EP, et al. Recommendations for reducing radiation exposure in myocardial perfusion imaging. *J Nucl Cardiol.* 2010;17:709-718.

Cerqueira MD, Weissman NJ, Dilsizian V, et al. Standardized myocardial segmentation and nomenclature for tomographic imaging of the heart: a statement for healthcare professionals from the Cardiac Imaging Committee of the Council on Clinical Cardiology of the American Heart Association. *Circulation.* 2002;105:539-542.

Chikamori T, Yamashina A, Hida S, Nishimura T. Diagnostic and prognostic value of BMIPP imaging. *J Nucl Cardiol.* 2007;14:111-125.

Conversion coefficients for use in radiological protection against external radiation: adopted by the ICRP and ICRU in September 1995. *Ann ICRP.* 1996;26:1-205.

Cullom SJ, Case JA, Bateman TM. Electrocardiographically gated myocardial perfusion SPECT: technical principles and quality control considerations. *J Nucl Cardiol.* 1998;5:418-425.

DePuey EG, Bommireddipalli S, Clark J, Leykekhman A, Thompson LB, Friedman M. A comparison of the image quality of full-time myocardial perfusion SPECT vs wide beam reconstruction half-time and half-dose SPECT. *J Nucl Cardiol.* 2011;18:273-280.

DePuey EG, Bommireddipalli S, Clark J, Thompson L, Srour Y. Wide beam reconstruction "quarter-time" gated myocardial perfusion SPECT functional imaging: a comparison to "full-time" ordered subset expectation maximum. *J Nucl Cardiol.* 2009;16:736-752.

DePuey EG, Gadiraju R, Clark J, Thompson L, Anstett F, Shwartz SC. Ordered subset expectation maximization and wide beam reconstruction "half-time" gated myocardial perfusion SPECT functional imaging: a comparison to "full-time" filtered backprojection. *J Nucl Cardiol.* 2008;15:547-563.

DePuey EG, Garcia EV. Optimal specificity of thallium-201 SPECT through recognition of imaging artifacts. *J Nucl Med.* 1989;30:441-449.

DePuey EG, Guertler-Krawczynska E, Robbins WL. Thallium-201 SPECT in coronary artery disease patients with left bundle branch block. *J Nucl Med.* 1988;29:1479-1485.

Deutsch E, Bushong W, Glavan KA, et al. Heart imaging with cationic complexes of technetium. *Science.* 1981;214:85-86.

Di Carli MF, Dorbala S, Curillova Z, et al. Relationship between CT coronary angiography and stress perfusion imaging in patients with suspected ischemic heart disease assessed by integrated PET-CT imaging. *J Nucl Cardiol.* 2007;14:799-809.

Di Carli MF, Dorbala S, Meserve J, El Fakhri G, Sitek A, Moore SC. Clinical myocardial perfusion PET/CT. *J Nucl Med.* 2007;48:783-793.

Dorbala S, Vangala D, Sampson U, Limaye A, Kwong R, Di Carli MF. Value of vasodilator left ventricular ejection fraction reserve in evaluating the magnitude of myocardium at risk and the extent of angiographic coronary artery disease: a 82Rb PET/CT study. *J Nucl Med.* 2007;48:349-358.

Einstein AJ, Moser KW, Thompson RC, Cerqueira MD, Henzlova MJ. Radiation dose to patients from cardiac diagnostic imaging. *Circulation.* 2007;116:1290-1305.

Einstein AJ, Weiner SD, Bernheim A, et al. Multiple testing, cumulative radiation dose, and clinical indications in patients undergoing myocardial perfusion imaging. *JAMA.* 2010;304:2137-2144.

Elhendy A, van Domburg RT, Bax JJ, et al. Dobutamine-atropine stress myocardial perfusion SPECT imaging in the diagnosis of graft stenosis after coronary artery bypass grafting. *J Nucl Cardiol.* 1998;5:491-497.

Esteves FP, Raggi P, Folks RD, et al. Novel solid-state-detector dedicated cardiac camera for fast myocardial perfusion imaging: multicenter comparison with standard dual detector cameras. *J Nucl Cardiol.* 2009;16:927-934.

Faber TL, Cooke CD, Folks RD, et al. Left ventricular function and perfusion from gated SPECT perfusion images: an integrated method. *J Nucl Med.* 1999;40:650-659.

Flamen P, Bossuyt A, Franken PR. Technetium-99m-tetrofosmin in dipyridamole-stress myocardial SPECT imaging: intraindividual comparison with technetium-99m-sestamibi. *J Nucl Med.* 1995;36:2009-2015.

Fletcher GF, Balady GJ, Amsterdam EA, et al. Exercise standards for testing and training: a statement for healthcare professionals from the American Heart Association. *Circulation.* 2001;104:1694-1740.

Flotats A, Knuuti J, Gutberlet M, et al. Hybrid cardiac imaging: SPECT/CT and PET/CT. A joint position statement by the European Association of Nuclear Medicine (EANM), the European Society of Cardiac Radiology (ESCR) and the European Council of Nuclear Cardiology (ECNC). *Eur J Nucl Med Mol Imaging.* 2011;38:201-212.

Gal R, Grenier RP, Carpenter J, Schmidt DH, Port SC. High count rate first-pass radionuclide angiography using a digital gamma camera. *J Nucl Med.* 1986;27:198-206.

Gallagher BM, Ansari A, Atkins H, et al. Radiopharmaceuticals XXVII: 18F-labeled 2-deoxy-2-fluoro-D-glucose as a radiopharmaceutical for measuring regional myocardial glucose metabolism in vivo: tissue distribution and imaging studies in animals. *J Nucl Med.* 1977;18:990-996.

Gambhir SS, Berman DS, Ziffer J, et al. A novel high-sensitivity rapid-acquisition single-photon cardiac imaging camera. *J Nucl Med.* 2009;50:635-643.

Gao Z, Li Z, Baker SP, et al. Novel short-acting A2A adenosine receptor agonists for coronary vasodilation: inverse relationship between affinity and duration of action of A2A agonists. *J Pharmacol Exp Ther.* 2001;298:209-218.

Garcia EV, Faber TL. New trends in camera and software technology in nuclear cardiology. *Cardiol Clin.* 2009;27:227-236.

Garcia EV, Faber TL, Esteves FP. Cardiac dedicated ultrafast SPECT cameras: new designs and clinical implications. *J Nucl Med.* 2011;52:210-217.

Gerber TC, Carr JJ, Arai AE, et al. Ionizing radiation in cardiac imaging: a science advisory from the American Heart Association Committee on Cardiac Imaging of the Council on Clinical Cardiology and Committee on Cardiovascular Imaging and Intervention of the Council on Cardiovascular Radiology and Intervention. *Circulation.* 2009;119:1056-1065.

Germano G, Erel J, Kiat H, Kavanagh PB, Berman DS. Quantitative LVEF and qualitative regional function from gated thallium-201 perfusion SPECT. *J Nucl Med.* 1997;38:749-754.

Germano G, Erel J, Lewin H, Kavanagh PB, Berman DS. Automatic quantitation of regional myocardial wall motion and thickening from gated technetium-99m sestamibi myocardial perfusion single-photon emission computed tomography. *J Am Coll Cardiol.* 1997;30:1360-1367.

Gibbons RJ, Balady GJ, Beasley JW, et al. ACC/AHA guidelines for exercise testing: a report of the American College of Cardiology/American Heart Association Task Force on Practice Guidelines (Committee on Exercise Testing). *J Am Coll Cardiol.* 1997;30:260-311.

Gimelli A, Bottai M, Giorgetti A, et al. Comparison between ultrafast and standard single-photon emission CT in patients with coronary artery disease: a pilot study. *Circ Cardiovasc Imaging.* 2011;4:51-58.

Gottdiener JS, Mathisen DJ, Borer JS, et al. Doxorubicin cardiotoxicity: assessment of late left ventricular dysfunction by radionuclide cineangiography. *Ann Intern Med.* 1981;94:430-435.

Gould KL, Ornish D, Scherwitz L, et al. Changes in myocardial perfusion abnormalities by positron emission tomography after long-term, intense risk factor modification. *JAMA.* 1995;274:894-901.

Hambye AS, Delsarte P, Vervaet AM. Influence of the different biokinetics of sestamibi and tetrofosmin on the interpretation of myocardial perfusion imaging in daily practice. *Nucl Med Commun.* 2007;28:383-390.

Hatano T, Chikamori T, Usui Y, Morishima T, Hida S, Yamashina A. Diagnostic significance of positive I-123 BMIPP despite negative stress Tl-201 myocardial imaging in patients with suspected coronary artery disease. *Circ J.* 2006;70:184-189.

Hegge FN, Hamilton GW, Larson SM, Ritchie JL, Richards P. Cardiac chamber imaging: a comparison of red blood cells labeled with Tc-99m in vitro and in vivo. *J Nucl Med.* 1978;19:129-134.

Hendel RC, Bateman TM, Cerqueira MD, et al. Initial clinical experience with regadenoson, a novel selective A2A agonist for pharmacologic stress single-photon emission computed tomography myocardial perfusion imaging. *J Am Coll Cardiol.* 2005;46:2069-2075.

Henzlova MJ, Cerqueira MD, Mahmarian JJ, Yao SS. Stress protocols and tracers. *J Nucl Cardiol.* 2006;13:e80-e90.

Herzog BA, Buechel RR, Katz R, et al. Nuclear myocardial perfusion imaging with a cadmium-zinc-telluride detector technique: optimized protocol for scan time reduction. *J Nucl Med.* 2010;51:46-51.

Hesse B, Tagil K, Cuocolo A, et al. EANM/ESC procedural guidelines for myocardial perfusion imaging in nuclear cardiology. *Eur J Nucl Med Mol Imaging.* 2005;32:855-897.

Holly TA, Abbott BG, Al-Mallah M, et al. Single photon-emission computed tomography. *J Nucl Cardiol.* 2010;17:941-973.

Huang SC, Schwaiger M, Carson RE, et al. Quantitative measurement of myocardial blood flow with oxygen-15 water and positron computed tomography: an assessment of potential and problems. *J Nucl Med.* 1985;26:616-625.

Ishimaru S, Tsujino I, Takei T, et al. Focal uptake on 18F-fluoro-2-deoxyglucose positron emission tomography images indicates cardiac involvement of sarcoidosis. *Eur Heart J.* 2005;26:1538-1543.

Iskandrian AE, Bateman TM, Belardinelli L, et al. Adenosine versus regadenoson comparative evaluation in myocardial perfusion imaging: results of the ADVANCE phase 3 multicenter international trial. *J Nucl Cardiol.* 2007;14:645-658.

Kaufmann PA, Camici PG. Myocardial blood flow measurement by PET: technical aspects and clinical applications. *J Nucl Med.* 2005;46:75-88.

Klocke FJ, Baird MG, Lorell BH, et al. ACC/AHA/ASNC guidelines for the clinical use of cardiac radionuclide imaging—executive summary: a report of the American College of Cardiology/American Heart Association Task Force on Practice Guidelines (ACC/AHA/ASNC Committee to Revise the 1995 Guidelines for the Clinical Use of Cardiac Radionuclide Imaging). *Circulation.* 2003;108:1404-1418.

Knesaurek K, Machac J, Krynyckyi BR, Almeida OD. Comparison of 2-dimensional and 3-dimensional 82Rb myocardial perfusion PET imaging. *J Nucl Med.* 2003;44:1350-1356.

Kontos MC, Dilsizian V, Weiland F, et al. Iodofiltic acid I 123 (BMIPP) fatty acid imaging improves initial diagnosis in emergency department patients with suspected acute coronary syndromes: a multicenter trial. *J Am Coll Cardiol.* 2010;56:290-299.

Lazarenko SV, van der Vleuten PA, Tio RA, et al. Left ventricular volume assessment by planar radionuclide ventriculography evaluated by MRI. *Nucl Med Commun.* 2009;30:727-735.

Leppo JA, Meerdink DJ. Comparison of the myocardial uptake of a technetium-labeled isonitrile analogue and thallium. *Circ Res.* 1989;65:632-639.

Lertsburapa K, Ahlberg AW, Bateman TM, et al. Independent and incremental prognostic value of left ventricular ejection fraction determined by stress gated rubidium 82 PET imaging in patients with known or suspected coronary artery disease. *J Nucl Cardiol.* 2008;15:745-753.

Levin CS, Hoffman EJ. Calculation of positron range and its effect on the fundamental limit of positron emission tomography system spatial resolution. *Phys Med Biol.* 1999;44:781-799.

Levine MG, Ahlberg AW, Mann A, et al. Comparison of exercise, dipyridamole, adenosine, and dobutamine stress with the use of Tc-99m tetrofosmin tomographic imaging. *J Nucl Cardiol.* 1999;6:389-396.

Lubberink M, Harms HJ, Halbmeijer R, de Haan S, Knaapen P, Lammertsma AA. Low-dose quantitative myocardial blood flow imaging using 15O-water and PET without attenuation correction. *J Nucl Med.* 2010;51:575-580.

Machac J, Bacharach SL, Bateman TM, et al. Positron emission tomography myocardial perfusion and glucose metabolism imaging. *J Nucl Cardiol.* 2006;13:e121-e151.

Mack RE, Nolting DD, Hogancamp CE, Bing RJ. Myocardial extraction of Rb-86 in the rabbit. *Am J Physiol.* 1959;197:1175-1177.

Maddahi J, Mendez R, Mahmarian JJ, et al. Prospective multicenter evaluation of rapid, gated SPECT myocardial perfusion upright imaging. *J Nucl Cardiol.* 2009;16:351-357.

Massardo T, Gal RA, Grenier RP, Schmidt DH, Port SC. Left ventricular volume calculation using a count-based ratio method applied to multigated radionuclide angiography. *J Nucl Med.* 1990;31:450-456.

Massardo T, Jaimovich R, Lavados H, et al. Comparison of radionuclide ventriculography using SPECT and planar techniques in different cardiac conditions. *Eur J Nucl Med Mol Imaging.* 2007;34:1735-1746.

Moore SC, Kouris K, Cullum I. Collimator design for single photon emission tomography. *Eur J Nucl Med.* 1992;19:138-150.

Mullani NA, Goldstein RA, Gould KL, et al. Myocardial perfusion with rubidium-82. I. Measurement of extraction fraction and flow with external detectors. *J Nucl Med.* 1983;24:898-906.

Muller CE, Jacobson KA. Recent developments in adenosine receptor ligands and their potential as novel drugs. *Biochim Biophys Acta.* 2011;1808:1290-1308.

Muller P, Czernin J, Choi Y, et al. Effect of exercise supplementation during adenosine infusion on hyperemic blood flow and flow reserve. *Am Heart J.* 1994;128:52-60.

Murray JJ, Weiler JM, Schwartz LB, et al. Safety of binodenoson, a selective adenosine A2A receptor agonist vasodilator pharmacological stress agent, in healthy subjects with mild intermittent asthma. *Circ Cardiovasc Imaging.* 2009;2:492-498.

Nichols K, Dorbala S, DePuey EG, Yao SS, Sharma A, Rozanski A. Influence of arrhythmias on gated SPECT myocardial perfusion and function quantification. *J Nucl Med.* 1999;40:924-934.

Nichols K, Yao SS, Kamran M, Faber TL, Cooke CD, DePuey EG. Clinical impact of arrhythmias on gated SPECT cardiac myocardial perfusion and function assessment. *J Nucl Cardiol.* 2001;8:19-30.

Nitzsche EU, Choi Y, Czernin J, Hoh CK, Huang SC, Schelbert HR. Noninvasive quantification of myocardial blood flow in humans: a direct comparison of the [13N]ammonia and the [15O]water techniques. *Circulation.* 1996;93:2000-2006.

O'Keefe Jr JH, Bateman TM, Barnhart CS. Adenosine thallium-201 is superior to exercise thallium-201 for detecting coronary artery disease in patients with left bundle branch block. *J Am Coll Cardiol.* 1993;21:1332-1338.

Okumura W, Iwasaki T, Toyama T, et al. Usefulness of fasting 18F-FDG PET in identification of cardiac sarcoidosis. *J Nucl Med.* 2004;45:1989-1998.

Parkash R, deKemp RA, Ruddy TD, et al. Potential utility of rubidium 82 PET quantification in patients with 3-vessel coronary artery disease. *J Nucl Cardiol.* 2004;11:440-449.

Pavel DG, Zimmer M, Patterson VN. In vivo labeling of red blood cells with 99mTc: a new approach to blood pool visualization. *J Nucl Med.* 1977;18:305-308.

Ratib O, Phelps ME, Huang SC, Henze E, Selin CE, Schelbert HR. Positron tomography with deoxyglucose for estimating local myocardial glucose metabolism. *J Nucl Med.* 1982;23:577-586.

Ravizzini GC, Hanson MW, Shaw LK, et al. Efficiency comparison between 99m Tc-tetrofosmin and 99m Tc-sestamibi myocardial perfusion studies. *Nucl Med Commun.* 2002;23:203-208.

Rimoldi OE, Camici PG. Positron emission tomography for quantitation of myocardial perfusion. *J Nucl Cardiol.* 2004;11:482-490.

Sanchez-Crespo A, Andreo P, Larsson SA. Positron flight in human tissues and its influence on PET image spatial resolution. *Eur J Nucl Med Mol Imaging.* 2004;31:44-51.

Schelbert HR, Phelps ME, Huang SC, et al. N-13 ammonia as an indicator of myocardial blood flow. *Circulation.* 1981;63:1259-1272.

Schelbert HR, Wisenberg G, Phelps ME, et al. Noninvasive assessment of coronary stenoses by myocardial imaging during pharmacologic coronary vasodilation. VI. Detection of coronary artery disease in human beings with intravenous N-13 ammonia and positron computed tomography. *Am J Cardiol.* 1982;49:1197-1207.

Senthamizhchelvan S, Bravo PE, Esaias C, et al. Human biodistribution and radiation dosimetry of 82Rb. *J Nucl Med.* 2010;51:1592-1599.

Senthamizhchelvan S, Bravo PE, Lodge MA, Merrill J, Bengel FM, Sgouros G. Radiation dosimetry of 82Rb in humans under pharmacologic stress. *J Nucl Med.* 2011;52:485-491.

Sharir T, Ben-Haim S, Merzon K, et al. High-speed myocardial perfusion imaging initial clinical comparison with conventional dual detector anger camera imaging. *JACC Cardiovasc Imaging.* 2008;1:156-163.

Sharir T, Slomka PJ, Berman DS. Solid-state SPECT technology: fast and furious. *J Nucl Cardiol.* 2010;17:890-896.

Sharir T, Slomka PJ, Hayes SW, et al. Multicenter trial of high-speed versus conventional single-photon emission computed tomography imaging: quantitative results of myocardial perfusion and left ventricular function. *J Am Coll Cardiol.* 2010;55:1965-1974.

Slomka PJ, Hurwitz GA, Stephenson J, Cradduck T. Automated alignment and sizing of myocardial stress and rest scans to three-dimensional normal templates using an image registration algorithm. *J Nucl Med.* 1995;36:1115-1122.

Slomka PJ, Nishina H, Berman DS, et al. "Motion-frozen" display and quantification of myocardial perfusion. *J Nucl Med.* 2004;45:1128-1134.

Smits P, Corstens FH, Aengevaeren WR, Wackers FJ, Thien T. False-negative dipyridamole-thallium-201 myocardial imaging after caffeine infusion. *J Nucl Med.* 1991;32:1538-1541.

Steinberg JS, Wasserman AG. Radionuclide ventriculography for evaluation and prevention of doxorubicin cardiotoxicity. *Clin Ther.* 1985;7:660-667.

Sugihara IT, Yonekura Y, Miyazaki Y, Taniguchi Y. Estimation of cardiac output by first-pass transit of radiotracers. *Ann Nucl Med.* 1999;13:299-302.

Taillefer R, DePuey EG, Udelson JE, Beller GA, Benjamin C, Gagnon A. Comparison between the end-diastolic images and the summed images of gated 99mTc-sestamibi SPECT perfusion study in detection of coronary artery disease in women. *J Nucl Cardiol.* 1999;6:169-176.

Tamas E, Broqvist M, Olsson E, Franzen S, Nylander E. Exercise radionuclide ventriculography for predicting post-operative left ventricular function in chronic aortic regurgitation. *JACC Cardiovasc Imaging.* 2009;2:48-55.

Tilkemeier PL, Cooke CD, Ficaro EP, Glover DK, Hansen CL, McCallister Jr BD. American Society of Nuclear Cardiology information statement: standardized reporting matrix for radionuclide myocardial perfusion imaging. *J Nucl Cardiol.* 2006;13:e157-e171.

van Eijk CW. Inorganic scintillators in medical imaging. *Phys Med Biol.* 2002;47:R85-R106.

Venero CV, Heller GV, Bateman TM, et al. A multicenter evaluation of a new post-processing method with depth-dependent collimator resolution applied to full-time and half-time acquisitions without and with simultaneously acquired attenuation correction. *J Nucl Cardiol.* 2009;16:714-725.

Votaw JR, White M. Comparison of 2-dimensional and 3-dimensional cardiac 82Rb PET studies. *J Nucl Med.* 2001;42:701-706.

Weich HF, Strauss HW, Pitt B. The extraction of thallium-201 by the myocardium. *Circulation.* 1977;56:188-191.

Wilson RF. Assessing the severity of coronary-artery stenoses. *N Engl J Med.* 1996;334:1735-1737.

Yalamanchili P, Wexler E, Hayes M, et al. Mechanism of uptake and retention of F-18 BMS-747158-02 in cardiomyocytes: a novel PET myocardial imaging agent. *J Nucl Cardiol.* 2007;14:782-788.

Yamagishi H, Shirai N, Takagi M, et al. Identification of cardiac sarcoidosis with (13)N-NH(3)/(18)F-FDG PET. *J Nucl Med.* 2003;44:1030-1036.

Yu M, Guaraldi MT, Mistry M, et al. BMS-747158-02: a novel PET myocardial perfusion imaging agent. *J Nucl Cardiol.* 2007;14:789-798.

CHAPTER 6

Vascular Ultrasound

Tharakeswara K. Bathala

Ultrasound is the most popular noninvasive imaging technique for evaluation of the vascular system. Vascular ultrasound has significant advantages. It provides comprehensive anatomic and flow details of the vascular system, particularly the peripheral vessels. It is easily available, is cost effective when compared with the other vascular imaging methods, and involves no ionizing radiation. However, the diagnostic yield is highly dependent on the expertise of the operator. The patient's body habitus often limits the quality of the examination and visibility of the vessels, especially the intraabdominal vasculature. Certain anatomic and pathologic characteristics of the vessels, such as vessel tortuosity, multifocal tandem atherosclerotic stenosis, and extensive vascular calcifications, pose limitations for the use of vascular ultrasound.

Vascular ultrasound has two basic components: conventional B-mode ultrasonography, which provides morphologic information about the lumen and vessel wall; and Doppler ultrasonography, which displays flow direction and velocity of red blood cells (RBCs).

■ PHYSICAL PRINCIPLES

Ultrasound is a high-frequency sound (by definition, >20,000 Hz, but medical ultrasound imaging frequencies range from 2 to 15 MHz) produced by piezoelectric effect by the elements within the ultrasound transducer. Modern ultrasound machines are equipped with multi-element transducers, with each element having its own circuit. Each transducer is designed to work best at given range of frequencies. The frequency of the transducer depends on the thickness of the piezoelectric element and the voltage applied to the piezoelectric element. The transducers vary by shape (linear or sector), physical functioning principle (mechanical or electronic), and the range of frequencies of the ultrasound beam emitted. The ultrasound frequency determines the depth of penetration and the resolution of the image.

Ultrasound interacts with tissues as it propagates and returns. As an ultrasound wave passes through the tissues, a fraction of it is converted to heat, and a fraction is converted to reflected or scattered ultrasound. The transducer receives and converts the reflected or scattered ultrasound from tissues into electric signals that can then be amplified, analyzed, and displayed to provide both an anatomic image and flow information.

Each ultrasound image is made up of image lines. Each image line is formed by hundreds of grayscale pixels based on the information in the reflected and scattered waves from the tissues. Strong reflectors are depicted by white pixels, and weak reflectors are represented as dark shades of gray. Thus, in B-mode imaging, the vessel wall, which is a strong reflector, appears bright, whereas intravascular blood flow is anechoic because the RBCs are very small and have a very low backscattering coefficient.

Doppler ultrasonography is based on the principle of the Doppler effect. When a wave is reflected from a moving target, the frequency of the perceived wave is different from that of the transmitted wave. This difference in frequency is known as the Doppler shift. The magnitude of the shift depends on the relative motion between the source and the receiver of the sound. The frequency of the perceived wave increases when the source moves toward the receiver, whereas it decreases when the source moves away from the receiver (Fig. 6-1). The direction of the Doppler shift depends on whether the motion is toward or away from the receiver.

In vascular imaging, the Doppler signal is generated by the blood cells that backscatter the transmitted ultrasound wave. Because of relatively low numbers of white blood cells and small size of platelets, the RBCs are generally assumed to be responsible for scattering of ultrasound by blood. Individual RBCs act as point scatterers because their mean diameter is much smaller than the wavelength of the ultrasound.

The Doppler equation is formulated as follows (Fig. 6-2):

$$f_D = f - f_r = 2 f v \cos \theta / c$$

Where f_D is the Doppler shift frequency f is the frequency of the transmitted ultrasound wave, v is the relative velocity of the moving target with respect to the transducer, and c is the speed of sound in the tissue (on average, 1540 m/second); θ is the angle of the direction of the moving target with respect to the transducer. This angle is 0 degrees when the target is moving head-on toward the transducer, and it is 90 degrees when the target is moving parallel to the transducer surface. Factor 2 represents two equal successive Doppler shifts that simply are added together. The first Doppler shift occurs when sound is received by the moving RBCs from the stationary transmitting transducer, and the second occurs when

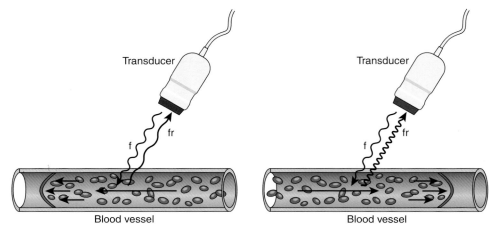

Figure 6-1 Doppler frequency shift. Blood moving away from the probe *(left)* results in decreased perceived frequency (fr) compared with the transmitted frequency (f). When the blood is moving toward the probe *(right)*, the perceived frequency increases.

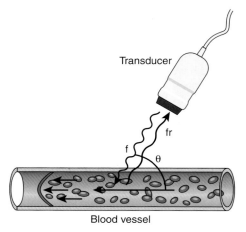

Figure 6-2 Doppler interrogation of a blood vessel with laminar flow.

sound is received by the stationary transducer from the RBCs that now act as a moving source as they reradiate sound back toward the transducer.

The Doppler signal is proportional to frequency shift (f_D). According to the equation, the Doppler frequency shift is directly proportional to the transmitted ultrasound frequency. Thus, higher-frequency transducers are preferred for Doppler studies. Because the rate of attenuation of the ultrasound beam is directly proportional to the transmitted frequency, higher-frequency ultrasound transducers have poor signal from deeper tissues because of high beam attenuation. Conversely, lower-frequency ultrasound transducers have better signal from deeper tissues. Scatterers smaller than the ultrasound wavelength are not good reflectors. For example, RBCs have poor scatter intensity at lower ultrasound frequencies (the wavelength is inversely proportional to the frequency). According to the Rayleigh theory of wave scattering, the scattered intensity increases with the fourth power of the ratio of scatterer (RBC) size to wavelength. For higher ultrasound frequencies with shorter wavelengths, the scattering from RBCs increases. Thus, 8-MHz ultrasound gives the strongest signal from the carotid arteries 2 cm deep under the fat and muscle in

the neck; 3.5-MHz ultrasound has good penetration and gives the strongest echo from the renal arteries 10 cm deep under the muscle and fat in the abdomen.

The Doppler signal also depends on the angle between the direction of motion and the axis of the ultrasound beam. The Doppler shift is maximum and so is Doppler signal when the blood flow is parallel (*cos θ* is equal to 1) to the ultrasound beam and is zero when the blood flow is at right angles (*cos 90* is equal to 0) to the ultrasound beam. In clinical practice, the ultrasound beam is aligned to make a 30- to 60-degree angle with the arterial lumen to obtain a reliable Doppler signal. Other important factors that affect Doppler signal are the velocity and number of the blood cells in the sample volume.

The two main types of Doppler ultrasound equipment in clinical use today are continuous wave Doppler and pulsed wave Doppler. In continuous wave Doppler, the probe contains two piezoelectric crystals, one to transmit the ultrasound wave continuously and the other to receive from the sensitive region of the beam (which is at the intersection of the transmitted and returning beams) continuously. The equipment usually operates at one continuous frequency. Continuous wave Doppler simultaneously analyzes many returning signals from multiple vessels in the line of the beam and thus has no range or depth information. It does not provide directional information about the flow, nor does it have axial resolution. The operator must distinguish veins and arteries by flow characteristics alone because the images provide only qualitative information (magnitude of Doppler shift). Continuous wave Doppler is resistant to aliasing and is more sensitive to slow flow than is pulsed wave Doppler. In current practice, continuous wave Doppler is used in cardiac examinations and in pressure studies for evaluating the peripheral arteries.

Newer ultrasound devices use the pulsed wave Doppler ultrasound technique. As the name suggests, the pulsed wave Doppler ultrasound probe transmits short bursts of ultrasound at regular intervals and receives them as they return. This system measures the phase shift in the received signal by using the mathematical process of autocorrelation. It obtains phase shift information by sampling the same sample volume multiple times and analyzing the echoes. The information obtained by measuring the phase shift is almost the same as that obtained by measuring the frequency shift, with certain limitations. In contrast to continuous wave Doppler systems, pulsed wave Doppler ultrasound provides information about the velocity and direction of flow. In addition, pulsed wave Doppler allows precise control over range in tissue (depth) and sample volume. The range in tissue at which Doppler signals are detected can be controlled simply by changing the length of time the system waits after sending a pulse before it changes to receiver mode. The location of the sample volume within the area of interest is guided by real-time B-mode imaging. This combination of real-time B-mode imaging and pulsed Doppler technique is known as duplex scanning. Color Doppler and spectral Doppler devices use pulsed wave Doppler techniques to process information that can provide flow characteristics such as velocity and direction.

Color Doppler translates Doppler phase shift information containing velocity details from an area of interest into color-coded images. Two basic colors are used to specify the direction of flow in the area of interest, and this color display is usually superimposed on the conventional B-mode image. Typically, blue represents positive flow, which is toward the heart, whereas copper represents negative flow, which is away from the heart. The depth and width of the Doppler interrogation in the area of interest are usually defined by the user and are known as the color window. This technique is particularly useful for identifying the location of abnormal velocity and for mapping the extent of flow in anatomic regions for stenosis, aneurysm, or turbulence.

Spectral Doppler is another form of pulsed wave Doppler that analyzes Doppler frequency shift information from a specific area within a vessel and displays it as a function of time. The focal area interrogated by spectral Doppler is known as the range gate (sample volume). The spectrum of velocities of blood cells within the range gate is displayed in a waveform on a two-dimensional display with time on the x-axis and frequency on the y-axis. Depending on the direction of flow, spectrum is deflected on either side of the x-axis (baseline). In clinical practise, positive Doppler frequency shifts (blood moving toward the probe) are displayed above the baseline, and negative Doppler shifts (blood moving away from the probe) are displayed below the baseline. The amplitude of each velocity component is depicted as grayscale brightness of the spectral waveform. It takes approximately 64 to 128 pulses per scan line to calculate the spectral Doppler shift. The maximum possible pulse repetition frequency (PRF) and maximum recordable Doppler shift depend on the depth of the range gate. The new ultrasound pulse should not be emitted before all information from the previous pulse is received, for optimal quantification of Doppler shifts. Thus, PRF should be at least twice the maximum velocity (or Doppler shift frequency) of blood within a vessel to display actual measurements without ambiguity. The Nyquist limit is the maximum Doppler shift frequency that can be measured without aliasing, usually less than PRF / 2. The spectral Doppler technique is used to quantify flow velocities and to identify abnormal blood flow.

The Doppler shift frequency may also be represented as an audible sound. It is qualitative: a higher pitch of the sound usually indicates a larger Doppler shift (or higher velocities). In addition, this frequency is independent of the direction of blood flow.

Power Doppler ultrasound is another Doppler technique that measures the amplitude of the Doppler frequency shift independent of the Doppler angle. The magnitude of the Doppler frequency shift is usually displayed with one color of varying brightness by the autocorrelation technique. Power Doppler ultrasound displays neither flow direction nor flow velocities. Because of its better signal-to-noise ratio, power Doppler is sensitive to slow flow velocities in small vessels.

B-flow imaging is a newer vascular imaging method that images blood vessels in B-mode without application of the Doppler principle. This technique measures the amplitude of scatterers in flowing blood to construct a grayscale image with shades of gray. B-flow imaging depicts the vessel lumen, plaque characteristics, and broad spectrum of velocities better than does color Doppler because of a higher frame rate and better special resolution. Nonapplication of the Doppler principle means that B-flow imaging is resistant to artifacts such as aliasing and overamplification of the signal. Because B-flow imaging is a B-mode technique, estimation of blood flow velocities and determination of flow direction are not possible.

Ultrasound contrast imaging uses microbubble contrast media to image blood vessels. The injected intravascular microbubbles act as nonlinear reflectors or scatterers of the ultrasound beam and can be imaged using B-mode and Doppler techniques.

Pearls and Pitfalls

- For spectral Doppler imaging, high PRF settings are used when high flow velocities are suspected. The PRF depends on the depth of the range gate: the closer the range gate to the transducer, the higher the maximum PRF that can be used; the shorter the depth of the range gate, the higher the maximum PRF that can be used.
- Color Doppler imaging provides visual representation of flow direction and areas of increased velocities. Quantification and accurate flow characteristics are best evaluated with spectral Doppler techniques.
- The most important advantage of power Doppler imaging is improved flow sensitivity because of an increased signal-to-noise ratio and the ability to use a low PRF. The Doppler signal is independent of the angle of insonation. Aliasing is not seen in power Doppler imaging because the amplitude is independent of flow direction. Power Doppler imaging lacks velocity and flow direction information. It is prone to flash artifact secondary to tissue motion, especially in a low-PRF setting.

■ PROBLEM SOLVING: IMAGE OPTIMIZATION

Optimal image acquisition in vascular ultrasound depends on two main factors: ultrasound technique and instrumentation. Ultrasound technique largely relies on the individual sonographer's skill and experience. Adoption of good technique and a standard imaging protocol with sound knowledge of anatomy and vascular hemodynamics can yield better images. A good practice is to image blood vessels in the B-mode, to visualize normal anatomy and pathologic features, before color Doppler is performed for qualitative assessment of blood flow and flow abnormalities. Finally, spectral Doppler imaging is used to assess vascular flow quantitatively. Most modern ultrasound Doppler equipment is configured to image various specific anatomic regions with predetermined scan parameters. However, proper instrument selection and knowledge of the scanning parameters as detailed here are crucial for optimal vascular ultrasound imaging.

1. Transducer frequency determines the depth of view and the strength of the Doppler signal.
2. Gain is the amplitude of the received signals over the total length of the ultrasound beam. B-mode gain increases the overall brightness of the image and helps display contrast among various tissues. The color and spectral Doppler gain determines the sensitivity to detect flow in a given sample volume.
3. Time gain compensation (TGC) allows step-up or step-down amplification of sound from various depths to compensate for the effect of attenuation.
4. The focal zone is the point of greatest intensity at which the width of the ultrasound beam is at its narrowest and has best lateral resolution.
5. High-pass filter removes unwanted frequencies (generated from vessel wall and adjacent soft tissue motion) below a set frequency limit.
6. The baseline is the center of the spectral Doppler display, and it corresponds to a zero Doppler shift or zero velocity. The baseline and velocity scale should be adjusted in such a way that the entire spectrum of waveform is visible in a single frame.
7. The angle of insonation is the angle at which the ultrasound beam intersects the blood flow. The Doppler frequency increases as the ultrasound beam becomes more aligned to the flow direction.
8. Sample volume is the site in which the ultrasound beam interrogates the blood cells in the area of interest. In color Doppler technique, the size, shape, and location of the sample volume determine where the color display of the Doppler frequency shift will occur. Sample volume in spectral Doppler imaging determines the segment of vessels to be sampled for spectral analysis.
9. PRF determines the rate at which the transducer generates the ultrasound pulse. In clinical practise, low PRF is used to detect low velocities, and high PRF is used for detection of high velocity. In addition, the deeper the sample volume is in the tissue, the lower the PRF should be to detect slow flow.

Pearls: General Scanning Technique

- Select the appropriate probe frequency and footprint based on the anatomic region.
- Always start scanning blood vessels in the B-mode first and then follow with color and spectral Doppler imaging.
- Select an acoustic window where the target vessels are in the most superficial plane and are visible through soft tissues of uniform density, such as muscle.
- Position the focal zone just deep to the area of interest for better lateral resolution.
- In B-mode, try to examine the vessel in a plane perpendicular to the vascular lumen for better visualization of the vessel wall, plaques, or thrombus.
- Optimize the gain setting in such a way that no noise is seen within the lumen on B-mode imaging, filling of color is uniform within the lumen on color Doppler imaging, and no noise is noted in the spectral display.
- Keep the sample volume (color box) small to the area of interest in color Doppler imaging to achieve a higher frame rate.
- Steer the sample volume or "heel and toe" the transducer to insonate the vessel of interest at an angle of up to 60 degrees.
- Use a high-frequency transducer to increase the Doppler shift if low-velocity flow is suspected.
- In spectral Doppler imaging, set the wall filter at the minimum level to detect low velocities and set it at a high level to omit wall motion artifact.

Doppler Artifacts

Artifacts result from inadequate transducer and image acquisition settings, anatomic factors, and hemodynamic changes. Various Doppler artifacts are listed in Table 6-1.

■ BLOOD VESSELS AND HEMODYNAMICS

Arterial Flow Dynamics

The systemic circulation is a closed-loop system in which the pressure wave generated by the left ventricle travels along the aorta, arteries, arterioles, capillaries, venules, and veins and finally reaches the right ventricle. Systemic pressure is highest at the left ventricle and decreases as it moves distally. Blood flows in the arteries because of the pressure gradient between the arterial and venous ends of the heart. The driving pressure for flow within a vessel is determined by its potential energy generated by left ventricular contraction that distends the vessel wall and the kinetic energy acquired by flow itself. The pulsatile arterial flow signal is a summation of forward flow from the left ventricle and reverse flow from tidal reflection (Fig. 6-3).

In most vessels, blood moves in concentric layers, a process known as laminar flow (Fig. 6-4). Flow is fastest in the center of the vessel and decreases toward the wall, and it becomes absent adjacent to the vessel wall. The profile for laminar flow is determined by frictional and inertial forces between the layers of blood and changes throughout the pulse cycle. Soon after the pressure wave propagates, flow begins as a result of the high-pressure–to–low-pressure gradient. Blood velocity increases uniformly across the vessel in early systole as fluid motion begins. As the pressure wave begins to propagate, however, a parabolic flow profile results from the friction induced on the fluid layer close to the vessel

Table 6-1   Doppler Artifacts

Artifacts	Identification	Solution	Comments
Aliasing: results when the velocity of blood exceeds one half of the pulse repetition frequency (Nyquist limit)	Color Doppler: velocities higher than Nyquist limit in a vessel code as reversed color. Spectral Doppler depicts higher velocities as if flow is reversed (wrapped around)	Increase pulse repetition frequency (velocity scale). Decrease probe frequency. Increase angle of insonation. Move baseline in spectral Doppler to see complete waveform	Only pulsed Doppler technique subject to aliasing. Aliasing potentially mistaken for flow reversal or turbulent flow
Spectral broadening: spectrum of velocities in a given sample volume determines degree of spectral broadening. Insonating angle >60 degrees and backscattered frequencies from various angles can lead to spectral broadening in normal vessel	Laminar flow with most RBCs traveling at constant uniform velocity have clear spectral window. Turbulent flow secondary to any cause such as stenosis has greater spectral broadening because of wide range of velocities in sample volume	Keep insonating angle at <60 degrees. Transducer with optimal aperture size. Decrease sample size	Spectral broadening an important sign to detect turbulent flow; avoiding false-positive spectral broadening secondary to technique and instrumentation can detect disease more accurately
Flow direction artifact seen when curved vessels examined by color Doppler	Absent color Doppler signal noted when flow is perpendicular (angle of insonation 90 degrees) to transducer. Curved or branching artery or vein in color window may encode two different colors depending on direction of flow with respect to transducer	Beam steering. Scanning vessel at different insonating angle or probe position	Angle of insonation and proper scanning plane essential for optimal Doppler signal detection
Mirror-image artifact seen when vessel is adjacent to highly reflective surface such as diaphragm and pleura-lung interface	In spectral Doppler, waveform seen on either side of baseline. It is seen with high receiver gain for detecting low-velocity flow. In B-mode and color Doppler, mirror image of vessel seen deep to the true vessel	Adjust insonating angle to <60 degrees and decrease receiver gain	Proper knowledge of anatomy around highly reflective surfaces can avoid misinterpretation of artifact
Side lobe or grating artifact is display of Doppler signal from area interrogated by weak side-lobe beam	Depending on signal strength and direction, artificial waveform can be displayed along main spectral waveform	Change probe position and insonating angle	

wall. A thin layer of blood with zero velocity seen adjacent to the vessel wall becomes thicker when flow velocity decreases or if the wall is irregular. This results in disturbed flow with segments of stationary or reversed flow. This phenomenon is seen at sites of arterial dilatation, curvature, branching, or bifurcation. Turbulent flow is a disturbed flow pattern with chaotic fluid movements and significant irreversible loss of energy. The disturbed flow and turbulence flow are seen at the entrance and exit of stenosis with a drop in arterial pressure in the downstream vessel.

Blood flow within the vascular system is a complex phenomenon. It is influenced by numerous factors such as cardiac function, vessel compliance, peripheral resistance, tone of vascular musculature, blood viscosity, pattern of branching and collateral vessels, vasoconstriction, vasodilation, exercise, and autoregulation. The dynamics of pulsatile flow change periodically over time with cardiac function, and phases of acceleration and deceleration vary in relation to changes in pressure. A uniform steady flow is maintained in the vessels as the pressure amplitude created by left ventricular contraction is reduced by compliance of the aorta and other large elastic arteries.

Another important factor that influences the movement of blood in the vascular system is peripheral resistance. Arterioles and capillaries located in the microcirculation control the resistance to blood flow in the arteries and determine how much blood flows through a particular anatomic region. These arterioles and capillaries have vast numbers of smooth muscle cells. By contracting or relaxing these muscles, arterioles can alter their diameter and thus change the resistance to flow. Two types of regulation exist, based on the anatomic region and physiologic needs of the body. Autoregulation maintains a constant blood flow (cerebral perfusion, renal vessels), whereas adaptive regulation varies the blood supply according to the demand (extremity vessels). Based on resistance, two distinct flow patterns are recognized: low–peripheral resistance flow and high–peripheral resistance flow. Low–peripheral resistance flow is characterized by continuous forward flow, which is inherently seen in arteries supplying the parenchymal organs and the brain. High–peripheral resistance flow is characterized by low, absent, or reversed flow during diastole and is seen in arteries supplying the limbs and the small intestine.

The pulsatile arterial flow demonstrates three typical wave patterns on Doppler spectrum imaging with

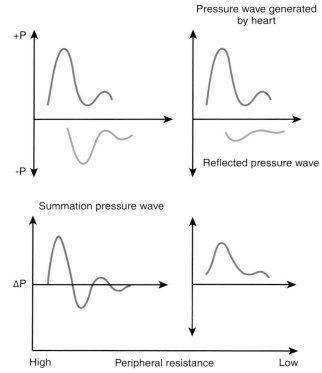

Figure 6-3 *Top,* Two pressure (P) waves with the same amplitude (above the baseline). The reflected pressure waves are depicted below the baseline. The *top left corner image* represents the pressure wave from a high–peripheral resistance vascular bed, and the *top right corner image* represents the pressure wave from a low–peripheral resistance vascular bed. *Bottom,* Summation pressure waves: high pulsatile wave with diastolic flow reversal in high-resistance arteries *(bottom left)* and low pulsatile wave with forward diastolic flow in low-resistance arteries *(bottom right).*

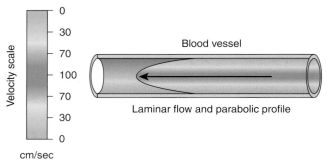

Figure 6-4 Laminar flow with parabolic profile in a blood vessel.

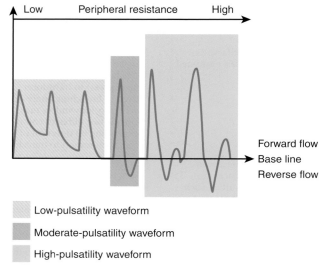

Figure 6-5 Typical spectral wave pattern.

each cardiac cycle that begin with systole and terminate at the end of diastole (Fig. 6-5). Low-pulsatility Doppler waveforms have a broad systolic peak and forward flow throughout diastole. Given that low-pulsatility waveforms are either above or below the Doppler spectrum baseline, they are also known as monophasic waveforms. The arteries with low peripheral resistance flow, such as the carotid, vertebral, and renal arteries (Fig. 6-6), have low-pulsatility waveforms in physiologically normal individuals. Moderate-pulsatility Doppler waveforms have a tall and sharp systolic peak with forward flow during all of diastole. The blood flow during diastole is relatively less than is the flow seen in low–peripheral resistance vessels because of moderate peripheral resistance. This pattern is typically seen in the external carotid artery (Fig. 6-7) and in the superior mesenteric artery during the fasting state. A dicrotic notch is a normal finding that results from closure of the aortic valve, with temporary cessation of forward flow, followed by resumption of forward flow driven by elastic rebound of the arterial wall. Moderate–peripheral resistance vessels also demonstrate a spectral wave pattern known as biphasic flow, which contains a single antegrade wave and a single retrograde wave in a cardiac cycle. High-pulsatility Doppler waveforms have narrow, tall, sharp systolic peaks and reversed or absent diastolic

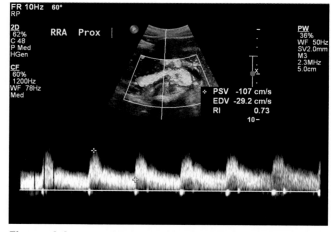

Figure 6-6 Longitudinal color and spectral Doppler image of the right renal artery (RRA) showing a low-resistance waveform with a significant amount of flow during diastole (monophasic flow). *CF,* ???; *EDV,* end-diastolic volume; *FR,* frequency; *Prox,* proximal; *PSV,* peak systolic velocity; *PW,* ???; *RI,* resistive index.

flow. This pattern is typically seen in peripheral arteries in the resting phase and is classically known as a triphasic waveform (Fig. 6-8), which consists of a sharp systolic peak (phase I), followed by brief flow reversal (phase II) and then by brief forward flow (phase III).

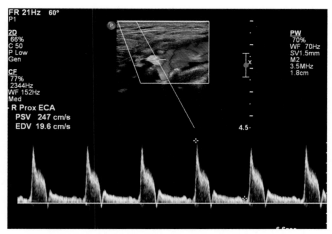

Figure 6-7 Longitudinal color and spectral Doppler image of the external carotid artery (ECA) showing a moderate-resistive waveform with minimal flow during diastole (biphasic flow). *EDV,* End-diastolic velocity; *FR,* frequency; *Prox,* proximal; *PSV,* peak systolic velocity.

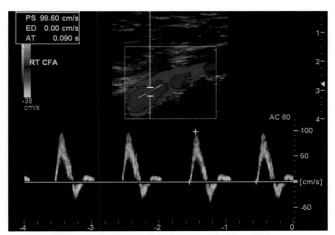

Figure 6-8 Longitudinal color and spectral Doppler image of the right common femoral artery (RT CFA) showing a high-resistive waveform with reversed flow during diastole (triphasic flow). *AC,* Angle correction; *AT,* acceleration time; *ED,* end-diastolic velocity; *PS,* peak systolic velocity.

Venous Hemodynamics

Venous flow to the heart is a passive process through intermittent contraction of adjacent muscles. In addition, the transmitted systolic pressure through the microcirculation maintains a slow forward pressure within the veins. Various factors influence the dynamics of venous flow. Vasodilatation with exercise increases venous return, and vasoconstriction secondary to cold or arterial insufficiency decreases venous return. Inspiration increases the intrathoracic pressure, which causes increased venous return from the upper limb and decreased return from the lower limb. Expiration decreases the intrathoracic pressure and leads to increased venous return from the lower limb but slow return from the upper limb. The Valsalva maneuver slows or stops venous flow by increasing intrathoracic and intraabdominal pressure. Right-sided heart events are transmitted to the central

veins such as the superior vena cava, brachiocephalic vein, inferior vena cava, and hepatic veins.

Spectral Waveform Analysis

The Doppler spectral waveform is a graphic display of the frequency shifts or velocities of all RBCs in the Doppler sample volume on the y-axis and time on the x-axis. The direction of flow relative to the ultrasound beam is displayed relative to the baseline. The amplitude of each velocity component (RBC) is represented as a shade of gray. The laminar flow pattern seen in normal arteries generates a thin waveform because most of the RBCs are traveling at certain constant velocity in the same direction. The clear area under this curve is called the spectral window. In disturbed flow, RBCs in the sample volume have less orderly and uniform flow, thus leading to spectral broadening or widening of the spectral waveform. This finding is seen at the areas of vascular bifurcation, curves, kinks, stenosis, and arteriovenous shunts.

The Doppler spectral waveform can be analyzed by qualitatively, either by visual inspection or by listening to the auditory signal for vascular flow abnormalities. More objective analysis can be performed by measuring peak systolic velocity (PSV), diastolic velocity, mean velocity, acceleration time, acceleration rate, and Doppler indices such as systolic-to-diastolic ratio, pulsatility index, and resistive index (Fig. 6-9).

■ VASCULAR DISEASE

Arterial Stenosis

Atherosclerosis is the most common disease that affects the arterial wall and causes arterial stenosis. Symptoms depend on the severity of stenosis and the reduction in the luminal diameter (Fig. 6-10). Stenosis becomes hemodynamically significant and causes symptoms when the vessel diameter is reduced by at least 50%. Abrupt narrowing of the vascular lumen is associated with an increase in blood flow velocity through the stenotic segment. In addition, the parabolic laminar flow profile changes to a plug profile at the stenotic segment and to disturbed or turbulent flow in the poststenotic segment. The spectral Doppler image displays these hemodynamic changes as high-resistance flow in the prestenotic segment, high-velocity flow with spectral broadening at the site of stenosis, and low-resistance monophasic flow with increased diastolic flow at the poststenotic segment (Figs. 6-11 and 6-12). A 50% decrease in luminal diameter, corresponding to a 75% decrease in cross-sectional area, results in a fourfold higher flow velocity. The PSV, end-diastolic velocity, and systolic velocity ratio (ratio of the PSV in the stenotic zone to the PSV in the normal zone proximal to the stenosis) are commonly used parameters to assess the degree of stenosis.

Aneurysm

Aneurysm results in an abnormal increase in the vessel diameter that leads to disturbed flow with decreased

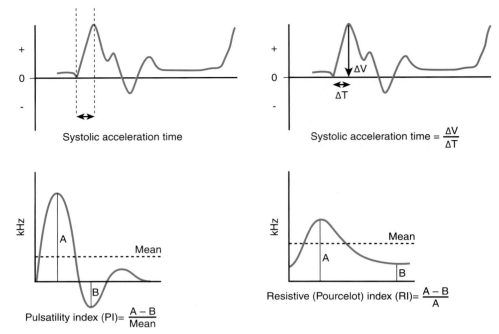

Figure 6-9 Doppler indices.

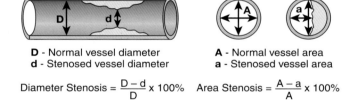

Figure 6-10 Methods to calculate the percentage of change in diameter and area in a diseased vessel.

velocities. Spectral Doppler imaging demonstrates a multiphasic spectrum with a mixed color spectrum resulting from the turbulent flow. Pseudoaneurysms have a communication with the arterial lumen through a narrow neck in which to-and-fro flow with a yin-yang pattern is seen within the aneurysm sac (Fig. 6-13).

Arteriovenous Shunts

Communication between the arteries and veins can be congenital, as in malformations, or iatrogenic or traumatic in origin. Because of the direct communication, the systolic pressure wave is directly transmitted to the venous end without any peripheral resistance, thereby leading to arterialization of the veins. Thus, afferent arterial flow demonstrates turbulent high-velocity flow throughout the cardiac cycle.

Steal Phenomenon

The vertebral arteries have antegrade flow during the entire cardiac cycle. In cases of subclavian artery stenosis proximal to the origin of the vertebral artery, blood flow may assume a retrograde pattern known as steal phenomenon to compensate for blood flow to the ipsilateral upper limb. End-diastolic flow is the first Doppler parameter to become abnormal in the vertebral arteries. As the steal phenomenon progresses, monophasic flow becomes biphasic and then is completely reversed (Fig. 6-14).

Venous Thrombosis and Venous Obstruction

Acute venous thrombus fills the lumen and distends the vein without compressibility and venous flow. Veins in the upstream venous system demonstrate stagnant or decreased flow, with loss of respiratory or cardiac modulation. Depending on the underlying cause and the patient's response to treatment, thrombus can propagate within veins or recanalize. Chronic venous thrombus causes partial or complete occlusion of the vein, with fibrotic changes and collateral vessel formation.

■ CONCLUSION

Vascular ultrasound is an important noninvasive imaging modality for evaluating vascular disease. B-mode and Doppler ultrasound techniques remain valuable tools in the assessment of vascular anatomy and hemodynamics. Pulsed Doppler is the most widely used ultrasound technique. Good scanning technique and optimal scan parameters are crucial for generating clinically relevant images. Most vascular flow abnormalities are diagnosed using Doppler ultrasound in conjunction with having a good understanding of vascular hemodynamics.

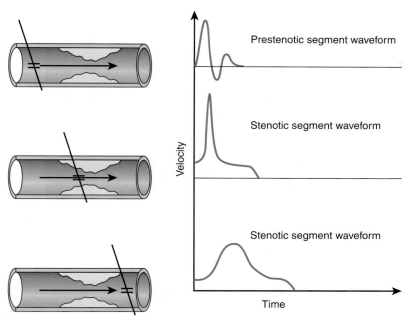

Figure 6-11 Changes in the spectral waveform at various segments of a diseased artery.

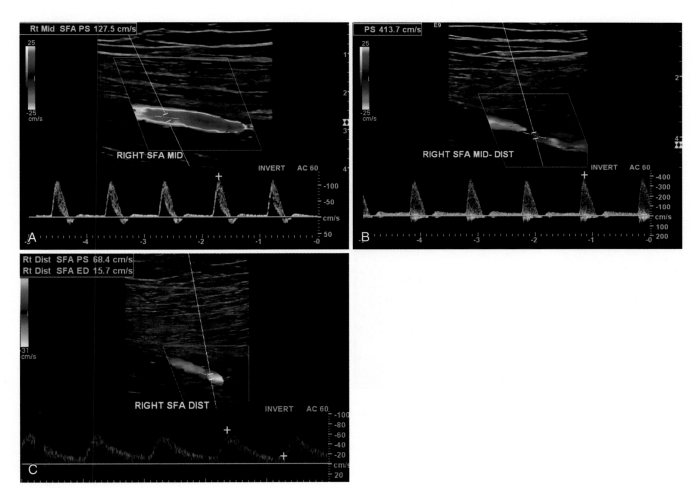

Figure 6-12 **A,** Longitudinal color and spectral Doppler image of the prestenotic femoral artery (SFA) showing a high-resistive waveform with reversed flow during diastole. **B,** Longitudinal color and spectral Doppler image of the stenotic segment femoral artery showing high-velocity turbulent flow with spectral broadening. **C,** Longitudinal color and spectral Doppler image of the poststenotic femoral artery showing a low-resistive waveform with forward flow during diastole. *AC,* angle correction; *DIST,* distal; *ED,* end-diastolic velocity; *MID,* middle; *PS,* peak systolic velocity.

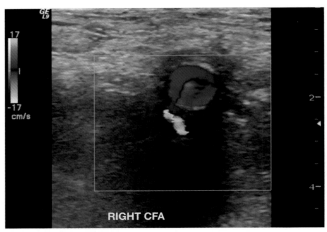

Figure 6-13 Axial color Doppler image of a pseudoaneurysm arising from the common femoral artery (CFA) showing typical to-and-fro flow with a yin-yang pattern.

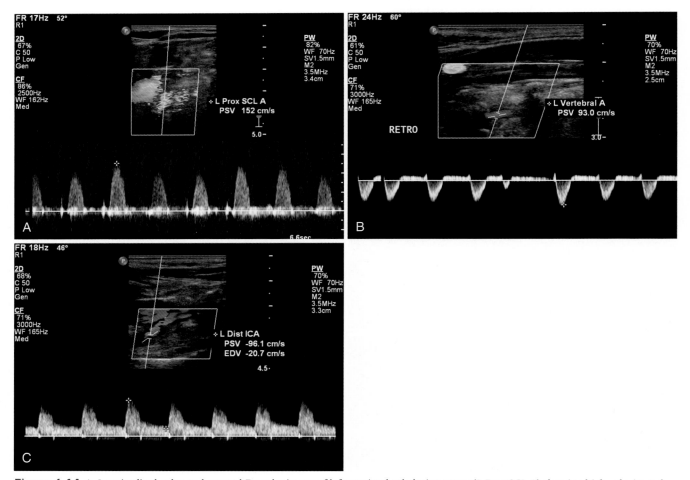

Figure 6-14 A, Longitudinal color and spectral Doppler image of left proximal subclavian artery (L Prox SCL A) showing high-velocity turbulent flow with spectral broadening suggestive of stenosis. **B,** Longitudinal color and spectral Doppler image of the left vertebral artery (L Vertebral A) showing reversed flow. **C,** Longitudinal color and spectral Doppler image of the left distal internal carotid artery (L Dist ICA) showing a low-resistant waveform with forward flow in diastole. Both the vertebral and carotid arteries show forward flow in physiologically normal individuals. In the presence of subclavian steal from proximal subclavian artery stenosis, flow in the vertebral artery reverses. *EDV,* end-diastolic velocity; *PSV,* peak systolic velocity.

Bibliography

Knighton RA, Priest DL, Zwiebel WJ, Lawrence PF, Miller FJ, Rose SC. Techniques for color flow sonography of the lower extremity. *Radiographics.* 1990;10:775-786.

Kruskal JB, Newman PA, Sammons LG, Kane RA. Optimizing Doppler and color flow US: application to hepatic sonography. *Radiographics.* 2004;24:657-675.

Liu JB, Merton DA, Mitchell DG, Needleman L, Kurtz AB, Goldberg BB. Color Doppler imaging of the iliofemoral region. *Radiographics.* 1990;10:403-412.

Pozniak MA, Zagzebski JA, Scanlan KA. Spectral and color Doppler artifacts. *Radiographics.* 1992;12:35-44.

Tahmasebpour HR, Buckley AR, Cooperberg PL, Fix CH. Sonographic examination of the carotid arteries. *Radiographics.* 2005;25:1561-1575.

CHAPTER 7

Computed Tomography Angiography (Vascular)

Avinash Kambadakone

Computed tomography angiography (CTA) is an exciting technology that allows noninvasive assessment of the vasculature. Over the past few decades, the use of CTA has grown tremendously due to the introduction of multidetector CT (MDCT), which enables acquisition of isotropic volumetric data. Technologic advances in MDCT, coupled with the advances in imaging workstations, have permitted high-quality multiplanar and three-dimensional (3-D) reformations that have opened new paradigms in the field of vascular imaging. As a consequence of these developments, MDCT angiography has superseded conventional catheter-based angiography as the preferred technique for diagnosis of cardiovascular disease. Ongoing innovations in MDCT technology, such as the introduction of dual energy CT (DECT), have further diversified the role of imaging in visualization and characterization of vascular abnormalities. MDCT angiography has thus positioned itself as an integral component in the multidisciplinary management of patients with cardiovascular disease not only by facilitating accurate diagnosis but also by enabling post-treatment follow-up.

The dramatic growth in the field of CTA began with the introduction of spiral or helical CT and achieved greater strides with MDCT, which allowed volumetric acquisition in a single breath hold. The advantages of MDCT over single detector CT include increased temporal and spatial resolution, decreased image noise, efficient x-ray tube use, and longer anatomic coverage, all of which help increase the diagnostic accuracy of the examination. Better z-axis resolution and larger scan volumes also result in improved multiplanar reconstruction in the coronal and sagittal planes. The reduced scanning time achieved by MDCT also helps reduce respiratory and motion artifacts. The development of electrocardiogram gating technology synchronized with CT data acquisition has enabled acquisition of high-resolution images of the heart and coronary arteries within a single breath hold and has thus eliminated motion artifacts. The superiority of MDCT has also been enhanced by improved image postprocessing techniques, which have expanded the role of modern day CTA to virtually all vascular territories. This chapter discusses the key concepts of MDCT angiography technique in the evaluation of vascular disease.

■ CATHETER VERSUS COMPUTED TOMOGRAPHY ANGIOGRAPHY

MDCT angiography offers several advantages over conventional catheter-based angiography. The first and foremost benefit is the noninvasive nature of CTA, which limits the morbidity associated with catheter angiography and often causes little patient discomfort. Several of the vascular complications related to catheter angiography (e.g., bleeding, groin hematoma, and vascular thrombosis) are not encountered with CTA. Second, whereas catheter-based angiography provides a limited luminal view of the blood vessels, the volumetric acquisition with MDCT allows clear anatomic definition of the lumen, as well as of mural thrombus, atherosclerotic plaque, vessel wall, and adjacent structures. The exoluminal information provided by MDCT is particularly important when dealing with complex vascular diseases such as for (1) identifying pseudoaneurysms, (2) allowing accurate delineation of true and false luminal flow in arterial dissections, (3) showing perigraft blood flow in aortic stent grafts, and/or (4) depicting hematoma in traumatic vascular injuries. Third, CTA provides excellent depiction of the atherosclerotic plaque complex and its composition (i.e., fibrofatty versus calcified) that can have significant ramifications in patient management. Fourth, the cross-sectional nature of CT data acquisition allows simultaneous assessment of the function and integrity of target organs supplied by the vessels. For example, CT allows detection of ischemic changes in the bowel wall in mesenteric ischemia and delineation of the extent of cerebral infarction in carotid occlusive disease. This additional assessment of end-organ perfusion allows the referring physician to make crucial clinical decisions and has contributed to the frequent use of CTA in routine practice.

■ COMPUTED TOMOGRAPHY ANGIOGRAPHY: BASIC CONCEPTS

The basic principle of CTA is similar to that of catheter angiography because it exploits the inherent ability of iodinated contrast material (CM) to absorb x-rays and thereby generate an attenuation difference between the vessel and surrounding structures. This enhancement or the increase in attenuation in a given vessel achieved following intravascular injection of iodinated CM is directly proportional to the iodine concentration. The central purpose of CTA is to achieve an adequate iodine concentration (and thus increased attenuation) within the vessel of interest to enable accurate delineation of the vascular anatomy and disease. However, in contrast to catheter angiography, which involves direct arterial injection of CM, CTA involves intravenous administration of the CM to obtain arterial or venous opacification. Thus, the contrast dynamics governing arterial opacification in CTA are different from those involved in catheter angiography. Moreover, arterial opacification in CTA is not a static process, but rather a dynamic one dependent on several interconnected factors broadly classified as (1) patient-related factors, (2) CM-related factors, and (3) technical parameters. The following sections discuss these factors in greater detail. However, given the wide range of CT technology available, the varying patient physiologic features, the different vascular territories, and the complex cardiovascular diseases encountered, no universal CTA strategy exists. The following discussion is intended as a guide for basic understanding of CTA technique.

Patient-Related Factors

In terms of contrast dynamics and the CTA technique, understanding the influence of patient-related factors is very important. Out of the several patient-related factors, the most relevant include patient body habitus and cardiac output. Certain other factors (e.g., renal function and venous access) are also key to obtain a diagnostically acceptable CTA study. The targeted vascular structure and clinical situation also are essential for planning a CTA examination.

Patient Body Habitus

During planning of CTA, the body habitus of a patient needs careful consideration because of its impact on contrast dynamics. The common measures used to estimate body habitus include the body weight and body mass index. The body weight and the magnitude of contrast enhancement in a CTA examination are inversely related to each other. Therefore, for a given dose of iodinated CM, large patients have a lower degree of contrast enhancement than do small patients. The contrast circulation time and the timing of contrast enhancement (e.g., arterial peak) are not affected by body weight for the most part. The volume and injection rate of the CM should be tailored to the patient's body weight (i.e., the CTA protocol should be different in large and small patients). When planning CM protocols in patients of large body weight, the following strategies are beneficial: (1) using a higher overall iodine dose (i.e., higher CM volume or concentration) to maintain a constant degree of contrast enhancement and (2) using a faster injection rate to augment the magnitude of contrast enhancement.

Cardiac Output

Cardiac output is a crucial factor affecting the CM circulation time and so determines the timing of contrast enhancement during CTA. Cardiac output governs the

following components of contrast dynamics: the time of CM bolus arrival, the peak arterial and parenchymal enhancement, and clearance of the CM from the circulation. The time duration between the injection of CM through an intravenous route and the peak arterial enhancement in the aorta are directly proportional to cardiac output. However, the magnitude of arterial enhancement is inversely related to cardiac output. Therefore, the degree of arterial enhancement is lower in patients with high cardiac output as compared with patients with low cardiac output. In addition, in patients with low cardiac output, an increased and prolonged magnitude of peak aortic enhancement results from the late peak arterial enhancement because of delayed arrival of the CM and the reduced clearance of the CM from circulation. Given the significant interpatient and intrapatient variability of cardiac output, the scan timing must be individualized for each patient. The scan timing can be tailored to each patient either by test bolus or through a bolus tracking technique (discussed in detail later).

Renal Function

Patients must be screened before CTA to assess for risk of CM-induced nephropathy. A detailed discussion of this disorder is beyond the scope of this chapter. Serum creatinine and (estimated glomerular filtration rate [eGFR]) should be routinely checked before CM use in high-risk patients such as those with diabetes, myeloma, sickle cell anemia, cardiac failure, or a personal or family history of renal disease. Patients with an eGFR of more than 60 mL/minute/1.73 m^2 receive the usual dose of intravenous CM. Patients with an eGFR between 30 and 60 mL/minute/1.73 m^2 are given intravenous hydration and a standard or reduced dose (pertinent to the clinical situation) of CM. Intravenous CM is not administered to patients with an eGFR of less than 30 mL/minute/1.73 m^2.

Intravenous Access

The routine use of power injectors for intravenous delivery of the CM in CTA requires appropriate venous access to maintain the desired injection rate and thus optimal iodine flux. Obtaining adequate intravenous access is crucial not only to sustain the high injection rate (i.e., ≤8 mL/second for cardiac CTA studies) for the intended iodine flux, but also to prevent unintended extravasation of the CM. For most diagnostic CTA studies with an injection rate of 3.5 mL/second, a 22-gauge intravenous cannula is sufficient. However, higher injection rates of 5, 7, or 10 mL/second mandate intravenous access of 20, 18, and 17 gauge, respectively. When a disparity exists between the size of the intravenous access and the desired injection rate, the scan delay and CM volume must be adjusted according to the timing of acquisition.

Contrast-Related Factors

A key determinant of a diagnostically acceptable CTA scan is an optimized CM administration protocol. The CM delivery technique must be tailored to the specific vascular structure being studied and the clinical question that needs to be answered. In addition, the timing of CTA data acquisition should be synchronized with the CM delivery technique to optimize arterial enhancement. Arterial opacification is a time-dependent phenomenon, and attenuation of the vessels can be altered by changing the injection parameters. The fundamental components of a CM administration protocol include the volume (milliliters) and injection rate (milliliters/second) of the CM, the injection duration (seconds), the scan delay (seconds), and the use of a saline flush.

Iodine Concentration

The iodine concentration of the CM directly affects the magnitude of peak contrast enhancement. With all factors kept constant (i.e., volume and injection rate of the CM and injection duration), increasing the iodine concentration increases the iodine delivery rate and results in a higher degree of peak enhancement and a prolonged duration of enhancement. The time to peak enhancement is not affected by the iodine concentration, however. Interest in the use of CM with high iodine concentrations ($\geq$350 mg iodine/mL) for various MDCT applications is growing. The use of CM with high iodine concentrations has enabled the use of lower CM volumes as compared with CM with low iodine concentrations. However, the decrease in CM volume shortens the duration of enhancement and thus necessitates the use of faster scanning to permit data acquisition in the arterial phase. Iodine concentration and injection rate have the same proportional effect on arterial enhancement, and hence use of higher iodine concentrations is a substitute for a higher injection rate when increased iodine delivery rate is desired. For example, increasing the CM injection rate from 4 to 5 mL/second and increasing the iodine concentration from 300 to 350 mg iodine/mL result in a rise in arterial enhancement by 45%.

Injection Rate

The degree of arterial enhancement is directly proportional to the rate of iodine administration (i.e., doubling the injection rate produces an enhancement response that is twice as strong). A faster injection rate is also associated with a shorter time to peak enhancement. The incremental increase in enhancement observed following faster injection plateaus beyond a certain limit for a given patient, however. Studies show that increasing the injection rate beyond 8 mL/second does not produce stronger enhancement because of pooling of the CM in the central venous system and CM reflux into the inferior vena cava. This limit might be reached at a slower injection (i.e., <8 mL/second), when patients have a low cardiac output or diminished right ventricular function. The injection rates in large patients should be faster than those in small patients when the injection duration and volume of the CM are kept constant. Another important concept pertaining to injection rate is the ability to separate out contrast enhancement phases during multiphasic scans by using faster injection rates. For example in multiphase MDCT examination of the liver, more optimal separation of arterial and portal venous phases is possible with a faster injection rate. The routinely recommended CM injection rate for CTA studies is approximately 5 mL/second, which allows

downregulation ($\leq$4 mL/second) and upregulation ($\geq$6 mL/second) according to the patient's physiology.

Injection Duration

The duration of CM injection affects both the timing and the magnitude of contrast enhancement and is determined by the CM volume and injection rate. The longer the injection duration is, the greater the amount of iodine mass deposited will be. This results in a continuous temporal increase in arterial enhancement caused by the cumulative effects of freshly arriving CM and recirculated CM. In patients with normal cardiac output, peak arterial contrast enhancement is achieved shortly after termination of CM injection. As the volume of the CM increases, so does the time required to reach the peak of arterial or parenchymal contrast enhancement.

Selecting the appropriate injection duration based on patient-related factors and the clinical objective of the scan is important. For longer scanning (e.g., evaluation of the aorta and iliac arteries), the injection duration should be increased to maintain optimal enhancement throughout the period of image acquisition. However, too long an injection duration is not beneficial because it can result in undesirable parenchymal and venous enhancement and also leads to wastage of the CM. A shorter injection duration often results in inadequate degree and duration of contrast enhancement. To obtain optimal arterial enhancement in large patients, the injection duration should be longer than that for small patients for a fixed injection rate. Adding a constant factor (3 or 4 seconds) to the injection duration with a fast injection rate is often beneficial, to widen the temporal window for acquisition during peak arterial enhancement.

Contrast Material Volume

The volume of the CM for diagnostically acceptable CTA is mainly determined by the intended degree of enhancement and the vessels to be scanned. It also depends on several factors, including patient body weight, iodine concentration, CM injection rate, and scan duration. Contrast enhancement of 250 to 300 HU has been suggested to be adequate for the diagnosis of numerous vascular disorders. Larger patients often require a higher iodine dose to achieve a degree of contrast enhancement comparable to small patients. Furthermore, the CM requirement can be reduced by up to 15 to 25 mL with the use of a saline flush.

The CM volume, the CM injection rate, and the injection duration are interrelated. Their relationship can be described by the following simple equation:

$$\text{CM volume (mL)} = \text{Injection flow rate (mL/second)} \times \text{Injection duration (seconds)}$$

For example, intravenous CM injection stated as "120 mL at 6 mL/second" is the same as "6 mL/second for 20 seconds." From the foregoing equation, it is easy to understand that increasing the injection rate at a fixed duration of injection results in delivery of a higher iodine dose, which, in turn, augments the magnitude of peak arterial enhancement for a wider temporal window. Alternatively, increasing the injection rate with a fixed CM volume results in a greater magnitude of arterial enhancement that occurs early and lasts for a shorter period. This mechanism is important to understand, to synchronize the speed of CT acquisition favorably with the CM injection rate (i.e., with faster CT scanners [64 MDCT and newer DECT scanners], a quicker injection rate is beneficial to obtain shorter but more intense arterial enhancement). With slower CT scanners, however, a slower injection rate is preferred, to obtain more prolonged arterial enhancement.

Saline Flush

After intravenous injection of the entire CM bolus, a portion of the CM remains idle in the injection tubing and the peripheral veins. Typically, this dead space volume of CM can range from 12 to 20 mL, depending on the patient's size, the caliber of venous access, and the length of the injection tubing. This situation not only leads to wastage of the CM but also limits the extent of contrast enhancement and can cause streak artifacts from the CM in the central veins such as the superior vena cava. For these reasons, the CM bolus is followed by a bolus of normal saline (~30 to 40 mL of 0.9% w/v of NaCl.), which is injected at the same rate as that of the CM bolus. This saline flush thrusts forward the tail of the injected CM in the injection tubing and peripheral veins into the central blood volume. Regular use of a saline flush has the following benefits: (1) improved degree of contrast enhancement, (2) reduced streak artifacts, (3) better efficiency of CM use, and (4) more importantly, ability to use less CM.

Technical Parameters

Scan Coverage

The scan length for CTA is based on the vessels to be evaluated and the clinical question to be answered. The length of the arterial tree to be included in the CTA determines the CM volume, injection rate, injection duration, and scan delay. Proper planning allows targeted CT examination encompassing only relevant anatomic areas and thus helps significantly reduce the radiation dose.

Scanning Parameters

Most CTA studies in adults are performed with a tube potential of 120 kVp. Tube potential has a complex relationship with image noise, CT attenuation values (image contrast), and radiation dose. A decrease in peak kilovoltage (kVp) increases the image noise and decreases the radiation dose, but it improves the image contrast. Scanning at low kVp (80 to 100 kVp) is particularly beneficial for CTA studies because it not only improves the image contrast but also helps reduce the volume of intravenous CM. To avoid inadvertently high image noise with low-kVp CT studies, tube current must be correspondingly raised. However, kVp reduction in the obese or large patients must be avoided to ensure an adequate signal-to-noise ratio for an image of acceptable diagnostic quality. Generally, the tube potential is optimized based on the patient's body weight. A lower kVp and milliampere setting is suitable for small patients, whereas obese patients usually require greater tube current and potential. Appropriate tube current

(milliampere) selection for CTA studies can be achieved either by fixed tube current or automated tube current modulation (ATCM) techniques. ATCM customizes the tube current delivery to the patient's size and tissue density and permits a significant reduction in radiation dose. The techniques and nomenclature of ATCM software available from various manufacturers differ. ATCM relies on operator-defined parameters, such as noise index with General Electric CT scanners and reference tube current–time product with Siemens CT scanners.

For CTA, thin slices are used for axial viewing (0.625- to 2.5-mm slice thickness). The reconstructions should be performed with a small field of view and should typically use soft or medium reconstruction algorithms (kernels) to minimize the noise in thin sections obtained with CTA. For routine CTA scanning, the fastest possible gantry rotation time should be used to minimize scan duration and CM dose (usually 0.5 seconds). In obese patients, however, a slower gantry rotation time is used to improve image quality (0.6 to 0.8 seconds). CTA scanning is ideally performed with the patient holding his or her breath at the end of inspiration.

Other Parameters

Unenhanced CT is generally acquired before CTA and is helpful to (1) detect hematoma in the surrounding structures during traumatic and nontraumatic vascular injuries, (2) demonstrate intramural hematoma in aortic aneurysms, (3) assess coronary calcium score before coronary CTA for risk stratification, and (4) detect endoleak following aortic stent graft by identifying the location of calcification within the aneurysmal sac (Fig. 7-1). In view of the limited diagnostic value of these unenhanced scans, they should be acquired with low-dose protocols to limit the total radiation dose to the patient. During CTA of the abdomen and pelvis, positive oral CM is avoided because it limits postprocessing of axial data while generating the 3-D images. Water or neutral oral CM does not hinder the postprocessing of CTA data sets and is frequently used. In addition, neutral oral CM in the abdomen also permits simultaneous evaluation of the bowel wall and lumen.

Scan Delay

The scan delay for CTA (i.e., the period between the start of CM injection and the beginning of CT data acquisition) depends on the injection rate, the injection duration, the CM arrival time, and the scanning duration. In general, peak arterial enhancement is observed immediately following the cessation of CM injection. A faster injection rate and a shorter injection duration result in earlier peak arterial enhancement, whereas a slower injection rate and a longer injection duration result in later peak enhancement. The scan delay is similar to the CM transit time, which represents the time interval from the beginning of CM injection to the CM arrival in the aorta (usually ranging from 12 to 40 seconds). The scan delay must be individualized, based on the vessels being evaluated. In certain circumstances, such as the peripheral run-off CTA, it is essential to scan with longer delay so that the scan does not outrun the CM bolus. Because of the high degree of interpatient

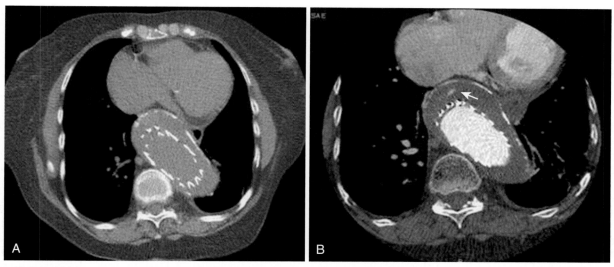

Figure 7-1 Multidetector computed tomography (MDCT) axial images in a 54-year-old man presenting with an enlarging aneurysmal sac after aortic stent graft placement. **A,** The initial unenhanced CT image demonstrates absence of any calcification within the aneurysm sac outside the stent graft. **B,** An arterial phase MDCT image demonstrates an endoleak *(arrow)*. The unenhanced CT scan permits differentiation of enhancing endoleaks from calcification.

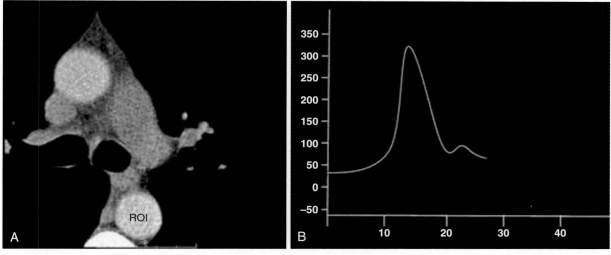

Figure 7-2 Test bolus technique. A, Snapshot image of the dynamic series of axial computed tomography (CT) images obtained after injection of a test bolus of the contrast material followed by a saline chaser. When the intravascular enhancement peaks in the reference artery (e.g., the descending aorta), the scan is stopped. A region of interest is placed over the descending aorta to obtain the time attenuation curve (**B**) and determine the time for peak aortic enhancement. The time it took to reach the peak enhancement from the time of injection of the contrast material is the time delay for CT angiography study. *ROI,* Region of interest.

and intrapatient variability of circulation time, two techniques are commonly used to determine the scan delay for CTA studies: the test bolus method and the automatic bolus triggering method. The basic premise of both these techniques involves the placement of a region of interest (ROI) in a vessel just proximal to the organ of interest (e.g., the ascending aorta for coronary CTA). The scan delay is then estimated based on the time required for the vessel in question to achieve a predetermined attenuation value.

Test Bolus

The test bolus technique involves scanning at two different time points. The first scan is performed with a small test bolus of CM, which is then followed by the actual CTA study (second scan) (Fig. 7-2). The initial scan consists of a low-dose dynamic contrast-enhanced study obtained at a predetermined (single nonincremental) location after injection of a small test bolus (usually 15 to 20 mL injected at the same rate as that of the planned CTA). An ROI is then placed on a reference vessel within the acquired CT series to determine the time taken for peak arterial enhancement. The actual CTA study with the complete dose of CM follows subsequently. This technique is a reliable and accurate method for estimation of scan delay, particularly for coronary CTA studies. The main disadvantage of this technique is the need for an additional dose of CM, and this can have workflow implications in a busy MDCT setting.

Automated Bolus Triggering

The automated bolus triggering technique does not entail the administration of a test bolus. In this technique, a circular ROI is first placed on a target vessel on a noncontrast CT image (Fig. 7-3). This is followed by injection of the full dose of CM. A series of low-dose, nonincremental scans is obtained at the region of the target vessel during simultaneous monitoring of the attenuation within the ROI. When a predefined enhancement (HU) threshold or trigger level is reached, the actual scan begins. In view of the nature of the triggering process, a slight delay is often introduced before the actual scanning begins because of several factors, such as the CT scanner type, the location of the preliminary scan in relation to the organ of interest, and the time for prerecorded breath-holding instructions. Despite the minimal delay, this technique is very robust and practical for routine use. Because it eliminates the need for a test bolus injection, the total CM dose is reduced.

■ COMPUTED TOMOGRAPHY ANGIOGRAPHY: POSTPROCESSING TOOLS

As discussed previously, a major contributor to the escalating use of CTA has been the tremendous growth in the development of postprocessing techniques. In addition, advances in 3-D workstations have allowed more efficient management and interpretation of the large volume of axial CTA data obtained from the newer MDCT scanners. Multiplanar reformations (MPRs) and 3-D reconstructions of the CTA data set not only allow evaluation of the vascular structures from various angles and planes but also enables faster and easier interpretation. Despite the availability of very high-quality 3-D data sets, the assessment of

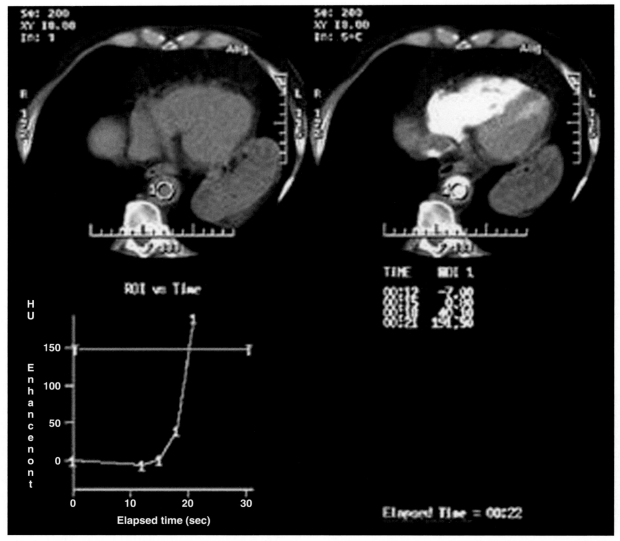

Figure 7-3 Automatic bolus triggering for computed tomography angiography. The snapshot figure shows the placement of the region of interest (ROI) cursor in the descending aorta and acquisition of sequential images during dynamic contrast injection. When the attenuation in the ROI reaches a preset value of 100 HU or on visualization of adequate opacification of the descending aorta by the technologist, the scan begins. The time attenuation curve is also shown which demonstrates the tracing of the vascular enhancement in Hounsfield units versus time.

axial images remains crucial to the accurate diagnostic interpretation of vascular abnormalities. In addition, a review of the axial data set is important for assessment of nonvascular abnormalities and for identification of artifacts. A brief outline of the various postprocessing techniques is provided here. A detailed description of these techniques is beyond the scope of this chapter.

The isotropic volumetric MDCT data obtained from a CTA examination can be reconstructed and viewed using coronal and sagittal MPRs, curved planar reformations (CPR), maximum intensity projection (MIP), volume rendering techniques (VR), and virtual angioscopy (Figs. 7-4 to 7-6). Whereas the reformatted images provide details of the vascular anatomy in different planes, the MIP and VR images offer 3-D angiographic images of the vasculature. These techniques are therefore particularly valuable to evaluate branch vessel involvement. The MIP technique displays the maximum intensity voxel values along a particular projection from the given 3-D volume data. However, a drawback of this technique is the time-consuming process of removing bones and other hyperdense structures because they often overlap and obscure the vessels of interest. Other disadvantages are the unintentional removal of vessels adjacent to bony structures and lack of depth information. VR techniques, conversely, preserve spatial depth details, do not need bone removal, and require minimal postprocessing by the operator. VR techniques are particularly suited for rapid and interactive viewing of the peripheral arterial, peripancreatic, and renal arterial data sets. One of the main limitations of both MIP and VR techniques is that vessel wall calcifications and stents completely obscure visualization of the vessel lumen. Therefore, in the presence of calcified plaques, wall calcifications, or endoluminal stents, axial data sets and two-dimensional MPRs are more reliable. CT virtual angioscopic views have been found particularly beneficial in evaluation of the intraabdominal aorta, in which they allow excellent depiction of the 3-D relationship of the stents with the branch vessel ostia, particularly the renal arteries.

■ FUTURE DIRECTIONS

CT detector technology has developed dramatically since the introduction of the 4-slice CT scanner in 1998. Currently, the preferred MDCT technology is the 64-slice MDCT scanner. The detector widths in the currently available 64-slice CT scanners range from 2.8 to 4 cm. The existing 64-slice MDCT technology is sophisticated enough to meet routine and advanced expectations of radiologists and physicians alike. Nevertheless, a limitation of the 64-slice scanners lies in their limited craniocaudal coverage, which ranges from 3.2 to 4 cm. This limitation has led to the proliferation of newer CT scanners with wider detector arrays that eliminate the need for spiral scanning and can achieve a "single-shot" scan. The 128-slice scanner has coverage of 8 cm, whereas the 320-slice dynamic volume CT scanner has detector coverage of 16 cm, which makes it possible to scan the entire heart without table motion and within a single heartbeat. Wide area detector CT allows for greater length scanning in the z-axis direction that brings about temporal uniformity and eliminates step or misregistration artifacts.

The other major advance in CT scanner technology that has revolutionized the field of cardiovascular

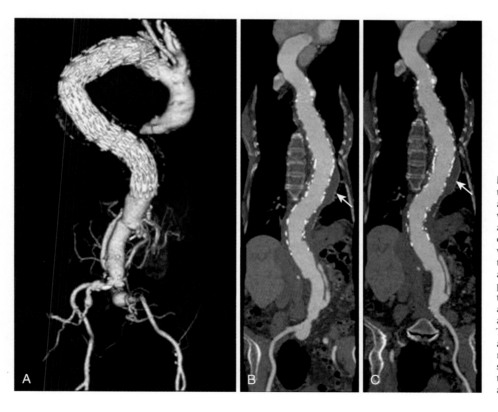

Figure 7-4 Multidetector computed tomography (MDCT) images from a CT angiographic study in a patient with stent graft placement for an aortic aneurysm. **A,** Volume rendering demonstrates the entire extent of the aorta with the metallic stent (white), the aortic lumen (pink), and the thrombosed aneurysm (dark red). **B** and **C,** Curved planar reformations through the aortic arch, the descending thoracic and abdominal aorta and the right iliac artery (**B**), and the left iliac artery (**C**). The curved planar reformatted images allow clear delineation of the contrast material–opacified aortic lumen, the stent graft, and the thrombosed portions (*arrow*) of the thoracoabdominal aneurysm outside the stent graft.

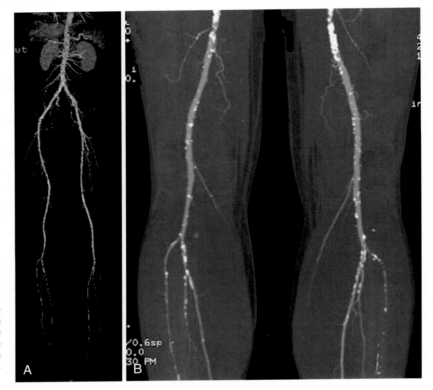

Figure 7-5 Volume rendered (VR) and maximum intensity projection (MIP) images from a 63-year-old man with peripheral arterial disease. **A,** The anteroposterior VR image allows visualization of the arterial tree from the abdominal aorta to the ankle vessels and provides an excellent overview of the complex anatomy. **B,** The anteroposterior MIP image in the same patient demonstrates excellent visualization of the severely diseased arteries of the leg.

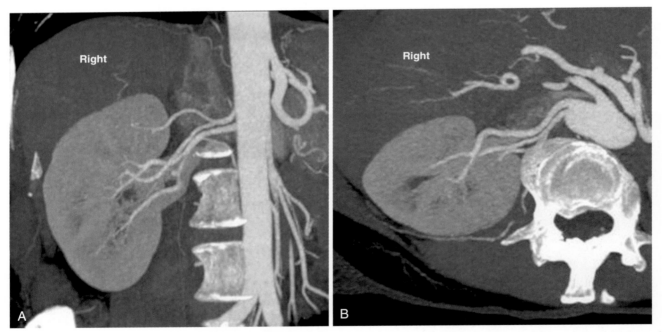

Figure 7-6 Multidetector computed tomography (MDCT) angiographic images in a 34-year-old man undergoing renal donor protocol CT. Coronal (**A**) and axial (**B**) maximum intensity projection images demonstrate the arterial anatomy of the right kidney. The depiction of the two renal arteries on the right side is excellent. The preoperative depiction of the arterial anatomy is valuable to a transplant surgeon for surgical planning.

imaging is Dual Source CT (DSCT). DSCT contains two sets of x-ray tube and detector arrays, which are arranged in a single gantry perpendicular (90 degrees) to each other in the x-y plane. DSCT has three main advantages over the single source scanners, depending on the mode of scan acquisition. Operating the two tubes at different tube potentials allows dual energy

scanning and thus has applications for tissue differentiation. When the two x-ray tubes are used in unison at equal tube potentials, the resultant increased photon flux permits scanning of larger patients with acceptable noise. The third, and most thoroughly explored, capability of DSCT is improved temporal resolution achieved by the use of two x-ray tubes. By using the

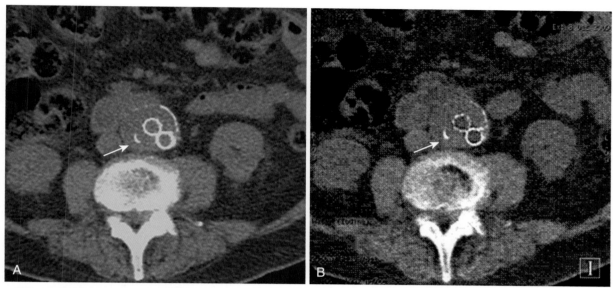

Figure 7-7 Dual energy computed tomography (CT) images in a 52-year-old man with an aortic stent graft. **A,** The axial true unenhanced image demonstrates a focus of calcification *(arrow)* in the thrombosed aneurysmal sac outside the stent graft. Dual energy CT angiography was later performed (not shown here). **B,** The virtual noncontrast CT image generated from the dual energy CT acquisition shows excellent depiction of the calcification *(arrow)* with image quality comparable to that of the true noncontrast image.

two tubes at identical kVp levels, one can acquire images using data from only 90 degrees of gantry rotation instead of the conventional 180-degree data required for the single source CT. The resultant temporal resolution of only 83 msec is particularly advantageous in coronary artery imaging. Dual energy scanning (i.e., simultaneous scanning using two different energies) can also be performed using single source CT by rapid voltage and milliampere modulation. This technique may achieve dual energy processing using projection data acquired in both axial and helical modes, unlike the image-based, dual energy processing of DSCT. Theoretically, this technique permits accurate material decomposition and monochromatic CT image display, which should potentially facilitate more precise tissue characterization and substantially decrease image artifacts. Dual energy CT can also generate virtual unenhanced CT images from the contrast-enhanced CT images acquired in the dual energy mode.

The more recently introduced 64-detector row (128-slice) vascular CT scanner allows dual source imaging with a very high helical pitch. This permits fast acquisition including large volume acquisition in the z-axis and allows coronary artery CTA in a single heartbeat when the heart rate is less than 60 to 65 beats/minute and regular. Dual energy CT has several clinical applications in vascular imaging. In patients with aortic aneurysms with stent graft placement, the virtual unenhanced CT images obviate the need for a noncontrast scan, thus reducing the total radiation exposure to the patient (Fig. 7-7). In addition, the monochromatic images (e.g., 50 keV) generated from dual energy spectral acquisition could help reduce the total iodinated dose of CM. The material decomposition capabilities of dual energy CT permit faster removal of calcific plaques in large vessels and bony structures during reconstruction of CTA examinations, particularly in the region of the skull

base. An exciting potential application of dual energy CTA is the improved differentiation of plaque composition, although further research is needed.

■ COMPUTED TOMOGRAPHY VENOGRAPHY

CT evaluation of the venous system, or CT venography, has several applications, although they are limited as compared with CT arteriography. The applications include (1) evaluation of peripheral veins for deep venous thrombosis, (2) evaluation of pulmonary vein anatomy, (3) evaluation of the hepatic veins and inferior vena cava in Budd-Chiari syndrome or venous thrombosis, and (4) portal vein evaluation in portal hypertension. The venous system of the abdomen is accurately assessed in routine abdominal and pelvic CT scans, which are acquired in the portal venous phase (60 to 70 seconds after CM injection). For evaluation of the inferior vena cava, scanning can be performed either in the portal phase or in the equilibrium phase (90 to 120 seconds).

■ CONCLUSION

Because of advances in MDCT technology, CTA has emerged as the preferred imaging investigation for the evaluation of cardiovascular disorders. As the technology continues to evolve, clinicians will need to understand the basic concepts governing contrast dynamics in a CTA study. A fundamental understanding is necessary for planning strategies to design optimal and effective CTA protocols. A CTA protocol designed after careful consideration of the patient's physiology, contrast factors, and MDCT technology is more likely to result in a diagnostically acceptable and accurate CTA examination.

Bibliography

Achenbach S, Anders K, Kalender WA. Dual-source cardiac computed tomography: image quality and dose considerations. *Eur Radiol.* 2008;18:1188-1198.

Awai K, Hori S. Effect of contrast injection protocol with dose tailored to patient weight and fixed injection duration on aortic and hepatic enhancement at multidetector-row helical CT. *Eur Radiol.* 2003;13:2155-2160.

Bae KT. Peak contrast enhancement in CT and MR angiography: when does it occur and why? Pharmacokinetic study in a porcine model. *Radiology.* 2003;227:809-816.

Bae KT. Principles of contrast medium delivery and scan timing in MDCT. In: Kalra M, Saini S, Rubin G, eds. *MDCT: From Protocols to Practice.* Milan: Springer; 2008:10-24.

Bae KT, Heiken JP, Brink JA. Aortic and hepatic peak enhancement at CT: effect of contrast medium injection rate—pharmacokinetic analysis and experimental porcine model. *Radiology.* 1998;206:455-464.

Bae KT, Heiken JP, Brink JA. Aortic and hepatic contrast medium enhancement at CT. Part I. Prediction with a computer model. *Radiology.* 1998;207:647-655.

Bae KT, Heiken JP, Brink JA. Aortic and hepatic contrast medium enhancement at CT. Part II. Effect of reduced cardiac output in a porcine model. *Radiology.* 1998;207:657-662.

Bae KT, Seeck BA, Hildebolt CF, et al. Contrast enhancement in cardiovascular MDCT: effect of body weight, height, body surface area, body mass index, and obesity. *AJR Am J Roentgenol.* 2008;190:777-784.

Bae KT, Tao C, Gurel S, et al. Effect of patient weight and scanning duration on contrast enhancement during pulmonary multidetector CT angiography. *Radiology.* 2007;242:582-589.

Berland LL, Lee JY. Comparison of contrast media injection rates and volumes for hepatic dynamic incremented computed tomography. *Invest Radiol.* 1988;23:918-922.

Brink JA. Contrast optimization and scan timing for single and multidetector-row computed tomography. *J Comput Assist Tomogr.* 2003;27(suppl 1):S3-S8.

Brink JA. Use of high concentration contrast media (HCCM): principles and rationale—body CT. *Eur J Radiol.* 2003;45(suppl 1):S53-S58.

Cademartiri F, Mollet N, van der Lugt A, et al. Non-invasive 16-row multislice CT coronary angiography: usefulness of saline chaser. *Eur Radiol.* 2004;14:178-183.

Cademartiri F, Nieman K, van der Lugt A, et al. Intravenous contrast material administration at 16-detector row helical CT coronary angiography: test bolus versus bolus-tracking technique. *Radiology.* 2004;233:817-823.

Cahir JG, Freeman AH, Courtney HM. Multislice CT of the abdomen. *Br J Radiol.* 2004;77(spec 1):S64-S73.

Calhoun PS, Kuszyk BS, Heath DG, Carley JC, Fishman EK. Three-dimensional volume rendering of spiral CT data: theory and method. *Radiographics.* 1999;19:745-764.

Chambers TP, Baron RL, Lush RM. Hepatic CT enhancement. Part II. Alterations in contrast material volume and rate of injection within the same patients. *Radiology.* 1994;193:518-522.

Dorio PJ, Lee Jr FT, Henseler KP, et al. Using a saline chaser to decrease contrast media in abdominal CT. *AJR Am J Roentgenol.* 2003;180:929-934.

Fleischmann D. CT angiography: injection and acquisition technique. *Radiol Clin North Am.* 2010;48:237-247, vii.

Fleischmann D. High-concentration contrast media in MDCT angiography: principles and rationale. *Eur Radiol.* 2003;13(suppl 3):N39-N43.

Fleischmann D. How to design injection protocols for multiple detector-row CT angiography (MDCTA). *Eur Radiol.* 2005;15(suppl 5):E60-E65.

Fleischmann D. Use of high-concentration contrast media in multiple-detector-row CT: principles and rationale. *Eur Radiol.* 2003;13(suppl 5):M14-M20.

Fleischmann D, Kamaya A. Optimal vascular and parenchymal contrast enhancement: the current state of the art. *Radiol Clin North Am.* 2009;47:13-26.

Fleischmann D, Rubin GD. Quantification of intravenously administered contrast medium transit through the peripheral arteries: implications for CT angiography. *Radiology.* 2005;236:1076-1082.

Flohr TG, McCollough CH, Bruder H, et al. First performance evaluation of a dual-source CT (DSCT) system. *Eur Radiol.* 2006;16:256-268.

Freeny PC, Gardner JC, von Ingersleben G, Heyano S, Nghiem HV, Winter TC. Hepatic helical CT: effect of reduction of iodine dose of intravenous contrast material on hepatic contrast enhancement. *Radiology.* 1995;197:89-93.

Furuta A, Ito K, Fujita T, Koike S, Shimizu A, Matsunaga N. Hepatic enhancement in multiphasic contrast-enhanced MDCT: comparison of high- and low-iodine-concentration contrast medium in same patients with chronic liver disease. *AJR Am J Roentgenol.* 2004;183:157-162.

Garcia PA, Bonaldi VM, Bret PM, Liang L, Reinhold C, Atri M. Effect of rate of contrast medium injection on hepatic enhancement at CT. *Radiology.* 1996;199:185-189.

Garcia PA, Genin G, Bret PM, Bonaldi VM, Reinhold C, Atri M. Hepatic CT enhancement: effect of the rate and volume of contrast medium injection in an animal model. *Abdom Imaging.* 1999;24:597-603.

Geleijns J, Salvado Artells M, de Bruin PW, Matter R, Muramatsu Y, McNitt-Gray MF. Computed tomography dose assessment for a 160 mm wide, 320 detector row, cone beam CT scanner. *Phys Med Biol.* 2009;54:3141-3159.

Graser A, Johnson TR, Chandarana H, Macari M. Dual energy CT: preliminary observations and potential clinical applications in the abdomen. *Eur Radiol.* 2009;19:13-23.

Haage P, Schmitz-Rode T, Hubner D, Piroth W, Gunther RW. Reduction of contrast material dose and artifacts by a saline flush using a double power injector in helical CT of the thorax. *AJR Am J Roentgenol.* 2000;174:1049-1053.

Han JK, Choi BI, Kim AY, Kim SJ. Contrast media in abdominal computed tomography: optimization of delivery methods. *Korean J Radiol.* 2001;2:28-36.

Heiken JP, Brink JA, McClennan BL, Sagel SS, Crowe TM, Gaines MV. Dynamic incremental CT: effect of volume and concentration of contrast material and patient weight on hepatic enhancement. *Radiology.* 1995;195:353-357.

Hopper KD, Mosher TJ, Kasales CJ, TenHave TR, Tully DA, Weaver JS. Thoracic spiral CT: delivery of contrast material pushed with injectable saline solution in a power injector. *Radiology.* 1997;205:269-271.

Kalra M, Rubin G. MDCT angiography of peripheral arterial disease. In: Kalra M, Saini S, Rubin G, eds. *MDCT: From Protocols to Practice.* Milan: Springer; 2008:250-262.

Kalra M, Rubin G. MDCT angiography of the thoracic aorta. In: Kalra M, Saini S, Rubin G, eds. *MDCT: From Protocols to Practice.* Milan: Springer; 2008:225-235.

Kirchner J, Kickuth R, Laufer U, Noack M, Liermann D. Optimized enhancement in helical CT: experiences with a real-time bolus tracking system in 628 patients. *Clin Radiol.* 2000;55:368-373.

Kormano M, Partanen K, Soimakallio S, Kivimaki T. Dynamic contrast enhancement of the upper abdomen: effect of contrast medium and body weight. *Invest Radiol.* 1983;18:364-367.

Kumamaru KK, Hoppel BE, Mather RT, Rybicki FJ. CT angiography: current technology and clinical use. *Radiol Clin North Am.* 2010;48:213-235, vii.

Lee CH, Goo JM, Ye HJ, et al. Radiation dose modulation techniques in the multidetector CT era: from basics to practice. *Radiographics.* 2008;28:1451-1459.

Maher MM, Kalra MK, Sahani DV, et al. Techniques, clinical applications and limitations of 3D reconstruction in CT of the abdomen. *Korean J Radiol.* 2004;5:55-67.

Mori S, Endo M, Obata T, et al. Clinical potentials of the prototype 256-detector row CT-scanner. *Acad Radiol.* 2005;12:148-154.

Mori S, Endo M, Obata T, Tsunoo T, Susumu K, Tanada S. Properties of the prototype 256-row (cone beam) CT scanner. *Eur Radiol.* 2006;16:2100-2108.

Platt JF, Reige KA, Ellis JH. Aortic enhancement during abdominal CT angiography: correlation with test injections, flow rates, and patient demographics. *AJR Am J Roentgenol.* 1999;172:53-56.

Prokop M. General principles of MDCT. *Eur J Radiol.* 2003;45(suppl 1):S4-S10.

Rogalla P, Kloeters C, Hein PA. CT technology overview: 64-slice and beyond. *Radiol Clin North Am.* 2009;47:1-11.

Rubin GD. Cardiac CT technologies: what is important. In: *Abdominal Radiology Course 2009.* Maui, HI: Society of Gastrointestinal Radiology; 2009.

Rydberg J, Buckwalter KA, Caldemeyer KS, et al. Multisection CT: scanning techniques and clinical applications. *Radiographics.* 2000;20:1787-1806.

Saini S. Multi-detector row CT: principles and practice for abdominal applications. *Radiology.* 2004;233:323-327.

Schindera ST, Nelson RC, Yoshizumi T, et al. Effect of automatic tube current modulation on radiation dose and image quality for low tube voltage multidetector row CT angiography phantom study. *Acad Radiol.* 2009;16:997-1002.

Schoellnast H, Tillich M, Deutschmann HA, et al. Abdominal multidetector row computed tomography: reduction of cost and contrast material dose using saline flush. *J Comput Assist Tomogr.* 2003;27:847-853.

Schoellnast H, Tillich M, Deutschmann HA, et al. Improvement of parenchymal and vascular enhancement using saline flush and power injection for multiple-detector-row abdominal CT. *Eur Radiol.* 2004;14:659-664.

Schoellnast H, Tillich M, Deutschmann MJ, Deutschmann HA, Schaffler GJ, Portugaller HR. Aortoiliac enhancement during computed tomography angiography with reduced contrast material dose and saline solution flush: influence on magnitude and uniformity of the contrast column. *Invest Radiol.* 2004;39:20-26.

Singh AK, Hiroyuki Y, Sahani DV. Advanced postprocessing and the emerging role of computer-aided detection. *Radiol Clin North Am.* 2009;47:59-77.

Small WC, Nelson RC, Bernardino ME, Brummer LT. Contrast-enhanced spiral CT of the liver: effect of different amounts and injection rates of contrast material on early contrast enhancement. *AJR Am J Roentgenol.* 1994;163:87-92.

Suzuki H, Oshima H, Shiraki N, Ikeya C, Shibamoto Y. Comparison of two contrast materials with different iodine concentrations in enhancing the density of the aorta, portal vein and liver at multi-detector row CT: a randomized study. *Eur Radiol.* 2004;14:2099-2104.

Suzuki H, Shibamoto Y, Oshima H, Takeuchi M, Ito M, Hara M. Comparison of 2 contrast materials with different iodine concentrations in 3-dimensional computed tomography angiography of the hepatic artery at multi-detector-row computed tomography: a randomized study. *J Comput Assist Tomogr.* 2007;31:840-845.

Udayasankar U, Momin Z, Small W. 3-D post-processing: principles and practical applications. In: Kalra M, Saini S, Rubin G, eds. *MDCT: From Protocols to Practice.* Milan: Springer; 2008:65-82.

van Hoe L, Marchal G, Baert AL, Gryspeerdt S, Mertens L. Determination of scan delay time in spiral CT-angiography: utility of a test bolus injection. *J Comput Assist Tomogr.* 1995;19:216-220.

Wang L, Menias C, Bae K. Mesenteric and renal CT angiography. In: Kalra M, Saini S, Rubin G, eds. *MDCT: From Protocols to Practice.* Milan: Springer; 2008:120-137.

CHAPTER 8

Magnetic Resonance Angiography: Technique

Constantine A. Raptis, Kathryn J. Fowler, and Vamsi R. Narra

Today, imagers are presented with more options than ever before for imaging vascular structures throughout the body. This is in part due to the evolution of magnetic resonance angiography (MRA), which has benefitted from advances in sequence design, scanner technology, and contrast development to evolve as a powerful clinical tool. The purpose of this chapter is to provide an overview of noncontrast and contrast-enhanced (CE) MRA techniques.

Before doing so, however, some of the relative strengths and weaknesses of MRA in comparison with its main noninvasive counterpart, computed tomography angiography (CTA), should be considered. MRA, unlike CTA, is performed without ionizing radiation, an increasingly important advantage given the growing movement to reduce medical radiation exposure. An additional advantage of MRA over CTA is that gadolinium-based contrast materials (GBCMs) are not nephrotoxic and thus are suitable for patients with borderline or at-risk renal function. Patients with severe chronic renal dysfunction (glomerular filtration rate <30), as well as all patients with acute renal failure, should not be given GBCMs because of the risk of nephrogenic systemic fibrosis (NSF), a life-threatening disease resulting in fibrosis of the skin, joints, eyes, and internal organs. In patients who have severe renal dysfunction requiring dialysis, CTA with iodinated contrast material is a better choice than MRA with gadolinium contrast. From an image quality standpoint, MRA provides high contrast resolution. Although the spatial resolution of MRA with extracellular GBCMs is typically lower than that of CTA, newer blood pool contrast materials allow for acquisition of higher–spatial resolution sequences with isotropic voxels that can be reconstructed in an infinite number of planes. Some additional limitations of MRA include longer acquisition times, poor suitability for patients with claustrophobia, and incompatibility with certain implanted medical devices.

■ NONCONTRAST MAGNETIC RESONANCE ANGIOGRAPHY

Although noncontrast MRA techniques have long been available, they were largely relegated to second-line status after the introduction of CE MRA in the mid-1990s. In more recent years, however, interest in noncontrast MRA has been renewed, mainly because of the identification of the relationship between GBCMs and NSF. Fortunately, this increased need has also been met with advances in scanner and sequence design that have resulted in improvements in existing noncontrast MRA techniques, as well as the development of several newer and promising techniques. The following is a discussion of the many available noncontrast techniques used clinically in MRA. The techniques can be simplistically divided into sequences that create bright-blood signal resulting from inflow and those that exploit the lack of signal associated with flow voids.

Bright-Blood Noncontrast Magnetic Resonance Angiography

Bright-blood MRA techniques are all similar in that they produce images in which the signal of the blood is bright relative to background signal. Several of these methods, such as time of flight (TOF) and phase contrast (PC) MRA, rely on the motion of protons in blood to induce signal relative to stationary protons of background tissues. Although other techniques are not directly reliant on flow, they exploit the differential signal of blood during systole and diastole to create angiographic images, as is done in electrocardiogram (ECG)-gated fast spin echo (FSE) MRA. Yet further removed from reliance on flow, balanced steady-state free precession (bSSFP) sequences display bright-blood pool signal solely as a result of its fluid nature. Finally, quiescent interval single shot (QISS) MRA relies on a combination of gating and the fluid nature of blood to create a robust and novel approach to noncontrast MRA.

Time of Flight Imaging

TOF MRA produces images of blood vessels by taking advantage of the differences between flowing and stationary protons. The first step in TOF MRA is the saturation of the imaging section with repeated excitation pulses. Provided the pulses are administered fast enough so that tissues cannot regain their signal (i.e., the repetition time [TR] is sufficiently shorter than the T1 of the tissues), the result is background saturation. Flowing blood outside the saturated section can then enter the imaging plane with full magnetization, thus allowing for high signal relative to the saturated background. To distinguish between arteries and veins entering the section of interest from different directions, saturation bands can be used. The saturation band should be placed such that the protons to be saturated encounter the band before they enter the section to be imaged. For example, a saturation band should be placed toward the abdomen to null venous signal on MRA of the chest. Moreover, to mitigate signal loss from flow-related dephasing, additional positive and negative lobed gradients may be necessary.

Several important imaging parameters can alter image quality in TOF MRA. Using a longer TR can increase the signal from the blood by allowing greater inflow of vascular protons, but at the expense of longer imaging times and increased background signal. Minimizing the echo time (TE) can reduce signal loss within vessels that can be caused by dephasing from complex flow. Increasing the flip angle helps to suppress background signal and increase apparent signal from the inflowing protons; typical flip angles in TOF MRA are between 25 and 60 degrees. Decreasing the slice thickness allows for faster imaging with a shorter TR, but anatomic coverage is diminished. Cardiac gating can also improve image quality by reducing the effects of pulsatile flow, but it requires longer imaging times. Finally, magnetization transfer and fat saturation pulses can be applied to decrease background signal and increase the contrast-to-noise ratio further, although the acquisition time is increased.

TOF MRA can be performed as a two-dimensional (2-D) or three-dimensional (3-D) acquisition. Three-dimensional acquisitions have the advantage of allowing for high–spatial resolution isotropic imaging, but they are more prone to blood saturation effects resulting from in-plane flow and have limited anatomic coverage.

Imaging of the intracranial vessels is the most common clinical application for 3-D TOF MRA. Two-dimensional TOF MRA is preferred for body and peripheral applications, in which sections can be obtained perpendicular to the vessels of interest. Although 2-D TOF MRA can be used to image any vessel of interest, some common clinical applications of 2-D TOF MRA include noncontrast venous imaging and imaging of the tibial and pedal arteries.

Although TOF MRA is the most widely used noncontrast MRA technique, it suffers from several important limitations. One limitation of TOF MRA is long acquisition times. Another limitation is the possibility of overestimating stenoses in regions of turbulent flow as a result of spin dephasing. Probably the greatest limitation of TOF MRA from an imaging standpoint is loss of signal from saturation of in-plane (with 2-D imaging) or in-slab (with 3-D imaging) flow. In-plane saturation and in-slab saturation are problems especially in tortuous vessels or in vessels with a normal course that travel parallel to the imaging plane (Fig. 8-1). A classic example is loss of signal in the proximal anterior tibial artery in a 2-D TOF acquisition as it arises laterally from the popliteal artery and travels for a short segment in a relatively horizontal plane.

Phase Contrast Imaging

PC angiography is based on the phase shift that occurs in flowing protons when gradients of equal strength but opposite polarity are applied in succession. The first gradient dephases the spins of all protons (both flowing blood and stationary background tissues), whereas the second rephases the spins of stationary or background

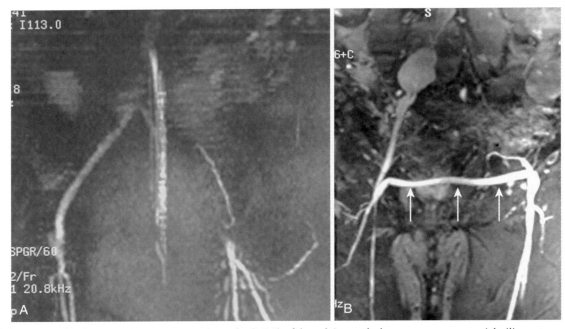

Figure 8-1 **A,** Time of flight magnetic resonance angiography (MRA) of the pelvic vessels demonstrates a patent right iliac system and severely diseased left iliac system with patent proximal femoral systems bilaterally. **B,** Contrast-enhanced MRA of the same patient confirms these findings but also demonstrates a patent femoral-femoral bypass graft *(arrows)*. The graft was not seen on the time of flight examination because it travels in a horizontal fashion and was subject to in-plane saturation. Before any MRA examination, the examiner should determine whether the patient has any grafts that need to be included in the field of view. Knowledge of the course of these grafts is particularly important in time of flight examinations in which in-plane saturation effects are a concern.

protons only. This net phase accumulation in the flowing protons, or phase shift, can then be used to calculate flow velocities, with flow velocity directly proportional to the phase shift. In PC MRA, angiographic images reflect the absolute velocity of each voxel, irrespective of flow direction. Saturation bands can be used to eliminate flow from unwanted directions. Key advantages of PC MRA are the excellent background suppression resulting in a relatively high contrast-to-background ratio and the ability to determine flow velocity.

PC MRA has several limitations. One problem with PC MRA, particularly in 3-D acquisitions, is that data acquisition is time consuming. In addition, turbulent flow distal to a stenosis can result in intravoxel dephasing and signal loss, which may overestimate degree of stenosis. Because the flow-uncompensated images are subtracted from the flow-compensated images, PC MRA is susceptible to motion. Given these and other technical limitations, PC MRA is not often used as a primary angiographic technique.

The PC technique, however, is more often used as a supplement to other MRA methods for the purpose of flow quantification. An example is gradient measurement across the aortic valve in patients with aortic stenosis. In these applications, velocity encoded flow quantification images are created, in which signal intensity is directly proportional to the accumulated phase shift, which ranges from −180 to +180 degrees. Typically, flow in the same direction as the bipolar gradient is depicted as bright pixels, whereas flow in the opposite direction is depicted as dark pixels. A user-defined parameter, the encoding velocity, represents the maximum measurable velocity, which corresponds to the 180-degree phase shift. When velocities higher than this value are encountered, aliasing occurs, and flow is represented as taking place in the opposite direction. Thus, the examiner must select a value that is higher than the maximum velocity to be encountered. However, selecting values far higher than the maximum encountered velocities results in decreased sensitivity to slow flow, particularly near the edge of the lumen (Fig. 8-2).

Electrocardiogram-Gated Fast Spin Echo Magnetic Resonance Angiography

On T2-weighted images, arteries and veins have high signal during diastole because of slower flow within their lumina. During systole, however, faster flow in the arteries causes spin dephasing, which results in luminal flow void. Using ECG-gated or peripheral pulse wave–gated 3-D partial Fourier FSE sequences, images can be obtained in both systole and diastole. The systolic images, with bright veins only, can be subtracted from the diastolic images with bright arteries and veins, to produce a composite angiographic image in which only arteries are bright. This approach is the basis of ECG-gated FSE MRA, also known by various proprietary names: Fresh Blood Imaging (FBI, Toshiba), NATIVE SPACE (Siemens), TRANCE (Philips), and DeltaFlow (GE).

Although in principle this technique appears simple, the application requires some knowledge and oversight on the part of the MRA examiner. To perform ECG-gated FSE MRA, a 2-D ECG preparatory scan is required before data acquisition, to determine the trigger delays for systole and diastole. A second 2-D preparatory scan may be acquired to determine the best flow-spoiling gradient pulses to increase dephasing (signal loss) within the arteries of interest. The MRA data themselves are typically acquired using partial Fourier and parallel imaging techniques to reduce scan time and consequent motion related artifacts. Data are acquired every second to third R-R interval, to allow for sufficient T1 recovery.

Although not routinely used in clinical practice, 3-D ECG-gated FSE MRA has many potential applications. Thoracic aortic imaging can be performed using this method. To reduce the T2-blurring effect, one phase encoding direction should be oriented as parallel as possible to the direction of flow in the aorta. To avoid wraparound artifact in the coronal plane, superior and inferior presaturation bands can be applied. Because venous contamination is not a concern when imaging a vessel as large as the aorta, only the diastolic acquisition needs to be acquired, hence reducing imaging time. Three-dimensional ECG-gated FSE MRA also has applications in peripheral MRA. In contradistinction to thoracic aortic applications, the frequency encoding direction is oriented parallel to the direction of flow in peripheral applications to improve systolic flow spoiling. Flow spoiling in the arteries can be further enhanced by additional readout gradient pulses. Because of its sensitivity to slow flow, ECG-gated FSE MRA is a useful noncontrast technique for the imaging of small peripheral vessels such as those found in the calf, foot, and hand (Fig. 8-3).

ECG-gated FSE MRA has several important limitations. Although scan times are less than with other noncontrast MRA techniques, they are still long; each systolic and diastolic acquisition typically takes 1 to 3 minutes, for total scan times of 2 to 6 minutes. With long sampling windows in each cardiac cycle, motion artifacts and blurring can be difficult problems to overcome. The imaging technique is also complex, requiring physician monitoring because of the use of preparatory scans to determine optimal timing of systolic and diastolic phases, as well as the amount of flow-spoiling gradient pulses. Timing of the systolic and diastolic phases can be extremely difficult, particularly in distal vessels in the setting of upstream stenoses, which result in dampening of arterial waveforms. Patients with arrhythmias are particularly difficult to image with ECG-gated FSE MRA as a result of an inability to time systole and diastole reasonably. Finally, because the final MRA images are achieved by subtraction, vessel wall abnormalities can be missed.

Balanced Steady-State Free Precession Imaging

bSSFP sequences (Balanced Gradient Echo, True-FISP (Siemens, Munich), FIESTA (GE, Fairfield, CT), balanced-FFE (Philips, Amsterdam), TrueSSFP (Toshiba, Tokyo) use a free precession gradient echo sequence with balanced gradients in all directions that results in images that have both T1 and T2 weighting. Although the contrast mechanisms for bSSFP sequences are complex, the important result is that image contrast is determined

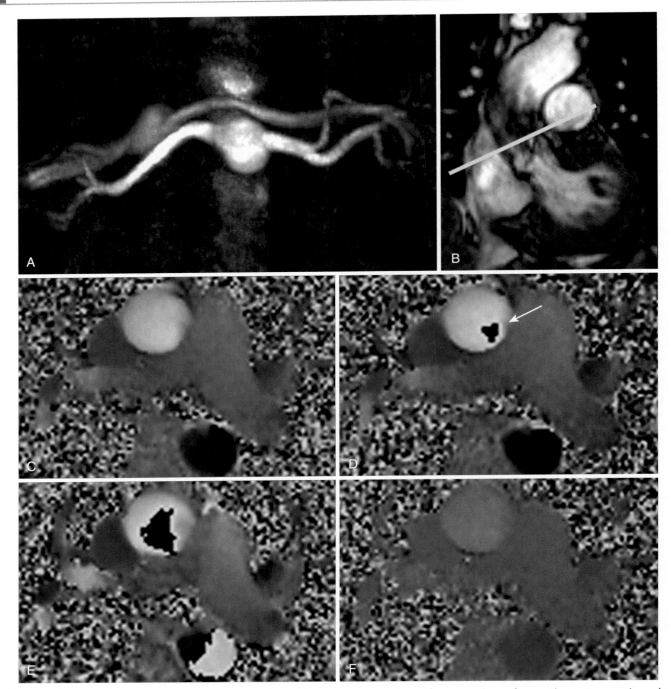

Figure 8-2 Although phase contrast techniques are rarely used for purely angiographic applications as in renal magnetic resonance angiography performed with phase contrast technique (**A**), they are routinely used for flow quantification. Typically, a balanced steady-state free precession cine sequence (**B**) is first obtained in the plane of the vessel of interest, in this case the ascending aorta. The velocity encoded phase contrast sequence is then obtained in a plane perpendicular to the dephasing jet or direction of flow, approximately 1 cm above its origin. The examiner should select a velocity encoding gradient (Venc) that is just higher than the maximum flow velocity. **C**, An optimal Venc is selected, which depicts forward flow as bright and reverse flow as dark. **D**, The Venc is slightly low, resulting in a small focus of aliasing *(arrow)* within the center of the ascending aorta. **E**, The Venc is far too low, resulting in extensive aliasing. **F**, When the Venc is too high, the velocity encoded image appears washed out and has decreased accuracy, particularly with regard to slower flow.

by differences in the T2*/T1 ratio of the imaged tissues. Given that liquid compartments, muscle, fat, and other body tissues have different T2*/T1 ratios, MR images with strong contrast can be produced. Unlike TOF MRA and PC MRA, blood within vessels appears bright as a result of its fluid composition, independent of flow

direction. The degree of vessel brightness is related to the flip angle used. For bSSFP sequences, the ideal flip angle is greater than 70 degrees. bSSFP sequences can be acquired very rapidly and are particularly well suited for cine imaging. Because the background signal in bSSFP sequences is high, additional preparatory pulses to

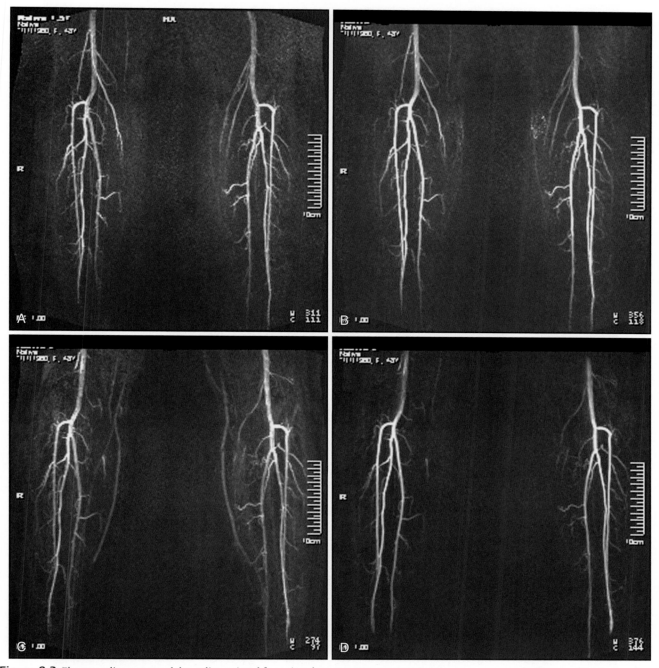

Figure 8-3 Electrocardiogram-gated three-dimensional fast spin echo noncontrast magnetic resonance angiography images of the lower extremities using the NATIVE SPACE technique. **A** and **B,** Images were obtained at 1.5 T, with magnetization transfer and fat saturation pulses applied in **B. C** and **D,** Images were obtained at 3 T, with magnetization transfer and fat saturation pulses applied in **D.** Note the increased contrast-to-noise ratio after application of the magnetization transfer and fat saturation pulses, an effect even more pronounced at 3 T.

suppress fat or other background tissues are often used. Arterial spin labeling can also be implemented to increase the contrast-to-background ratio of the images. One important limitation of bSSFP sequences, susceptibility to field heterogeneities, can be mitigated by increasing the bandwidth and hence the readout time, thus allowing the user to decrease the TR as much as possible. Another option for decreasing field heterogeneities is to use localized shimming to obtain a more homogeneous magnetic field.

Although bSSFP sequences are widely incorporated into body and cardiac imaging protocols, several applications are specifically directed at MRA (Fig. 8-4). ECG-gated breath-hold bSSFP is an excellent choice for noncontrast evaluation of the aorta. In aortic applications, stacked single shot bSSFP sequences can be used in conjunction with bSSFP cine images to evaluate flow dynamics and luminal disease including dissection flaps. Because of the relative speed of acquisition, non–breath-hold, nongated bSSFP can be

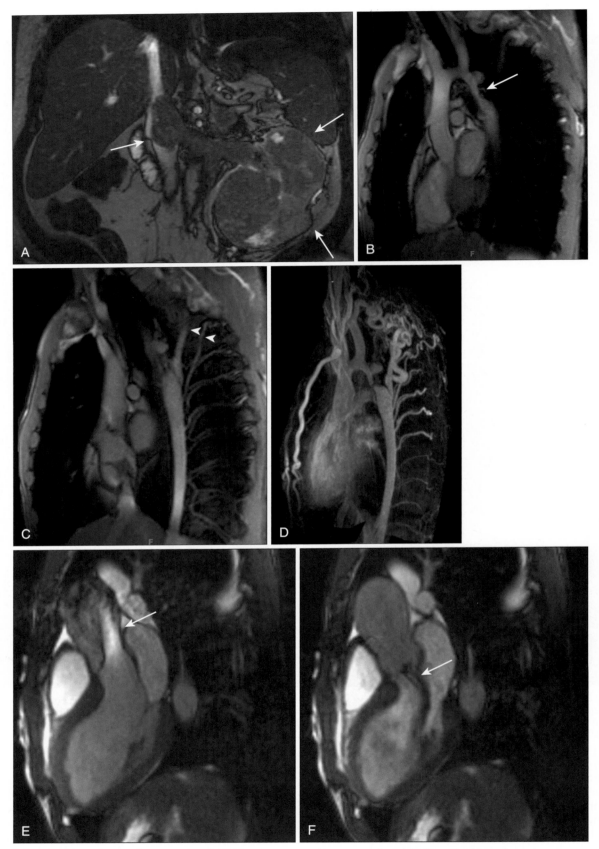

Figure 8-4 Balanced steady-state free precession (bSSFP) sequences provide a means for bright-blood imaging of vascular structures without contrast. **A,** This bSSFP image demonstrates a large renal cell cancer *(arrows)* invading the left renal vein and inferior vena cava. **B** and **C,** A post-ductal coarctation *(arrow)* with associated enlarged intercostal collateral vessels *(arrowheads)* is visible. These images can be compared with a maximum intensity projection **(D)** from the contrast-enhanced magnetic resonance angiography portion of the examination in the same patient. Because it is relatively fast, bSSFP sequences can be acquired with retrospective gating and displayed as cine images. Images in systole **(E)** and in diastole **(F)** from a bSSFP cine sequence of a patient with a bicuspid valve demonstrate dephasing jets of aortic stenosis and regurgitation *(arrows)*.

a salvage sequence for evaluating dissection or aneurysm in the hospital or emergency room setting when dealing with patients who are unable to cooperate with breath-holding instructions. bSSFP with respiratory and ECG-gating has also been used in whole heart coronary angiography. These coronary MRA techniques often use preparatory pulses to suppress background fat and myocardial signal. Breath-hold bSSFP sequences can also be used to evaluate the abdominal and pelvic vasculature, including renal arterial disease.

Quiescent Interval Single Shot Technique

A newer noncontrast MRA technique introduced by Edelman et al in 2010, QISS MRA, has shown great promise and clinical applicability. QISS MRA is ECG gated and begins with a slice selective radiofrequency (RF) pulse applied to set the magnetization of tissues within the selected slice to zero. After a tracking saturation pulse eliminates venous signal, the quiescent interval occurs, coinciding with the systolic inflow of arterial blood. During this quiescent interval, following an RF fat saturation pulse and RF catalyzation pulse to force the magnetization of the in-plane spins toward the steady state value, a single shot 2-D bSSFP is used to image the arterial spins. The arterial spins are imaged during diastole because flow is slow or minimal. The process is repeated for each subsequent slice in sequential fashion.

QISS MRA has several advantages over other noncontrast techniques. The most important is that QISS MRA is relatively fast and easy to use. Unlike the other techniques, which are often technically demanding and require case-by-base adjustments, QISS MRA is relatively easy to use "out of the box," with little modification required for use in individual patients. In contrast to 3-D ECG-gated FSE MRA, QISS MRA is less sensitive to precise timing because the relatively long duration of the quiescent interval provides a sizeable window for the bSSFP data to be acquired. Consequently, no preparatory sequences are required, thus greatly simplifying data acquisition. QISS MRA also has the potential to perform well in patients with arrhythmias who present significant challenges with TOF and 3-D ECG-gated FSE MRA. In addition, because it uses a single shot acquisition without subtraction, QISS is less sensitive to motion, a problem inherent to TOF and 3-D ECG-gated FSE MRA. Finally, although it is flow dependent, QISS MRA is sensitive to many different flow velocities, down to 10 cm/second. This feature is particularly advantageous in imaging patients with significant peripheral vascular disease because, unlike TOF, QISS MRA is less prone to overestimate degrees of stenosis. Although it is a new technique, because of its ease of use and excellent image quality, QISS MRA shows great promise in imaging peripheral vascular disease in patients who cannot receive contrast agents (Fig. 8-5).

Dark-Blood Imaging Techniques

Although they are not used to produce angiographic images, dark-blood (or black-blood) imaging techniques are often helpful in the assessment of intraluminal or intramural vascular abnormalities. Unlike bright-blood techniques, in which the goal is to increase signal within the lumen, dark-blood techniques aim to eliminate it. In most spin echo sequences, the lumina of vessels with flowing blood are dark. This is because flowing protons are exposed only to the 90-degree excitation pulse, not to the refocusing pulse, as they flow out of the imaging slice before it occurs. Consequently, they have no signal, and a flow void image is produced with the vessel. This flow void phenomenon can be used in image interpretation to determine vessel patency. Vessels that are occluded or have very slow flow do not produce flow voids and thus appear bright. Care must be taken when evaluating tortuous vessels, because in-plane flow does not always produce flow voids. Moreover, the flow void on spin echo sequences does not always result in complete intraluminal signal loss. For example, sections of the vessel imaged during diastole may have some bright signal as a result of slow flow or entry-exit phenomena. One possible solution for decreasing the intraluminal signal on a spin echo sequence is to increase the TE and thereby allow additional time for protons to exit the imaged section. Thinner slices can also be used to create a shorter path for blood protons to exit the slice. Another option is to use an upstream saturation band to eliminate further signal from blood flowing into the section.

Double inversion recovery is an additional technique that can be used to further decrease intraluminal signal in dark-blood images. In double inversion recovery technique, two consecutive 180-degree pulses are applied. The first pulse is nonselective and is applied to the entire imaging volume, thus inverting all spins. The second pulse is slice selective and returns all stationary spins in the slice to their equilibrium positions. Blood flowing into the imaging slice experiences only the first nonselective inversion pulse and subsequently reaccumulates its longitudinal magnetization according to its T1 relaxation time. The imaging data are then acquired during diastole, which is timed to coincide with the inversion time of blood (~650 msec), at which point the blood has no signal. Because double inversion recovery technique is an ECG-gated, sequential slice sequence, it is not particularly time efficient, although useful anatomic coverage can be acquired in one breath hold by using an appropriate slice thickness.

Dark-blood imaging, particularly with double inversion recovery techniques, has important applications in vascular imaging, especially of the aorta. Luminal abnormalities such as dissection flaps can often be identified on dark-blood sequences, although they are usually better depicted on either postcontrast gradient echo or noncontrast bSSFP sequences. In the setting of dissection, however, dark-blood sequences have an important role in detecting slow or absent flow within the false lumen. The most important benefit of dark-blood sequences in imaging of the aorta is for evaluation of intramural hematoma, which appears as smooth crescentic increased signal along the affected wall of the vessel. With gadolinium-enhanced images, the intramural hematoma may blend with signal in the lumen, thereby potentially limiting detection (Fig. 8-6).

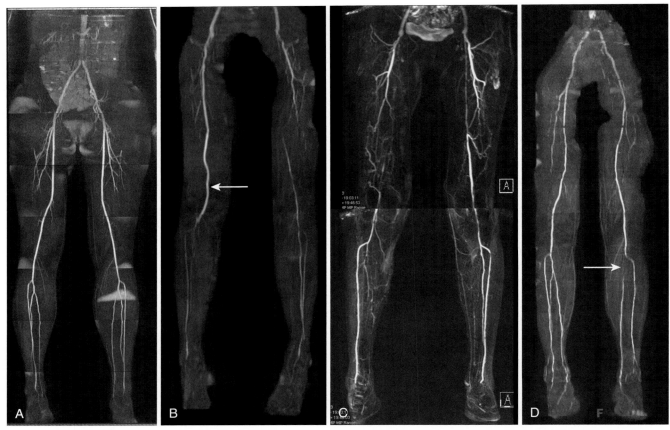

Figure 8-5 A, Multistation quiescent interval single shot (QISS) magnetic resonance angiography (MRA) in a normal patient. This examination used nine stations. **B,** QISS MRA in a different patient was performed to demonstrate patency of a right femoral-popliteal artery bypass graft *(arrow).* **C,** This patient's contrast-enhanced MRA performed several years before revascularization is shown for comparison. **D,** A third patient demonstrates a severely diseased proximal left posterior tibial artery *(arrow),* a finding that was correlated with segmental lower extremity pressure measurements.

■ CONTRAST-ENHANCED MAGNETIC RESONANCE ANGIOGRAPHY

Despite the many advances and growing clinical utility of noncontrast MRA techniques, CE MRA is a superior method and should be considered a first-line imaging technique in suitable patients. CE MRA is faster, flow independent, and does not suffer from many of the artifacts seen with noncontrast MRA techniques. CE MRA provides for an excellent contrast-to-noise ratio and renders angiographic images that both radiologists and clinicians are comfortable interpreting. Furthermore, with technical advances in sequence design, scanners, coils, and contrast agents, CE MRA can be optimized for high–spatial and temporal resolution imaging. In the subsequent sections, the contrast materials, sequences, acquisition techniques, and postprocessing methods used in CE MRA are discussed.

Gadolinium-Based Contrast Materials

Extracellular Materials
Whereas noncontrast MRA techniques rely on blood motion and fluid composition to differentiate vascular signal from background, CE MRA uses the injection of a paramagnetic gadolinium chelate as a contrast material to shorten the T1 and T2 relaxation times of blood by disrupting spin lattice and spin spin interactions, respectively. These effects make the T1 significantly less than that of fat, which is the brightest surrounding tissue. Blood can then be imaged directly with a T1-weighted sequence, independent of the direction of flow and with decreased sensitivity to turbulent flow. As a result, CE MRA sequences can be acquired with only a few slices oriented to capture the longitudinal course of the vessel of interest, thus allowing for larger anatomic coverage in a shorter time.

Extracellular GBCMs are chelates of the gadolinium ion (Gd^{3+}) with other ligands (e.g., DTPA in gadobenate dimeglumine; Multihance, Bracco Diagnostic, Inc., Milan, Italy) that form small-molecular-weight contrast materials. After injection, extracellular GBCMs have an intravascular residence of a few minutes (intravascular half-lives of ~100 seconds), and this property allows for imaging in multiple vascular phases. Because extracellular agents diffuse into the interstitial tissues and equilibrate among the intravascular, extravascular, and extracellular compartments fairly rapidly, MRA sequences using extracellular agents must be relatively fast to provide an adequate contrast-to-background ratio.

In comparison with iodinated contrast agents, gadolinium chelates have a lower rate of adverse events and

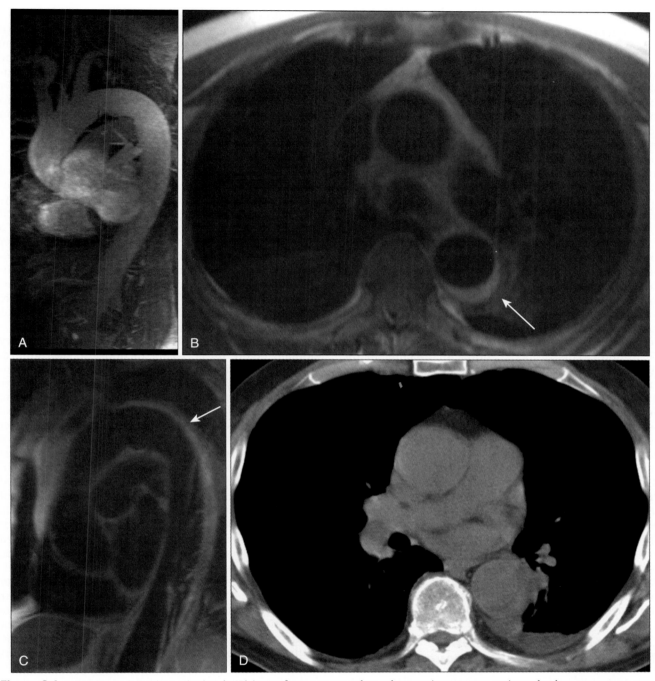

Figure 8-6 **A,** Maximum intensity projection (MIP) image from contrast-enhanced magnetic resonance angiography demonstrates no appreciable abnormality in the aorta in this patient presenting with chest pain. Black-blood axial (**B**) and sagittal (**C**) HASTE images, however, demonstrate thickening of the wall of the descending aorta *(arrows)* with a smooth inner border, a finding consistent with an intramural hematoma. **D,** These findings were also demonstrated on a noncontrast computed tomography examination as a hyperattenuating crescent in the wall of the descending aorta. Black-blood imaging can be very useful in evaluating for mural abnormalities such as intramural hematoma. This example also demonstrates lack of visualization of the wall of vessels as a pitfall of MIP images.

no nephrotoxicity at clinically used doses. Therefore, these agents are a good choice in patients with borderline or at-risk renal function. As stated earlier, patients with severe chronic renal dysfunction (glomerular filtration rate <30), as well as all patients with acute renal failure, should not be given GBCMs because of the risk of nephrogenic systemic fibrosis (NSF). Because no proven treatment exists for NSF, prevention of this disease is paramount. Therefore, all patients presenting for CE MRI of any kind should have a serum creatinine measured before the examination.

Blood Pool Materials

Whereas extracellular GBCMs diffuse out of the intravascular space and allow only a few minutes for CE MRA to be performed, blood pool agents are larger molecules designed to have an extended intravascular residence. At present, the only blood pool agent that is approved by the U.S. Food and Drug Administration and available in the United States is gadofosveset trisodium (Ablavar). Gadofosveset trisodium has a lipophilic side chain, which results in reversible transient noncovalent binding to albumin. This interaction leads to the formation of a larger molecule with slower tumbling, a property that enhances the paramagnetic effectiveness of gadolinium. This feature, in turn, increases T1 relaxivity by four to five times compared with standard extracellular agents at 1.5 T. The results of improved T1 relaxivity are greater achievable contrast-to-noise ratios and hence lower recommended contrast doses with gadofosveset trisodium (0.03 mmol/kg) than with standard extracellular GBCMs (0.1 mmol/kg). Gadopentate dimeglumine, an extracellular GCBM, also exhibits some in vivo protein binding that results in increased signal for CE MRA, but this interaction is weak, and gadopentate dimeglumine is not considered a true blood pool agent.

The noncovalent binding of gadofosveset trisodium to albumin also results in prolonged intravascular residence, with an intravascular half-life of approximately 28 minutes. This property allows for imaging in the "steady state," during which contrast enhancement of the arteries and veins is relatively equal. The steady state can last for up to 60 minutes, thus permitting the use of longer sequences with higher spatial resolution and isotropic voxels. Steady-state imaging can also be exploited for examinations requiring multiple or provocative patient positions such as MRA for thoracic outlet or popliteal artery entrapment syndrome (Fig. 8-7). Additional vascular territories can also be imaged during the steady state; for example, the pelvic and proximal lower extremity veins can be imaged for deep venous thrombosis after CE MRA sequences of the pulmonary vasculature are obtained to evaluate for pulmonary embolism. Finally, the longer window afforded by steady-state imaging yields greater forgiveness for common problems encountered during MRA examinations, such as patient motion, missed contrast bolus, or an inadequate field of view (FOV).

Contrast-Enhanced Magnetic Resonance Angiography Sequences

Sequences used for CE MRA must have several important characteristics to produce angiographic-quality images with a high contrast-to-noise ratio. First, the sequence must be fast. Speed is essential when imaging the chest and upper abdomen, in which the entire sequence must be acquired in one breath hold and thus is typically less than 25 seconds, preferably less than 15 seconds. The sequence also must be fast enough such that in a multistation examination, all stations can be acquired during the arterial phase (i.e., fast enough to chase the bolus). If the sequence is too long, venous contamination can make vessel interpretation difficult, particularly in the extremities. In addition, the sequence must have one center of k-space for the entire volume of data, thus allowing for the arrival of the peak of the contrast bolus

to be timed to coincide with the center of k-space. In addition to speed and timing issues, a CE MRA sequence must be heavily T1 weighted to take advantage of the induced T1 relaxivity of the blood and maximize the contrast-to-noise ratio. The background signal of angiographic sequences can also be suppressed, further increasing the contrast-to-noise ratio. Finally, within the limitations of sequence duration, spatial resolution should be maximized.

k-Space

Before any discussion of technique, the importance of central k-space to the concept of CE MRA must be mentioned. Unlike CTA, which obtains data in a slice-by-slice manner, the three-dimensional gradient recalled echo (3-D GRE) sequences used in CE MRA acquire a full 3-D volume in the frequency domain before Fourier transform reconstruction. This difference may be advantageous in that slight motion is distributed throughout the entire volume of data in 3-D MRA sequences, thus limiting its effects. The converse is also true; severe motion occurring during a short portion of the 3-D MRA volume is distributed throughout the entire image set.

Acquisition of the full 3-D volume in the frequency domain before image reconstruction also has implications for bolus timing. To begin to understand bolus timing in CE MRA, one must recognize that the periphery of k-space determines spatial resolution and edge detail, whereas the center of k-space dominates image contrast. Consequently, for CE MRA, the acquisition of the center of k-space must be timed with the peak contrast bolus. If the center of k-space is acquired far too early, the worst case situation will result, in which the vessel will contain no contrast material. If the center of k-space is acquired during the edges of the bolus geometry in the vessel of interest (i.e., early during rapid upslope or late during rapid downslope), ringing or banding artifact will occur in the vessels. Finally, if the center of k-space is acquired too late, contamination from venous structures will occur, and this is unwanted for pure arterial phase images.

Another essential factor to understand for proper timing of CE MRA is the phase encoding order of the 3-D GRE sequence. Two phase encoding orders for data acquisition in CE MRA are widely available. Linear or sequential k-space filling is the standard acquisition. With linear phase encoding, the center of k-space occurs near the midpoint of data acquisition. Consequently, bolus timing must be calculated so the peak bolus coincides with one half the sequence duration (or time to center of k space). Unlike linear k space encoding, with centric encoding, the center of k-space is acquired at the beginning of the scan. Centric encoding can be performed as an elliptical variant with two phase encoding directions. In elliptical phase ordering, the acquisition of the center of k-space is concentrated into a shorter time at the beginning of the scan. Although centric and elliptically ordered sequences allow for simpler timing and are less prone to artifacts from incomplete breath holds, timing must be precise because these sequences are more prone to artifacts related to rapid changes in the concentration of gadolinium during the early acquisition of the center of k-space.

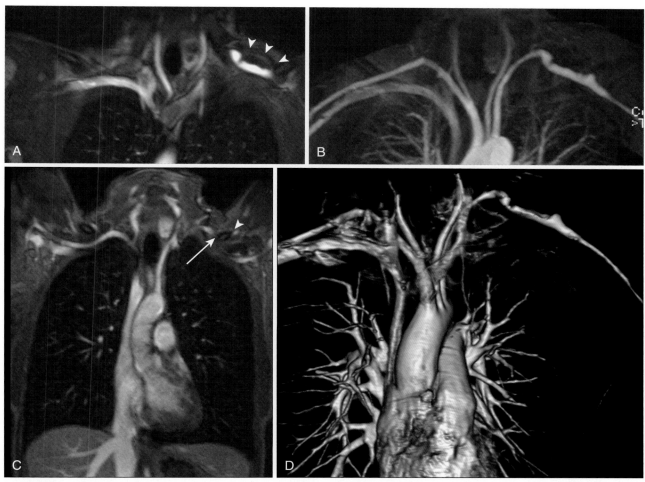

Figure 8-7 With the patient's arms adducted, coronal contrast-enhanced three-dimensional (3-D) gradient recalled echo images (**A**), maximum intensity projection (**B**), and 3-D volumetric reconstructed images (**C**) demonstrate narrowing of the left subclavian artery at the thoracic inlet with a partially thrombosed poststenotic aneurysm *(arrowheads)*. **D,** In the steady-state phase with the arms up, one sees complete occlusion of the left subclavian artery *(arrow)* as it passes below the left clavicle *(arrowhead)*. This patient underwent a surgical procedure to repair the pseudoaneurysm and relieve the obstruction. This study was performed with only 6 mL of gadofosveset trisodium, a blood pool gadolinium-based contrast material. When using a blood pool agent for multiposition examinations such as this for thoracic outlet syndrome, only one injection is required, given the extended intravascular residence.

Three-Dimensional Spoiled Gradient Recalled Echo Sequences

Aside from imaging small parts and small vascular malformations, most angiographic imaging requires multistation examinations and depiction of several vascular territories. Three-dimensional GRE sequences are commonly used for MRA because they provide a well-balanced combination of speed, signal-to-noise, background suppression, and spatial resolution. TR (usually <5 msec) and TE (usually <3 msec) are kept at a minimum, and flip angles typically range from 25 to 45 degrees. Because of the low TR and TE, 3-D GRE sequences are inherently T1 weighted. Background suppression is added in the form of RF spoiling, in which repeated RF pulses are applied to the tissue. If the flip angle is large enough, background tissues do not have time to recover their longitudinal magnetization sufficiently and thus become saturated; this situation, in turn, increases the vessel contrast-to-noise ratio. Additional techniques for background suppression can be applied to improve the contrast-to-noise ratio further,

including fat suppression and magnetization transfer. Fat suppression is particularly useful in abdominal and pelvic CE MRA to most clearly distinguish vessels and organs from surrounding background fat.

In certain instances, particularly when imaging the chest, abdomen, and pelvis, increased background signal is desirable, to allow evaluation of the organs or surrounding tissues. The volume-interpolated breath-hold examination (VIBE) represents a modification of the 3-D GRE sequence to meet these needs. By reducing the flip angle to 10 to 15 degrees and changing to a symmetric readout in the KY direction, background tissue signal is increased. With its excellent depiction of both vessel and background anatomy, the VIBE sequence has become commonly used for dynamic postcontrast chest, abdominal, and pelvic MRI examinations. VIBE sequences are particularly useful in angiographic applications when a question of mural enhancement or enhancement of intraluminal tumor thrombus exists (Fig. 8-8). High-resolution VIBE images may also be useful in depicting anatomy of vascular malformations,

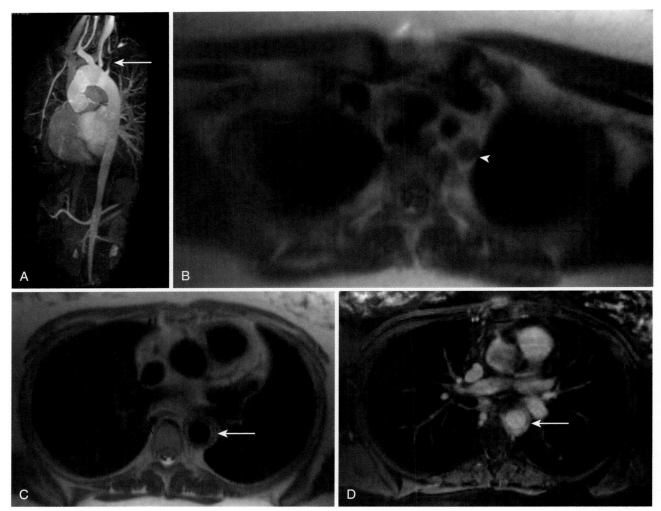

Figure 8-8 A, This maximum intensity projection image from contrast-enhanced magnetic resonance angiography demonstrates irregular narrowing of the left subclavian artery *(arrow)* and the left common carotid artery. **B** and **C,** Corresponding noncontrast black-blood HASTE images demonstrate associated wall thickening of the left subclavian artery *(arrowhead)* and descending aorta *(arrow)* in this patient with Takayasu arteritis. To evaluate disease acuity, interrogation of vascular wall enhancement can be helpful. This is best done with a sequence that has increased background contrast, thus allowing the wall to be seen. **D,** This postcontrast volume-interpolated breath-hold examination image depicts avid enhancement of the wall of the descending aorta *(arrow)*.

as an adjunct to traditional GRE sequences, particularly when blood pool GBCMs are used.

Partial Fourier and parallel imaging techniques can be added to the 3-D GRE sequences used in CE MRA to decrease scan times or allow for the acquisition of higher–spatial resolution data in acceptable scan times. Partial Fourier techniques, sometimes referred to as "partial NEX" or "half-scan," take advantage of the relative symmetry of k-space by acquiring just more than half of k-space and then synthesizing the remaining part by complex conjugation. The result is an increase in speed, with the unavoidable tradeoff of increased noise and some blurring of the image. Parallel imaging techniques use the signal from several coil arrays to reduce the data set acquired in the phase encoding direction of k-space. Stated differently, when an acceleration factor of 2 is used, every other phase encoding step is acquired.

The missing data from the phase encoding steps that were not sampled are mathematically extrapolated from the data collected and the information from the coils. Consequently, the maximum increase in speed is proportional to the number of coils used. Parallel imaging techniques can be applied in image space after Fourier transform (through sensitivity encoding [SENSE]) or in k-space (generalized auto calibrating partially parallel acquisition [GRAPPA]). Another parallel imaging technique, simultaneous acquisition of spatial harmonics (SMASH), uses combinations of component coil signals in an RF coil array to substitute for omitted gradient steps, and it ultimately results in up to a fourfold reduction in imaging time. Although parallel imaging techniques are powerful tools that do not affect spatial resolution, their main disadvantage is the reduction in signal-to-noise ratio by a factor of approximately the square root of the acceleration factor multiplied by a geometry factor. In CE MRA, however, loss of even up to 55% of the signal-to-noise ratio is relatively well tolerated secondary to the high baseline contrast-to-noise ratio facilitated by the administered GBCM.

Partition dimensions (slice thickness, matrix size, and FOV) used in 3-D GRE sequences for CE MRA are determined by the requirements of the imaging protocol and the vascular territory being imaged. For imaging of larger vessels such as the thoracic aorta, large ranges of anatomic coverage are required, and thus a slice thickness of 1.5 to 2.5 mm is acceptable. This is in contradistinction to imaging of the small vessels of the extremities, for which submillimeter voxel sizes are essential to diagnose stenoses. Although the goal is to achieve the smallest possible voxel size while still performing the scan in an acceptable time with appropriate coverage, a general rule is that the spatial resolution in all planes should be no less than approximately one third the diameter of the vessel of interest. When possible, consideration should be given to the benefits of prescribing isotropic voxels because they allow for distortion-free reconstruction of the acquired source images.

Contrast Injection and Bolus Timing

Gadolinium-Based Contrast Agent Dose and Injection Rate

In arterial first-pass CE MRA, the general goals are to increase the intraarterial signal and to optimize the contrast-to-noise ratio. These goals are accomplished by maximizing the concentration of the GBCM in the artery of interest during the acquisition of the center of k-space. Because arterial gadolinium concentration is proportional to injection rate and cardiac output, increasing the injection rate has the potential to increase vascular signal. However, important tradeoffs must be considered when increasing injection rates. Faster injections with the same total dose of gadolinium and volume of administered contrast result in tighter bolus geometry that is more difficult to time precisely to the center of k-space. Although slower injection rates do not deliver as high an arterial gadolinium concentration, they have more uniform and wider bolus geometry, thus making them easier to time and causing fewer artifacts. Typically, an injection duration of approximately 50% to 70% of the overall acquisition time is used because injecting contrast material during the acquisition of the periphery of k-space is not generally necessary. In patients of normal size, this approach results in a contrast injection rate of approximately 2 mL/second with a contrast dose of 0.1 to 0.2 mmol/kg of an extracellular GBCM.

As previously mentioned, because of the higher T1 relaxivity of blood pool GBCMs such as gadofosveset trisodium, the recommended dose for blood pool GBCMs in angiographic applications is 0.03 mmol/kg. This dose results in a smaller injected volume of contrast and tighter bolus geometry, which can, in turn, lead to issues with bolus timing. To mitigate the effect of the smaller injected volume, lower rates of injection (1 mL/second) are typically used to widen the bolus geometry. In lieu of lowering the injection rate of a blood pool GBCM, another option is to dilute the contrast in saline solution to a larger volume. Given the high relaxivity of blood pool GBCMs, the contrast-to-noise ratio is still excellent despite the lower

injection rate or diluted volume. Finally, following injection of any type of GBCM, a chaser of at least 20 to 30 mL of saline solution should be administered to propagate the bolus centrally.

Timing the Bolus
SCAN DELAY USING TIME TO PEAK ESTIMATE
Several different schemes can be used to determine appropriate bolus timing. One method is to use a scan delay. When a scan delay is used in a linear phase encoded 3-D GRE acquisition, the following formula is used:

$$\text{Scan delay} = \text{Time to peak} + (\text{Injection duration} / 2) - (\text{Time to center of k-space})$$

For centric phase encoded acquisitions, the scan delay is calculated by the following formula:

$$\text{Scan delay} = \text{Time to peak} + (\text{Injection duration} / 2)$$

A few seconds can be added to these scan delays to decrease the chance of ringing artifact, which can occur when the center of k-space is acquired during the rapid rise of the contrast peak.

To use the formulas for scan delay, the time to peak must be determined. The simplest method of determining the time to peak is the "best guess" method, in which the time to peak is estimated based on a general assessment of the patient's age, size, and cardiac output. The time from the antecubital vein to the abdominal aorta can be estimated at 15 seconds for a healthy young patient, at 20 to 25 seconds for an older healthy patient, at 30 to 35 seconds for patients with a large aneurysm or cardiac disease, and at 45 to 50 seconds for patients with severe cardiac dysfunction. Clearly, using the best guess method is prone to error because patient factors are widely variable and difficult to assess. This method should be used only for linear phase encoded sequences, given that these acquisitions are less sensitive to timing errors.

A more reproducible method for determining time to peak is use of a test bolus. With a test bolus, a small volume (1 to 2 mL) of contrast is injected at the same rate as that planned for the full examination, followed by a 20-mL saline chaser. Imaging after the injection is then performed with a rapidly repeated (at least one image per 2 seconds) single slice low spatial resolution 2-D gradient echo sequence including the vessel of interest. The time to peak can then be determined by visually examining the resultant images or by using region of interest analysis. Use of a test bolus is more accurate than the best guess method, but it does add significantly to the overall examination time. Additionally, with blood pool GBCMs, the test bolus can be particularly problematic because even the very small doses of contrast administered for the test bolus can lead to venous contamination on future acquisitions.

AUTOMATED BOLUS DETECTION
Automated bolus detection uses a fast gradient echo sequence combined with software that measures the signal intensity of the vessel of interest, usually the

aorta, before and during contrast administration. This sequence has high temporal resolution on the order of approximately 20 msec, thus ensuring that the bolus is not missed. The signal intensity during contrast administration is compared with that at baseline, and when a predetermined threshold is met, breath-holding commands commence, and a centric 3-D GRE sequence is run to obtain the angiographic data. Typically, the trigger threshold is set approximately 20% higher than baseline, to allow time for the breath hold to take place during the leading edge of the bolus in the vessel of interest and then for the center of k-space to be obtained at the peak. Automated bolus detection has the advantage of being relatively simple to use and, unlike the timing bolus technique, does not require an additional acquisition. Potential pitfalls of this technique involve placing the region of interest in the wrong location or patient motion that moves the volume outside the vessel of interest. In addition, the patient must hold his or her breath rather quickly because not much time elapses between the trigger and the onset of the 3-D GRE data collection.

FLUOROSCOPIC TRIGGERING

In MR fluoroscopic triggering, fast 2-D gradient refocused images that include the vessel of interest are acquired and then rapidly reconstructed in near real time for the operator to follow the contrast bolus manually. The operator can then manually initiate breath-hold instructions and the acquisition of a centric phase ordered 3-D GRE sequence at the time of his or her choosing. When using MR fluoroscopic triggering, a useful approach is to include vasculature proximal to the vessel of interest such that the breath hold and scan initiation can be completed by the time the contrast material reaches the vessel of interest. Given that this technique requires a well-trained operator who understands both the imaged anatomy and contrast dynamics, this method has a short but steep learning curve. MR fluoroscopic triggering can be particularly valuable in patients with complex or asymmetric flow patterns. In addition, patients who have slow vascular flow, or an aneurysm that could limit flow, are well suited to this technique because it allows the operator to wait for filling of the vessels distal to the aneurysm.

Time-Resolved Magnetic Resonance Angiography

Time-resolved MRA involves the repeated sampling of a volume of tissue at multiple consecutive time points to allow the examiner to follow the distribution of the administered contrast over time. Unlike traditional 3-D CE MRA, time-resolved MRA does not require timing of the bolus. Image acquisition is begun, often simultaneous to or preceding the contrast bolus, and images are acquired for a preset number of cycles to incorporate the necessary vascular phases. This technique can prove to be an effective means of imaging vascular beds that contain rapidly enhancing veins or to evaluate patients in whom bolus timing is difficult secondary to reduced or inconsistent cardiac output. As a general rule, temporal resolution must be shorter than 10 seconds to isolate the arterial phase, and preferably significantly faster.

Standard 3-D GRE sequences can be modified to maximize temporal resolution, thus providing one means of performing time-resolved MRA. This is typically done by using a combination of decreasing spatial resolution, limiting anatomic coverage, applying a rectangular FOV, reducing TR, or implementing the partial Fourier or parallel imaging techniques described previously. Of course, these modifications of 3-D GRE sequences to improve temporal resolution come with tradeoffs in signal-to-noise ratio (SNR) and spatial resolution, and additional postcontrast acquisitions with conventional 3-D GRE sequences may be beneficial, to provide better anatomic detail.

Although modified 3-D GRE sequences as described earlier may provide some measure of improved temporal resolution and can image multiple vascular phases, fully sampled 3-D GRE sequences have temporal limitations that usually preclude detailed assessment of contrast kinetics, determination of flow direction in complex vessels, and assessment of structures or lesions with short arterial-venous transit times such as high-flow peripheral vascular malformations. Newer techniques using k-space sharing yield further improvements in temporal resolution with relative preservation of spatial resolution and allow more detailed assessment of contrast kinetics and distribution. In the most basic terms, k-space sharing techniques acquire the central and peripheral portions of k-space at different time points and ultimately share these data between time points for full reconstructions. For example, time-resolved imaging with stochastic trajectories (TWIST) alternates acquisition of the central ellipsoid and peripheral portions of k-space in a radial manner based on the distance from the center of k-space and later synthesizes full volumes.

In another technique, four-dimensional time-resolved angiography using keyhole (4-D–TRAK), the center ellipsoid keyhole of k-space is sampled at each time point, whereas the periphery is sampled only at the last time point and is then used to reconstruct all previous time points. In time-resolved imaging of contrast kinetics (TRICKS), the center of k-space is continuously oversampled and interleaved with peripheral blocks of k-space. This is similar to the time-resolved echo-shared angiographic technique (TREAT), in which the continuously resampled center of k-space is interleaved with peripheral lines of k-space. With all these techniques, the entirety of k-space is not sampled at all time points, and hence speed is greatly accelerated, with subsecond temporal resolution possible. Even faster acceleration can be achieved through additional sharing of the center of k-space among different time points. Although SNR can be decreased in applications with very high temporal resolution, the size of the central portion of k-space can be controlled by the user, thus allowing for tradeoffs between temporal resolution and SNR (Fig. 8-9).

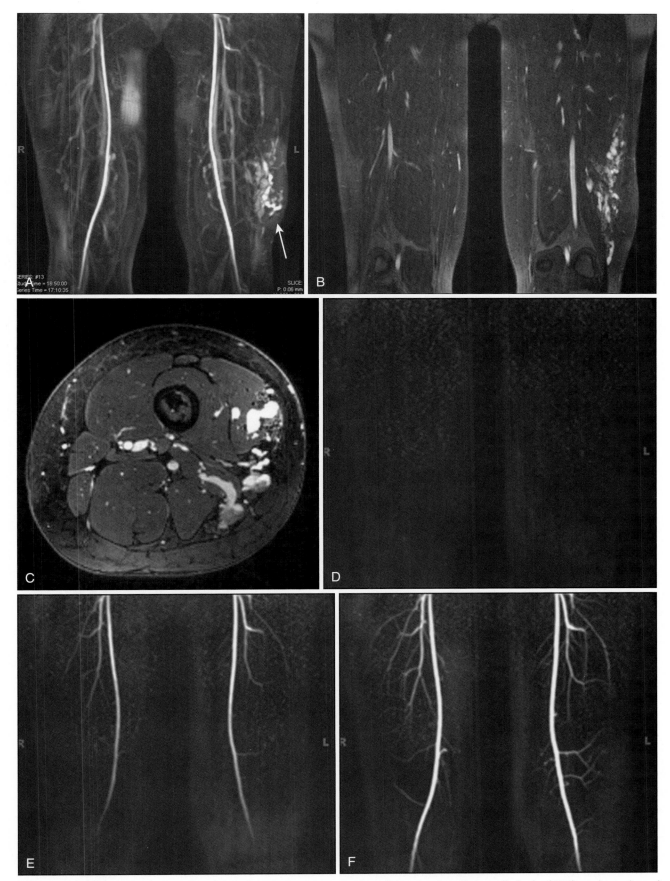

Figure 8-9 Although contrast-enhanced magnetic resonance angiography three-dimensional gradient recalled echo (GRE) maximum intensity projection (**A**), high-resolution GRE (**B**), and axial volume-interpolated breath-hold examination (**C**) images of this slow-flow vascular lesion *(arrow)* in the left thigh are useful for determining the relationship of the lesion with surrounding vessels, bones, and muscles, the time-resolved sequences performed with the time-resolved imaging with stochastic trajectories technique (**D** to **L**) best depict the vascular supply of the lesion. On the earlier arterial phases, the lesion is not seen, but it slowly enhances during the venous phases, an appearance characteristic of a slow-flow vascular lesion.

Continued

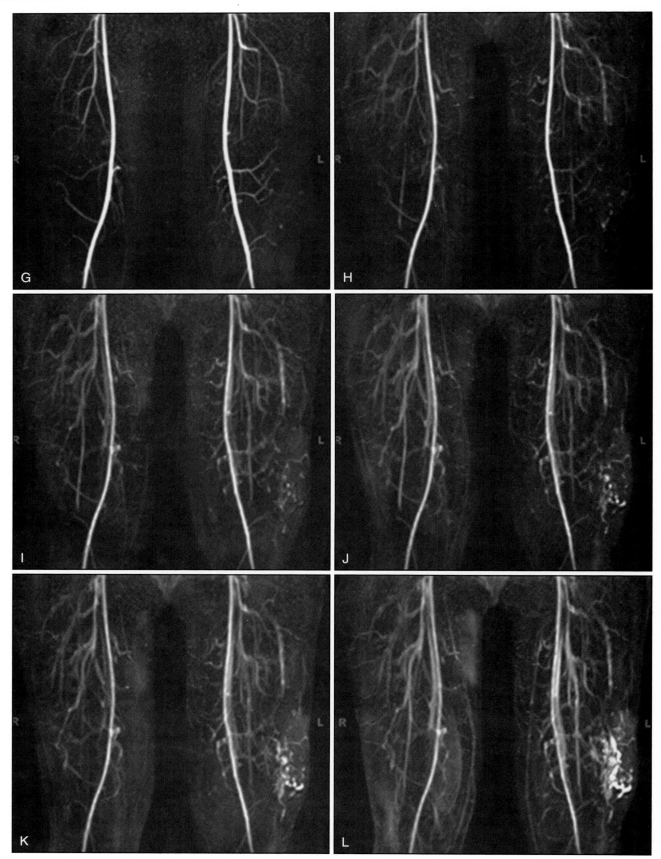

Figure 8-9, cont'd For legend see p.145

Magnetic Resonance Angiography Data Postprocessing

Postprocessing is a core component of MRA interpretation and is essential for conveying results to referring clinicians, most of whom do not have the time to assess the source images carefully. In addition, many referral clinicians are more accustomed to viewing conventional angiography or CTA images and thus are more comfortable reviewing postprocessed MRA images than the source images themselves. Before reviewing the different postprocessing techniques, any abnormality detected on the postprocessed images should be confirmed on the source images.

Subtraction

Subtraction images are routine components of MRA examinations and often are automatically performed by the scanner software. To obtain subtraction images, a precontrast mask 3-D GRE sequence is obtained with the exact parameters that will be used in the postcontrast CE MRA images. The mask data set can subsequently be digitally subtracted from the postcontrast data set to remove background signal and greatly improve the contrast-to-noise ratio. For example, subtracting the mask from the arterial phase can produce an image set that depicts essentially only the arteries. To depict the veins primarily, one would subtract the arterial phase from a later, more delayed venous phase. Subtracted images are beneficial in CE MRA because they allow the reader to focus primarily on the vasculature. The main problem with subtracted images is that they require consistent positioning to avoid spatial misregistration. This problem can be particularly significant in the chest and upper abdomen, where spatial misregistration can result from different breath holds. Finally, as mentioned earlier, findings depicted on subtracted images must be confirmed on the source data set.

Maximum Intensity Projection

The maximum intensity projection (MIP) provides a powerful means of presenting MRA data. In a MIP, the highest intensity voxel in each projection ray perpendicular to the viewing plane becomes a pixel on the final image. MIP images can be depicted in any projection, and a composite of multiple projections can be created to allow the reader to rotate the image. This feature is important because structures may overlap on MIP images in one projection, but they may be distinguished from each other in another projection.

MIP postprocessing is particularly useful in CE MRA because the signal within the vessels is much brighter than background signal and dominates the postprocessed images. MIP images often function as a general map of the vasculature and are particularly well adapted to tracking tortuous vessels that course in and out of a single plane. Furthermore, clinicians are often more comfortable interpreting MIP images, which more closely resemble conventional angiograms.

The most important artifact that affects MIP images in CE MRA occurs when background stationary tissue (fat, hemorrhage, metallic susceptibility) or a superimposed vessel has as high or higher signal intensity than the vessel of interest. When this occurs, the unwanted signal not in the vessel of interest can be mapped to the projection image and causes an apparent discontinuity in the vessel of interest. Subvolume, or partial volume, MIP images can overcome this problem. In subvolume MIP images, the user selects only a certain thickness of the source images in the reconstructed volume. This approach allows the exclusion of structures in the background that may obscure visualization of the underlying vessels. The subvolume MIP images can then be scrolled through at the desired thickness to view the full volume.

Multiplanar Reconstruction

Multiplanar reconstruction (MPR) is an essential component of MRA interpretation. At the viewing workstation, the source data can be reconstructed in any plane, thus allowing the reader to gain a 3-D understanding of the imaged volume. Unlike MIP images, which are affected by overlapping structures, MPR data sets are not projections and provide thin, scrollable images for the reader. Oblique MPR data sets are essential when measuring vascular structures because they allow for measurements to be obtained orthogonal to the long axis of the vessel. For particularly tortuous vessels, curved MPR data sets can be obtained. In curved MPRs, the reader selects the midpoint of the vessel over its entire course, and the image is reconstructed along that axis. This allows a tortuous vessel to be visible to the reader on a single image. Curved MPR data sets are useful for obtaining complex sets of measurements in vessels, as are often used in planning aortic endovascular stent repair. MPR data sets in CE MRA examinations can suffer from distortion caused by the use of nonisotropic voxels. Although isotropic voxels are ideal for the purposes of MPR, they may not be possible in many cases in which compromise is often made by increasing slice thickness while maintaining high in-plane resolution to accommodate imaging a larger FOV within an acceptably short time frame. The longer intravascular residence of blood pool agents provides one potential means of overcoming this problem because these agents allow for longer, higher-spatial resolution sequences with isotropic voxels to be performed during the steady state after initial first-pass arterial images using faster sequences are obtained. MPR of the high-resolution steady-state sequences can be of particularly high quality as a result of the small source data set voxels and the absence of distortion.

Shaded Surface Display

In shaded surface display (SSD), the user selects a minimum signal intensity threshold and discards data that are lower than this threshold. The remaining data are rendered into a 3-D surface representation and are illuminated with a virtual light source. The result is an image that appears somewhat 3-D and, because of the light source, conveys some degree of depth perception. The user must select a minimum threshold that is high enough to exclude unwanted background structures but not so high that it removes portions of the vessels that are to be displayed. Although SSD techniques have some

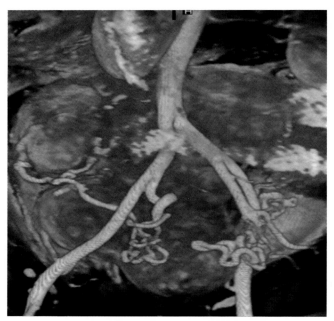

Figure 8-10 Surface rendered image of a contrast-enhanced volume-interpolated breath-hold examination sequence demonstrates markedly tortuous uterine vessels in this patient with large uterine fibroids. Although characterizing stenoses with postprocessed techniques is not advisable, these techniques can be useful for displaying tortuous vessels in a single image.

use in displaying complex anatomy, their main utility is in providing clinicians with a more understandable depiction of imaging findings (Fig. 8-10). Vessel characterization, and in particular stenosis grade, should not be evaluated on SSD images because partial volume effects on the edges of vessels can overestimate areas of narrowing.

Volume Rendering

The fundamental difference between volume rendering (VR) techniques and SSD and MIP techniques is that every voxel contributes to image reconstruction in VR techniques. Whereas data lower than thresholds are discarded in SSD and only the maximum values are represented in MIP, VR assigns each volume an opacity value between 0% and 100%. These values can then be rendered into volumetric representations of the tissues of interest. Unlike threshold techniques, in which a binary system based on an intensity threshold determines whether a voxel lies within an organ or vessel of interest, the opacity scale of VR techniques allow for better delineation of the interfaces and relationships among tissues. Vendors have developed a multitude of algorithms and software packages for VR postprocessing, with a wide range of user-controlled values that contribute to the appearance of the final product. For example, cut-plane techniques allow the user to strip away overlying structures; this approach can be useful for delineating the location of vessel ostia along the interior surface of the vessel. Interrogation of the vessel lumen can also be performed by virtual angioscopy, which allows for a fly-through of the vessel of interest (Fig. 8-11).

Magnetic Resonance Angiography Pitfalls and Artifacts

Bolus Timing Related

CONTRAST ARRIVING TOO EARLY

Accurate bolus timing is critical in CE MRA because the presence of the paramagnetic contrast agent within the vascular space allows for the creation of images in which the vascular signal dominates. As discussed earlier in the section on bolus timing, when the center of k-space is acquired during the rapid upslope or downslope of the contrast peak in the vessel of interest, ringing (also known as banding or Maki) artifact can occur (Fig. 8-12). This artifact greatly degrades image quality and, depending on its severity, can make images uninterpretable. Ringing artifact is more common with centric ordered acquisitions in which the acquisition of the center of k-space is triggered too soon, a problem often amplified in patients with decreased cardiac output or a large aneurysm upstream from the vascular bed of interest.

Ringing artifact can be prevented or mitigated in various ways. The acquisition of back-to-back 3-D GRE sequences after triggering is one solution. Typically, if the first acquisition has ringing artifact, the second one will not, even if it may suffer from some venous enhancement. When scan delay methods are used, whether by best guess or a timing bolus, linear phase encoded sequences are more forgiving and can be used to prevent ringing artifact. Additionally, adding a few extra seconds to the scan delay may be helpful because being a bit late with the contrast bolus is better than being too early in CE MRA. When using automated triggering, increasing the threshold value for triggering or instituting a short delay before triggering the centric ordered 3-D GRE sequence can help prevent ringing artifact. This delay can be lengthened to accommodate large upstream aneurysms or slow flow.

Because of its real-time nature, fluoroscopic MR triggering allows the user to assess the contrast peak visually, but it requires an experienced user and may not be practical for examinations not monitored by a physician. One nearly fail-safe method to prevent ringing artifact that is particularly useful in patients with unreliable or complex flow is to acquire the first-pass images as part of a high–temporal resolution time-resolved sequence such that the arterial phase is captured multiple times. This approach may be useful during single station MRA but would require protocol modifications to allow for contrast washout during multistation examinations.

VENOUS CONTAMINATION

Venous contamination occurs when the center of k-space is acquired too long after contrast administration, at which point contrast has arrived in the veins. In larger vascular beds, typically extending to the elbows in the upper extremities and the knees in the lower extremities, venous contamination may not inhibit correct interpretation of the source data, although the MIP images are compromised by overlapping venous contamination. Peripheral to the knees and elbows, however, even

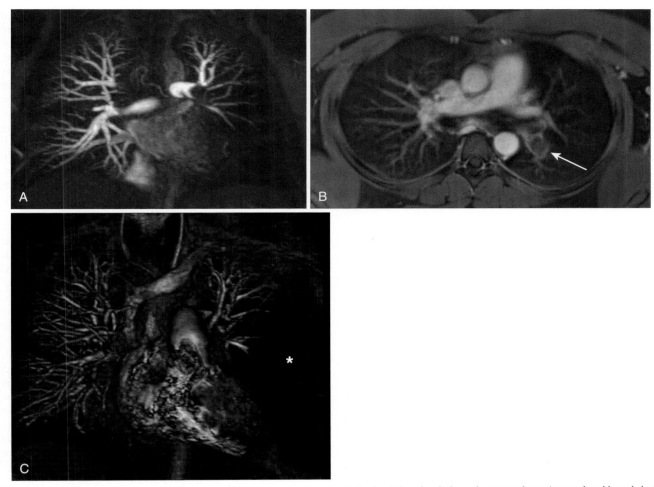

Figure 8-11 Coronal contrast-enhanced three-dimensional gradient recalled echo (**A**) and radial steady-state volume-interpolated breath-hold examination (**B**) images demonstrate a filling defect in the left main pulmonary artery consistent with a pulmonary embolism *(arrow)*. Although these images are sufficient for diagnosis, the cut-plane volume rendered image (**C**) can be used as an adjunct to the source images to display the perfusion defect *(asterisk)*. Postprocessing techniques such as volume rendering often are not necessary for interpretation, but they can highlight certain abnormalities and make the images easier to interpret for referring clinicians.

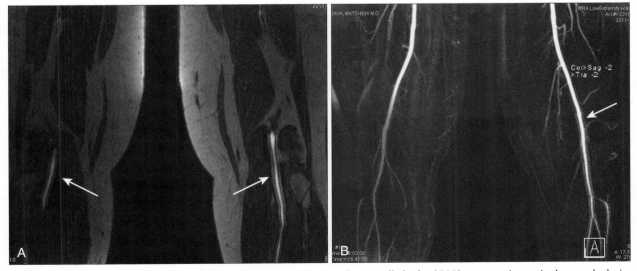

Figure 8-12 When the center of k-space of the three-dimensional (3-D) gradient recalled echo (GRE) sequence is acquired too early during the upstroke of the contrast bolus, a characteristic artifact that goes by the name of ringing, banding, or Maki artifact can arise. Ringing artifact *(arrows)* is shown in these 3-D coronal GRE (**A**) and maximum intensity projection (**B**) images from a lower extremity runoff.

assessment of the source images can be difficult because of the small size of the vessels and the close relationship to the adjacent veins, which are typically more numerous than their arterial counterparts.

In the chest and abdomen, venous contamination is prevented by proper bolus timing. In the extremities, where proper timing is both more difficult and critical secondary to the smaller caliber of the vessels, several modifications can be made to prevent venous contamination. One possibility is to use a thigh or upper arm inflatable cuff to increase the arteriovenous transit time and provide a longer window before venous contamination occurs. When using a thigh cuff, one potential problem is pseudoocclusion resulting from compression from the cuff. This problem may be particularly important in patients with femoral popliteal grafts, in whom lower inflation pressures are recommended. Additionally, patient movement after cuff inflation may result in motion artifact. To minimize the effects of patient movement, the cuff should be inflated before the mask images, to help ensure consistent positioning throughout the examination.

Several modifications to peripheral MRA protocols can also help prevent venous contamination. In standard bolus chase lower extremity runoff examinations, the bolus is timed to the first station (abdomen and pelvis) and then is chased as rapidly as possible inferiorly to the calves. Although this method often works without venous contamination, the station most at risk for venous contamination is the most distal calf station, which is also the station most severely affected by venous contamination. To mitigate this problem, hybrid MRA protocols have been developed. In hybrid peripheral MRA protocols, the bolus of extracellular GBCM is split, and the distal calf station is imaged first, either with multiple full volume 3-D GRE acquisitions or with a time-resolved sequence. For timing of the calf station, the bolus is triggered from the popliteal artery. In this split bolus method, the second half of the bolus is then used for a standard bolus chase technique from the proximal station downward.

Blood pool agents can also be used in hybrid MRA protocols, but important modifications must be made to limit potential venous contamination from the first injection on sequences obtained after the second injection. The most important modification is to use a minimum of contrast for the first injection. Diagnostic time-resolved MRA of the calf vessels can be obtained using only 1 to 2 mL of a blood pool agent. The remainder of the prescribed contrast bolus can then be used for the second injection as part of a standard bolus chase MRA. Subtraction techniques can also be used on the sequences obtained after the second injection to further reduce the effects of any venous contamination from the first injection.

SLOW OR ASYMMETRIC FLOW

Patients with slow or asymmetric flow can present a particularly difficult timing problem. For example, patients with severe congestive heart failure may have very slow transit times that delay the contrast bolus. Large aneurysms or severe stenoses upstream from a vascular bed

of interest can also delay flow distally. If scan delay or automated bolus triggering is used in these patients, an often helpful approach is to place the region of interest in and not upstream from the vascular bed of interest. As mentioned previously, adding an additional delay to the calculated scan delay or trigger point can also help prevent ringing artifact. MR fluoroscopy can be particularly helpful in these cases because the examiner can visually observe the contrast arriving in the target vessel of interest and trigger the scan appropriately. If flow is significantly complex, as may be encountered in a patient with a complex vascular malformation, time-resolved sequences can be performed to ensure that enhancement of downstream vascular beds is captured.

WHEN VENOUS ENHANCEMENT IS WANTED

Although modifications are made to arterial phase images to prevent venous contamination, venous enhancement can be used to advantage when a detailed examination of the veins is necessary. With extracellular GBCMs, the venous phase is usually easily captured with several back-to-back 3-D GRE acquisitions of the imaging volume. To increase the contrast-to-noise ratio in the veins further, the arterial phase can be subtracted from the venous phase. When available, blood pool GBCMs are the optimal choices for venous imaging. With their extended intravascular residence, the steady state or venous phase for blood pool agents can be captured for up to an hour and with high-resolution sequences that are particularly beneficial when imaging complex venous anatomy. The use of blood pool GBCMs also obviates the need for timing to the venous phase (Fig. 8-13).

Pseudostenosis

Pseudostenosis, as its name suggests, refers to a situation in which the vessel caliber appears narrowed as a result of artifact. Pseudostenoses arise in several important circumstances. One such case was mentioned previously in the discussion of vessel occlusion secondary to cuff overinflation. Another particularly common form of pseudostenosis can arise from susceptibility artifacts from adjacent metallic stents, prostheses, and surgical clips. With a proper examination of the source images or longer TE noncontrast sequences, the characteristic blooming artifact can usually be appreciated. When in doubt, conventional radiographs or CT scans can be obtained to determine the location of metallic material precisely.

When the subclavian artery is investigated, dense gadolinium in the adjacent subclavian vein can cause pseudostenosis secondary to a T2* effect. A similar problem can also arise in the carotid system during jugular injections. This problem is easily prevented by injecting on the contralateral side of a suspected abnormality. If an abnormality is possible on either side, contrast material should be injected on the right side because this prevents dense contrast from traveling through the left brachiocephalic veins and potentially leading to a T2* effect on the aortic arch branches. Delayed sequences in the venous phase after dense gadolinium has cleared from the subclavian vein should

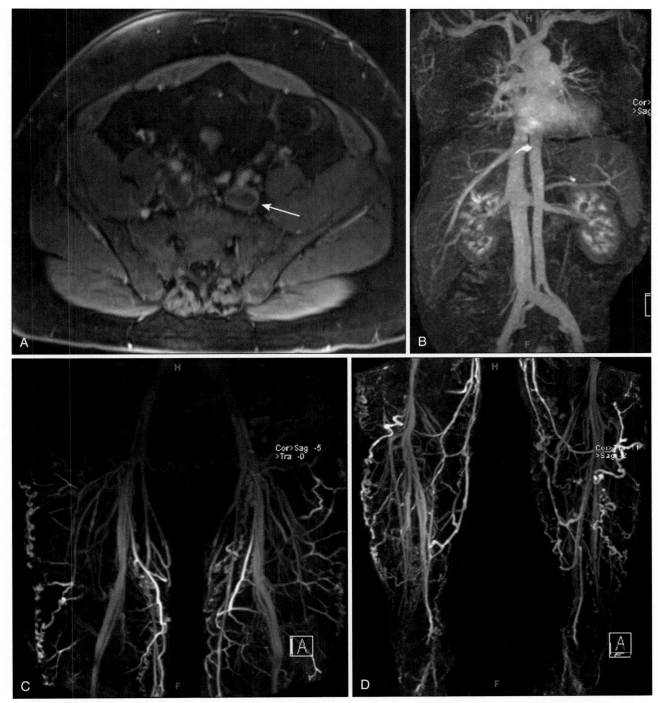

Figure 8-13 For venous imaging, use of a blood pool agent can be advantageous because it obviates the need for timing. In addition, because of the steady state, images can be easily obtained at multiple stations and with longer higher-resolution sequences if necessary. **A,** This blood pool gadolinium-based contrast agent–enhanced axial volume-interpolated breath-hold examination image of the pelvic vessels demonstrates bilateral common iliac thrombosis *(arrow)* in this patient with factor V Leiden deficiency. **B to D,** This whole body magnetic resonance venogram was performed after administration of a blood pool agent in this patient with extensive venous varicosities to look for thrombi; none were found.

also be performed to allow for adequate imaging of the artery on the side ipsilateral to the injection. Blood pool GBCMs can be particularly helpful in this regard, given their prolonged steady state. Blood pool GBCMs are also helpful in patients with a central venous stenosis that results in pooling of contrast in collateral vessels, a problem that can result in extensive T2* artifact. The

steady state allows for redistribution of the blood pool GBCM and imaging of the collateral network.

Pseudostenoses can also complicate postprocessed MIP images. One instance in which pseudostenosis occurs on MIP images is when brighter soft tissue is included in the volume for the MIP. This phenomenon, sometimes referred to as T1 shine through, leads to an apparent vessel discontinuity if the vascular signal is not the brightest signal in the projection ray. Inflamed soft tissue with early enhancement or particularly bright fat can be a source of this problem. Subvolume MIP images can also result in pseudostenoses if the entire vessel is not included in the volume for the MIP. This can be an issue with tortuous vessels, particularly in the renal and iliac beds. Pseudostenoses from MIP images are usually readily discernible after review of the source images and underscore the need to corroborate all suspected abnormalities carefully with the source images.

Pitfalls Related to Field of View

Assigning appropriate FOV in CE MRA studies is essential to accurate vessel depiction. The most commonly encountered artifact related to FOV is wraparound or aliasing. Aliasing occurs when the FOV is too small in the phase encoding direction. Three-dimensional acquisitions have two phase encoding directions. With lower extremity runoff examinations, one phase encoding direction is from left to right. To decrease the coverage volume and help prevent wrap artifact, the patient's arms should be placed over the head if possible or at least out of the imaged volume. The second phase encoding direction in 3-D acquisitions is in the slice direction (front to back for coronally acquired images). To prevent wrap in this direction, the FOV should be adequately large, or slice oversampling should be added.

Given the relatively stringent time restraints involved with arterial MRA, the FOV is often acquired coronal to the vessel of interest and cropped to exclude any excess tissues. With peripheral MRA, the FOV is often slanted to the course of the vessel and is not acquired in skin-to-skin fashion. As a result, in tortuous vascular beds, such as the renal and iliac systems, portions of the vessels may be inadvertently excluded from the imaging volume. To allow for the smallest FOV for coronal acquisitions in bolus chase peripheral runoff CE MRA, the patient's legs should be elevated such that the posteriorly coursing popliteal arteries are included in the same plane as the femoral arteries. Another relatively infrequent, but important, situation in which FOV can exclude a structure of interest occurs in femoral-femoral bypass grafts that course anteriorly. The best protections against exclusion of vessels from the FOV are careful assessment of the spatial localizers and knowledge of any vascular grafts. Review of the source images should promptly detect exclusion of a portion of a vessel and prevent misinterpretation.

Another important point regarding FOV relates to multistation examinations, such as arterial runoffs, in which the designation in the z-direction becomes important to both image quality and speed. Maximizing the z-direction (craniocaudal) FOV to acquire the fewest number of stations possible and, one hopes, avoid venous contamination is tempting. This approach is particularly of interest to clinicians who are primarily using short-bore magnets. However, magnetic field heterogeneities result in a warped appearance of the ends of the image when the FOV is stretched to the maximum dimension (Fig. 8-14). The result is a poorly interpretable study. A superior approach is to assign

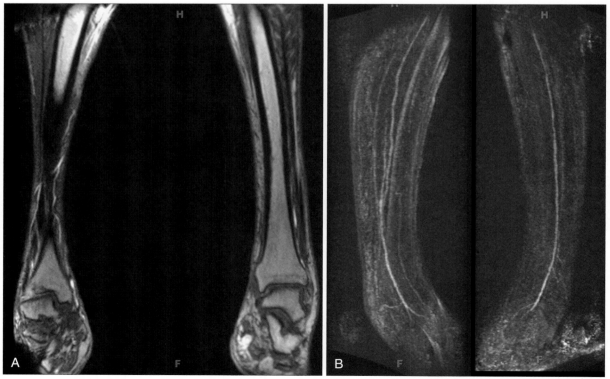

Figure 8-14 In multistation examinations, increased z-axis coverage can reduce the number of stations required, but it also runs the risk of warping artifact. Three-dimensional gradient recalled echo source (**A**) and maximum intensity projection (**B**) images show artifactual warping or bowing of the lower extremities resulting from magnetic field inhomogeneities at the periphery of the field of view.

shorter z-direction FOV and add additional stations to the examination, even though in some instances the study may contain four or five stations. Maximizing speed, optimizing bolus timing, and using blood pressure cuffs can all help avoid venous contamination in this situation.

Phase Ghosting

Occasionally, phase ghosting from the wall of a vessel can project into its lumen and can simulate a dissection flap. This can be a problem in the ascending aorta, in which robust pulsation can create this artifact. When phase ghosting is suspected in the aorta, one potential troubleshooting technique is to perform noncontrast cine bSSFP images through the level of interest. Cine bSSFP sequences are not affected by pulsation artifact and are excellent at depicting dissection flaps and their motion. If the suspected phase ghost is not seen on the cine bSSFP images, it can be assumed to be artifactual and not a true dissection (Fig. 8-15).

Extraluminal Abnormalities

With subtraction, MIP, or even arterial phase images in which intraluminal vascular signal dominates, abnormalities outside the opacified portion of the lumen can be missed. One example of this problem arises with nonvisualization of a large aneurysm sac that is filled with mural thrombus. Large aneurysms can usually be detected on source images, in which the vessel wall contour can be better defined. Detection of intramural hematoma is particularly difficult on 3-D GRE sequences and is essentially impossible on MIP images unless the hematoma is large and greatly distorts the luminal caliber. Evaluation for intramural hematoma highlights the need for the inclusion of noncontrast sequences tailored to answer specific questions in MRA protocols. In the example of intramural hematoma, thoracic dissection protocols should include noncontrast black-blood and bSSFP sequences because these sequences provide excellent assessment of the vessel wall. For assessment of possible enhancement within the vessel wall, as may be desired in patients with aortitis or vasculitis, acquisition of postcontrast VIBE sequences increases background and therefore vessel wall signal, thus allowing for more detailed evaluation. Diffusion sequences may also play a role in evaluating vasculitis.

Breathing Artifact

Respiratory motion can result in significant artifact in CE MRA examinations, particularly images involving the chest and abdomen. In the 3-D GRE sequences, ghosting occurs in the phase encoding directions, whereas blurring occurs in the direction of the motion. Fortunately, advances in scanner technology and sequence design allow acquisitions with adequate spatial resolution to be performed in a single breath hold. In patients who have difficulty holding their breath even for shorter times, centric reordered sequences are more forgiving in terms of respiratory motion artifact. The reason is that the 3-D GRE sequences used in CE MRA are most sensitive to breathing motion during the acquisition of the center of k-space, and with this occurring nearer to the onset of the breath hold in the use of centric phase ordered sequences, breathing artifact will be minimized if the patient begins shallow respiration during the later acquisition of the periphery of k-space. Assessing the patient's breath-holding capability before the examination can aid the operator in determining when to modify standard protocols. In addition, the operator should review the breath-holding instructions and their importance with the patient before the examination, to maximize compliance and breath-hold quality.

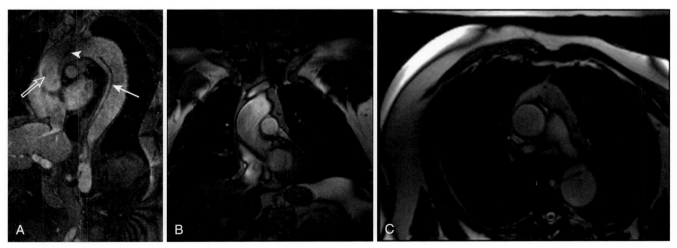

Figure 8-15 A, This contrast-enhanced coronal three-dimensional (3-D) gradient recalled echo (GRE) image demonstrates a dissection flap in the descending aorta *(solid arrow)* and additional linear hypointensity in the ascending aorta *(arrowhead)* that was worrisome for an additional component of the flap. To evaluate the ascending aorta, balanced steady-state free precession (bSSFP) cine sequences (**B and C**) were performed, and they did not demonstrate a flap in the ascending aorta. The finding seen in the ascending aorta in **A** is a phase ghost from the wall of the ascending aorta. Note the additional phase ghost from the pulmonary artery *(open arrow* in **A**). This case highlights two important points. First, questionable dissection flaps detected on contrast-enhanced magnetic resonance angiography images can be corroborated with bSSFP cine images at the same level to evaluate their validity. Second, 3-D GRE images have two phase encoding directions, in this case right-to-left and through plane. Phase ghost artifacts occur in phase encoding directions and are a particular problem in vessels with extensive pulsation, as is seen in the ascending aorta.

Overestimation of Stenosis

Although CE MRA is less sensitive to flow-related dephasing related to turbulent flow downstream of stenoses than are noncontrast MRA techniques, some dephasing and signal loss do occur. These issues can lead to overestimation of stenosis severity, a problem that is more significant in vessels of smaller caliber. MIP images can also lead to overestimation of stenosis because the edge of a vessel can be obscured by noise projected from the background. Source images should always be used to grade stenosis severity in CE MRA.

Bibliography

Blackham KA, Passalacqua MA, Sandhu GS, et al. Applications of time-resolved MR angiography. *AJR Am J Roentgenol.* 2011;196:W613-W620.

Blockley NP, Jiang L, Gardener AG, et al. Field strength dependence of R1 and R2* relaxivities of human whole blood to ProHance, Vasovist, and deoxyhemoglobin. *Magn Reson Med.* 2008;60:1313-1320.

Bremerich J, Bliecen D, Reimer P. MR Angiography with blood pool contrast agents. *Eur Radiol.* 2007;17:3017-3024.

Edelman RR, Sheehan JJ, Dunkle E, et al. Quiescent-interval single-shot unenhanced magnetic resonance angiography of peripheral vascular disease: technical considerations and clinical feasibility. *Magn Reson Med.* 2010;63:951-958.

Ersoy H, Rybicki FJ. MR Angiography of the lower extremities. *AJR Am J Roentgenol.* 2008;190:1675-1684.

Fuchs F, Laub G, Othomo K. TrueFISP: technical considerations and cardiovascular applications. *Eur J Radiol.* 2003;46:28-32.

Griffin M, Grist TM, François CJ. Dynamic four-dimensional MR angiography of the chest and abdomen. *Magn Reson Imaging Clin N Am.* 2009;17:77-90.

Hartung MP, Grist TM, François CJ. Magnetic resonance angiography: current status and future directions. *J Cardiovasc Magn Reson.* 2011;13:19.

Ivancevic MK, Geerts L, Weadock WJ, et al. Technical principles of MR angiography methods. *Magn Reson Imaging Clin N Am.* 2009;17:1-11.

Kramer H, Nikolaou K, Sommer W, et al. Peripheral MR angiography. *Magn Reson Imaging Clin N Am.* 2009;17:91-100.

Larkman DJ, Nunes RG. Parallel magnetic resonance imaging. *Phys Med Biol.* 2007;52:R15-R55.

Lee VS, Martin DJ, Krinsky GA, et al. Gadolinium-enhanced MR angiography: pitfalls and Artifacts. *AJR Am J Roentgenol.* 2000;175:197-205.

Malcolm PN, Craven P, Klass D. Pitfalls and artefacts in performance and interpretation of contrast-enhanced MR angiography of the lower limbs. *Clin Radiol.* 2010;65:651-658.

Maki JH, Chenevert TL, Prince MR. Contrast-enhanced MR angiography. *Abdom Imaging.* 1998;23:469-484.

Maki JH, Wang M, Wilson GJ. Highly accelerated first-pass contrast-enhanced magnetic resonance angiography of the peripheral vasculature: comparison of gadofosveset trisodium with gadopentetate dimeglumine contrast agents. *J Magn Reson Imaging.* 2009;30:1085-1092.

Miyazaki M, Lee VS. Nonenhanced MR angiography. *Radiology.* 2008;248:20-43.

Morita S, Masukawa A, Suzuki K, et al. Unenhanced MR angiography: techniques and clinical applications in patients with chronic kidney disease. *Radiographics.* 2011;31:E12-E33.

Nishimura DG. Time-of-flight MR angiography. *Magn Reson Med.* 1990;14:194-201.

Nissen JC, Attenberger UI, Fink C, et al. Thoracic and abdominal MRA with gadofosveset: influence of injection rate on vessel signal and image quality. *Eur Radiol.* 2009;19:1932-1938.

Sakamoto I, Sueyoshi E, Uetani M. MR imaging of the aorta. *Magn Reson Imaging Clin N Am.* 2010;18:43-55.

Scheffler K, Lehnhardt S. Principles and applications of balanced SSFP techniques. *Eur Radiol.* 2003;13:2409-2418.

Vogt FM, Goyen M, Debatin JF. MR angiography of the chest. *Radiol Clin North Am.* 2003;41:29-41.

Zhang H, Maki JH, Prince MR. 3D contrast-enhanced MR angiography. *J Magn Reson Imaging.* 2007;25:13-25.

CHAPTER **9**

Catheter Angiography (Vascular)

Sandeep S. Hedgire and Sanjeeva P. Kalva

Catheter angiography refers to x-ray imaging of the blood vessels while contrast material is injected through an introducer (needle, catheter, or sheath) positioned within the vessel of interest. First developed by the Portuguese physician and neurologist Egas Moniz at the University of Lisbon in 1927, catheter angiography became popular with the introduction of a percutaneous arterial catheterization technique by Sven Ivan Seldinger in 1953. This technique, known as the Seldinger technique, eliminated the need for surgical exposure of the vessel before catheterization. Later, in 1964, Charles Dotter introduced the idea of catheter-directed therapy during the first femoral angioplasty. During the next 2 decades, catheter angiography flourished as the sole minimally invasive diagnostic tool for localization and characterization not only of vascular disease but also of other conditions such as neoplasms. With more recent developments in noninvasive vascular imaging techniques such as duplex ultrasound, computed tomography angiography (CTA), and magnetic resonance angiography (MRA), the role of catheter angiography in the diagnosis of vascular and nonvascular disease is diminishing. However, it still remains the gold standard for vascular imaging to which all other imaging modalities are compared. Despite its invasiveness, catheter angiography exceeds all other currently available noninvasive vascular imaging tests in providing the best temporal and spatial resolution for assessing the blood vessels. In addition, it is an integral part of all therapeutic vascular interventions.

The practice of angiography involves performing the procedure, as well as preprocedure patient evaluation, selection of appropriate hardware and technical parameters during the procedure, and appropriate postprocedure care. This chapter covers the basic principles and techniques of catheter angiography.

◼ PREPROCEDURAL CLINICAL ASSESSMENT

Clinical assessment of patients before catheter angiography is required, to obtain the following information:
1. Why does the patient require catheter angiography? Can the required information be obtained from other noninvasive vascular imaging studies? What additional information can catheter angiography provide if other noninvasive vascular imaging studies are already available? What level of selective angiography is required to answer the clinical question?
2. Can the patient tolerate catheter angiography? If pharmacoangiography is planned, can the patient tolerate the pharmacologic stress?
3. Is a therapeutic intervention planned? Is such therapeutic intervention better than or at least equal to the available alternatives?
4. Was the patient educated and informed about the procedure, anticipated risks, and benefits?

Preprocedure assessment involves personal interaction with the patient or the family (especially if the patient is incapacitated) to obtain relevant medical history, perform physical examination, discuss the procedure, and obtain informed consent. Table 9-1 summarizes the checklist for preprocedure assessment.

◼ INDICATIONS

Current indications for diagnostic catheter angiography are limited. Vascular diseases involving large and medium-size vessels can be well studied with duplex ultrasound, CTA, or MRA. The following are the current indications for catheter angiography:
1. Assessment of small arteries
   a. Detection of microaneurysms or steno-occlusive patterns in small arteries (e.g., in suspected inflammatory arteritis, noninflammatory arterial diseases such as fibromuscular dysplasia, and idiopathic or congenital microaneurysms)
   b. Assessment of the distal arterial bed in patients with extensive peripheral arterial disease
   c. Assessment of microvascular obstruction in patients with thromboembolic disease, thromboangiitis, frostbite, and other small vessel diseases
   d. Assessment of smaller arterial anatomy before tissue transplantation
2. Assessment of flow dynamics
   a. Assessment of flow dynamics in patients with steal syndromes, arteriovenous fistulas or malformations, and tumoral shunting
   b. Assessment of flow dynamics of collaterals in arterial and veno-occlusive diseases
   c. Assessment of intravascular pressure to ascertain the hemodynamic significance of an obstructive lesion

Table 9-1 Patient Assessment Before Catheter Angiography

Medical History and Chart Review	History of present illness (the need for angiography) Relevant past medical history (especially about cardiac and renal function, hypertension, thromboembolic disease, bleeding diathesis, acute inflammatory disorders) Evidence of atherosclerotic disease (stroke, myocardial infarction, atheroemboli) History of bleeding disorders Allergies (especially to angiographic contrast materials) Current medications (especially metformin, which must be stopped 24 hr before and 48 hr after angiography, anticoagulants, and antiplatelet agents) Review of all available vascular imaging studies and vascular surgical procedures Previous laboratory results
Physical Examination	General cognition assessment to assess whether patient can provide informed consent Assessment of airway (for conscious sedation) Assessment of lungs, heart, peripheral pulses, and neurologic system (especially if supradiaphragmatic vessels or spinal arteries must be catheterized) Assessment of vascular access site
Laboratory Workup	Coagulation parameters: prothrombin time (PT), activated partial thromboplastin time (APTT), international normalized ratio (INR) Complete blood count: hematocrit, platelet count, white blood cell count Inflammatory markers (especially when angiography is planned in patients with inflammatory vasculitis; angiography not recommended if inflammatory markers are elevated in patients with active vasculitis) Renal function: estimated glomerular filtration rate, serum creatinine Liver function: required if hepatic arterial or portal venous interventions planned or if patient is clinically suspected to have hepatic dysfunction Electrocardiography: required in patients >70 yr old and in every patient who is undergoing pulmonary angiography Assessment of left ventricular ejection fraction: required as part of regular workup in patients with clinical signs of heart failure or any patient with significant cardiac history or pulmonary hypertension and in patients >70 yr old
Patient Instructions	Nothing by mouth for 6-8 hr before the procedure: required if conscious sedation planned for the angiography; otherwise, nothing by mouth for 3 hours before the procedure Clear liquids: can be consumed until 2 hr before the procedure Withholding medications: except for anticoagulants, patients receive their regular medications; insulin and antidiabetic medications may be reduced to half the regular dose if needed before angiography; warfarin (Coumadin) stopped ≥3 days before procedure to allow the INR to be at ≤1.5; low-molecular-weight heparins may be stopped 12 hr before procedure; metformin stopped 24 hr before procedure and restarted 48 hr later
Informed Consent	Informed consent obtained from patient or health care proxy after explaining procedure, anticipated risks, and benefits Estimated radiation dose and its effects discussed, in addition to other risks of angiography (see section on complications)

d. Assessment of dynamic vascular occlusion secondary to arterial or venous compression from adjacent bony or muscular structures
3. Assessment of arterial supply or venous drainage of a tissue or tumor
   a. Accurate delineation of tumoral vascular supply, especially to assess the contribution of parasitized blood vessels
   b. Assessment of venous drainage, which may be of paramount importance in patients with venous obstruction or when venous sampling is required in a suspected hormone-secreting tumor
4. Assessment of in-stent stenosis, especially in small vessels
5. Assessment of arteries and veins for vessel patency, course, and caliber when the information provided by other noninvasive modalities is inadequate
6. Accurate localization of a bleeding source when the information provided by other imaging modalities is inadequate
7. As part of pharmacoangiography
8. As part of therapeutic interventions on blood vessels

■ CONTRAINDICATIONS

Severe allergic reactions to contrast materials, lack of vascular access, and active inflammatory vascular disease are relative contraindications to angiography.

■ TECHNIQUE

Catheter angiography involves intravascular access, selection of the vessel of clinical interest, injection of contrast material into the vascular territory with simultaneous x-ray imaging, and safe removal of intravascular devices used for angiography. A brief review of these steps is provided in this section.

Premedication

Catheter angiography involves injection of contrast materials, which have the propensity to stimulate H_1 and H_2 histamine receptors, with subsequent development of allergic reactions. Other considerations include the risk of nephrotoxicity and cardiotoxicity associated with the contrast material. As such, premedication of patients with H_1- and H_2-receptor blockers (e.g., diphenhydramine and ranitidine) and adequate intravenous (IV) hydration (half-normal saline at 1 mL/kg/hour) are often recommended. Other renoprotective drugs such as N-acetylcysteine (Mucomyst, 600 mg twice a day, started at least 12 to 24 hours before the procedure) and sodium bicarbonate (150 mEq of sodium bicarbonate mixed in 850 mL of 5% dextrose in water [D5W] administered intravenously at 3 mL/kg 1 hour before the procedure and 6 hours after the procedure) may be given, although the superiority of these drugs over hydration is questioned. Adequate precautions should be taken not to overhydrate patients with poor left ventricular ejection fraction. Antibiotics are not required for diagnostic catheter angiography.

Patients with known allergy to contrast materials or who are at risk of contrast material–related allergic reactions should receive appropriate premedication (regimen 1:50 mg of oral prednisone 13 hours, 7 hours, and 1 hour before the procedure and 50 mg of oral diphenhydramine 1 hour before the procedure; or regimen 2: 125 mg IV methylprednisone, 50 mg of IV diphenhydramine, and 20 mg of IV famotidine just before angiography). Oral benzodiazepines such as midazolam are useful to alleviate anxiety in some patients. Conscious sedation may be used for diagnostic angiography.

Choice of Contrast Material

Currently, iodinated, nonionic, low-osmolar (iopamidol or iohexol) or iso-osmolar (iodixanol) contrast materials are typically used for catheter angiography. Although no maximum dose is suggested, doses in excess of 300 mL of contrast material should be avoided during angiography. Patients with renal failure or who are at risk of renal failure may benefit from alternative contrast materials such as carbon dioxide (CO_2). Understanding the compressibility and buoyancy of CO_2 during angiography is important. In addition, the use of CO_2 as contrast material during angiography requires digital subtraction angiography (DSA) and special image acquisition parameters. CO_2 is contraindicated for angiography of supradiaphragmatic arteries, given the risk of possible neurologic complications.

Selection of Hardware

Vascular access needles, guidewires, dilators, sheaths, and catheters are the basic tools for catheter angiography. The most commonly used vascular access needles are 18 gauge in diameter and range from 2.25 to 5 inch in length. They permit insertion of 0.038- or 0.035-inch helical spring guidewires. These needles have a central sharp stylet (the double wall puncture needles) that puncture the vessels through both the walls. The stylet is removed, and the needle is slowly withdrawn. The intravascular location of the needle tip is confirmed by visibility of blood at the needle hub (Fig. 9-1). Vascular access needles without a stylet are also available, and these allow single wall puncture. A 21-gauge micropuncture needle is helpful in minimizing vessel trauma and is often preferred in patients with prolonged prothrombin time or activated partial thromboplastin time. A 21-gauge micropuncture needle permits the passage of

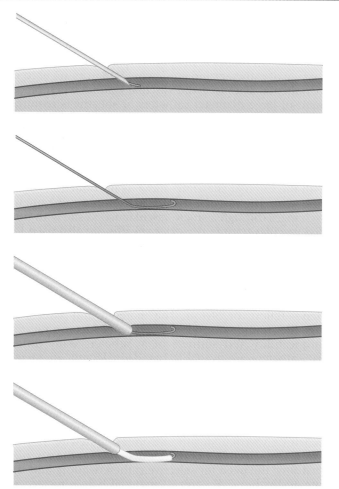

Figure 9-1 Modified Seldinger technique. Illustration demonstrates the technique of vascular access. *Top to bottom:* A hollow needle is used to puncture the anterior wall of the vessel, and a guidewire is inserted through the needle once the intravascular location of the needle is confirmed by visualization of blood dripping at the hub of the needle. Next, the wire is fixed, and the needle is removed. During this step, firm pressure is applied over the puncture site to avoid hematoma formation. Then, a sheath is introduced over the wire. Finally, the selected catheter is introduced through the sheath to enter the vessel of interest.

a 0.018-inch guidewire. Then the puncture is upsized to a larger sheath.

Guidewires are available in various diameters (0.010 to 0.038 inch) and lengths (≤300 cm) and are made of different materials. The selection of a guidewire depends on the catheter inner diameter, the need for exchange of a catheter, the flexibility and torque required, and the anatomy of the vessels being catheterized. Typically, a guidewire is made of an outer wire wrapped around a central stiff core with a safety wire in between them. The tapering of the core wire at the distal end of the wire determines its floppiness. A major breakthrough in guidewire technology was the development of nitinol-based hydrophilic guidewires, which allow greater torque and are kink resistant. These hydrophilic guidewires are used in conjunction with catheters to facilitate selective arterial catheterization. Their use through access needles should be avoided. The tip of the guidewires may be straight, angled, curved, or shapeable.

Dilators are tapered short catheters that help to displace the soft tissues at the puncture site to facilitate easy passage of catheters and guidewires. Dilators are used in incremental sizes to avoid vascular trauma when placement of large diameter catheters or sheaths is required at the vascular access site.

Vascular sheaths are plastic cannulas with a smooth, open distal end and a hemostatic valve at the proximal end. A side arm at the proximal end allows period flushing to prevent clot formation. A dilator is provided with the vascular sheath to allow its introduction over a guidewire. The vascular sheaths permit multiple catheter exchanges through a single vascular access site with limited vascular trauma. Vascular sheaths are also used for foreign body retrieval, introduction of nontapering catheters or intravascular stents, and limiting of the tortuosity of vessels to permit adequate catheter maneuvers. The sheaths are available in various diameters and lengths.

Catheters are composed of polyurethane, polyethylene, Teflon, or Nylon. The material and associated metallic frame around the polymer determine the torqueability and stiffness of a catheter. Many different catheters are available based on length, diameter, shape, tip configuration, and location and number of distal holes. The length of the catheters varies between 30 and 110 cm. The outer diameter (in French size) and the diameter (in inches) of the end hole are mentioned on the package insert and serve as a guide to choose the matching vascular sheath and inner guidewire, respectively. The selection of catheter depends on the vascular anatomy, the need for selective catheterization, and the rate and volume of contrast material being injected to opacify the vessel of interest. Catheters with a reverse curve allow selective catheterization of a cranially directed vessel that arises from a caudally oriented vessel. Microcatheters can be placed through the diagnostic catheters to superselect distal arteries. Microcatheters range in size from 1.7 to 3 French and allow passage of a 0.010- to 0.025-inch guidewires.

Vascular Access Site Preparation

The selected vascular access site should be free of local infection and should be cleaned with povidone-iodine or chlorhexidine. The entire region should be draped with sterile sheets. Local anesthesia (1% lidocaine with or without sodium bicarbonate) is provided after the vascular access site is confirmed by palpation of the artery, the bony landmarks are identified on fluoroscopy, or the vessel is identified on ultrasound examination. A small skin incision is made before the vessel is accessed with a vascular access needle. The subcutaneous tissues are dissected with a clamp to allow subsequent easy passage of a vascular sheath.

Obtaining Vascular Access

The selection of a vascular access site depends on the accessibility of the vessel for percutaneous catheterization, the patency of the vessel being accessed, the healthiness of the overlying skin and soft tissues, and the ability to catheterize the vessel of clinical interest selectively. Vessels may be accessed in an antegrade (in the direction of blood flow) or retrograde manner (against the direction of blood flow), depending on the need to catheterize the required arterial bed. The original technique of percutaneous vascular catheterization as described by Seldinger is still followed by some angiographers; however, a modified Seldinger technique with a single wall puncture using a hollow needle is more often used (see Fig. 9-1). The accessed artery is palpated, and the needle is advanced at a 45- to 65-degree angulation toward the artery. The intraarterial location of the needle is confirmed by the pulsatile flow through the hub of the needle. A guidewire is advanced through the needle, and the needle is exchanged for a dilator and then for a hemostatic sheath. The advantages and disadvantages of various arterial access sites are listed in Table 9-2. Nonpalpable arteries may be difficult to access; direct visualization with ultrasound during access is highly recommended in such cases. When ultrasound is not available, bony landmarks and arterial calcifications on fluoroscopy may be useful for arterial access (Fig. 9-2).

Venous access, conversely, requires use of anatomic landmarks or image guidance because the veins are not palpable. The location of veins in relation to the arteries (e.g., the femoral vein is medial to the femoral artery) may also help access the vein. The vein is commonly punctured by using a sharp needle without a stylet. A syringe maintaining suction is attached to the needle while the needle is advanced toward the vein. This technique is helpful to assess the intravascular location of the needle tip because the low venous pressure may not allow free flow of blood through the needle. Commonly accessed veins are the common femoral, internal jugular, subclavian, basilic, and saphenous veins.

Catheterization of Vessels of Interest

Selective arterial catheterization requires either direct percutaneous access to the artery (e.g., lumbar aortic access to study the distal abdominal aorta or common femoral artery access to study the ipsilateral lower extremity arteries) or selection of the vessel of interest with a catheter through arterial access. Aortography is performed with positioning of a multiside hole catheter (pigtail or Omni Flush catheter) at the desired location (ascending aorta, aortic arch, and thoracic or abdominal aorta) (Fig. 9-3) for studying the respective segments of the aorta and the branch vessels.

Selective cannulation requires appropriately shaped catheters and guidewires. In general, great vessels of the aortic arch can be selected with long catheters having a short, 45-degree angulated tip (Berenstein or Davis catheters). When the aortic arch is dilated, a catheter with secondary and tertiary curves (Newton, Bentson, Headhunter, Mani, Simmons catheters) proximal to the distal angled tip is very helpful. Selective visceral artery cannulation requires catheters that are supported by the opposite wall of the aorta and an acute angle at the tip of the catheter (Cobra, Rim, SOS, Lev, Renal

Table 9-2   Arterial Access Sites: Advantages and Disadvantages

Arterial Access Site	Advantages	Disadvantages
Common femoral artery	First choice Easy palpation Large vessel Fewer and easy to manage complications	Challenging access in patients with severe atherosclerosis or obesity Challenging access in pulseless artery Long path for remote targets (e.g., distal forearm) Restricted mobility after angiography
Brachial artery	Second choice Usually disease free, unlike common femoral artery Access to most targeted vessels Great access to arteries that emanate from descending aorta in an acute, caudal angle	Tendency to thrombosis Patient discomfort from arm board Long tortuous route for catheter manipulation Risk of stroke
Axillary artery	Large vessel Short distance from aorta	Hematoma possibly leading to brachial plexopathy Uncomfortable patient position
Subclavian artery	Large vessel Short distance from aorta Easy access to distal vessels	Potential pneumothorax Difficult compression High risk of hematoma, especially with large catheters Most difficult to access, requires experience
Radial artery	Easy access Facilitating early patient discharge	Long working distance for lower limb arteries Hand ischemia from thrombosis Nerve damage

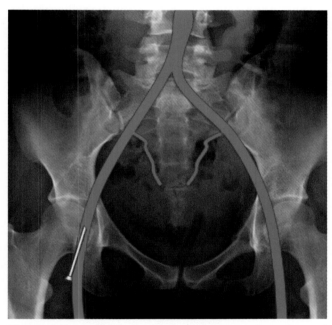

Figure 9-2 Using bony landmarks for obtaining femoral arterial access. The schematic illustration superimposed on the radiograph shows the site of arterial access in the right side of the groin.

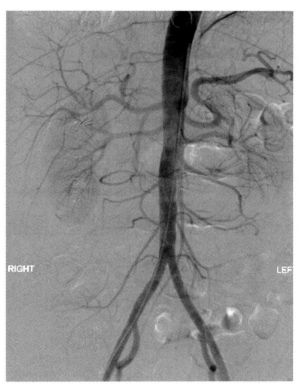

Figure 9-3 Digital subtraction angiography of the abdominal aorta with a pigtail catheter positioned in the proximal abdominal aorta shows a normal course and caliber of the abdominal aorta and its branches.

Double Curve catheters). Reversed curve catheters are highly useful for selective catheterization of acutely angulated vessels arising from the aorta. The aortic bifurcation can be crossed with any of the visceral catheters or a reverse curve catheter. The selection of an artery is greatly aided by identifying the location of the ostium in relation to the parent artery and the direction and course of the proximal segment of the artery being catheterized. Selection of appropriate catheters and guidewires is of paramount importance for selective arterial catheterization.

Intraarterial pressure measurements can be obtained by attaching the catheter to a manometer. Intravascular ultrasound–guided flow velocity and pressure measurement devices are also available. In addition, Doppler measurements through intravascular ultrasound catheters provide information about flow velocity and flow direction.

Injection of Contrast Material

Injection of contrast material should be tailored to the clinical information required. The injected dose (iodine concentration, volume and rate of contrast material injection) depends on multiple factors including those dependent on the catheter (diameter of the inner lumen, number of distal holes, ability to withstand high pressures), the vessels being cannulated (aorta versus radial artery), the flow dynamics of the distal arterial bed (slow flow versus high flow), the volume of the distal arterial bed (small volume as in the forearm arteries versus large volume as in the splenic artery), and the desire to study the venous system in addition to the arteries (especially in mesenteric arterioportography). In general, the rate of injection of the iodinated contrast material should be able to replace one third of the regional blood flow per second to provide adequate opacification of the arteries on DSA. The volume of the contrast material is highly dependent on flow dynamics (cardiac output, presence of arteriovenous communications in the distal arterial bed, volume of the distal arterial bed) and the need to study the venous phase of the arterial injection. Commonly used contrast material injection rates and volumes for various vessels are listed in Table 9-3.

Imaging (Digital Subtraction Angiography)

DSA has largely replaced film screen imaging. Digital angiography without subtraction is integral to DSA imaging and can be turned on anytime (Fig. 9-4).

Current imaging systems provide acquisition rates up to 30 frames per second during fluoroscopy and 10 to 15 frames per second during DSA. Higher frame rates ($\leq$30 frames per second) can be obtained with cine angiography. This is the reason that catheter angiography remains the best imaging modality for providing the highest temporal resolution that is often required to assess the flow dynamics of fast-flowing blood, as in arteriovenous communications and other situations with high flow rates. At present, most DSA systems acquire images at 1024 × 1024 matrix (some newer systems allow 2048 × 2048 matrix) to permit the best spatial resolution compared with CTA (512 × 512 matrix) or MRA (usually 256 × 256 or 512 × 512 matrix). The addition of subtraction during catheter angiography allows accurate delineation of small vessels by improving contrast resolution (Fig. 9-5). During subtraction, the first image (the mask, which is acquired before the administration of contrast material) is subtracted from the subsequent images (these are acquired during or after the administration of the contrast material), thus leading to contrast material–only images.

Some of the newer systems have many options to aid selective catheterization. The roadmap technique displays the previously acquired angiographic image over the real-time fluoroscopic image while subtracting the background and thus displaying the catheter or wire in relation to the angiographic image. Similar to the roadmap technique, the image overlay technique allows display of a DSA run over the fluoroscopic image to allow

Table 9-3 Commonly Used Contrast Material Injection Rates During Selective Vascular Catheterization

Vessel	Rate (mL/sec)	Volume (mL)
Ascending aorta	20-30	30-40
Aortic arch	20-30	30-40
Descending thoracic aorta	20-30	20-30
Abdominal aorta	15-20	20-30
Carotid artery	4-8	8-10
Subclavian artery	4-6	10-15
Bronchial artery	1-2	4-8
Intercostal artery	1-2	4-10
Celiac artery	5-7	30-40
Superior mesenteric artery	5-7	30-40
Inferior mesenteric artery	4-5	15-30
Renal artery	4-5	10-15
Femoral artery	4-5	10-15
Inferior vena cava	20-30	30-40
Left or right pulmonary artery	20-30	35-45

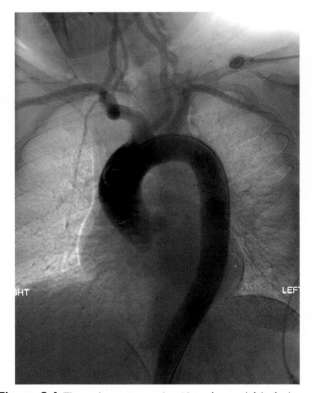

Figure 9-4 Thoracic aortography. Note the partial inclusion of the background. This feature is part of digital subtraction angiography wherein the initial image (mask) is superimposed on the image with partial transparency.

the visual representation of the catheters or wires in relation to the previously acquired DSA image. Rotational angiography systems allow three-dimensional reconstruction of vessels, a feature that is highly desirable for assessing the origin and direction of branch vessels, the size and neck of aneurysms, and the tortuosity and overlap of branch vessels (Fig. 9-6). Newer flat panel technology systems allow cone beam computed tomography (CT) acquisition during angiography. This is very helpful in selective catheterization of tumor feeding arteries, assessment of tumoral arterial supply, and anatomy of intracranial aneurysms and arteriovenous malformations. These systems allow incorporation of CT or magnetic resonance data in to the angiography systems, provide image fusion capabilities, and assist during fluoroscopically guided biopsy or selective cannulation. Other advances include color-coded display of the angiographic image, with each color representing flow direction or apparent flow velocity (Fig. 9-7).

Image acquisition should be tailored to the clinical question. Although higher frame rates and prolonged acquisition provide extensive information, they often result in a high radiation dose to the patient. Unless high flow dynamics are important to image, angiographic acquisition at three to four frames per second during arterial imaging and at one to two frames during venous imaging is sufficient for most clinical indications.

Removal of the Vascular Access Sheath

The arterial access sheaths or catheters should be removed immediately after the procedure unless the examiner wishes to reimage the patient within 24 hours or the coagulation parameters do not permit adequate hemostasis. Manual compression remains the preferred technique for hemostasis, although many arterial closure devices are popular among angiographers. These devices may be desirable in patients who cannot lie still after the procedure or in patients with a coagulation system disorder. Patients should be followed up for 4 to 6 hours after angiography to observe for access site complications. Renal function tests may be repeated in patients with poor renal function. Any contrast-induced nephropathy must be treated adequately to prevent chronic renal failure.

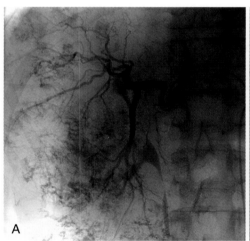
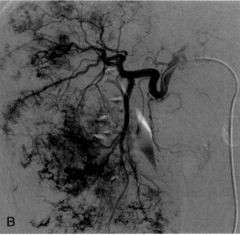

Figure 9-5 A, Selective right hepatic angiogram demonstrating tumor vascularity. **B,** Note improved visualization of smaller vessels on digital subtraction angiography.

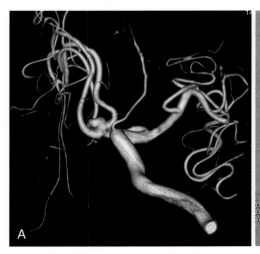
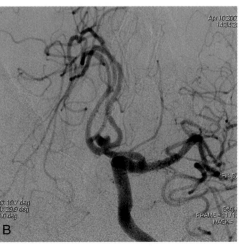

Figure 9-6 Three-dimensional rotation angiography (**A**) and digital subtraction angiography (**B**) demonstrate a wide neck anterior communicating artery aneurysm. Three-dimensional angiography is highly useful to localize the neck of a complex aneurysm, separate overlying branch vessels, and identify tumoral vascular supply. This technique can be combined with cone beam computed tomography.

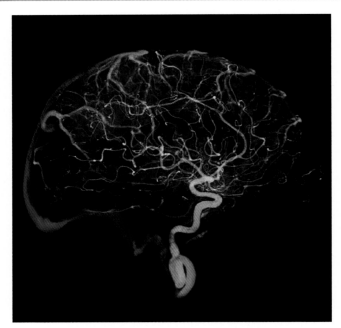

Figure 9-7 Color-coded subtraction angiography of the internal carotid artery. Note the differential color representation of the arterial, capillary, and venous flow. (Courtesy of Siemens Medical, Erlangen, Germany.)

■ LIMITATIONS

The main limitation of catheter angiography is that the vessel wall cannot be directly imaged with this technique. Imaging of the vessel wall and mural plaque or thrombosis can be improved with newer technical advances in DSA systems that incorporate cone beam CT and with the use of intravascular ultrasound. In addition, this test is invasive and is associated with a low but definite incidence of complications.

■ COMPLICATIONS

Catheter angiography is not devoid of complications. Procedure-related complications include access site hematoma (<1% for common femoral artery), infection (<0.01% for common femoral artery), pseudoaneurysm or arteriovenous malformation (<1% for common femoral artery), and arterial injury leading to thrombosis or dissection (<1% for common femoral artery). Arterial injuries (dissection, rupture, intramural hematoma, thrombosis) during selective arterial catheterization are rare, but they can occur in diseased vessels or in patients who have received anti–vascular endothelial growth factor inhibitors or tyrosine kinase inhibitors for cancer therapy. Other complications include atheroembolism, which is common in older patients with extensive atherosclerotic disease, fractures of catheters or guidewires, and distal embolization of catheter or wire fragments. Catheter thrombosis and distal embolism can occur with prolonged catheterization. Adequate, intermittent flushing of the catheter and systemic heparinization help reduce the incidence of this complication.

■ CONCLUSION

Catheter angiography is a safe and highly effective imaging test for assessment of vascular disease. It remains the gold standard to which all other vascular imaging tests are compared. Its ability to assess vascular disease and flow dynamics is unparalleled. Catheter angiography is an integral part of all types of endovascular and open vascular surgical therapies.

Bibliography

Back MR, Caridi JG, Hawkins Jr IF, Seeger JM. Angiography with carbon dioxide (CO_2). *Surg Clin North Am.* 1998;78:575-591.

Cope C. Minipuncture angiography. *Radiol Clin North Am.* 1986;24:359-367.

Gailloud P, Oishi S, Murphy K. Three-dimensional fusion digital subtraction angiography: new reconstruction algorithm for simultaneous three-dimensional rendering of osseous and vascular information obtained during rotational angiography. *AJNR Am J Neuroradiol.* 2005;26:908-911.

Heran NS, Song JK, Namba K, Smith W, Niimi Y, Berenstein A. The utility of DynaCT in neuroendovascular procedures. *AJNR Am J Neuroradiol.* 2006;27:330-332.

Levin DC, Schapiro RM, Boxt LM, Dunham L, Harrington DP, Ergun DL. Digital subtraction angiography: principles and pitfalls of image improvement techniques. *AJR Am J Roentgenol.* 1984;143:447-454.

Rösch J, Keller FS, Kaufman JA. The birth, early years, and future of interventional radiology. *J Vasc Interv Radiol.* 2003;14:841-853.

Siegelman SS, Caplan LH, Annes GP. Complications of catheter angiography: study with oscillometry and "pullout" angiograms. *Radiology.* 1968;91:251-253.

Turski PA, Stieghorst MF, Strother CM, Crummy AB, Lieberman RP, Mistretta CA. Digital subtraction angiography "road map." *AJR Am J Roentgenol.* 1982;139:1233-1234.

CHAPTER 10

When to Choose What Test (Cardiac)

Venkatesh L. Murthy and Ron Blankstein

Many symptoms and signs encountered in the course of clinical care may raise concern for cardiac dysfunction. These manifestations may include chest pain or discomfort, dyspnea, exercise intolerance, edema, syncope, and palpitations. Combined, these complaints account for a substantial share of presentations in both inpatient and outpatient settings. When the clinician strongly suspects a cardiac origin, imaging tests can play a central role in confirming or excluding suspected diagnoses and in selecting among potential therapies or procedures. In some cases, even when other causes may be more likely, imaging tests may be helpful in excluding rarer but potentially life-threatening (i.e., "cannot miss") cardiac conditions.

Although many different cardiac imaging tests are available to clinicians, each discussed in detail elsewhere in this book, not every test is equally effective in all clinical circumstances and for all questions. Tests have differing strengths, limitations, availability, costs, and contraindications. Subsequently, decision making regarding the most optimal test for a given patient is complex, particularly because no published guidelines are available to use for selecting among the available testing options. Choosing the right test for the right patient requires an understanding of both the clinical question at hand and the technical aspects of the multiple available testing options.

Cardiac imaging tests can be used to evaluate disorders of nearly every aspect of cardiac anatomy and physiology, including estimating cardiac chambers size and function, identifying myocardial scar or infiltration, assessing valvular function, identifying and characterizing cardiac masses, and evaluating the presence and size of pericardial effusions. Because the most frequent indication for cardiac imaging is evaluation of suspected coronary stenosis or ischemia, most of this chapter focuses on this indication. Suspected coronary stenosis or ischemia accounts for a large proportion of cardiac testing, and given the availability of many different testing options, the decision regarding which test to use is most complex.

The purpose of this chapter is to provide a framework for selecting the most optimum test. As such, the discussion answers the following questions:

1. Should a cardiac imaging test be performed?
2. What is the best means to evaluate symptomatic patients with known or suspected CAD?
   a. What is the best method to determine the pretest probability of disease?
   b. What are the available testing options?
   c. What are the advantages of anatomic versus physiologic methods?
   d. What are the advantages of exercise stress over pharmacologic stress agents?
   e. When is an imaging test needed in addition to exercise treadmill testing alone?
3. What is the best means of assessing cardiac risk in asymptomatic individuals?
4. In imaging for noncoronary indications, how does one choose between echocardiography and cardiovascular magnetic resonance (CMR)?

■ SHOULD A CARDIAC IMAGING TEST BE PERFORMED?

Although advances in cardiovascular imaging have greatly improved the ability to diagnose and treat various clinical conditions, the rising cost of testing has generated concern regarding the potential overuse of such procedures. To address these issues, and in recognition of the limited evidence on the clinical effectiveness of imaging, multiple medical specialty societies, including the American College of Cardiology and the American College of Radiology, developed appropriate use criteria (AUC). These criteria, which describe clinical situations in which an imaging test may or may not be appropriate, are available for all the major noninvasive cardiovascular tests. Even though the AUC are intended to facilitate more efficient allocation of health care resources in cardiovascular imaging, they have notable limitations. First, the AUC approach is primarily opinion based because of the paucity of data linking cardiovascular imaging with patient outcomes. Second, some reports have shown that the use of AUC does not lead to a consistent decline in the use of tests deemed inappropriate. Third, the AUC for each imaging modality were developed separately, and as such, they cannot be used for choosing the best test among the numerous testing options that may be available for a given patient. Indeed, for any given patient with a clinical question, several different testing options may be considered appropriate. The American College of Radiology's AUC use an approach in which a clinical situation (e.g., suspected congenital heart disease in the adult) is discussed and various imaging modalities are rated according to their potential appropriateness. However, the clinical situations are broad categories and are not further refined, and the imaging tests are not weighted against each other or against nonimaging tests.

In deciding whether to obtain a cardiac imaging test for a particular patient, the first step is to define the clinical question at hand (Box 10-1). Next, clinicians must decide whether the test has the potential to alter subsequent patient management (e.g., initiation of a new therapy, referral for further testing or procedures). Tests that confirm a known diagnosis or that identify a condition for which no changes in treatment are anticipated may not be necessary. A more challenging question is this: How likely is an imaging test to provide new information or to answer the clinical question at hand? In some instances, this may be difficult to determine, and a consultation between clinicians and imaging experts may be beneficial for deciding whether further testing would be beneficial.

WHAT IS THE BEST MEANS TO EVALUATE SYMPTOMATIC PATIENTS WITH SUSPECTED CORONARY ARTERY DISEASE?

In most patients with suspected coronary artery disease (CAD), the main goal of testing is to exclude the presence of CAD as the cause of symptoms. Selection of the optimal imaging modality for a given patient requires careful consideration of the strengths and weakness of each modality, as well as patient-related factors (e.g., body habitus, conditions that may be contraindications to some forms of testing). Finally, because many modalities can assess other ancillary questions, knowing all the potentially relevant clinical questions for each patient is helpful. Unfortunately, even though a large body of experience exists for most imaging modalities, few direct comparative studies have been conducted.

Figure 10-1 is a decision-making algorithm that can be used in selecting specific tests in patients with suspected CAD. Any such algorithm should serve merely as an initial guide, and clinical judgment, institutional experience, and patient preferences are all important factors that must be considered. A key principle, however, is that the first step in deciding which test to obtain is to determine the pretest probability of flow-limiting (i.e., obstructive) CAD.

BOX 10-1 Reasons for Obtaining a Cardiac Imaging Study

Diagnosis
- Determine the cause of the patient's symptoms.
- Exclude a cardiac condition as a potential cause of the symptoms.

Prognosis
- Establish the prognosis (i.e., risk of future cardiovascular events or death).

Treatment
- Determine the need, intensity, and type of therapy.
- Determine the potential benefit of cardiac procedures.
- Evaluate the response to therapy.

Pretest Probability of Disease

Because the diagnostic accuracy of different tests may be affected by the prevalence of disease, the clinician must first determine the pretest probability of obstructive disease. The presence of coronary artery stenosis or even myocardial ischemia does not necessarily imply that the patient's symptoms have a cardiac origin because an alternative pulmonary, gastrointestinal or musculoskeletal source may also coexist and be the actual cause of the patient's complaints. This possibility underscores the importance of estimating the pretest probability or, in Bayesian formalism, the prior probability. Only by consideration of a patient's pretest probability of CAD can a clinician evaluate whether a positive result is more likely to be a true-positive or a false-positive result. In the context of a high pretest likelihood of underlying disease, a negative test result may not be sufficient to exclude underlying disease. On the other end of the spectrum, evaluation of patients with an extremely low pretest probability of disease may result in excessive testing costs, particularly given the high frequency of false-positive results. Thus, to maximize diagnostic accuracy and minimize testing costs, the clinician must restrict testing to patients with an appropriate (e.g., low to intermediate) pretest probability of disease.

Several methods have been developed to estimate a given symptomatic patient's pretest probability of obstructive CAD based on age, gender, symptoms, and comorbid conditions. Most common among these are the Diamond and Forrester Score and the Duke Clinical Score (Table 10-1). These methods are limited in that they were both developed decades ago (1979 and 1983, respectively) and may no longer reflect contemporary patient populations who are referred for noninvasive imaging.

Alternatively, many clinicians rely on clinical intuition and experience to compose a pretest probability. Regardless of whether a formal score or an informal estimation is used, formulation of a patient's pretest probability is an important step in the decision to pursue further testing, in the choice of testing modality, and in the interpretation and application of the test results.

What Are the Available Testing Options?

Nearly every imaging modality used in cardiovascular imaging can be used for evaluating patients who exhibit signs or symptoms suggestive of coronary ischemia. Broadly, these modalities can be divided into anatomic and functional approaches (Table 10-2). Anatomic methods include invasive coronary angiography (ICA) and coronary computed tomography angiography (CTA). In contrast, functional methods employ the concept of stress testing, which refers to a focus on the identification of electrical, perfusion, or contractile abnormalities induced by exercise or pharmacologic stress.

Anatomic Methods
INVASIVE CORONARY ANGIOGRAPHY
To date, quantitative analysis of ICA images has generally been considered the "gold standard" for assessment

of CAD. The threshold of 50% or greater stenosis is considered hemodynamically significant in the left main coronary artery, and the threshold of 70% or greater stenosis is considered hemodynamically significant in all other vessels. More recently, investigators have recognized that not all lesions that are visually estimated to cause stenosis truly result in hemodynamic significance. Further, some lesions that are lower than these thresholds may indeed be functionally significant. Consequently, evaluating the hemodynamic significance of CAD is helpful for determining whether potential symptoms are the result of ischemia. Moreover, determining the amount of ischemia can be used to identify which patients are most likely to benefit from coronary revascularization. The gold standard for determining the hemodynamic significance of a particular coronary lesion is to calculate the fractional flow reserve (FFR) by using invasive pressure wires; an FFR of less than 0.8 indicates a hemodynamically significant lesion. However, FFR is an invasive technique that is relatively cumbersome and subsequently is underused. Nevertheless, the landmark Fractional Flow Reserve versus Angiography in Multi-vessel Evaluation (FAME) study showed that, in comparison with visual estimations of stenosis, a strategy of measuring coronary FFR during adenosine infusion with a pressure wire led to fewer coronary revascularizations, better outcomes, and lower cost.

Other invasive intravascular imaging modalities such as intravascular ultrasound (IVUS) and optical coherence tomography (OCT) can improve plaque identification and quantification. Although these modalities are invasive and costly, they offer the opportunity to characterize plaque composition and, perhaps, plaque stability more clearly. These features likely have substantial prognostic significance beyond stenosis severity.

Although ICA and newer catheter-based methods afford the most definitive anatomic diagnoses, they

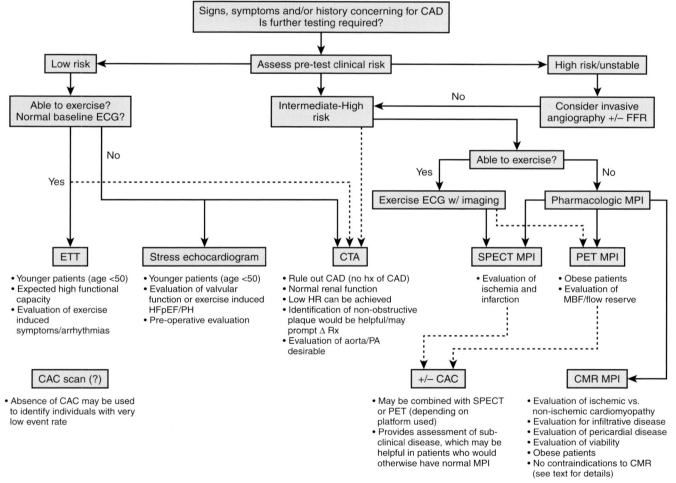

Figure 10-1 Example of a flow chart depicting a decision algorithm for test selection for patients with suspected obstructive coronary artery disease. Several modalities may be useful for any given clinical situation, and thus clinical judgment and local expertise should be incorporated into decision making. For each modality *(shaded boxes)*, compelling indications or reasons that could be used to favor that particular examination are listed. *Dashed lines* represent alternatives. *CAC,* Coronary artery calcification; *CAD,* coronary artery disease; *CMR,* cardiovascular magnetic resonance; *CTA,* computed tomography angiography; *Δ,* change in; *ECG,* electrocardiogram; *ETT,* exercise tolerance testing; *FFR,* fractional flow reserve; *HFpEF,* heart failure with preserved ejection fraction; *HR,* heart rate; *hx,* history; *MBF,* myocardial blood flow; *MPI,* myocardial perfusion imaging; *PA,* pulmonary artery; *PET,* positron emission tomography; *PH,* pulmonary hypertension; *Rx,* treatment; *SPECT,* single-photon emission computed tomography.

Table 10-1 Methods Used to Estimate the Pretest Probability of Coronary Artery Disease Among Symptomatic Patients

	Diamond and Forrester Method	Duke Clinical Score
Population used to derive score	Combination of (1) symptomatic patients referred for invasive angiography and (2) autopsy studies	Symptomatic patients referred for invasive angiography
Prediction factors	Chest pain type Gender Age	Chest pain type Gender Age Smoking Hyperlipidemia Diabetes Previous myocardial infarction (q-waves on electrocardiogram) ST-T wave changes on electrocardiogram
Risk score predicts	≥50% stenosis	≥75% stenosis
Risk categories	Low (<10%) Intermediate (10-90%) High (>90%)	Low (<30%) Intermediate (30-70%) High (>70%)

Data from Wasfy MM et al. *Am J Cardiol.* 2012;109:998-1004.

Table 10-2 Tests Used to Evaluate Patients With Known or Suspected Coronary Artery Disease

Physiology and Function	Anatomy
Exercise treadmill testing (no imaging) Exercise treadmill testing with imaging • Nuclear MPI • Echocardiography Pharmacologic testing with imaging • Dobutamine stress echocardiogram • Pharmacologic nuclear MPI • Pharmacologic cardiac magnetic resonance MPI • Pharmacologic myocardial CTP (investigational)	Coronary artery calcium scoring Coronary computed tomography angiography Invasive coronary angiography

CTP, Computed tomography perfusion; *MPI,* myocardial perfusion imaging.

require invasive procedures with associated costs and risks. Thus, in most stable patients who do not have a very high pretest likelihood of obstructive CAD, noninvasive testing strategies are preferred.

When to Choose Invasive Coronary Angiography. ICA is the test of choice in unstable patients because of the ability to proceed immediately to therapeutic intervention on ischemia-causing lesions. ICA may also be an appropriate choice in patients with a high (i.e., >90%) pretest probability of obstructive CAD. Even among high-risk patients, however, an initial evaluation of ischemia may be helpful to identify the "culprit lesion" when multiple obstructive lesions are identified. Finally, ICA may rarely be required in patients who cannot exercise and who have contraindications to both vasodilators and dobutamine (e.g., a patient with critical aortic stenosis and asthma who cannot exercise).

Although ICA may be more complicated in patients with large body habitus, adequate results can be obtained. Obesity-related complications are primarily related to vascular access and bleeding, although image quality may also be reduced. The need for iodinated contrast mandates careful consideration of renal function, as well as risk factors for contrast-induced nephropathy.

CORONARY COMPUTED TOMOGRAPHY ANGIOGRAPHY

Coronary CTA offers a noninvasive approach to visualize the presence of both calcified and noncalcified coronary atherosclerosis and can detect coronary stenosis with high diagnostic accuracy. In particular, CTA has an excellent negative predictive value (~95%) and can thus be used to exclude the presence of obstructive CAD. Conversely, CTA has a lower positive predictive value for identifying the presence of coronary stenosis, in part because of the potential to overestimate the severity of stenosis when extensive coronary artery calcifications (CACs) are present. As is also true for ICA, the presence of anatomic stenosis does not always imply the presence of ischemia. Therefore, patients who are found to have moderate to severe coronary stenosis often require further evaluation to assess the functional significance of disease.

Advantages of CTA include rapid examination time and high accuracy in excluding the presence of plaque or stenosis. Unlike functional techniques, which can identify only flow-limiting lesions, CTA can identify the presence of nonobstructive plaque, which may result in intensification of lifestyle or medical therapies in some subgroups of patients. Another potential advantage of CTA is the ability to provide an alternative explanation for the patient's symptoms (e.g., pulmonary disease, disease of the aorta).

When to Choose Computed Tomography Angiography. Compared with ICA, CTA avoids the need for an invasive procedure, but it does not eliminate exposure to ionizing radiation or the need for iodinated contrast material. CTA should be considered in symptomatic patients with a low to intermediate pretest likelihood of obstructive disease. Other useful indications for CTA include the following: (1) clarification of inconclusive stress test results; (2) suspected anomalous origin of the coronary arteries; and (3) acute chest pain in selected patients. CTA is not useful in high-risk patients or those with known CAD because the presence of severe CACs may lower the accuracy of the examination or may render the study uninterpretable for evaluating the severity of stenosis. Contraindications to CTA include renal dysfunction, morbid obesity, inability to breath-hold, elevated heart rate, and abnormal heart rhythms.

CTA can identify nonobstructive (i.e., subclinical) lesions, which are unlikely to cause symptoms but are associated with a higher risk of future events. Ultimately, one goal of CTA is to identify high-risk plaques that may be more likely to rupture and lead to future adverse events. Nevertheless, even if such high-risk lesions could be reliably identified, additional research is required to determine the optimal treatment strategy in for such patients.

Physiologic Methods

Physiologic methods of coronary evaluation are based on the identification of signs of myocardial ischemia induced by exercise or pharmacologic stress. The most basic signs are changes on the electrocardiogram (ECG) that indicate myocardial ischemia. Other methods rely on identification of deficits in relative perfusion in areas downstream of coronary stenosis by using a radiotracer or other marker of blood flow. Alternatively, significant ischemia results in regional myocardial systolic dysfunction, which can be directly visualized with functional imaging during stress. The advantage of these methods is that they transcend the weak relationship between the degree of stenosis on anatomic assessment and functional significance. However, most physiologic methods cannot identify lesions that do not cause ischemia but may still have adverse prognostic significance.

STRESS ECHOCARDIOGRAPHY

Stress echocardiography protocols are based on the identification of stress-induced wall motion abnormalities following exercise or pharmacologic stress. Advantages of stress echocardiography include widespread availability, portability, lower cost than nuclear and magnetic resonance imaging (MRI) techniques, absence of ionizing radiation, and the ability to evaluate parameters of ventricular and valvular function during the test. Patients with poor acoustic windows (e.g., obese patients and those with obstructive lung disease) may have reduced image quality, which can lower the diagnostic accuracy of the examination. In such cases, image quality may be improved by administration of echocardiographic contrast agents that enhance endocardial delineation. The accuracy of this examination may also be reduced in patients with resting wall motion abnormalities (e.g., prior infarction, severe left ventricular dysfunction, right ventricular pacing, prior cardiac surgery).

When to Choose Stress Echocardiography. Stress echocardiography may be particularly useful in younger patients, in whom radiation exposure may have greater adverse consequences. This technique is also useful in evaluating for exercise-induced dyspnea in patients with valvular heart disease or suspected exercise-induced heart failure with preserved ejection fraction or pulmonary hypertension, although special protocols and expertise are required for such examinations.

NUCLEAR METHODS

Modern nuclear methods include single-photon emission computed tomography (SPECT) and positron emission tomography (PET). These methods are based on the identification of relative differences in myocardial perfusion. Technetium-99m agents are the most commonly used radiotracers and provide excellent image quality. SPECT can be performed in conjunction with exercise or pharmacologic stress. As with most modalities, image quality can be compromised by obesity. This situation can be ameliorated, in part, by performing stress and rest studies on separate days, to allow for increased radiotracer doses. Furthermore, newer-generation SPECT cameras can improve image quality in obese patients.

The primary limitation of SPECT methods is the prevalence of artifacts from breast or diaphragmatic attenuation or excess hepatic or gastrointestinal tracer uptake. These artifacts can be reduced by the application of attenuation correction techniques. Less commonly, underestimation of the extent of coronary disease can result from a global or balanced reduction in myocardial perfusion, typically in patients with significant left main or three-vessel coronary disease (Fig. 10-2).

PET imaging provides improved image quality, fewer artifacts, and decreased radiation exposure, albeit at increased financial cost. Although exercise imaging is possible using nitrogen-13 ammonia, this technique requires the presence of a cyclotron in close proximity. Rubidium-82 is more frequently employed because it can be produced with a generator and thus does not require a cyclotron. However, because of the very short half-life (76 seconds) of rubidium-82, exercise studies are not possible. Fluorine-18–containing tracers, which are currently in advanced clinical trials, will offer further improvements in image quality while also increasing clinical availability. Finally, PET methods also allow quantification of absolute myocardial perfusion during stress and rest. Data from Murthy et al (2011) suggests that this information has substantial prognostic value beyond conventional risk markers and visual assessment of myocardial perfusion Murthy, et al. Circulation 2011. 124:2215-24 (Fig. 10-3).

MAGNETIC RESONANCE IMAGING

CMR provides high-resolution imaging of cardiac structure, function, and morphology without any radiation exposure. When obstructive CAD is suspected, analysis of myocardial perfusion defects during pharmacologically induced vasodilation and under resting conditions can be used to identify areas of ischemia, whereas late enhancement imaging can be used to identify areas of prior infarction. When areas of prior infarction are identified, the transmural extent of scar can be used to assess the degree of viable myocardium and predict the degree of expected functional recovery when coronary revascularization is being considered. Although vasodilator perfusion imaging is generally preferred, the administration of dobutamine may be used to assess for stress-induced wall motion abnormalities.

Advantages of CMR include the ability to obtain high-quality images, even among overweight patients, and the capacity to visualize many other cardiac conditions, thus enabling a customized protocol that can answer multiple clinical questions during a single examination. For example, CMR can assess left and right ventricular function, provide quantitative information on pulmonic and systemic blood flow (i.e., Qp/Qs ratio), and evaluate for the presence of infiltrative heart disease, such as sarcoidosis, amyloidosis, or hemochromatosis.

Like echocardiography, CMR allows concurrent assessment of the pericardium and cardiac valves. The addition of angiographic sequences to assess the great vessels is straightforward. Angiographic imaging of the coronary arteries is also possible, but it does not yet have the performance characteristics of ICA or CTA. MRI also

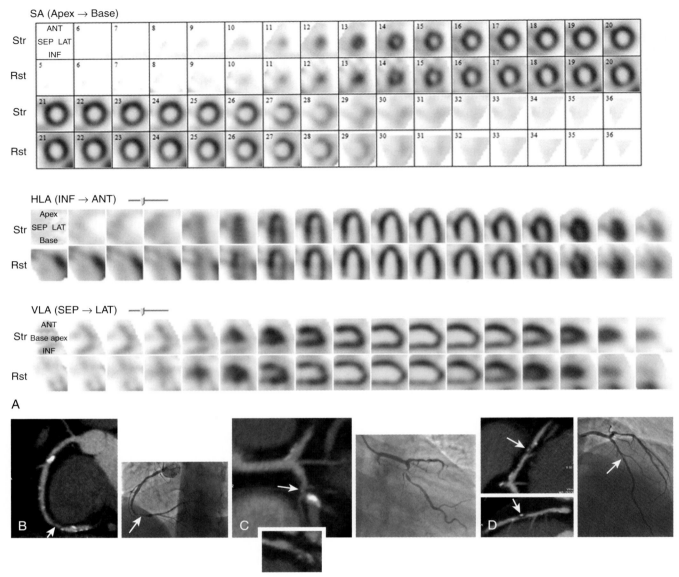

Figure 10-2 A 66-year-old man with hypertension and hyperlipidemia was referred for exercise single-photon emission computed tomography (SPECT) for evaluation of atypical chest pain. The patient exercised for 5 minutes and 44 seconds (7 metabolic equivalents) on a standard Bruce protocol without ischemic electrocardiographic changes and stopped because of dyspnea. Rest-stress SPECT images (*bottom,* **A**) showed no evidence of exercise-induced ischemia. Because of recurring symptoms, computed tomography angiography was performed, and it showed greater than 70% stenosis in a multivessel distribution (*bottom:* **B,** right coronary artery; **C,** left anterior descending coronary artery; and **D,** left circumflex coronary artery). Invasive coronary angiography confirmed the presence of stenosis in all three epicardial vessels. Discrepant results, in which anatomic imaging shows obstructive coronary artery disease although no perfusion defects are identified, are common and most often represent lesions that are not flow limiting. Less frequently, however, a balanced reduction in flow (e.g., balanced ischemia) secondary to three-vessel disease may be result in false-negative results of myocardial perfusion imaging. *ANT,* Anterior; *HLA,* horizontal long-axis view; *INF,* inferior; *LAT,* lateral; *Rst,* rest; *SA,* short-axis view; *SEP,* septum; *Str,* stress; *VLA,* vertical long-axis view.

allows identification of myocardial scar and fibrosis, quantification of systolic function, and assessment of regional strain and dyssynchrony.

The primary limitations of CMR are availability and cost. Some patients may have difficulty tolerating CMR studies because of claustrophobia, although this problem can be ameliorated with pretreatment with anxiolytic medications, as well as use of a larger-bore magnet, when available. CMR cannot be performed in patients with some implanted ferromagnetic objects (e.g., pacemakers). Because of the rare but potentially

life-threatening complication of nephrogenic systemic fibrosis, administration of gadolinium-based contrast media (which is required only for some types of CMR studies) is contraindicated in patients with a creatinine clearance of 30 mL/minute or less and is discouraged in patients with less severe renal impairment. Finally, many CMR sequences depend on ECG gating and require repeated breath holding. Thus, image quality may be reduced in patients with highly irregular heart rhythms (e.g., frequent premature ventricular contractions) or in patients who cannot perform sufficient

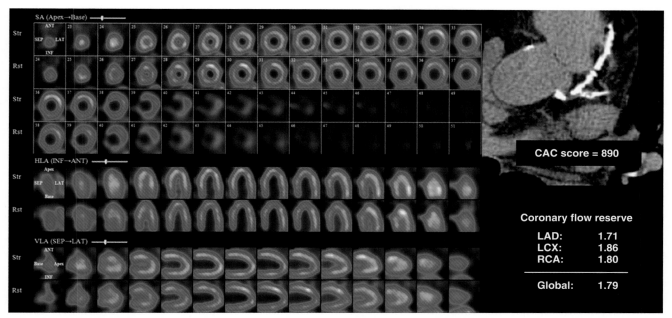

Figure 10-3 Rubidium-82 positron emission tomography stress-rest myocardial perfusion imaging *(left)* from a 72-year-old man with history of hypertension and atypical chest pain showed no evidence of ischemia or infarction. However, extensive coronary artery calcification (CAC) was present (Agatston score of 890), and quantitative assessment of myocardial perfusion was decreased. In this patient, the presence of severe CAC and impaired coronary flow reserve implied a substantially higher risk of future cardiac events. As a result, these findings prompted medical and lifestyle therapies. *ANT,* Anterior; *HLA,* horizontal long-axis view; *INF,* inferior; *LAD,* left anterior descending coronary artery; *LAT,* lateral; *LXC,* left circumflex coronary artery; *RCA,* right coronary artery; *Rst,* rest; *SA,* short-axis view; *SEP,* septum; *Str,* stress; *VLA,* vertical long-axis view.

breath holds. However, myocardial perfusion imaging is less dependent on the ECG signal and thus can be performed even if heart rhythm abnormalities are present.

When Is Exercise Favored Over Pharmacologic Stress?

Exercise tolerance testing (ETT), usually performed with graded treadmill exercise, can be coupled with ECG and imaging assessments of myocardial ischemia. In general, patients who can exercise should undergo exercise rather than pharmacologic stress testing. ETT provides important data on functional capacity and exercise-induced symptoms and thus integrate data on overall cardiac, pulmonary, peripheral vascular, and musculoskeletal physiology. Patients who can achieve 10 metabolic equivalents (METS) or more in the absence of ECG changes are extremely unlikely to have any ischemia and have an excellent prognosis. ETT may be particularly useful when arrhythmia is a known or suspected contributor to the patient's symptoms. In special circumstances, ETT may be coupled with analysis of exhaled gases to determine whether a patient's exercise intolerance is the result of pulmonary disease, myocardial ischemia, or skeletal myopathies. However, the widely used Bruce exercise protocol may be too challenging for older patients and patients with significant arthritis or other skeletal abnormalities. In these cases, exercise protocols may be tailored to patients' needs. The major disadvantage of this approach is that, without standardized protocols, a reliable estimate of a patient's exercise capacity may be difficult to obtain.

When Are Pharmacologic Tests Preferred Over Exercise? And Which One?

Pharmacologic stress is chosen over exercise for four reasons. First, exercise may be unsafe in some patients, such as those who have disorders of gait or balance. Second, in patients with left bundle branch block, the resulting ventricular dyssynchrony may induce artifacts (i.e., false-positive perfusion defects in septum). Although the additional data obtained during exercise assessment may outweigh the loss of diagnostic precision in some cases. Third, patients whose exercise tolerance is already known to be inadequate (i.e., patients unable to achieve ≥85% of age-predicted maximal heart rate) need to undergo pharmacologic stress testing. In these patients, a potential alternative is to initiate testing with exercise and convert to pharmacologic stress if needed. Fourth, patients who may benefit from an imaging modality (e.g., cardiac MRI, rubidium PET) that cannot readily be coupled with exercise may be best served with pharmacologic stress testing.

Once the decision to employ pharmacologic stress is made, the agent must be selected (Table 10-3). The two primary mechanisms are as follows: (1) causing coronary vasodilatation and therefore leading to preferentially higher flow in areas supplied by normal vessels and relatively lower perfusion downstream of significant coronary lesions; and (2) increasing myocardial oxygen demand by increasing heart rate and myocardial contractility. Most agents currently in use employ the first mechanism. These include dipyridamole, adenosine, and regadenoson. These agents work by similar mechanisms and, as a consequence, have similar limitations. All should be used with caution in patients with bronchospastic disease and should not be used in the setting of active wheezing. Vasodilators should be avoided in the setting of recent methylxanthine use, including caffeine and theophylline. Finally, all these agents decrease conduction through the atrioventricular node and should be avoided in patients with high-degree heart block.

Dobutamine is the only stress agent whose primary mechanism is induction of myocardial ischemia by increasing heart rate and contractility. As such, this agent should be used with caution in patients with marginal clinical stability or a history of tachyarrhythmias. Further, because outright ischemia (as opposed to relative perfusion deficits) may be induced by administration of dobutamine, this drug should not be used in patients with active or recent myocardial infarction. Another critical limitation of dobutamine is that an adequate level of stress may be difficult to achieve in patients taking concomitant beta-adrenergic blocking medications. This concern may be addressed either by instructing the patient to discontinue the beta-blocker medications for the test or by adding

atropine (which should be avoided in patients with urinary retention or closed angle glaucoma). The primary advantage of dobutamine over vasodilator stress agents is that it more closely approximates the physiologic features of exercise. However, whereas dobutamine is usually preferred for testing modalities that assess for stress-induced wall motion abnormalities (i.e., stress echocardiogram, CMR), vasodilators are preferred for myocardial perfusion imaging, because of better patient tolerability and higher accuracy. Nonetheless, dobutamine can also be used to assess for stress-induced perfusion abnormalities.

When Is an Imaging Test Necessary?

Because of limited sensitivity of ETT alone, an imaging test should be considered in all patients who have intermediate to high pretest probability of obstructive CAD, except possibly when the test is not obtained to evaluate ischemia, and the only required clinical information pertains to exercise-induced symptoms, arrhythmias, or exercise capacity. In patients with underlying left bundle branch block, exercise alone may not be sufficient because the ECG will be uninterpretable for any ischemic changes. In such situations, careful consideration should be given to a vasodilator stress test or

Table 10-3 Overview of Exercise and Pharmacologic Stress Testing

	Mechanism	Contraindications	Warnings	Dosing	Antagonist
Exercise	Increased heart rate and contractility	Unstable ventricular arrhythmias Hypertrophic cardiomyopathy with outflow obstruction	Caution with gait instability, after myocardial infarction, and in severe valvular disease	Various graded treadmill, bicycle, and ergometer protocols	Intravenous beta-adrenergic blocking agents (e.g., metoprolol, 5 mg slow IVP)
Inotropes					
Dobutamine	Sympathomimetic beta$_1$-adrenergic agonist: increased heart rate and contractility beta$_2$-adrenergic agonist (weak): peripheral vasodilation	Unstable ventricular arrhythmias	Caution after myocardial infarction and in hypertrophic cardiomyopathy with obstruction May result in rapid ventricular response in setting of atrial fibrillation May induce hypotension in hypovolemia	10 mcg/kg/min × 4 min 20 mcg/kg/min × 4 min 30 mcg/kg/min × 4 min 40 mcg/kg/min × 4 min (until 85% of age predicted maximum heart rate achieved)	Intravenous beta-adrenergic blocking agents (e.g., metoprolol, 5 mg slow IVP)
Vasodilators					
Adenosine	Adenosine A1 and A2 receptor agonist	Bronchospastic lung disease High-grade atrioventricular block (second or third degree) (unless pacemaker present) Sinus node dysfunction (unless pacemaker present)	Caution in unstable angina, autonomic dysfunction, hypovolemia, recent stroke or transient ischemic attack, and severe stenotic valvular disease May cause profound vasodilation with subsequent hypotension	142 mcg/kg/min IV × 4 min	Aminophylline, 1 mg/kg
Dipyridamole	Increased extracellular adenosine by inhibiting reuptake and degradation	Similar to above	Similar to adenosine Caution in severe hepatic impairment	140 mcg/kg/min IV × 6 min	Aminophylline, 1 mg/kg
Regadenoson	Adenosine A2A receptor agonist	Similar to above	Similar to adenosine Uncertain dosing in severe renal impairment	0.4 mg IVP	Aminophylline, 1 mg/kg

IV, Intravenously; *IVP,* by intravenous push.

CTA because exercise may exacerbate ventricular dysynchrony leading to false positive results. All patients undergoing pharmacologic stress testing should have concurrent imaging.

In contrast, in patients with low pretest probability, an imaging test may be unnecessary. For these patients, an exercise treadmill test with ECG may be adequate to demonstrate the absence of significant myocardial ischemia. Although ETT is widely recognized to have low sensitivity (~65%), the presence of high exercise tolerance, which is associated with an excellent prognosis and a low likelihood of ischemia, may be sufficient. Although this issue is controversial in the United States, some international guidelines (e.g., the National Institute for Clinical Health and Excellence guidelines in the United Kingdom) advise against the use of ETT alone for evaluating symptomatic patients.

■ HOW SHOULD ASYMPTOMATIC INDIVIDUALS BE RISK STRATIFIED?

Although most of this chapter focuses on the diagnosis and risk stratification of patients with signs or symptoms suggestive of coronary ischemia, even larger populations of patients are at risk of complications of CAD, such as myocardial infarction or death, but do not exhibit overt signs or symptoms. Many of these patients would benefit from more aggressive medical therapy or perhaps from coronary revascularization.

As discussed earlier, the first step for patients with symptoms should be to estimate the pretest likelihood of complications of CAD. Various tools exist for this purpose, including the Framingham Risk Score and the Reynolds Risk Score. For patients at extremely low pretest risk, additional testing is unlikely to be of benefit. Similarly, for patients at very high pretest risk, aggressive medical treatments without further testing may be reasonable. For patients at intermediate risk (5% to 20% 10-year risk), however, further testing may avoid unnecessary treatment, decrease treatment complications, and possibly result in lower overall costs.

The ideal test for asymptomatic patients with no prior CAD would have low cost, be risk free, and could accurately identify both high-risk and low-risk patients beyond traditional risk factors, thus providing the ability to reclassify risk across clinically meaningful categories. Although virtually every imaging modality discussed earlier has been used to evaluate asymptomatic individuals, more recent guidelines published by the American College of Cardiology and the American Heart Association recommended against the use of ETT, nuclear stress testing, and stress echocardiography for such populations. Nevertheless, in select high-risk cohorts (patients with known peripheral vascular disease, patients with human immunodeficiency virus infection, and higher-risk diabetic patients), perfusion imaging may be reasonable, to assess for clinically silent ischemia, particularly if such information would be used to intensify medical therapies or pursue coronary revascularization.

Data on the potential role of CAC screening using cardiac computed tomography (CT) have grown substantially. A CAC scan offers a quick, inexpensive, and highly reproducible method to estimate the presence or absence of calcified coronary atherosclerosis. This test does not require any intravenous contrast and is performed during a single breath hold. In patients with CAC, the Agatston score can be used to quantify the severity of disease as mild (<100), moderate (100 to 400), or severe (>400).

The absence of CAC in an asymptomatic adult is associated with an excellent long-term prognosis (mortality rate of ~1% over 10 years), and it could be useful to identify patients in whom lifestyle therapies may be pursued while more expensive medical therapies are deferred. In contrast, patients with severe CACs (e.g., score >300) have a nearly tenfold increased risk of adverse coronary events. In two large population studies (the Multi-Ethnic Study of Atherosclerosis and the Heinz-Nixdorf study) examining the value of CAC beyond traditional risk markers, CAC scanning was shown to improve model discrimination and result in improved reclassification of patients into the appropriate clinical risk groups. Other studies showed that CAC scanning may lead to improvement in some risk factors by intensification of lifestyle and medical therapies.

Although the early detection of coronary atherosclerosis with CAC imaging may enhance risk prediction, the potential benefits of CAC scanning must be weighed against the potential risks of exposure to ionizing radiation. When appropriate techniques are employed, the mean effective radiation dose associated with a CAC scan is approximately 1.0 mSv. Table 10-4 compares radiation doses of various imaging modalities. Given the paucity of prospective randomized data demonstrating the clinical effectiveness of CAC scanning, the routine widespread screening of patients is not recommended at this time. Nevertheless, CAC scanning may be considered among selected patients at low to intermediate risk in whom additional therapy is being considered.

■ CARDIAC IMAGING FOR NONCORONARY INDICATIONS

Evaluation of known or suspected CAD represents the most common indication for cardiac imaging, but many other disorders can be evaluated with echocardiography,

Table 10-4 Estimated Effective Radiation Dose of Various Cardiac Imaging Tests

Test	Effective Dose (mSv)
Coronary artery calcium score	1
Cardiac CT angiography	1-12
SPECT thallium-201 and technetium-99m	~20
SPECT technetium-99m sestamibi*	11.3
PET rubidium-82[†]	~4
PET nitrogen-13 ammonia[‡]	2.4
Invasive coronary angiography	4-8

CT, Computed tomography; *PET*, positron emission tomography; *SPECT*, single-photon emission computed tomography.
*Assuming injected activity of 10 mCi at rest and 27.5 mCi during stress.
[†]Assuming injected activity of 50 mCi at rest and 50 mCi during stress.
[‡]Assuming injected activity of 15 mCi at rest and 15 mCi during stress.

cardiac CT, and MRI. Broadly, these conditions include disorders of the myocardium, cardiac valves, and pericardium, as well as infections and tumors involving cardiac structures (Table 10-5).

Imaging for Disorders of the Myocardium

Heart Failure

Signs and symptoms of ventricular systolic dysfunction include pedal and pulmonary edema, jugular venous distention, and dyspnea. Although the most common causes of ventricular systolic dysfunction are myocardial ischemia and infarction related to coronary atherosclerosis, various other nonischemic cardiomyopathies may lead to ventricular dysfunction. Examples include genetic mutations, viral infections, infiltrative heart disease (e.g., sarcoidosis, hemochromatosis), and treatment with cardiotoxic drugs.

Echocardiography remains the mainstay of routine evaluation of myocardial structure and function. However, CMR is generally considered to provide more precise estimates of ventricular dimensions and systolic function. Furthermore, CMR may be particularly helpful when assessing for various nonischemic conditions. For example, the pattern of late gadolinium enhancement

Table 10-5   Cardiac Imaging for Noncoronary Indications

Diagnosis	Signs and Symptoms	Modality	Findings
Heart failure	Dyspnea Pulmonary edema Pedal edema Jugular venous distention	Echocardiography	Chamber dimensions Systolic function Regional wall motion abnormalities Valvular dysfunction (gold standard) Diastolic function
		Cardiac MRI	Chamber dimensions (gold standard) Systolic function (gold standard) Regional wall motion abnormalities Valvular dysfunction Diastolic function Myocardial scar/infiltration (gold standard)
		Cardiac CT	Differentiation of ischemic from nonischemic causes
Valvular disease	Murmur Dyspnea Palpitations Chest pain	Echocardiography	Chamber dimensions Systolic function Quantification of valvular regurgitation (gold standard) Quantification of valvular stenosis (gold standard)
		Cardiac MRI	Chamber dimensions (gold standard) Systolic function (gold standard) Quantification of valvular regurgitation Quantification of valvular stenosis
		Cardiac CT	Planning for transcatheter aortic valve replacement or implantation Planimetry of left-sided valve orifices for stenosis and regurgitation Prosthetic valve endocarditis (paravalvular leak, pseudoaneurysms)
Pericardial disease	Dyspnea Pulmonary edema Pedal edema Jugular venous distention Hypotension Tachycardia Pericardial knock	Echocardiography	Pericardial effusion Diastolic filling velocity (gold standard) Respirophasic septal shift (gold standard) Respirophasic variation in transvalvular velocities (gold standard)
		Cardiac MRI	Pericardial effusion Pericardial thickness or morphology (gold standard) Pericardial enhancement (gold standard) Pericardial adhesions
		Cardiac CT	Pericardial effusion Pericardial thickness Pericardial calcification (gold standard) Pericardial enhancement
Cardiac mass	Embolization Dyspnea Chest pain Murmur	Echocardiography	Mass size and location Mass morphology
		Cardiac MRI	Mass size and location Mass morphology Mass vascularity or perfusion (gold standard) Thrombus (gold standard)
		Cardiac CT	Mass size and location Mass morphology Mass vascularity or perfusion Pulmonary embolization

CT, Computed tomography; *MRI*, magnetic resonance imaging.

on CMR can be used to differentiate between myocardial infarction and nonischemic causes with fibrosis (e.g., hypertrophic and dilated cardiomyopathies), infiltration (e.g., sarcoidosis, hemochromatosis, and amyloidosis), or inflammation (e.g., myocarditis).

Increasing numbers of patients with heart failure have preserved systolic function (i.e., heart failure with preserved ejection fraction). For these patients, echocardiography plays an important role in the identification and quantification of diastolic filling abnormalities because of the superior temporal resolution of this technique. Strain measures using either tissue Doppler imaging or speckle-tracking methods can often identify subtle abnormalities of systolic function in these patients. Although CMR can also be used to assess diastolic function, these methods are more cumbersome and less well studied than corresponding echocardiographic techniques.

Hypertrophic Cardiomyopathy

Echocardiography remains the first-line method for identification and characterization of hypertrophic cardiomyopathy. Its high temporal resolution and Doppler capabilities allow characterization of left ventricular outflow obstruction at rest or in response to provocations, such as Valsalva maneuver or exercise. Echocardiography allows quantification of septal thickness, which carries prognostic value and is an important consideration in patients evaluated for prophylactic defibrillator implantation. CMR, however, provides more robust quantification of wall thickness because of better endocardial delineation, and better differentiation of the left and right ventricles along the septum. In addition, CMR adds the ability to quantify fibrosis with late gadolinium enhancement, which is associated with adverse prognosis and increased arrhythmia risk.

Arrhythmogenic Right Ventricular Dysplasia and Cardiomyopathy

Mutations of the desmosome, a cell-cell adhesion complex, result in abnormalities of the myocardium, skin, and hair. In its earliest stages, arrhythmogenic right ventricular cardiomyopathy usually affects the right ventricle, but it may also involve the left ventricle. Although abnormalities of right ventricular size and function may be identifiable on echocardiography, CMR allows for improved visualization of the right ventricle. Thus, CMR is better suited for assessing for right ventricular size and function, as well as focal wall motion abnormalities or microaneurysms, which are important features of this disease. Fibrofatty infiltration of the myocardium can also be characterized by CMR, although this finding is no longer part of the diagnostic criteria, and in the absence of right ventricular dilatation or dysfunction, it is nonspecific.

Valvular Disorders

The superior temporal resolution and ability to characterize transvalvular velocities with Doppler imaging have established the role of echocardiography in the evaluation of valvular disorders. In particular, transesophageal echocardiography can be useful in evaluating mitral valve disease (in part because of the posterior location of this valve), and it offers insight into the mechanism of valvular dysfunction, prognosis, and choice of optimal treatment (i.e., repair versus replacement). Nonetheless, MRI methods have improved precision in the quantification of chamber volumes and systolic function, both important criteria in therapeutic decision making regarding the timing of valve repair or replacement. When evaluation by echocardiography is limited or when a discrepancy is noted among the clinical impression, echocardiographic findings, or data from other modalities (i.e., invasive catheterization), CMR can quantify transvalvular velocities and regurgitant volumes using phase contrast techniques. However, such an assessment is most robust for the aortic and pulmonic valves, which generally have a more laminar flow profile. Because of turbulence and eccentricity, CMR flow analysis for mitral and tricuspid valve disease is more challenging.

Although underrecognized, the use of cardiac CT can also provide precise anatomic visualization of the mitral and aortic valves. When image quality is insufficient on echocardiography or CMR, or when CT is already being performed for the evaluation of the coronary arteries, useful anatomic data can be obtained for assessing valvular disease. For example, planimetry of the aortic valve orifice during systole can allow precise quantification of aortic valve area. Similarly, a flail mitral valve leaflet can be visualized in individuals who have mitral regurgitation. One especially useful application of CT is in evaluating the function of prosthetic valves because extensive artifacts are often present on both echocardiographic and CMR images in such cases. Whenever the cardiac valves are evaluated by CT, multiphase acquisition, in which data are obtained throughout the cardiac cycle, is needed, but results in higher radiation exposures.

Pericardial Disorders

The most common disorders of the pericardium are pericardial effusion, pericarditis, and pericardial constriction. Pericardial effusions may result from many different disorders, ranging from trauma to tumors to autoimmune disorders. Large and rapidly growing effusions may result in pericardial tamponade, causing impaired cardiac diastolic filling and, in severe cases, hemodynamic collapse. Because of its rapid availability and ability to characterize physiologic changes preceding hemodynamic compromise, echocardiography is the initial modality of choice. Size and morphology of pericardial effusions can also be characterized with a gated CT or MRI scan. MRI may be most useful when a mass or pericardial inflammation is also suspected.

In pericardial constriction, the pericardium is thickened and fibrosed, thus preventing complete filling of the cardiac chambers. This disorder may be caused by adhesions related to prior cardiac surgery, but can also result from radiation therapy or from infectious, inflammatory, or infiltrative disorders. Most cases of pericardial constriction are associated with increased pericardial thickness. This measurement can be accurately made by either MRI or CT. Whereas CT has better spatial resolution and the ability to identify pericardial calcifications

(calcifications can also be detected on radiographs or by fluoroscopy), MRI can be used to assess for pericardial late enhancement, a finding that signifies the presence of fibrosis or inflammation. Tagging techniques can be helpful in identifying pericardial adhesions, which at times may be present even when pericardial thickness is normal.

Echocardiography can provide important hemodynamic data regarding respiratory changes in the filling of the left and right ventricles. This information can be used to assess exaggerated interventricular dependence, as well as the attenuated relationship between intrapleural pressures and the cardiac chambers observed in this condition. In addition, tissue Doppler assessment can be used to assess the longitudinal motion of the mitral valve annulus, a parameter that is helpful in distinguishing constriction from restriction. No single imaging finding can confirm the diagnosis of pericardial constriction, and integrating data from multiple modalities may be beneficial when this diagnosis is in question, particularly given that treatment may involve high-risk surgical pericardiectomy.

Masses and Infections

Although primary tumors of the myocardium are rare, metastatic disease may involve the myocardium, cardiac valves, or pericardium. Initial characterization is usually with echocardiography, although CT and MRI allow better delineation of tumor size, involvement of neighboring structures, and vascularity. Echocardiography may be helpful when masses impair valvular function. Postcontrast MRI with high inversion times can be useful in distinguishing tumor from thrombus (Fig. 10-4).

How to Choose Between Echocardiography and Cardiac Magnetic Resonance Imaging

In choosing between CMR and echocardiography, the clinician must first ensure that the patient does not have any contraindications to CMR, as discussed earlier. In general, for most conditions that can be evaluated with either modality (e.g., left ventricular function), echocardiography should be the initial choice, mostly because of its lower cost. CMR may then be considered in rare situations in which images provided by echocardiography are insufficient. As discussed previously, conditions that are more suitable for evaluation using echocardiography include assessment of valvular function and evaluation of diastolic dysfunction. Conversely, CMR offers improved contrast resolution and a superior ability to characterize different types of tissues, and thus it is more useful for evaluating patients with known or suspected infiltrative heart disease or cardiac masses. However, echocardiography has better spatial and temporal resolution and therefore may be better for evaluating small, highly mobile structures such as small vegetations.

Finally, in evaluating certain conditions such as pericardial constriction, CMR and echocardiography may be complementary, and integrating data from both modalities may be useful. For example, CMR may provide information on pericardial thickness and enhancement, as well as evaluate for possible adhesions (using tagging sequences), whereas echocardiography may provide important hemodynamic information by assessing for respiratory changes in transvalvular flow.

■ PEARLS AND PITFALLS

1. Before choosing among different tests, the clinician should first establish whether any testing is required.
2. Choosing the right test for the right patient requires an understanding of both the clinical question at hand and the technical aspects of the multiple available testing options.
3. Consultation between clinicians and imaging experts may be helpful in selecting the most beneficial testing strategy, particularly when uncertainty exists about test options or whether a given test will answer the clinical question.
4. Institutional experience and expertise are important determinants of diagnostic accuracy and should be integrated in deciding which test to choose.
5. When evaluating symptomatic patients with suspected CAD, the clinician should always consider the pretest probability of obstructive CAD first. In high-risk patients (or those who have known CAD), a functional test such as perfusion imaging or assessment of wall motion abnormalities during stress is preferred.
6. Most asymptomatic patients without known CAD do not require any stress testing. In selected individuals, however, a CAD scan may be helpful in establishing future risk of cardiovascular disease and thus the potential benefit of preventive therapies.

Echocardiography

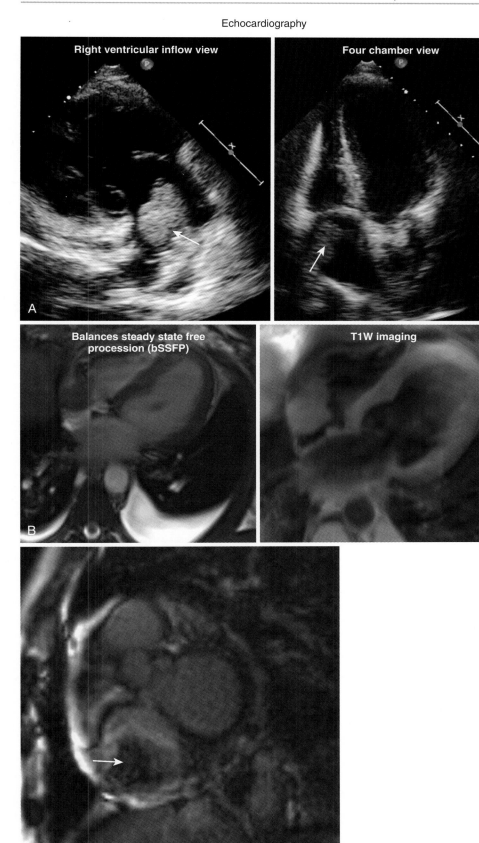

Figure 10-4 Example of CMR confirming the diagnosis of an atrial thrombus. **A,** This 48-year-old woman with a history of ovarian cancer was found to have a large right atrial mass *(arrow)* on echocardiography after she had a long-term central venous catheter. The differential diagnosis for this finding included thrombus and tumor. **B,** Subsequently, the patient was referred for cardiovascular magnetic resonance (CMR) for further evaluation. CMR showed a mobile mass adjacent to the lateral wall of the right atrium. The mass was isointense to myocardium on T1- (T1W) and T2-weighted images and did not enhance on a first-pass perfusion study or with late gadolinium enhancement. **C,** In addition, the mass was nulled when it was imaged using a long inversion time, a characteristic consistent with the presence of thrombus *(arrow)*.

Bibliography

Amsterdam EA, Kirk JD, Bluemke DA, et al. Testing of low-risk patients presenting to the emergency department with chest pain: a scientific statement from the American Heart Association. *Circulation.* 2010;122:1756-1776.

Blankstein R, Devore AD. Selecting a noninvasive imaging study after an inconclusive exercise test. *Circulation.* 2010;122:1514-1518.

Blankstein R, Di Carli MF. Integration of coronary anatomy and myocardial perfusion imaging. *Nat Rev Cardiol.* 2010;7:226-236.

Bourque JM, Holland BH, Watson DD, Beller GA. Achieving an exercise workload of > or = 10 metabolic equivalents predicts a very low risk of inducible ischemia: does myocardial perfusion imaging have a role? *J Am Coll Cardiol.* 2009;54:538-545.

Douglas PS, Garcia MJ, Haines DE, et al. ACCF/ASE/AHA/ASNC/HFSA/HRS/SCAI/SCCM/SCCT/SCMR 2011 appropriate use criteria for echocardiography: a report of the American College of Cardiology Foundation Appropriate Use Criteria Task Force, American Society of Echocardiography, American Heart Association, American Society of Nuclear Cardiology, Heart Failure Society of America, Heart Rhythm Society, Society for Cardiovascular Angiography and Interventions, Society of Critical Care Medicine, Society of Cardiovascular Computed Tomography, and Society for Cardiovascular Magnetic Resonance Endorsed by the American College of Chest Physicians. *J Am Coll Cardiol.* 2011;57:1126-1166.

Earls JP, White RD, Woodard PK, Abbara S, et al. ACR Appropriateness Criteria chronic chest pain: high probability of coronary artery disease. *J Am Coll Radiol.* 2011;8:679-686.

Gibbons RJ, Balady GJ, Bricker JT, et al. ACC/AHA 2002 guideline update for exercise testing: summary article. A report of the American College of Cardiology/American Heart Association Task Force on Practice Guidelines (Committee to Update the 1997 Exercise Testing Guidelines). *J Am Coll Cardiol.* 2002;40:1531-1540.

Hendel RC, Berman DS, Di Carli MF, et al. ACCF/ASNC/ACR/AHA/ASE/SCCT/SCMR/SNM 2009 appropriate use criteria for cardiac radionuclide imaging: a report of the American College of Cardiology Foundation Appropriate Use Criteria Task Force, the American Society of Nuclear Cardiology, the American College of Radiology, the American Heart Association, the American Society of Echocardiography, the Society of Cardiovascular Computed Tomography, the Society for Cardiovascular Magnetic Resonance, and the Society of Nuclear Medicine. *Circulation.* 2009;119:e561-e587.

Koh AS, Blankstein R. Selecting the best noninvasive imaging test to guide treatment after an inconclusive exercise test. *Curr Treat Options Cardiovasc Med.* 2012;14:9-23.

Mammen L, White RD, Woodard PK, et al. ACR Appropriateness Criteria on chest pain suggestive of acute coronary syndrome. *J Am Coll Radiol.* 2011;8:12-18.

Murthy VL, Naya M, Foster CR, et al. Improved cardiac risk assessment with noninvasive measures of coronary flow reserve. *Circulation.* 2011;124:2215-2224.

Taylor AJ, Cerqueira M, Hodgson JM, et al. ACCF/SCCT/ACR/AHA/ASE/ASNC/SCAI/SCMR 2010 appropriate use criteria for cardiac computed tomography: a report of the American College of Cardiology Foundation Appropriate Use Criteria Task Force, the Society of Cardiovascular Computed Tomography, the American College of Radiology, the American Heart Association, the American Society of Echocardiography, the American Society of Nuclear Cardiology, the Society for Cardiovascular Angiography and Interventions, and the Society for Cardiovascular Magnetic Resonance. *Circulation.* 2010;122:e525-555.

ANATOMY

CHAPTER 11

Cardiovascular Anatomy and Pathology on Radiography

Stephen W. Miller and James Kin Ho Woo

To lay the foundation for a discussion of thoracic cardiovascular disease, this chapter begins with an introductory review of anatomy on the chest radiograph. Central venous catheters are then used to illustrate vascular anatomy further and aid in recognition of malposition. Radiographic clues to abnormalities of the thoracic aorta and pulmonary vasculature are reviewed. Finally, pathologic appearances of the heart and pericardium are examined.

■ NORMAL CARDIOVASCULAR ANATOMY ON THE CHEST RADIOGRAPH

Normal posteroanterior (PA) and lateral chest radiographs, as well as relevant computed tomography (CT) correlations, are shown in Figure 11-1. On the PA radiograph, the cardiovascular structures visible in the mediastinum are those that produce interfaces with the lungs. Along the right aspect of the cardiomediastinal silhouette, from superior to inferior, the margins of the right innominate vein, superior vena cava (SVC), right pulmonary artery, right atrial appendage, right atrium, and inferior vena cava (IVC) are visible. Along the left aspect of the cardiomediastinal silhouette, from superior to inferior, the left subclavian artery, aortic arch, aortopulmonary window, main and left pulmonary artery, and left ventricle are visible. Other cardiovascular structures and interfaces that can usually be seen on the radiograph include the azygoesophageal recess, azygos vein, and descending aorta.

On the lateral radiograph, the anterosuperior margin of the right ventricular wall and right ventricular outflow tract are visible adjacent to the retrosternal airspace. The IVC, lateral wall of the left ventricle, and aorta form interfaces with the lung. The right pulmonary artery is usually visible as an oval opacity anterior to the right upper lobe bronchus, whereas the left pulmonary artery can be seen coursing over the left upper lobe bronchus.

The normal locations of the cardiac valves can be approximated on radiography. On the lateral radiograph, the phrase "PAM watches TV" can be helpful in remembering the location of the valves with respect to each other. Because of the fibrous continuity of the aortic and mitral valves, these valves should always be in close proximity to each other.

■ VENOUS ANATOMY AND NORMAL AND MALPOSITIONED CENTRAL VENOUS CATHETERS

Chest radiographs are frequently obtained to confirm the position of central venous catheters and to exclude complications associated with line insertion. The course and tip position of the catheter allow the examiner to infer whether the vessel in which it travels is a specific vein or artery or whether it is extravascular in location.

Innominate, Subclavian, and Internal Jugular Veins

The right subclavian vein joins the right internal jugular vein to form the right innominate vein. Of these vessels, only the right lateral aspect of the innominate vein may be visible on the radiograph because an interface is created between the vein and the right upper lobe. In contrast, the left subclavian vein joins the left internal jugular vein, but the left innominate vein is not visible. The right and left innominate veins join to form the SVC. The relationships of these veins are demonstrated in Figure 11-2. Peripherally inserted central catheters (PICCs) are commonly malpositioned in the internal jugular or left innominate vein (Fig. 11-3).

The medial aspect of the subclavian veins should parallel the medial third of the clavicles, as should catheters in the subclavian veins. A catheter inserted into the right subclavian artery courses more medially into the mediastinum, with a less vertical course than expected from a catheter in the right subclavian vein. A catheter inserted into the left subclavian artery courses inferolaterally to the aortic arch instead of crossing the mediastinum in the left innominate vein, as expected (Fig. 11-4). The subclavian vein courses between the first rib and the clavicle, anterior to the subclavian artery. Rarely, a catheter inserted into the subclavian vein can fracture as a result of repetitive compression of the catheter between the first rib and the clavicle, with migration of the distal fragment.

The internal jugular veins have a relatively vertical course, and catheters should also have a vertical orientation. A catheter inserted into the common carotid artery courses medially toward the aortic arch and is vertical in orientation (Fig. 11-5).

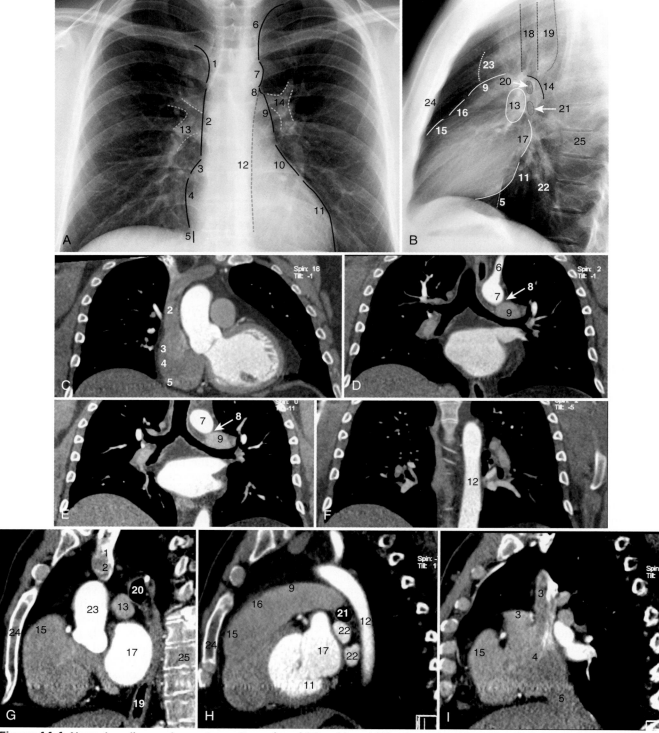

Figure 11-1 Normal cardiovascular anatomy. Posterolateral (**A**) and lateral (**B**) radiographs with computed tomography (CT) correlation. **C** to **I**, Coronal and sagittal oblique CT reformats demonstrate structures corresponding to the interfaces seen on the radiographs. *1*, Right innominate vein; *2*, superior vena cava; *3*, right atrial appendage; *4*, right atrium; *5*, inferior vena cava; *6*, left subclavian artery; *7*, aortic knob; *8*, aortopulmonary window; *9*, main pulmonary artery; *10*, left atrial appendage; *11*, left ventricle; *12*, descending aorta; *13*, right pulmonary artery; *14*, left pulmonary artery; *15*, right ventricle; *16*, right ventricular outflow tract; *17*, left atrium; *18*, trachea; *19*, esophagus; *20*, right main bronchus; *21*, left main/upper lobe bronchus; *22*, left lower lobe pulmonary veins; *23*, ascending aorta; *24*, body of sternum; *25*, spine.

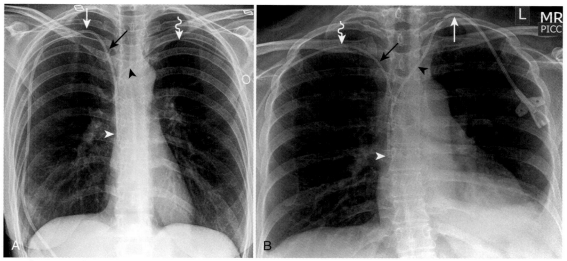

Figure 11-2 Systemic venous anatomy in the upper thorax. A, Right internal jugular (IJ) dual lumen catheter courses superior to the medial clavicle *(white arrow)* before coursing inferiorly into the right innominate vein *(black arrow)* and into the superior vena cava (SVC; *white arrowhead*). Left peripherally inserted central catheter (PICC) parallels the medial left clavicle *(squiggly arrow)* in the left subclavian vein and courses into the left innominate vein *(black arrowhead)* to the origin of the SVC. **B,** A different patient with a right PICC parallels the medial right clavicle *(squiggly arrow)* in the right subclavian vein and courses into the right innominate vein *(black arrow)* with the tip at the origin of the SVC. The left IJ line courses superior to the medial clavicle *(white arrow)* before continuing in the left innominate vein *(black arrowhead)* and into the SVC *(white arrowhead)*.

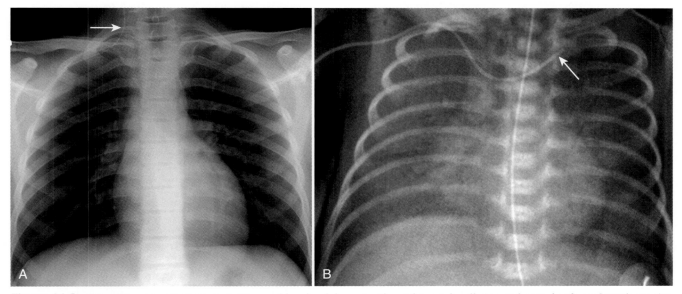

Figure 11-3 Malpositioned catheters. A, A 16-year-old male adolescent with a right peripherally inserted central catheter (PICC) coursing superiorly into the right internal jugular vein *(arrow)* instead of inferomedially into the right innominate vein. **B,** A 2-week-old infant with a right PICC coursing leftward, superolaterally across the mediastinum in the left innominate vein *(arrow)*, instead of into the superior vena cava.

Superior Vena Cava

The inferior margin of the SVC is at the SVC–right atrial junction or cavoatrial junction and is indicated by a convex bump that usually corresponds to the right atrial appendage. Because the right atrial appendage abuts the SVC to form this convex bump and they are in the same approximate coronal plane, this landmark is not usually affected by lordotic or antilordotic positioning. When visible, this convex bump is the most reliable marker of the cavoatrial junction, and the termination of the SVC is usually less than 1 cm inferior to this level.

A left-sided SVC occurs when the left superior cardinal vein caudal to the innominate vein fails to regress in embryologic development. The left SVC can be difficult to see on the chest radiograph, and it usually appears as a vertical interface projected over the aortic arch. The superior margin of the left SVC is formed by the left subclavian and jugular veins. The left SVC usually drains into the great cardiac vein in the left atrioventricular groove and then becomes the coronary sinus. In most cases, the left innominate vein persists between the two SVCs. Rarely, the right SVC regresses, and the left SVC is the only route for

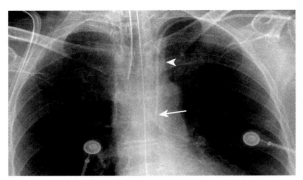

Figure 11-4 Attempted left subclavian vein catheter insertion. Instead of paralleling the left medial clavicle and crossing the mediastinum, the catheter courses superior to the medial left clavicle and then points inferiorly along the left aspect of the superior mediastinum in the expected course of the left subclavian artery *(arrowhead)* with the tip in the proximal descending aorta *(arrow)*.

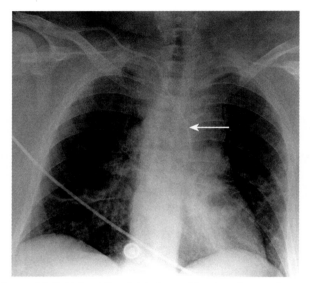

Figure 11-5 Malpositioned right internal jugular vein central venous catheter. The catheter *(arrow)* courses inferomedially into the mediastinum along the expected course of the right common carotid artery and right innominate artery with the tip in the descending aorta.

drainage of blood from the upper body. The presence of a left SVC can be inferred by the vertical course of a catheter along the left aspect of the mediastinum (Fig. 11-6). Occasionally, an anomalous left innominate vein or an anomalous pulmonary vein can mimic a left SVC (Fig. 11-7).

Inferior Vena Cava

The lateral margin of the suprahepatic IVC is visible on the frontal radiograph as a short line inferior to the right heart border. On the lateral radiograph, the posterior margin of the IVC is visible adjacent to the posteroinferior margin of the left ventricle.

Azygos Vein

The azygos vein ascends in the posterior mediastinum along the right anterior aspect of the spine, drapes

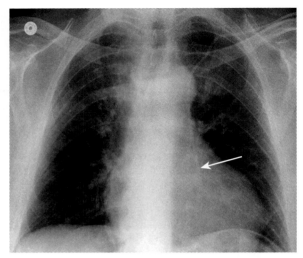

Figure 11-6 Malpositioned left peripherally inserted central catheter (PICC). Left PICC in the left superior vena cava with the tip *(arrow)* in the expected location of the coronary sinus.

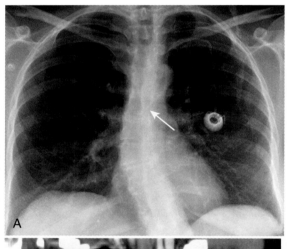

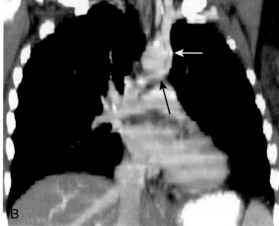

Figure 11-7 Anomalous accessory left innominate vein. **A,** Left subclavian vein Port-A-Cath *(arrow)* courses inferiorly, mimicking a left superior vena cava (SVC), but then courses rightward and inferolaterally to the SVC within an anomalous accessory left innominate vein. **B,** Computed tomography coronal reformat confirms the anomalous left innominate vein *(arrows)*. A normally located left innominate vein was also present (not shown).

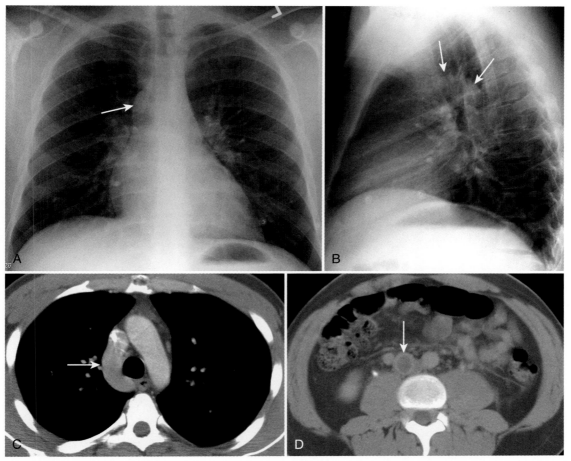

Figure 11-8 Dilated azygos vein secondary to inferior vena cava (IVC) thrombosis. **A,** Posterolateral radiograph shows dilatation of the azygos vein *(arrow)*. **B,** The azygos vein *(arrows)* can be seen coursing over the right mainstem bronchus on the lateral radiograph. **C,** Contrast-enhanced axial computed tomography (CT) confirms dilatation of the azygos vein *(arrow)*. **D,** Contrast-enhanced axial CT through the abdomen demonstrates a low-attenuation filling defect in the IVC *(arrow)* consistent with thrombus.

over the right mainstem bronchus, and drains into the posterior wall of the SVC. On a frontal radiograph, the normal azygos vein can be identified as an oval or round opacity in the right tracheobronchial angle and is usually less than 1 cm in maximal dimension. Enlargement of the azygos vein can be seen in the setting of volume overload or in any condition that impedes the return of blood to the heart through the SVC or IVC such as SVC obstruction or IVC thrombosis (Fig. 11-8). Azygos continuation of an interrupted IVC (Fig. 11-9) may be as large as and mistaken for a right aortic arch. A common normal variant is the presence of an azygos fissure (Fig. 11-10). In this developmental variant, the azygos vein takes a more superior and lateral course through the lung before it crosses over the right mainstem bronchus and empties into the SVC. Malpositioned catheters in the azygos vein have a characteristic appearance on the frontal chest radiograph with a small, superiorly directed curve of the distal tip (Fig. 11-11). On a lateral radiograph, a catheter in the SVC takes an approximate 90-degree turn posteriorly to enter the azygos vein.

Other Smaller Left-Sided Veins

The left second superior intercostal vein may be visible on the frontal chest radiograph as the vein courses anteriorly over the superolateral aspect of the aortic arch and appears as the so-called aortic nipple. If a catheter enters the left internal mammary vein and then the second superior intercostal vein, it can also have a classic appearance similar to a catheter in the azygos vein with a small, superiorly directed curve of the tip.

Occasionally, a left-sided catheter may not follow the course of the left innominate vein but takes a relatively vertical course. A left-sided SVC may be present, but malposition in a normal vein such as the left internal mammary vein (Fig. 11-12) or left pericardiophrenic vein should also be considered, especially when the distal catheter does not course into the coronary sinus or right atrium. The left internal mammary vein is a tributary of the left innominate vein and runs immediately left of and posterior to the sternal body. On a lateral radiograph, the catheter is anterior to a catheter in a left SVC and also paralleling the sternum. Patients usually

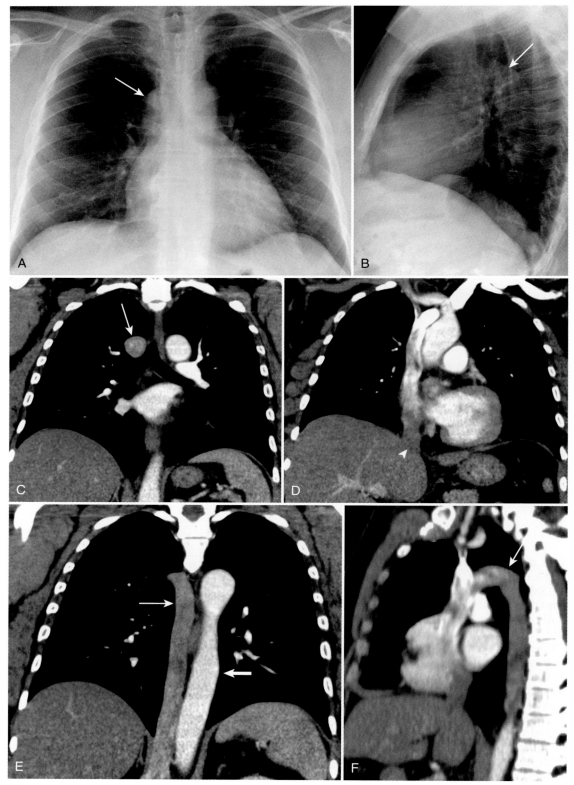

Figure 11-9 Azygos continuation of an interrupted inferior vena cava (IVC) in a 53-year-old man. **A,** Posterolateral radiograph shows a dilated azygos vein *(arrow)*. **B,** The azygos vein *(arrow)* can be seen draping over the right mainstem bronchus on the lateral radiograph. **C** to **E,** Coronal computed tomography reformats confirming the dilated azygos vein **(C)**, the expected location of the interrupted IVC **(D,** *arrowhead),* and the continuation of the dilated azygos vein *(arrow)* parallel to the thoracic aorta *(thick arrow)* **(E)**. **F,** Sagittal oblique reformat showing the dilated azygos *(arrow)* draining into the superior vena cava.

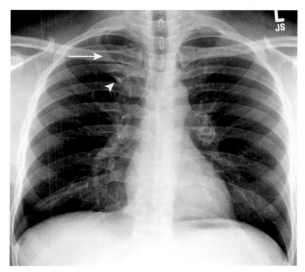

Figure 11-10 **Azygos fissure.** Incidental azygos vein *(arrowhead)* and azygos fissure *(arrow)*.

have two or three pericardiophrenic veins, and on the left side, these veins can outline the contour of the cardiomediastinal silhouette (Fig. 11-13).

Extravascular Catheters and Complications

Catheters that do not conform to the expected course of a known artery or vein must be suspected to be extravascular in location (Fig. 11-14). In addition to malposition, a high suspicion of complications of catheter insertion including pneumothorax and hemorrhage aids in detection. Mediastinal widening caused by hemorrhage may be easier to detect by comparison with prior radiographs.

■ THORACIC AORTA

The normal left aortic arch produces an oval opacity to the left of the spine at the level of T4 that is commonly referred to as the aortic knob. The descending aorta creates a vertically oriented linear interface with the left upper and lower lobes as it descends adjacent to the left aspect of the spine. On the frontal radiograph, the

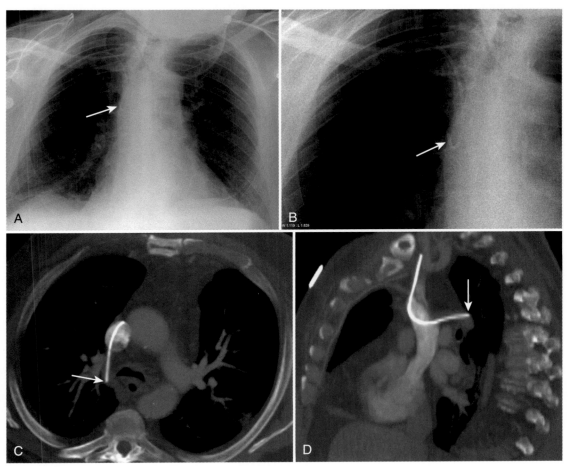

Figure 11-11 Malpositioned right peripherally inserted central catheter (PICC) in the azygos vein. Chest radiograph **(A)** and coned, magnified image **(B)** demonstrate the right PICC tip *(arrow)* curling and pointing superiorly, thus indicating that it is in the azygos vein *(arrow)*. Computed tomography axial **(C)** and sagittal **(D)** images confirm malposition *(arrows)* in the azygos vein.

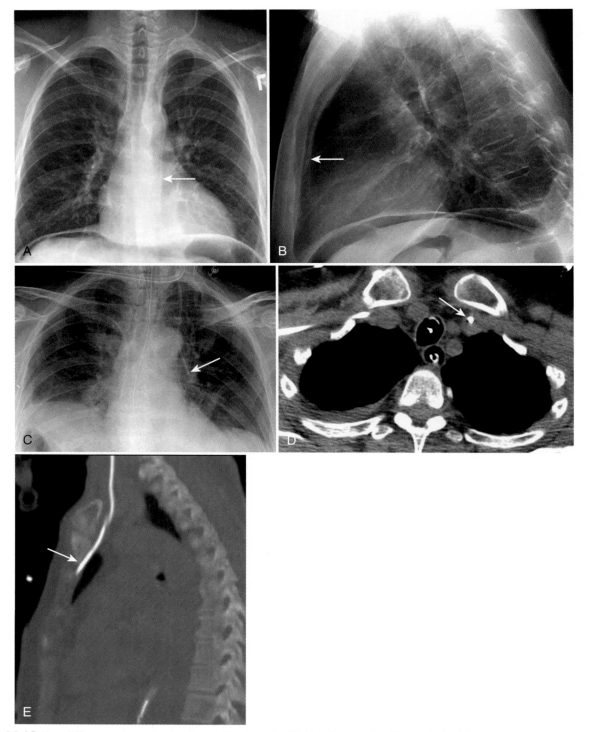

Figure 11-12 Two different patients with left internal jugular vein (LIJV) catheter malpositioned in the left internal mammary vein (LIMV). Frontal (**A**) and lateral (**B**) chest radiographs demonstrate the catheter *(arrows)* coursing along the left superior mediastinum in the expected course of the LIJV, through the left innominate vein, into the origin of the LIMV, and immediately posterior to the sternum. Free intraperitoneal air is also noted. **C**, A second patient demonstrates slightly different appearance to the catheter *(arrow)* as it enters the LIMV, but it is confirmed to be in the LIMV on computed tomography (**D** and **E**).

ascending aorta is usually not visible, except in the setting of older patients who have unfolding of the thoracic aorta, aortic dilatation, or, occasionally, aortic stenosis.

On the lateral radiograph, the anterior margin of the ascending aorta creates an interface with lung in the retrosternal space. The aortic arch and descending aorta are vaguely visible but are better delineated when patients have atherosclerosis and concomitant calcification.

Left Aortic Arch

The most common aortic arch variant is the common origin of the right innominate and left common carotid arteries, the so-called bovine arch (bovines do not actually have this aortic branching morphology). This aortic arch variant is typically not visible on radiography, although occasionally it can cause widening of a narrow superior mediastinum. The second most common aortic arch variant is independent origin of the left vertebral artery from the aortic arch, between the left common carotid artery and the left subclavian artery. The third

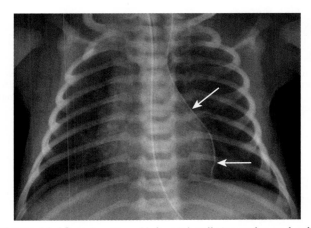

Figure 11-13 Malpositioned left peripherally inserted central catheter (PICC) in the pericardiophrenic vein. A PICC *(arrows)* inserted in a left scalp vein of an infant courses along the left cardiomediastinal contour in a left pericardiophrenic vein.

most common aortic arch variant, the left aortic arch with retroesophageal aberrant right subclavian artery, occurs in approximately 1% of the population.

On the frontal radiograph, the aberrant right subclavian artery is occasionally visible as a mediastinal mass distorting the normal superior mediastinal contour (Fig. 11-15). On the lateral radiograph, the aberrant subclavian artery (left or right) may appear as an oval opacity indenting the posterior aspect of the esophagus in the upper thorax. Rarely, the aberrant subclavian artery may cross the mediastinum between the esophagus and trachea or anterior to the trachea. If the origin of the aberrant subclavian artery is dilated, it is called a diverticulum of Kommerell.

If a predominantly right-sided superior mediastinal mass crosses the mediastinum and appears to arise from the aortic arch, the possibility of an aberrant right subclavian artery aneurysm should be considered (Fig. 11-16).

Right Aortic Arch

If the normal left aortic arch is absent and a mass in the right paratracheal region is identified, the examiner should consider the possibility of a right aortic arch (Fig. 11-17). The right aortic arch causes slight leftward deviation of the trachea and esophagus as it passes to the right. Then it descends along the right aspect of the spine, crosses to the left at the level of the right pulmonary artery, and continues its descent into the abdomen on the left side. Thus, the descending aortic interface is visible initially on the right in the upper mediastinum and then on the left in the inferior thorax.

Right aortic arch with mirror-branching morphology is a mirror image of the left aortic arch. The order of branches, from anterior to posterior, is as follows: left innominate artery, right common carotid artery, and right subclavian artery. Right aortic arch with aberrant left subclavian artery branches is as follows, from anterior to posterior: left common carotid artery, right common carotid artery, right subclavian artery, and left subclavian artery. In conjunction with the ligamentum arteriosum, the right aortic arch with aberrant left subclavian artery produces a vascular ring around the

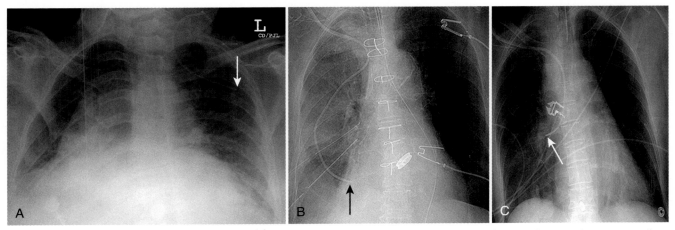

Figure 11-14 Malpositioned central venous catheters. A to C, These catheters *(arrows)* do not conform to a known vein or artery and are extravascular in location.

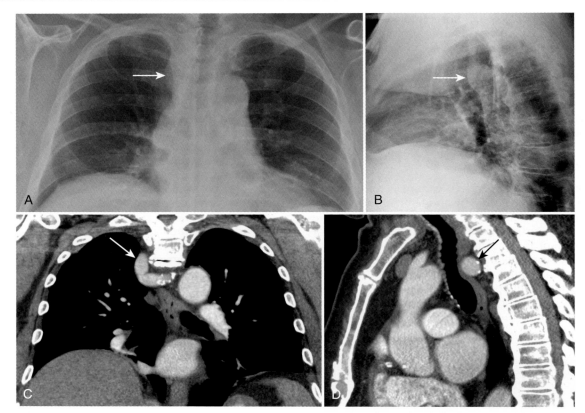

Figure 11-15 A 75-year-old man with a tortuous aberrant right subclavian artery (RSCA). **A,** The aberrant RSCA *(arrow)* appears as a convex bulge in the right superior mediastinum. **B,** The aberrant RSCA *(arrow)* takes a retroesophageal course and indents the posterior wall of the esophagus. **C,** Computed tomography (CT) coronal reformat confirms the finding and also demonstrates some calcification *(arrow)* in the proximal aberrant RSCA. **D,** CT sagittal reformat better depicts the retroesophageal location of the aberrant RSCA *(arrow)*.

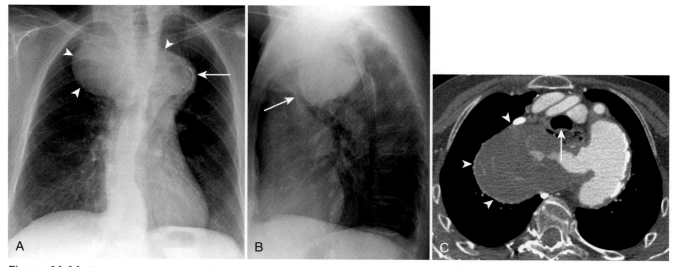

Figure 11-16 Aneurysmal aberrant right subclavian artery. **A,** Posterolateral radiograph demonstrates a well-defined mass *(arrowheads)* extending from the right lung apex and superior mediastinum to the aortic knob *(arrow)*. The contiguous border with the aorta and calcification suggestive of atherosclerosis leads the reader to the correct diagnosis. **B** and **C,** The trachea *(arrows)* and esophagus are anteriorly deviated by the mostly thrombosed aberrant right subclavian artery aneurysm *(arrowheads)*.

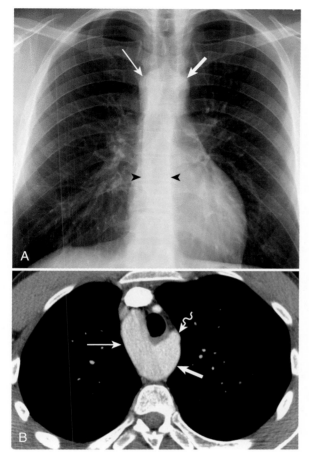

Figure 11-17 A 30-year-old man with a right aortic arch, aberrant left subclavian artery and diverticulum of Kommerell. **A,** Posterolateral radiograph demonstrates the absence of the aortic knob and a convex opacity representing the right aortic arch *(thin arrow)*. The right and left para-aortic stripes *(arrowheads)* are also visible as the aorta crosses from right to left in the midthorax. **B,** A smaller convex opacity in the left paratracheal region *(thick arrow arrow in A)* corresponds to a diverticulum of Kommerell *(thick arrow)* at the origin of the aberrant left subclavian artery *(squiggly arrow)* on computed tomography.

esophagus and can result in dysphagia, although most patients are asymptomatic. In contrast, the mirror right aortic arch has a ductus arteriosus that connects the left subclavian artery to the left pulmonary artery in front of the trachea and does not result in a vascular ring. More than 95% of patients with right aortic arch with mirror branching also have congenital heart disease. Fewer than 2% of patients with right aortic arch with aberrant left subclavian artery have congenital heart disease. Forty percent of patients with truncus arteriosus and 25% of patients with tetralogy of Fallot (TOF) have a right aortic arch with mirror-branching morphology.

Double Aortic Arch

Double aortic arch occurs when the ascending aorta divides into left and right aortic arches. This abnormality can be suspected on the frontal radiograph in patients with bilateral paratracheal masses indenting

the lateral aspects of the trachea; these masses represent the aortic arches (Fig. 11-18). The right aortic arch is usually larger and more superior than the left aortic arch. The arches join up posterior to the trachea and esophagus. On an esophagogram, the aortic arches that cause indentation of both sides of the contrast column can be seen. Classically, the more superior indentation results from the right aortic arch, whereas the more inferior indentation is caused by the left aortic arch. Thus, this complete vascular ring can also result in dysphagia or dyspnea.

Aortic Aneurysms

Fusiform aortic aneurysms are usually true aneurysms (i.e., all three layers of the vessel wall confine the aneurysm). Fusiform aortic aneurysms can be difficult to exclude on radiography unless the margins of the aorta are well visualized. In a young patient, visualization of the ascending aortic contour on the frontal radiograph should raise the possibility of an ascending aortic aneurysm or other aortic disease. The maximal diameters in the adult of the ascending aorta, aortic arch, and descending aorta are 4, 3, and 2 cm, respectively. An aneurysm is classically defined as present when the vessel is larger than 50% of its upper limit of normal. However, the ascending aorta is usually practically classified as aneurysmal when it is greater than 4.5 cm in maximal diameter and ectatic if it is between 4 and 4.5 cm. In addition to aortic dilatation, aortitis or inflammation of the aortic wall can cause tortuosity of the aorta.

Saccular aneurysms are usually pseudoaneurysms (i.e., not all three layers of the vessel wall surround the aneurysm). Saccular aneurysms can be identified as focal outpouchings of the aortic contour on radiography. Saccular aneurysms of the descending aorta (Fig. 11-19) are usually easier to visualize than are those arising from the aortic arch. Saccular aneurysms may be secondary to infections (also referred to as mycotic aneurysms, although fungal organisms are not the only etiologic agent) (Fig. 11-20) or trauma.

Acute aortic syndromes such as aortic dissection or intramural hematoma can cause nonspecific widening of the mediastinum, but this finding is not sensitive.

Aortic Coarctation

Aortic coarctation is a developmental anomaly that is thought to occur because of a small amount of tissue from the ductus arteriosum that migrates onto the descending aorta and constricts, as does the ductus arteriosus after birth. The coarctation usually occurs distal to the left subclavian artery origin, although occasionally it can be between the origin of the left common carotid artery and that of the left subclavian artery.

On the frontal radiograph, the constricted segment of the descending aorta appears as an indentation in the lateral interface of the descending aorta that produces the so-called figure 3 sign (Fig. 11-21). Sixty percent of patients with coarctation have an abnormal radiographic contour of the aorta. The superior convexity, or

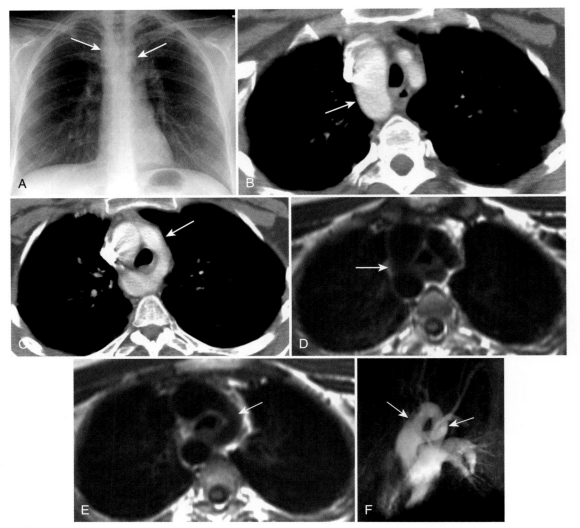

Figure 11-18 Double aortic arch. Frontal radiograph (**A**) shows oval opacity *(arrows)* in the right paratracheal region representing the right aortic arch indenting the right lateral wall of the distal trachea and oval opacity in the left paratracheal region representing the left aortic arch. Axial computed tomography (**B** and **C**) and magnetic resonance imaging (MRI) (**D** and **E**) demonstrate a right aortic arch that is more superior and larger than the left aortic arch *(arrows)*. **F,** Three-dimensional MRI demonstrates another view of the double aortic arch *(arrows)*.

top half of the 3, is the aorta proximal to the coarctation and may not be visible in children. The inferior convexity, or bottom half of the 3, is the aorta distal to the coarctation and represents poststenotic dilatation.

Because of the flow-limiting coarctation, blood is directed into the aortic branches and takes a circuitous route to the descending thoracic aorta through the internal mammary arteries and retrograde flow in the intercostal arteries. Increased blood flow through the intercostal arteries causes these vessels to be enlarged and results in bilateral inferior rib notching because the intercostal arteries run in the neurovascular groove at the inferior aspect of each rib. Because the first and second intercostal arteries are supplied by the subclavian arteries, the first and second ribs do not demonstrate notching. In contrast, intercostal arteries supplied by the descending aorta can serve as collateral vessels. In other words, the path of blood from the aorta proximal to the coarctation to the aorta distal to the coarctation

is as follows: subclavian artery to internal mammary artery to retrograde flow in intercostal artery to descending thoracic aorta.

A small notch near the costovertebral joint is normal, so pathologic rib notching is more likely if the notching is more lateral. Superior rib notching can occur if tortuosity of an intercostal artery is significant enough to affect the superior aspect of an adjacent rib. Rib notching is rarely seen in patients less than 6 years old. It is more commonly seen with increasing age, so it is usually visible in adults. Whether the notching is minimal or deep, involves few or many ribs, depends on the amount of collateral flow through the intercostal arteries.

Unilateral rib notching can be seen if the coarctation is proximal to a subclavian artery origin. For example, when the coarctation is located proximal to the left subclavian artery origin, rib notching is right sided only because the left-sided intercostal arteries are protected from the increased collateral flow. If the patient has an

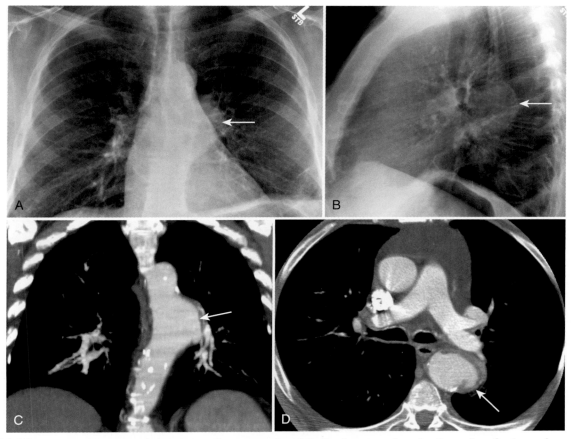

Figure 11-19 Saccular aneurysm of the descending aorta. A and **B,** On the posterolateral radiograph, a focal round mass *(arrows)* obscures the descending aortic interface and is well seen posterior to the left hilum on the lateral radiograph. **C** and **D,** Contrast-enhanced computed tomography images confirm the presence of a saccular aneurysm *(arrows)* arising from the descending aorta.

aberrant right subclavian artery distal to the coarctation, then rib notching will be left sided only.

Aortic coarctation is commonly associated with Turner syndrome, bicuspid aortic valve with stenosis and regurgitation, patent ductus arteriosus, and ventricular septal defects.

Aortic Pseudocoarctation

Aortic pseudocoarctation occurs when the morphology is similar to that of a classic coarctation but without a flow-limiting obstruction. The aorta is kinked at the isthmus (the segment of aorta between the distal subclavian artery origin and the narrowing), but no significant pressure gradient is identified. The aortic arch usually follows a more superior and elongated course and may course above the level of the clavicles (Fig. 11-22). In addition, the figure 3 sign may be present. However, no rib notching is seen in pseudocoarctation because the absence of a significant obstruction precludes the need for collateral flow. Magnetic resonance imaging (MRI) is helpful in differentiating between a true coarctation and a pseudocoarctation.

Aortic Calcification

Atherosclerotic, calcified plaques in the thoracic aorta can be visible on frontal and lateral radiographs. Aortic calcification detected on the radiograph is associated with an increased risk of cardiovascular events. A diffusely calcified thoracic aorta can be a contraindication to any surgical procedure that requires cross-clamping of the aorta.

■ PULMONARY VASCULATURE

Approach to Pulmonary Vascularity

Pulmonary vascularity is difficult to analyze. The significant variability in interpretation results from the complex overlapping pattern of pulmonary arteries and veins on the frontal radiograph. Segmental analysis can help with classification of pulmonary vascular patterns. The pulmonary vasculature is divided into the following three areas, and each area is analyzed separately:
■ Main pulmonary artery
■ Hilar pulmonary arteries
■ Parenchymal arteries and veins

Main Pulmonary Artery

The main pulmonary artery is located inferior to the aortopulmonary window and medial to the left hilum. It usually has a straight contour or may be mildly convex in children and young women. Enlargement of this

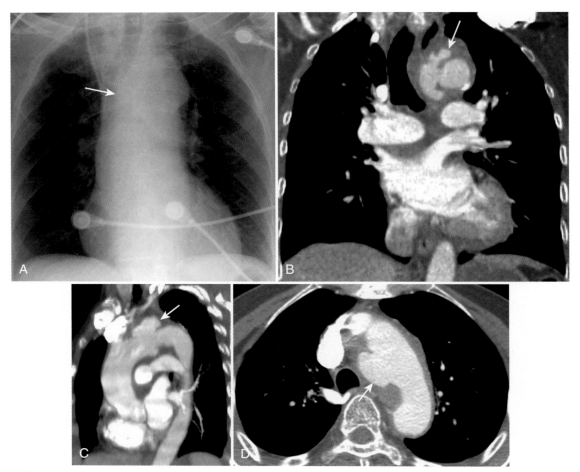

Figure 11-20 Infectious pseudoaneurysm of the aortic arch. A, Frontal radiograph demonstrates widening of the superior mediastinum, enlargement of the aortic knob and rightward deviation of the intrathoracic trachea *(arrow)*. **B,** Coronal computed tomography (CT) reformat shows an irregular collection of contrast *(arrow)* between the trachea and aortic arch. **C** and **D,** Sagittal oblique maximum intensity projection and axial CT show the pseudoaneurysm *(arrows)* relative to the aortic arch.

segment is one of the earliest signs of pressure or volume overload in the main pulmonary artery.

Hilar Pulmonary Arteries

The next segment to enlarge after the main pulmonary artery comprises the hilar pulmonary arteries. This segment corresponds to the right and left main, right interlobar, and left descending pulmonary arteries. On the frontal radiograph, pulmonary hypertension is suggested by enlargement of the right interlobar artery greater than 16 mm in diameter, from its lateral margin to the lateral wall of the bronchus intermedius. Smooth enlargement suggests pulmonary artery enlargement, whereas lobulation suggests hilar lymphadenopathy. On the lateral radiograph, the right and left pulmonary artery diameters should approximately be less than the tracheal air column diameter in a physiologically normal patient.

Parenchymal Arteries and Veins

In an upright patient, a gravity-dependent gradient of blood flow occurs from superior to inferior, with the smallest pulmonary arteries near the lung apices and the largest pulmonary arteries near the lung bases. At the hilum, the pulmonary artery is approximately the same diameter as the adjacent bronchus. In the upper lung zones, the pulmonary arteries are approximately 85% of the adjacent bronchial diameter. In the lower lung zones, the pulmonary arteries are approximately 30% larger than the adjacent bronchial diameter. In a prone or supine patient, the nondependent arteries are smaller than the dependent arteries. Both pulmonary arteries and veins should be well defined in the normal patient.

Patterns of Pulmonary Vascularity

Using segmental analysis, the examiner should decide which of the following patterns of pulmonary vascularity is present on the chest radiograph:

- Normal
- Decreased
- Increased or high-output state
- Pulmonary arterial hypertension
- Pulmonary venous hypertension

Normal Pulmonary Vascularity

Normal appearance of the main and hilar pulmonary arteries and parenchymal arteries and veins is discussed earlier in the description of segmental analysis.

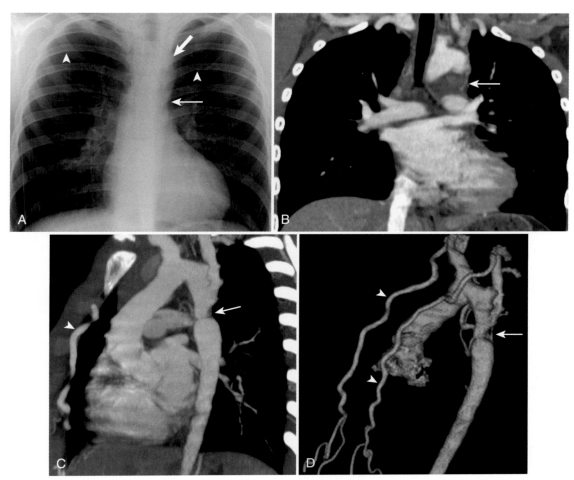

Figure 11-21 Aortic coarctation in a 12-year-old boy. **A,** Frontal chest radiograph demonstrates a notch *(arrow)* in the descending aorta that produces a so-called 3 sign. The aortic knob *(thick arrow)* is more superiorly located than usual, so a large aortopulmonary window is present. Bilateral inferior rib notching is also present *(arrowheads)*. **B,** Computed tomography (CT) coronal reformat shows the increased space *(arrow)* between the aortic arch and main pulmonary artery. **C,** CT sagittal maximum intensity projection confirms narrowing of the aorta distal to the left subclavian artery takeoff *(arrow)*. Note the enlarged internal mammary artery *(arrowhead)*. **D,** CT three-dimensional image shows another view of the coarctation *(arrow)* and enlarged internal mammary arteries *(arrowheads)*.

Decreased Pulmonary Vascularity

Decreased pulmonary vascularity is the most difficult pattern to detect because of the significant overlap in radiographic appearance with normal pulmonary vascularity. The main pulmonary artery segment may be concave, a finding suggesting a small main pulmonary artery. The hilar pulmonary artery segments may appear smaller than the adjacent bronchi, and the parenchymal arteries and veins are small from the lung apices to the lung bases. The lung may also appear hyperlucent.

Diffusely decreased pulmonary vascularity may be secondary to decreased blood volume (e.g., in shock), poor right ventricular function (e.g., in tamponade) or right-to-left shunts associated with pulmonic stenosis. Cyanotic congenital heart diseases with decreased pulmonary vascularity include TOF, single ventricle, tricuspid atresia, pulmonary valve atresia and Ebstein anomaly. The differential diagnosis of decreased pulmonary vascularity is listed in (Box 11-1).

Decreased pulmonary vascularity localized to a single lobe is easier to appreciate because normal lung can be used as a comparison. Focal lesions such as peripheral pulmonary embolus, congenital branch stenosis, Takayasu arteritis, destroyed lung secondary to pneumonia, air trapping, abscess, or bulla may result in localized decreased pulmonary vascularity.

Increased Pulmonary Vascularity or High-Output State

The size of the main, hilar, and parenchymal pulmonary arteries and veins reflect the pressure, flow, and volume of blood in the lungs. In a high-output state, the heart has increased cardiac output secondary to increased stroke volume and heart rate. The increased cardiac output causes all the pulmonary segments to be enlarged. The main pulmonary artery segment is convex, the hilar pulmonary arteries are enlarged, and the parenchymal arteries and veins are also enlarged from the lung apices to the lung bases. The parenchymal arteries and veins tend to be ill-defined.

In a high-output state, patients can have (1) increased blood flow in both the pulmonary and systemic circulation or (2) increased blood flow in the pulmonary

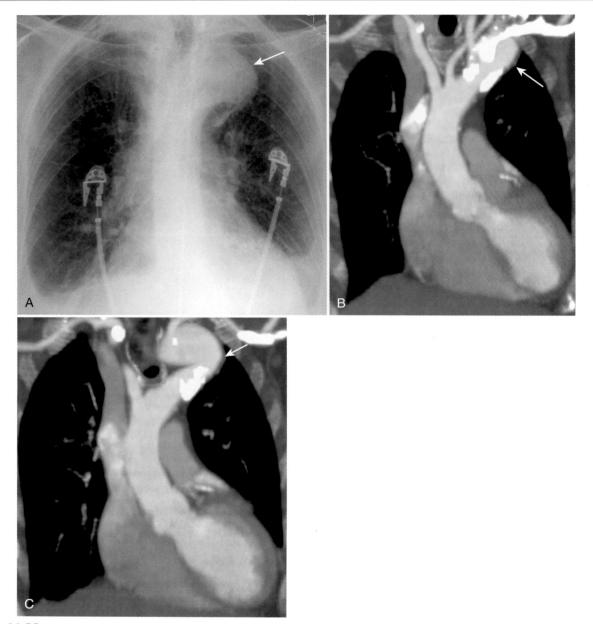

Figure 11-22 Aortic pseudocoarctation in a tortuous, atherosclerotic aorta. **A,** Frontal radiograph demonstrates an aortic knob *(arrow)* projecting at the level of the clavicles. Small bilateral pleural effusions and mild interstitial pulmonary edema is also present. **B,** Coronal maximum intensity projection (MIP) shows the elongated ascending aorta coursing much higher than would normally be expected *(arrow)*. **C,** Coronal MIP slightly more posterior to **B** shows the kink *(arrow)* (the MIP makes the left subclavian artery appear to originate distal to the kink, but **B** shows that it arises from the ascending aorta).

circulation only. Enlargement of the vascular pedicle is evidence of increased blood flow in both the pulmonary and systemic circulations. The width of the vascular pedicle is an estimate of systemic circulation blood volume and should be greater than 6 cm in patients with increased blood flow in both the pulmonary and systemic circulations. It is less than 6 cm in physiologically normal patients or in patients with increased blood flow in the pulmonary circulation only. High-output states with increased blood flow in both the pulmonary and systemic circulations are often the result of metabolic or endocrine disorders or changes such as pregnancy, thyrotoxicosis, pheochromocytoma, or right-to-left shunts from arteriovenous malformations and fistulas.

Increased blood flow in the pulmonary circulation is usually appreciated only when flow in the pulmonary circulation is twice as great as in the systemic circulation. The vascular pedicle in this high-output state tends to be normal. This constellation of findings suggests a left-to-right shunt such as an atrial septal defect (Fig. 11-23). Increased pulmonary vascularity can be seen in the setting of the cyanotic and acyanotic congenital heart diseases listed in Box 11-2.

BOX 11-1   Differential Diagnosis of Decreased Pulmonary Vascularity

Congenital Hypoplastic Pulmonary Arteries
Cyanotic Congenital Heart Disease
- Tetralogy of Fallot (10% of all congenital heart disease)
- Single ventricle (1%)
- Tricuspid atresia (0.8%)
- Pulmonary valve atresia (0.7%) with or without a ventricular septal defect
- Ebstein anomaly (0.3%)

By Location
- Diffuse hypoplasia
- Segmental stenosis
- Main pulmonary artery (supravalvular pulmonary stenosis)
- Bifurcation of right and left pulmonary artery
- Branch or peripheral pulmonary arteries

By Disease
- Williams syndrome
- Noonan syndrome
- Ehlers-Danlos syndrome
- Cutis laxa
- Alagille syndrome (biliary hypoplasia and vertebral anomalies)

Acquired Small Pulmonary Arteries
Central Obstruction
- Emboli
- Neoplasm

Hilar Obstruction
- Emboli
- Takayasu arteritis
- Rubella

Precapillary Obstruction
- Air trapping diseases (e.g., emphysema and Swyer-James syndrome)

Pulmonary Arterial Hypertension

Pulmonary arterial hypertension is present when the pulmonary systolic pressure greater than 30 mm Hg and the mean pulmonary arterial pressure is greater than 20 mm Hg. The numerous causes of pulmonary arterial hypertension are listed in Box 11-3.

The earliest sign of pulmonary arterial hypertension on radiography is enlargement of the main pulmonary artery segment. Chronic pulmonary arterial hypertension also causes enlargement of the hilar pulmonary artery segment. However, the parenchymal arteries and veins remain normal in size and are also well defined, unlike in the high-output state. The gradient of small vessels at the lung apices and large vessels at the lung bases is preserved.

Eisenmenger syndrome occurs in adults when pulmonary vascular resistance increases to the point that the pulmonary arterial pressure is greater than systemic arterial pressure. In this setting, a left-to-right shunt reverses and becomes a right-to-left shunt. Radiographically, the

main and hilar pulmonary artery segments are markedly enlarged and aneurysmal (Fig. 11-24). However, the hilar pulmonary artery segment rapidly tapers to the periphery with a so-called pruned tree appearance, with fewer arterial branches than would normally be expected. The parenchymal arteries also are tortuous and serpiginous.

Pulmonary Venous Hypertension

Pulmonary venous pressure is equivalent to the left atrial pressure and is measured using a pulmonary artery catheter balloon, which is wedged in a pulmonary artery such as the right interlobar pulmonary artery or right lower lobe pulmonary artery. This pressure is also referred to as the pulmonary capillary wedge pressure (PCWP).

Pulmonary edema is the result of excessive fluid in the interstitial and alveolar compartments of the lung. Pulmonary edema can be classified as cardiogenic or noncardiogenic (also known as permeability edema). Cardiogenic pulmonary edema is most often caused by left ventricular failure or acute mitral regurgitation. Permeability edema is secondary to disruption of the alveolar-capillary membrane and has numerous causes such as acute respiratory distress syndrome, neurologic injury, aspiration, cirrhosis, renal failure, and drug reaction. In permeability edema, the PCWP is normal.

In physiologically normal people, the PCWP is less than 12 mm Hg. Normally, the edges of the pulmonary veins are well defined, and multiple secondary branches are visible. In the midlung, halfway between the hilum and the cortex, the average size of vessels is 4 to 8 mm, and at least five to eight arteries can be seen at the right lung base. A gravity-dependent gradient occurs, with greater blood flow and volume to the lung bases. The four stages of pulmonary venous hypertension resulting from cardiogenic pulmonary edema are listed in Box 11-4.

The first sign and stage of pulmonary venous hypertension consists of vascular redistribution with enlarged pulmonary veins at the lung apices and small pulmonary veins at the lung bases (Fig. 11-25). The PCWP is usually between 12 and 18 mm Hg in patients with pulmonary venous hypertension. Because blood returning to the left atrium faces increased resistance and thus pressure, the lower pressure upper lobe veins dilate and appear to increase in number to accommodate the blood. The apparent increase in number of upper lobe veins is likely secondary to better visibility when dilated.

In the second stage, fluid escapes from the pulmonary veins into the pulmonary interstitium, thus making it thicker than normal. Radiographically, this finding appears as ill-defined pulmonary veins, peribronchial cuffing (end-on appearance of a thickened bronchus), and Kerley B and Kerley A lines. Kerley B lines are perpendicular, thickened interlobular septa in the subpleural lung. Kerley A lines are 3 to 5 cm long, approximately 1 mm thick, and represent distended lymphatic vessels in the central part of the lung. The PCWP is usually between 18 and 24 mm Hg in patients with interstitial pulmonary edema.

In the third stage, interstitial fluid pours into the alveolar space, with resulting confluent, ill-defined airspace opacities on the radiograph. Classically, the airspace

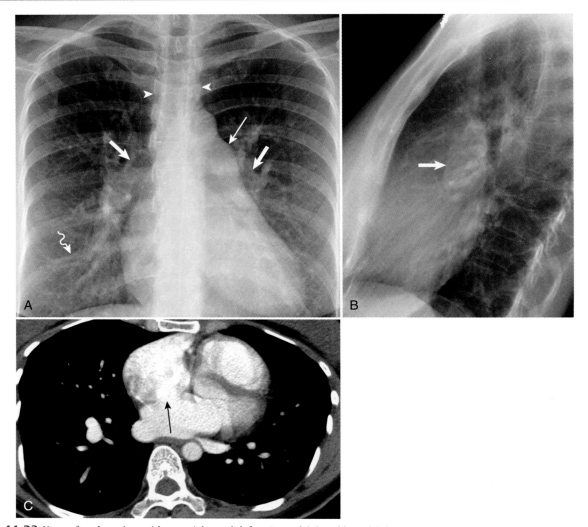

Figure 11-23 Young female patient with an atrial septal defect. Frontal (**A**) and lateral (**B**) radiographs show a convex main pulmonary artery segment *(arrows)*, enlarged hilar segment *(short arrows)* and mildly enlarged parenchymal pulmonary arteries and veins *(squiggly arrow)*. The vascular pedicle is normal in size *(arrowheads)*, and the parenchymal arteries remain well-defined. Computed tomography (**C**) shows a large secundum atrial septal defect *(arrow)*.

---

opacities are perihilar and symmetric in location, and they create a so-called bat-wing appearance. This finding is usually more severe in the lung bases than the apices. Airspace edema can appear asymmetric because of underlying lung disease, patient positioning, or a superimposed process such as papillary muscle rupture from myocardial infarction resulting in right upper lobe pulmonary edema from acute mitral regurgitation. The PCWP is usually between 24 and 30 mm Hg in patients with airspace pulmonary edema.

The fourth stage is the result of chronic pulmonary venous hypertension, which can eventually cause pulmonary arterial hypertension with dilatation of the main and hilar pulmonary artery segments. However, the parenchymal veins remain large at the lung apices and small at the lung bases. Rarely, red blood cells can extrude from the pulmonary arteries, deposit in the parenchyma, calcify, and cause parenchymal calcification.

As pulmonary edema is treated, usually with diuretics, a therapeutic lag may occur between the radiographic

---

BOX 11-2   Differential Diagnosis of Pulmonary Overcirculation (Presence or Absence of Cyanosis Is Helpful in Narrowing the Diagnosis)

Acyanotic (Left-to-Right Shunts)
- Ventricular septal defect (VSD)
- Atrial septal defect (ASD)
- Patent ductus arteriosus (PDA)
- Atrioventricular septal defect (AVSD; also known as endocardial cushion defect [ECD] or atrioventricular canal)

Cyanotic
- Transposition of the great arteries (TGA)
- Total anomalous pulmonary venous return (TAPVR)
- Truncus arteriosus (TA)
- Single ventricle

appearance and the PCWP, with pulmonary edema persisting for hours to days despite a normalizing PCWP. In the resorption phase of pulmonary edema, the correlation between the radiographic appearance of pulmonary edema and PCWP is poor. In this setting, the radiographic appearance is a better marker of the degree of fluid in the lungs.

Pulmonary Emboli

The chest radiograph may be abnormal in pulmonary embolism but in a nonspecific way. For example, the radiograph may demonstrate pleural effusion, atelectasis, cardiomegaly, or even normal features. However, in the appropriate clinical setting, certain findings can be more specific, especially if they are seen in the context of an otherwise unremarkable chest radiograph. Occasionally, pulmonary hemorrhage or infarction secondary to pulmonary embolus can manifest radiographically as a wedge-shaped peripheral opacity, the Hampton hump. The pulmonary embolus obstructs the distal segmental or subsegmental artery, and the subtending lung becomes opacified by hemorrhage or infarction. If a pulmonary embolus is large and more centrally located, the subtending lung can appear more lucent as a result of focal oligemia or attenuated vessels from lack of blood flow, the Westermark sign. The vascular obstruction from the embolus can also cause enlargement of a major pulmonary artery, the Fleischner sign.

BOX 11-3   Differential Diagnosis of Pulmonary Arterial Hypertension

Precapillary Causes
- Chronic pulmonary emboli
- Peripheral pulmonary stenosis
- Hypoplastic pulmonary arteries

Capillary Causes
- Primary pulmonary hypertension
- Diffuse interstitial lung disease (e.g., emphysema, pulmonary fibrosis)
- Obstructive lung disease (e.g., obstructive sleep apnea)
- Diffuse airspace disease such as pneumonia, neoplasm, atelectasis or pneumonectomy
- Eisenmenger syndrome (sequela of left-to-right shunt)

Postcapillary Causes
- Pulmonary veno-occlusive disease
- Cor triatriatum
- Mitral stenosis
- Left ventricular failure
- Obstructing masses
- Aortic stenosis
- Aortic coarctation
- Fibrosing mediastinitis
- Restrictive cardiomyopathy (e.g., amyloidosis, sarcoidosis)

BOX 11-4   Stages of Pulmonary Venous Hypertension

- Pulmonary venous redistribution
- Interstitial pulmonary edema
- Alveolar pulmonary edema
- Hemosiderosis

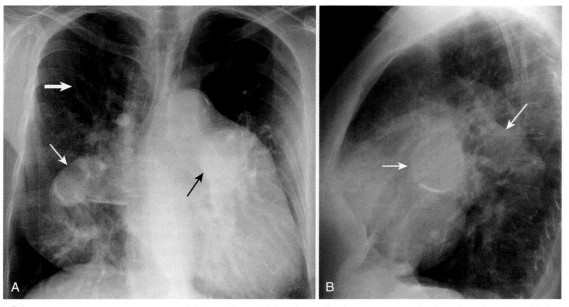

Figure 11-24 Eisenmenger syndrome. Frontal (**A**) and lateral (**B**) radiographs demonstrate markedly enlarged main and hilar pulmonary arteries *(black and white thin arrows)* with small peripheral pulmonary arteries *(thick arrow)* and mural pulmonary arterial calcification.

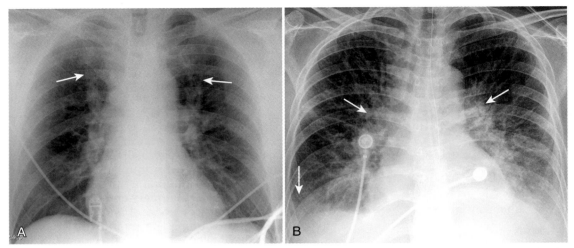

Figure 11-25 Stages of pulmonary venous hypertension. A, Stage 1. Frontal radiograph demonstrates redistribution with relative enlargement of the pulmonary veins in the upper lobes *(arrows)* and smaller veins in the lower lobes. **B,** Stages 2 and 3. Frontal radiograph shows bilateral perihilar airspace edema, engorgement of the perihilar vessels, peribronchial cuffing and Kerley B lines *(arrows).*

Proximal Interruption of the Pulmonary Artery

Proximal interruption of the right or left pulmonary artery is a rare anomaly that is thought to result from abnormal development of the main pulmonary arteries from the proximal sixth aortic arches during the first 16 weeks of gestation. The pulmonary artery is referred to as interrupted because the pulmonary arterial network within the lung parenchyma remains intact. However, the arterial supply is usually from hypertrophied systemic collateral vessels such as intercostal, bronchial, or internal mammary arteries or anomalous arteries arising from the descending thoracic aorta. Usually, the mediastinal segment of the right or left pulmonary artery is absent, and a hilar segment of the pulmonary artery remains. The tracheobronchial tree is normal. The aortic arch is usually contralateral to the side of the interrupted pulmonary artery. Interruption of the left pulmonary artery is associated with congenital heart defects, most commonly TOF. Approximately 10% of patients with proximal interruption of the pulmonary artery present with hemoptysis caused by rupture of thin-walled collateral arteries and may need embolization.

On the frontal radiograph, ipsilateral volume loss with hypoplastic lung, a small hemithorax, elevation of the hemidiaphragm, shift of the cardiomediastinal silhouette, and a small hilum are visible (Fig. 11-26). In the lung periphery, a fine reticular pattern may result from the presence of transpleural collateral arteries. In the lung centrally, a reticular pattern may be caused by larger tortuous collateral arteries. If the ipsilateral intercostal arteries are enlarged, ipsilateral rib notching may also be present. The contralateral artery is often enlarged because of increased blood flow to the contralateral lung. On the lateral radiograph, the retrosternal airspace may be hyperlucent and expanded secondary to hyperinflation and herniation of the contralateral upper lobe.

The differential diagnosis of the radiographic appearance includes hypoplastic lung, hypogenetic lung syndrome, and Swyer-James syndrome. Hypoplastic lung is generally not radiographically distinguishable because the ipsilateral pulmonary artery may be very hypoplastic and mimic an interrupted pulmonary artery. Visualization of an ipsilateral anomalous pulmonary vein, known as the scimitar vein, suggests hypogenetic lung syndrome. Swyer-James syndrome is postobstructive bronchiolitis affecting one lung, and it can be differentiated on the basis of hyperinflation and air trapping on expiration, as well as bronchiectasis.

Pulmonary Artery Sling

Pulmonary artery sling occurs in patients with an aberrant origin of the left pulmonary artery from the right pulmonary artery. The left pulmonary artery courses between the trachea and the esophagus, instead of taking its normal course anterior to the trachea. This aberrant course of the left pulmonary artery produces a "sling" around the right mainstem bronchus and carina that can have variable effect. Although some patients remain asymptomatic, others can develop severe, long-segment tracheal and bronchial stenosis requiring airway reconstruction. Complete cartilage rings are often present in the trachea. The main cause of morbidity in pulmonary artery sling is from large airway disease.

Pulmonary artery sling is usually not detectable on the frontal radiograph. Indirect signs of pulmonary artery sling include right-sided air trapping or opacity (from inadequate clearance of fetal fluid) or lobar emphysema resulting from a stenotic right mainstem or right upper lobe bronchus. The carinal angle is usually increased and has an inverted T shape. On the lateral radiograph, the aberrant left pulmonary artery can appear as an oval opacity between the trachea and esophagus (Fig. 11-27). This finding is usually better

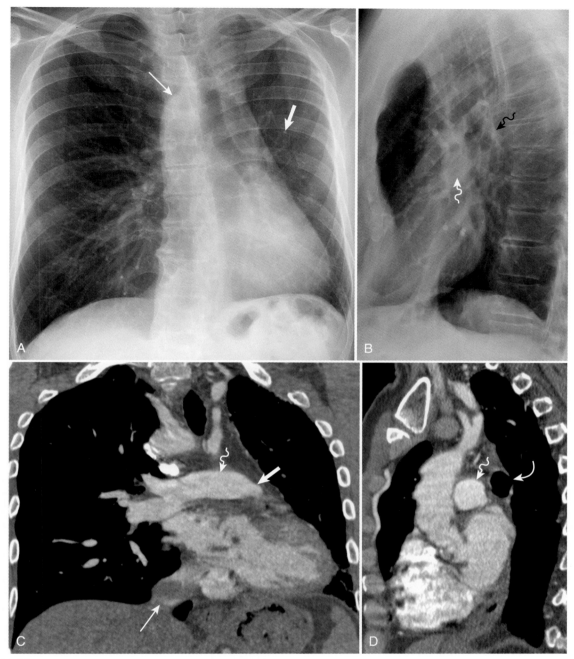

Figure 11-26 A 55-year-old man with proximal interruption of the left pulmonary artery. **A,** Frontal radiograph demonstrates a hypoplastic left lung, leftward mediastinal shift, right aortic arch *(arrow),* and absence of the left aortic arch. The left-sided pulmonary vessels *(thick arrow)* are diminutive and "lace-like" compared with the right lung. **B,** Lateral radiograph shows absence of the left main pulmonary artery that would be expected to course over the left mainstem bronchus *(black squiggly arrow).* **C** and **D,** Computed tomography coronal and sagittal reformats confirm interruption of the left pulmonary artery. Main pulmonary artery, *thick arrow;* right pulmonary artery, *white squiggly arrow;* right mainstem bronchus, *curved arrow;* inferior vena cava, *black arrow.*

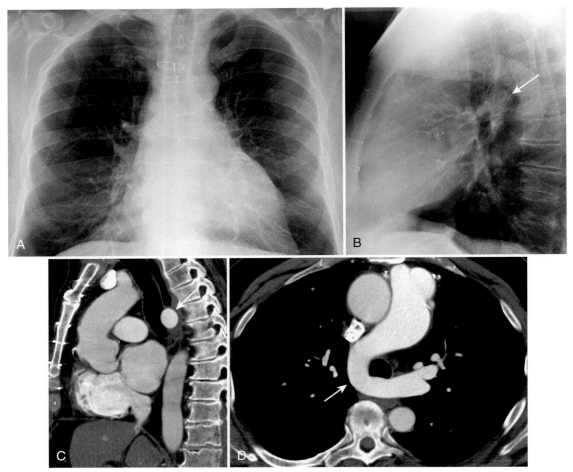

Figure 11-27 A 63-year-old man with incidentally discovered pulmonary artery sling. **A,** Clear lungs, prior sternotomy, and surgical clips from coronary artery bypass grafting are seen. **B,** Lateral radiograph demonstrates an oval opacity *(arrow)* posterior to the trachea and indenting the anterior esophagus. **C,** Sagittal computed tomography (CT) reformat confirms that the oval opacity in **B** corresponds to the left pulmonary artery *(arrow)*. **D,** Axial CT image shows the left pulmonary artery *(arrow)* arising from the right pulmonary artery and coursing posterior to the trachea and anterior to the esophagus.

appreciated on an esophagogram, with indentation of the anterior aspect of the esophagus by the left pulmonary artery. Rarely, a left aortic arch with an aberrant right subclavian artery can course between the trachea and esophagus, but in this anomaly, the opacity or indentation is more superiorly located.

Hypogenetic Lung Syndrome Hypogenetic lung syndrome, also known as congenital pulmonary venolobar syndrome or scimitar syndrome, is right sided in most cases. Approximately half these patients are asymptomatic, whereas the remainder have recurrent infections. Associated findings include congenital heart defects (25%), bronchogenic cysts, and vertebral anomalies. The features are hypoplastic lung, hypoplastic pulmonary artery, and partial anomalous pulmonary venous return to an infracardiac vein, usually the subdiaphragmatic IVC.

On radiography, if the pulmonary hypoplasia is marked, the right hemithorax may be small, with ipsilateral mediastinal shift and diaphragmatic elevation. If the pulmonary hypoplasia is mild, volume loss may be difficult to appreciate. The anomalous draining vein usually curves inferomedially and becomes larger as it drains into the IVC, with a resulting left-to-right shunt. The vein resembles a Turkish sword called a scimitar (Fig. 11-28). Shunt vascularity may be present, depending on the size of the left-to-right shunt.

■ HEART

Cardiomegaly

Evaluation of heart size by radiography can be performed subjectively or quantitatively and both methods have similar sensitivity (0.45) and specificity (0.85) for cardiomegaly. The objective method requires division of the widest transverse cardiac diameter by the widest inner thoracic diameter, with a ratio less than 0.5 being normal. Neonates are allowed to have a slightly larger cardiothoracic ratio, with less than 0.6 being normal. The correlation of heart size and size of the cardiac silhouette is degraded and limited by numerous factors including projection, degree of inspiration, and, to a lesser extent, upright versus supine positioning and intravascular volume status.

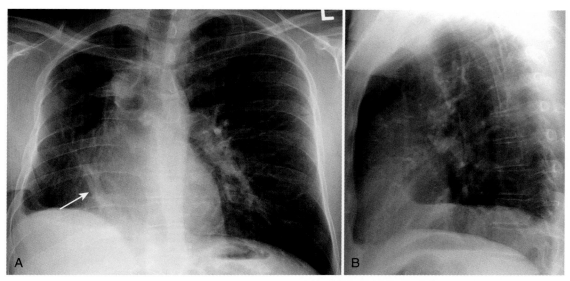

Figure 11-28 Hypogenetic lung syndrome. A, Frontal radiograph demonstrates a small right hemithorax with hypoplastic right lung, ipsilateral mediastinal shift, decreased intercostal spaces, and elevated right hemidiaphragm. The anomalous draining vein (scimitar, *arrow*) has an inferomedial orientation, unlike other pulmonary veins. **B,** Lateral radiograph demonstrates elevated right hemidiaphragm and small right pulmonary artery. The scimitar vein is not well seen.

The difference in transverse heart diameter between systole and diastole is less than 1 cm, and thus the phase of the cardiac cycle has a minimal effect on the cardiothoracic ratio. Left atrial or right ventricular enlargement does not affect the cardiothoracic ratio unless it is severe because these two chambers are not reflected in the transverse dimension. Given that the left ventricle is border forming, enlargement eventually results in a larger cardiac silhouette and an increased cardiothoracic ratio.

Right Atrium

The right atrium lateral wall produces a smooth interface with the right middle lobe that tends to be convex to the right. On expiration, the right atrial contour become rounders and also shifts to the right. Abnormalities of the myocardium, pericardium, right middle lobe, or right atrium itself can focally distort the right atrial contour (Fig. 11-29).

Right atrial enlargement is difficult to appreciate by radiography because of the significant variability of the right atrial contour even among physiologically normal people. Right atrial enlargement can occasionally be suspected when it is severe or when the right atrium is disproportionately enlarged compared with the rest of the heart. Radiographic signs of right atrial enlargement are listed in Box 11-5. Right atrial enlargement is often secondary to tricuspid stenosis or regurgitation, atrial fibrillation, dilated cardiomyopathy, atrial septal defect, or Ebstein anomaly (Fig. 11-30).

Right Ventricle

The right ventricle is not border forming on the frontal radiograph. Indirect signs can be seen in the setting of severe right ventricular enlargement as it contacts the posterior aspect of the sternum, thus pushing the heart in a clockwise direction (think of a CT scan). The left atrial appendage is rotated posteriorly and no longer forms part of the left heart border on the frontal radiograph. As a result, the left heart border has a long convex curvature that extends inferiorly from the main pulmonary artery. In extremely severe right ventricular enlargement, the entire left heart border may represent the right ventricle.

On the lateral radiograph, right ventricular enlargement should be suspected if the most superior aspect of the right ventricle is greater than one third of the distance from the sternodiaphragmatic angle to the intersection of the trachea and sternum. If right ventricular enlargement is present, the diagnosis of left ventricular enlargement may not be possible. Thus, evaluation of right ventricular size on the lateral radiograph should be performed before evaluation of left ventricular size.

Left Atrium

Dilatation of the left atrium is most commonly acquired and is secondary to mitral stenosis or regurgitation, left ventricular failure, or left atrial myxoma. Congenital causes such as ventricular septal defect, patent ductus arteriosus, and hypoplastic left heart may also result in left atrial enlargement. Several radiographic signs that may indicate moderate or severe left atrial enlargement are listed in Box 11-6.

Left atrial appendage convexity indicates chronic rheumatic disease with predominant mitral stenosis (Fig. 11-31). The left atrial appendage is usually spared in mitral regurgitation, which results in predominant enlargement of the left atrial body.

Chronic rheumatic disease can cause left atrial calcification, which usually involves the body but spares the interatrial septum. On radiography, the calcification

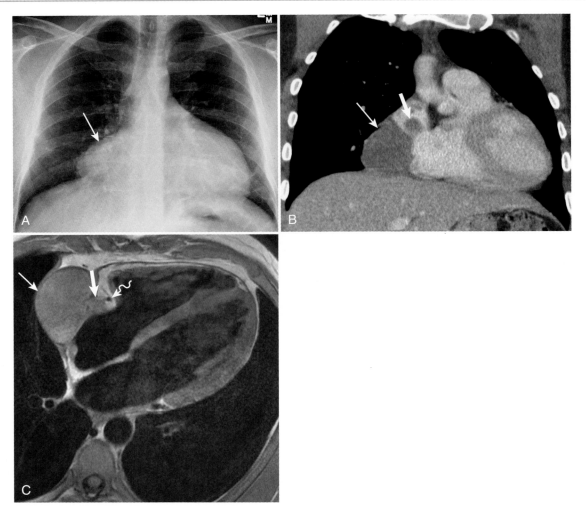

Figure 11-29 A 37-year-old man with cardiac angiosarcoma. **A,** Frontal radiograph demonstrates an abnormal round, smooth convex mass *(arrow)* that focally obscures the right atrial contour with an obtuse angle at the superior vena cava–right atrial junction. Pulmonary vessels can be seen through this mass. **B,** Coronal computed tomography reformat confirms a soft tissue mass *(arrow)* that is contiguous with and invading the right atrium *(thick arrow)*. **C,** Magnetic resonance imaging axial T1-weighted black-blood image shows the homogeneous T1-weighted mass of intermediate signal intensity *(arrow)* also invading the right atrioventricular groove *(thick arrow)*, adjacent to the right coronary artery *(squiggly arrow)*.

BOX 11-5   Radiographic Signs of Right Atrial Enlargement

Frontal
- Displacement of the right atrial border several centimeters to the right of the spine
- Conspicuous superior convexity near the superior vena cava–atrial junction

Lateral
- Horizontal interface with the lung superior to the right ventricle (right atrium normally not visible on the lateral projection)
- Posterior displacement of the heart behind the inferior vena cava mimicking left ventricular enlargement

is usually thin, curvilinear, eggshell in morphology but more nodular when it involves the left atrial appendage. Left atrial calcification is associated with atrial fibrillation. Rarely, left atrial neoplasms such as myxomas may also calcify.

Left Ventricle

The etiologic approach to left ventricular enlargement is listed in Box 11-7. Enlargement of the left ventricle is suggested by displacement of the left cardiac border laterally, posteriorly, or inferiorly and rounding of the cardiac apex. Inferior displacement can cause inversion of the diaphragm, and the inferior cardiac border can appear in the gastric air bubble. Radiographic differentiation between left ventricular hypertrophy and left ventricular dilatation is not possible.

After a left anterior descending coronary artery territory myocardial infarction, a true aneurysm of the apex or left ventricular anterior wall can form. The aneurysm

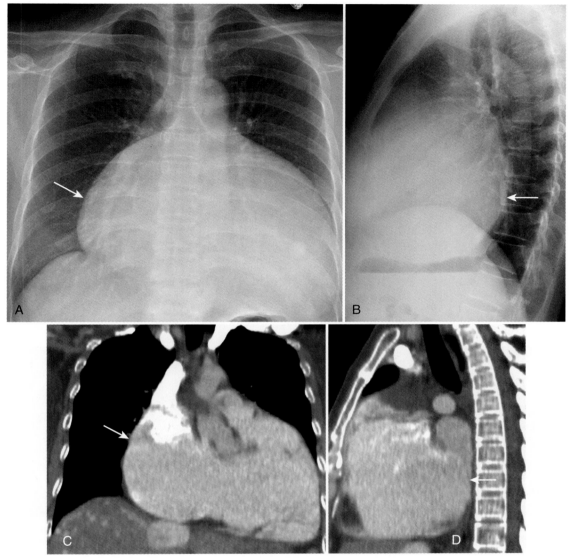

Figure 11-30 Two different adults with Ebstein anomaly. Frontal (**A**) and lateral (**B**) radiographs with corresponding computed tomography coronal (**C**) and sagittal (**D**) reformats show an enormous, globular heart with massively dilated right atrium *(arrows)*. The right atrium lateral margin is several centimeters to the right of the spine and the posterior margin projects posterior to the inferior vena cava, thus mimicking left ventricular enlargement on the sagittal reformat. In addition to Ebstein anomaly, the differential diagnosis for a so-called wall-to-wall heart includes pericardial effusion, dilated cardiomyopathy, and tricuspid atresia.

BOX 11-6   Radiographic Signs of Left Atrial Enlargement

- Double density (two superimposed convex densities) to the right of the spine
- Double density to the left of the spine as the left atrium extends into the left lower lung zone
- Splaying of the carina
- Posterior displacement of the esophagus on the esophagogram
- Superior displacement of the left mainstem bronchus on the frontal radiograph and posteriorly on the lateral radiograph
- Convexity of the left atrial appendage segment at the left heart border

is a segment of akinetic or dyskinetic, well-defined, thin-walled, fibrotic myocardium. On radiography, the left ventricular aneurysm is visible when it is lined by thin, curvilinear calcification that conforms to the expected location of the left ventricle (Fig. 11-32). When myocardial calcification cannot be differentiated from pericardial calcification by radiography, further imaging is warranted.

Cardiac Valves

The most common cause of valvular disease worldwide is rheumatic heart disease, the sequela of an acute systemic inflammatory response to group A streptococcal infection. Chronic inflammation causes valvular deformity that can affect any valve, although the mitral and

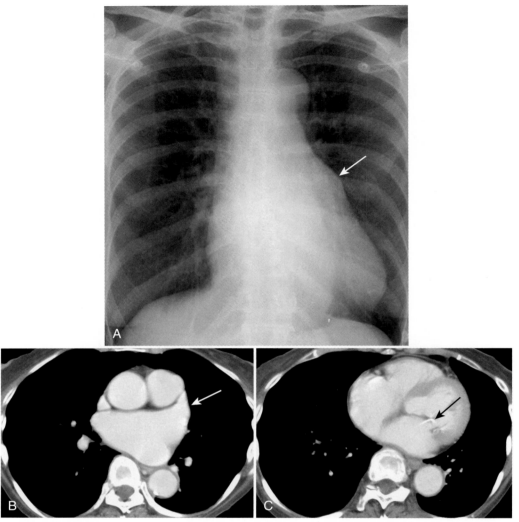

Figure 11-31 Left atrial enlargement secondary to mitral stenosis. A, Frontal radiograph shows an abnormal convexity *(arrow)* along the left cardiac border. **B,** Computed tomography axial image confirms enlargement of the left atrial appendage *(arrow).* **C,** The stenotic mitral valve is partially calcified *(arrow).*

BOX 11-7   Causes of Left Ventricular Enlargement

Pressure Overload
- Hypertension
- Aortic stenosis

Volume Overload
- Aortic regurgitation
- Mitral regurgitation
- Ventricular septal defects

Wall Abnormalities
- Left ventricular aneurysm
- Hypertrophic cardiomyopathy

---

aortic valves have the most severe involvement. Endocarditis and degenerative and congenital diseases also affect the cardiac valves. The end point of these valvular diseases is stenosis, insufficiency (regurgitation), or both. On radiography, valve disease may manifest as abnormal proximal or distal chamber size or calcification of the valve itself.

The general location of the valves can be predicted on radiography based on knowledge of the location of the cardiac chambers. When the cardiac chambers become markedly distorted secondary to disease, specific valve location is much more difficult to predict. Radiographic visualization of native valves is not possible unless the valve or annulus is calcified.

On the lateral radiograph, a line drawn from the junction of the diaphragm and the sternum to the carina passes through the aortic valve. The mitral valve is located posterior to this line, whereas the tricuspid and pulmonic valves are generally anterior to the line.

Aortic Valve
Of all the cardiac valves, only aortic valve calcification seen by radiography is correlated with aortic stenosis. When chronic rheumatic disease is the cause of aortic valve calcification, the mitral valve is also usually calcified. If only the aortic valve is calcified, other

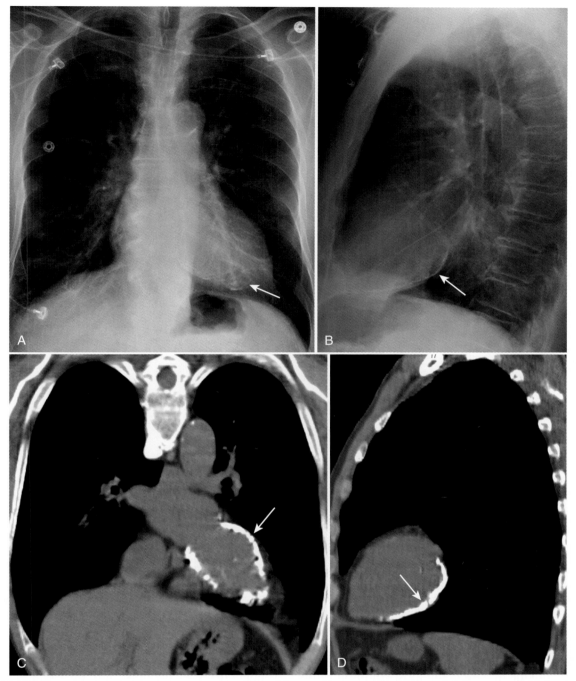

Figure 11-32 Calcified left ventricular aneurysms. A 79-year-old man with a remote large posteroinferior myocardial infarction. Frontal (**A**) and lateral (**B**) radiographs demonstrate thin, curvilinear calcification *(arrows)* along the posteroinferior margin of the left heart that could also be pericardial in location. Computed tomography coronal oblique (**C**) and sagittal (**D**) reformatted images show that the calcification is myocardial rather than pericardial in location, thus confirming a left ventricular aneurysm *(arrows)*.

possibilities such as bicuspid aortic valve or infective endocarditis should be considered in a patient less than 70 years old. Otherwise, age-related degenerative aortic valve calcification is the most common cause. In this setting, associated atherosclerotic calcification of the aorta and coronary arteries is also seen.

On radiography, aortic valve calcification is usually best visualized on the lateral radiograph as a short segment of coarse calcification angulated from anteroinferior to posterosuperior (Fig. 11-33). The aortic valve is usually located anterosuperior to the mitral valve.

As aortic stenosis progresses, increased transvalvular pressure gradient is required to force an equivalent amount of blood through the narrowed aortic valve orifice. As a result, compensatory concentric left ventricular hypertrophy occurs. Poststenotic aortic dilatation is also seen in approximately 25% of patients with severe aortic stenosis.

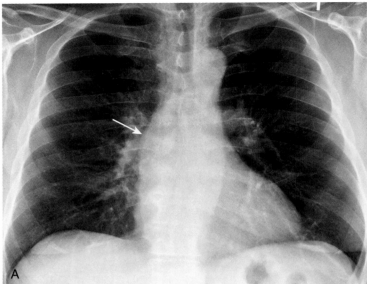

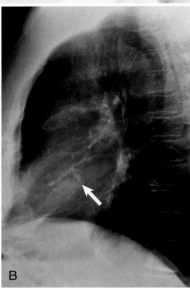

Figure 11-33 Aortic stenosis in a 60-year-old man with a bicuspid aortic valve. **A,** Frontal radiograph demonstrates a convexity along the right mediastinal border consistent with a dilated ascending aorta *(arrow)*. **B,** Lateral radiograph demonstrates a severely calcified aortic valve *(thick arrow)* that raises the possibility of aortic stenosis.

Mitral Valve

Chronic rheumatic disease is the most common cause of mitral leaflet calcification. Other causes, including infective endocarditis or neoplasms involving the mitral valve, can rarely cause leaflet calcification. Severe calcification of the mitral valve is associated with stenosis, although stenosis may also occur in the absence of calcification.

On radiography, mitral leaflet calcification initially appears as fine speckled calcification and later coalesces into larger, amorphous calcification.

The mitral annulus is a band of tissue to which the mitral valve leaflets are attached. Mitral annular calcification (MAC) is fibrous, degenerative calcification of the mitral annulus. In the Multiethnic Study of Atherosclerosis trial of men and women 45 to 84 years of age, MAC was significantly associated with increasing age, female gender, diabetes mellitus, and increased body mass index, with an overall prevalence of 9%. In rare cases, the calcification can cause heart block by extending into the ventricular myocardium or may cause mitral stenosis and regurgitation by extending onto the mitral valve leaflets. MAC is also associated with aortic stenosis and hypertension, likely because of increased strain on the mitral valve apparatus.

On radiography, severe MAC appears as coarse, amorphous calcification in the shape of an oval ring or reverse letter C separating the left atrium and left ventricle (Fig. 11-34). The mitral valve is usually oriented vertically between the left atrium and left ventricle, posteroinferior to the aortic valve, and posterior and to the left of the tricuspid valve.

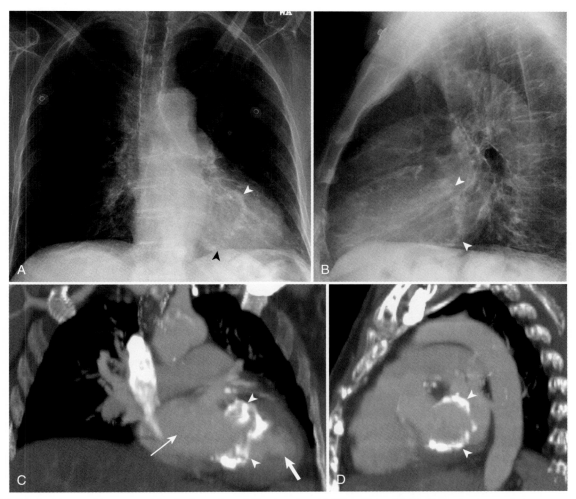

Figure 11-34 An 80-year-old woman with mitral annular calcification. Frontal (**A**) and lateral (**B**) radiographs demonstrate coarse, amorphous calcification in the expected location of the mitral annulus. Coronal (**C**) and sagittal (**D**) maximum intensity projections confirm the finding. Mitral annular calcification, *arrowheads*; left atrium, *arrow*; left ventricle, *thick arrow*. (Courtesy of Dr. Carol Wu, Massachusetts General Hospital, Boston.)

Pulmonic Valve

The pulmonic valve is the least common cardiac valve to be replaced. Pulmonic stenosis is congenital in 95% of cases and is usually an isolated abnormality. Pulmonic stenosis is also one of the lesions seen in TOF. After TOF repair, the pulmonic regurgitation that is often present results in right ventricular hypertrophy and eventually right ventricular dilatation and failure. More recently, pulmonic valve replacement in patients who have undergone remote TOF repair has been performed to reverse right ventricular disease and preserve ventricular function (Fig. 11-35). Pulmonic regurgitation is also commonly seen in patients with pulmonary hypertension, connective tissue disorders such as Marfan syndrome, and absence of the pulmonary valve in TOF.

Acquired pulmonic stenosis is rare, but it may be caused by rheumatic heart disease or carcinoid syndrome. In carcinoid syndrome, metastatic carcinoid to the liver produces vasoactive substances that escape hepatic degradation and gain access to the systemic circulation. The pathophysiology is not well understood, but fibrous carcinoid plaque is deposited on the endocardial surface of the valve leaflets, right atrium, right ventricle, chordae tendineae, and papillary muscles. The predominant results at the tricuspid valve are insufficiency and a lesser degree of stenosis. At the pulmonic valve, the predominant lesion is stenosis. The combination of tricuspid annuloplasty and pulmonic valve replacement raises the likelihood of carcinoid heart disease (Fig. 11-36).

On radiography, poststenotic dilatation of the main and left pulmonary arteries can be seen (Fig. 11-37). The right pulmonary artery is thought to be normal in size because the turbulent jet from the stenotic pulmonary valve is directed straight into the main and left pulmonary arteries, rather than into the right pulmonary artery. Right ventricular hypertrophy is also usually present, with opacification of the retrosternal airspace. The pulmonic valve is usually vertically oriented between the right ventricular outflow tract and the main pulmonary artery, superior to the aortic valve.

Tricuspid Valve

Tricuspid stenosis is most commonly the result of rheumatic heart disease, but it is also seen in infectious

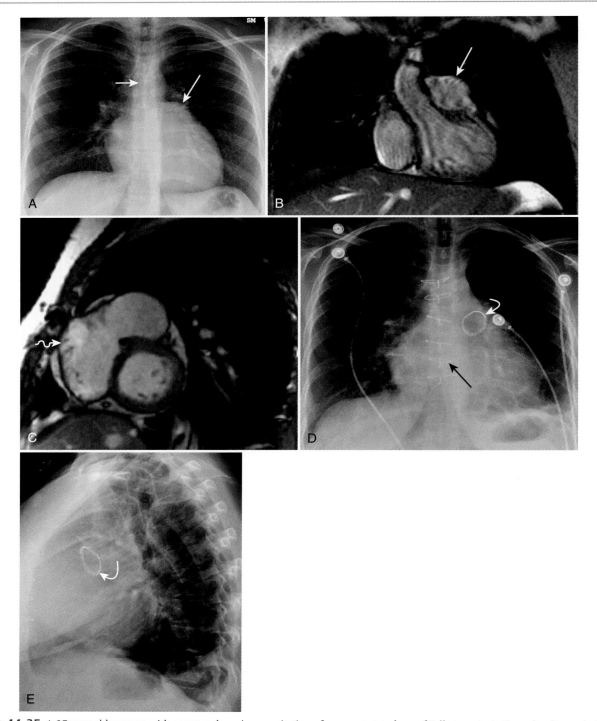

Figure 11-35 A 27-year-old woman with severe pulmonic regurgitation after remote tetralogy of Fallot repair. **A,** Frontal radiograph demonstrates a convex, enlarged main pulmonary artery *(arrow)*. Small sternotomy wires *(short arrow)* also indicate remote pediatric surgery. **B,** Magnetic resonance imaging (MRI) coronal FIESTA localizer shows the enlarged main pulmonary artery *(arrow)*. **C,** MRI sagittal FIESTA also shows enlarged right ventricle *(squiggly arrow),* right ventricular outflow tract, and pulmonary artery. **D** and **E,** Frontal and lateral radiographs show pulmonic valve replacement *(curved arrow)* and repeated sternotomy *(black arrow)*.

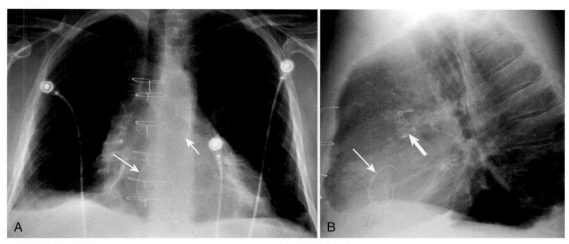

Figure 11-36 Carcinoid heart disease. Windowed frontal (**A**) and lateral (**B**) radiographs demonstrate tricuspid annuloplasty *(arrows)* and rare pulmonic valve replacement *(short and thick arrows)*. Small right pleural effusion is also present.

endocarditis, congenital tricuspid atresia, and carcinoid syndrome. On radiography, right atrial dilatation is the predominant finding.

Tricuspid regurgitation is commonly secondary to right ventricular and tricuspid annular dilatation, which are, in turn, secondary to pulmonary arterial hypertension. Other less common causes of tricuspid regurgitation include rheumatic heart disease, infectious endocarditis, Ebstein anomaly, and carcinoid syndrome.

The tricuspid valve is vertically oriented between the right atrium and the right ventricle, located to the right of and anterior to the mitral valve. To bring the leaflets closer together for optimal coaptation and reduction of regurgitation, an annuloplasty ring is inserted (Fig. 11-38). The ring appears narrower on the frontal radiograph and is seen en face on the lateral radiograph. The ring is incomplete to reduce the risk of heart block.

■ PERICARDIUM

Pericardial Effusion

Pericardial effusions have numerous causes, including congestive heart failure, collagen vascular diseases, and infectious, metabolic, neoplastic, and iatrogenic conditions, as well as Dressler syndrome. Pericardial effusions cause globular enlargement of the cardiac silhouette on the frontal radiograph (Fig. 11-39). This appearance has been historically termed the water-bottle heart. If that image is not familiar, one may want to think of it as a chicken on a fence, in which the cardiomediastinal silhouette looks like a chicken, and the diaphragm is the fence. On the lateral radiograph, the classic finding of pericardial effusion is seen posterior to the sternum, the so-called Oreo cookie sign, in which the pericardial fluid is outlined between the mediastinal and epicardial fat.

Pericardial Calcification

Pericardial calcification is the sequela of chronic inflammation. Worldwide, the most common cause is

Mycobacterium tuberculosis infection, or tuberculosis. In the United States and Canada, the most common causes are postoperative, viral, and uremic pericarditis. On radiographs, pericardial calcification may appear as thin eggshell calcification or dense, amorphous curvilinear calcification conforming to the cardiac silhouette (Fig. 11-40). Differentiation from myocardial calcification, such as in the setting of prior myocardial infarction or calcification within a ventricular pseudoaneurysm, is important. Because the pericardium extends up the ascending aorta, calcification seen in this region is helpful in confirming that the calcification is pericardial. Moreover, calcification distributed around the atrial chambers or both ventricular chambers suggests pericardial calcification. Although pericardial calcification is often present in the setting of constrictive physiology, pericardial constriction may be absent with excessive calcification, or it may be present with no calcification and simply pericardial thickening or fibrosis. MRI can be used as a problem-solving tool to determine whether pericardial constriction is present.

Pneumopericardium

Air within the pericardial space is seen most commonly after cardiac surgery. However, it can also be seen in the setting of penetrating trauma, tracheoesophageal fistulas, or bacterial pericarditis. Differentiation from pneumomediastinum can be difficult. If the air conforms to the shape of the cardiac silhouette or if the parietal pericardium can be seen as a line separate from the remainder of the silhouette, then air is likely within the pericardial space (Fig. 11-41). Rarely, pneumopericardium can cause cardiac tamponade.

Congenital Absence or Defects of the Pericardium

Absence of the pericardium may be congenital, or it may result from surgical resection. Congenital absence of the parietal pericardium is usually partial, with variable

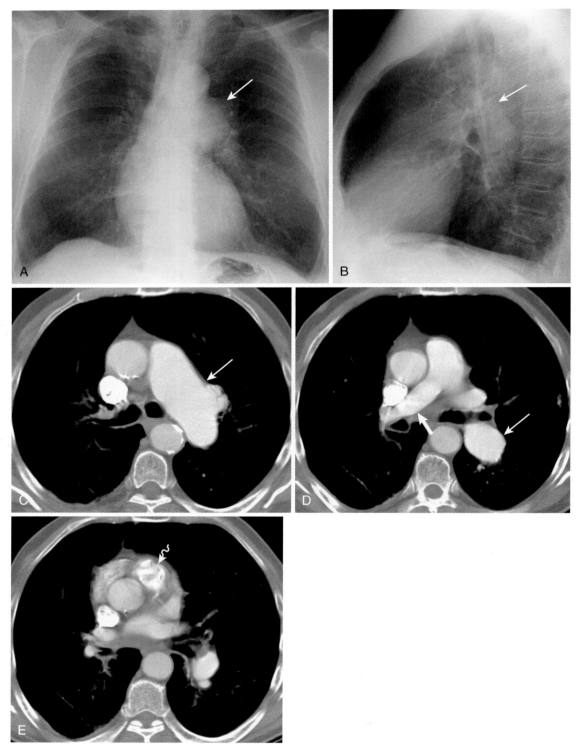

Figure 11-37 Pulmonic valve stenosis. A to D, Frontal and lateral radiographs demonstrate unilateral enlargement of the left pulmonary artery *(arrows)* and normal size right pulmonary artery *(thick arrow)*. E, The pulmonic valve has coarse calcification *(squiggly arrow)*.

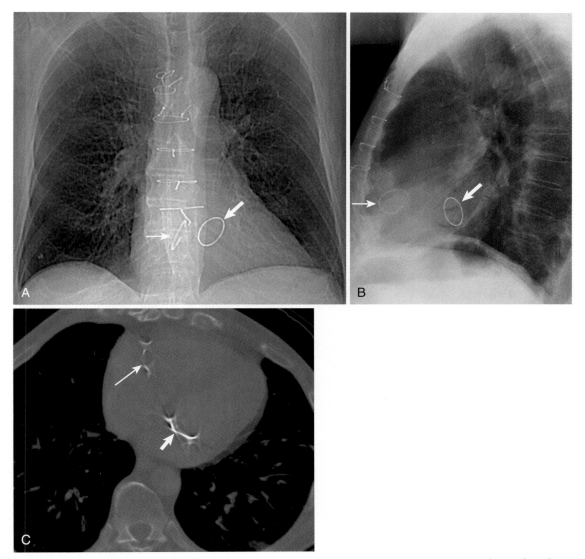

Figure 11-38 Tricuspid annuloplasty and mitral valve replacement A and B, Frontal and lateral radiographs windowed to visualize the valve prostheses more clearly demonstrate tricuspid annuloplasty ring (*arrows*) and mitral valve replacement (*thick arrows*). C, Computed tomography with bone windows confirms the location of the valve prostheses. Tricuspid annuloplasty ring, *arrow*; mitral valve replacement, *thick arrow.*

location of the defect. The most common location for the defect is over the left atrial appendage and adjacent pulmonary artery. Complete absence of the pericardium is extremely rare, and partial defects overlying the SVC, right atrium, or along the diaphragm are uncommon. Twenty percent of patients have associated congenital heart defects such as atrial septal defect, patent ductus arteriosus, or TOF or mediastinal anomalies such as bronchogenic cysts or pulmonary sequestration.

Findings on radiography depend on the location of the defect. A pericardial defect may appear as a conspicuous lucent notch in the aortopulmonary window as lung is interposed between the aorta and the main pulmonary artery. If the patient has a diaphragmatic pericardial defect, lung can be seen between the heart and the diaphragm. The heart is also often rotated to the left in patient with left-sided pericardial defects, with resulting levocardia and elongation or convexity of the left cardiac contour.

Patients with partial absence of the pericardium are at risk for herniation of a part of the heart (e.g., the left atrial appendage) through the defect and subsequent strangulation. Patients with larger defects (congenital, postsurgical such as after left pneumonectomy), tears (after trauma), or complete absence of the pericardium are at risk of cardiac luxation or torsion of the heart into the left hemithorax. Cardiac luxation is a surgical emergency because the left side of the heart can be compressed between the ascending and descending aorta at the level of the mitral valve, and this compression can result in shock. Cardiac luxation is difficult to diagnose by radiography, and a high degree of suspicion after trauma or left pneumonectomy is needed. Clues to the diagnosis on radiography include levocardia, air or lung between the heart and the diaphragm, pneumomediastinum, pneumopericardium, and left pneumothorax.

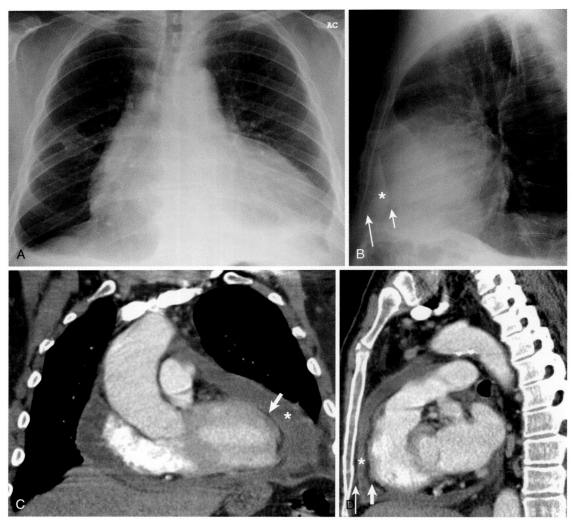

Figure 11-39 A 66-year-old man with a large pericardial effusion. **A,** Frontal radiograph demonstrates globular enlargement of the cardiac silhouette. Small bilateral pleural effusions are also present. **B,** Lateral radiograph shows the so-called Oreo cookie sign. The vertical dense band represents the pericardial fluid (white creamy center of the cookie), whereas the adjacent vertical lucent stripes anteriorly and posteriorly represent the mediastinal fat and epicardial fat, respectively (chocolate cookie sides of the cookie). **C** and **D,** Coronal and sagittal computed tomography reformats confirm the pericardial effusion and also demonstrate enhancement of both the parietal and visceral pericardium. Pericardial effusion, *asterisks;* mediastinal fat, *arrows;* epicardial fat, *thick arrows.*

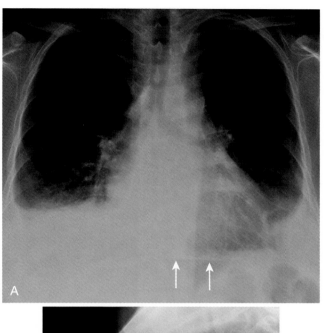

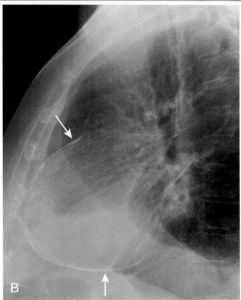

Figure 11-40 Pericardial calcification. A 48-year-old woman with dyspnea and small to moderate bilateral pleural effusions. **A,** Frontal radiograph has been windowed to accentuate the linear coarse calcification along the inferior pericardium *(arrows)*. **B,** Lateral radiograph better demonstrates the curvilinear coarse calcification *(arrows)* that extends from the inferior pericardium, along the pericardium adjacent to the anterior free wall of the right ventricle to the superior pericardial recess anterior to the ascending aorta.

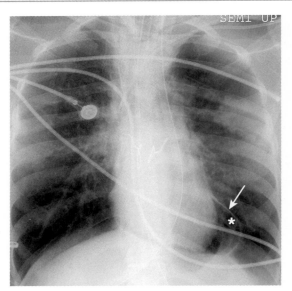

Figure 11-41 A 22-year-old woman after bilateral lung transplantation for cystic fibrosis. The parietal pericardium *(arrow)* is elevated laterally, and air is seen within the pericardial space *(asterisk)*.

Bibliography

Castañer E, Gallardo X, Rimola J, et al. Congenital and acquired pulmonary artery anomalies in the adult: radiologic overview. *Radiographics.* 2006;26:349-371.

Chen JJ, Manning MA, Frazier AA, et al. CT angiography of the cardiac valves: normal, diseased, and postoperative appearances. *Radiographics.* 2009;29:1393-1412.

Gluecker T, Capasso P, Schnyder P, et al. Clinical and radiologic features of pulmonary edema. *Radiographics.* 1999;19:1507-1531.

Hunter TB, Taljanovic MS, Tsau PH, et al. Medical devices of the chest. *Radiographics.* 2004;24:1725-1746.

Kimura-Hayama ET, Meléndez G, Mendizábal AL, et al. Uncommon congenital and acquired aortic diseases: role of multidetector CT angiography. *Radiographics.* 2010;30:79-98.

Lawler LP, Corl FM, Fishman EK. Multi–detector row and volume-rendered CT of the normal and accessory flow pathways of the thoracic systemic and pulmonary veins. *Radiographics.* 2002;22:S45-S60.

McLoud TC, Boiselle PM. *Thoracic Radiology: The Requisites.* ed 2 Philadelphia: Mosby; 2010.

Miller SW, Abbara S, Boxt L. *Cardiac Radiology: The Requisites.* ed 3 Philadelphia: Mosby; 2009.

McMahon MA, Squirrell CA. Multidetector CT of aortic dissection: a pictorial review. *Radiographics.* 2010;30:445-460.

Sebastià C, Quiroga S, Boyé R, et al. Aortic stenosis: spectrum of diseases depicted at multisection CT. *Radiographics.* 2003;23:S79-S91.

CHAPTER 12

Cardiac Anatomy on Computed Tomography

Victoria L. Mango and Jill E. Jacobs

Evaluation of cardiac computed tomography (CT) images requires a thorough understanding of normal cardiac anatomy and common anatomic variants. Technologic advances, including electrocardiographically gated multidetector CT scanners, submillimeter collimation, and gantry rotation times shorter than 0.35 seconds, allow image acquisition with high temporal resolution and isotropic voxels. This makes noninvasive, motion-free imaging throughout the cardiac cycle and a comprehensive examination of the heart possible. The use of postprocessing techniques, including multiplanar reformation (MPR), maximum intensity projection (MIP), volume rendering (VR), curved reformation, and cine imaging, enables detailed evaluation of cardiac structures. Given the broad application of cardiac CT to various clinical situations, the use of standard terminology to describe and localize cardiac structures and coronary segments is essential for accurate communication of examination results. This chapter reviews the normal cardiac anatomy on CT and common anatomic variants.

■ CARDIAC CHAMBERS: RIGHT HEART

The right atrium (RA) is positioned anteriorly and to the right, to form the inferior right heart border. The inferior vena cava (IVC), superior vena cava (SVC), and coronary sinus (CS) empty deoxygenated blood into the RA. The RA consists of three parts: the vestibule, the appendage, and the venous part, also known as the sinus venosus.

The sinus venosus is the smooth portion of the posterolateral RA wall located between the openings of the SVC and IVC. The crista terminalis, a prominent fibromuscular ridge formed by the junction of the sinus venosus and primitive RA, separates the smooth muscle fibers of the sinus venosus posteriorly from the trabeculated muscle fibers of the atrial appendage anteriorly (Fig. 12-1). The crista terminalis varies in size and thickness in different individuals and is significant in several forms of atrial tachyarrhythmias that may necessitate catheter-guided radiofrequency ablation. The crista terminalis gives rise to the pectinate muscles, which fan out anteriorly. The septum spurium, the largest anterior pectinate muscle arising from the crista terminalis, is prominent in most patients and should not be mistaken for an intraatrial mass. The crista terminalis corresponds externally with the terminal groove, also known as the

sulcus terminalis, a fat-filled groove on the epicardial side of the atrium containing the sinoatrial (SA) node and the terminal segment of the SA nodal artery. The inferior border of the crista terminalis near the IVC orifice is indistinct. The superior aspect of the crista terminalis arches anterior to the SVC orifice and extends to the anterior interatrial groove, where it merges with the Bachmann bundle, a flat band of muscle fibers bridging the anterosuperior margin of the interatrial groove. The Bachmann bundle, the largest anatomic and preferential interatrial electrical connection, facilitates rapid interatrial conduction and maintains physiologic, synchronous atrial contraction.

The right atrial appendage (RAA) is typically pyramidal, with a wider base and slightly larger pectinate muscles compared with the left atrial appendage (LAA), which has a narrower, finger-like appearance (Fig. 12-2). These features aid differentiation between the two appendages when situs is questioned. The RA vestibule is a smooth muscular rim that surrounds the tricuspid orifice.

The RA also contains electrophysiologically significant structures such as the SA node and atrioventricular (AV) node. The SA node is located within the subepicardium, at the superior cavoatrial junction, extending from the SVC along the crista terminalis toward the IVC. It penetrates the crista terminals musculature to lie in the subendocardium. The SA node surrounds the SA nodal artery, which is centrally located in 70% of cases. In catheter-guided radiofrequency ablation, CT is used to measure the crista terminalis thickness and demonstrate the approximate location of the SA nodal artery in the nodal tissue. The Koch triangle lies in the RA at the orifice of the CS and is significant because its midportion contains the compact AV node (fast pathway) and its base contains the slow pathway.

The eustachian valve is located at the junction of the RA and IVC and, in utero, directs inflowing blood from the IVC toward the foramen ovale. The eustachian valve is variably developed and may be large and muscular. This valve usually inserts medially onto the eustachian ridge, which forms the border between the CS and the oval fossa. The eustachian valve free border continues as the tendon of Todaro, which runs in the musculature of the eustachian ridge. The thebesian valve is located at the CS entrance into the RA and prevents blood reflux into the CS (Fig. 12-3). The thebesian valve usually

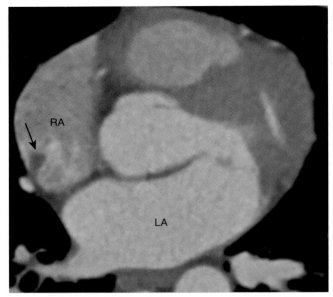

Figure 12-1 Axial computed tomography image at the level of the crista terminalis (*arrow*), a prominent fibromuscular ridge formed at the junction of the sinus venosus and primitive right atrium (RA). *LA*, Left atrium.

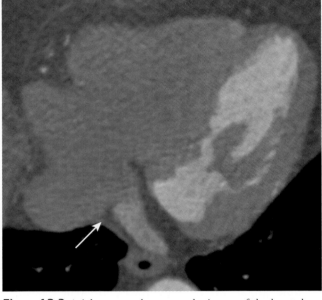

Figure 12-3 Axial computed tomography image of the heart demonstrates the thebesian valve (*arrow*) at the coronary sinus entrance into the right atrium.

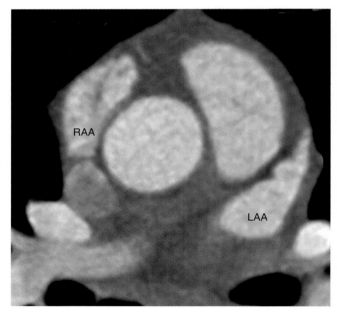

Figure 12-2 Short-axis view at the level of the atrial appendages demonstrating the pyramid-shaped right atrial appendage (RAA) with slightly larger pectinate muscles. The left atrial appendage (LAA) demonstrates a narrower, finger-like appearance and slightly smaller pectinate muscles.

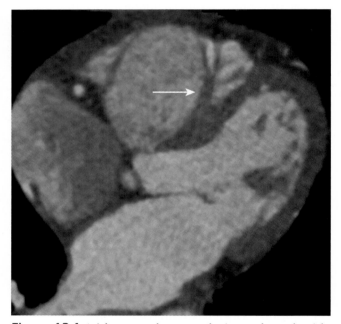

Figure 12-4 Axial computed tomography image shows the right ventricular moderator band (*arrow*), a muscular band extending from the right side of the interventricular septum to the anterior papillary muscle base.

consists of a thin semilunar fold in the anteroinferior ostium rim.

The right ventricle (RV) is the most anteriorly located cardiac chamber and has a characteristic heavily trabeculated apex, papillary muscles, and septomarginal bands. A distinguishing element of the RV is the moderator band, also known as the trabecula septomarginalis or septomarginal trabeculation, which is a muscular band extending from the interventricular septum to the anterior papillary muscle base (Fig. 12-4). The moderator band is part of the right bundle branch conduction system and contains the right AV bundle (also known as His bundle), along with one or more arteries supplied by the left coronary artery system. The moderator band artery most commonly originates from the second anterior septal artery from the left coronary system. Additional connections between the moderator band artery and the right marginal artery or right ventricular branches (which originate from the right coronary artery) create a potential protective anastomotic network between the right and left coronary systems.

The RV conus (also known as the right ventricular outflow tract [RVOT] or infundibulum), a smooth muscular infundibulum located directly inferior to the pulmonary valve (PV), provides the outflow tract for blood from the RV through the PV into the main pulmonary artery. In complex cases, the RV may be differentiated from the left ventricle (LV) by identification of the moderator band, the heavily trabeculated apex of the RV, a well-developed infundibulum, septal papillary muscles, and lack of fibrous continuity of the AV valve and outflow tract. RV short-axis diameter is measured on axial CT images at the level of the tricuspid valve (TV) as the maximum distance between the endocardial surfaces of the free wall and the septal wall. The maximum diastolic minor axis value for the RV on average measures 41.3 mm (± 6.8). An increased RV/LV diameter ratio in the setting of pulmonary embolism of greater than 1 can be seen as a result of right-sided heart strain, and a ratio greater than 1.5 may indicate severe strain and is associated with poorer prognosis.

■ CARDIAC CHAMBERS: LEFT HEART

The left atrium (LA) is located posteriorly to the left and, similar to the RA, consists of three parts: a vestibule, an appendage, and a venous portion. Although many common variants of pulmonary venous anatomy are recognized, as described later in the pulmonary vein subsection, the superior and inferior right and left pulmonary veins typically drain into the posteriorly located venous component of the LA. Most of the atrium is smooth walled, including the venous component, the vestibule, and the septum. The LA vestibular component surrounds the mitral valve (MV) orifice. The trabeculated LAA is derived from the primitive atrium and arises from the superolateral aspect of the LA, thus projecting anteriorly over the proximal left circumflex (LCx) artery. The LAA is more tubular and finger-like in shape, compared with the pyramidal RAA, and it has a narrower base. The LAA is a potential site for thrombus formation because of the narrow neck connecting it to the LA, although unmixed blood and contrast material in the LAA can mimic a thrombus or mass on CT. Compared with the RAA, the LAA pectinate muscles are smaller, (Fig. 12-5). These muscles are continuous fibers oriented parallel to each other within the LAA and should not be mistaken for thrombus. Normal LA area (excluding the LAA and pulmonary veins) is less than 20 cm². An area of 20 to 29 cm² is mildly enlarged, an area 30 to 40 cm² is moderately enlarged, and one greater than 40 cm² is severely enlarged. The superior wall or dome of the LA is thickest, measuring 3.5 to 6.5 mm, whereas the anterior LA wall, just behind the aorta, is thin and vulnerable to tear.

The LV is located posterior and left lateral to the RV and, although thick walled, lacks the heavy trabeculations of the RV. The LV demonstrates fine trabeculations and two papillary muscles, anterolateral and

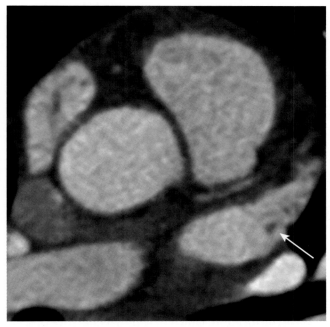

Figure 12-5 Axial computed tomography image shows the trabeculated left atrial appendage (LAA) along the superolateral aspect of the left atrium with smaller pectinate muscles (*arrow*). Although the LAA can be a site for thrombus formation, the pectinate muscle fibers or unmixed blood and contrast material should not be mistaken for thrombus.

posteromedial, which are in continuity with the ventricular myocardium. The posteromedial papillary muscle arises from the LV lateral wall. The papillary muscles function as part of the MV apparatus to ensure proper functioning of the MV leaflets. The LV myocardium has an anterior and inferior wall best visualized on paraseptal (or vertical) long-axis views, and the septal, apical, and lateral walls are best visualized on the four-chamber (or horizontal long-axis) views. The short-axis views enable assessment of the basal (closest to the MV), middle, and apical portions of the LV myocardium. The LV short-axis diameter is measured on axial CT images at the level of the MV as the maximum distance between the endocardial surfaces of the free wall and septal wall. The maximum diastolic minor axis value for the LV on average measures 42.0 mm (± 6.5). The LV is normally thin at the very apex (1 to 2 mm), even in abnormally thick-walled hearts (apical thin point). The outflow of the LV is by the LV outflow tract (LVOT), through the aortic valve into the aorta.

■ CARDIAC VALVES

The excellent spatial resolution of multidetector row CT enables visualization of valve leaflet anatomy, chordae tendineae, and papillary muscles. Valve motion and function can be assessed semiquantitatively with CT, and for patients with single left-sided valve dysfunction, CT can be used to calculate regurgitant volume and orifice size. CT is advantageous with better spatial resolution than magnetic resonance imaging for detailed leaflet anatomy and for accurate and reproducible evaluation

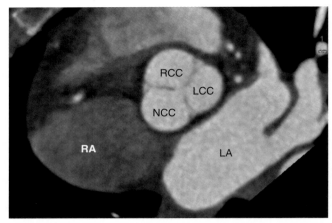

Figure 12-6 Short-axis computed tomography image demonstrating the trileaflet aortic valve. The right coronary cusp (RCC) is located most anteriorly, the left coronary cusp (LCC) most superiorly, and the noncoronary cusp (NCC) closest to the interatrial septum. The commissures *(arrows)* are the areas where two leaflets come together. *LA,* Left atrium; *RA,* right atrium.

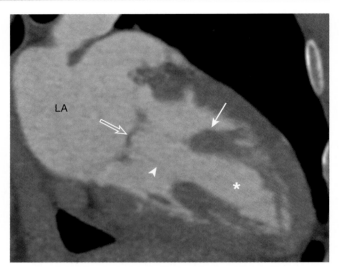

Figure 12-7 Vertical long-axis computed tomography image demonstrating the mitral valve leaflets (*open arrow*), papillary muscles (*arrow*), and chordae tendineae (*arrowhead*). *LA,* Left atrium; *asterisk,* left ventricle.

of valve calcification, which may be degenerative or seen in association with valve stenosis. Valve prostheses are usually well visualized with CT; however, depending on the type of valve replacement, streak artifacts resulting from metallic components may limit leaflet assessment.

Aortic Valve

The aortic valve separates the LVOT from the ascending aorta and is composed of an annulus, cusps, and commissures (the area where two leaflets come together). This valve has no associated papillary muscles or chordae tendineae. The aortic valve is trileaflet and has right, left, and noncoronary (posterior) cusps (Fig. 12-6). The right coronary cusp is located most anteriorly, the left coronary cusp most superiorly, and the noncoronary cusp most posteriorly, closest to the interatrial groove. The aortic cusps are half-moon shaped; thus, the aortic valve is also known as a semilunar valve. When closed, each cusp forms a pocket-like outpouching that opens into the ascending aorta and directs blood into the sinuses of Valsalva during diastole. The right and left coronary arteries arise from the right and left cusps, respectively. The aortic cusps are separated by three aortic commissures, roughly equally spaced around the valve annulus. The MV and aortic valve demonstrate fibrous continuity with each other, a feature that may assist in identifying the LV in patients with complex congenital heart disease.

Mitral Valve

The MV separates the LA and LV. It is the only bileaflet cardiac valve and is composed of anterior and posterior leaflets. The MV and its apparatus consist of an annulus, two leaflets, two commissures, two papillary muscles, and several chordae tendineae (linear fibrous bands) (Fig. 12-7). Direct fibrous continuity occurs between the MV and the aortic valve through the MV annulus, a saddle-shaped fibrous ring embedded in the myocardium. This structure anchors the MV leaflets in continuity

with the aortic annulus through three fibrous trigones, or intervalvular fibrosa. The MV annulus boundaries are normally not well visualized on cardiac CT; however, calcification is a common abnormality that permits its visualization. The free edges of the mitral leaflets are connected to the anterolateral and posteromedial LV papillary muscles through the chordae tendineae. During systole, the LV myocardium and papillary muscles contract, thus tugging on MV leaflets to ensure complete MV closure and to prevent prolapse.

The posterior leaflet is divided into three scallops. The most cephalad (or anterolateral) scallop is called P1, the most caudal (or posteromedial) scallop is P3, and the scallop in between is P2. The opposing portions of the anterior leaflet are A1, A2, and A3. P1 is adjacent to the anterolateral commissure and is closest to the aorta (anterior).

Tricuspid Valve

The TV separates the RA from the RV and, similar to the MV, is composed of leaflets, an annulus, commissures, papillary muscles, and chordae tendineae. The TV has three leaflets, the anterior, posterior, and septal leaflets, connected to the papillary muscles of the RV by chordae tendineae. In contrast to the fibrous continuity of the MV and the aortic valve, the TV is separated from the PV by the crista supraventricularis, a muscular ridge, and the RVOT (or infundibulum). The TV also has a direct connection to the interventricular septum, unlike the MV. In patients with complex congenital heart disease, these findings may aid in distinguishing the TV from the MV.

Pulmonary Valve

The PV (also known as the pulmonic valve or right semilunar valve) divides the RVOT from the main pulmonary artery. The PV is also trileaflet and consists of right, left, and anterior leaflets. The PV is located anterior, superior, and to the left of the aortic valve. It is separated from the TV by the RVOT and the crista supraventricularis.

■ CORONARY ARTERIES

The coronary arteries are normally located along the surface of the heart and are surrounded by epicardial fat. The four major coronary arteries are the right coronary artery (RCA) and the three components of the left coronary system: the left main (LM) artery and its branches, the left anterior descending (LAD) artery, and the LCx coronary artery. The size of the coronary arteries correlates with ventricular mass, body size, and gender; women have smaller coronary artery cross-sectional areas compared with men. Normal coronary artery diameters established by catheter angiography, which accounts for only luminal diameter, are, on average, approximately 3 mm in female patients and 4 mm in male patients. Knowledge of normal coronary artery size and configuration aids identification of coronary artery abnormalities such as ectasia, aneurysm (dilatation >1.5 times the diameter of the adjacent normal coronary artery), or stenosis.

Left Coronary Arteries

The LM artery originates from the left sinus of Valsalva and courses a variable distance, usually 3 to 20 mm, before typically giving rise to the LAD and LCx arteries. The LAD (also known as the ramus interventricularis anterior) courses anterolaterally in the epicardial fat of the anterior interventricular groove to the cardiac apex (Fig. 12-8). The branches of the LAD artery include diagonal branches and septal perforating arteries. The laterally located diagonal branches supply the anterior LV free wall, whereas the medially located septal perforator branches penetrate the myocardium to supply most of the anterior interventricular septum, the AV bundle, and the proximal bundle branch. The diagonal branches and septal perforator branches are numbered from proximal to distal origin as they arise from the LAD artery. The LAD artery normally supplies the cardiac apex; however, if the LAD is small, the posterior descending artery (PDA) can extend around the apex to supply one third of the anterior interventricular septum. Rarely, in less than 0.5% of cases, the LM artery is absent, and the LAD and LCx arteries arise directly and separately from the left CS (Fig. 12-9). In approximately 15% of the population, a ramus intermedius (RI) artery arises in the crotch between the LAD and LCx arteries, with resulting trifurcation of the LM artery (Fig. 12-10). The RI artery courses laterally, similar to the first diagonal branch of the LAD artery, to supply the LV free wall.

The other major branch of the LM artery is the LCx artery (occasionally called the ramus circumflexus), which courses in the left AV groove and gives rise to obtuse marginal (OM) branches, also called lateral or marginal branches. Together, the LCx artery and OM branches supply the LV free wall and a variable portion of the anterolateral LV papillary muscle. OM branches are numbered sequentially from the most proximal origin

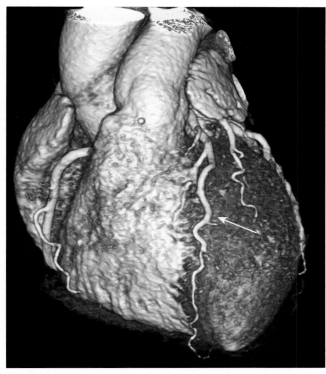

Figure 12-8 Volume-rendered image of the anterior heart shows the left anterior descending artery *(arrow)* coursing anterolaterally in the anterior interventricular groove between the right and left ventricles.

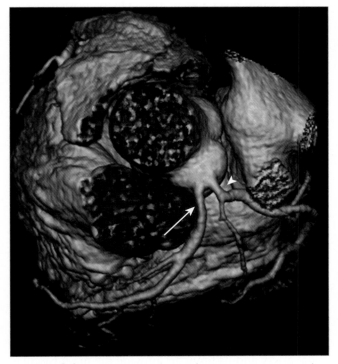

Figure 12-9 Volume-rendered view shows an uncommon variant of an absent left main artery with the left anterior descending *(arrow)* and left circumflex *(arrowhead)* arteries arising separately from the left coronary sinus.

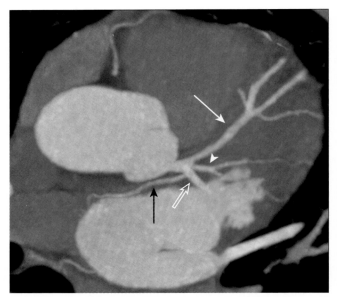

Figure 12-10 Axial maximum intensity projection image of the left main artery trifurcation into the left anterior descending (LAD, *white arrow*), ramus intermedius (RI) *(arrowhead)*, and left circumflex (LCx, *open arrow*) arteries. The RI arises in the crotch between the LAD and LCx and courses laterally to supply the left ventricular free wall. The sinoatrial nodal artery *(black arrow)* arises from the proximal LCx, which is an occasionally encountered normal variant.

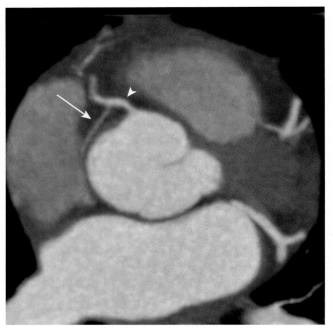

Figure 12-11 Axial maximum intensity projection image of the sinoatrial nodal artery *(arrow)* arising from the proximal right coronary artery *(arrowhead)* in the typical location.

to the most distal as they arise from the LCx artery. In most patients (i.e., with right-dominant coronary artery systems), the LCx artery terminates at the obtuse margin of the heart. In a left-dominant or codominant system, the LCx artery gives rise to the PDA or posterolateral (PL) branches.

Right Coronary Arteries

The RCA (or arteria coronaria dextra) arises from the right sinus of Valsalva. It runs rightward, posterior to the pulmonary outflow tract, then caudally in the right AV groove, and curves posteriorly at the acute margin of the RV to the crux of the heart. The crux of the heart is the point where the AV groove transects the interventricular septum along the posterior surface of the heart, to form a cross. In 50% to 60% of the population, the most proximal branch of the RCA is the conus artery, which supplies the RVOT (conus arteriosus) and forms anastomoses with the LAD arterial circulation through the circle of Vieussens. In the remaining population, the conus artery originates directly from the right CS. The SA nodal artery is usually a single branch arising from the proximal RCA (60% of the population) or LCx artery (40%) (see Fig. 12-10; Fig. 12-11). Regardless of origin, the SA nodal artery courses along the anterior interatrial groove toward the superior cavoatrial junction, where the course becomes variable, either anterior (precaval) or posterior (retrocaval), to enter the SA node. The SA nodal artery and its branches provide the main vascular supply of the Bachmann bundle.

Additional multiple anterior ventricular branches from the RCA supply the RV free wall. The largest of

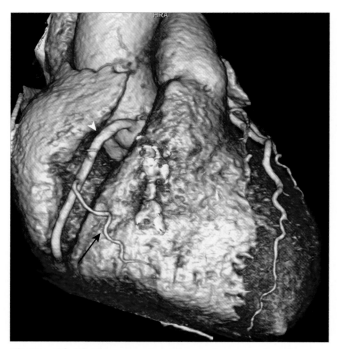

Figure 12-12 Volume-rendered image demonstrating the acute marginal branch *(arrow)* arising from the midright coronary artery *(arrowhead)* to supply the right ventricular anterior free wall.

these branches is the acute marginal branch, located at the junction of the middle and distal RCA (Fig. 12-12). In most patients (i.e., with right-dominant coronary artery systems), the distal RCA divides into the PDA (also known as the ramus interventricularis posterior) and posterior LV branch (PL or PLV, or ramus posterolateralis dexter).

The AV nodal artery arises from the dominant coronary artery system. Usually, the AV nodal artery originates from the apex of proximal PLV and penetrates the base of the posterior interatrial septum at the level of the crux of the heart. This artery provides branches to the posterior interventricular septum, interatrial septum, AV node, and penetrating His bundle.

Coronary Artery Dominance

Coronary artery dominance is defined by the coronary artery that gives rise to the PDA and PL branch. Variable dominance rates are reported; right dominance occurs in 70% to 85% of the population, left dominance in 8 to 10%, and codominance between the RCA and LCA in the remainder. In a right-dominant heart, the PDA originates from the RCA and extends down the posterior interventricular groove, and at least one other PLV branch arises from the distal RCA, to supply the diaphragmatic wall of the LV. In a left-dominant heart, the left coronary system supplies the entire LV, with the LCx artery continuing to the crux of the heart and giving rise to both the PDA and PLV branch. In these cases, the RCA tends to be diminutive relative to the LCx artery, and it typically tapers and terminates near the acute margin of the heart. In a codominant coronary artery system, portions of the LV diaphragmatic surface are supplied by branches of both the RCA and the LCx artery. The length of the distal RCA is inversely proportional to the length of the LCx artery along the inferior aspect of the heart.

Coronary Artery Segmentation

Coronary artery segmentation is a classification scheme used to divide the coronary arteries into segments based on specific anatomic structures and arterial branches. This systematic nomenclature facilitates reproducible reporting and standardized communication of the precise location of coronary artery disease. Although various nomenclatures are used, an 18-segment coronary model has been adapted for coronary CT angiography (CCTA) (Fig. 12-13).

Left Coronary Artery Segmentation

When this segmentation model is used, the LM segment extends from the left coronary artery ostium to the bifurcation into the LAD and LCx arteries (or trifurcation if an RI artery is present). The LAD artery is divided into proximal, middle, and distal segments. The proximal LAD artery extends from the left main bifurcation to the first large septal or diagonal branch (depending on which is most proximal). The mid-LAD artery begins at the end of the proximal LAD artery and extends to where the artery forms an acute angle, which may coincide with the second septal perforator origin. Alternatively, the middle and distal LAD artery segments are distinguished at the halfway point between the first septal perforator and the heart apex. The distal LAD artery extends from the mid-LAD artery to its termination.

The LCx artery is divided into proximal and distal segments, based on the OM branches. The proximal LCx branch extends from its origin at the LM artery to the origin of the first OM branch. The distal LCx artery extends from the first OM branch to the end of the vessel or, in a left-dominant system, to the PDA origin and PLV branch.

Right Coronary Artery Segmentation

The RCA is divided into proximal, middle, and distal segments. The proximal RCA extends from the right coronary artery ostium to half the distance to the acute margin of the heart. The mid-RCA extends from the end of the proximal RCA to the acute heart margin. The distal RCA courses along the posterior AV groove, from the acute margin of the heart to the PDA origin (in a right-dominant coronary artery system).

■ CARDIAC VEINS

The major components of the cardiac venous system include the CS, middle cardiac vein, great cardiac vein, and anterior and posterior interventricular veins (Fig. 12-14). The cardiac venous system anatomy can be quite variable, but the CS is the most constant structure. The CS is approximately 45 mm long and 10 to 12 mm in diameter. The CS runs along the left AV groove along the inferior aspect of the heart before it empties into the RA. The middle cardiac vein, also known as the posterior interventricular vein, is the first branch of the CS and courses in the posterior interventricular groove from the cardiac base to the apex. The next two branches of the CS are the posterior vein of the LV (PVLV, also known as the posterolateral vein), and the left marginal vein. The left marginal vein courses along the lateral border of the LV. After these branches, the CS becomes the great cardiac vein, which courses in the lateral left AV groove with the LCx artery. It continues in the anterior interventricular groove with the LAD artery, as the anterior interventricular vein, from the base of the heart toward the apex.

Variability in cardiac venous anatomy usually results from absence of the PVLV or the left marginal vein, with 55% of the population having the PVLV and 83% having the left marginal vein. Knowledge of this variability is particularly important in evaluation of patients before cardiac resynchronization therapy because the left marginal vein and PVLV are often the target veins for pacemaker lead placement. If a suitable vein for transvenous placement of an LV pacer lead cannot be identified on cardiac CT angiography, surgical placement may be required.

The vein of Marshall drains into the CS and is located within a fold of pericardium (the ligament of Marshall), the remnant of the embryonic left SVC. In most people, the ligament of Marshall is almost obliterated. It remains patent in 0.3% of the population as an isolated malformation, a persistent left SVC, which drains into the CS.

■ PULMONARY VEINS

Detailed knowledge of pulmonary vein anatomy is important because ectopic electrical foci at the venous ostia may cause atrial fibrillation or tachycardia, or both.

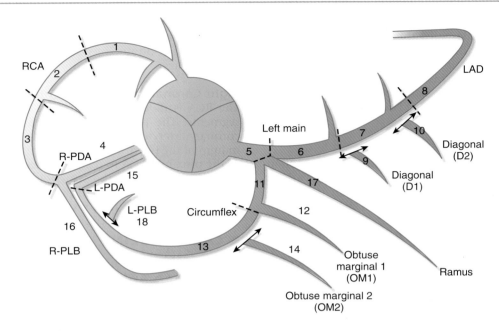

Segment	Abbreviation	Description
Proximal RCA	pRCA	Ostium of the right coronary artery (RCA) to one half the distance to the acute margin of heart
Mid-RCA	mRCA	End of the proximal RCA to the acute margin of heart
Distal RCA	dRCA	End of the mid-RCA to the origin of the posterior descending artery (PDA)
PDA-RCA	R-PDA	PDA from the RCA
PLB-RCA	R-PLB	Posterior lateral branch (PLB) from the RCA
LM LCx	LM	Ostium of the left main coronary artery (LM) to the bifurcation of the left anterior descending artery (LAD) and the left circumflex artery (LCx)
Proximal LAD	pLAD	End of the LM to the first large septal or first diagonal (D1) branch, whichever is most proximal
Mid-LAD	mLAD	End of the proximal LAD to one half the distance to the apex
Distal LAD	dLAD	End of the mid-LAD to the end of the LAD
Diagonal 1	D1	First diagonal branch (D1)
Diagonal 2	D2	Second diagonal branch (D2)
Proximal LCx	pCx	End of the LM to the origin of the first obtuse marginal (OM1) branch
OM1	OM1	First OM1 traversing the lateral wall of the left ventricle
Mid and distal LCx	LCx	Traveling in the atrioventricular groove, distal to the OM1 branch to the end of the vessel or origin of the L-PDA (left PDA)
OM2	OM2	Second obtuse marginal branch (OM2)
PDA-LCx	L-PDA	PDA from the LCx
Ramus intermedius	RI	Vessel originating from the LM between the LAD and LCx in case of a trifurcation
PLB-L	L-PLB	PLB from the LCx

Figure 12-13 Society of Cardiovascular Computed Tomography coronary segmentation diagram. *Dashed lines* represent divisions among the RCA, LAD, and LCx and the end of the posterior left ventricular branch (LMPLB 5 PLV) Additional nomenclature may be added (e.g., D3,R-PDA2, SVG [saphenous vein graft], mLAD). (From Raff GL, Abidov A, Achenbach S, et al. SCCT guidelines for the interpretation and reporting of coronary computed tomographic angiography. *J Cardiovasc Comput Tomogr.* 2009;3:127, copyright 2009, Elsevier; with permission.)

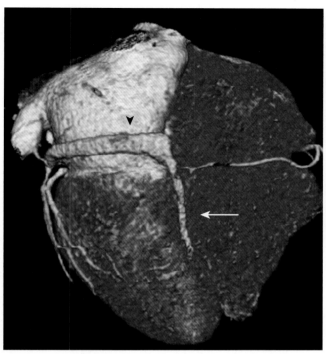

Figure 12-14 Volume-rendered image of the inferior surface of the heart shows the coronary sinus (*arrowhead*) in the region of the atrioventricular groove and middle cardiac vein (also known as the posterior interventricular vein) (*arrow*).

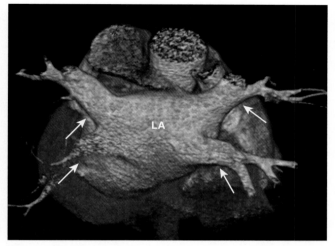

Figure 12-15 Volume-rendered view of the left atrium (LA) demonstrates the typical pulmonary vein configuration with two right pulmonary veins and two left pulmonary veins (*arrows*), each draining through separate ostia into the LA.

Therapies are directed at these foci with radiofrequency catheter ablation to either eliminate the foci or encircle and electrically isolate the pulmonary veins. Depiction of pulmonary vein anatomy with CT facilitates an anatomically based radiofrequency catheter ablation procedure by providing a map of pulmonary vein size and ostial diameter, number, location, and anatomic variants, in addition to LA dimensions, presence or absence of LA thrombus, and relationship between the esophagus and the posterior LA wall.

Typically, patients have two right pulmonary veins and two left pulmonary veins, each draining through separate ostia into the LA (Fig. 12-15). Variations in pulmonary vein number, ostial diameter, and shape are common. Additional pulmonary venous ostia are more commonly seen on the right side, usually a separate right middle pulmonary vein ostium located between the superior and inferior right pulmonary venous ostia. Solitary pulmonary venous ostia are more commonly seen on the left side.

■ **PERICARDIUM**

The heart is enveloped by the pericardium, a paperthin structure of varying thickness normally measuring 2 mm or less. The pericardium is composed of two layers, the tough outer parietal layer and the inner more delicate serous layer. The parietal layer attaches to the sternum and proximal great vessels. Most of the ascending aorta, pulmonary trunk, portions of the SVC, IVC, and most of the pulmonary veins are intrapericardial. The serous layer lines the fibrous pericardium and outer surface of the heart and great vessels. The pericardium lining the heart surface is called the visceral pericardium or epicardium. On CT, the pericardium usually appears to be a thin line of tissue delineated by low-attenuation mediastinal fat and epicardial fat. The pericardial sac contains a small amount of fluid, normally between 15 and 50 mL. Recesses and sinuses are formed at the junctions of the visceral and parietal pericardium and are continuous with the pericardial cavity. Multidetector CT has improved visualization of pericardial sinuses and recesses, which may vary in shape with increased pericardial fluid. Familiarity with the normal pericardial anatomy is necessary to prevent misdiagnosis of the pericardial recesses as mediastinal or hilar disease, including aortic dissection, mediastinal mass, pericardial cyst, thymic cyst, thymus or mediastinal, or hilar lymphadenopathy.

The three main sites of pericardial recess origin are the transverse sinus, the oblique sinus, and the pericardial cavity proper. The transverse sinus is located cranial to the LA and posterior to the ascending aorta or pulmonary trunk and gives rise to several recesses extending between the major vessels and the atrium. These include the superior aortic recess, the inferior aortic recess, and the right and left pulmonic recesses. The superior aortic recess has three subdivisions: anteriorly between the ascending aorta and pulmonary trunk with a characteristic triangular shape, posteriorly directly behind the ascending aorta with a characteristic crescent shape, and a right lateral extension between the SVC and the ascending aorta. The anterior and posterior subdivisions of the superior aortic recess are in continuity. Fluid within the normal superior pericardial recess can mimic an intramural hematoma or aortic dissection; however, recognition of continuity with the pericardial space and simple fluid attenuation can aid identification as a normal recess. The inferior aortic recess is a caudal extension from the transverse sinus between the aortic root and the RA. The right and left pulmonic recesses extend inferolaterally from the transverse sinus, caudal to the pulmonary arteries.

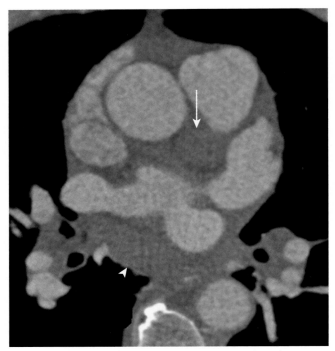

Figure 12-16 Axial computed tomography image in a patient with a pericardial effusion demonstrates fluid filling the pericardial recesses. Fluid is seen in the transverse sinus *(arrow)* and the oblique sinus *(arrowhead).*

The oblique sinus is located posterior to the LA and inferior to the transverse sinus and is in continuity with the subcarinal region (Fig. 12-16). This sinus is the most posterior pericardial space from which the posterior pericardial recess arises and extends superiorly, posterior to the right pulmonary artery and medial to the bronchus intermedius. Recesses originating from the pericardial cavity proper include the postcaval recess and the left and right pulmonary venous recess. The postcaval recess is located posterolateral to the SVC. The left and right pulmonary venous recesses are located between the respective superior and inferior pulmonary veins.

■ CONCLUSION

Precise evaluation of cardiac CT images requires a detailed understanding of normal cardiac anatomy and common anatomic variants. The use of standard termi-

nology is essential for accurate anatomic description and communication of examination results.

Bibliography

Austen WG, Edwards JE, Frye RL, et al. A reporting system on patients evaluated for coronary artery disease. *Circulation.* 1975;51(suppl 4):3-40.

Collomb D, Paramelle PJ, Calaque O, et al. Severity assessment of acute pulmonary embolism: evaluation using helical CT. *Eur Radiol.* 2003;13:1508-1514.

Ghay B, Ghuysen A, Bruyere PJ, et al. Can CT pulmonary angiography allow assessment of severity and prognosis in patients presenting with pulmonary embolism? What the radiologist needs to know. *Radiographics.* 2006;26:23-40.

Jacobs JE. Computed tomographic evaluation of the normal cardiac anatomy. *Radiol Clin North Am.* 2010;48:701-710.

Jongloed MRM, Dirksen MS, Bax JJ, et al. Atrial fibrillation: multi-detector row CT of pulmonary vein anatomy prior to radiofrequency catheter ablation-initial experience. *Radiology.* 2005;234:702-709.

Lang RM, Bierig M, Devereux RB, et al. Recommendations for chamber quantification: a report from the American Society of Echocardiography's Guidelines and Standards Committee and the Chamber Quantification Writing Group, developed in conjunction with the European Association of Echocardiography, a branch of the European Society of Cardiology. *J Am Soc Echocardiogr.* 2005;18:1440-1463.

O'Brien JP, Srichai MB, Hecht EM, et al. Anatomy of the heart at multidetector CT: what the radiologist needs to know. *Radiographics.* 2007;27:1569-1582.

O'Leary SM, Williams PL, Williams MP, et al. Imaging of the pericardium: appearances on ECG-gated 64-detector row cardiac computed tomography. *Br J Radiol.* 2010;83:194-205.

Ozmen CA, Akpinar MG, Akay HO, et al. Evaluation of pericardial sinuses and recesses with 2-, 4-, 16-, and 64-row multidetector CT. *Radiol Med.* 2010;115:1038-1046.

Pannu HK, Flohr TG, Corl FM, et al. Current concepts in multi-detector row CT evaluation of the coronary arteries: principles, techniques, and anatomy. *Radiographics.* 2003;23:S111-S125.

Raff GL, Abidov A, Achenbach S, et al. SCCT guidelines for the interpretation and reporting of coronary computed tomographic angiography. *J Cardiovasc Comput Tomogr.* 2009;3:122-136.

Saremi F, Channual S, Krishnan S, et al. Bachmann bundle and its arterial supply: imaging with multidetector CT-implications for interatrial conduction abnormalities and arrhythmias. *Radiology.* 2008;248:447-457.

Saremi F, Krishnan S. Cardiac conduction system: anatomic landmarks relevant to interventional electrophysiologic techniques demonstrated with 64-detector CT. *Radiographics.* 2007;27:1539-1567.

Schoenhagen P, Halliburton SS, Stillman AE, et al. Noninvasive imaging of coronary arteries: current and future role of multi-detector row CT. *Radiology.* 2004;232:7-17.

Schoepf UJ, Zwerner PL, Savino G, et al. Coronary CT angiography. *Radiology.* 2007;244:48-63.

Vogel-Claussen J, Pannu H, Spevak PJ, et al. Cardiac valve assessment with MR imaging and 64-section multi-detector row CT. *Radiographics.* 2006;26:1769-1784.

Yang F, Minutellio RM, Bhagan S, et al. The impact of gender on vessels size in patients with angiographically normal coronary arteries. *J Interv Cardiol.* 2006;19:340-344.

CHAPTER 13

Cardiac Anatomy on Magnetic Resonance Imaging

Jonathan D. Dodd and Ronan Kileen

Cardiac magnetic resonance (CMR) imaging allows high-contrast, spatial, and temporal resolution imaging of the heart and related structures. The absence of ionizing radiation and the greater contrast and temporal resolution when compared with multidetector computed tomography are significant benefits of CMR. By combining different imaging sequences, cardiac abnormalities can be identified with high diagnostic accuracy. An understanding of the normal anatomic structures is of paramount importance to allow the reader to recognize such pathologic processes.

Using CMR, images may be acquired in any orientation, but typically the tomographic method of image display similar to that used in echocardiography is employed (Fig. 13-1). This involves bisecting the heart with a single slice in a particular plane and then viewing adjacent parallel slices. The three most common imaging planes used are the short-axis view, the horizontal long-axis (or four-chamber) view, and the vertical long-axis (or two-chamber) view. In the short-axis view, the left ventricle is imaged perpendicular to a line from the apex to the center of the mitral valve apparatus. In the horizontal long axis-view, the lateral walls of both ventricles are sliced in such a way that both atria and ventricles are visible on the same image. In the vertical long-axis view, the plane bisects the left ventricular apex and the center of the mitral valve orifice.

■ ORIENTATION OF THE HEART

The heart is located within the middle mediastinum between the lungs. The heart lies obliquely within the chest cavity, with the interventricular septa angled approximately at 45 degrees to the transaxial plane. The atrioventricular valves (mitral and tricuspid) are at right angles to the interventricular septum. The right atrium is anterior and inferior to the left atrium, and the right ventricle forms the majority of the anterior border of the heart. The left atrium is the most posterior chamber.

■ PERICARDIUM

The pericardium envelops the heart within the middle mediastinum and consists of two components, the fibrous pericardium and the serosal pericardium. The fibrous pericardium, the outer component, is made of tough connective tissue and is not attached to the heart itself. Superiorly, the fibrous pericardium is continuous with the adventitia of the great vessels, and inferiorly, it is continuous with the central tendon of the diaphragm. Anteriorly, it is attached to the posterior surface of the sternum. The serosal pericardium has visceral and parietal layers. The visceral layer is attached to the myocardium and great vessels and forms the epicardium. A reflection of the visceral layer connects the epicardium with the parietal serous pericardium, which is adherent to the fibrous pericardium. These reflections also give rise to the transverse and oblique sinuses, which are potential spaces. The transverse sinus lies posterior to the aorta and pulmonary trunk and anterior to the atria. The oblique sinus is a cul de sac that lies posterior to the left atrium. Several pericardial recesses are also formed that may become visible on CMR if they contain fluid (Fig. 13-2). The postcaval recess is located posterior to the junction of the right atrium and the superior vena cava (SVC) and lies between the right pulmonary artery and the right superior pulmonary vein (Fig. 13-3). The right and left pulmonary venous recesses lie between the superior and inferior pulmonary veins on either side. The superior aortic recess (superior pericardial recess) extends from the transverse sinus to the right of and posterior to the ascending aorta and anterior to the proximal right pulmonary artery. The inferior aortic recess extends inferiorly from the transverse sinus between the ascending aorta and the right atrium.

Clinical Pearl

The fibrous pericardium cannot stretch. As a result, hemopericardium from a ruptured ascending aorta causes cardiac tamponade and can be rapidly fatal unless treated.

■ RIGHT ATRIUM

The right atrium has a posterior smooth-walled venous component, a muscular anterior component, and a right atrial appendage. The venous component receives the inferior vena cava (IVC), the SVC, and the coronary sinus. It is separated from the anterior component by a smooth internal muscular ridge called the crista terminalis that correlates with the embryonic location of the right venous valve (Fig. 13-4). The IVC drains into the inferior aspect of the posterior right atrium. At the

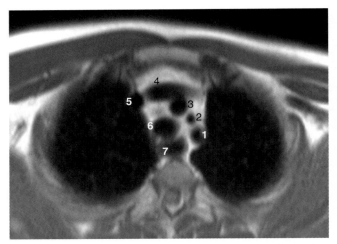

Figure 13-1 Axial black-blood axial image just above the level of the aortic arch. *1*, Left subclavian artery; *2*, left common carotid artery; *3*, innominate artery; *4*, left brachiocephalic vein; *5*, right brachiocephalic vein; *6*, trachea; *7*, esophagus. A bovine arch occurs when the left common carotid artery arises from the innominate artery. A level slightly below this image would have the right and left brachiocephalic veins merge to form the superior vena cava.

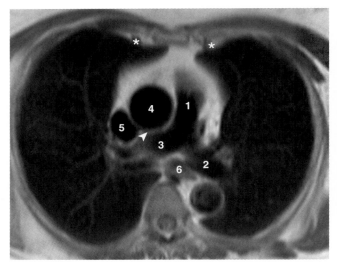

Figure 13-2 Axial black-blood axial image at the level of the main pulmonary artery. *1*, Main pulmonary artery; *2*, left pulmonary artery; *3*, right pulmonary artery; *4*, ascending aorta; *5*, superior vena cava; *6*, esophagus. Note also the location of the internal mammary vessels *(asterisks)*; scrutinizing these vessels is important because they are a common location for lymph node metastases (especially from breast cancer). Note also the transverse pericardial recess *(arrowhead)*. This should not be mistaken for lymphadenopathy, and it may be quite prominent.

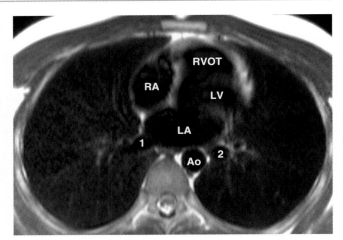

Figure 13-3 Axial black-blood axial image at the level of the left atrium. *1*, Right inferior pulmonary vein; *2*, left inferior pulmonary vein. Scrutinizing the pulmonary vein ostia carefully after pulmonary vein ablation is important to exclude pulmonary vein stenosis. *Ao*, Aorta (descending); *LA*, left atrium; *LV*, left ventricle; *RA*, right atrium; *RVOT*, right ventricular outflow tract.

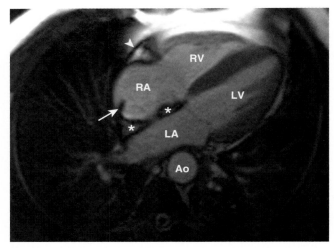

Figure 13-4 Steady-state free precession image in the four-chamber view at the level of the left ventricle (LV). The crista terminalis *(arrow)* is an embryonic ridge in the right atrium (RA; normal structure) that can be mistaken for thrombus or tumor. Note the normal pericardium *(arrowhead)* anterior to the right atrioventricular groove; it should not exceed 4 mm in thickness. Note also lipomatous hypertrophy of the interatrial septum *(asterisks)* showing a characteristic dumbbell-shaped appearance with sparing of the fossa ovalis. *Ao*, Aorta (descending); *LA*, left atrium; *RV*, right ventricle.

anterior and right lateral aspect of the IVC orifice is the eustachian valve or eustachian ridge. This valve is a fold of endocardium that is much larger in utero, at which time it serves to direct oxygenated blood returning from the placenta through the foramen ovale in the interatrial septum and into the left atrium. This anatomic configuration makes transeptal puncture easier using an IVC approach. The eustachian valve is continuous inferiorly with the valve of the coronary sinus (thebesian valve), which covers the lower part of the orifice of the coronary sinus. The thebesian valve may be complete, incomplete

or fenestrated, or absent. The coronary sinus lies within the left atrioventricular groove and drains into the right atrium medial and superior to the IVC orifice (Fig. 13-5). The pectinate muscles extend from the crista terminalis into the right atrial appendage, which is a broad-based triangular structure that extends around the anterior and right lateral aspect of the ascending aorta.

The interatrial septum separates the left atrium from the right atrium and usually bows into the right atrium because of slightly higher pressure in the left side of the heart. On the right side of the interatrial septum is the fossa ovalis. A peripheral muscular limbus with a central depression above and to the left of the orifice of the IVC

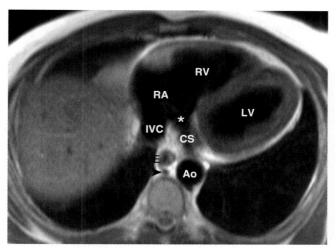

Figure 13-5 Axial black-blood axial image at the level of the coronary sinus (CS). The CS lies within the left atrioventricular groove and drains into the right atrium (RA) medial and superior to the inferior vena cava (IVC) orifice. Occasionally, the thebesian valve (*asterisk*) may be seen at its ostium with the RA. If the CS appears particularly enlarged, assess images for a left-sided superior vena cava, or possibly an unroofed CS or a coronary artery–to–CS fistula. The azygos vein (*arrowhead*) is a small vein in the posterior mediastinum. If it is enlarged, assess images for azygos continuation of the IVC. *Ao*, Aorta (descending); *E*, esophagus; *LV*, left ventricle; *RV*, right ventricle.

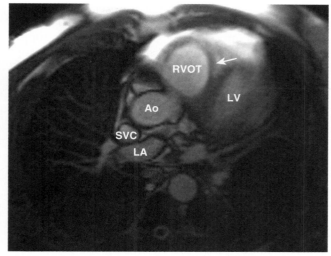

Figure 13-6 Axial steady-state free precession image at the level of the right ventricular outflow tract (RVOT). The supraventricular muscular ridge extends from the interventricular septum to the right ventricular free wall and upward to the RVOT. This crest is made up of three bands: septal, parietal, and infundibular. The parietal band (*arrow*) is often visualized on cardiac magnetic resonance imaging. *Ao*, Aorta (ascending); *LA*, left atrium and right superior pulmonary vein; *LV*, left ventricle; *SVC*, superior vena cava.

represents the valve of the fossa ovalis. A small slit may be present at the superior aspect of the valve that allows communication with the left atrium. This is called a patent foramen ovale and is present in one third of people.

The normal area of the right atrium, viewed on the four-chamber view during ventricular systole and as measured on CMR, is 21 cm². The upper limit of normal is 24 cm².

Clinical Pearl

Patent foramen ovale may be complicated by paradoxical embolism.

■ RIGHT VENTRICLE

The right ventricle lies directly posterior to the sternum and forms the majority of the anterior border of the heart. It is a complex structure. The right ventricle may be subdivided as follows: an inflow component, which extends from the annulus of the tricuspid valve to the origins of the papillary muscles; a trabeculated component, which extends toward the apex; and the infundibulum (also known as the right ventricular outflow tract or conus), which is a smooth-walled muscular channel that extends toward the pulmonary valve (Fig. 13-6). The normal right ventricular end-diastolic volumes are 190 ± 33 mL in boys and men and 148 ± 35 mL in girls and women. The normal end-systolic volumes are 78 ± 20 mL in boys and men and 56 ± 18 mL in girls and women. The supraventricular crest, which separates the pulmonary and tricuspid valves, is a thick, muscular ridge that extends from the septum to the right ventricular free wall. This crest is made up of three bands: septal, parietal, and infundibular. These bands may appear as distinct structures. Near

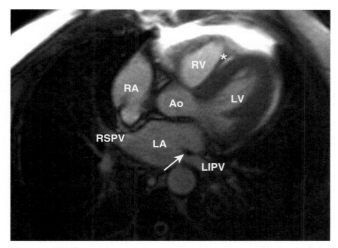

Figure 13-7 Steady-state free precession image at the level of the right ventricle (five-chamber view). Note the moderator band (*asterisk*) in the right ventricle (RV). The warfarin (Coumadin) ridge (*arrow*) is a normal soft tissue ridge between the left inferior pulmonary vein and the left atrial wall. *Ao*, Aorta (ascending); *LA*, left atrium; *LIPV*, left inferior pulmonary vein; *LV*, left ventricle; *RA*, right atrium; *RSPV*, right superior pulmonary vein and middle lobe pulmonary vein.

the apex, the septal band extends to the anterior papillary muscle of the tricuspid valve as the moderator band, so named because it was thought to prevent overdistention of the ventricular apex (Fig. 13-7).

The tricuspid valve has anterior, septal, and posterior cusps. The largest is the anterior cusp, which attaches to the atrioventricular junction at the posterior and lateral aspect of the supraventricular crest and extends to the membranous septum. The valve is oriented vertically, almost in the sagittal plane.

Typically, two large papillary muscles are present in the right ventricle (anterior and posterior), with a smaller septal muscle. The papillary muscles supply chordae tendineae to the corresponding cusps they support. The septal cusp is the smallest and is relatively immobile because it is tethered to the septum directly by chordae tendineae. During valve opening, the two larger cusps move into the right ventricle without significant septal cusp motion.

The pulmonary valve has three semilunar cusps. In the fetus, an anterior cusp, a posterior cusp, and a septal cusp are present. Adults have two anterior and one posterior cusp. These cusps are often very thin and require high-resolution imaging to be evaluated with CMR.

Clinical Pearl

A useful image plane for visualizing the pulmonary valve cusps is the right ventricular outflow tract view.

■ LEFT ATRIUM

The left atrium is the most posterior heart chamber and is smaller than the right atrium. The walls of the left atrium (3 mm) are thicker than are those of the right atrium (1 mm). The left atrium receives a variable number of pulmonary veins at its posterolateral aspects, but typically it has four dominant veins. Two right (superior and inferior) and two left (superior and inferior) pulmonary veins are present. The inferior pulmonary veins are oriented horizontally, and the superior pulmonary veins are oriented anterosuperiorly. The orifices of the pulmonary veins lie at the posterolateral aspect of the left atrium. The left superior and inferior pulmonary veins frequently have a common orifice. The left atrial appendage extends from the roof of the left atrium to the left of the pulmonary trunk and contains all the pectinate muscles of the left atrium. The left atrial appendage is typically shaped like a finger, is larger and longer than the right atrial appendage, and has a narrower neck. Its shape can be variable, however, and may frequently be bilobar or trilobar. This consideration is important when evaluating the appendage for thrombus because some components may be difficult to assess with echocardiography. The coronary sinus courses in the left atrioventricular groove before it drains into the right atrium. The esophagus and descending thoracic aorta are posterior in relation to the left atrium, and disease in either of these structures may affect the left atrium. Similarly, the esophagus and descending thoracic aorta may become damaged because of their close proximity to the left atrium during pulmonary vein ablation.

The normal area of the left atrium, as seen on the four-chamber view during ventricular systole and as measured on CMR, is 21 cm^2. The upper limit of normal is 24 cm^2.

Clinical Pearls

Myocardial sleeves extend into the proximal pulmonary veins and cause the pulmonary vein orifices to contract during systole. These sleeves may act as a trigger for atrial fibrillation, which is amenable to catheter ablation.

■ LEFT VENTRICLE

The left ventricle is designed to provide pulsatile flow to the highly pressurized systemic arterial system. The wall of the left ventricle is approximately three times thicker (8 to 11 mm) than that of the right ventricle and is usually thinnest at the apex (1 to 2 mm), a site referred to as the apical thin point (a normal structure) (Fig. 13-8). The left atrioventricular valve is called the mitral valve. During diastole, blood flows across the mitral valve from the left atrium into the left ventricle. During systole, the mitral valve leaflets close, and blood is expelled into the systemic circulation through the aortic valve. Unlike the tricuspid and pulmonary valves, the mitral and aortic valves are in fibrous continuity through the intervalvular fibrosa. The left ventricular wall is trabeculated, although less so than the right ventricle, and these trabeculations are finer than those of the right ventricle and are more developed toward the apex, with a smoother proximal septum. The normal end-diastolic left ventricular volumes on CMR are 160 ± 29 mL in boys and men and 135 ± 26 mL in girls and women. The normal end-systolic volumes are 50 ± 16 mL in boys and men and 42 ± 12 mL in girls and women (Fig. 13-9).

The mitral valve, similar to the tricuspid valve, has a supporting annulus and valve cusps, which are attached to chordae tendineae and papillary muscles. The orifice of the mitral valve is smaller than that of the tricuspid valve, with a mean circumference of 9.0 cm in boys and men compared with the mean tricuspid valve circumference of 11.4 cm in boys and men. The geometry of the mitral valve is complex, and the supporting fibrocollagenous annulus allows significant changes in the conformation of the valve throughout the cardiac cycle. The mitral valve is considered bicuspid, with an anterior and posterior cusp or leaflet. A continuous veil is attached around the orifice, with two deep indentations that form the commissure with valve leaflet coaptation. The anterior leaflet is smaller than the posterior leaflet and covers one third of the orifice; the posterior leaflet covers the remainder. The posterior valve leaflet may have additional indentations that divide it into three crescentic scallops, with the largest in the middle of the cusp.

Within the left ventricle are anterolateral and posteromedial papillary muscles that give rise to chordae tendineae, usually from the apical one third of the muscle. The chordae tendineae typically arise as a single stem and then divide into branches that attach to the corresponding valve cusps. Chordae tendineae may also arise from the ventricular wall and attach to the mitral valve cusps. These are called basal chordae. False chordae are a common anatomic variant that are present in up to 50% of people. They are chordae tendineae that do not attach to the mitral valve cusps but instead connect two papillary muscles, a papillary muscle to the ventricular wall, or two ventricular walls together. Chordae tendineae attaching the mitral valve to the septum are abnormal and may be associated with atrioventricular septal defects.

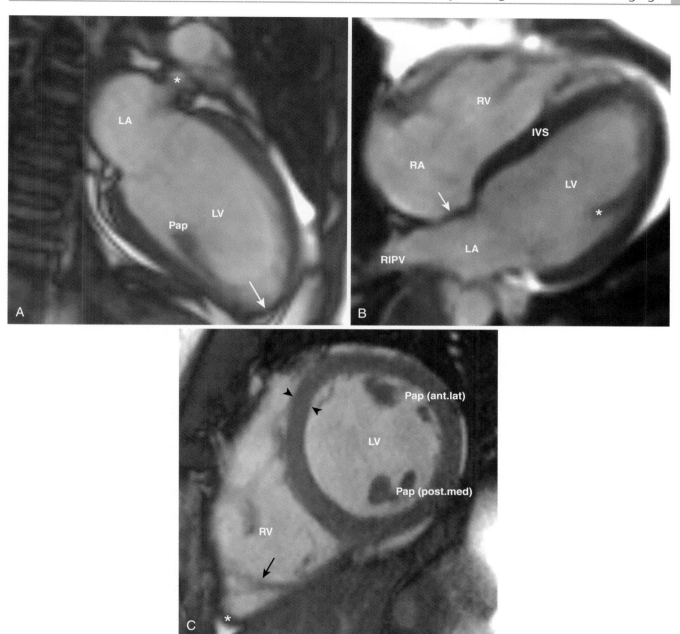

Figure 13-8 Steady-state free precession (SSFP) images in the typical standardized image planes acquired during cardiac magnetic resonance imaging (vertical long-axis, horizontal long-axis, and short-axis views). Vertical long-axis view (**A**) shows the apical thin point *(arrow)*, a normal structure that can help differentiate normal from apical variant hypertrophic cardiomyopathy. Note also the left atrial appendage *(asterisk)*; it should be scrutinized to exclude thrombus. The horizontal long-axis view (**B**) demonstrates the anterolateral papillary muscle *(asterisk)*. Note also the interatrial septum *(arrow)*, which can appear very thin on SSFP sequences and should not be mistaken for a shunt. The left ventricular short-axis view (**C**) shows the anterolateral (ant. lat.) and posteromedial (post. med.) papillary muscles of the left ventricle. The end-diastolic left ventricular wall should measure less than 12 mm *(arrowheads)*. The ratio of the anteroseptal wall to the posterolateral wall is normally less than 1.3 to 1.5. Note how much more trabeculated the right ventricle is compared with the left ventricle. Some of the trabeculations may be quite thick *(arrow)* and should not be mistaken for the right ventricular free wall *(asterisk)*. *IVS,* Interventricular septum; *LA,* left atrium; *LV,* left ventricle; *Pap,* papillary muscle; *RA,* right atrium; *RIPV,* right inferior pulmonary vein; *RV,* right ventricle.

The aortic valve has three semilunar cusps and, as in the pulmonary valve, no complete cartilaginous ring supporting the cusps. Instead, the aortic valve has a semilunar fibrous attachment. The anterior and right cusp is called the right coronary cusp, the left posterior cusp is called the left coronary cusp, and the right posterior cusp is caller the noncoronary cusp. The sinuses

of Valsalva extend superior to the level of the aortic cusps and give the aortic root a clover-leaf appearance when it is viewed axially. At the superior limit of the sinuses is the sinotubular ridge or junction. The aortic walls thin at the level of each sinus and are less than one fourth the thickness of the sinotubular ridge. The diameter of the aortic root at the level of the sinuses is

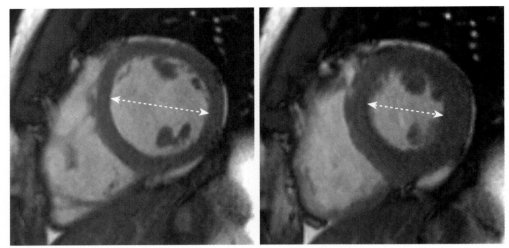

Figure 13-9 Steady-state free precession left ventricular short-axis images in end-diastole *(left)* and end systole *(right)*. The end-diastolic mean diameters are 50.2 mm (upper 95% confidence interval, 58.5 mm) for male patients and 45.6 mm (upper 95% confidence interval, 51.1 mm) for female patients.

up to two times larger than the size of the ascending aorta. The closed aortic valve has a triradiate appearance (Mercedes Benz sign). Because the pressure in the ventricle exceeds that of the systemic circulation, the aortic valve opens passively. The combination of increased pressure in the left ventricle and the fibroelastic walls of the upper portions of the sinuses allows the radius of the aortic sinuses to increase by approximately 16% during left ventricular systole. The commissures move apart, and the aortic valve opens with a triangular orifice because the valve cusps do not oppose the sinus walls. The aortic sinuses form vortices during valve opening and have been shown experimentally to reduce aortic regurgitation.

Clinical Pearls

In clinical practice, the examiner should provide not just absolute measurements of left ventricular volumetrics but also measurements normalized for age and body surface area.

■ CORONARY ARTERIAL ANATOMY

See Chapter 37.

■ CORONARY VENOUS ANATOMY

The coronary sinus, the anterior cardiac veins, and the small cardiac veins drain the heart. Most veins drain into the coronary sinus, which lies in the left posterior atrioventricular groove. The coronary sinus receives venous blood from the great, middle, and small cardiac veins, the oblique vein of the left atrium, and the posterior vein of the left ventricle. The anterior cardiac veins drain the anterior part of the right ventricle before passing into the right atrioventricular groove. They form a vein called the anterior marginal vein, which typically drains directly into the right atrium. Numerous small cardiac veins are also present that drain directly into all cardiac

chambers but most frequently into the right atrium and the right ventricle.

Clinical Pearls

A large coronary sinus may be a clue to the presence of a left-sided SVC. A persistent left-sided SVC usually courses inferiorly between the left atrium and the left superior pulmonary vein before it drains into the coronary sinus.

■ PULMONARY ARTERY

The pulmonary artery is approximately 5 cm in length and in diameter should be smaller than or equal to the adjacent ascending aorta. The mean diameter of the pulmonary artery is 2.7 cm, with the upper limit of normal between 3.3 and 3.5 cm. The pulmonary artery sits within the visceral pericardium. The fibrous pericardium fuses with the adventitia of the pulmonary arteries. The left pulmonary artery continues in the direction of the main pulmonary artery and travels over the left main bronchus and into the left hilum. The right pulmonary artery angles acutely to the right and posteriorly along the roof of the left atrium before it enters the right hilum. The ascending aorta and the SVC lie anterior to the right pulmonary artery.

■ AORTA

The thoracic aorta commences at the level of the aortic valve and is divided into ascending aorta, the aortic arch, and the descending aorta. The ascending aorta is further divided into tubular and sinus portions. The sinus component is described with the aortic valve in the section on the left ventricle. The tubular component extends from the sinotubular junction to the origin of the brachiocephalic trunk. The diameter of the tubular component increases with age and is larger in male than in female patients. The upper limits of the normal diameter of the ascending aorta, when measured in the transaxial plane from side to side (rather than from anterior to posterior) orthogonal to the expected long axis of the arch and at the level of the main pulmonary artery, are 36 mm for boys and mens and 33.5 mm for girls and women. The aortic arch begins to the right at the upper border of the second right sternocostal joint and arches posteriorly and to the left past the left lateral aspect of the trachea, to lie to the left of T4. The aortic arch typically gives rise to three branches. The first branch is the innominate artery (or brachiocephalic trunk), which divides into the right subclavian and right common carotid arteries. The second branch is the left common carotid artery, and the third branch is the left subclavian artery.

This normal pattern is present in about 70% of people. The most common variation is common origin of the left common carotid artery and the innominate artery; less often, the common carotid artery arises directly from the innominate artery (see Fig. 13-1). These two variations are frequently referred to as a bovine-type arch, although technically this term is a misnomer because cattle do not usually have this arch anatomy. Common origin of the left common carotid artery and left innominate artery is more common in blacks (25%) than in whites (8%) and has an overall incidence of 13%. Origin of the left common carotid artery from the innominate artery is also more common in blacks (10%) than in whites (5%) and has an overall incidence of 9%.

The descending thoracic aorta begins just distal to the left subclavian artery origin, usually near the lower border of T4, and ends at the lower border of T12. It is initially to the left of midline but moves anterior to the vertebral column as it descends within the posterior mediastinum. The descending thoracic aorta gives rise to bronchial arteries (usually one right and two left) and paired intercostal arteries.

Clinical Pearl

The term bovine arch is a misnomer. Cattle have a single common brachiocephalic trunk arising from the aorta that gives rise to both subclavian arteries and a bicarotid trunk.

■ SUPERIOR VENA CAVA

The SVC is formed by the union of the innominate veins behind the lower border of the first right rib. The left innominate vein is much longer than the right innominate vein because it must cross the midline, anterior to the aortic arch, to form the SVC. The SVC is valveless and descends vertically before it enters the right atrium at the level of the third right costal cartilage. The SVC lies anterior to the right pulmonary artery, and the inferior half of the SVC is covered with fibrous pericardium. The azygos vein arches anteriorly at the level of T4, over the right pulmonary artery, to drain into the SVC. In 1% of people, the azygos vein fails to migrate superiorly over the lung apex and instead invests itself within the right upper lobe, surrounded by the pleural layers, to forming an azygos fissure. The lung contained medially within the azygos fissure is termed an azygos lobe.

Clinical Pearl

An enlarged azygos vein may be a clue to the presence of azygos continuation of the IVC.

Bibliography

Fuster V, Alexander RW, O'Rourke RA, eds. *Hurst's The Heart.* 11th ed. New York: McGraw-Hill; 2004:45-87.

Kwong R. *Cardiovascular Magnetic Resonance Imaging.* Totowa, NJ: Humana; 2008:79–113.

Standring S, ed. *Gray's Anatomy: The Anatomical Basis of Clinical Practice.* 39th ed. New York: Churchill Livingstone; 2005:977-1057.

CHAPTER 14

Cardiac Anatomy on Coronary Angiography

Joo Heung Yoon, Brian G. Hynes and Ik-Kyung Jang

Tremendous advances in understanding of the circulatory system stemmed from the groundbreaking work of Claude Bernard, a French physiologist who performed cardiac catheterization of an equine heart in 1844. However, only with Wilhelm Konrad Röentgen's revolutionary discovery of x-rays in Germany in 1895 did direct imaging of the heart in vivo became feasible. The first human in vivo cardiac catheterization was performed in 1929 by the German urologist Werner Forssmann, who put a urethral catheter into the right cardiac chambers through his own antecubital vein. Subsequently, the era of percutaneous invasive cardiology was introduced by Andreas Gruentzig in 1977.

In the clinical setting, coronary angiography is performed to visualize coronary endoluminal vascular anatomy in assessing for the presence (and burden) or absence of coronary artery disease. Information about the luminal obstructive pattern and collateral pattern can also be obtained. Conventional invasive coronary angiography remains the standard procedure in the evaluation of anatomic coronary disease, although it has limitations. In vivo structural and physiologic evaluations such as intravascular ultrasound (IVUS) and fractional flow reserve have expanded the clinical usefulness of invasive diagnostic cardiac catheterization.

This chapter provides a clinically oriented review of coronary anatomy as assessed with cardiac angiography. Normal coronary anatomy as assessed with conventional coronary angiography is reviewed, as are common coronary artery anomalies.

■ NORMAL CORONARY ANATOMY

Two coronary ostia arise from the proximal aorta; the left main coronary artery (LMCA) comes out of the left coronary sinus, and the right coronary artery (RCA) originates from the right coronary sinus, located slightly lower than the LMCA ostium. The LMCA is further divided into the left anterior descending (LAD) coronary artery and the left circumflex (LCx) coronary artery. The LMCA, LAD, and LCx arteries and their branches comprise the left coronary system, and the RCA belongs to the right coronary system (Fig. 14-1). Depending on the vessel sizes and collateral vessels, the posterior (inferior wall) side of the heart can be supplied by different arteries. Hence, the coronary blood flow system can be referred to as either left dominant

(both the posterior descending and posterior left ventricular branches originate from the LCx artery; 15% of cases) or right dominant (both branches take off from the RCA; 60% to 85% of cases). In addition, codominance (balanced distribution) of the arteries (the posterior descending branch comes from the RCA, and the posterior left ventricular branch derives from the LCx artery) is found in less than 20% of cases. Normally, the arteries run through grooves of the epicardial surface of the heart.

Common Views for Coronary Angiography

Horizontally, the x-ray plane can be positioned in the midline (anteroposterior [AP] view), from the patient's left side (left anterior oblique [LAO] view) or right side (right anterior oblique [RAO] view). Perpendicular angles are either cranial (downward view from the head of the patient) or caudal (upward view from the foot of the patient) (Fig. 14-2). No fixed sequence of order in visualization is used because each patient may have different indications for coronary angiography. However, the angiographer usually begins with an evaluation of the left coronary system and then proceeds to right coronary angiography. When left heart catheterization is indicated (i.e., to assess left ventricular end-diastolic pressure), this should be carried out before contrast administration.

The following practical angiography sequence is routinely used:
1. RAO caudal for the LMCA, proximal LAD artery, and LCx artery
2. RAO cranial for the middle and distal portions of the LAD artery
3. LAO cranial for the middle and distal portions in an orthogonal position
4. LAO caudal ("spider view") for the LMCA, proximal LAD artery, and LCx artery
5. LAO caudal for the proximal RCA
6. AP or LAO cranial for the distal RCA, posterior descending artery (PDA), and posterior left ventricular branch

Table 14-1 summarizes commonly used views for each coronary artery segment. However, additional views can be obtained in case of overlapping or unclear images.

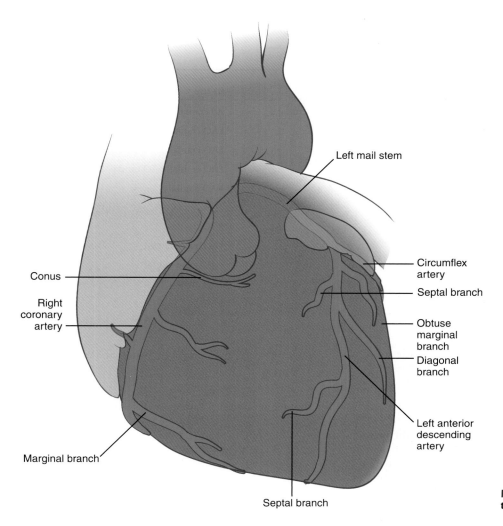

Figure 14-1 Schematic drawing of the coronary arteries.

Left mail stem

Circumflex artery

Septal branch

Obtuse marginal branch

Diagonal branch

Left anterior descending artery

Septal branch

Conus

Right coronary artery

Marginal branch

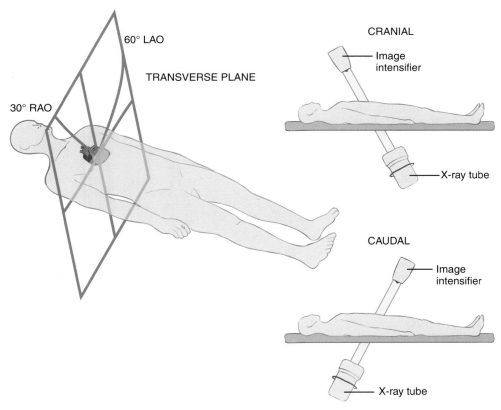

60° LAO

TRANSVERSE PLANE

30° RAO

CRANIAL

Image intensifier

X-ray tube

CAUDAL

Image intensifier

X-ray tube

Figure 14-2 Fluoroscopic planes for cardiac catheterization. *LAO*, Left anterior oblique; *RAO*, right anterior oblique.

Table 14-1   Common Angiographic Views for Coronary Artery

Coronary Artery Branches and Segments	At Origin	In the Course
LMCA	AP cranial, RAO caudal, LAO cranial, LAO caudal	AP cranial, LAO caudal
Proximal LAD	LAO cranial, RAO cranial, AP caudal	LAO cranial, LAO caudal, RAO cranial
Mid-LAD	LAO cranial, RAO cranial	LAO cranial, LAO caudal, RAO cranial
Distal LAD	AP cranial, RAO cranial	LAO cranial, LAO caudal, RAO cranial
Diagonal	LAO cranial, RAO cranial	RAO cranial
Proximal LCx	RAO caudal, LAO caudal	LAO caudal
OM	RAO caudal, LAO caudal	RAO caudal
Proximal RCA	LAO	LAO, right lateral
Mid-RCA	RAO, LAO	LAO, right lateral
Distal RCA	LAO cranial	LAO cranial
PDA	LAO cranial	RAO
Posterior left ventricular	RAO cranial	RAO cranial

Modified from Fuster V, O'Rourke RA, Walsh RA et al, eds. *Hurst's the Heart.* 12th ed. New York: McGraw-Hill; 2008.

AP, Anteroposterior; *LAD,* left anterior descending; *LAO,* left anterior oblique; *LCx,* left circumflex; *LMCA,* left main coronary artery; *OM,* obtuse marginal; *PDA,* posterior descending artery; *RAO,* right anterior oblique; *RCA,* right coronary artery.

Segmental Nomenclature of the Coronary Artery System

The Coronary Artery Surgery Study (CASS) classification system of the coronary artery tree was developed by the CASS, Thrombolysis in Myocardial Infarction (TIMI), and Bypass Angioplasty Revascularization Investigation (BARI) study groups in 1992. The entire coronary arterial network is divided into 29 anatomic segments. Figure 14-3 illustrates three coronary arteries and their major branches. Numbers 1 through 8 denote the RCA and its branches. The LAD and LCx arteries are detailed in numbers 12 to 17, and 18 to 23, respectively.

Assessment of Coronary Artery Blood Flow

One of the most widely used methods to quantify the coronary angiographic blood flow is the TIMI flow grading system developed by the TIMI group in 1987. Although the trial itself was designed to compare the efficacy of intravenous streptokinase and recombinant-plasminogen activator in achieving reperfusion, this classification was found to be useful in quantifying the flow of diseased coronary arteries (Table 14-2).

The complexity of coronary artery disease can be assessed using the SYNTAX score, which was developed in an effort to provide an evidence base for determination of best treatment options. An online calculator and tutorial with a detailed description can be found online at www.syntaxscore.com.

■ PROBLEM SOLVING: COMBINING CARDIAC ANGIOGRAPHY WITH OTHER IMAGING MODALITIES

For the most part, coronary angiography is limited to detailing large epicardial artery blood flow. Assessing

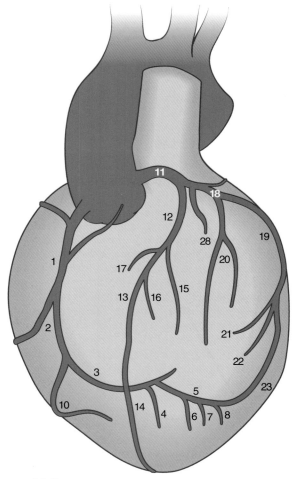

Figure 14-3 The Coronary Artery Surgery Study segmental classification of the coronary arteries.

Table 14-2   Thrombolysis in Myocardial Infarction Classification of Coronary Blood Flow

Grade 0 (no perfusion)	No antegrade flow occurs beyond the point of occlusion.
Grade 1 (penetration with minimal perfusion)	The contrast material passes beyond the area of obstruction, but it "hangs up" and fails to opacify the entire coronary bed distal to the obstruction for duration of the cine run.
Grade 2 (partial perfusion)	The contrast material passes across the obstruction and opacifies the coronary bed distal to the obstruction. However, the rate of entry of contrast material into the vessel distal to the obstruction or its rate of clearance from the distal bed (or both) is perceptibly slower than its entry into or clearance from comparable areas not perfused by the previously occluded vessel (e.g., the opposite coronary artery or the coronary bed proximal to the obstruction).
Grade 3 (complete perfusion)	Antegrade flow into the bed distal to the obstruction occurs as promptly as antegrade flow into the bed proximal to the obstruction, and clearance of contrast material from the involved bed is as rapid as clearance from an uninvolved bed in the same vessel or the opposite artery.

Modified from Sheehan FH, Braunwald E, Canner P, et al. The effect of intravenous thrombolytic therapy on left ventricular function: a report on tissue-type plasminogen activator and streptokinase from the Thrombolysis in Myocardial Infarction (TIMI Phase I) trial. *Circulation*. 1987;75:817-829.

myocardial perfusion defects (ischemia or infarction) with other noninvasive imaging modalities plays a crucial role in guiding revascularization therapy. The American Heart Association suggested a 17-segment system of regional wall distribution map for 2-dimensional echocardiography (Fig. 14-4, *A*) and for single photon emission computed tomography (SPECT) nuclear cardiology study (see Fig. 14-4, *B*).

■ **PROBLEM SOLVING: ANGIOGRAPHIC VISUALIZATION OF INDIVIDUAL CORONARY ARTERY AND ITS BRANCHES**

Because the coronary arteries form a globelike three-dimensional structure around the myocardium, each segment must be visualized at a specific angle. Moreover, because of the eccentricity of the obstruction, a different angle is often required to visualize the same segment of artery to obtain a clearer picture. Orthogonal views are desired to exclude significant stenosis, given the potential limitation of underestimation of eccentric stenoses and foreshortening of vessels.

Left Main Coronary Artery

The LMCA originates from the left coronary sinus. Studies showed that the average length of the LMCA measures approximately 3 to 6 mm, with a wide variation of 0 to 15 mm. The average diameter of the LMCA is approximately 4.5 mm, but it can vary from 3 to 6 mm, depending on gender and ethnicity. Table 14-3 shows anatomic variations in coronary artery diameter by gender. Several studies showed that the LMCA diameter is 75% to 91% smaller in women than in men. The LMCA runs behind the right ventricular outflow tract (RVOT), between the pulmonary trunk and the left atrium. At the distal end, it bifurcates to the LAD and LCx arteries. In approximately 30% of the population, the intermediate branch (ramus intermedius) exists between the LAD and LCx arteries. This intermediate artery usually follows the course of a high obtuse marginal (OM) branch of the LCx artery.

Standard views for the LMCA include the RAO caudal and AP views (Fig. 14-5, *A* and *B*), in addition to the LAO caudal view. The LAO caudal view is very useful for

separating the distal LMCA in cases of overlapping vessels (see Fig. 14-5, *C*).

Left Anterior Descending Coronary Artery

The LAD artery arises from the LMCA, crosses beneath the left atrial appendage, and travels down the anterior interventricular sulcus to feed the majority of the anterior wall of the left ventricle and ventricular septum. The average diameter of the proximal LAD artery is 3.5 to 3.6 mm in men and 2.9 to 3.2 mm in women. In general, women tend to have a 15% to 20% smaller diameter compared with men. The diameter of the LAD artery tapers gradually as it runs distally (see Table 14-3). Approximately 80% to 90% of population will exhibit left coronary dominance wherein the LAD artery wraps around the apex and runs in the inferior interventricular groove on the back of the heart (Fig. 14-6, *A*). In contrast, only 40% to 50% of the LAD artery goes beyond the apex in case of right dominance because the RCA supplies the apical territory with its PDA branch (see Fig. 14-6, *B*).

Along the course of the LAD artery, side branches of two major types can be seen: the diagonal (D) and septal (S) (or perforating) branches (Fig. 14-7). In general, the diagonal branches are larger, longer, and have more angular takeoff from the LAD artery. Diagonal arteries run across between the interventricular and AV grooves and supply the anterior left ventricular free wall, the anterolateral mitral papillary muscle, and part of the anterior right ventricular wall. The septal branches are usually smaller, shorter, and form almost perpendicular angles to the LAD artery. These perforating branches enter the septum and deliver blood to the apical and anterior two thirds of the interventricular septum. The first septal perforating branch perfuses the His bundle and the proximal left bundle branch.

Left Circumflex Coronary Artery

The LCx artery arises at an almost perpendicular angle from the LMCA and runs behind the left atrial appendage toward the posterior surface of the heart. The average diameter of the proximal LCx artery is 3.1 to 3.4 mm in men and 2.6 to 2.9 mm in women. Along its course,

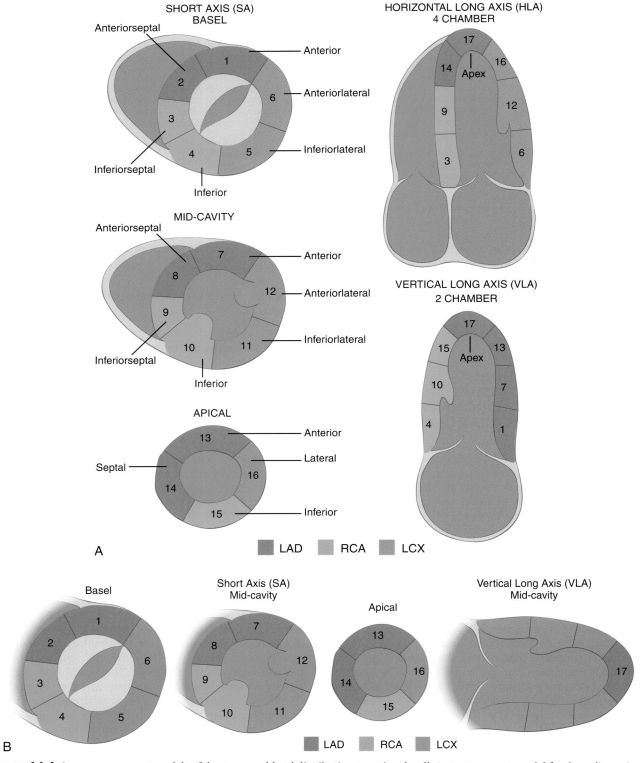

Figure 14-4 Seventeen-segment models of the coronary blood distribution to regional wall. **A,** A 17-segment model for the 2-dimensional transthoracic echocardiography. **B,** A 17-segmental model for the nuclear stress test. *LAD,* Left anterior descending artery; *LCx,* left circumflex artery; *RCA,* right coronary artery.

Table 14-3   Angiographic Coronary Artery Diameter by Location and Gender

	Dodge et al	MacAlpin et al	Others
LMCA (mm)	4.5 ± 0.5 (men) 3.9 ± 0.4 (women)	4.3 ± 0.6 (men) 3.5 ± 0.7 (women)	
Proximal LAD (mm)	3.6 ± 0.5 (men) 3.2 ± 0.5 (women)	3.5 ± 0.5 (men) 2.9 ± 0.4 (women)	3.3 ± 0.5 (Kimball et al)
Mid-LAD (mm)	2.3 ± 0.4 (men) 2.2 ± 0.5 (women)	2.0 ± 0.4 (men) 1.8 ± 0.2 (women)	
Distal LAD (mm)	1.1 ± 0.4 (men) 0.9 ± 0.3 (women)		
Proximal LCx (mm)*	3.4 ± 0.5 (men) 2.9 ± 0.6 (women)	3.1 ± 0.7 (men) 2.6 ± 0.6 (women)	
Proximal RCA (mm)†	3.9 ± 0.6 (men) 3.3 ± 0.6 (women)	3.4 ± 0.7 (men) 3.0 ± 0.5 (women)	

Data from Dodge JT Jr, Brown BG, Bolson EL, et al. Lumen diameter of normal human coronary arteries; influence of age, sex, anatomic variation, and left ventricular hypertrophy or dilation. *Circulation.* 1992;86:232-246; MacAlpin RN, Abbasi AS, Grollman JH, et al. Human coronary artery size during life: a cinearteriographic study. *Radiology.* 1973;108:567-576; and Kimball BP, LiPreti V, Buis, et al. Comparison of proximal left anterior descending and circumflex coronary artery dimensions in aortic valve stenosis and hypertrophic cardiomyopathy. *Am J Cardiol.* 1990;65:767-771..
LAD, Left anterior descending; *LCx,* left circumflex; *LMCA,* left main coronary artery; *RCA,* right coronary artery.
*Measured from the segment proximal to the first obtuse marginal branch.
†Measured from the segment proximal to the first acute marginal branch.

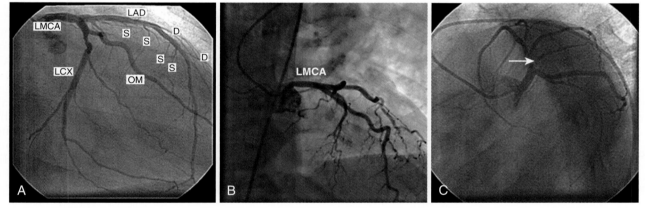

Figure 14-5 Variable angiographic views of the left main coronary artery (LMCA). **A,** Right anterior oblique caudal view visualizes the LMCA. The proximal left anterior descending (LAD) and left circumflex (LCx) arteries are also seen. **B,** Anteroposterior cranial view to visualize the LMCA. **C,** Left anterior oblique caudal "spider" view to visualize the LMCA and the proximal LAD. The intermediate branch (ramus) is also seen *(arrow)*.

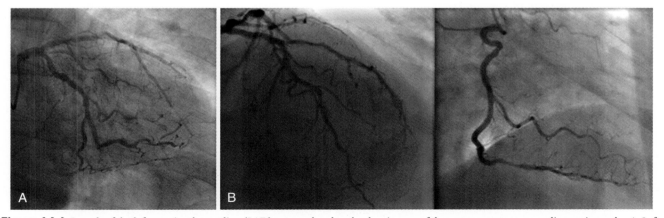

Figure 14-6 Length of the left anterior descending (LAD) artery related to the dominance of the coronary artery on cardiac angiography. **A,** Left-dominant coronary artery system. **B,** Right-dominant coronary artery system *(left panel,* the LAD and the left circumflex (LCx) arteries; *right panel,* the right coronary artery). Compare the length of the LAD in the right-dominant system with the left-dominant system in **A.**

it gives off OM branches, which run in between the anterior and posterior left ventricular free wall. These branches follow the obtuse angle of the surface and supply the posterolateral wall of the left ventricle. Usually, two or three OM branches can be seen on a coronary angiogram. They can be numbered from proximal to distal, as follows: the anterolateral branch (OM1), the OM branch (OM2), and the posterior left ventricular branch (OM3) (Fig. 14-8).

In approximately 60% to 85% of population, the LCx artery is nondominant. In this case, the RCA supplies the inferior side of the heart with the PDA. In 7% to 20%, the LCx artery supplies the posterior descending branch

of the RCA (left dominance). When the LCx artery supplies territories normally supplied by the RCA, it gives rise to the atrioventricular (AV) node branch. In approximately 40% of those left-dominant cases, the LCx artery is also responsible for the (SA) node.

Right Coronary Artery

The RCA arises from the right coronary cusp. It travels down the right atrial appendage groove, which connects to the right AV groove. The average diameter of the proximal RCA is 3.4 to 3.9 mm in men and 3.0 to 3.3 mm in women. The conus branch, which is the first branch arising from the RCA, runs anteriorly to supply the infundibulum. In approximately 50% of the population, this branch takes off directly from the right ostium. The conus branch supplies the RVOT and creates an anastomosis with an analogous branch of the LAD artery (circle of Vieussens). The acute marginal branches originate from the RCA to supply the right ventricular free wall. The PDA supplies the posterior third of the interventricular septum, which is drained by the middle cardiac vein. At the distal RCA, the PDA and distal posterior left ventricular branches arise in the right-dominant heart. Those arteries then supply the basal and middle inferior walls, as well as the base of the inferior septum.

The RCA provides blood flow to many components of the conduction system. In approximately 60% of cases, the SA node is supplied by the RCA. However, this artery may also arise from the LCx artery (35% to 40%) or even directly from the aorta (1%). The SA nodal artery may then take three different routes (precaval, postcaval, or pericaval) around the superior vena cava to reach the SA node. In the right-dominant system, the PDA and posterior left ventricular branches give smaller branches to the conduction system, including the AV node, His bundle, right bundle branch, and posterior portion of the left bundle branch (Fig. 14-9).

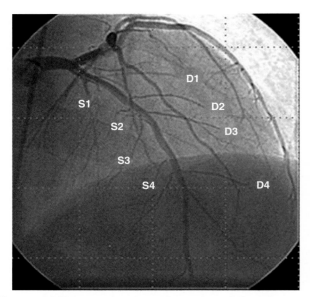

Figure 14-7 Diagonal and septal branches of the left anterior descending (LAD) artery. From the anteroposterior cranial projection, the LAD shows two types of branches: diagonal (D1, D2, D3, D4) and septal (S1, S2, S3, S4).

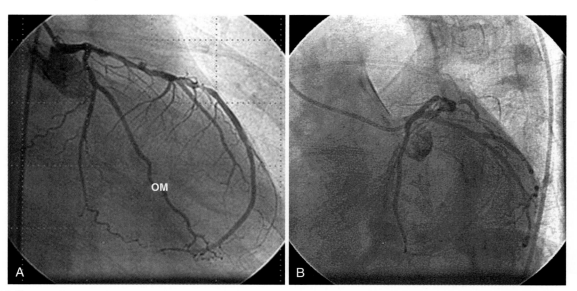

Figure 14-8 The left circumflex (LCx) coronary artery. A, Right anterior oblique caudal view, showing obtuse marginal (OM) branches of the LCx artery. **B,** Left anterior oblique caudal view.

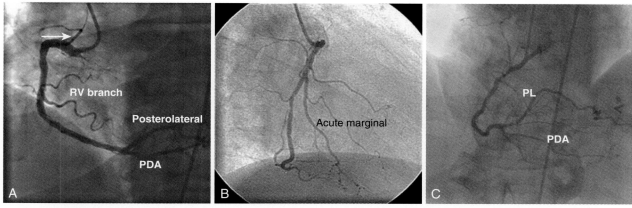

Figure 14-9 The right coronary artery (RCA). **A,** The conus branch *(arrow)* and the posterior descending artery (PDA) of the RCA are seen on this left anterior oblique projection of the right-dominant coronary system. The PDA, shown in the right lower side of the x-ray plane, supplies the inferior and posterior wall. *RV,* Right ventricular. **B,** The acute marginal branch is clearly seen in the right anterior oblique view. **C,** Anteroposterior cranial view of the RCA shows the PDA and posterior left ventricular (PL) branch.

■ PROBLEM SOLVING: VISUALIZATION OF ANOMALOUS CORONARY ARTERIES ON CORONARY ANGIOGRAPHY

Angelini et al defined a coronary anomaly as any coronary artery pattern seen only rarely in the general population (i.e., <1% of cases). Defining features of an anomalous artery may relate to number of ostia or proximal course, as well as a host of other deviations from patterns commonly encountered in the physiologically normal population (Box 14-1). Although the incidence of coronary anomalies encountered during conventional coronary angiography ranges from 0.6% to 1.6%, data indicate that they may account for almost 12% of deaths in high school and college athletes in the United States. Similar data from the American Heart Association suggest that coronary anomalies may be responsible for up to 19% of cases of sudden cardiac death (SCD) in athletes. The exact pathophysiologic mechanism for anomaly-induced SCD remains unclear, although certain abnormal anatomic features have been associated with myocardial ischemia resulting from possible compression, torsion, or vasospasm of the anomalous coronary artery. Investigators have postulated that this situation, in turn, may precipitate syncope or malignant arrhythmias. Approximately 80% of adults with coronary anomalies are asymptomatic. The incidental finding of a morphologically abnormal coronary artery on cardiac angiography may present a dilemma resulting from the continued uncertainty of the clinical significance of coronary anomalies with regard to morbidity and risk of SCD. This chapter contains a brief overview of the more commonly encountered coronary anomalies.

Many noninvasive diagnostic methods can also be used to evaluate coronary anomalies. Transesophageal echocardiography may detect these anomalies in some cases, but the diagnostic yield is very low. Contrast-enhanced computed tomography may provide detailed information of the coronary arterial tree because of the high spatial resolution. Magnetic resonance imaging is

---

BOX 14-1   Classification of the Anomalous Coronary Artery

Anomaly of Origin and Course
- Absence of left main trunk (separate left anterior descending and left circumflex artery ostia)
- Anomalous location of coronary ostium
- Anomalous location of coronary ostium, outside normal coronary aortic sinuses*
- Anomalous origination of coronary ostium from opposite coronary sinus† or noncusped (posterior) sinus
- Single coronary artery

Anomaly of Intrinsic Coronary Artery Anatomy
- Congenital ostial stenosis or atresia
- Coronary ectasia or aneurysm
- Coronary hypoplasia
- Intramural coronary artery (myocardial bridging)
- Intercoronary communication

Anomaly of Coronary Termination
- Coronary artery fistula

Modified from Angelini P. Coronary artery anomalies. *Circulation.* 2007;115:1296-1305.
*Examples including anomalous left coronary artery from the pulmonary artery (ALCAPA) or right coronary artery from the pulmonary artery (Bland-White-Garland syndrome).
†In cases of opposite origin, the subclassifications of anomaly depend on the course of the coronary artery: interarterial, prepulmonic, retroaortic, and subpulmonic (septal).

also a valuable modality without the associated radiation exposure of CT.

During conventional coronary angiography, the presence of a coronary anomaly should be suspected when multiple attempts to find the coronary ostium when using standard catheters are unsuccessful, or when one of the coronary systems can be visualized with substantial dominance supplying the entire myocardium. Nonselective angiography performed using a pigtail catheter and power injector positioned in the aortic root often helps identify arteries that appear to be missing. In this section, details pertaining to the angiographic features

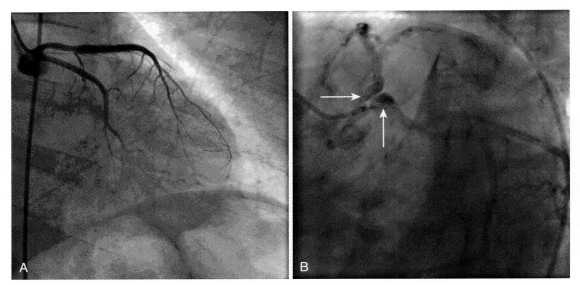

Figure 14-10 Separate origin of the left anterior descending (LAD) and left circumflex (LCx) coronary arteries from the left coronary sinus. **A,** Left heart catheterization shows only the LAD and LCx arteries without a common trunk. The proximal part of the LAD is diseased and was previously treated with a stent. **B,** Left anterior oblique caudal view shows that the LAD and LCx arteries originate *(arrows)* from two separate ostia, without forming the left main coronary artery.

of some more common anomalies are illustrated. Box 14-1 summarizes the classification of coronary anomalies developed by Angelini et al.

Anomalies of the Origin and Course

Absence of the Left Main Coronary Artery (Separate Origin of the Left Anterior Descending and Left Circumflex Arteries from the Left Coronary Sinus)

Absence of the LMCA is one of the most common (~30% of all anomalies) types of coronary anomaly, and it is often accompanied by aortic valve disease and dominance of the left coronary artery (Fig. 14-10). With the separate ostia in the left sinus of Valsalva, a true LMCA is absent. This anomaly is best visualized in the LAO caudal projection, with contrast injection into the left sinus. The investigator should be mindful of this anomaly, to ensure complete angiography of the left system. Because no other anomalies in distribution of coronary blood flow are present, this feature is not thought to result in myocardial ischemia.

Aortic Origin of the Coronary Ostium

The origin of the left coronary system may be located above the left coronary sinus. An example is high takeoff of the LMCA (Fig. 14-11). Defining this anomaly can sometimes be challenging, and measurement can be difficult. Muriago et al compared the height of the coronary ostium with the depth of the coronary sinus and defined a high takeoff anomaly as one in which the location of the coronary ostium is higher than 120% of the depth of the coronary sinus. The angiographer should suspect this anomaly when a thorough search of the left coronary sinus shows no coronary ostium. Aortography usually facilitates identification of the artery. High takeoff

has been associated with SCD, although this association is extremely rare. This anomaly may have implications for the cardiac surgeon with regard to aortic clamping or vein graft placement during operation.

Anomalous Location of the Coronary Ostium Outside Normal Coronary Sinuses

This rare syndrome, which occurs in 1 in 300,000 live births and is also known as Bland-White-Garland syndrome, is characterized by the origin of the left coronary system from the pulmonary artery. An example is an anomalous left coronary artery from the pulmonary artery (ALPACA) (Fig. 14-12). Prompt surgical reconstruction of a dual blood supply is given a class I recommendation. The deoxygenated blood runs through the coronary artery system, and this syndrome is among the most common causes of myocardial ischemia and infarction in children, with mortality rates of up to 90% at 12 months. The clinical manifestations are variable and may represent global dysfunction. These features include a continuous murmur, angina, mitral regurgitation, cardiac arrhythmias, myocardial ischemia, and SCD.

Similarly, the origin of the RCA from the pulmonary artery has also been described. It is frequently not symptomatic and is usually an incidental finding during imaging, operation, or autopsy. Different management strategies have been introduced, but single bypass of the RCA may be preferred.

Anomalous Origin of the Coronary Ostium from the Opposite Coronary Sinus or the Noncusped (Posterior) Sinus

This anomaly is diagnosed when the ostium of one coronary artery is found in the cusp other than its inherent location. Four patterns of this anomaly are possible: (1) the RCA from the left coronary sinus; (2) the LMCA

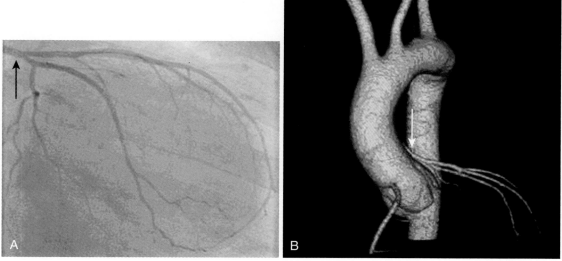

Figure 14-11 Aortic origin of the left main coronary artery (high takeoff). **A,** Cardiac angiography of the anomalous origin of the left main coronary artery (LMCA) from the ascending aorta. The LMCA *(arrow)* and distribution of the left coronary system otherwise look unremarkable. **B,** Three-dimensional reconstructed computed tomography scan image of the aortic arch. The LMCA is originating from the ascending aorta, above the coronary sinus *(arrow)*. The right coronary artery is at its normal level. (From Purvis M, Dunphy T. Anomalous origin of the left main coronary artery from the ascending aorta. *J Invasive Cardiol.* 2008;20:681-682.)

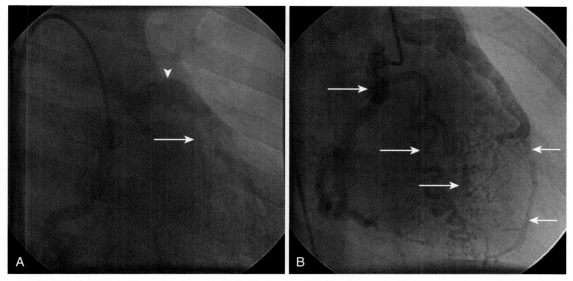

Figure 14-12 Anomalous left coronary artery from the pulmonary artery (ALCAPA). **A,** An angiogram of a 16-year-old patient who developed cardiac arrest at school. On an echocardiogram, a severely dilated right coronary artery was found. Cardiac angiography showed the left coronary system *(arrow)* originating from the pulmonary artery *(arrowhead)*. The patient underwent an emergency left main coronary artery ligation procedure with saphenous vein graft from the aorta to the middistal left anterior descending (LAD) artery. **B,** Another cardiac angiogram of a patient with ALCAPA. Note the highly tortuous right coronary artery and its branches *(longer arrows)*, with collateral vessels supplying the left side of the heart. The contrast material also fills the pulmonary trunk and anomalous left coronary system. The normal-looking distal LAD artery is seen on the right lower part of the image *(shorter arrows)*. This patient underwent elective single coronary artery bypass graft surgery with a left internal mammary artery graft, with ligation of the anomalous coronary artery at its pulmonary artery origin.

from the right coronary sinus; (3) the LAD artery or LCx branch from the right coronary sinus; and (4) the LAD artery, LCx artery, or RCA originating from the noncoronary sinus (posterior side). In addition, this anomaly of origination usually takes four different routes in returning back to the inherent myocardium, depending on the location of adjacent structures (the aorta and pulmonary trunk). They are as follows: (1) interarterial course (the RCA or LMCA runs between the aorta and the pulmonary trunk); (2) prepulmonic course (runs on the anterior side of the pulmonary artery); (3) retroaortic course (runs behind the aorta); and (4) subpulmonic course (runs beneath the RVOT). The last three courses (prepulmonic, retroaortic, and subpulmonic) are regarded as benign, but the interarterial course should be managed with caution because it is associated with SCD in 30% of cases.

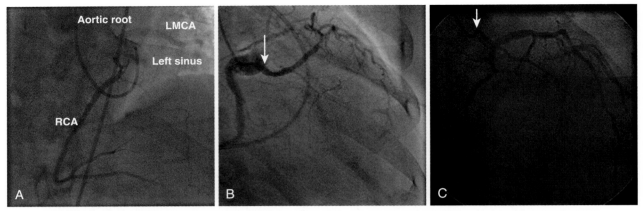

Figure 14-13 Anomalous origination of the coronary ostium from ectopic coronary sinuses. A, Anomalous origination of the right coronary artery (RCA) from the left coronary sinus. The contrast injection into the left coronary sinus reveals both the left main coronary artery (LMCA) and the RCA. **B,** The right coronary angiogram reveals the left coronary system *(arrow)* from the right sinus of Valsalva. **C,** Ectopic origin of the both coronary arteries from the noncusped (posterior) sinus. Left coronary angiography demonstrates a diseased left anterior descending and left circumflex arteries on the right anterior oblique caudal plane. Note the rotation of the catheter toward the posterior cusp to engage the left main ostium *(arrow).*

In a series of autopsy studies, this interarterial course of the coronary artery was found in approximately 80% of the athletes with SCD and an anomalous coronary artery. Traditionally, investigators have offered dynamic closure mechanisms as an explanation. Two possible mechanisms are as follows: (1) the increased cardiac output hinders coronary flow by closing down at the sharp bend of the ostium; or (2) the acute angle of origination can be kinked between the pulmonary artery and the dilated aorta, especially during exertion. Using IVUS, Angelini et al further suggested intramural proximal intussusception of the ectopic artery at the aortic root area as the culprit cause of SCD. Younger patients are more vulnerable to SCD, whereas older patients may have different manifestations (dyspnea, syncope, dizziness, palpitations, or angina).

The origin of the RCA from the left coronary sinus is reported to occur in approximately 0.03% to 0.17% of patients undergoing coronary angiography. Among those patients, the interarterial course is most common (~30% of the patients). Figure 14-13, *A*, shows the anomalous origination of the RCA from the left coronary sinus.

The LMCA may also originate from the right coronary sinus in approximately 0.1% of patients undergoing coronary angiography. In most (75%) cases, the artery follows an interarterial course. This anomaly may be suspected when blood flow to the left lateral wall appears absent during contrast injection of the left coronary system. Especially in the RAO plane, this interarterial course of the LMCA can be seen as a dot-on-end pattern on the anterior surface of the aorta during the aortogram.

A branch of the LMCA, either the LAD or LCx artery, can originate from the right coronary sinus in approximately 0.32% to 0.67%. Usually, this type of anomalous origin takes a subaortic course, without causing significant risk of SCD. The LCx artery originating from the right coronary sinus is the most common anomaly. During coronary angiography, the proximal portion of the LAD artery may appear unusually long. Contrast injection of the right coronary system may then reveal a long LCx artery crossing the aorta toward the left lateral wall (see Fig. 14-13, *B*, which shows abnormal LCx artery origin from the right coronary sinus).

Rarely, the ostia of the coronary arteries can be found in the noncoronary sinus (see Fig. 14-13, *C*). This type of ectopic origin is not usually associated with clinical symptoms or perfusion abnormalities. During cardiac angiography, the examiner should pay additional attention when attempted injection of the left and right sinus of Valsalva fails to visualize both arterial systems or shows only one system without evidence of global distribution or an extensive collateral network. Further catheter readjustment and rotation to the posterior coronary cusp may enable visualization of both coronary systems.

Single Coronary Artery

The occurrence of a single coronary artery, in which just one artery arises from the aorta and divides into all three major branches, has also been linked to SCD during strenuous physical activity (Fig. 14-14). In coronary angiography, this anomaly is defined as a combination of the agenesis of one (left or right) coronary system and complete dominance of the other remaining system over the whole myocardium. No clear-cut criteria are available to classify the single coronary artery, but the investigator can follow the angiographic classification suggested by Lipton et al As a first step, the ostium of the coronary artery is labeled "R" or "L," depending on its location of origin from the right or left coronary sinus, respectively. Then the coronary artery is divided into three groups by its distribution. In group I, one coronary artery covers the whole myocardium without making a side branch to assume the normal position of the inherent coronary artery. Group II starts from the left or right sinus of Valsalva, but the artery runs across the base of the heart to mimic the distribution of the inherent coronary artery. A group III single coronary artery shows a separate origin of the LAD and LCx arteries from the proximal portion of the RCA. In this system

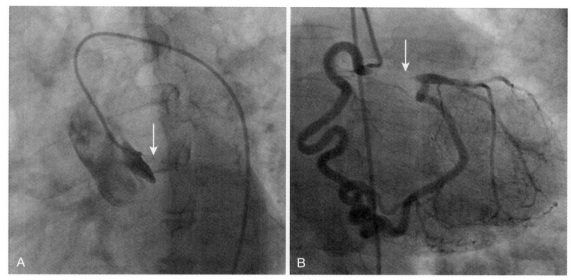

Figure 14-14 Single coronary artery. A, Attempted selective left main coronary artery (LMCA) angiography demonstrates a rudimentary LMCA. Only a thin line of contrast *(arrow)* is shown despite the proper positioning of the catheter. **B,** Catheterization of the right coronary system revealed a large-caliber, tortuous right coronary artery that supplies the entire myocardium and gives branches to the proximal LMCA through the large left circumflex artery.

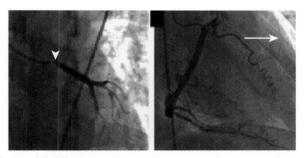

Figure 14-15 Coronary ostial stenosis. The left main coronary artery shows severe ostial stenosis *(left, arrowhead)*. The left coronary system receives collateral flow from the right coronary artery and its branches *(right, arrow)*. The ostial stenosis resulted from extensive Takayasu arteritis in a young female. (From Bansal N, Wang N, Choo D, et al. Ostial left main stenosis due to Takayasu arteritis: multimodality imaging and surgical ostioplasty. *Echocardiography.* 2011;28:E5-E8.)

of nomenclature, the last abbreviations, "A," "B," and "P." refer to anterior, between, and posterior, respectively. This system classifies the relationship between the coronary artery and adjacent structures (i.e., aorta and pulmonary trunk).

Anomaly of Intrinsic Coronary Artery Anatomy

Congenital Ostial Stenosis or Atresia

Ostial stenosis is reported in approximately 0.13% to 0.25% of cardiac angiograms (Fig. 14-15). This lesion can be acquired by pathologic changes of the coronary and aortic arch structures including aortitis (by syphilis or Takayasu disease), or it can be a complication of radiation therapy. Usually, coronary artery bypass graft (CABG) surgery is the preferred revascularization strategy.

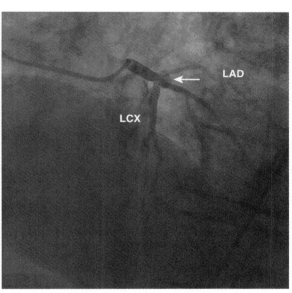

Figure 14-16 Coronary ectasia. Coronary angiography shows aneurysmal change *(arrow)* at the bifurcation of the left anterior descending (LAD) and left circumflex (LCx) arteries.

Coronary Ectasia or Aneurysm

Coronary ectasia or aneurysm refers to an abnormal (1.5 times or more) dilatation of a segment of the coronary artery (Fig. 14-16). The incidence of isolated ectasia is approximately 0.2% to 1.2%. However, this anomaly is sometimes acquired, and pathologic ectasia can be seen at the site of atherosclerosis because of the remodeling process of the diseased coronary artery. The most commonly involved coronary artery is the RCA. Figure 14-16 shows the typical angiographic appearance.

Coronary Hypoplasia

Congenital coronary artery hypoplasia disease is a rare finding, characterized by underdevelopment of one

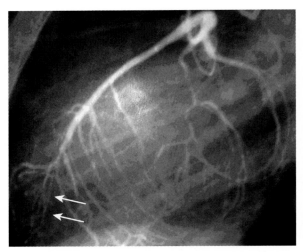

Figure 14-17 Coronary hypoplasia. Left anterior oblique view shows a hypoplastic distal left anterior descending artery *(arrows).* The septal branches are covering the base of the interventricular septum, whereas diagonal branches are lacking. (From Amabile N, Fraisse A, Quilici J. Hypoplastic coronary artery disease: report of one case. *Heart.* 2005;91:e12.)

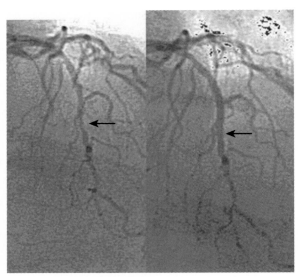

Figure 14-18 Intramural coronary artery (myocardial bridging). Coronary angiography shows rhythmic, phase dependent *(left,* systolic; *right,* diastolic) compression of the midleft anterior descending artery *(arrows).*

or more major branches of the coronary arteries with decreased diameter or length (Fig. 14-17). This anomaly is strongly associated with SCD in children or young adults during intense physical activity. Narrowing of the artery and the resultant demand ischemia likely provoke the fatal arrhythmia resulting in SCD. This anomaly can also be seen in conjunction with the anomalous origin of a coronary artery from the opposite sinus. In this specific anomalous pattern, congenital coronary hypoplasia is formed by intramural intussuscepted portion in the proximal part embedded in the aortic wall. For those affected, cardiac angiography shows clear diagnostic images. Patients often require CABG surgery or heart transplantation.

Intramural Coronary Artery (Myocardial Bridging)

Intramural coronary artery, a rather common anomaly largely confined to the mid-LAD artery, has a reported incidence of 0.5% to 12% during routine coronary angiography (Fig. 14-18). The coronary artery segment normally runs on the epicardial surface. However, where myocardium overlies the coronary artery, a bridge is created between the muscle layers. During angiography, systolic compression of the affected segment is evident. Myocardial bridging has been linked to angina, ventricular dysfunction, arrhythmia, and SCD. Although the intima under the myocardium is thought to be less prone to atherosclerosis, the proximal portion of the bridge may be more susceptible to disease, largely as a consequence of altered hemodynamics. The clinical significance of this anomaly is unclear. Because normally only 15% of coronary flow occurs during systole, the contribution of myocardial bridge itself in causing demand ischemia may not be significant. In patients with progressive atherosclerosis in the proximal segment of the myocardial bridge, however, the myocardial bridge may be linked to myocardial ischemia, especially in conditions of increased myocardial oxygen demand.

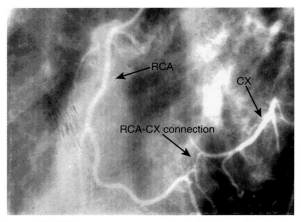

Figure 14-19 Intercoronary communications. Intercoronary communications *(arrows)* between the right coronary artery (RCA) and the left circumflex (Cx) artery are found. (From Atak R, Güray U, Akin Y. Intercoronary communication between the circumflex and right coronary arteries: distinct from coronary collaterals. *Heart.* 2002;88:29.)

To evaluate the degree of compression further, IVUS or intracoronary Doppler measurement of flow velocity may be used.

Definitive therapy is unclear because no randomized clinical trials of this anomaly have been conducted. Proposed management options include medical therapy (beta-blockers, calcium channel antagonists, avoidance of nitrates), angioplasty with stenting, and surgical interventions (CABG or focal myotomy).

Intercoronary Communications

Sometimes, one coronary artery can be connected to another by an anomalous vessel (Fig. 14-19). This anomaly should be differentiated from a watershed territory supplied by nearby collateral vessels. Injection of the left coronary system may result in back-filling of the

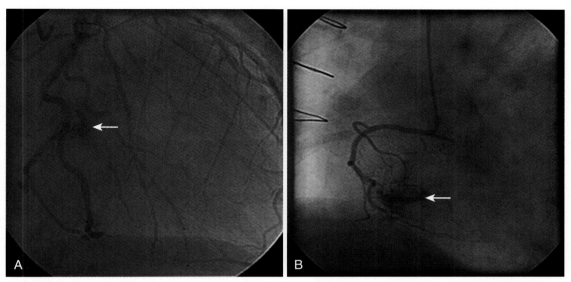

Figure 14-20 Coronary artery fistulas. A, Right lateral view of the left coronary system has a left circumflex (LCx) artery–left ventricle fistula. The midportion of the LCx artery gives a "puff" of contrast material to the adjacent left ventricle *(arrow)*. **B,** Left anterior oblique caudal view of the right coronary system revealed a right coronary artery (RCA)–right ventricle (RV) fistula. The distal RCA continues to the RV *(arrow)*, thus leaving the contrast material inside the RV.

RCA. Conversely, a right coronary system can show slow retrograde filling into the LCx or LAD artery. The perfusion scan may detect a functional defect in these regions without any angiographic evidence of coronary artery occlusions.

Anomaly of Coronary Termination

Coronary Artery Fistula

Coronary artery fistula is a rare congenital coronary anomaly (0.1% to 0.2% of routine angiograms) characterized by a single branch of coronary artery draining into a nearby chamber of the heart (Fig. 14-20). Fistulas may be single or multiple. They may arise from either coronary system and terminate in any cardiac chamber, as well as in the superior vena cava or pulmonary artery. The most common type of this anomaly arises from the RCA (60% of cases) and empties into the right ventricle. The next most frequently encountered type involves drainage of the LAD artery into the pulmonary trunk. In these types of fistula, a left-to-right shunt is formed to create a high-cardiac output state. Because of the low pressure of the right heart system, the LAD artery territory normally is not significantly affected by the deoxygenated blood flow from the right pulmonary artery. The clinical significance of this finding is uncertain. However, if any fistula tract is connected to the left ventricle, increased left ventricular end-diastolic volume may result. The region supplied by the anomalous artery may be exposed to a steal phenomenon of flow that creates a functional ischemic zone. A long-term (11-year) follow-up study of small coronary fistulas showed no clinical consequences or change in fistula size. Based on these findings, this anomaly can be regarded as benign in patients without superimposed coronary atherosclerosis.

Patients with large coronary artery fistulas usually are usually recognized even before the defect is visualized with the coronary angiography. Exertional dyspnea, continuous murmur, and symptoms of congestive heart failure usually occur during childhood or adolescence. Large fistulas have been reported to induce SCD, and they usually require surgical repair rather than percutaneous embolization.

Other Coronary Anomaly Related to Structural Change

Dextrocardia

Dextrocardia has been reported to occur in approximately 1 in 12,000 live births and is characterized by the abnormal positioning of the heart within the right thoracic cavity, with the apex directed to the right (Fig. 14-21). Dextrocardia can be further classified into three categories, depending on other organ abnormalities. *Situs solitus* refers to the heart position on the right side without any other visceral organ involvement. Because the aortic arch still lies on the left side of the thoracic cavity, situs solitus heart morphologically resembles congenitally corrected transposition of the great vessels. *Situs inversus*, slightly more common than situs solitus, involves total reversal of all thoracoabdominal organs. A right-sided aorta is found approximately 80% of patients with situs inversus. Kartagener syndrome, also known as immotile cilia syndrome (a triad of sinusitis, azoospermia, and bronchiectasis), is a clinical manifestation of situs inversus. Finally, *situs ambiguus* refers to the subgroup that does not fall into the previous two groups. Asplenia or polysplenia is usually seen in this group. Despite the striking morphologic change, the prevalence of the atherosclerosis is not different from that of the general population.

Although no specific anomaly of the coronary artery system is linked with this structural mirror image, angiography may be challenging with regard to catheter

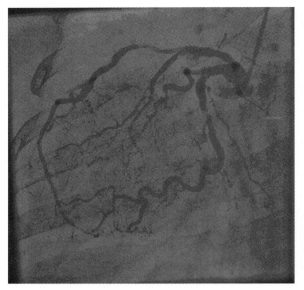

Figure 14-21 Dextrocardia. The left coronary system is shown on the right side of the thoracic cavity. The left heart catheter is rotated toward the right side to engage into the left main ostium. The rim of the rib cage is shown on the *left side of the image.*

positioning. Monitoring rhythm with right-sided electrocardiography is helpful in rapid recognition of ischemia during cardiac catheterization. Angiographic views can also be altered to the opposite side to facilitate an understanding of the structure. Blankenship et al suggested counterdirectional rotation when advancing the catheter, to achieve good apposition and visualization of the coronary structure.

■ CONCLUSION

A thorough understanding of normal coronary anatomy is an integral component of successful coronary angiography. This provides the angiographer with vital information enabling the diagnosis or exclusion of coronary artery disease. Correlating the findings from coronary angiography with other noninvasive modalities to assess both anatomic and functional aspects of the coronary artery disease is also important. Anomalous coronary artery disease, although rare, can be life-threatening, and the diagnosis and treatment are often challenging.

Bibliography

Aciero LJ. *The History of Cardiology*. London: Parthenon; 1994.
Algeria JR, Herrmann J, Holmes DR, et al. Myocardial bridging. *Eur Heart J.* 2005;26:1159-1168.
Amabile N, Fraisse A, Quilici J. Hypoplastic coronary artery disease: report of one case. *Heart.* 2005;91:e12.
Angelini P. Coronary artery anomalies: an entity in search of an identity. *Circulation.* 2007;115:1296-1305.
Angelini P. Functionally significant versus intriguingly different coronary artery anatomy: anatomo-clinical correlation in coronary anomalies. *G Ital Cardiol.* 1999;29:607-615.
Angelini P. Normal and anomalous coronary arteries: definitions and classification. *Am Heart J.* 1989;117:418-434.
Atak R, Güray U, Akin Y. Intercoronary communication between the circumflex and right coronary arteries: distinct from coronary collaterals. *Heart.* 2002;88:29.

Balm DS. *Grossman's Cardiac Catheterization, Angiography, and Intervention.* 7th ed. Philadelphia: Lippincott Williams & Wilkins; 2006.
Bansal N, Wang N, Choo D, et al. Ostial left main stenosis due to Takayasu arteritis: multimodality imaging and surgical ostioplasty. *Echocardiography.* 2011;28:E5-E8.
Blankenship JC, Ramires JA. Coronary arteriography in patients with dextrocardia. *Cathet Cardiovasc Diagn.* 1991;23:103-106.
Burke AP, Farb A, Virmani R, et al. Sports-related and non-sports-related sudden cardiac death in young adults. *Am Heart J.* 1991;121:568-575.
Cademartiri F, La Grutta L, Malagò R, et al. Prevalence of anatomical variants and coronary anomalies in 543 consecutive patients studied with 64-slice CT coronary angiography. *Eur Radiol.* 2008;18:781-791.
Cerqueira MD, Weissman NJ, Dilsizian V, et al. Standardized myocardial segmentation and nomenclature for tomographic imaging of the heart: a statement for healthcare professional from the Cardiac Imaging Committee of the Council on Clinical Cardiology of the American Heart Association. *Circulation.* 2002;105:539-542.
Chaitman BR, Lesperance J, Saltiel J, et al. Clinical, angiographic, and hemodynamic findings in patients with anomalous origin of the coronary arteries. *Circulation.* 1976;53:122-131.
Cheitlin MD, MacGregor J. Congenital anomalies of coronary arteries: role in the pathogenesis of sudden cardiac death. *Herz.* 2009;34:268-279.
Cheitlin MD, De Castro CM, McAllister HA. Sudden death as a complication of anomalous left coronary origin from the anterior sinus of Valsalva: a not-so-minor congenital anomaly. *Circulation.* 1974;50:780-787.
Chen JP. Repeat right transradial percutaneous coronary intervention in a patient with dextrocardia: the right approach to the right-sided heart. *Catheter Cardiovasc Interv.* 2007;69:223-226.
Chiu CZ, Shyu KG, Cheng JJ, et al. Angiographic and clinical manifestations of coronary fistulas in Chinese people: 15-year experience. *Circ J.* 2008;72:1242-1248.
Dodge JT, Brown BG, Bolson EL, et al. Lumen diameter of normal human coronary arteries; influence of age, sex, anatomic variation, and left ventricular hypertrophy or dilation. *Circulation.* 1992;86:232-246.
Fox C, Davies MJ, Webb-Peploe MM. Length of left main coronary artery. *Br Heart J.* 1973;35:796-798.
Fuster V, O'Rourke RA, Walsh RA, et al, eds. *Hurst's the Heart.* 12th ed. New York: McGraw-Hill; 2008.
Hobbs RE, Millit HD, Raghavan PV, et al. Coronary artery fistulae: a ten-year review. *Cleve Clin Q.* 1982;49:191-197.
Hountis P, Dedeilias P, Vourlakou C, et al. Isolated bilateral coronary artery ostial stenosis in aortitis syndrome. *Hellenic J Cardiol.* 2010;51:472-474.
Ilia R, Rosenshtein G, Weinstein JM, et al. Left anterior descending artery length in left and right coronary artery dominance. *Coron Artery Dis.* 2001;12:77-78.
Kim SY, Seo JB, Do KH, et al. Coronary artery anomalies: classification and ECG-gated multi-detector row CT findings with angiographic correlation. *Radiographics.* 2006;26:317-334.
Kimball BP, LiPreti V, Buis, et al. Comparison of proximal left anterior descending and circumflex coronary artery dimensions in aortic valve stenosis and hypertrophic cardiomyopathy. *Am J Cardiol.* 1990;65:767-771.
Kronzon I. Length of the left main coronary artery: its relation to the pattern of coronary arterial distribution. *Am J Cardiol.* 1974;34:787-789.
Lipton MJ, Barry WH, Obrez I, et al. Isolated Single coronary artery: diagnosis, angiographic classification, and clinical significance. *Radiology.* 1979;130:39-47.
MacAlpin RN, Abbasi AS, Grollman JH, et al. Human coronary artery size during life: a cineateriographic study. *Radiology.* 1973;108:567-576.
Maron BJ, Thompson PD, Puffer JC, et al. Cardiovascular preparticipation screening of competitive athletes: a statement for health professionals from the Sudden Death Committee (Clinical Cardiology) and Congenital Cardiac Defects Committee (Cardiovascular Disease in the Young), American Heart Association. *Circulation.* 1996;94:850-856.
Muriago M, Sheppard MN, Ho SY, et al. Location of the coronary arterial orifices in the normal heart. *Clin Anat.* 1997;10:297-302.
Nicholson WJ, Schuler B, Lerakis S, et al. Anomalous origin of the coronary arteries from the pulmonary trunk in two separate patients with a review of the clinical implications and current treatment recommendations. *Am J Med Sci.* 2004;328:112-115.
Pritchard CL, Mudd JG, Barner HB, et al. Coronary ostial stenosis. *Circulation.* 1975;52:46-68.
Roberts WC, Siegel RJ, Zipes DP. Origin of the right coronary artery from the left sinus of Valsalva and its functional consequences: analysis of 10 necropsy patients. *Am J Cardiol.* 1982;49:863-868.
Ropers D, Gehling G, Pohle K, et al. Anomalous course of the left main or left anterior descending coronary artery originating from the right sinus of Valsalva identification of four common variations by electron beam tomography. *Circulation.* 2002;105:e42-e43.
Scanlon PJ, Faxon DP, Audet AM, et al. ACC/AHA Guideline for Coronary Angiography: a report of the American College of Cardiology/American Heart Association Task Force on Practice Guidelines (Committee on Coronary Angiography). Developed in collaboration with the Society for Cardiac Angiography and Interventions. *J Am Coll Cardiol.* 1999;33: 1756-1824.
Schmitt R, Froehner S, Brunn J, et al. Congenital anomalies of the coronary arteries: imaging with contrast-enhanced, multidetector computed tomography. *Eur Radiol.* 2005;15:1110-1121.

Serruys PW, Onuma Y, Garg S, et al. Assessment of the SYNTAX score in the Syntax study. *EuroIntervention*. 2009;5:50-56.

Sheehan FH, Braunwald E, Canner P, et al. The effect of intravenous thrombolytic therapy on left ventricular function: a report on tissue-type plasminogen activator and streptokinase from the Thrombolysis in Myocardial Infarction (TIMI Phase I) trial. *Circulation*. 1987;75:817-829.

Sheifer SE, Canos MR, Weinfurt KP, et al. Sex differences in coronary artery size assessed by intravascular ultrasound. *Am Heart J*. 2000;139:649-653.

Taylor AJ, Byers JP, Cheitlin MD, et al. Anomalous right or left coronary artery from the contralateral coronary sinus: "high-risk" abnormalities in the initial coronary artery course and heterogeneous clinical outcomes. *Am Heart J*. 1997;133:428-435.

Topol EJ. *Textbook of Interventional Cardiology*. 5th ed. Philadelphia: Saunders; 2008.

Van Camp SP, Bloor CM, Mueller FO, et al. Nontraumatic sports death in high school and college athletes. *Med Sci Sports Exerc*. 1995;27:641-647.

Yamanaka O, Hobbs RE. Coronary artery anomalies in 126,595 patients undergoing coronary arteriography. *Cathet Cardiovasc Diagn*. 1990;21: 28-40.

Yildiz A, Okcun B, Peker T, et al. Prevalence of coronary artery anomalies in 12,457 adult patients who underwent coronary angiography. *Clin Cardiol*. 2010;33:E60-E64.

SECTION II

CHAPTER 15

Vascular Anatomy and Variants

Avinash Kambadakone

Diseases of the vascular system encompass a wide range of pathologic conditions with myriad clinical presentations. Appropriate diagnosis and management of these disorders require accurate depiction of the vascular anatomy, its variants, and pathologic abnormalities. Precise assessment of the vascular anatomy has been facilitated by an array of imaging techniques that provide accurate and excellent illustration of the arterial and venous structures. Technologic advances in noninvasive imaging techniques such as multidetector computed tomography (MDCT) and magnetic resonance imaging have opened new paradigms in vascular imaging and have limited the need for invasive catheter angiography. A sound knowledge of vascular anatomy and its variants is crucial for successful practice of vascular imaging. Although detailed description of vascular anatomy and its variants is beyond the scope of this chapter, this discussion describes the salient aspects of vascular anatomy and their variants.

■ HEAD AND NECK

Arterial System

Common Carotid artery

The common carotid arteries (CCAs) represent the main arterial supply of the head and neck (Fig. 15-1). Both CCAs have a similar course and branching pattern within the head and neck but differ in their origin. Whereas the right CCA arises from the brachiocephalic trunk, the left CCA originates from the arch of the aorta. Each CCA divides into two main branches at the level of the upper border of the thyroid cartilage: the external carotid artery (ECA) and the internal carotid artery (ICA).

EXTERNAL CAROTID ARTERY

The ECA supplies a greater portion of the neck, the face, and the external portion of the soft tissues of the head (Fig. 15-2). After its origin from the CCA, the ECA has a curved course and terminates by dividing into the maxillary and superficial temporal arteries. Each ECA has eight branches in the head and neck that can be divided as follows: medial branch (ascending pharyngeal), anterior branches (superior thyroid, lingual, and facial), posterior branches (occipital and posterior auricular), and terminal branches (superficial temporal and maxillary).

INTERNAL CAROTID ARTERY

The ICA constitutes the main vascular supply to a greater portion of the brain and the orbital structures (Fig. 15-3). It also supplies a portion of the forehead and the nose. After its origin from the CCA, the ICA has a tortuous course before its termination within the cranial cavity. The ICA has been divided into the following four portions, based on its course: the cervical portion, petrous portion, cavernous portion, and supraclinoid portion. The cervical portion of the ICA does not give any branches. Each ICA gives off the following branches: cervical portion (no branches), petrous portion (caroticotympanic artery and artery of the pterygoid canal), cavernous portion (hypophyseal, cavernous, anterior meningeal, and ophthalmic branch), and supraclinoid portion (anterior cerebral, middle cerebral, posterior communicating, and choroidal branch).

Intracranial Circulation

The brain derives its arterial supply from the ICA (through the anterior cerebral artery [ACA] and middle cerebral artery [MCA]) and the vertebral arteries (Fig. 15-4). The ACA arises from the supraclinoid portion of the ICA and runs medially into the longitudinal fissure over the corpus callosum (Fig. 15-5). The right and left ACAs communicate with each other through the anterior communicating artery (ACOM). The ACA gives several branches to the medial portion of the cerebral hemispheres and ends at the posterior aspect of the corpus callosum by anastomosing with the posterior cerebral arteries (PCAs). The MCA, the largest terminal branch of ICA, runs laterally in the sylvian fissure and divides into several branches that supply the lateral portion of the cerebral hemispheres (Fig. 15-6). The posterior communicating artery (PCOM) branch of the ICA runs posteriorly and communicates with the PCA, which is a branch of the basilar artery. The PCOM gives off several branches, which supply the medial surface of the thalami and the walls of the third ventricle. The anterior choroidal branch of the ICA supplies the hippocampus and the tela choroidea and choroid plexus of the third ventricle.

Vertebrobasilar System

The two vertebral arteries on each side along with the basilar artery together form the vertebrobasilar system, which supplies posterior portion of the brain, the

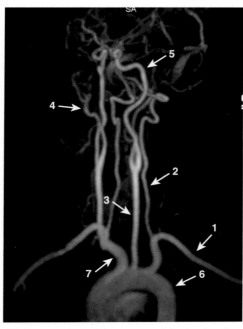

Figure 15-1 Normal arterial anatomy of the head and neck using maximum intensity projection display following magnetic resonance angiography of the head and neck. *1,* Left subclavian artery; *2,* left vertebral artery; *3,* left common carotid artery; *4,* right external carotid artery; *5,* left internal carotid artery; *6,* aorta; and *7,* brachiocephalic trunk.

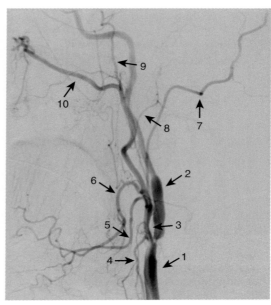

Figure 15-2 Normal anatomy and branches of the external carotid artery seen on catheter angiography of the common carotid artery in a 69-year-old man with transient ischemic attacks. Severe stenosis of the internal carotid artery origin is visible. *1,* Common carotid artery; *2,* internal carotid artery; *3,* external carotid artery; *4,* superior thyroid artery; *5,* lingual artery; *6,* facial artery; *7,* occipital artery; *8,* posterior auricular artery; *9,* superficial temporal artery; and *10,* maxillary artery.

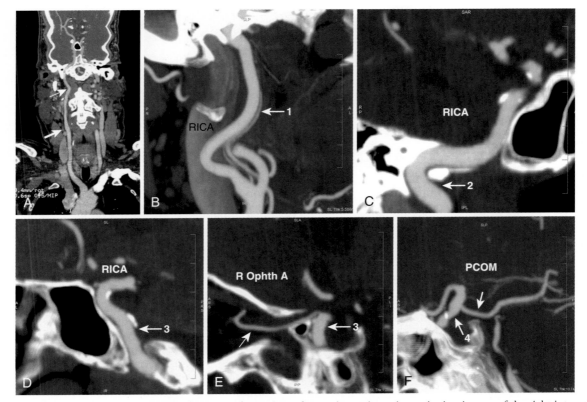

Figure 15-3 Multiple multidetector computed tomography angiography maximum intensity projection images of the right internal carotid artery (RICA). **A,** Coronal curved multiplanar reformatted images shows the entire extent of the RICA *(thin arrow)* from the common carotid artery *(thick arrow)* to its bifurcation into the anterior cerebral and middle cerebral arteries in the cranium. **B** to **F,** Coronal and sagittal multiplanar reformatted images show the various portions of the RICA. *1,* Cervical portion; *2,* petrous portion; *3,* cavernous portion; and *4,* supraclinoid portion. The ophthalmic artery *(thin arrow)* is branch of the cavernous portion of the RICA **(E),** and the posterior communicating artery (PCOM) is a branch of the supraclinoid portion of the RICA **(F).**

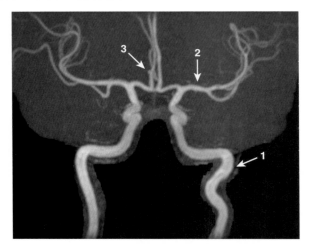

Figure 15-4 Normal arterial branches of the bilateral internal carotid artery using maximum intensity projection display following magnetic resonance angiography of the brain. *1,* Internal carotid artery; *2,* middle cerebral artery; and *3,* anterior cerebral artery.

cerebellum, and the brainstem (Fig. 15-7). The vertebral arteries arise from the first portion of the subclavian artery on each side. After originating from the subclavian artery, they course for a short interval in the neck and then enter the foramen transversarium of the cervical vertebral bodies. Within the foramen transversarium, the vertebral arteries course cranially in a vertical direction and reach the base of the skull, where they curve to enter the posterior fossa through the foramen magnum and are located anterior to the brainstem. The two vertebral arteries unite at the region of the medulla to form the basilar artery. The basilar artery then courses anterior to the pons and terminates by branching into two PCAs on each side. The vertebrobasilar system has the following branches: the posterior inferior cerebellar artery, which arises from the vertebral artery; the anterior inferior cerebellar artery, which arises from the basilar artery; the superior cerebellar artery; the pontine arteries; and the PCAs (Fig. 15-8).

Circle of Willis
The circle of Willis is a tangle of arteries at the base of the brain that forms a crucial anastomotic network between the ICA and the vertebrobasilar arterial systems.

Figure 15-5 Normal arterial branches of the anterior cerebral artery (ACA). **A,** Sagittal multidetector computed tomography (MDCT) angiographic maximum intensity projection (MIP) image of the ACA demonstrates its course *(arrows)* longitudinally around the corpus callosum. **B,** Coronal MDCT angiographic MIP image of the bilateral ACA *(arrows)* shows its paramedian course.

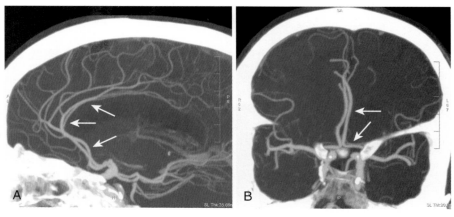

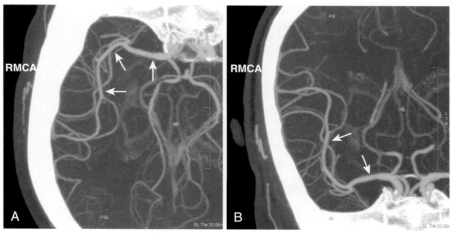

Figure 15-6 Normal arterial branches of the right middle cerebral artery (RMCA). Axial **(A)** and coronal **(B)** multidetector computed tomography angiographic maximum intensity projection images of the RMCA demonstrate its course *(arrows)* laterally and superiorly around the sylvian fissure.

The circle of Willis is formed anteriorly by the ACA and the ACOM and posteriorly by the PCA and the PCOM (Fig. 15-9).

Venous System

The venous system of the brain consists of the cerebral and cerebellar veins, which drain into the cranial venous sinuses located within the dura mater. These veins are extremely thin because they lack a muscular wall, and they do not have any valves.

Cerebral Veins

The cerebral veins are broadly classified into the external group (superior cerebral, inferior cerebral, and middle cerebral vein) and the internal group (internal cerebral vein and vein of Galen). The superior cerebral vein drains the superior, lateral, and medial surfaces of the cerebral hemispheres and drains into the superior sagittal sinus. The middle cerebral vein is situated in the sylvian fissure and drains into the cavernous or the sphenoparietal sinus. The middle cerebral vein is connected

to the superior sagittal sinus through the great anastomotic vein of Trolard and the transverse sinus through the posterior anastomotic vein of Labbe. The inferior cerebral vein drains the basal portion of the cerebral hemispheres and drains into the superior cerebral veins, middle cerebral veins, or the basal veins. The basal vein is formed by the union of the anterior cerebral vein, the deep middle cerebral vein, and the inferior striate veins. The basal vein travels backward and terminates in the internal cerebral vein. The internal cerebral veins drain the deep parts of the cerebral hemispheres and are formed at the interventricular foramen by the union of the terminal and choroid veins. The internal cerebral veins run backward and, after receiving the basal veins on each side, unite to form the great cerebral vein of Galen. The great cerebral vein ends in the anterior portion of the straight sinus.

Cerebellar Veins

The cerebellar veins consist of the superior and inferior cerebellar veins. The superior cerebellar veins drain into the straight sinus, the transverse sinus, and the superior

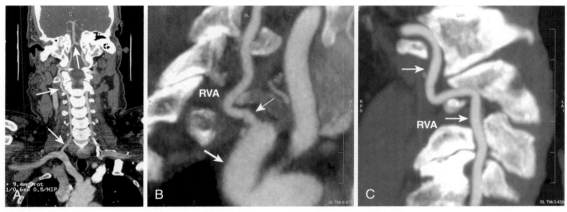

Figure 15-7 Multiple multidetector computed tomography angiography maximum intensity projection (MIP) images of the right vertebral artery (RVA). **A,** Coronal curved multiplanar reformatted image shows the entire extent of the RVA *(arrows)* from its origin from the subclavian artery up to the union of the two vertebral arteries to form the basilar artery. **B,** Coronal MIP image shows the origin of the RVA *(thin arrow)* from the subclavian artery *(thick arrow)*. **C,** Coronal MIP image demonstrates the course of the RVA *(arrows)* within the foramen transversarium.

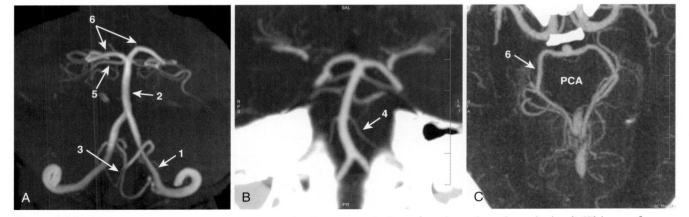

Figure 15-8 Normal arterial anatomy of the vertebrobasilar system. A, Coronal maximum intensity projection (MIP) image of a magnetic resonance angiography study of the vertebral and basilar arteries. Coronal **(B)** and axial **(C)** MIP images of a multidetector computed tomography angiography study show the vertebral and basilar artery branches. *1,* Vertebral artery; *2,* basilar artery; *3,* posterior inferior cerebellar display; *4,* anterior inferior cerebellar artery; *5,* superior cerebellar artery; and *6,* posterior cerebral artery (PCA).

petrosal sinus, whereas the inferior cerebellar veins drain into the transverse, superior petrosal, and occipital sinuses.

Dural Sinuses

The dural sinuses are venous channels draining the brain. These sinuses are positioned within the two layers of dura mater and are devoid of any valves (Fig. 15-10). The superior sagittal sinus begins at the foramen cecum, travels backward within the convex portion of the midline falx cerebri, and continues as the transverse sinus (usually right). The superior sagittal sinus is triangular in section; it gradually widens as it travels backward from its origin and receives drainage from the superior cerebral veins and diploic veins. Numerous communications exist between the superior sagittal sinus and the veins of the nose and scalp. The inferior sagittal sinus is situated within the posterior half of the free margin of the falx cerebri and terminates in the straight sinus. The straight sinus is located at the line of junction of the falx cerebri situated with the tentorium cerebelli. It begins at the posterior portion of the inferior sagittal sinus, extends backward, and continues as

the transverse sinus (the opposite side to the transverse sinus formed by superior sagittal sinus). The straight sinus receives the great cerebral vein and the superior cerebellar veins and communicates with the confluence of sinuses.

The transverse sinus begins at the internal occipital protuberance. On the right side, the transverse sinus usually is a continuation of the superior sagittal sinus, whereas on the left side, it is a continuation of the straight sinus. Each transverse sinus passes laterally and anteriorly along the attached margin of the tentorium cerebelli, curves medially and inferiorly, and continues as the sigmoid sinus before it terminates in the internal jugular vein at the jugular foramen. The transverse sinus formed by the superior sagittal sinus is larger than that formed by the straight sinus. The transverse sinuses receive drainage from the superior petrosal sinuses and from the inferior cerebral and inferior cerebellar veins. The occipital sinus is situated along the attached margin of the falx cerebelli and joins the confluence of the sinuses. The confluence of the sinuses refers to the dilated distal portion of the superior sagittal sinus that is lodged on the internal occipital protuberance. The

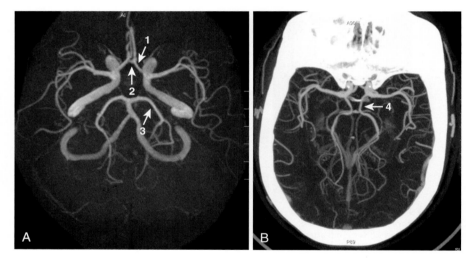

Figure 15-9 Arterial anatomy of the circle of Willis. Magnetic resonance angiography maximum intensity projection (MIP) image **(A)** and multidetector computed tomography angiography MIP image **(B)** show the arterial anatomy of the circle of Willis. The circle of Willis is formed anteriorly by the anterior cerebral artery and the anterior communicating artery and posteriorly by the posterior cerebral artery and the posterior communicating artery. 1, Anterior cerebral artery; 2, anterior communicating artery; 3, posterior cerebral artery; and 4, posterior communicating artery.

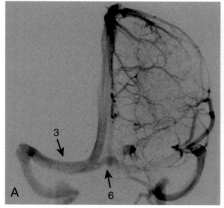 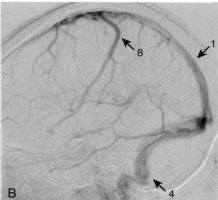 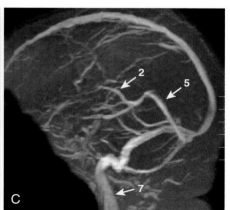

Figure 15-10 Dural venous sinuses. A and **B,** Coronal and sagittal views from a cerebral angiogram in the venous phase demonstrate the dural sinuses. **C,** Sagittal maximum intensity projection image from a magnetic resonance venogram demonstrates the dural sinus anatomy. *1,* Superior sagittal sinus; *2,* inferior sagittal sinus; *3,* transverse sinus; *4,* sigmoid sinus; *5,* straight sinus; *6,* confluence of sinuses; *7,* internal jugular vein; and *8,* superior cerebral vein.

confluence of sinuses gives rise to the transverse sinus and receives blood from the occipital sinus.

The cavernous sinuses are placed on either side of the body of the sphenoid bone and have a reticulate structure traversed by numerous filaments. The cavernous sinuses contain the ICA and abducent nerve along the medial wall, and several cranial nerves (oculomotor, trochlear, and trigeminal nerve) course along the lateral wall. The cavernous sinuses receive blood from the superior ophthalmic vein and the sphenoparietal sinus, and they communicate with the transverse sinus through the superior petrosal sinus. The bilateral cavernous sinuses communicate through two intercavernous sinuses situated anterior and posterior to the hypophysis cerebri. The superior ophthalmic vein begins at the inner angle of the orbit as the nasofrontal vein and communicates with the angular vein. The inferior ophthalmic vein begins in the floor of the orbit and joins the pterygoid venous plexus before it ends in the cavernous sinus. The superior petrosal sinus connects the transverse sinus with the cavernous sinus and receives cerebellar venous drainage. The inferior petrosal sinus connects the cavernous sinus with the superior bulb of the internal jugular vein and receives venous drainage from the pons, medulla, and cerebellum.

Vertebral Venous System

The vertebral venous plexuses drain the venous blood from the vertebral column, the spinal meninges, and the surrounding musculature. The intercommunicating vertebral venous plexuses are categorized as external (outside vertebral canal) and internal (inside vertebral canal). The external vertebral venous plexuses have anterior and posterior groups that drain the vertebral bodies and posterior vertebral elements, respectively. The external venous plexuses freely communicate with the basivertebral and intervertebral veins. The internal vertebral venous plexuses have paired anterior and posterior groups that receive blood from the bones and spinal medulla. The cranial most portion of the internal venous plexuses forms a complex network of veins at the foramen magnum that communicate with the vertebral veins, the basilar plexus, and the occipital sinus. The internal and external vertebral venous plexuses drain into the intervertebral veins, which terminate in the vertebral, intercostal, lumbar, and lateral sacral veins at the corresponding levels. The spinal medulla is drained by two median longitudinal and four lateral longitudinal veins that form a plexus over the spinal medulla. These veins end in the intervertebral veins at the corresponding level, and at the base of the skull they communicate with the vertebral veins, the inferior cerebellar veins, or the inferior petrosal sinuses.

■ THORAX

Arterial System

The major arterial structures within the thorax are the aorta and the pulmonary arteries.

Aorta

The intrathoracic portion of the aorta includes the ascending aorta, the arch of aorta, and the descending aorta up to the aortic hiatus in the diaphragm, beyond which it continues as the abdominal aorta.

ASCENDING AORTA

The ascending aorta begins at the upper part of the left ventricle at the ventricular outflow tract, and its origin is termed the aortic root. The aortic root is situated to the right and posterior relative to the subpulmonary infundibulum. The ascending aorta at its origin has three bulbous dilatations called the aortic sinuses that correspond to the segments of the aortic valve. It then ascends for a short distance and continues as the arch of the aorta. The branches of the ascending aorta include the right and left coronary arteries, which arise in the region of the aortic sinuses.

AORTIC ARCH

The aortic arch curves backward and to the left to continue as the descending thoracic aorta. The three principal branches of the arch of aorta are the brachiocephalic trunk, the left CCA, and the left subclavian artery (Fig. 15-11). The brachiocephalic trunk is the largest branch and divides into the right CCA and the right subclavian artery.

DESCENDING THORACIC AORTA

The descending thoracic aorta descends along the left side of the vertebral column and continues as the abdominal aorta at the aortic hiatus of the diaphragm. The descending thoracic aorta primarily has the following branches: the visceral branches, which include the bronchial, esophageal, mediastinal, and pericardial arteries, and the parietal branches, which include the subcostal, superior phrenic, and posterior intercostal arteries.

VARIANTS

The most common anatomic variant of the aortic arch branching is known as the bovine aortic arch. In this variant, the left CCA originates directly from the brachiocephalic trunk, instead of arising from the aortic arch (Fig. 15-11). This configuration of aortic arch branching has no clinical relevance. Another common variant is the aberrant origin of the right subclavian artery from the aortic arch, rather than from the brachiocephalic trunk (Fig. 15-13). Occasionally, the left vertebral artery can have an anomalous origin from the aortic arch instead of arising from the subclavian artery.

Right-sided aortic arch is an anatomic variant in which the ascending aorta arches to the right and descends along the right half of the vertebral column. Two types of right-sided aortic arch are recognized. The first type is the right-sided aortic arch with a mirror image branching pattern. In this case, the left brachiocephalic trunk arises as the first branch of the aortic arch and divides into the left CCA and the left subclavian artery (see Fig. 15-11). In the second type, the right-sided aortic arch is associated with an aberrant left subclavian artery (Fig. 15-12). These anatomic variants can form a vascular

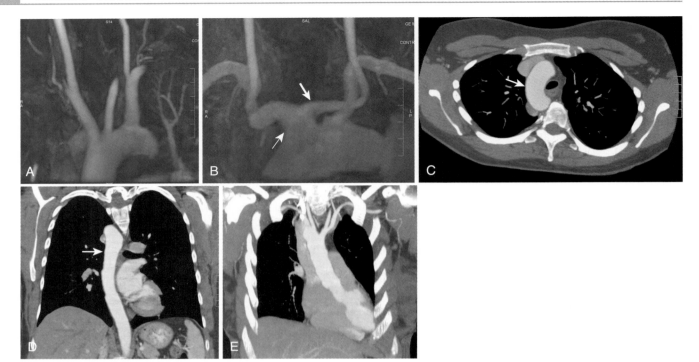

Figure 15-11 Aortic arch and its variants. A, Normal three-vessel left-sided aortic arch. **B,** Coronal maximum intensity projection image of a magnetic resonance angiogram shows a bovine arch configuration with the left common carotid artery *(thick arrow)* taking origin from the brachiocephalic trunk *(thin arrow)*. **C to E,** Multiplanar reformatted multidetector computed tomography images show a right-sided aortic arch *(arrow)* with a mirror image branching pattern.

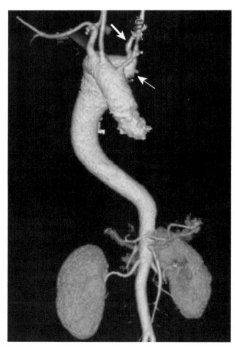

Figure 15-12 Right-sided aortic arch with aberrant left subclavian artery. Maximum intensity projection images from a multidetector computed tomography angiogram show a right-sided aortic arch and an aberrant left subclavian artery *(thick arrow)* arising from the dilated portion of the descending aorta (diverticulum of Kommerell) *(thin arrow)*.

ring and can cause symptoms resulting from airway or esophageal compression. Right-sided aortic arch with mirror image branching pattern is most often associated with a congenital cardiac anomaly, usually tetralogy of Fallot, whereas right aortic arch with aberrant left subclavian artery is rarely associated with a congenital cardiac defect.

The most common clinical recognized cause of a vascular ring is double aortic arch. In this condition, the ascending aorta divides into right and left arches on either side of trachea. One of the arches is usually dominant, most commonly the right. Associated cardiac congenital anomalies can occur, including tetralogy of Fallot, transposition of the great arteries, coarctation of the aorta, ventricular septal defect, and patent ductus arteriosus.

Pulmonary Artery

The main pulmonary artery is the principal vessel that carries deoxygenated blood from the right ventricle to the lungs. The main pulmonary artery continues from the right ventricular outflow tract to the left of the ascending aorta and divides into the right and left pulmonary arteries. The right pulmonary artery continues to the pulmonary hilum and courses behind the ascending aorta and superior vena cava (SVC) before it divides into two branches. The left pulmonary artery, which is shorter and smaller than the right, courses in front of descending aorta before it divides into two branches.

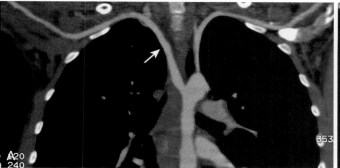

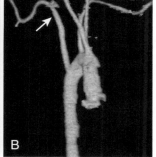

Figure 15-13 Aberrant right subclavian artery. Coronal curved reformatted multidetector computed tomography image (**A**) and coronal maximum intensity projection image (**B**) show the aberrant origin and course of the right subclavian artery *(arrow)* from the descending thoracic aorta.

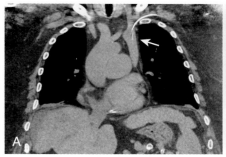

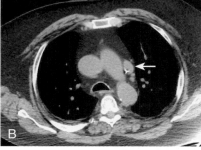

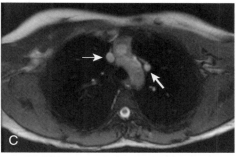

Figure 15-14 Left-sided superior vena cava (SVC). Coronal multidetector computed tomography (MDCT) image (**A**) and axial MDCT image (**B**) show a left-sided superior vena cava completely replacing the right-sided SVC *(arrow)*. **C,** Axial T2-weighted magnetic resonance angiogram in a different patient shows a left-sided SVC *(thick arrow)* and a normally placed right SVC *(thin arrow)*.

Venous System

Brachiocephalic Veins

The major venous structures within the thorax are the brachiocephalic veins and the pulmonary veins. The brachiocephalic veins are formed by the union of the internal jugular veins and the subclavian veins and are devoid of any valves. The right and left brachiocephalic veins join at the right border of sternum to form the SVC. The right brachiocephalic vein also receives venous blood from the right vertebral vein, the right internal mammary, and the right inferior thyroid vein. The left brachiocephalic vein receives venous blood from the left vertebral, left internal mammary, left inferior thyroid and the left highest intercostal veins. These tributaries accompany the corresponding arteries. The highest intercostal vein or the superior intercostal vein (right and left) receives blood from the upper 3-4 intercostal spaces. The right superior intercostal vein drains into the azygos vein, whereas the left drains into the left brachiocephalic vein. The visceral venous branches (bronchial, esophageal, and mediastinal veins) follow the accompanying arteries and drain either into the brachiocephalic veins or the azygos venous system.

Superior Vena Cava

The SVC forms the main draining vein for the upper half of the body and has no valves. SVC is formed from the union of brachiocephalic veins and ends in the upper part of the right atrium. The SVC also receives drainage from the azygos, small pericardial, and mediastinal veins. The left brachiocephalic vein may have separate drainage into the heart, and in such situations it is called the left SVC and drains into the coronary sinus (Fig. 15-14).

Azygos Vein

The azygos vein carries the venous blood from the posterior walls of the thorax and abdomen into the SVC. The azygos system, which has imperfect valves, is the main alternate pathway for venous drainage when either the SVC or the inferior vena cava (IVC) is blocked. The azygos vein begins in the abdomen as the ascending lumbar vein and enters the thorax through the aortic hiatus in the diaphragm. After ascending along the right side of vertebral column, it arches anteriorly and enters into the SVC. The azygos vein receives drainage from the right subcostal and right intercostal veins (including the right superior intercostal vein). Before its termination into the SVC, the azygos vein receives drainage from the hemiazygos vein, the right bronchial vein, and the esophageal, mediastinal, and pericardial veins.

Hemiazygos and Accessory Hemiazygos veins

Similar to the azygos venous system on the right side, drainage on the left side is provided by the hemiazygos and accessory hemiazygos veins. The hemiazygos vein begins as the left ascending lumbar vein in the abdomen. After ascending into the thorax, the hemiazygos vein terminates in the azygos vein. The hemiazygos vein receives drainage from the lower four or five intercostal veins, the left subcostal vein, and the esophageal and mediastinal veins. The accessory hemiazygos vein receives drainage from the intercostal veins not drained by the superior intercostal vein and ends in the azygos or hemiazygos vein.

■ ABDOMEN AND PELVIS

Arterial System

Abdominal Aorta

The abdominal portion of the descending aorta commences at the diaphragmatic hiatus for the aorta and divides into two common iliac arteries at the level of the L4 vertebral body (Fig. 15-15). The abdominal aorta has four unpaired branches (celiac, superior mesenteric, inferior mesenteric, and middle sacral) and five paired branches (middle suprarenal, renal, testicular or ovarian, inferior phrenic, and lumbar).

Celiac Trunk

The celiac trunk is the artery of the foregut, and it consists of a short segment that arises from the anterior aspect of the aorta at the level of the L1 vertebral body (Fig. 15-16). The celiac trunk has three branches: the left gastric, common hepatic, and splenic artery. The dorsal pancreatic artery may arise as a fourth branch from the proximal celiac artery. The common hepatic artery divides into the gastroduodenal artery and the proper hepatic artery. The proper hepatic artery bifurcates into the right and left hepatic arteries and supplies the hepatobiliary system. The splenic artery has the following branches: the pancreatic, short gastric, and left gastroepiploic arteries. The gastroduodenal artery gives off the superior pancreaticoduodenal artery and continues as the right gastroepiploic artery.

Superior Mesenteric Artery

The superior mesenteric artery (SMA) is the artery of the midgut, and it arises from the front of aorta below the celiac trunk at the level of the lower border of L1 vertebral body (Fig. 15-17). The SMA supplies the entire small bowel (except the proximal duodenum) and the large colon up to the proximal half of transverse colon. The branches of the SMA include the inferior pancreaticoduodenal, intestinal, middle colic, ileocolic, and right colic arteries. The superior and inferior pancreaticoduodenal arteries form the collateral pathway between the celiac trunk and the SMA.

Inferior Mesenteric Artery

The inferior mesenteric artery (IMA) is the artery of the hindgut, and it arises from the aorta at the level of the L3 vertebral body (Fig. 15-18). The IMA supplies the large colon distal to the proximal half of transverse colon and the greater part of the rectum. The branches of IMA include the left colic, sigmoid, and superior rectal arteries. The colonic branches of the SMA and IMA anastomose with each other and form a vascular arcade close to the bowel wall called the marginal artery of Drummond. The arc of Riolan refers to another vascular arcade that is closer to the root of the colonic mesentery and that connects the middle colic branch of the SMA with the IMA.

Renal Arteries

The two renal arteries arise from the lateral aspect of aorta at the level of the L1-L2 intervertebral disk. The

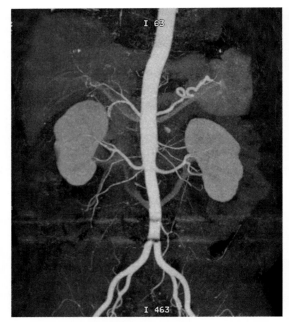

Figure 15-15 Abdominal aorta. Coronal maximum intensity projection image from a multidetector computed tomography angiogram shows the abdominal aorta and its branches.

right renal artery passes behind the IVC (Fig. 15-19). The inferior suprarenal artery arises from the corresponding renal artery.

Variants

Variations in celiac artery anatomy can be seen in more than 40% of patients (Fig. 15-20). The most common variant is a replaced right hepatic artery from the SMA (15% of patients). This anatomic variant has important implications for pancreatic surgical procedures. The proper right hepatic artery is anterior to the right portal vein, whereas the replaced right hepatic artery is posterior to the main portal vein. This placement increases the risk of injury if the anatomic variant is not identified. Another common variant is the replaced left hepatic artery from the left gastric artery (8% of patients). In addition to these anatomic variants, accessory hepatic arteries can be present and reinforce the arterial supply of the liver. Identification and differentiation of replaced and accessory hepatic arteries are essential to prevent vascular injury. In up to 2% of patients, the common hepatic artery can originate from the SMA. Occasionally, the celiac artery and the SMA can have a common origin. Extremely rarely, a common origin of the celiac artery, SMA, and IMA has been described. A single renal artery supplies each kidney in more than 75% of cases. Accessory renal arteries, which may arise from the aorta or the common iliac arteries and supply a portion of the kidney in addition to the main renal artery, are seen in up to 20% of cases (Fig. 15-21).

Common Iliac Arteries

The common iliac artery divides into the external iliac and internal iliac arteries (Fig. 15-22). The external iliac artery supplies the lower limbs, whereas the internal iliac artery

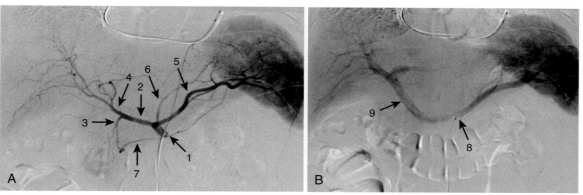

Figure 15-16 Catheter angiogram demonstrating the celiac artery and its branches. **A,** Arterial phase of a catheter angiogram showing the celiac artery branches. **B,** Venous phase showing the splenic vein joining the portal vein. *1,* Celiac artery; *2,* common hepatic artery; *3,* gastroduodenal artery; *4,* proper hepatic artery; *5,* splenic artery; *6,* left gastric artery; *7,* left gastroepiploic artery; *8,* splenic vein; and *9,* portal vein.

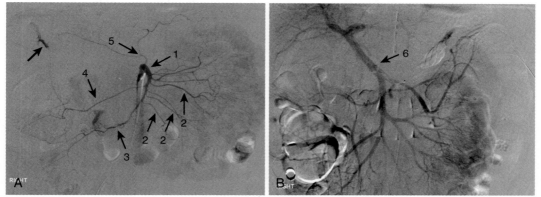

Figure 15-17 Catheter angiogram demonstrating the superior mesenteric artery and its branches. **A,** Arterial phase of the catheter angiogram showing the superior mesenteric artery branches. Active extravasation of contrast material occurs at the hepatic flexure of the colon *(thick arrow).* **B,** Venous phase showing the superior mesenteric vein joining the portal vein. *1,* Superior mesenteric artery; *2,* small intestinal branches; *3,* ileocolic artery; *4,* right colic artery; *5,* middle colic artery; and *6,* superior mesenteric vein.

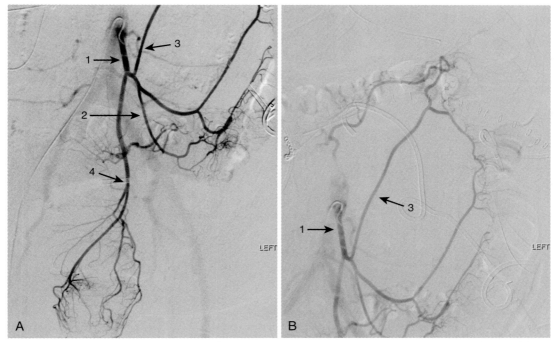

Figure 15-18 Catheter angiogram demonstrating the inferior mesenteric artery and its branches. **A and B,** Arterial phase of the catheter angiogram shows the inferior mesenteric artery and its branches. *1,* Inferior mesenteric artery; *2,* sigmoid artery; *3,* left colic artery; and *4,* superior rectal artery.

supplies the pelvic structures. The common iliac artery gives off small branches to the peritoneum, the psoas muscle, and the ureters. The internal iliac artery (also called the hypogastric artery) has two main branches: the anterior trunk and the posterior trunk. The anterior trunk has the following branches: the umbilical, inferior vesical, middle rectal, obturator, internal pudendal, inferior gluteal, uterine, and vaginal arteries. The posterior trunk has three branches: the iliolumbar, lateral sacral, and superior gluteal arteries. In the pelvis, the external iliac artery has the inferior epigastric and deep circumflex iliac branches.

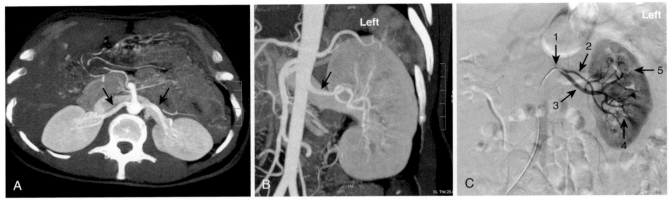

Figure 15-19 Renal artery and its branches. Axial (**A**) and coronal (**B**) maximum intensity projection images from a multidetector computed tomography angiogram showing the renal arteries *(arrows)*. **C,** Catheter angiogram image of the left renal artery showing the branching pattern of the renal artery. *1,* Main renal artery; *2,* inferior segmental renal artery; *3,* superior segmental renal artery; *4,* interlobar artery; and *5,* arcuate artery.

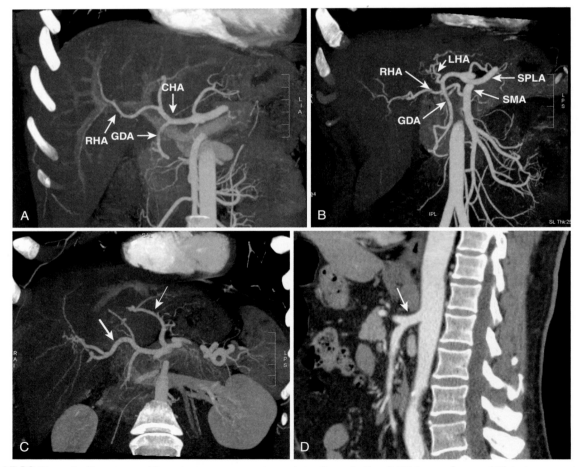

Figure 15-20 Normal celiac artery and its variants seen on maximum intensity projection (MIP) images from multidetector computed tomography angiography in different patients. **A,** Coronal MIP image shows the normal origin of hepatic artery from celiac artery (CA). *CHA,* Common hepatic artery; *GDA,* gastroduodenal artery; *RHA,* right hepatic artery. **B,** Replaced RHA arising from the superior mesenteric artery (SMA). The left hepatic artery (LHA) arises from the celiac artery. *SPLA,* Splenic artery. **C,** Replaced LHA arising from the left gastric artery *(thin arrow)*. The RHA arises from the celiac artery *(thick arrow)*. **D,** Common origin of the celiac trunk and the SMA from the aorta *(arrow)*.

Venous System

Inferior Vena Cava

The veins of the abdomen and pelvis accompany the corresponding arteries. The IVC is the chief venous channel that drains the lower half of the body. The IVC is formed from the union of the common iliac veins at the level of the L5 vertebra. The IVC ascends along the right side of the vertebral column and continues within the posterior surface of the liver before it terminates in the right atrium.

VARIANTS

In cases of left-sided IVC, the IVC runs along the left side of the aorta up to the level of left renal vein and then crosses to its usual position on the right side. Rarely, duplication of infrarenal portion of the IVC can occur (Fig. 15-23). In rare cases, patients may have complete transposition, which is often accompanied by complete transposition of the thoracic and abdominal viscera. In cases of the azygos continuation of the IVC, the IVC joins the azygos vein, which becomes enlarged and drains into the SVC, thus forming the only source of drainage of venous supply from the lower half of the body (Fig. 15-24).

Common Iliac Veins

The common iliac veins are formed by the union of the external and internal iliac veins opposite the sacroiliac joint. The shorter right common iliac vein is lateral to the right common iliac artery, whereas the left common iliac vein lies medial to the corresponding artery. The external iliac vein is the cranial extension of the femoral vein and receives the inferior epigastric, deep circumflex iliac, and pubic veins. The internal iliac vein runs along the internal iliac artery and has tributaries corresponding to its branches. An exception is the iliolumbar vein, which usually joins the common iliac vein. The lumbar

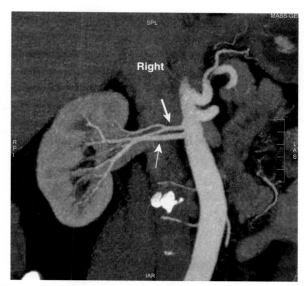

Figure 15-21 Accessory right renal artery. Coronal maximum intensity projection image from a multidetector computed tomography angiogram shows the accessory right renal artery *(thick arrow)* supplying the upper pole of right kidney. The main renal artery *(thin arrow)* supplies the rest of the kidney.

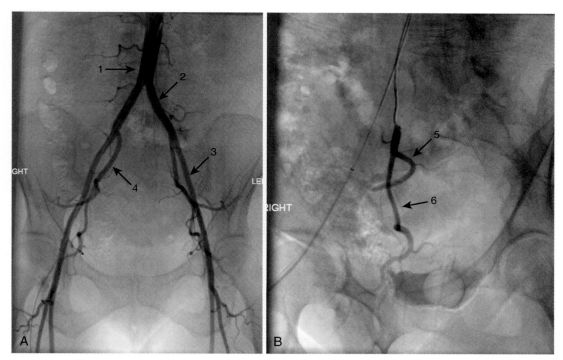

Figure 15-22 Common iliac artery and its branches seen on catheter angiogram. **A,** Aortogram shows the common iliac artery and its branches. **B,** Selective catheter injection of the internal iliac artery shows the anterior and posterior branches of the internal iliac artery. *1,* Aorta; *2,* common iliac artery; *3,* external iliac artery; *4,* internal iliac artery; *5,* posterior division of internal iliac artery; and *6,* anterior division of the internal iliac artery.

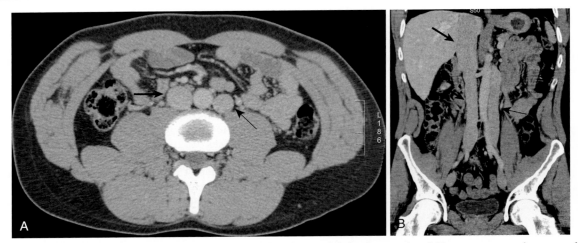

Figure 15-23 Duplicated inferior vena cava (IVC). Axial **(A)** and coronal **(B)** reformatted multidetector computed tomography images show duplicated IVC *(thin arrows)* to the left of the aorta, in addition to the normally placed right IVC *(thick arrows)*.

veins (four total) on each side join to form the ascending lumbar vein, which drains into the common iliac, iliolumbar, or azygos or hemiazygos veins.

Visceral Venous System

Both renal veins drain into the IVC (the left renal vein is longer than the right). The left renal vein also receives drainage from the left gonadal vein, the left inferior phrenic vein, and the left suprarenal vein. The right suprarenal vein drains into the IVC. The hepatic veins constitute the venous drainage of the liver consist of the right, middle, and left hepatic veins. The main hepatic veins open into the intrahepatic portion of the IVC (Fig. 15-25). Smaller hepatic venous branches from the caudate lobe drain directly into the IVC. Several visceral venous plexuses are found around the pelvic organs. The hemorrhoidal plexus surrounds the rectum and communicates with the vesical plexus in men and with the uterovaginal plexus in women. Three hemorrhoidal veins arise from the hemorrhoidal plexus: the superior, which drains into the inferior mesenteric vein (part of the portal system); the middle, which drains into the internal iliac vein; and the inferior, which drains into the internal pudendal vein. The hemorrhoidal plexus forms a site of free communication between the portal and systemic venous systems. The paired spermatic (testicular) veins, which drain the testis and the epididymis, begin as the pampiniform plexus around the spermatic cord. The right spermatic vein drains into the IVC, whereas the left spermatic vein drains into the left renal vein. The spermatic veins have valves. The corresponding ovarian veins in women also have a similar pattern of termination.

VARIANTS

Variations in hepatic vein anatomy are quite common, and knowledge of this variant anatomy is crucial in the planning of liver operations, including transplantation procedures. A common variant is an accessory or replaced inferior right hepatic vein, which can drain

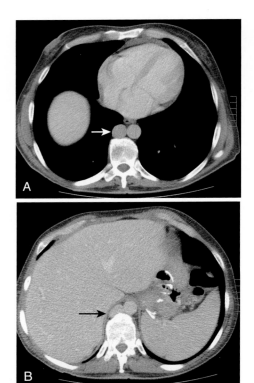

Figure 15-24 Azygos continuation of the inferior vena cava (IVC). The infrarenal IVC continues as the azygos vein before it terminates into the superior vena cava. **A,** Axial contrast-enhanced multidetector computed tomography (MDCT) image shows the dilated azygos vein *(arrow)* to the right of aorta. **B,** Axial contrast-enhanced MDCT image shows the absent intrahepatic portion of the IVC and the prominent azygos vein *(arrow)* posterior to the diaphragmatic crura.

separately into the IVC caudal to the drainage of the main right hepatic vein into the IVC. Portal vein variations are also common, the most common of which is trifurcation of the main portal vein into a left portal vein and the anterior and posterior branch of the right portal vein.

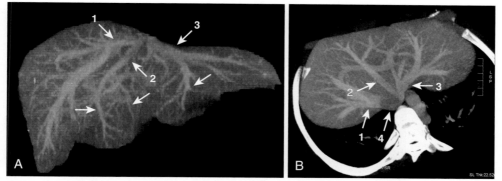

Figure 15-25 Hepatic vein anatomy. A, Volume-rendered image of the hepatic venous anatomy shows the intrahepatic tributaries of the hepatic veins *(unnumbered arrows)*. B. Axial maximum intensity projection image from the multidetector computed tomography angiogram shows the three hepatic veins joining the inferior vena cava. *1,* Right hepatic vein; *2,* middle hepatic vein; *3,* left hepatic vein; and *4,* inferior vena cava.

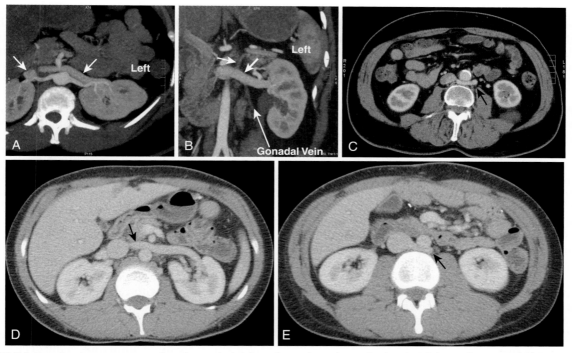

Figure 15-26 Renal vein anatomy and variants. A, Axial maximum intensity projection (MIP) image from a multidetector computed tomography (MDCT) angiogram shows the normal course of the left renal vein *(thick arrow)* anterior to the aorta before joining the inferior vena cava *(thin arrow)*. B, Coronal MIP image from an MDCT angiogram shows the left adrenal vein *(arrowhead)* and the left gonadal vein draining into the left renal vein *(thick arrow)*. C, Axial MDCT image shows the variant retroaortic left renal vein *(arrow)* coursing posterior to the aorta. D and E, Axial MDCT images show the circumaortic left renal vein *(arrows)*.

The common variations of renal vein anatomy often involve the left renal vein. Circumaortic left renal vein, the most common variant, occurs in 5% to 7% of patients, and in this variation, two left renal veins course anterior and posterior to the aorta (Fig. 15-26). In retroaortic left renal vein, (2% to 3% of cases), patients have only one renal vein coursing posterior to the aorta.

Portal Venous System

The portal venous system constitutes the major venous drainage pathway for the abdominal viscera. The main vein of the portal system is the portal vein, which is formed by confluence of the splenic and superior mesenteric veins (Fig. 15-27). The portal vein ramifies within the hepatic hilum into right and left branches, which ultimately drain into the hepatic sinusoids. Hepatic venous tributaries then convey this venous blood into the IVC. The right branch of the portal vein receives the blood from the gallbladder in the form of cystic vein. The coronary vein, which receives tributaries from stomach and esophageal veins, drains into the portal vein at the confluence of the splenic and superior mesenteric veins. The splenic vein receives tributaries from short gastric veins, the left gastroepiploic vein, the pancreatic veins, and the inferior mesenteric veins, which course along their corresponding arteries. The inferior mesenteric vein begins as the superior hemorrhoidal vein originating from the hemorrhoidal

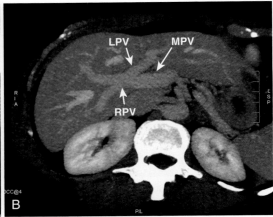

Figure 15-27 Portal venous anatomy. Coronal (**A**) and axial (**B**) maximum intensity projection images show the formation and branching pattern of the portal vein. *1,* Superior mesenteric vein; *2,* splenic vein; and *3,* main portal vein (*MPV*); *LPV,* left portal vein; *RPV,* right portal vein.

plexus. The inferior mesenteric vein receives tributaries from the sigmoid veins and left colic vein. The superior mesenteric vein has tributaries, which run along the corresponding arteries and include the ileocolic, right colic, and middle colic veins and the intestinal veins. The right gastroepiploic vein and the pancreaticoduodenal vein also drain into the superior mesenteric vein.

Portosystemic Collateral Vessels

Portosystemic collateral vessels are present between the portal circulation and the systemic venous system. These collateral vessels become prominent at times of portal venous obstruction or portal venous hypertension. The sites of portosystemic communications include the following: the lower esophagus, between the gastric veins (portal) and the esophageal veins (systemic); the retroperitoneum, between the left renal vein (systemic) and the veins of the stomach and pancreas (portal); the umbilicus, between the abdominal wall veins (systemic) and the paraumbilical vein (portal); the veins of Retzius, which connect the intestinal veins to the IVC and its retroperitoneal branches; and the lower rectum, which includes the inferior mesenteric vein and the hemorrhoidal veins draining into internal iliac veins.

■ UPPER LIMBS

Arterial System

The subclavian arteries constitute the main arterial supply of the upper limbs. On the right side, the subclavian artery arises from brachiocephalic trunk; on the left side, it arises from the arch of the aorta. The subclavian artery has the following branches: the vertebral artery, the thyrocervical trunk, the costocervical trunk, the internal mammary artery, and the dorsal scapular artery.

The subclavian artery continues as the axillary artery beyond the outer border of the first rib. The axillary artery is divided into three parts and has the following branches: the first part (the highest thoracic artery), the second part (the thoracoacromial and lateral thoracic arteries), and the third part (the subscapular, posterior humeral circumflex, and anterior humeral circumflex arteries). The axillary artery continues as the brachial artery beyond the teres major muscle (Fig. 15-28).

The brachial artery terminates by dividing into the radial and ulnar arteries. The branches of the brachial artery include the deep brachial (profunda brachii), the superior ulnar collateral, the inferior ulnar collateral, and muscular branches. The radial artery has several branches in the forearm (the radial recurrent, palmar carpal, and superficial palmar branches), two branches in the wrist (dorsal carpal and first dorsal metacarpal), and three branches in the hand (princeps pollicis, radialis indicis, and deep palmar arch). The ulnar artery also has several branches in the forearm (anterior recurrent, posterior recurrent, common interosseous, and muscular), two branches in the wrist (palmar carpal and dorsal carpal), and at the level of hand it contributes to the superficial palmar arch and deep palmar arch.

Venous System

The venous drainage of the upper limb is constituted by the deep and superficial venous system. These two systems communicate with each other frequently and contain numerous valves. The superficial veins are placed immediately beneath the integument between the two layers of superficial fascia. Both sets are provided with valves, which are more numerous in the deep veins than in the superficial veins.

The superficial veins of the upper limb are as follows: the digital, metacarpal, cephalic, basilic, and median veins. The digital and metacarpal veins form a venous network on the dorsal and palmar aspect of the hand. The cephalic vein begins on the radial side of the dorsal venous network and ascends along the radial aspect of the forearm and arm (Fig. 15-29). The cephalic vein ultimately drains into the axillary vein just below the clavicle. The cephalic vein communicates with the basilic vein through the median basilic vein in the front of the elbow. The basilic vein begins in the ulnar part of the dorsal venous network and ascends along the ulnar side of the forearm and the medial aspect of the arm. The basilic vein runs deep at the midportion of the arm and continues as the axillary vein. The axillary vein is an extension of the basilic vein and continues into the neck as the subclavian vein. The subclavian vein unites with the internal jugular vein to form the brachiocephalic vein.

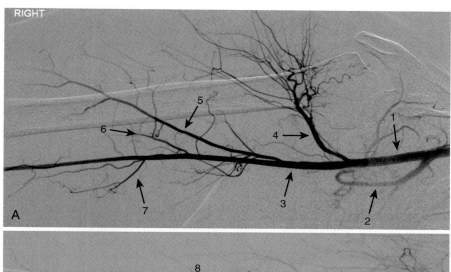

RIGHT

A

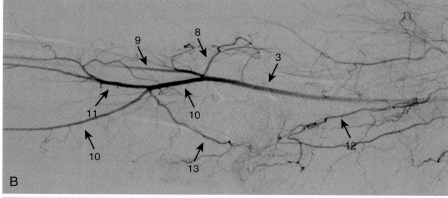

B

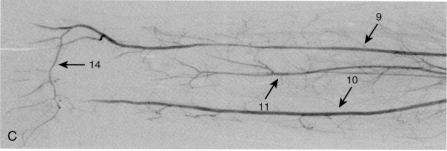

C

Figure 15-28 Upper limb arterial anatomy. A to C, Catheter angiogram images show the arterial anatomy to the upper limb. *1*, Axillary artery; *2*, subscapular artery; *3*, brachial artery; *4*, anterior and posterior circumflex humeral arteries; *5*, profunda branchial artery; *6*, muscular branches; *7*, superior ulnar collateral artery; *8*, radial recurrent artery; *9*, radial artery; *10*; ulnar artery; *11*, interosseous artery; *12*, inferior ulnar collateral artery; *13*, ulnar recurrent artery; and *14*, deep palmar arch.

The subclavian vein receives tributaries from the external jugular vein and, at the junction with the internal jugular vein, receives the thoracic duct on left side and right lymphatic duct on right side. The deep veins of the upper limb accompany the corresponding arteries and constitute their venae comitantes. The superficial and deep volar arterial arches are each accompanied by a pair of venae comitantes that constitute, respectively, the superficial and deep volar venous arches and receive the veins corresponding to the branches of the arterial arches.

■ LOWER LIMBS

Arterial System

The external iliac artery forms the main arterial supply of the lower limbs and continues as the femoral artery beyond the inguinal ligament (Fig. 15-30). The femoral artery continues as the popliteal artery beyond the

adductor canal and divides into two branches: the tibioperoneal trunk and the anterior tibial artery. The branches of the femoral artery include the superficial epigastric, superficial circumflex iliac, superficial and deep external pudendal, highest genicular, muscular, and profunda femoris arteries (Fig. 15-31). The profunda femoris artery is the largest branch of the femoral artery, and it has the following branches: the lateral and medial circumflex femoral arteries, four perforating branches, and the muscular branches.

The popliteal artery is a continuation of the femoral artery in the popliteal fossa, and it terminates by dividing into the anterior tibial artery and tibioperoneal trunk. The tibioperoneal trunk divides into the posterior tibial artery and peroneal artery. The genicular branches of the popliteal artery form a complex network of vessels around the knee joint. The anterior tibial artery gives off the following branches: the anterior and posterior tibial recurrent, anterior medial,

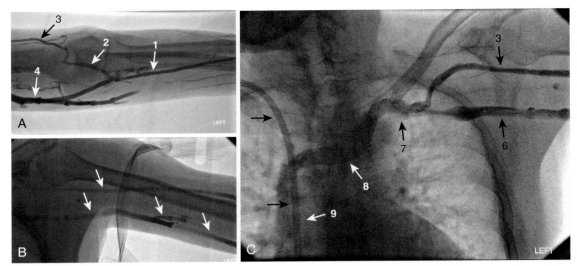

Figure 15-29 Venous anatomy of the upper limbs. A to C, Diagnostic upper limb venograms obtained in different patients show the anatomy of the upper limb veins. *1,* Median antebrachial vein; *2,* median antecubital vein; *3,* cephalic vein; *4,* basilic vein; *5,* brachial vein; *6,* axillary vein; *7,* subclavian vein; *8,* brachiocephalic vein; and *9,* superior vena cava (SVC). A hemodialysis catheter *(unnumbered arrows)* is seen in the right brachiocephalic vein and the SVC.

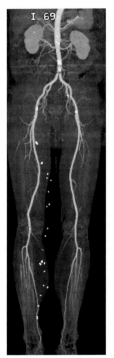

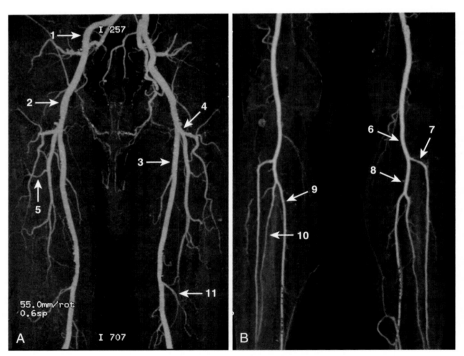

Figure   15-30 Coronal   maximum intensity projection image from a multidetector computed tomography angiogram shows the arterial anatomy of abdominal aorta and the bilateral lower limbs.

Figure 15-31 A and **B,** Coronal maximum intensity projection images from multidetector computed tomography angiograms show the bilateral lower limb arteries and their anatomy. *1,* External iliac artery; *2,* common femoral artery; *3,* superficial femoral artery; *4,* profunda femoris artery; *5,* perforating arteries; *6,* popliteal artery; *7,* anterior tibial artery; *8,* tibioperoneal trunk; *9,* posterior tibial artery; *10,* peroneal artery; and *11,* genicular artery.

and anterior lateral malleolar arteries. The anterior tibial artery continues as the dorsalis pedis artery and divides finally into the first dorsal metatarsal and the deep plantar arteries. The posterior tibial artery has the following branches: the fibular, posterior medial malleolar, medial calcaneal, and lateral and medial plantar arteries (Fig. 15-32). An interesting rare variant of lower limb arterial vasculature is the persistent sciatic artery (Fig. 15-33). Persistent sciatic artery is anatomically an extension of the internal iliac artery that takes the course of the inferior gluteal artery through the greater sciatic foramen and runs on the posterior aspect of the adductor magnus in the thigh to continue as the popliteal artery in the knee. It has anastomotic communications with the perforating vessels of the profunda femoris artery along its course.

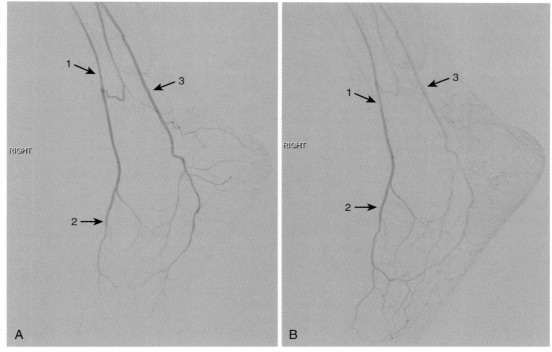

Figure 15-32 Distal arteries of the foot and leg. A and **B,** Catheter angiogram images show the distal arteries of the foot. *1,* Anterior tibial artery; *2,* dorsalis pedis artery; and *3,* posterior tibial artery.

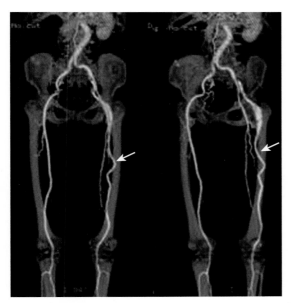

Figure 15-33 Coronal maximum intensity projection computed tomography image demonstrating persistent sciatic artery *(arrows)* on the left side.

Venous System

As in the upper limb, the venous system of the lower limb is formed by the deep and the superficial venous system. The principal superficial veins of the lower extremity are the small saphenous veins and the great saphenous vein (GSV). The small saphenous vein originates from the lateral aspect of the foot and ascends up to the knee. The small saphenous vein terminates by draining into the popliteal vein or joins the GSV through a Giacomini vein or the deep muscular veins. The GSV originates in the medial aspect of the foot, passes anterior to the medial malleolus, and then ascends medially to terminate in the common femoral vein at the groin crease. This junction is called the saphenofemoral junction. Before its termination into the common femoral vein, the GSV receives the superficial inferior epigastric, superficial external pudendal, and superficial circumflex iliac veins. The superficial veins communicate with the deep veins of the calf and thigh through the perforating veins. The perforating veins usually have venous valves that prevent reflux of blood from the deep veins into the superficial system. The perforating veins are frequently constant and include the perforators in the midthigh (Hunter), in the distal thigh (Dodd), at the knee (Boyd), and at the distal medial calf and ankle (Cockett). The deep veins of the lower limb, often paired, accompany the corresponding arteries and include the popliteal vein and the femoral vein in the thigh and the anterior tibial, posterior tibial, and peroneal veins in the leg.

Bibliography

Abraham V, Mathew A, Cherian V, Chandran S, Mathew G. Aberrant subclavian artery: anatomical curiosity or clinical entity. *Int J Surg.* 2009;7:106-109.

Alsenaidi K, Gurofsky R, Karamlou T, Williams WG, McCrindle BW. Management and outcomes of double aortic arch in 81 patients. *Pediatrics.* 2006;118:e1336-e1341.

Baptista-Silva JC, Verissimo MJ, Castro MJ, Camara AL, Pestana JO. Anatomical study of the renal veins observed during 342 living-donor nephrectomies. *Sao Paulo Med J.* 1997;15:1456-1459.

Donnelly LF, Fleck RJ, Pacharn P, Ziegler MA, Fricke BL, Cotton RT. Aberrant subclavian arteries: cross-sectional imaging findings in infants and children referred for evaluation of extrinsic airway compression. *AJR Am J Roentgenol.* 2002;178:1269-1274.

Ellis H. The superficial veins of the leg. *Br J Hosp Med (Lond)*. 2006;67:M186-M187.

Ellis H. The superficial veins of the leg. *Br J Hosp Med (Lond)*. 2009;70:M164-M165.

Erbay N, Raptopoulos V, Pomfret EA, Kamel IR, Kruskal JB. Living donor liver transplantation in adults: vascular variants important in surgical planning for donors and recipients. *AJR Am J Roentgenol*. 2003;181:109-114.

Gray H. The Arteries. In: Gray H, ed. *Anatomy of the Human Body*. 20th ed. Philadelphia: Lea & Febiger; 1918.

Gray H. The veins. In: Gray H, ed. *Anatomy of the Human Body*. 20th ed. Philadelphia: Lea & Febiger; 1918.

Hamper UM, DeJong MR, Scoutt LM. Ultrasound evaluation of the lower extremity veins. *Radiol Clin North Am*. 2007;45:525-547, ix.

Kanne JP, Godwin JD. Right aortic arch and its variants. *J Cardiovasc Comput Tomogr*. 2010;4:293-300.

Layton KF, Kallmes DF, Cloft HJ, Lindell EP, Cox VS. Bovine aortic arch variant in humans: clarification of a common misnomer. *AJNR Am J Neuroradiol*. 2006;27:1541-1542.

Mandell VS, Jaques PF, Delany DJ, Oberheu V. Persistent sciatic artery: clinical, embryologic, and angiographic features. *AJR Am J Roentgenol*. 1985;144: 245-249.

Nonent M, Larroche P, Forlodou P, Senecail B. Celiac-bimesenteric trunk: anatomic and radiologic description—case report. *Radiology*. 2001;220:489-491.

Richard 3rd HM, Selby Jr JB, Gay SB, Tegtmeyer CJ. Normal venous anatomy and collateral pathways in upper extremity venous thrombosis. *Radiographics*. 1992;12:527-534.

Stepansky F, Hecht EM, Rivera R, et al. Dynamic MR angiography of upper extremity vascular disease: pictorial review. *Radiographics*. 2008;28:e28.

Winston CB, Lee NA, Jarnagin WR, et al. CT angiography for delineation of celiac and superior mesenteric artery variants in patients undergoing hepatobiliary and pancreatic surgery. *AJR Am J Roentgenol*. 2007;189:W13-W19.

CHAPTER 16

Comparative Anatomy

Carlos Andres Rojas and Suhny Abbara

This chapter illustrates basic cardiovascular anatomy using multiple imaging modalities for correlation. Examples of normal anatomy in standard planes are given, as well as a few examples of abnormal cardiac anatomy with corresponding appearances on various imaging techniques. The goal of this chapter is to help the reader, who may be familiar with one or two cardiac imaging modalities, recognize the orientation and identify the anatomy in other imaging techniques.

First, this chapter reviews the cardiovascular borders on standard posteroanterior (PA) and lateral views of the chest and correlates these borders with coronal and sagittal reconstruction of computed tomography (CT) of the chest (Figs. 16-1 and 16-2). The figures show matching colored dotted lines on both CT and chest radiography that outline the respective border-forming structures that result in differential attenuation in chest radiography.

From there, the chapter reviews and depicts the basic standard echocardiographic projections. Several figures illustrate the orientation of the echocardiographic planes and the probe orientation on CT volume-rendered three-dimensional (3-D) reconstruction of the chest (see Figs. 16-13 to 16-16). Illustration of the basic standard echocardiographic projections and their corresponding CT and magnetic resonance imaging (MRI) images is also performed (Figs. 16-3 to 16-12).

Finally, conventional angiographic projections and their coronary CT angiogram correlations are shown (Figs. 16-17 to 16-26). The hope is that this chapter will facilitate an understanding of the anatomy and orientation of the heart and great vessels as seen in these various imaging modalities.

■ CHEST RADIOGRAPH

The cardiovascular silhouette in chest radiography is the result of multiple superimposed structures. The examiner must recognize the normal structures that comprise the cardiovascular borders in both standard posteroanterior (PA) and lateral projections. On the PA view, the right cardiac border has three border-forming segments: the superior vena cava (SVC) or ascending aorta, the right atrium (RA), and the inferior vena cava (IVC). The left cardiac border has four segments: the distal aortic arch or knob (arch is a commonly used misnomer because the aortic contour usually is distal to the left subclavian artery origin, thus making this segment

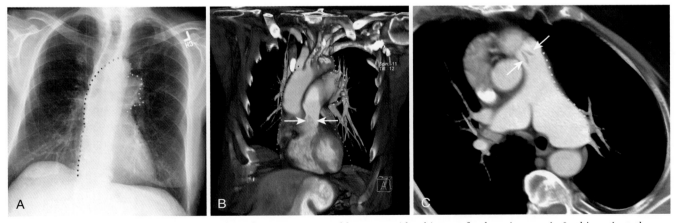

Figure 16-1 **A,** Posteroanterior (PA) view of the chest in a 27-year-old woman with a history of pulmonic stenosis. In this patient, the cardiovascular silhouette on the PA view of the chest is composed of the inferior vena cava *(dark red dotted line),* right atrium *(orange dotted line),* ascending aorta *(purple dotted line),* aortic arch *(green dotted line),* left pulmonary artery *(yellow dotted line),* left atrial appendage *(red dotted line),* and left ventricle *(blue dotted line).* The left pulmonary artery is abnormally enlarged secondary to pulmonic stenosis. In the setting of pulmonic stenosis, the direction of flow results in asymmetric poststenotic dilatation of the left pulmonary artery. Coronal **(B)** and axial oblique **(C)** CT volume-rendered images of the chest in the same patient demonstrate thickening of the pulmonic valve leaflets *(arrows)* and preferential dilatation of the left pulmonary artery.

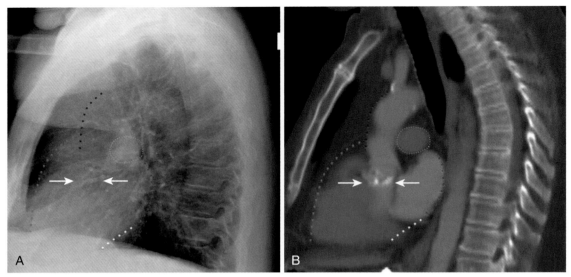

Figure 16-2 A, Lateral view of the chest in a 85-year-old woman with critical aortic stenosis. The cardiovascular silhouette on the lateral view consists of the right ventricle and right ventricular outflow tract *(blue dotted line)*, ascending aorta *(purple dotted line)*, right pulmonary artery *(yellow dotted oval)*, left atrium *(red dotted line)*, and left ventricle *(white dotted line)*. The left and main pulmonary arteries are not well depicted in this view. Abnormal calcifications are noted on the lateral view of the chest in the expected location of the aortic valve *(arrows)*. **B,** Corresponding coronal reconstruction of a nongated computed tomography image with contrast in the same patient confirms the presence of aortic valve calcifications *(arrows)* in this patient with known severe aortic stenosis.

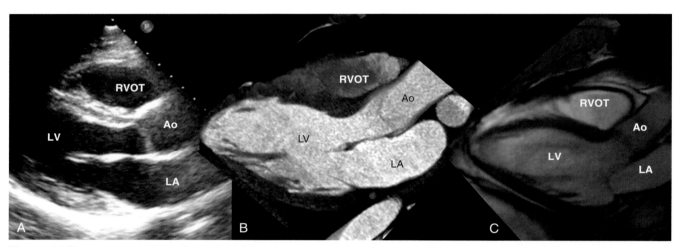

Figure 16-3 Transthoracic echocardiographic left parasternal long-axis view **(A)** and corresponding computed tomography **(B)** and magnetic resonance imaging **(C)** images in the same plane. This projection allows visualization of the left ventricle (LV; anteroseptal and inferolateral walls), right ventricle/right ventricular outflow tract (RVOT), left atrium (LA), mitral and aortic valves, LV outflow tract, aortic root, and coronary sinus. It is a good projection to assess mitral and aortic disease when using color Doppler imaging. The left parasternal long-axis view is one of the standard views to assess left ventricular function, chamber size and LV wall thickness. Its limitations include poor visualization of the apex (echocardiography only). *Ao,* Aorta; *RVOT,* right ventricular outflow tract.

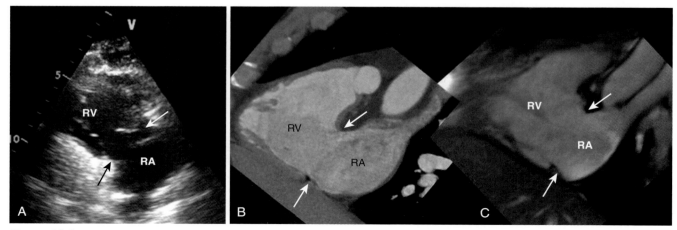

Figure 16-4 Transthoracic echocardiographic parasternal right ventricular inflow view **(A)** and corresponding computed tomography **(B)** and magnetic resonance imaging **(C)** images in similar planes. This projection allows visualization of the right ventricle (RV), right atrium (RA), tricuspid valve *(arrows)*, and coronary sinus drainage into the RA. It is a good projection to assess the severity of tricuspid regurgitation with color Doppler imaging.

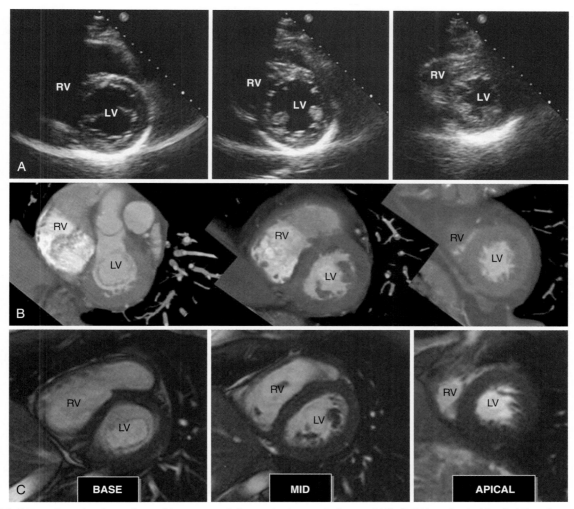

Figure 16-5 Transthoracic echocardiographic parasternal short-axis views at the base, middle (MID), and apical levels **(A)** and corresponding computed tomography **(B)** and magnetic resonance imaging **(C)** images in the same planes. These projections allow assessment of left and right ventricular segmental wall motion. It is also a good additional projection to assess the mitral valve leaflets and apparatus. The apical region is commonly difficult to assess because of interposition of the lung. *LV,* Left ventricle; *RV,* right ventricle.

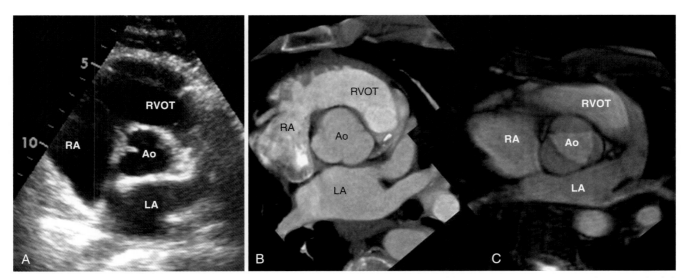

Figure 16-6 Transthoracic echocardiographic parasternal short-axis view of the aortic valve **(A)** and corresponding computed tomography **(B)** and magnetic resonance imaging **(C)** images in the same plane. This projection allows visualization of the aortic valve, right atrium (RA), left atrium (LA), interatrial septum, right ventricular outflow tract (RVOT), and proximal pulmonary artery. The origins of the coronary arteries can occasionally be visualized. *Ao,* Aorta.

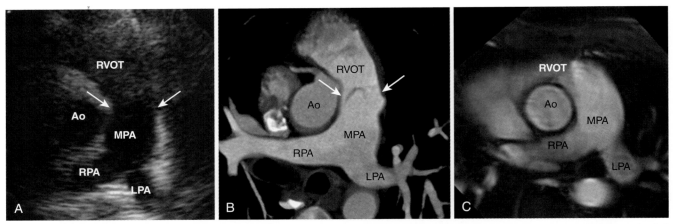

Figure 16-7 Transthoracic echocardiographic parasternal right ventricular outflow view (**A**) and corresponding computed tomography (**B**) and magnetic resonance imaging (**C**) images in the same plane. This projection allows assessment of the proximal pulmonary artery (PA) and the PA bifurcation. It is an important view to evaluate PA enlargement in patients with pulmonary hypertension and to assess for patent ductus arteriosus. *Ao*, Aorta; *LPA*, left pulmonary artery; *MPA*, main pulmonary artery; *RPA*, right pulmonary artery; *RVOT*, right ventricular outflow tract.

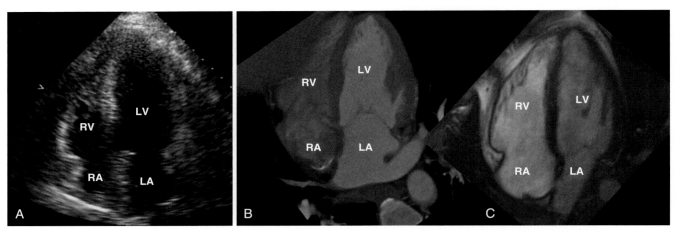

Figure 16-8 Transthoracic echocardiographic apical four-chamber view (**A**) and corresponding computed tomography (**B**) and magnetic resonance imaging (**C**) images in the same plane. This projection allows visualization of all four chambers of the heart and the interatrial septum. It is an essential projection for the determination of left ventricular volumes and left ventricular ejection fraction (biplane Simpson method). It also allows physiologic evaluation of mitral valve function, particularly mitral stenosis, because of optimal (parallel) alignment of the blood flow and the Doppler beam. The apical four-chamber view also allows assessment of LV apical function. *LA*, Left atrium; *LV*, left ventricle; *RA*, right atrium; *RV*, right ventricle.

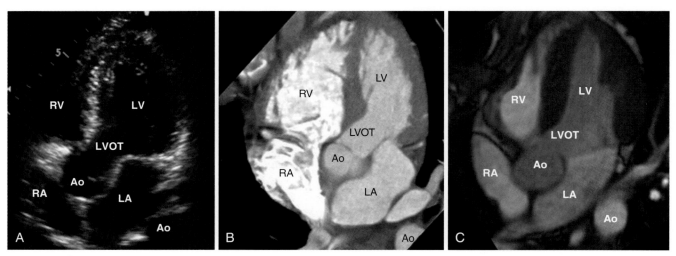

Figure 16-9 Transthoracic echocardiographic apical five-chamber view (**A**) and corresponding computed tomography (**B**) and magnetic resonance imaging (**C**) images in the same plane. A five-chamber view is a modified four-chamber view that includes the aortic outflow tract and portions of the aortic root. It allows evaluation of aortic regurgitation and stenosis using Doppler imaging. Appropriate alignment of aortic stenosis jets is needed for optimal assessment. This is the ideal view to assess left ventricular outflow tract (LVOT) obstruction disorders, such as hypertrophic obstructive cardiomyopathy and subaortic membrane. *Ao*, Aorta; *LA*, left atrium; *LV*, left ventricle; *RA*, right atrium; *RV*, right ventricle.

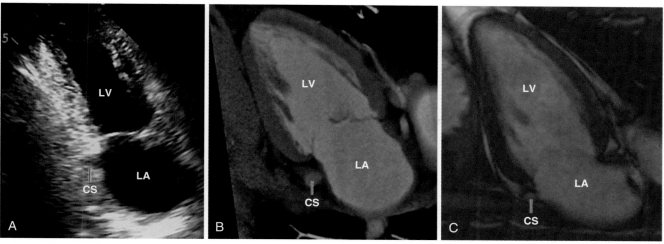

Figure 16-10 Transthoracic echocardiographic apical two-chamber view **(A)** and corresponding computed tomography **(B)** and magnetic resonance imaging **(C)** images in the same plane. This projection allows visualization of the left atrium (LA), left ventricle (LV), and coronary sinus (CS). It is essential for the determination of left ventricular volumes (biplane Simpson method). It is a complementary view for assessment of mitral valve disease. The apical two-chamber view is the only view including the entire inferior and anterior LV walls.

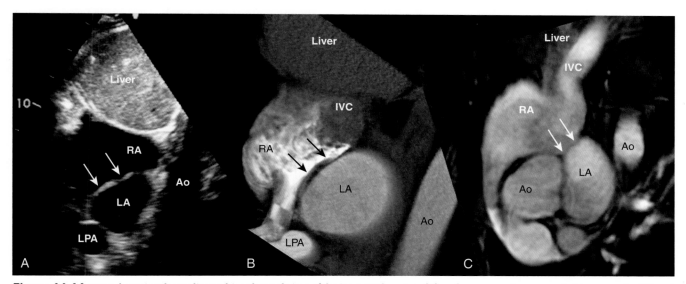

Figure 16-11 Transthoracic echocardiographic subcostal view of the interatrial septum **(A)** and corresponding computed tomography **(B)** and magnetic resonance imaging **(C)** images in the same plane. This projection is a good echocardiographic projection to evaluate the interatrial septum *(arrows)*. Shunts can be assessed with color Doppler imaging or with intravascular contrast. *Ao,* Aorta; *IVC,* inferior vena cava; *LA,* left atrium; *LPA,* left pulmonary artery; *RA,* right atrium.

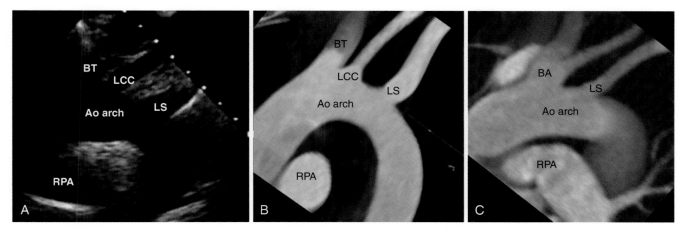

Figure 16-12 Transthoracic echocardiographic suprasternal long-axis view of the aortic arch (Ao arch) **(A)** and corresponding computed tomography **(B)** and magnetic resonance imaging **(C)** images in the same plane. This is an important projection for assessment of aortic disorders, such as aneurysms, dissection, and coarctation. Notice the bovine arch (BA) configuration in **C**, with the brachiocephalic trunk (BT) and the left common carotid (LCC) artery sharing a common origin. *LS,* Left subclavian artery; *RPA,* right pulmonary artery.

technically the proximal descending aorta), the main pulmonary artery, the left atrial appendage, and the left ventricle (LV). On the lateral view, the anterior cardiac border has three segments: the right ventricle (RV), the right ventricular outflow tract (RVOT) and main pulmonary artery, and the ascending aorta. On the lateral view, the posterior cardiac margin has two segments: the LV and the left atrium. The right pulmonary artery can be seen as a density anterior to the tracheal, or more correctly the main stem bronchial, lucency.

■ ECHOCARDIOGRAPHY

Two-dimensional echocardiography is a relatively inexpensive, readily available technique to evaluate the cardiac morphology and function. Grayscale images are obtained from four standard transducer positions: parasternal, apical, subxiphoid (subcostal), and suprasternal (Figs. 16-13 to 16-16). Usually, the LV is displayed on the left side, and the apex appears on the top of the image.

Eighteen standard projections are routinely obtained on transthoracic echocardiography. Eight of them are obtained in the parasternal projection, and they are the long-axis view, the RV inflow view, the LV outflow view, three short-axis views of the LV (base, middle, and apical), the short-axis view of the aortic valve and RV outflow, and a view of the pulmonary artery bifurcation. From the apical projection, three views are routinely obtained: a four-chamber view, a five-chamber view, and a two-chamber view.

The subcostal projection is particularly useful in patients with poor precordial windows. From a subcostal projection, images of the IVC and hepatic veins (tricuspid regurgitation, pulmonary hypertension, restrictive right-sided filling, and constrictive pericarditis produce distinct Doppler signals in the hepatic veins), RA inflow, RV and LV inflow, LV, aorta, and RV outflow tract are typically obtained. The subcostal is the best projection to evaluate the entirety of the atrial septum. From the suprasternal projection, images in the long axis and short axis of

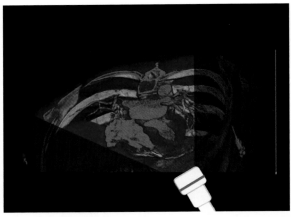

Figure 16-14 Transthoracic apical four-chamber view illustrated on a three-dimensional computed tomography volume-rendered image. Apical images are obtained by placing the transducer at the point of maximal apical impulse.

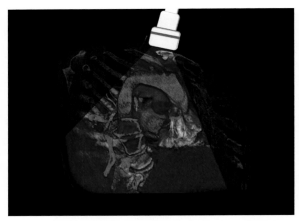

Figure 16-15 Computed tomography volume-rendered image depicts the suprasternal technique used in transthoracic echocardiography when obtaining suprasternal long-axis view obtained. Images are acquired by placing the transducer in the suprasternal notch.

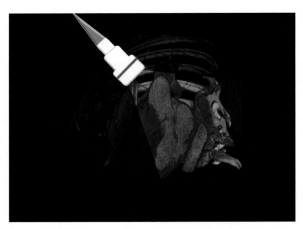

Figure 16-13 Computed tomography volume-rendered image depicts the left parasternal window and imaging plane illustrated on a three-dimensional volume-rendered computed tomography angiography image. Left parasternal images are obtained by placing the transducer in the left parasternal region at the level of the third to fourth intercostal space.

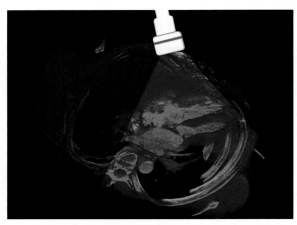

Figure 16-16 Computed tomography volume-rendered image depicts the subcostal projection used in transthoracic echocardiography with a subcostal four-chamber view obtained. Subcostal images are obtained by placing the transducer in the right subcostal or subxiphoid region.

the aorta are obtained to include views of the SVC and pulmonary arteries. For more detail, and examples of each of the standard projection, see Chapter 1. Several standard-plane echocardiographic images and multiplanar reformations of coronary CT angiography (CTA) and MRI images in corresponding planes are demonstrated in Figures 16-3 to 16-12.

Catheter Angiography

Catheter angiography is a minimally invasive procedure with diagnostic and therapeutic implications. The nomenclature of the standard projections used during evaluation of the coronary arteries is relative to the position of the image intensifier with respect to the patient. Examples of the angiographic projections and the corresponding CTA image planes are given in Figures 16-17

to 16-26. For example, in a right anterior oblique (RAO) projection, the patient's anterior right side is closer to the image intensifier and farther away from the x-ray source. The same concept applies to the cranial or caudal angulations, with the image intensifier closer to the patient's head in a cranial projection. The basic standard projections used are AP, RAO, and left anterior oblique (LAO), with various degrees of craniocaudal angulation to visualize different coronary segments more clearly. For more details on angiographic projections and the resulting views, see Chapters 2 and 14.

■ MAGNETIC RESONANCE IMAGING AND COMPUTED TOMOGRAPHY

Cardiac MRI and CT are cross-sectional modalities that allow unrestricted user definition of any plane imaginable. CTA uses isovolumetric voxels that allow superior 3-D volume rendering and creation of any imaging plane during image analysis without repeat imaging of the patient. Many MRI pulse sequences can be prescribed in any plane; once the patient has left the scanner, however, only the planes that were prospectively acquired are available. The exceptions are 3-D MRI angiography and other 3-D acquisitions that are becoming available. Detailed descriptions of cross-sectional CT and MRI anatomy of the heart can be found in Chapters 12 and 13. In this chapter, CT and MRI are used for the purpose of correlation and are presented in in standard echocardiographic planes and angiographic projections.

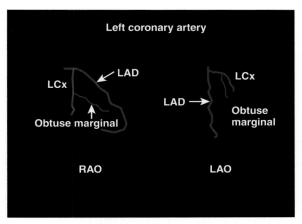

Figure 16-17 Illustration of the usual layout of the left coronary arterial system in the right anterior oblique (RAO) and left anterior oblique (LAO) projections. Various degrees of cephalocaudal angulations are commonly obtained to visualize the different coronary segments more clearly. *LAD,* Left anterior descending coronary artery; *LCx,* left circumflex coronary artery.

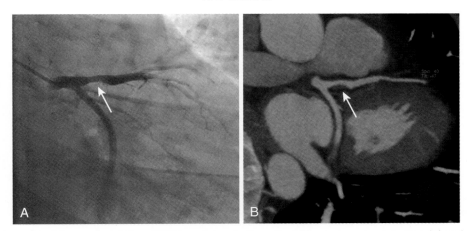

Figure 16-18 Angiographic right anterior oblique (RAO) caudal projection after left coronary artery injection **(A)** and a corresponding computed tomography (CT) maximum intensity projection (MIP) image **(B)** demonstrate the presence of a noncalcified plaque in the proximal left anterior descending coronary artery with approximately 40% luminal narrowing *(arrows)*. An angiogram is a pure luminogram and as such does not visualize the atheroma. CT does show the luminal narrowing, but it also shows the underlying cause of the obstructive lesion, a noncalcified atherosclerotic plaque in this case.

RAO CRANIAL

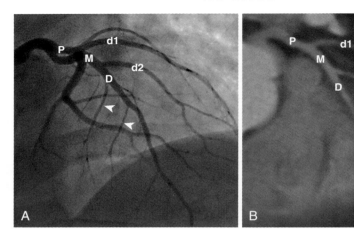

Figure 16-19 Angiographic right anterior oblique (RAO) cranial projection **(A)** and a corresponding computed tomography volume-rendered image **(B)** demonstrate the normal appearance of the proximal (P), middle (M), and distal (D) left anterior descending coronary artery (LAD) and the presence of two diagonal branches (d1, d2). Notice the nearly perpendicular origin of the septal perforator branches *(arrowheads)*, which help identify the LAD.

LAO CAUDAL

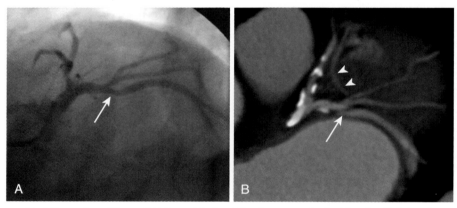

Figure 16-20 Angiographic left anterior oblique (LAO) caudal view (also known as the "spider view") **(A)** and a corresponding computed tomography (CT) volume-rendered image **(B)** demonstrate a 30% lesion in the middle left circumflex (LCx) coronary artery *(arrows)*. The volume-rendered CT image demonstrates a large amount of calcified plaque in the left main coronary artery and a moderate amount of scattered calcified plaque in the proximal left anterior descending coronary artery and LCx. The volume-rendered image overestimates the degree of luminal narrowing in the middle LCx; therefore, this type of reconstruction should not be used for diagnostic purposes. Incidentally noted is the great cardiac vein *(arrowheads)* on the CT image **(B)**.

LAO CRANIAL

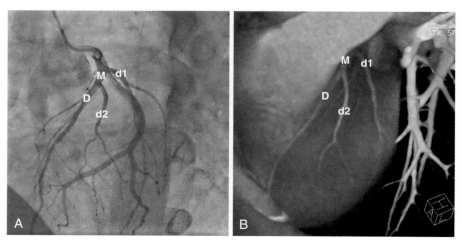

Figure 16-21 Angiographic left anterior oblique (LAO) cranial view **(A)** and a corresponding computed tomography volume-rendered image **(B)** demonstrate the normal appearance of the middle (M) and distal (D) left anterior descending coronary artery and two diagonal branches (d1, d2).

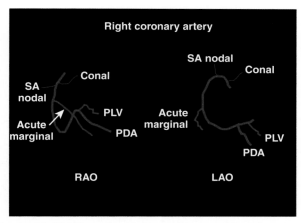

Figure 16-22 Illustration of the usual layout of the right coronary system in the right anterior oblique (RAO) and left anterior oblique (LAO) projections. *PDA*, Posterior descending artery; *PLV*, posterior left ventricular branch; *SA nodal*, sinoatrial nodal branch

RAO

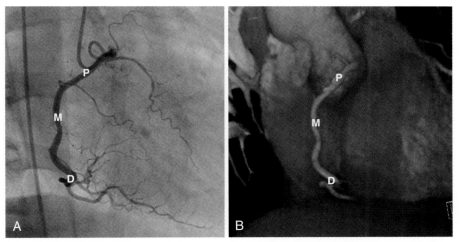

Figure 16-23 Angiographic right anterior oblique (RAO) view **(A)** of the right coronary artery (RCA) and a corresponding computed tomography volume-rendered image **(B)** demonstrate the normal appearance of the proximal (P), middle (M), and distal (D) segments of the RCA.

RAO

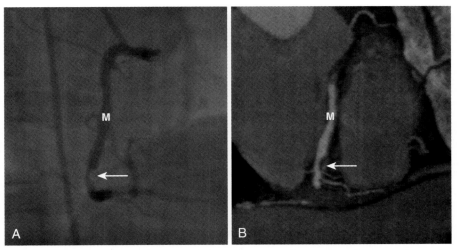

Figure 16-24 Angiographic right anterior oblique (RAO) view **(A)** and a corresponding computed tomography maximum intensity projection image **(B)** demonstrate a 70% lesion in the distal middle (M) segment of the right coronary artery *(arrows)*.

LAO

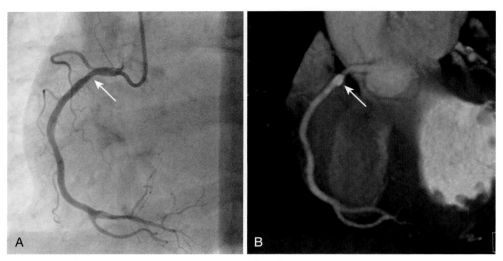

Figure 16-25 Angiographic left anterior oblique (LAO) projection **(A)** and a corresponding computed tomography volume-rendered image **(B)** demonstrate a 20% lesion in the proximal segment of the right coronary artery *(arrows)*. The CT volume-rendered image **(B)** demonstrates a small amount of calcified plaque, which limits the evaluation of the lumen on volume-rendered images.

LAO

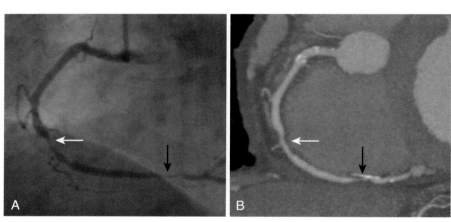

Figure 16-26 Angiographic left anterior oblique (LAO) view **(A)** and a corresponding computed tomography (CT) maximum intensity projection image **(B)** demonstrate a 70% lesion in the distal midsegment of the right coronary artery (RCA) *(white arrows)* and a high 90% stenosis in the distal RCA *(black arrows)*. The CT maximum intensity projection image **(B)** demonstrates a moderate amount of calcified plaque near the distal RCA lesion.

Bibliography

Angelini P. Normal and anomalous coronary arteries: definitions and classification. *Am Heart J.* 1989;117:418-434.

Austen WG, Edwards JE, Frye RL, et al. A reporting system on patients evaluated for coronary artery disease. *Circulation.* 1975;51(suppl 4):3-40.

Cerqueira MD, Weissman NJ, Dilsizian V, et al. Standardized myocardial segmentation and nomenclature for tomographic imaging of the heart: a statement for healthcare professional from the cardiac imaging committee of the council on clinical cardiology of the American Heart Association. *Circulation.* 2002;105:539-542.

Jacobs JE. Computed tomographic evaluation of the normal cardiac anatomy. *Radiol Clin North Am.* 2010;48:701-710.

Lang RM, Bierig M, Devereux RB, et al. Recommendations for chamber quantification: a report from the American Society of Echocardiography's Guidelines and Standards Committee and the Chamber Quantification Writing Group, developed in conjunction with the European Association of Echocardiography, a branch of the European Society of Cardiology. *J Am Soc Echocardiogr.* 2005;18:1440-1463.

O'Brien JP, Srichai MB, Hecht EM, et al. Anatomy of the heart at multidetector CT: what the radiologist needs to know. *Radiographics.* 2007;27:1569-1582.

Pannu HK, Flohr TG, Corl FM, et al. Current concepts in multi-detector row CT evaluation of the coronary arteries: principles, techniques, and anatomy. *Radiographics.* 2003;23:S111-S125.

Raff GL, Abidov A, Achenbach S, et al. SCCT guidelines for the interpretation and reporting of coronary computed tomographic angiography. *J Cardiovasc Comput Tomogr.* 2009;3:122-136.

Saremi F, Krishnan S. Cardiac conduction system: anatomic landmarks relevant to interventional electrophysiologic techniques demonstrated with 64-Detector CT. *Radiographics.* 2007;27:1539-1567.

Schoepf UJ, Zwerner PL, Savino G, et al. Coronary CT angiography. *Radiology.* 2007;244:48-63.

Standring S, ed. *Gray's Anatomy: The Anatomical Basis of Clinical Practice.* 39th ed, New York: Churchill Livingstone; 2005:977-1057.

Vogel-Claussen J, Pannu H, Spevak PJ, et al. Cardiac valve assessment with MR imaging and 64-section multi-detector row CT. *Radiographics.* 2006;26:1769-1784.

DEVICES

CHAPTER 17

Cardiac Valves

Vikram Venkatesh and Suhny Abbara

■ HISTORY

Since their inception in the 1950s, cardiac valve prostheses have undergone remarkable improvements, yet their fundamental construction has remained largely unchanged. The prosthetic cardiac valve is inextricably linked to the development of extracorporeal circulation, which was also being designed during the same period, in the early 1950s. The use of extracorporeal circulation permitted the delivery of cardioplegia to arrest cardiac motion temporarily for placement of valvular prostheses, among other indications.

The first artificial valve was placed by Dr. Charles Hufnagel in the descending thoracic aorta for the treatment of a patient with aortic insufficiency. Although this effort was only minimally successful, rapid advances in the field led to the first successful artificial valve implantation, which was performed in 1960 by Dr. Dwight Harken and involved placing a caged ball valve in a subcoronary position. Since that initial surgical procedure, cardiac valves have been placed in situ in hundreds of thousands of patients worldwide. A concomitant decrease in mortality has also occurred, from almost 20% in the early years of cardiac valve implantation to less than 2% in most centers worldwide today.

More than 70 different types of both mechanical and bioprosthetic valves have been placed since the inception of valve replacement surgery. In practice, however, only a few valves are commonly used at present, and these include the Starr-Edwards ball valve, the Omniscience, Omnicarbon, and Medtronic Hall tilting disk valves, and the St. Jude and Carbomedics bileaflet valves.

■ IMAGING

Imaging of cardiac valve prostheses has been an integral part of evaluation since the mechanical valve itself was first introduced. Knowledge of the different valve prostheses allows the cardiac imager to make an accurate determination about the function and placement of the valve prosthesis, either mechanical or bioprosthetic.

Initial evaluation of valve prostheses was limited to the use of radiographs and was largely confined to anatomic delineation. With the advent of more advanced echocardiographic techniques, as well as improvements in computed tomography (CT) imaging and magnetic resonance imaging (MRI), however, noninvasive prosthetic valvular

assessment became possible. More invasive imaging in terms of both anatomic delineation and function is also possible with cardiac catheterization.

Caged Ball Valves

The caged ball valve was the original mechanical heart valve. Over the years, several iterations have provided variations on the theme of a ball in a cage. Various attempts have been made in each of these designs to develop better cage mechanisms by using different alloys such as titanium and by altering the configuration of the cage itself, such as incorporating double cages. The ball within the cage was also changed several times to incorporate different alloys and different combinations of nylon and silicone in attempts to reduce ball variance. A significant improvement in ball technology occurred when the silicone ball was heat cured, a process that essentially eliminated variance, which was one of the main problems of the earlier designs.

Hufnagel Aortic Ball Valve

The first valvular prosthesis placed by Dr. Hufnagel was a methacrylate ball contained in a methacrylate tube. The ball sat in the proximal portion of the tube in diastole, and three outpouchings opened during systole and allowed for unidirectional flow of blood across the valve. The valve was placed in the descending aorta and was designed for use in patients with aortic insufficiency.

More than 200 individuals received the Hufnagel prosthesis. No anticoagulation was used. Hufnagel ball valves recovered 30 years after implantation showed no wear. The prosthesis remained essentially untouched from its original design, except for the replacement of the methacrylate ball with a hollow nylon ball that was coated in silicone to reduce valve noise.

Harken-Soroff Ball Valve

Originally introduced in 1960, the Harken-Soroff ball valve consisted of a Magovern turtleneck sewing ring covered by a Dacron skirt to facilitate easy insertion. Approximately 2300 patients had Harken valves inserted in the late 1960s and early 1970s. The operative mortality and long-term risk of thrombosis were both reported to be approximately 7%. The valve itself was found to suffer from variance and disk wear. At the time of its inception, it had a significantly lower rate of complication than the Starr-Edwards valve.

Bahnson Fabric Cusp Valve

Originally introduced in 1960, the Bahnson valve consisted of Teflon knit aortic cusps. Anywhere from one to three cusps could be replaced with this design. Although the initial evaluation of the efficacy of the valve was successful, ultimately the valve was limited by stiffening and tearing of the leaflets, which often occurred within the first 24 months because of fibrin deposition and ingrowth of connective tissue.

Magovern-Cromie Ball Valve

Originally introduced in 1962, the Magovern-Cromie ball valve (Pemco, Cleveland, Ohio) consisted of a caged ball valve apparatus that offered the distinct advantage of sutureless fixation with a pin system. The valve was in production from the early 1960s to 1980 and is no longer routinely used. The valve offered the benefit of allowing replacement with relatively short cardiopulmonary bypass times, an advantage at the time when cardiopulmonary bypass technology was at an early stage. In a 13-year follow-up study, the main identified risk was thromboembolic disease. A report from Magovern in 1989 delineated his experience with the procedure and found an 11% rate of isolated aortic valve replacement (AVR) and a relatively low risk of postoperative complications. In his 25-year review, Magovern was able to conclude that the valve was both safe and durable.

Smelloff-Cutter (SCDK) Ball Valve

Originally introduced in 1964, the Smelloff-Cutter ball valve incorporated a double cage design to hold the ball more in the equator of the apparatus. Long-term efficacy of this valve also proved to be quite good. At 25 years, the rates of valvular dysfunction, reoperation, and endocarditis were reported to be 1.16%, 1.16%, and 0.2%, respectively, per patient-year. Furthermore, no surviving patient deteriorated over the reported time in his or her functional New York Heart Association classification. Current reports have noted intact Smelloff-Cutter valves up to 37 years after implantation that are in good condition. The longest reported valve duration was 43 years; however, at that point the valve had to be retired because of lipid infiltration and pannus formation.

DeBakey-Surgitool Valve

The DeBakey-Surgitool valve was introduced in 1967. It was on the market from 1969 to 1978, and approximately 3300 valves were implanted worldwide. The valve represented progress in technology given that it was the first valve to introduce pyrolytic carbon, which provided superior durability and biocompatibility. Ultimately, the valve was discontinued because of its propensity for strut fracture; however, case reports have noted valve durability for more than 30 years.

Braunwald-Cutter Valve

The Braunwald-Cutter caged ball apparatus was first introduced in 1960. The original design incorporated flexible Teflon-coated chordae tendineae. Unfortunately, in the initial offering, the mitral and aortic fabric prostheses became stiff and immobile. Recovered specimens demonstrated covering and infiltration with a tightly adherent layer of fibrous connective tissue. The model was then revised and was reissued in 1968 with struts covered with a knit Dacron tubing and an inflow ring covered with ultrathin polypropylene mesh fabric. This second model was found to suffer from significant cloth and poppet wear, particularly in the aortic position. In several instances, the poppet escaped from the apparatus and embolized. Mitral position valves had better outcomes, likely because of the lower pressures in this position.

Starr-Edwards Valve

The Starr-Edwards valve (Edwards Lifesciences, Irvine, Calif.) was introduced in 1960. The design was much the same as that of other caged ball valves. Between the initial introduction of this valve in 1960 and 1982, several modifications were made to achieve greater stability. These included changing the original Lucite cage to a metal cage and changing the ball from silicone to a hollow satellite ball. Eventually, this ball was replaced with a heat-cured ball that all but eliminated the problem of variance (Figs. 17-1 and 17-2). The fundamental construction of this valve has remained essentially unchanged for more than 30 years.

In intermediate-term follow-up at approximately 8 years, 95% of patients had only New York Heart Association class I or class II symptoms. Same study had no reports of valve thrombosis or late valve-related deaths. In a larger study, Orszulak et al reported on 1100 patients who underwent valve replacement with the 1260 Starr-Edwards valve. This study demonstrated the absence of thromboemboli and of anticoagulant-related bleeding at 5 years to be 90.8% and 98.7%, respectively. Survival from all-cause mortality in this patient population was 76.6%, 59.6%, 44.9%, and 31.2%, at 5, 10, 15, and 20 years, respectively, including operative mortality in this study with median age of 57 years at the time of implantation.

Case reports of the Starr-Edwards valve more than 30 and even 40 years after implantation show excellent durability and no structural valve degeneration. Furthermore, these valves are generally free of thromboembolic or bleeding complications related to anticoagulation.

The initial imaging strategy in the evaluation of the Starr-Edwards valve is typically echocardiography. Comprehensive data on Doppler echocardiographic assessment of the function of the normal Starr-Edwards mitral valve prosthesis are available. Detection of complications related to Starr-Edwards valves is also the typical starting point for evaluation, with reasonable detection rates. Echocardiography has been used to detect cloth tears, thrombosis, and paravalvular regurgitation. Transesophageal echocardiography is typically more sensitive for the detection of complications than is transthoracic echocardiography. Cardiac CT and MRI are potential problem-solving tools to delineate complications seen on echocardiography more clearly or to look for complications in patients when reasonable clinical suspicion exists. Reports of detection of complications related specifically to the Starr-Edwards valve have not been published. The reader is referred to the later section on complication detection for a discussion of the current literature on this subject.

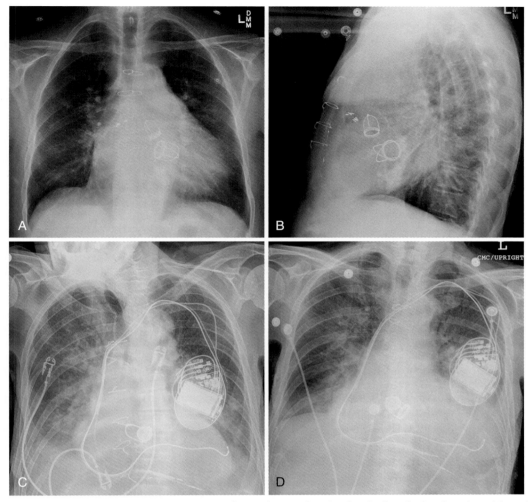

Figure 17-1 Posteroanterior (**A**) and lateral (**B**) radiographs of normal Starr-Edwards valves in the mitral and aortic positions. **C** and **D**, Radiographs of another patient with an aortic Starr-Edwards valve with the metallic ball in the closed (**C**) and open (**D**) positions.

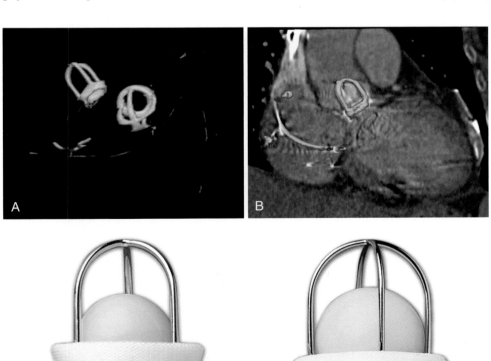

Figure 17-2 Aortic and mitral Starr-Edwards valves on computed tomography. **A**, Three-dimensional volume-rendered reconstruction shows three-pronged aortic and four-pronged mitral Starr-Edwards valves. **B**, Three-dimensional reconstruction with the normally seated aortic Starr-Edwards valve in the open position. Photograph of the three-pronged aortic valve prosthesis (**C**) and the four-pronged mitral valve prosthesis (**D**). (Photographs courtesy Edwards Lifesciences, Irvine, Calif.)

Tilting Disk Valves

The 1960s saw the development of tilting disk valves. These valves have also undergone several design changes since the first clinically available valve in 1969. The typical design of a tilting disk valve is a circular disk that opens and closes and is controlled by a metal strut. Typically, the valve consists of a metal ring covered by fabric. The disk is made of pyrolytic carbon because of the superior longevity and biocompatibility of this material. The main advantage of the tilting disk design is the ability to allow restoration of central blood flow, as opposed to the ball in cage design.

Björk-Shiley Valve

The Björk-Shiley valve (Shiley, Irvine, Calif.) was the first of the low-profile tilting disk valves to be introduced. Two types of valves were marketed. A flat disk model (Fig. 17-3) was introduced in 1969, and a convexoconcave design was subsequently marketed in 1975. In total, approximately 300,000 flat disk valves were inserted in both the mitral and aortic positions, and approximately 86,000 convexoconcave valves were implanted in the same positions. The convexoconcave design was developed to improve flow across the valve, but it led to strut fracture in approximately 2% of cases. This complication

led to a class action law suit and also necessitated prophylactic replacement in several patients.

In the early valves, the disk material was made of Delrin, which is an acetal resin. Initially, this compound was thought to provide stability for more than 50 years of use. However, over time, the disk became susceptible to distortion from steam absorption. Subsequent cases of valve deformity and dysfunction were reported. The valve was revised to change the disk to pyrolitic carbon in 1971, but the initial version was sold until 1979. The popular flat pyrolytic disk model was found to suffer from an increased risk of thrombosis, and therefore the convexoconcave model was subsequently introduced (see Fig. 17-3).

The Björk-Shiley convexoconcave disk was constrained within the device by inlet and outlet struts. Although the inlet strut was integral to the device, the outlet strut was welded to the apparatus. The purported mechanism was excessive force during closing of the disk that was almost 10 times the force experienced during disk opening. The stresses on the outlet strut were greater than the strut wire's fatigue endurance limit. The resulting complications proved catastrophic. Fractures of the valve's outlet struts resulted in escape of the disk, which led to consequent embolization, massive regurgitation, and often death. Sixty- and 70-degree models were introduced. The 70-degree model was withdrawn from the market in

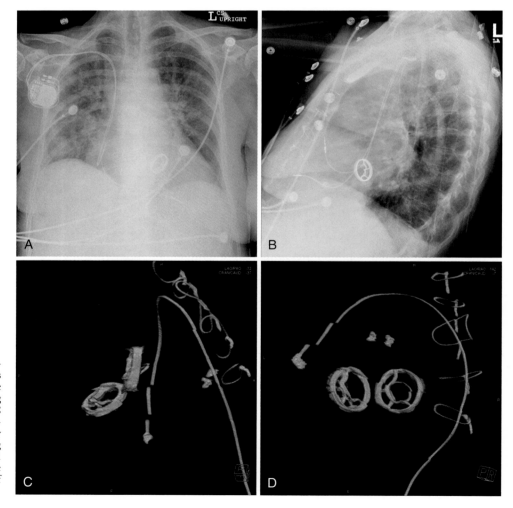

Figure 17-3 **A** and **B**, Postero-anterior and lateral radiographs of a Björk-Shiley valve. Note the appearance of the normal tilting disk valve in the mitral position. **C** and **D**, Three-dimensional volume-rendered computed tomography appearance of Björk-Shiley tilting disk valves placed in both the mitral and tricuspid positions. Note the single tilting disk configuration of the prosthesis.

1983, and the 60-degree model was withdrawn in 1986. The withdrawal of these devices from the market posed a significant risk to the roughly 86,000 patients who had already undergone valve replacement, and therefore reoperation was considered in a subset of patients.

The epidemiologic data identified four factors that contributed to valve failure: opening angle, valve size, mitral position, and young age. Several iterations of decision support about which patients should receive prophylactic valve replacement have been made. A second study concluded in 1998 allowed updating of the guidelines. A 25-year follow-up study on findings after valve replacement is now available. Based on the study by Blot et al, it appears that, in most patients, the risks of reoperation far outweigh the benefits. However, outlet strut fractures do continue to occur even 25 years later. Guidelines have been developed to identify the small percentage of patients who would be expected to have a gain in life expectancy should reoperative surgery be performed. These patients are mainly young men. The risks of outlet strut fracture tend to decrease with increasing age.

Some research on imaging of strut fracture related to these valves has been conducted. O'Neill et al demonstrated that strut fractures can be visualized using high-resolution cineradiography; however, this technique was unable to visualize all strut fractures. This finding led the authors of that study to conclude that although the risk of strut fracture is not entirely eliminated by cineradiographic screening, it can be reduced. In practice, the decision to reoperate is guided mainly by epidemiologic study. No reports of CT or MRI screening to identify those patients at risk of strut fracture have been published.

Medtronic Hall Valve

Originally introduced in 1977, the Medtronic Hall (Medtronic, Inc., Minneapolis, Minn) valve represented an improvement on the tilting disk valves of the day. The design incorporates a Pyrolite disk with a small central hole or perforation. The disk perforation slides over a guidewire, to tilt to the open position (Figs. 17-4 and 17-5). The housing for the disk is made of titanium with a Teflon sewing ring. In contrast to the Björk-Shiley valve, the Medtronic Hall valve contains no welds. In the aortic position, the valve opens to 75 degrees. To date, more than 300,000 of these valves have been placed, and the valve is still in production today. The valve roots originated in Norway, and is the most commonly placed tilting disk valve in the United States.

Long-term follow-up is available for up to 25 years. In their report of a 25-year experience Svennevig et al found no report of mechanical failure of the valve in their cohort of 816 patients. Furthermore, the rates of complication were 1.5% per patient-year for thromboembolic complications, 0.7% per patient-year for warfarin-related bleeding, and 0.16% per patient-year for endocarditis. In another study, Butchart et al found results similar to those of the study by Svennevig et al, with linearized rates of valve-related late death for AVR, mitral valve replacement (MVR), and double valve replacement of 0.8%, 0.9%, and 1.1% annually, respectively. The rates of adverse events were up to 0.04% per year for valve thrombosis, up to 4.0% for all cases of thromboembolism, up to 0.8% per

year for stroke, up to 1.6% for major hemorrhage, and up to 0.7% for prosthetic endocarditis, depending on the position of valve replacement. In contrast, in a smaller study of ethnic Koreans, Cho et al found higher rates of thrombus and pannus formation than reported in the foregoing studies; these complications were attributed to smaller valve sizes implanted in their patients compared with the others.

The goal of the Medtronic Hall design was to improve on previous tilting disk designs, with the aim of improving durability and hemodynamic performance and reducing thrombogenicity. The results of these long-term studies show that these aims have largely been achieved.

The Medtronic Hall valve has also proven to possess superior hemodynamic characteristics, which are intrinsic measures of valve performance. Echocardiographic assessment showed that the hemodynamic performance of the Medtronic Hall valve was significantly better than that of Björk-Shiley and Starr-Edwards prostheses of the same size. Moreover, in 29- or 31-mm prostheses, the hemodynamic parameters were similar to those of native mitral valves. Furthermore, Buthcart et al found that in those patients whose dominant lesion was aortic stenosis without coronary disease, survival was almost identical to that of the age- and sex-matched general population for the first 7.5 years.

The flow characteristics of the Medtronic Hall valve offer relief of transvalvular gradients and therefore allow left ventricular (LV) mass regression after AVR. Furthermore, optimal blood flow across the valve is also thought to reduce the risk of thrombus deposition and platelet activation, thus accounting for the relatively low rates of valve thrombosis. The Medtronic Hall valve has been shown to have superior hemodynamic performance compared with the St. Jude or Monostrut mechanical valves in patients with valves smaller than 20 mm. When these valves are optimally placed, less turbulent flow in comparison with the bileaflet design may contribute to the trend toward greater LV mass regression that has been reported with the Medtronic Hall valve.

CT studies of the Medtronic Hall valve itself are limited. However, in a previous study, investigators showed, using electron beam CT analysis, that Medtronic Hall valve implantation allowed for a reduction in LV mass in patients with small aortic roots.

Lillehei-Kaster, Omniscience, and Omnicarbon Valves

The Lillehei-Kaster valve (Lillehei-Kaster Medical, Inner Grove Heights, Minn.) was first issued in 1970. It was the first of the tilting disk valves to use a Pyrolite disk; the previous valves had all used Delrin as the disk material. The Omniscience and Omnicarbon valves were developed from the original Lillehei-Kaster valve. The Omniscience valve replaced the retaining rails with earlike guards, and the device was made with a much lower profile. The disk housing is made of titanium, and the disk is Pyrolite. The Omnicarbon valve is essentially identical to the Omniscience valve, but it contains a full Pyrolite housing and disk apparatus.

These valves remain in production today, and more than 100,000 of them have been inserted. In a 20-year

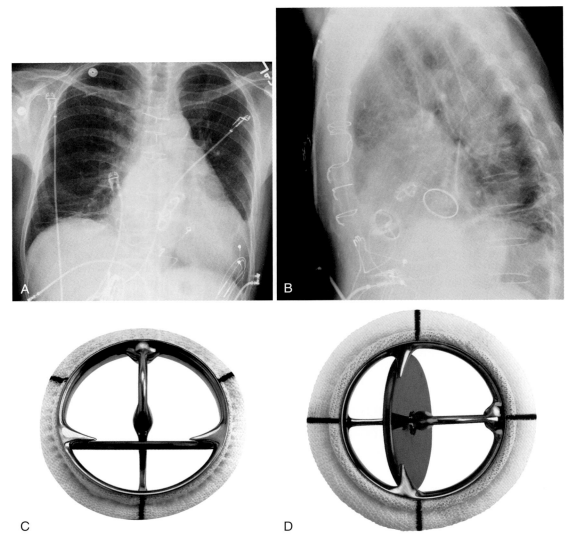

Figure 17-4 A, Posteroanterior radiograph of Medtronic Hall valves demonstrates normally seated single tilting disk valvular prostheses in the mitral and aortic positions. **B,** Lateral radiograph shows that the mitral prosthesis is in the open position, whereas the aortic prosthesis is in the closed position. **C** and **D,** Photographs of the Medtronic Hall Top Hat prosthesis for aortic and mitral valves in the open position. (Courtesy of Medtronic, Inc., Minneapolis, Minn. Copyright Medtronic, Inc. Medtronic Hall Valve Medtronic, Inc. Printed with permission.)

review of their experience with the Omniscience valve, Misawa et al found that the rate of thromboembolic complication was only 0.8%, with an identical rate of hemorrhagic complication. Teijeira reported on 200 Omniscience valve replacements and also found that 12-year thromboembolism-free and anticoagulation-free rates were approximately 80%. Nonstructural prosthetic valve dysfunction rates were 0.6%. In another study, Edwards et al reported a risk of thromboembolism of 0.2% to 1.3% and a risk of systemic embolic events of 1.57% to 2.90% per patient-year. Reports of these valves have had varied results and have been the source of considerable debate in the literature.

Monostrut Valve
The Monostrut valve (Shiley) contains two struts that are connected by machine to the housing, to reduce the chance of strut fracture. In a comparative study with the Carbomedics bileaflet valve, investigators reported a 0.2%

per year risk of thromboembolism and a 0.6% per year risk of anticoagulation-related bleeding. In this study of 200 patients, no difference was noted between the Monostrut tilting disk valve and the Carbomedics valve.

Bileaflet Valves
The general design of the bileaflet valve consists of two semicircular disks that rotate about struts in the valve housing. These valves are in theory more hemodynamically sound; however, they are also susceptible to backflow. They are also generally less thrombogenic and require a lower amount of anticoagulation. Several models of this type of valve are available, and the most important are reviewed here.

St. Jude Medical Valve
The St. Jude valves (St. Jude Medical, Inc., St. Paul, Minn) are the best known and most widely used of the

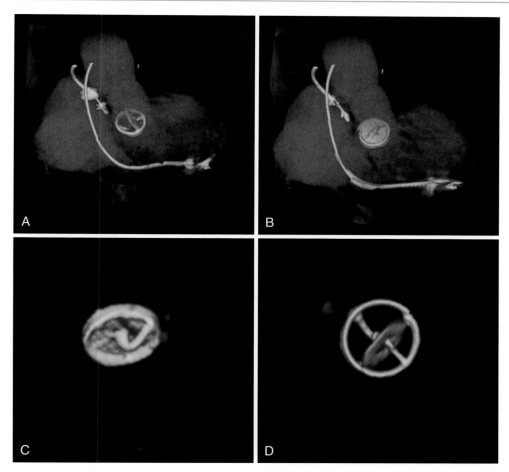

Figure 17-5 Three-dimensional volume-rendered computed tomography images of an aortic position Medtronic Hall valve in the open (**A**) and closed (**B**) positions. Coned-in views demonstrate the relationship of the flange and disk in the closed (**C**) and open (**D**) positions in an orthogonal projection.

bileaflet valves (Figs. 17-6 and 17-7). Originally introduced in 1977, the valve consists of a Pyrolite housing with a sewing ring and Pyrolite hemidisks. The initial design concept was to have peripheral hinges. During the development stages, however, the inventors realized that this design was impractical, and the hinges were therefore moved to be more central in location. This configuration leaves a small central opening in the valve. To date, more than 1.3 million of these valves have been implanted, predominantly in the aortic and mitral valve positions.

The safety profile of these valves has been extensively studied. In a 945-patient study, Toole et al reported their 25-year experience with 537 aortic valves and 408 mitral valves. In this follow-up study, in which the 5-, 10-, 15-, and 20-year results had also previously been reported, all patients underwent single valve replacement. The study did not find a single structural failure of the valve. In the AVR group, 20% of all-cause mortality deaths were found to be valve related, of which bleeding and thromboembolism accounted for 78%, whereas in the MVR group, 14% of deaths were found to be valve related, of which bleeding and thromboembolism accounted for 89%. These findings translate to a 1.9% per patient-year risk of thromboembolism and a 3.0% per patient-year risk of bleeding in the AVR group. In the MVR group, the rate of thromboembolism was 3.2% per patient-year, and the rate of bleeding was 2.3% per patient-year.

In another large study by Khan et al, the main findings were that individuals with the St. Jude valve were significantly more likely to die as a result of non–valve-related complications, and 84% to 91% of these patients had not died of valve-related causes at 10 years. The overall survival was 42% to 43% at 10 years. In their study of 399 patients (4328 patient-years) with MVR, 471 with AVR, and 130 with double (mitral and aortic) valve replacement, thromboembolism rates were 2.4/100, 2.5/100, and 3.2/100 patient-years, for MVR, AVR, and double valve replacement, respectively, whereas the rates of hemorrhage were 1.9/100, 2.0/100, and 2.3/100 patient-years for MVR, AVR, and double valve replacements, respectively.

Another study by Remadi et al, reported in 2001, evaluated MVRs and found that actuarial survival (only from valve-related mortality) was 83% at 10- to 19-year follow-up. The overall survival rate in this group of 446 patients was 63%, a finding once again implying that many patients died of causes other than valve-related mortality. No structural dysfunction was observed during the follow-up period. The most frequent complications were related to anticoagulants, at 1% per patient-year, and the valve thrombosis rate was low, at 0.2% per patient-year.

Data are now also available for reoperation using the St. Jude valvular prosthesis for redo open heart surgery valve replacement. The two most common indications for redo open heart surgery are a new requirement for coronary artery bypass grafting and replacement of a

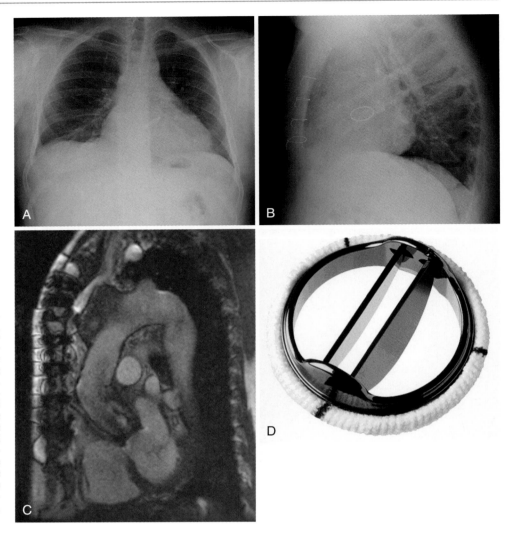

Figure 17-6 St. Jude Medical posteroanterior and lateral radiographs. **A** and **B,** Normal appearance of the bileaflet St. Jude Medical valve in the aortic position. Although the valve leaflets are radiopaque, they are not seen as well as the disk. **C,** Magnetic resonance imaging appearance of the St. Jude valve showing susceptibility related to the valve prosthesis with dephasing related to flow artifact across the valve. **D,** Photograph of the St. Jude Regent bileaflet prosthesis for correlation. (Photograph courtesy of St. Jude Medical, Inc., St. Paul, Minn.)

previously implanted bioprosthetic valve. The operative morbidity of redo sternotomy, even in the best of hands, is higher than that of the primary sternotomy. If a third sternotomy is required, the risk increases even further; therefore, valve selection at the outset is of paramount importance. In their study, Emery et al demonstrated that in patients with redo sternotomy, the St. Jude valve continued to provide a low incidence of valve-related events. No valve-related structural degeneration was noted that would have led to a repeat replacement of the St. Jude valve, and thromboembolic- and anticoagulant- related hemorrhage remained the most important consideration influencing postoperative valve-related morbidity.

Noninvasive techniques for assessment of valve morphology and function are limited. Echocardiographic assessment of mechanical valvular prosthetic function using Doppler techniques to measure gradients has a role. This method can be combined with cinefluoroscopic evaluation to achieve a reasonable assessment of valvular mechanical function. The type of valvular prosthesis can often be ascertained using cinefluoroscopy. Furthermore, the disk opening angle can be assessed using cinefluoroscopy, which, in combination with transesophageal echocardiography for the detection of pannus, can be used to distinguish among structural failure, pannus formation, and valve-prosthesis mismatch.

Investigators are establishing gradient measurements by means of phase contrast MRI; however, normative value determination is still in the experimental stages. The role of CT imaging to establish valvular mechanical dysfunction is discussed in the later section on complications.

Carbomedics Valve

The Carbomedics valve (Carbomedics, Austin, Tex.) was introduced in 1986. Although this valve resembles the St. Jude valve in its construction, it has a housing that can be rotated within the sewing ring. Subsequent to the original design, the company designed a Top Hat Carbomedics valve that could be used for implantation in patients with small aortic roots. The modification in the Top Hat device involved only the sewing ring. To date, more than 500,000 Carbomedics valves have been implanted worldwide.

Long-term follow-up results of the Carbomedics valve are sparse. In a 10-year comparison study, Bryan et al demonstrated relative equivalency of the St. Jude valve and the Carbomedics valve and found that the Carbomedics valve

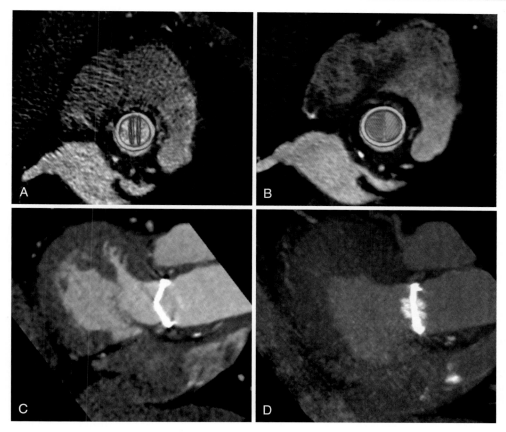

Figure 17-7 Three-dimensional volume-rendered computed tomography of a St. Jude valve in the aortic position. En face projection of a St. Jude valve in the closed (**A**) and open (**B**) positions. Maximum intensity projection of the St. Jude valve demonstrates normal closing (**C**) and opening (**D**) angles of the hemidisks.

had a 95% rate of freedom from valve-related mortality. The thromboembolism- and anticoagulation-related complication rates in this study were 1.1% and 2.3%, respectively, not statistically significantly different from the St. Jude valve. The Carbomedics valve also has the favorable hemodynamics expected from the bileaflet valve design.

In another study, Roedler et al demonstrated essentially no difference in valve-related complications between the traditional Carbomedics valve and the Top Hat valve. The same publication also mentioned the possibly advantageous features of the Sorin Mitroflow (Sorin Biomedica, Saluggia, Italy) valve. Kandemir et al also demonstrated results similar to those of the previously described studies and showed that both the St. Jude and Carbomedics valves had excellent intermediate-term results.

Sorin Bicarbon Valve

Introduced in 1990, the Sorin Bicarbon valve (Sorin Biomedica) represents another in the list of bileaflet valves. In a study of 1900 patients who were followed up to 15 years, Azarnoush et al confirmed a positive experience with this valve from their previously reported 5- and 10- year experience. The rate of valve-related thrombosis showed actuarial freedom at 15 years of 99.6% (98.6% to 99.9%) or 0.81% per patient-year. Hemorrhage related to anticoagulant treatment occurred in 293 cases, a finding that translated to 1.46% per patient-year, and the risk of endocarditis was 0.22% per patient-year. The hemodynamic profile of this valve has also shown to be favorable, much like the others in this category, with good LV mass regression.

Edwards MIRA Valve

The Edwards MIRA bileaflet valve (Edwards Lifesciences, Inc., Irvine, Calif) was introduced in 1998. It is composed of the main body of the Sorin mechanical prosthesis, with a swing ring that is comparable to that of the Starr prosthesis. Data on outcomes related to this valve are sparse; however, initial results of the Edwards MIRA valve also demonstrate a favorable risk profile. The design of the valve itself incorporates a thicker sewing ring than other valvular designs and thus offers better surgical visualization at the time of insertion. The valve also demonstrates favorable hemodynamics.

Bioprosthetic Valves

The ratio of mechanical to bioprosthetic valve implantation is approximately 55% to 45%, with the number of bioprosthetic valves increasing because of reduced risk of thrombogenicity and better durability than previous designs. Bioprosthetic valves can generally be classified into human-derived and animal-derived valves. Human-derived valves can be autografts or allografts. Autografts represent a patient's native valve that is, in essence, transposed from one location to the other, as in the Ross procedure (pulmonary artery to aortic position, and artificial replacement of the less critical pulmonary artery). Allografts are harvested from cadaveric donors. Animal-derived valves are generally porcine aortic valves, or alternatively, they can be fashioned from bovine pericardial tissues. These grafts are often referred to as xenografts or heterografts.

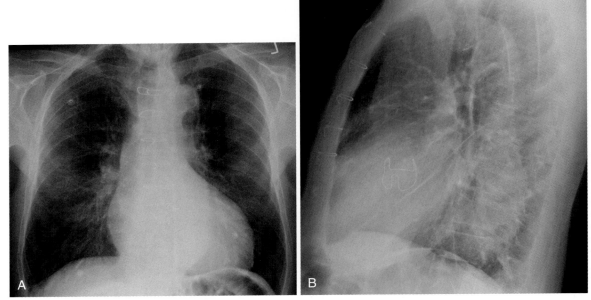

Figure 17-8 A, Posteroanterior radiograph of the Carpentier-Edwards stented valvular prosthesis demonstrates the normal appearance of the housing. B, The lateral radiograph demonstrates a well-seated valve with the stent struts pointing in the flow direction.

Grafts can be both stented and stentless. Stented grafts are more common and employ a housing over which the appropriate valve can be fixed. The disadvantage of these systems is that the stent itself can compromise the valve orifice area. In response to this concern, stentless valves have been developed that can be sewn in without the housing present in the stented valves.

Stented Bovine Pericardial Valves

CARPENTIER-EDWARDS PERIMOUNT VALVE

The Carpentier-Edwards bovine pericardial valve (Edwards Lifesciences, Irvine, Calif.) is a common bioprosthetic valve (Figs. 17-8 and 17-9). This stented aortic valve prosthesis is made of bovine pericardium. The Carpentier-Edwards bovine pericardial valve was originally introduced in 1981; however, it did not become available clinically in the United States until 1991. The long-term hemodynamic performance of this valve has been well established, with effective long-term transvalvular gradients and no significant change in the orifice areas with time. At 17 years, approximately 13% of the patients with these valves have progressed to severe aortic regurgitation. In the short term, similar results have been found in the mitral position as well.

In long-term studies, similar to other bioprosthetic valves, the Carpentier-Edwards valve is also susceptible to structural deterioration. Rates of freedom from structural valve deterioration at 18 years are 39% for recipients less than 60 years old and 66% for recipients more than 60 years old. In terms of complications, the 10-year actuarial survival rates were 69%, 58%, and 38% for AVR, AVR, and double valve replacement, respectively. The 14-year actuarial freedom rates from events after AVR are 88% for thromboembolism, 92% for endocarditis, 72% for reoperation, and 80% for structural dysfunction of the valve.

SORIN MITROFLOW VALVE

The Sorin Mitroflow valve (Sorin Biomedica) is a commonly used pericardial bioprosthesis (Fig. 17-10). Originally introduced in 1982, the Mitroflow valve consists of a single bovine pericardial sheet mounted on a Delrin sewing ring. The unique design is considered to optimize the orifice area of the prosthesis, which is designed especially for supra-annular placement. As with other bioprosthetic valves, the Mitroflow valve is recommended for an older patient population. The Mitroflow valve design is slightly different from that of other valves because the pericardial sheet is mounted on the outside of the stent to maximize the effective orifice area. In their study, Bleiziffer et al demonstrated that for larger Mitroflow valves, the mean transvalvular gradient was excellent (<15 mm Hg); however, for smaller valves, the transvalvular gradient was only adequate (19 mm Hg). Furthermore, the effective orifice area was satisfactory even for small prostheses.

Long-term studies of the complications of the Mitroflow valve are available. These studies recommend placing this particular valve in patients who are more than 70 years old and, more convincingly, in more than 75 years old. In their 19-year follow-up, Minami et al demonstrated that in patients less than 75 years old, rates of freedom from endocarditis, tear, and valve degeneration are high only in the first 5 years, beyond which the risk of valve explantation increases. In patients older than 75 years, the safety data at fifth to tenth year are also more favorable than in younger patients. This reason is thought to be that more active, younger patients exert more force on the pericardial tissue valve apparatus. In this study, the 15-year rate of freedom from endocarditis was 92%, the freedom rate from embolism was 83%, the freedom rate from bleeding was 94%, and the freedom rate from structural valve deterioration was 63%. Similarly, a multicenter Italian study also demonstrated a 65% rate of

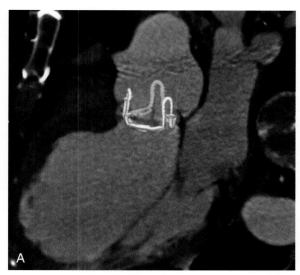

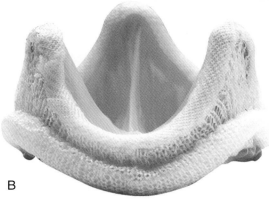

Figure 17-9 **A,** Three-dimensional reconstruction of the Carpentier-Edwards valve demonstrating the stent housing in the appropriate position. Note the normal trileaflet valve appearance crafted from bovine pericardium in the center. **B,** Note the correlation of the three-pronged stented housing of the bovine pericardial valve on the accompanying photograph. (Photograph courtesy of Edwards Lifesciences Irvine, Calif.)

freedom from structural valve deterioration at 18 years, a finding consistent with other published literature.

Stented Porcine Valves

HANCOCK VALVE
Several stented porcine valves have been introduced. The Medtronic Hancock standard and the Carpentier-Edwards porcine standard were the original first-generation valves. The common-second generation porcine valves are the Hancock II (Fig. 17-11) and the Carpentier-Edwards supra-annular valve.

The Hancock II prosthesis is a commonly placed bioprosthetic valve. The Hancock valves are made of porcine heterograft material. The initial Hancock valve was introduced in 1972 and was subsequently replaced by the Hancock II prosthesis, which is a lower-profile valve. Introduced in 1982, the Hancock II is a second-generation porcine aortic valve fixed with a buffered 0.625% glutaraldehyde solution in two stages: an initial stage of low pressure and a late stage of physiologic pressure. It is also chemically treated with sodium dodecyl sulfate to prevent calcification. The stent of this bioprosthesis is made

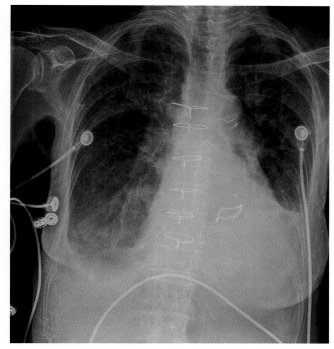

Figure 17-10 Anteroposterior radiograph demonstrates the Sorin Mitroflow valve in the aortic position. Note the irregular appearance on plain film similar to a lemon-type configuration that is a characteristic imaging feature.

of Delrin (DuPont, Wilmington, Del) instead of polypropylene, as in the stent of the original Hancock valve, to prevent creeping.

The long-term durability of this valve has proven to be quite good. In their 25-year experience in patients mostly more than 60 years old, Valfre et al (2010) reported excellent rates of freedom from reoperation of 86.8% and 61.9% for AVR and MVR, respectively. The overall survival rate in this population was generally lower because the patients in this study (as well as other studies) were older, with average age of 64 years. In this study, the Kaplan-Meier late survival rate for AVR was 23.3% at 20 years and 16.2% for MVR at 19 years. David et al also reported similar long-term survival results with survival at 20 and 25 years of 19.2% and 6.7%, respectively. In this study, the rate of freedom from structural valve deterioration at 20 years was 63.4% in the entire cohort; however, it was only 29.2% in patients younger than 60 years, a finding underscoring the importance of appropriate patient selection for valve placement. Forty-one episodes of endocarditis were encountered, and the freedom rate from endocarditis was 94.5% at 20 years. No episodes of valve thrombosis were reported, but several patients had thromboembolic complications. In a direct comparison with the Carpentier-Edwards Perimount valve, the results demonstrated excellent long-term durability in both valves and similar long-term clinical performance.

CARPENTIER-EDWARDS SUPRA-ANNULAR VALVE
The Carpentier-Edwards supra-annular valve is a second-generation porcine valvular prosthesis. The valve was introduced in 1981 and is currently recommended for patients more than 70 years old and in patients 61 to

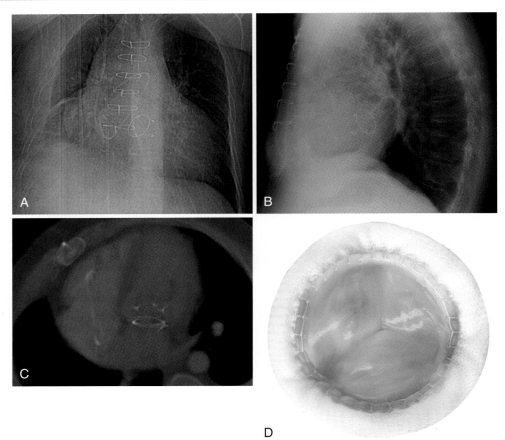

Figure 17-11 **A,** Posteroanterior computed tomography (CT) scout image of the Hancock standard valve demonstrates the stent housing with three radiopaque circles denoting the normal stent housing. **B,** Lateral radiograph demonstrates the three radiopaque circles denoting the stent housing. **C,** Maximum intensity projection images from a chest CT scan of the same patient once again denote the characteristic three radiopaque markers. **D,** Photograph of the Hancock II valve. (Photograph courtesy of Medtronic, Inc., Minneapolis, Minn. Copyright Medtronic, Inc. Hancock II Bioprosthesis Medtronic, Inc. Printed with permission.)

70 years old in whom comorbidities may compromise life expectancy. The valve was designed for supra-annular implantation to optimize hemodynamics. In their long-term follow-up study, Jamieson et al found that the rate of overall actual cumulative freedom from reoperation at 18 years was 85.0%, and the rate of freedom from valve-related mortality was 89%. The actual freedom rates from structural valve deterioration at 18 years were 90.5% for patients 61 to 70 years old and 98% for patients more than 70 years old. Corbineau et al found similar results, with low rates of structural valve deterioration in patients in whom the valve was implanted after 60 years of age.

Stentless Valves

Stentless bioprosthetic valves were created in response to the need to develop bioprosthetic valve systems that would allow maximization of effective orifice area. The ultimate goal of these bioprostheses is to allow for more rapid and greater regression of LV mass. The stentless valves were developed in response to ongoing concern that the stented valves diminished effective orifice area by virtue of the stent itself. The stent leads to turbulent flow even though the hemodynamic profiles of most bioprosthetic valves are favorable, as previously described. Furthermore, the initial structural valve degeneration typically occurs near the stent struts. Theoretically, these valves would offer benefit in patients with smaller aortic roots.

These theoretical disadvantages would be obviated by a stentless valve system. However, placement of stentless valve systems is considerably more technically challenging than implanting a stented system. In several studies, investigators showed that perioperative mortality is similar despite longer cross-clamping and extracorporeal circulation times.

The two stentless systems that have been available for a significant time are the Toronto Stentless system and the Medtronic Freestyle valve. Bach et al demonstrated good hemodynamic performance of these valves in their study encompassing 21 centers. However, this study did not compare those valves with stented bioprostheses. The investigators concluded that the Freestyle valve offers good hemodynamics and a rate of freedom from structural valve deterioration that is similar to those of other available bioprostheses. In contrast, following their up to 8-year experience, which demonstrated excellent initial results in terms of both hemodynamics and structural valve deterioration, a 12-year follow-up study was performed by the same group and by David et al. This research demonstrated that although survival rates were similar to those of the general population, valve durability was suboptimal in many of those patients. Patients whose valve implantation when they were less than 65 years old had a rate of freedom from structural valve deterioration of only 52%. Similar results were reported by Desai et al, who found that despite initial favorable results, at medium-term follow up, structural valve deterioration became an issue.

The theoretical advantages of greater effective orifice area and better hemodynamic performance have not yet been substantiated in the literature; varying reports range from improved performance to worse performance. Moreover, although the stented systems are typically implanted in an annular position, the stentless system can be implanted employing various techniques that may have affected the outcomes of these studies. In their meta-analysis, Payne et al concluded that the stentless valves had not demonstrated benefit in terms of LV mass regression or postoperative mean gradients, but the stentless valves did appear to display superior hemodynamics with regard to peak gradients. The overall hemodynamic results of these valves remain in question.

In summary, the stentless valves appear to offer theoretical advantages as compared with their stented counterparts. These valves have the theoretical advantages both of better hemodynamic performance and of less structural deterioration. However, in 10-year follow-up studies, these valves were not shown to improve hemodynamic performance or to result in decreased structural deterioration.

■ COMPLICATIONS

The most common complications related to mechanical prosthetic valves include thromboembolism and anticoagulation-related hemorrhage. Additional complications include pannus formation, infective endocarditis, paraprosthetic leak, and valvular dehiscence. Mechanical failure (e.g., stuck valve leaflets) is a less common complication. The reader is referred to the earlier discussions of the individual valves for discussion of thrombosis and hemorrhage rates, as well as for valve specific complications such as disk escape and isolated structural valve failure.

In terms of bioprosthetic valves, complications include valve degeneration from calcification, pannus formation, infective endocarditis, and valve thrombosis. The reader is referred to the earlier discussion of specific valves for descriptions of the complication rates of valve thrombosis.

Pannus and Thrombus

Pannus formation can occur on both bioprosthetic and mechanical heart valves. Pannus is the growth of host tissue on the prosthesis. It can be thought of as part of the normal healing process related to prosthetic implantation; however, it can cause complications when this growth becomes overexuberant. Although a small amount of pannus can be beneficial in preventing thrombosis along the suture line, excessive pannus formation may result in restricted leaflet function, which may lead to decreased opening area of the valve or to regurgitation if the leaflet freezes in the open position. Additionally, excessive pannus can create a nidus for superimposed thrombus formation and subsequent systemic embolization. The formation of pannus may be more important in stentless systems, in which pannus formation can directly infiltrate the valve.

Thrombus formation is the most common cause of failure of mechanical heart valves; however, it is infrequently seen in patients receiving optimal anticoagulation. Bioprostheses are not routinely anticoagulated and

are therefore preferred in older patients, in whom the risk of anticoagulation often outweighs the benefit of longevity afforded by mechanical prostheses. The risk of thrombosis is similar in patients who are appropriately anticoagulated and in those with bioprostheses.

Imaging studies of valvular pannus and thrombus formation have shown that CT can provide both direct and indirect evidence of these complications. Indirect corollary for pannus and thrombus formation can be seen in the setting of a valve with restricted opening (see the discussion of valvular prosthesis functional assessment). Direct visualization of pannus and thrombus is often a challenging diagnosis that requires contribution from both echocardiography and cinefluoroscopy. Cardiac CT may offer the simultaneous ability to examine directly for pannus and thrombus and also for the indirect effects by functional imaging. It can provide incremental benefit in some patients. Both pannus and thrombus can manifest as low-density lesions on or adjacent to the valve cusps. Although the density of the masses adjacent to prostheses can often be attributed to pannus or thrombus, higher attenuation (>200 HU) may be suggestive more of thrombus formation than of pannus formation.

Valvular Calcification

In bioprostheses, valvular calcification is also a recognized complication and contributes to decreased longevity of the valve. The presence of calcification is the most common cause of sterile valvular degeneration. Indeed, cuspal degeneration can occur from both calcific and noncalcific complications. Calcific sterile degeneration can manifest in several ways, including cusp tears on the calcified valve leaflet, regurgitation secondary to incomplete coaptation (Fig. 17-12), and stenosis resulting from exuberant calcification. The mechanism behind calcification on bioprosthetic valves is thought to be a chemical interaction between aldehyde groups phospholipids and circulating calcium ions.

The more common areas for valvular calcification include the commissural and basal areas of the cusp, which are the areas of highest stress during function. Cardiac CT can detect subtle calcifications on bioprosthetic valve leaflets as the initial manifestation of valvular degeneration before loss of valvular function (Fig. 17-13). The clinical implication of these findings is uncertain and has not been elucidated in the cardiac CT literature. Functional assessment of valve opening and the orifice area may also yield beneficial data points (Fig. 17-14). Closer clinical follow-up may or may not be warranted.

Valvular Prosthesis Functional Assessment

Functional assessment of valvular function has become increasingly more feasible with cinematic CT acquisition. Valvular function can be compared with cinefluoroscopy to determine whether stuck valve leaflets are present by ascertaining the possibility of abnormal opening angles. Furthermore, valve orifice area can be compared with manufacturer specifications to aid in

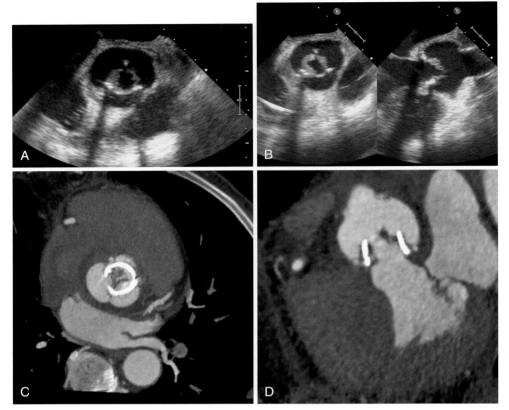

Figure 17-12 Prosthetic valve stenosis. This patient developed marked thickening of his Carpentier-Edwards aortic valve leaflets several years after implantation. Preoperative (**A**) and intraoperative (**B**) echocardiographic images demonstrate valve leaflet thickening, which is also seen by computed tomography imaging. **C**, Note the incomplete coaptation of the valvular orifice with closure that indicates insufficiency or regurgitation. In the open position (**D**), the restricted valve leaflet opening and doming indicate stenosis.

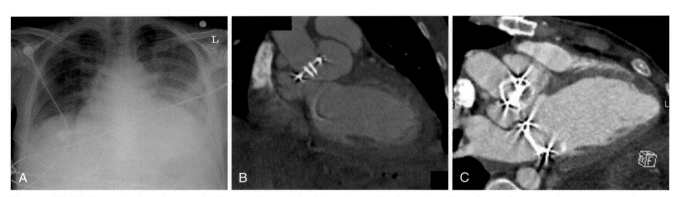

Figure 17-13 Paravalvular abscess. A, Chest radiograph in this patient with chest pain after valve replacement demonstrates pulmonary edema with bilateral effusions and atelectasis of the left lower lobe. No mass is seen in the mediastinum. Computed tomography images in the same patient demonstrate dehiscence of the aortic valve prosthesis from the annulus with a subvalvular leak resulting in pseudoaneurysms (**B** and **C**); these images also show a well-seated valve prosthesis in the mitral position.

determination of impaired function. The role of cardiac CT in the assessment of valvular heart disease may offer future potential based on initial studies.

Infective Endocarditis, Vegetations, and Pseudoaneurysm

Echocardiography and clinical criteria have long been the primary means of identifying those at risk of infectious endocarditis. The Duke criteria were originally proposed in 1994 and subsequently modified in 2000. The echocardiographic manifestations of disease include oscillating luminal mass on valve or supporting structures, in the path of regurgitant jets, on implanted

material or in the absence of an alternative anatomic explanation. Other echocardiographic manifestations include abscess cavities, new partial dehiscence of a prosthetic valve, or new valvular regurgitation. By using the combination of pathologic features, clinical criteria, and imaging findings, examiners can classify patients as having definite, possible, or absence of endocarditis.

The role of cardiac CT and MRI in the delineation of infective endocarditis is continually evolving. Cardiac CT can aid in the delineation of valvular vegetations and may also aid in the delineation of abscesses (see Figs. 17-13 and 17-14; Fig. 17-15). Newer scanners offer better spatial and temporal resolution and allow better

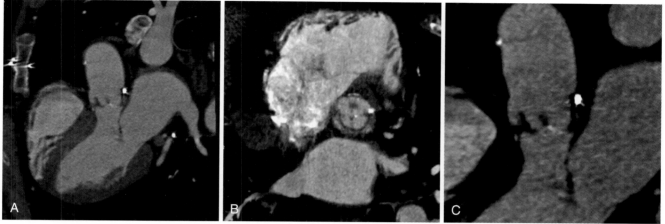

Figure 17-14 Computed tomography with contrast enhancement in long-axis (**A**), short-axis (**B**), and long-axis close-up (**C**) views. This patient has a mildly abnormally functioning bioprosthetic valve. The valve leaflets demonstrate subtle calcification. The thickening of the valve leaflets is also associated with this structural valve deterioration. At this stage, valvular gradients were only mildly elevated. In the close-up image (**C**), the valvular calcification is better seen.

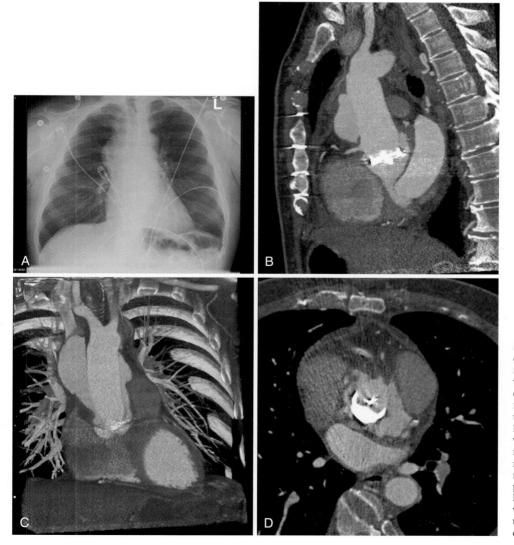

Figure 17-15 Paravalvular pseudoaneurysm on computed tomography (CT). This patient presented with symptoms suggestive of endocarditis. **A,** Chest radiograph reveals mediastinal widening localizing to the area of the ascending aorta. **B,** CT demonstrates a mechanical valve with a paravalvular defect resulting in a large pseudoaneurysm that occupies most of the mediastinum. Maximum intensity projection (**C**) demonstrates the large size of the pseudoaneurysm, whereas the axial image (**D**) shows the site of the leak adjacent the left coronary artery.

delineation of infective complications at lower radiation doses. Feuchtner et al showed that, in their study of 37 patients, 29 of whom had endocarditis at surgery, cardiac CT (64-slice CT scanner) had a high correlation with both intraoperative findings and transesophageal echocardiography. When compared with surgery, CT detection of vegetations had sensitivity of 96%, specificity of 97%, positive predictive value of 96%, and negative predictive value of 97%, whereas for abscesses and pseudoaneurysms, sensitivity was 100%, specificity was 100%, positive predictive value was 100%, and negative predictive value was 100%. In correlation with surgery, CT did miss some of the small abscesses (<4 mm). Additionally, cardiac CT could delineate coronary anatomy preoperatively. Furthermore, in their study, the number of patients with preexisting valvular prosthesis was not reported, and therefore the data for this subset of the population are uncertain.

In a separate study by Gahide et al of encompassing 19 consecutive patients over a 4-year period, the experience using both 16-slice and 64-slice CT scanners demonstrated that, for vegetations on the aortic valves, sensitivity, specificity, positive predictive value, and negative predictive value were 71.4%, 100%, 100%, and 55.5%, respectively. When considering valves with vegetations larger than 1 cm, these parameters were 100%. The sensitivity, specificity, positive predictive value, and negative predictive value of multidetector CT in depicting aortic valve pseudoaneurysms was 100%, 87.5%, 91.7%, and 100%, respectively. When considering extension of the aortic valve pseudoaneurysms into the intervalvular fibrous body, all these parameters were 100%. Once again, however, in their study, only 2 of the 19 patients had bioprosthetic valves, although the rest had native valve endocarditis. Therefore, results should be approached cautiously in this subgroup of patients.

The diagnosis of infective endocarditis and its complications represents an exciting realm of possibility for cardiac CT imaging. The reported rates of sensitivity and specificity for detection of endocarditis lesions by transesophageal echocardiography, regarded as the best technique for depicting endocarditis complications, were 48% for abscesses as confirmed by surgery, with a higher miss rate in lesions on the posterior mitral leaflet. Cardiac ultrasound is potentially limited by lack of acoustic windows in patients with prosthetic valves, as well as those with calcification. Therefore, the superior initial reports of cardiac CT for complication detection are encouraging. Additional possibilities include identifying valvular dehiscence and planning potential intervention, although these roles have not been well elucidated in the literature (Fig. 17-16). Experiences

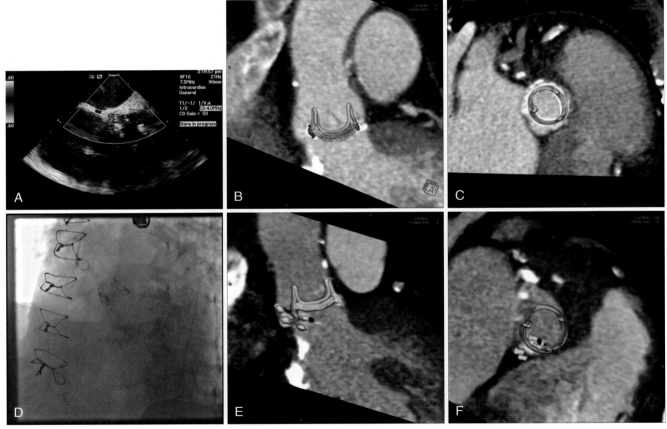

Figure 17-16 Valve dehiscence. A, Echocardiographic images demonstrate a jet of paravalvular contrast material on color Doppler images. **B** and **C,** Cardiac computed tomography (CT) images in modified three-chamber and axial views demonstrate a paravalvular dehiscence adjacent to the right sinus of Valsalva. The patient subsequently underwent cardiac catheterization, and the leak was closed with two occluder devices (**D**). **E** and **F,** Postprocedure three-dimensional cardiac CT images in similar projections demonstrate the occluder device in the position of the former paravalvular channel.

with newer-generation CT scanners for detecting endocarditis and its complications have yet to be reported but would be anticipated to be at least as good as results with older-generation scanners, given improved temporal and spatial resolutions, even as radiation doses have decreased.

Patient-Prosthesis Mismatch

Patient-prosthesis mismatch occurs when the implanted valve is effectively too small in relation to body size and therefore results in unexpectedly high transvalvular gradients. This complication is measured by using the effective orifice area indexed to patient size. The generally accepted threshold for patient-prosthesis mismatch in the aortic position is less than $0.85 \text{ cm}^2/\text{m}^2$, which is similar to that used in native aortic valves. For the mitral position, patient-prosthesis mismatch occurs when the orifice is less than $1.2 \text{ cm}^2/\text{m}^2$. Patient-prosthesis mismatch is common, occurring in 20% to 70% of AVRs and 30% to 70% of mitral prostheses.

Patient-prosthesis mismatch has predictably poor outcomes in terms of hemodynamic sequelae, manifested in terms of lack of LV mass regression and lack of recovery of LV function. The presence of mismatch is thought to be integrally related to early patient mortality. Patients with severe mismatch have a risk ratio of 11.4 compared with those with no mismatch. The sequelae of mismatch are even more pronounced in patients with concomitant LV dysfunction and even extend to affect long-term survival. Patient-prosthesis mismatch is best detected by Doppler echocardiography. No substantial studies addressing patient-prosthesis mismatch by cardiac CT or MRI have been published, although this could represent an area for future investigation.

Bibliography

Abdulali SA, Silverton NP, Schoen FJ, Saunders NR, Ionescu MI. Late outcome of patients with Braunwald-Cutter mitral valve replacement. Ann Thorac Surg. 1984;38:579-585.

Alton ME, Pasierski TJ, Orsinelli DA, Eaton GM, Pearson AC. Comparison of transthoracic and transesophageal echocardiography in evaluation of 47 Starr-Edwards prosthetic valves. J Am Coll Cardiol. 1992;20:1503-1511.

Anderson WA, Ilkowski DA, Eldredge J, et al. The small aortic root and the Medtronic Hall valve: ultrafast computed tomography assessment of left ventricular mass following aortic valve replacement. J Heart Valve Dis. 1996;5(suppl 3):S329-S335.

Aris A, Ramirez I, Camara ML, Carreras F, Borras X, Pons-Llado G. The 20 mm Medtronic Hall prosthesis in the small aortic root. J Heart Valve Dis. 1996;5:459-462.

Ayegnon KG, Aupart M, Bourguignon T, Mirza A, May MA, Marchand MA. 25-year experience with Carpentier-Edwards Perimount in the mitral position. Asian Cardiovasc Thorac Ann. 2011;19:14-19.

Azarnoush K, Laborde F, de Riberolles C. The Sorin Bicarbon over 15 year clinical outcomes: multicentre experience in 1704 patients. Eur J Cardiothorac Surg. 2010;38:759-766.

Bach DS, Kon ND, Dumesnil JG, Sintek CF, Doty DB. Ten-year outcome after aortic valve replacement with the freestyle stentless bioprosthesis. Ann Thorac Surg. 2005;80:480-486.

Bahnson HT, Hardesty RL, Baker Jr LD, Brooks DH, Gall DA. Fabrication and evaluation of tissue leaflets for aortic and mitral valve replacement. Ann Surg. 1970;171:939-947.

Bahnson HT, Spencer FC, Busse EF, Davis FW. Cusp replacement and coronary artery perfusion in open operations on the aortic valve. Ann Surg. 1960;152:494-503.

Balram A, Kaul U, Rama Rao BV, et al. Thrombotic obstruction of Björk-Shiley valves: diagnostic and surgical considerations. Int J Cardiol. 1984;6:61-73.

Banbury MK, Cosgrove 3rd DM, Thomas JD, et al. Hemodynamic stability during 17 years of the Carpentier-Edwards aortic pericardial bioprosthesis. Ann Thorac Surg. 2002;73:1460-1465.

Beiras-Fernandez A, Oberhoffer M, Kur F, Kaczmarek I, Vicol C, Reichart B. 34-year durability of a DeBakey Surgitool mechanical aortic valve prosthesis. Interact Cardiovasc Thorac Surg. 2006;5:637-639.

Biteker M, Gündüz S, Ozkan M. Role of MDCT in the evaluation of prosthetic heart valves. AJR Am J Roentgenol. 2009;192:W77.

Blais C, Dumesnil JG, Baillot R, Simard S, Doyle D, Pibarot P. Impact of valve prosthesis-patient mismatch on short-term mortality after aortic valve replacement. Circulation. 2003;108:983-988.

Blot WJ, Ibrahim MA, Ivey TD, Acheson DE, Brookmeyer R, Weyman A, Defauw J, Smith JK, Harrison D. Twenty-five-year experience with the Björk-Shiley convexoconcave heart valve: a continuing clinical concern. Circulation. 2005;111:2850-2857.

Bleiziffer S, Eichinger WB, Hettich IM, et al. Hemodynamic characterization of the Sorin Mitroflow pericardial bioprosthesis at rest and exercise. J Heart Valve Dis. 2009;18:95-100.

Bokros JC, Gott VL, La Grange LD, Fadall AM, Vos KD, Ramos MD. Correlations between blood compatibility and heparin adsorbtivity for an impermeable isotropic pyrolytic carbon. J Biomed Mater Res. 1969;3:497-528.

Borman JB, Brands WG, Camilleri L, et al. Bicarbon valve: European multicenter clinical evaluation. Eur J Cardiothorac Surg. 1998;13:685-693.

Borman JB, De Riberolles C. Sorin Bicarbon bileaflet valve: a 10-year experience. Eur J Cardiothorac Surg. 2003;23:86-92.

Bryan AJ, Rogers CA, Bayliss K, Wild J, Angelini GD. Prospective randomized comparison of Carbomedics and St. Jude Medical bileaflet mechanical heart valve prostheses: ten-year follow-up. J Thorac Cardiovasc Surg. 2007;133:614-622.

Buchart EG. Thrombogenesis and its management. In: Acar J, Bodnar E, eds. Textbook of Acquired Heart Valve Disease. London: ICR Publishers; 1995.

Butany J,LR. The failure modes of biological prosthetic heart valves. J Long Term Eff Med Implants. 2001;11:115-136.

Butchart EG, Li HH, Payne N, Buchan K, Grunkemeier GL. Twenty years' experience with the Medtronic Hall valve. J Thorac Cardiovasc Surg. 2001;121:1090-1100.

Byrne JG, Leacche M. Long-term follow-up of patients undergoing reoperative surgery with aortic or mitral valve replacement, using a St. Jude Medical prosthesis. J Heart Valve Dis. 2010;19:471-472.

Carrier M, Martineau JP, Bonan R, Pelletier LC. Clinical and hemodynamic assessment of the Omniscience prosthetic heart valve. J Thorac Cardiovasc Surg. 1987;93:300-307.

Chambers J, Rimington HM, Hodson F, Rajani R, Blauth CI. The subcoronary Toronto stentless versus supra-annular Perimount stented replacement aortic valve: early clinical and hemodynamic results of a randomized comparison in 160 patients. J Thorac Cardiovasc Surg. 2006;131:878-882.

Chan V, Kulik A, Tran A, et al. Long-term clinical and hemodynamic performance of the Hancock II versus the Perimount aortic bioprostheses. Circulation. 2010;14(suppl):S10-S16.

Chenot F,MP. Evaluation of anatomic valve opening and leaflet morphology in aortic valve bioprosthesis by using multidetector CT: comparison with transthoracic echocardiography. Radiology. 2010;255:377-385.

Cho YH, Jeong DS, Park PW, et al. Serial changes of hemodynamic performance with Medtronic Hall valve in aortic position. Ann Thorac Surg. 2011;91:424-431.

Cianciulli TE, Lax JA, Beck MA, et al. Cinefluoroscopic assessment of mechanical disc prostheses: its value as a complementary method to echocardiography. Heart Valve Dis. 2005;14:664-673.

Corbineau H, De La Tour B, Verhoye JP, Langanay T, Lelong B, Leguerrier A. Carpentier-Edwards supraannular porcine bioprosthesis in aortic position: 16-year experience. Ann Thorac Surg. 2001;71(suppl):S228-S231.

Cotrufo M, Renzulli A, Esposito V, et al. Intermediate term evaluation of Starr-Edwards ball valves in the mitral position. Tex Heart Inst J. 1985;12:43-47.

Crawford Jr FA, Kratz JM, Sade RM, Stroud MR, Bartles DM. Aortic and mitral valve replacement with the St. Jude Medical prosthesis. Ann Surg. 1984;199:753-761.

David TE, Armstrong S, Maganti M. Hancock II bioprosthesis for aortic valve replacement: the gold standard of bioprosthetic valves durability? Ann Thorac Surg. 2010;90:775-781.

David TE, Feindel CM, Bos J, Ivanov J, Armstrong S. Aortic valve replacement with Toronto SPV bioprosthesis: optimal patient survival but suboptimal valve durability. J Thorac Cardiovasc Surg. 2008;135:19-24.

De Carlo M, Milano AD, Nardi C, Mecozzi G, Bortolotti U. Serial Doppler echocardiographic evaluation of small-sized Sorin Bicarbon prostheses. J Thorac Cardiovasc Surg. 2003;126:337-343.

de Kerchove L, Glineur D, El Khoury G, Noirhomme P. Stentless valves for aortic valve replacement: where do we stand? Curr Opin Cardiol. 2007;22:96-103.

De Santo LS, De Feo M, Della Corte A, et al. A Starr-Edwards mitral prosthesis after 44 years of good performance. Int J Artif Organs. 2010;33:405-407.

Deleuze PH, Fromes Y, Khoury W, Maribas P, Lemaire S, Bical OM. Eight-year results of Freestyle stentless bioprosthesis in the aortic position: a single-center study of 500 patients. J Heart Valve Dis. 2006;15:247-252.

Dellgren G, Feindel CM, Bos J, Ivanov J, David TE. Aortic valve replacement with the Toronto SPV: long-term clinical and hemodynamic results. Eur J Cardiothorac Surg. 2002;21:698-702.

Desai ND, Merin O, Cohen GN, et al. Long-term results of aortic valve replacement with the St. Jude Toronto stentless porcine valve. Ann Thorac Surg. 2004;78:2076-2083.

DeWall R. Omniscience valves. *J Thorac Cardiovasc Surg.* 1984;88:1040.

DeWall R, Qasim N, Carr L. Evolution of mechanical heart valves. *Ann Thorac Surg.* 2000;69:1612-1621.

Dumesnil JG, Honos GN, Lemieux M, Beauchemin J. Validation and applications of indexed aortic prosthetic valve areas calculated by Doppler echocardiography. *J Am Coll Cardiol.* 1990;16:637-643.

Dumesnil JG, Pibarot P. Prosthesis-patient mismatch: an update. *Curr Cardiol Rep.* 2011;13:250-257.

Dunning J, Graham RJ, Thambyrajah J, Stewart MJ, Kendall SW, Hunter S. Stentless vs stented aortic valve bioprostheses: a prospective randomized controlled trial. *Eur Heart J.* 2007;28:2369-2374.

Durack D, Lukes AS, Bright DK. New criteria for diagnosis of infective endocarditis: utilization of specific echocardiographic findings: Duke Endocarditis Service. *Am J Med.* 1994;96:200-209.

Edmunds Jr LH. C. R. Guidelines for reporting morbidity and mortality after cardiac valvular operations. *J Thorac Cardiovasc Surg.* 1996;112:708-711.

Edwards MS, Clark RE, Cohn LH, Grunkemeier GL, Miller DC, Weisel RD. Results of valve replacement with Omniscience mechanical prostheses. *Ann Thorac Surg.* 2002;74:665-670.

Emery RW, Krogh CC, McAdams S, Emery AM, Holter AR. Long-term follow-up of patients undergoing reoperative surgery with aortic or mitral valve replacement using a St. Jude Medical prosthesis. *J Heart Valve Dis.* 2010;19:473-484.

Feuchtner GM, Stolzmann P, Dichtl W, et al. Findings, multislice computed tomography in infective endocarditis: comparison with transesophageal echocardiography and intraoperative findings. *J Am Coll Cardiol.* 2009;53:436-444.

Firstenberg MS, Morehead AJ, Thomas JD, et al. Short-term hemodynamic performance of the mitral Carpentier-Edwards PERIMOUNT pericardial valve: Carpentier-Edwards PERIMOUNT Investigators. *Ann Thorac Surg.* 2001;71(suppl):S285-S288.

Gahide G, Bommart S, Demaria R, et al. Preoperative evaluation in aortic endocarditis: findings on cardiac CT. *AJR Am J Roentgenol.* 2010;194: 574-578.

Glotzer TV, Tunick PA, Kloth H, Galloway AC, Kronzon I. Thrombosis of a Starr-Edwards tricuspid prosthesis: diagnosis by Doppler echocardiography and treatment with thrombolysis. *Am Heart J.* 1994;127:705-708.

Gödje O, FT. 25 years follow-up of patients after replacement of the aortic valve with a Smeloff-Cutter prosthesis. *Thorac Cardiovasc Surg.* 1996;44: 234-238.

Gott V, Alejo DE, Cameron DE. Mechanical heart valves: 50 years of evolution. *Ann Thorac Surg.* 2003;76:S2230-S2239.

Gulbins H, Reichenspurner H. Which patients benefit from stentless aortic valve replacement? *Ann Thorac Surg.* 2009;88:2061-2068.

Head SJ, Ko J, Singh R, Roberts WC, Mack MJ. 43.3-year durability of a Smeloff-Cutter ball-caged mitral valve. *Ann Thorac Surg.* 2011;91:606-608.

Hill EE, Herijgers P, Claus P, et al. Abscess in infective endocarditis: the value of transesophageal echocardiography and outcome: a 5-year study. *Am Heart J.* 2007;154:923-928.

Hsi DH, Ryan GF, Taft J, Arnone TJ. A 29-year-old Harken disk mitral valve: long-term follow-up by echocardiographic and cineradiographic imaging. *Tex Heart Inst J.* 2003;40:319-321.

Hufnagel CA. Reflections on the development of valvular prostheses. *Med Instrum.* 1977;11:74-76.

Hufnagel CA. Aortic plastic valvular prosthesis. *Bull Georgetown Univ Med Center.* 1951;5:128-130.

Hufnagel CA, Villegas PD, Nahas H. Experiences with new types of aortic valvular prostheses. *Ann Surg.* 1958;147:636-645.

Ikonomidis JS, Kratz JM, Crumbley 3rd AJ, et al. Twenty-year experience with the St. Jude Medical mechanical valve prosthesis. *J Thorac Cardiovasc Surg.* 2003;126:2022-2031.

ISTHMUS Investigators. The Italian study on the Mitroflow postoperative results (ISTHMUS): a 20-year, multicentre evaluation of Mitroflow pericardial bioprosthesis. *Eur J Cardiothorac Surg.* 2011;39:18-26.

Jamieson WR, Burr LH, Miyagishima RT, et al. Carpentier-Edwards supra-annular aortic porcine bioprosthesis: clinical performance over 20 years. *J Thorac Cardiovasc Surg.* 2005;130:994-1000.

Jamieson WR, Ling H, Burr LH, et al. Carpentier-Edwards supraannular porcine bioprosthesis evaluation over 15 years. *Ann Thorac Surg.* 1998;66(suppl): S49-S52.

Khan S, Chaux A, Matloff J, et al. The St. Jude Medical valve. Experience with 1000 cases. *J Thorac Cardiovasc Surg.* 1994;108(6):1010-1019.

Kleine P, Hasenkam MJ, Nygaard H, Perthel M, Wesemeyer D, Laas J. Tilting disc versus bileaflet aortic valve substitutes: intraoperative and postoperative hemodynamic performance in humans. *J Heart Valve Dis.* 2000;9: 308-312.

Konen E, Goitein O, Feinberg MS, et al. The role of ECG-gated MDCT in the evaluation of aortic and mitral mechanical valves: initial experience. *AJR Am J Roentgenol.* 2008;19:26-31.

Kratz JM, Crawford Jr FA, Sade RM, Crumbley AJ, Stroud MR. St. Jude prosthesis for aortic and mitral valve replacement: a ten-year experience. *Ann Thorac Surg.* 1993;56:462-468.

Kvitting JP, Dyverfeldt P, Sigfridsson A, et al. In vitro assessment of flow patterns and turbulence intensity in prosthetic heart valves using generalized phase-contrast MRI. *J Magn Reson Imaging.* 2010;31:1075-1080.

LaBounty TM, Agarwal PP, Chughtai A, Bach DS, Wizauer E, Kazerooni EA. Evaluation of mechanical heart valve size and function with ECG-gated 64-MDCT. *AJR Am J Roentgenol.* 2009;193:W389-W396.

Larmi TK, Kärkölä P. Shrinkage and degradation of the Delrin occluder in the tilting-disc valve prosthesis. *J Thorac Cardiovasc Surg.* 1974;68:66-69.

Leontyev S, Borger MA, Davierwala P, et al. Redo aortic valve surgery: early and late outcomes. *Ann Thorac Surg.* 2011;91:1120-1126.

Li JS, Sexton DJ, Mick N, et al. Proposed modifications to the Duke criteria for the diagnosis of infective endocarditis. *Clin Infect Dis.* 2000;30:633.

Loisance DY, Mazzucotelli JP, Bertrand PC, Deleuze PH, Cachera JP. Mitroflow pericardial valve: long-term durability. *Ann Thorac Surg.* 1993;56:131-136.

Luk A, Lim KD, Siddiqui R, et al. A Braunwald-Cutter valve: a mitral prosthesis at 33 years. *Cardiovasc Pathol.* 2010;19:e39-e42.

Maganti MR. Redo: vascular surgery in elderly patients. *Ann Thorac Surg.* 2009;87:521-525.

Magovern GJ, Cromie HW. Sutureless prosthetic heart valves. *J Thorac Cardiovasc Surg.* 1963;46:726-736.

Magovern GJ, Liebler GA, Cushing WJ, Park SB, Burkholder JA. A thirteen-year review of the Magovern-Cromie aortic valve. *J Thorac Cardiovasc Surg.* 1977;73:64-74.

Magovern GJ, Liebler GA, Park SB, Burkholder JA, Sakert T, Simpson KA. Twenty-five-year review of the Magovern-Cromie sutureless aortic valve. *Ann Thorac Surg.* 1989;48(suppl 3):S33-S34.

Marcus RH, Heinrich RS, Bednarz J, et al. Assessment of small-diameter aortic mechanical prostheses: physiological relevance of the Doppler gradient, utility of flow augmentation, and limitations of orifice area estimation. *Circulation.* 1998;98:866-872.

Mariscalco G, Cozzi GP, Gherli R, Sala A. Excellent durability of a Starr-Edwards mitral caged-ball-valve prosthesis over 34 years. *J Card Surg.* 2011;26:72.

Mehlman DJ, Resnekov L. A guide to the radiographic identification of prosthetic heart valves. *Circulation.* 1978;57:613-623.

Messmer BJ, Rothlin M, Senning A. Early disc dislodgment: an unusual complication after insertion of a Björk Shiley mitral valve prosthesis. *J Thorac Cardiovasc Surg.* 1973;65:386-390.

Mikhail AA. A scientific critique of an Omniscience clinical paper. *J Thorac Cardiovasc Surg.* 1984;88:307-310.

Minami K, Zittermann A, Schulte-Eistrup S, Koertke H, Körfer R. Mitroflow synergy prostheses for aortic valve replacement: 19 years' experience with 1,516 patients. *Ann Thorac Surg.* 2005;80:1699-1705.

Misawa Y, Taguchi M, Aizawa K, et al. Twenty-two year experience with the omniscience prosthetic heart valve. *ASAIO J.* 2004;50:606-610.

Moggio RA, Pooley RW, Sarabu MR, Christiana J, Ho AW, Reed GE. Experience with the Mitroflow aortic bioprosthesis. *J Thorac Cardiovasc Surg.* 1994;108:215-220.

Mohty D, Dumesnil JG, Echahidi N, et al. Impact of prosthesis-patient mismatch on long-term survival after aortic valve replacement: influence of age, obesity, and left ventricular dysfunction. *J Am Coll Cardiol.* 2009;53: 39-47.

Nihoyannopoulos P, Kambouroglou D, Athanassopoulos G, et al. Doppler haemodynamic profiles of clinically and echocardiographically normal mitral and aortic valve prostheses. *Eur Heart J.* 1992;13:348-355.

O'Neill WW, Chandler JG, Gordon RE, et al. Radiographic detection of strut separations in Björk-Shiley convexo-concave mitral valves. *N Engl J Med.* 1995;333:414-419.

Oparah SS, Keefe JF, Ryan TJ, Berger RL. Mitral valve replacement with a turtleneck-disc prosthesis. *J Thorac Cardiovasc Surg.* 1975;69:569-574.

Orszulak TA, Schaff HV, Puga FJ, et al. Event status of the Starr-Edwards aortic valve to 20 years: a benchmark for comparison. *Ann Thorac Surg.* 1997;63:620-626.

Payne DM, Koka HP, Karanicolas PJ, et al. Hemodynamic performance of stentless versus stented valves: a systematic review and meta-analysis. *J Card Surg.* 2008;23:556-564.

Pibarot P, Dumesnil JG. Hemodynamic and clinical impact of prosthesis-patient mismatch in the aortic valve position and its prevention. *J Am Coll Cardiol.* 2000;36:1131-1141.

Poirer NC, Pelletier LC, Pellerin M, Carrier M. 15-year experience with the Carpentier-Edwards pericardial bioprosthesis. *Ann Thorac Surg.* 1998;66(suppl):S57-S61.

Pollock SG, Dent JM, Simek CL, et al. Starr-Edwards valve thrombosis detected preoperatively by transesophageal echocardiography. *Cathet Cardiovasc Diagn.* 1994;31:156-157.

Reber D, Birnbaum DE, Tollenaere P, Eschenbruch E. Long-term results after aortic valve replacement with the Mitroflow pericardial valve. *J Cardiovasc Surg.* 1996;37(suppl 1):23-27.

Remadi JP, Baron O, Roussel C, et al. Isolated mitral valve replacement with St. Jude Medical prosthesis: long-term results: a follow-up of 19 years. *Circulation.* 2001;103:1542-1545.

Remadi JP, Marticho P, Nzomvuama A, Degandt A. Preliminary results of 130 aortic valve replacements with a new mechanical bileaflet prosthesis: the Edwards MIRA valve. *Interact Cardiovasc Thorac Surg.* 2003;2:80-83.

Roedler S, Czerny M, Neuhauser J, et al. Mechanical aortic valve prostheses in the small aortic root: Top Hat versus standard Carbomedics aortic valve. *Ann Thorac Surg.* 2008;86:64-70.

Sachdev M, Peterson GE, Jollis JG. Imaging techniques for diagnosis of infective endocarditis. *Cardiol Clin.* 2003;21:185-195.

Schoen FJ, Fernandez J, Gonzalez-Lavin L, Cernaianu A. Causes of failure and pathologic findings in surgically removed Ionescu-Shiley standard bovine pericardial heart valve bioprostheses: emphasis on progressive structural deterioration. *Circulation*. 1987;76:618-627.

Schoen FJ, Goodenough SH, Ionescu MI, Braunwald NS. Implications of late morphology of Braunwald-Cutter mitral heart valve prostheses. *J Thorac Cardiovasc Surg*. 1984;88:208-216.

Schoen FJ, Levy RJ. Tissue heart valves: current challenges and future research perspectives. *J Biomed. Mater Res*. 1999;65:439-465.

Schoen FJ, Titus JL, Lawrie GM. Durability of pyrolytic carbon-containing heart valve prostheses. *J Biomed Mater Res*. 1982;16:559-570.

Senning A. Fascia lata replacement of aortic valves. *J Thorac Cardiovasc Surg*. 1967;54:465-470.

Sezai A, Shiono M, Hata M, et al. 40 years' experience in mitral valve replacement using Starr-Edwards, St. Jude Medical and ATS valves. *Ann Thorac Cardiovasc Surg*. 2006;12:249-256.

Shapira Y, Feinberg MS, Hirsch R, Nili M, Sagie A. Echocardiography can detect cloth cover tears in fully covered Starr-Edwards valves: a long-term clinical and echocardiographic study. *Am Heart J*. 1997;134:665-671.

Si MS, Zapolanski A. A 37-year-old Smeloff-Cutter aortic valve. *Ann Thorac Surg*. 2009;87:628-629.

Siddiqui RF, Abraham JR, Butany J. Bioprosthetic heart valves: modes of failure. *Histopathology*. 2009;55:135-144.

Svennevig JL, Abdelnoor M, Nitter-Hauge S. Twenty-five-year experience with the Medtronic-Hall valve prosthesis in the aortic position: a follow-up cohort study of 816 consecutive patients. *Circulation*. 2007;116:1795-1800.

Symersky P, Budde RP, de Mol BA, Prokop M. Comparison of multidetector-row computed tomography to echocardiography and fluoroscopy for evaluation of patients with mechanical prosthetic valve obstruction. *Am J Cardiol*. 2009;104:1128-1134.

Tarzia V, Bottio T, Testolin L, Gerosa G. Extended (31 years) durability of a Starr-Edwards prosthesis in mitral position. *Interact Cardiovasc Thorac Surg*. 2007;6:570-571.

Teijeira FJ. Long-term experience with the Omniscience cardiac valve. *J Heart Valve Dis*. 1998;7:540-547.

Teshima H, Hayashida N, Enomoto N, et al. Detection of pannus by multidetector-row computed tomography. *Ann Thorac Surg*. 2003;75:1631-1633.

Teshima H, Hayashida N, Fukunaga S, et al. Usefulness of a multidetector-row computed tomography scanner for detecting pannus formation. *Ann Thorac Surg*. 2004;77:523-526.

Thubrikar MJ, Deck JD, Aouad J, Nolan SP. Role of mechanical stress in calcification of aortic bioprosthetic valves. *J Thorac Cardiovasc Surg*. 1983;86:115.

Thulin LI, Thilén UJ, Kymle KA. Mitroflow pericardial bioprosthesis in the aortic position: low incidence of structural valve deterioration in elderly patients during an 11-year follow-up. *Scand Cardiovasc J*. 2000;34:192-196.

Toledano D, Acar C. Usefulness of computed tomography scanning in the diagnosis of aortic prosthetic valve pannus. *J Heart Valve Dis*. 2010;19:665-668.

Toole JM, Stroud MR, Kratz JM, et al. Twenty-five year experience with the St. Jude Medical mechanical valve prosthesis. *Ann Thorac Surg*. 2010;89:1402-1409.

Valfrè C, Ius P, Minniti G, et al. The fate of Hancock II porcine valve recipients 25 years after implant. *Eur J Cardiothorac Surg*. 2010;38:141-146.

Verhoye JP, Abouliatim I, Lelong B, et al. Edwards MIRA bileaflet prosthesis in aortic position: midterm results of a prospective multi-centre study. *Interact Cardiovasc Thorac Surg*. 2007;6:458-461.

Von Der Emde JJ, Eberlein U, Breme JJ. Asymptomatic strut fracture in DeBakey-Surgitool aortic valves: incidence, management, and metallurgic aspects. *Tex Heart Inst J*. 1990;17:223-227.

Wann LS, Pyhel HJ, Judson WE, Tavel ME, Feigenbaum H. Ball variance in a Harken mitral prosthesis: echocardiographic and phonocardiographic features. *Chest*. 1977;72:785–777.

Yavari A, Spyropoulos A, Khawaja MZ, McWilliams ET. Paravalvular regurgitation of a Starr-Edwards mitral prosthesis depicted by real time three-dimensional transesophageal echocardiography. *Echocardiography*. 2008;25:1145-1146.

Zellner JL, Kratz JM, Crumbley 3rd AJ, et al. Long-term experience with the St. Jude Medical valve prosthesis. *Ann Thorac Surg*. 1999;68:1210-1218.

CHAPTER 18

Cardiac Devices

John P. Lichtenberger III, Gladwin Hui, Brett W. Carter, Carlos Jamis-Dow, and Suhny Abbara

The rapid evolution of devices in the diagnosis and treatment of cardiac disease poses a challenge to the imaging professional. Devices are often readily apparent on imaging, yet extrapolating their use from their appearance is not always straightforward. Understanding the expected appearance and function of cardiac devices is the first step to identifying clinically significant complications. Additionally, understanding the indications for cardiac devices can provide important clues to the patient's underlying cardiac disease if such clues are not provided in the clinical history.

■ INTRAAORTIC BALLOON PUMP

Background and Indications

The intraaortic balloon pump (IABP) or intraaortic counterpulsation balloon device is a 25-cm long inflatable balloon mounted along a catheter placed into the descending thoracic aorta through a transfemoral approach. Inflation of the balloon with carbon dioxide is coordinated with ventricular diastole to reduce left ventricular afterload and to augment coronary artery perfusion. This process both decreases the demand on cardiac function and increases myocardial oxygenation. This device is temporary and is usually indicated in the immediate postoperative setting after cardiac surgery or after an acute myocardial infarction until cardiac function has recovered. Other indications include cardiogenic shock, septic shock, and left ventricular failure.

Imaging

The tip of the IABP is ideally positioned approximately 3 cm distal to the expected location of the left subclavian artery in the descending thoracic aorta (Fig. 18-1). A radiopaque marker indicates the tip of the balloon pump. The position of this tip relative to the aortic knob (radiographic landmark representing the confluence of the aortic arch, left subclavian artery, and proximal descending thoracic aorta) is typically taken as a surrogate marker for the position of the left subclavian artery origin. Positioning the balloon too near the ostium of the left subclavian artery may predispose the patient to embolism to the brain. Positioning the balloon too distal in the descending thoracic aorta risks transient occlusion of the superior

mesenteric artery or renal arteries and subsequent ischemia or embolization.

Complications

The most common complications of IABP are vascular, including arterial perforation, dissection, visceral and limb ischemia, and peripheral embolization. Limb ischemia occurs in anywhere from 14% to 45% of patients. An IABP is an independent predictor of cerebrovascular accident in patients after percutaneous coronary procedures. Hemorrhage and infection of the groin access site are additional risks of this device.

■ IMPELLA

Background and Indications

The Impella Circulatory Support System (Abiomed, Inc., Danvers, Mass) is a percutaneously placed device inserted through the femoral artery and advanced across the left ventricular outflow tract to bypass left ventricular function. Once the device is in position, with the tip in the left ventricle, internal propellers siphon blood from the left ventricle to the aorta. This device is typically used for short-term hemodynamic support in the setting of left-sided heart failure.

Imaging

The Impella device is visible radiographically in the expected distribution of the left ventricular outflow tract and ascending aorta (Fig. 18-2). The curled tip of the device is meant to lie within the left ventricle and the outlet area in the ascending aorta.

■ TANDEMHEART

Background and Indications

The TandemHeart (CardiacAssist, Inc., Pittsburgh) is a continuous flow pump that directs blood from the left atrium to the systemic circulation and thus bypasses left ventricular function. Blood from the left atrium is accessed by passing an inflow cannula from the inferior vena cava to the right atrium and across the interatrial septum. This blood is transmitted to the systemic circulation

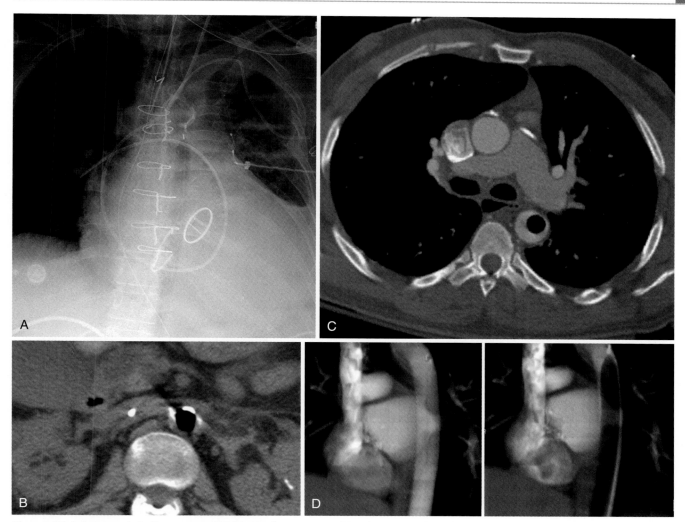

Figure 18-1 Intraaortic balloon pump (IABP). A and **B,** A 73-year-old male patient in heart failure with an IABP in place. The well-seated bal-loon is inflated in diastole to increase coronary artery perfusion and to decrease afterload, as confirmed on this anteroposterior chest radiograph (**A**) by the mechanical mitral valve in an open position. Axial computed tomography (CT) noncontrast image (**B**) shows the air-filled IABP within the aorta. **C** and **D,** IABP in a 62-year-old male patient. **C,** Axial diastolic image of a gated coronary CT angiogram shows an inflated IABP at the level of the pulmonary arteries. **D,** Systolic and diastolic sagittal oblique multiplanar reformations show a well-seated deflated IABP in systole *(left)* and an inflated IABP in diastole *(right).*

through the femoral arteries. This device is typically used for hemodynamic support in patients with cardiogenic shock and in patients requiring high-risk cardiac interventions who are not appropriate surgical candidates.

Imaging

The inflow cannula is visible on radiographs as it traversing the expected location of the interatrial septum (Fig. 18-3). The outflow cannulas are visible within the femoral arteries. The pump is not often imaged, external to the patient, and usually positioned about the thigh.

Complications

Complications of TandemHeart use include access site bleeding and hematoma, as well as the need for post-procedure transfusion.

■ VENTRICULAR ASSIST DEVICES

Background and Indications

Ventricular assist devices are implanted mechanical pump devices used to augment cardiac output in the setting of heart failure. These devices are typically used as a bridge to heart transplantation, by sustaining perfusion to other organs and helping to rehabilitate the patient before the surgical procedure. If the patient is not a candidate for heart transplantation, these devices may be the only treatment option. Types of ventricular assist devices include pulsatile and nonpulsatile extracorporeal devices, implantable devices, and the total artificial heart.

Implantable devices, the most common ventricular assist devices, are implanted in a preperitoneal pocket in the upper abdomen. This site is chosen for easy access in the case of bleeding and infection. The inflow conduit is connected to the left ventricular apex, thus diverting blood

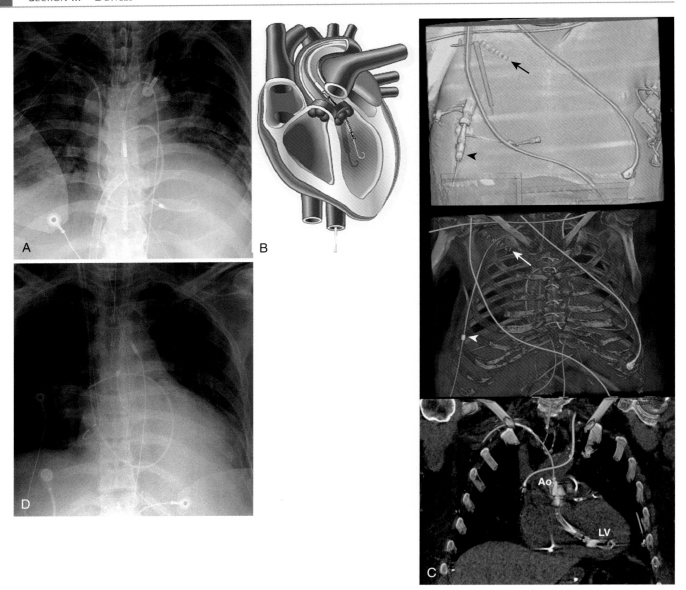

Figure 18-2 Impella device. A, Anteroposterior radiograph shows a well-seated Impella device through the transfemoral approach, which projects with its pigtail over the left ventricle (LV) cavity. **B,** Cartoon demonstrating the proper position of the device with the inflow portion in the LV and the outflow seated within the aorta. **C,** Computed tomography volume-rendered images show an Impella device through a subclavian artery access (*arrows* show skin staples at the cutdown site; the *arrowheads* points to the extracorporeal wire). Note the position of the pigtail within the LV and the outflow within the ascending aorta. **D,** Anteroposterior radiograph in a 38-year-old male patient with Lyme disease and sudden cardiac arrest shows a device seated too high within the ascending aorta. (**B,** Courtesy of Abiomed, Inc., Danvers, Mass.)

from the left ventricle to the device. The outflow conduit connects the device to the ascending aorta. The device contains internal valves to prevent reflux of blood back to the left ventricle, and an external power source drives forward blood flow. Whereas first-generation devices work by pulsatile pump (e.g., HeartMate, Novacor), second-generation devices use continuous flow. A newer design of ventricular assist device allows placement in the pericardial space, directly adjacent to the heart, above the diaphragm (HeartWare HVAD left ventricular assist device, HeartWare International, Inc., Framingham, Mass).

Imaging

On radiography, the mechanical device is easily identified, although often it is imaged only partially

(Fig. 18-4). The inflow conduit should project over the left ventricle, and the outflow conduit connecting to the ascending aorta is often not radiopaque. Computed tomography (CT) shows the device conduits and their insertion to the left ventricle and ascending aorta, although beam-hardening artifact may limit evaluation of the mechanical portions. The HeartWare HVAD left ventricular assist device is shown in Figure 18-4, *D*.

Complications

Device complications are related to device function or device placement. The risk of thromboembolic events necessitates anticoagulation while the device is in place. Pleural bleeding and pericardial bleeding are additional complications, and they should be suspected if the

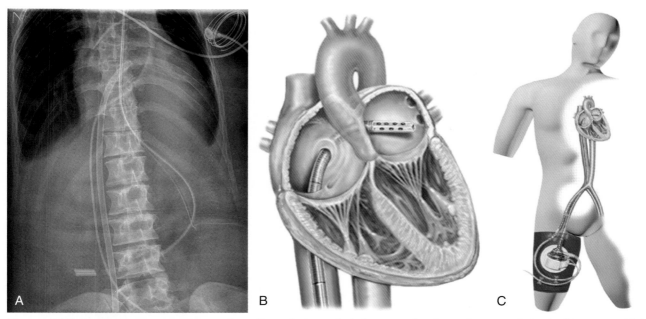

Figure 18-3 TandemHeart. A, Anteroposterior radiograph shows the inflow cannula of a TandemHeart device in this 26-year-old female patient in acute heart failure. The femoral outflow cannulas are not imaged. **B** and **C,** Graphics show the inflow cannula traversing the interatrial septum (**B**) and the entire device with the femoral outflow cannula (**C**). (**B** and **C,** Courtesy of CardiacAssist, Inc., Pittsburgh.)

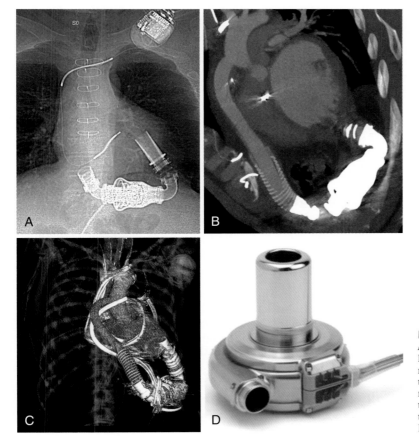

Figure 18-4 Left ventricular assist device (LVAD).
A, A 58-year-old male patient with heart failure and an LVAD in place on a scout image. **B,** The aortic conduit is not radiopaque and is better seen on oblique computed tomography (CT) with the LVAD implanted under the ribs. **C,** Three-dimensional reformatted CT image shows the entire device and ventricular insert. **D,** Photograph of the HeartWare HVAD LVAD. (**D,** Courtesy of HeartWare International, Inc., Framingham, Mass.)

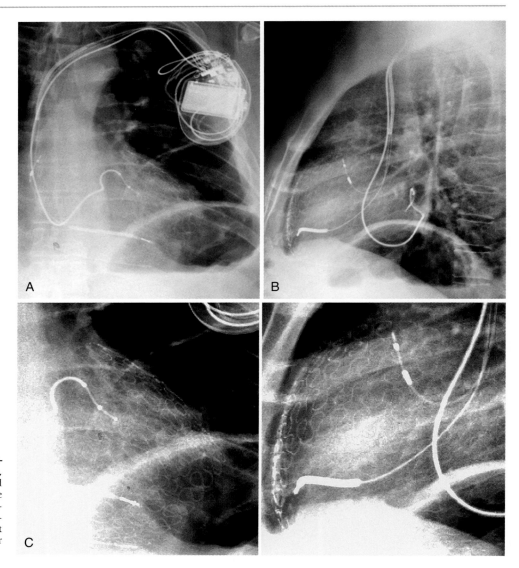

Figure 18-5 HeartNet (Paracor Medical, Inc., Sunnyvale, Calif). Posteroanterior (**A**), lateral (**B**), and zoomed (**C**) views of the chest in this patient with left ventricular failure show a wavy radiopaque mesh about the heart that acts as a restraint against further dilation of the ventricles.

cardiomediastinal contour suddenly changes or a large amount of pleural fluid suddenly accumulates. Hemoperitoneum and abscess formation are abdominal complications of device placement. Finally, device failure may lead to worsening heart failure symptoms and pulmonary edema.

Smaller patients may not be able to receive a ventricular assist device. If necessary, these devices may be positioned intraabdominally.

■ HEARTNET

Background and Indications

The Paracor HeartNet (Paracor Medical, Inc., Sunnyvale, Calif) is an investigational elastic ventricular restraint device developed for patients with heart failure in whom standard therapy has failed. The device is composed of nitinol mesh and is implanted around the ventricles through a minithoracotomy. The elasticity of the device is expected to reduce wall stress and to allow reverse ventricular remodeling.

Imaging

On chest radiographs, the HeartNet device appears as wavy radiopaque mesh around the ventricles (Fig. 18-5).

Complications

In a feasibility study of 21 patients with New York Heart Association functional class II or III heart failure, the device was successfully implanted in 20 patients. Atrial fibrillation occurred in 2 patients, and the 2 in-hospital deaths were not directly related to the device.

■ CARDIOMEMS HEART FAILURE PRESSURE MEASUREMENT SYSTEM

Background and Indications

The CardioMEMS heart failure pressure measurement system (CardioMEMS, Inc., Atlanta) uses microelectromechanical systems (MEMS) technology

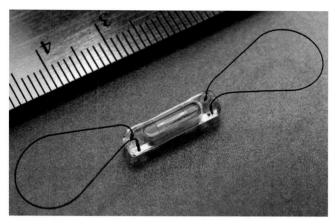

Figure 18-6 CardioMEMS. The device is implanted about the left pulmonary artery to monitor pulmonary arterial pressure in patients with heart failure. (Courtesy of CardioMEMS, Inc., Atlanta.)

to monitor pulmonary arterial pressure in patients with heart failure. The device, currently under investigation, consists of a radiopaque 15 mm × 3.5 mm wireless implantable sensor with nitinol anchoring loops (Fig. 18-6), as well as an external electronics module. The electronics module powers the sensor through transmitted radiofrequency energy and receives data from the sensor.

Imaging

The CardioMEMS device (see Fig. 18-6) is usually implanted in the left pulmonary artery and is visible on chest radiographs. Depending on its orientation, it may be more visible on the lateral or the frontal view. The nitinol anchoring loops are visible on CT scans but are not easily seen on radiographs.

Complications

Potential complications of the CardioMEMS device include those related to the implantation of the wireless sensor (infection, bleeding, and thrombosis).

■ C-PULSE

Background and Indications

The C-Pulse (Sunshine Heart, Inc., Eden Prairie, Calif) device is a non–blood-contacting extraaortic implantable counterpulsation pump designed for the treatment of moderate to severe heart failure. The device is implanted using a full open sternotomy-hemisternotomy approach or using a limited right parasternal thoracotomy incision, leaving the sternum intact, and is then secured around the ascending aorta and pneumatically driven by an external system controller.

Imaging

In chest radiographs, the C-Pulse device is visible as radiolucency around the ascending aorta, in both the frontal and lateral views (Fig. 18-7).

Complications

Device and drive-line infections have been reported with this device.

■ LEFT VENTRICULAR APICOAORTIC CONDUIT

Background and Indications

The apicoaortic conduit connects the left ventricle to the descending thoracic aorta. This conduit is typically used to bypass the aortic valve in patients with severe aortic stenosis when direct repair of the valve is precluded by contraindicated sternotomy (coronary bypass graft surgery) or severe ascending aortic calcification (porcelain ascending aorta). Alternatively, this device may be used when either the left ventricular outflow tract or the ascending aorta is hypoplastic, such as in congenital heart disease.

The conduit is connected between the left ventricular apex and the thoracic aorta, and an internal conduit valve prevents reflux of blood back to the left ventricle. Rarely, the outflow conduit is connected to a great vessel.

Imaging

The metallic ring of the apicoaortic conduit valve projects over the left lung base on frontal chest radiographs (Fig. 18-8). On the lateral chest radiograph, the metallic ring projects over the middle mediastinum, usually posterior to the cardiac silhouette. The conduit itself, however, may not be visible radiographically. CT best defines the anastomotic sites and course of the conduit. Electrocardiogram (ECG) gating provides the optimum evaluation of the inflow (ventricular) conduit. Alternatively, magnetic resonance angiography may demonstrate flow through the graft, although dephasing artifact from the valve may limit evaluation. Echocardiography does not show the course of the graft or its aortic insertion. However, because blood flow should preferentially enter the low-resistance graft, significant forward flow through the left ventricular outflow tract on echocardiography may be an indirect sign of graft occlusion.

Complications

The overall operative mortality rate in one series of apicoaortic conduit placements was 11%. Pseudoaneurysms of the conduit insertion and disruption of the conduit from the ventricular apex or aorta are life-threatening complications of this device. Conduit thrombosis or stenosis secondary to endothelial proliferation may result in device failure. The internal valve may fail, resulting in reflux of blood back to the left ventricle. The conduits may become infected or thrombogenic, and thrombus within the descending thoracic aorta has been reported.

■ OCCLUDER DEVICES

Septal Occluder

Defects in the septum dividing the atria (atrial septal defect [ASD], patent foramen ovale [PFO]) and ventricles

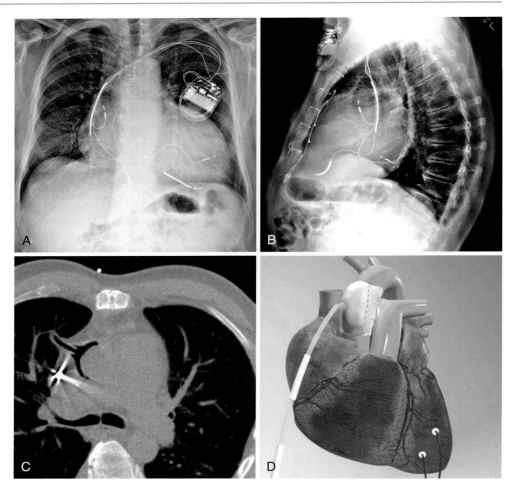

Figure 18-7 C-Pulse. This device is implanted about the extravascular ascending aorta through a median sternotomy, and it pneumatically inflates in diastole, similar to an IABP. Frontal (**A**), lateral (**B**), and computed tomography (**C**) images show the position of the device. **D,** Cartoon illustrating proper placement of the balloon cuff and epicardial sensing leads. (**D,** Courtesy of Sunshine Heart, Inc., Tustin, Calif.)

(ventricular septal defect [VSD], Gerbode defect) may be present in isolation or as a component of complex congenital heart disease. Alternatively, VSD may be acquired as a result of myocardial infarction, and atrial septal perforation may be necessary for some cardiac interventional procedures requiring access to the left side of the heart. These septal defects may lead to volume overload and shunt physiology. If large shunts are left untreated, pulmonary hypertension may occur, eventually leading to right–to-left shunt (Eisenmenger physiology) and the risk of paradoxical embolus. Evidence of significant left-to-right shunt (pulmonary to systemic blood flow ratio [QP/QS] >1.5 to 2) causing dilation of right heart chambers is the most common indication for closure of these defects. Transthoracic echocardiography is the modality of choice for evaluating septal defects, particularly in the pediatric population. Whereas percutaneous closure is the treatment of choice for ASD, surgical closure is the standard treatment for congenital VSD.

ASDs are present in 10% of congenital heart lesions in children and in 30% of congenital heart lesions in adults. Ostium secundum ASDs account for 75% of ASDs and are most amenable to percutaneous closure. Ostium primum and sinus venosus defects are much less common and are usually not suitable to percutaneous closure because of inadequate margins for attachment of the occluder or proximity to the atrioventricular valve. Amplatzer septal occluders (AGA Medical Corporation, Plymouth, Minn), most commonly used for percutaneous closure of ostium secundum ASDs, consist of preformed mesh and integral material (Fig. 18-9). These occluders are placed under transesophageal echocardiography guidance.

Although surgical correction is the standard treatment for VSDs, percutaneous closure has been performed with success in selected patients. Closure of acquired VSD may require a larger occluder device.

Amplatzer septal occluder devices are the most common, but other occluders are also available. The Gore HELEX septal occluder (Gore Medical, Flagstaff, Ariz) is a long nitinol wire with polytetrafluoroethylene (PTFE) fabric attached that spirals to form two circular disks (Fig. 18-10). The contour is considered less traumatic, and it creates less distortion of the septum before release. This device may become a suitable alternative for occlusion of smaller septal defects.

Complications

Malposition or dislodgment of the occluder is the most important complication of these devices. Thrombus formation associated with closure devices is rare but has been reported. A serious potential complication of ASD closure devices is erosion of the device through the atrial wall and possibly into the aortic root. Similarly, erosion of PFO

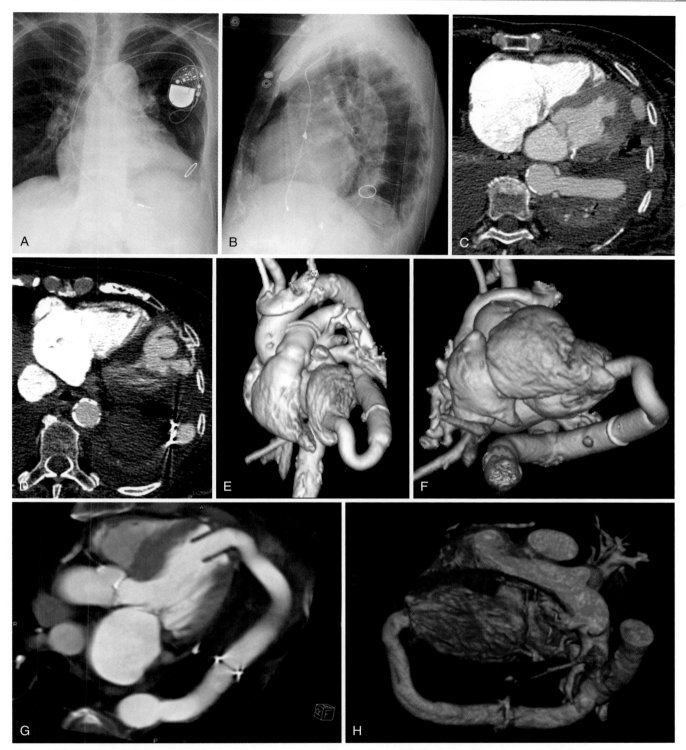

Figure 18-8 Left ventricular apicoaortic conduit. An 86-year-old woman with left ventricular failure has a metallic ring on posteroanterior (**A**) and lateral (**B**) radiographs of the chest that corresponds to the valve within a left ventricular apicoaortic conduit. **C** and **D**, Axial computed tomography (CT) images show the ventricular and aortic inserts. **E** and **F**, Three-dimensional reformatted images in the parasagittal oblique and axial planes show the conduit in its entirety. A different example of an apicoaortic conduit on a CT three-chamber view (**G**) and a three-dimensional volume-rendered image (**H**).

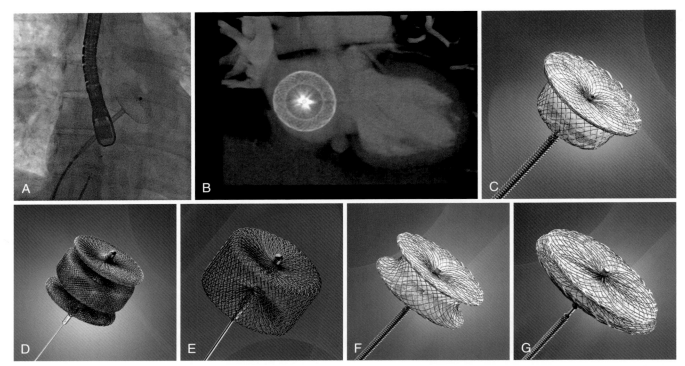

Figure 18-9 *Amplatzer occluder devices.* **A,** Fluoroscopic image from Amplatzer occluder device placement under transesophageal echocardiographic guidance. **B,** Reformatted computed tomography image shows the atrial septal occlusion device in place. **C** to **G,** Multiple types of Amplatzer occluder devices. (**C** to **G,** Courtesy of AGA Medical Corporation, Plymouth, Minn.)

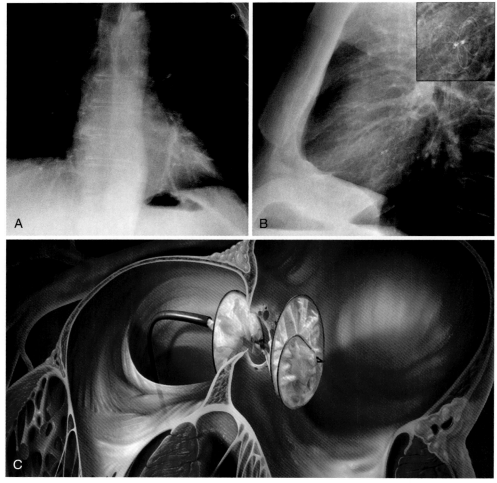

Figure 18-10 *Gore HELEX occluder.* Posteroanterior (**A**) and lateral (**B**) views of the chest show the metallic wire spiral of the occluder in this 62-year-old male patient with an atrial septal defect. **C,** Graphic shows placement of the occluder across an atrial septal defect. (**C,** Courtesy of Gore Medical, Flagstaff, Ariz.)

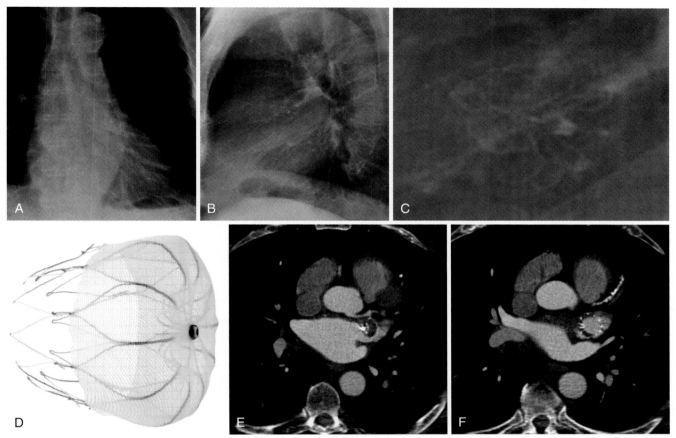

Figure 18-11 Watchman device. Posteroanterior (**A**), lateral (**B**), and coned-down lateral (**C**) images in this 86-year-old man with chronic atrial fibrillation show a Watchman device in position within the left atrial appendage. **D,** Photograph shows the nitinol frame and fabric cover, intended to reduce the risk of thromboembolism. **E** and **F,** Axial computed tomography with contrast demonstrates leak around a Watchman device. (**D,** Courtesy of Artitech, Minneapolis, Minn.)

closure devices has been reported. So far, no reports of Gore HELEX device erosion into the aortic root have been received. Complete heart block after Amplatzer membranous VSD occluder deployment has been reported.

Left Atrial Appendage Occluder Device

Background and Indications
Left atrial appendage occluder devices such as the Watchman (Artitech, Minneapolis, Minn) are percutaneously placed, permanently implanted trapping devices made of a self-expanding nitinol frame and a permeable polyester fabric cover. The devices are deployed into the left atrial appendage just distal to the ostium, to prevent thrombi from entering the circulation. Fixation barbs secure the device to the left atrial appendage wall. These devices are intended to reduce the risk of stroke and embolization of thrombus from the left atrial appendage in patients with atrial fibrillation who may have contraindications to or who may be at higher risk from lifelong anticoagulation. Studies have demonstrated the role of the left atrial appendage in atrial fibrillation–related stroke and have stated the noninferiority of these devices to warfarin therapy in the prevention of embolic events, depending on the operator's experience.

Imaging
When deployed successfully, the Watchman device occupies the left atrial appendage and excludes thrombus in the appendage from entering the left atrium (Fig. 18-11). ECG-gated cardiac CT may be the modality of choice for evaluating these devices, by demonstrating the lack of opacification of the left atrial appendage as well as possibly confirming device integrity.

Complications
Complications of device implantation include pericardial effusion possibly leading to pericardial tamponade, procedure-related stroke attributed to air embolism, device embolization , device-associated thrombus, and leakage around the device (see Fig. 18-11, *E* and *F*).

■ IMPLANTABLE LOOP RECORDERS

Background and Indications
Implantable loop recorders are small electronic devices capable of providing long-term continuous monitoring of arrhythmia. They can be automatically activated to record ECG information or triggered by the patient. The primary indication for placement of these devices is recurrent, unexplained syncope or events thought to be

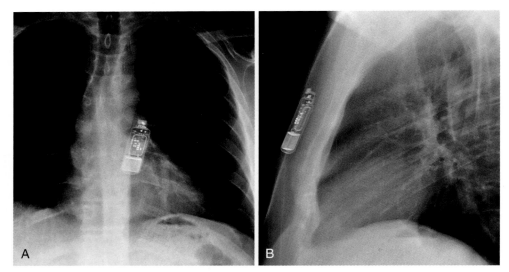

Figure 18-12 Implantable loop recorder. Posteroanterior (**A**) and lateral (**B**) radiographs in this 45-year-old male patient with syncope shows an implantable loop recorder in the normal position. This device is typically inserted under the skin below the left collar bone and continuously records electrocardiographic events.

related to cardiac arrhythmia. These devices are placed subcutaneously in the region of the left pectoral muscle and are retrievable. The battery life is approximately 2 years.

Imaging

Implantable loop recorders have a characteristic appearance on radiographs (Fig. 18-12). Although the recorders contain no lead wires or loops of electrical wires that would make them incompatible with magnetic resonance imaging (MRI), patients may feel movement of the device during MRI because it contains ferromagnetic components. Additionally, MRI has been reported to interfere with ECG data recorded by these devices, possibly producing artifactual arrhythmias or corrupting data previously recorded. Interpreting providers should be consulted before MRI is performed.

■ TRANSCATHETER AORTIC VALVE IMPLANTATION

Background and Indications

For patients with severe aortic stenosis, the traditional therapy is open heart surgical valve replacement. A newer technique, transcatheter aortic valve implantation or replacement (TAVI or TAVR), has been developed as an alternative, particularly for high-risk patients in whom surgical intervention is contraindicated. CT is a valuable tool for preprocedure assessment, by providing important information such as aortic root dimension, aortic valve area, and distance between coronary artery and annulus and by allowing proper selection of prosthesis size. In addition, CT also assesses the femoral vasculature for adequate access. The two approaches for TAVI are transfemoral and transapical. The two most widely used devices are the balloon-expandable Edwards SAPIEN valve (Edwards Lifesciences, LLC, Irvine, Calif) and the self-expanding CoreValve device (Medtronic, Minneapolis, Minn). Studies have shown improvement in left ventricular systolic function after the procedure.

Imaging

The Edwards SAPIEN Valve consists of a stainless steel stent, bovine pericardial leaflets, and a fabric sealing cuff. The CoreValve device consists of a nitinol (nickel titanium) alloy stent, with leaflets and sealing cuff constructed of porcine pericardial tissue. On imaging, a metallic stent with multiple struts can be seen at the level of the aortic valve (Fig. 18-13).

Complications

The most common complication of TAVI and TAVR is arterial injury at the peripheral access site. Other reported complications include myocardial ischemia and cardiogenic shock. The risks of stroke, atrioventricular block, and pacemaker dependence are low.

■ CARDIAC PACEMAKERS

Background and Indications

The first fully implantable cardiac pacemaker system was initially used in 1958, and since then, the utilization, effectiveness, and availability of cardiac pacemakers have greatly increased. Not only have the devices become smaller, but also they have become more affordable, durable, and technologically advanced. For example, most modern pacing systems are able to store information obtained from the ECG tracing for analysis. The most common clinical indication for pacemaker placement is symptomatic bradycardia or complete heart block. Other common indications include long QT syndrome and heart failure.

Modern pacemaker systems consist of a pulse generator, often termed the "box," and one or more leads or electrodes. The pulse generator consists of a lithium iodine cell and complementary metal oxide semiconductor (CMOS) enclosed in a titanium casing. Most devices demonstrate a radiopaque alphanumeric code indicating the model and manufacturer. Pacemaker leads consist of metal alloy conductors enclosed within

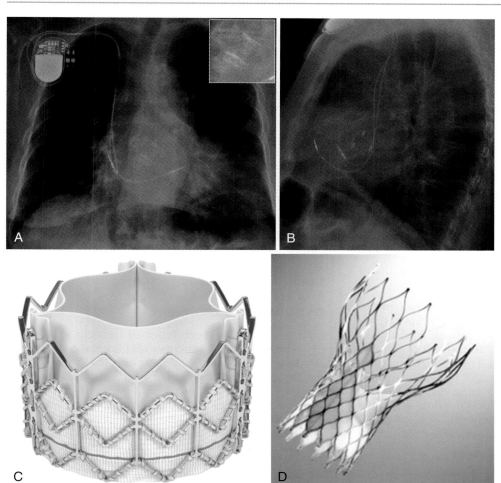

Figure 18-13 Frontal (**A**) and lateral (**B**) radiographs of a patient with a normally seated transcatheter aortic valve implantation (TAVI) device. **C** and **D**, Photographs of the two most common TAVI devices. **C**, Edwards SAPIEN valve. (**C**, Courtesy of Edwards Lifesciences, LLC, Irvine, Calif.) **D**, CoreValve. (**D**, Courtesy of Medtronic, Minneapolis, Minn.)

silicone or polyurethane sheaths. They are classified as either passive fixation or active fixation types, depending on tip configuration. The tips of passive fixation leads have multiple silicone barbs that allow anchorage to the heart. Active fixation leads are characterized by multiple screws at the tip that facilitate insertion into the myocardium.

The traditional method of pacemaker placement involved thoracotomy, although such an invasive procedure for placement of pacemaker systems is rarely performed today. The pulse generator is typically placed within the left infraclavicular region, but right infraclavicular, axillary, submammary, and abdominal positions may also be employed. Transvenous placement is the most commonly used technique today, and it usually involves infraclavicular subclavian and cephalic venous routes. For examples of normally placed devices and leads and for malpositioned devices, please also see Chapter 11. Other vessels, such as the internal jugular, brachial, and femoral veins, are less commonly used. Most pacemaker leads implanted today are bipolar, consisting of a cathode at the distal tip and an anode located approximately 1 to 3 cm from the tip. Unipolar pacing systems are less frequently encountered and consist of a cathode at the lead tip and the external pulse generator serving as an anode.

Confirmation of acceptable pulse generator and lead positions may be achieved by postprocedural chest radiographs or fluoroscopy, although no standard guidelines for performing these examinations after system placement are currently available. However, chest radiographs performed after the procedure can be used to evaluate for complications such as pneumothorax.

Single- and Dual-Chamber Pacing Systems

Pacemaker systems may be single or dual chamber, depending on the number of leads employed and their position within the heart. Single chamber systems involve the placement of a single pacemaker lead within either the right ventricle or the right atrium. Atrial fibrillation with sustained or intermittent slow ventricular response is the most common clinical indication for single chamber ventricular pacing, which is achieved by extending a single lead into the right ventricle so that the tip is near the apex. The frontal chest radiograph typically shows a single lead following the contour of the right heart border and terminating to the left of the spine. The lateral chest radiograph demonstrates the lead within the right ventricle anteriorly. The most common clinical indication for single chamber atrial pacing is sinus node disease characterized by a slow rate of discharge. The frontal chest radiograph demonstrates the lead following the contour of the right heart border and terminating in the expected position of the right atrial appendage. The lateral chest radiograph demonstrates the anterior direction of the lead, but in a more cephalad location than the right ventricular lead, consistent with placement in the right atrial appendage.

Dual chamber pacemakers, consisting of leads implanted within the right atrium and the right ventricle, may be used in cases of complete heart block characterized by persistent failure of conduction to the ventricles. A rate-responsive pacemaker may be employed in the case of concomitant sinus node disease. Chest radiographs show two leads, one terminating in the expected position of the right atrium anteriorly, usually in or near the atrial appendage, and the other terminating in the right ventricle near the apex.

Single Pass Pacing System

A single pass pacing system may be used in complete heart block when patients have a normal sinus response to exercise. This system consists of a single lead containing electrodes positioned approximately 15 cm from the lead tip that sense atrial signals. The lead tip terminates near the right ventricular apex and is used for pacing. Chest radiography demonstrates the radiopaque electrodes in the expected position of the atrium and the tip of the lead terminating in the right ventricle.

Biventricular Pacing Systems

Biventricular pacing systems are primarily used in patients with severe heart failure with conduction delays and desynchronized contractility who are refractory to medical therapy. Advanced chronic heart failure and a widened QRS complex are additional conditions in which biventricular pacing has shown benefit. In this system, leads are typically placed within the right atrium, right ventricle, and left ventricle, all of which are routinely visualized on chest radiography.

Placement of left ventricular pacing systems was previously achieved with thoracotomy or thoracoscopy. In such patients, chest radiography demonstrates the expected postsurgical changes and the lead extending along the surface of the heart. However, this procedure is rarely performed today, and most leads are placed percutaneously within the epicardial veins and advanced into a coronary vein through the coronary sinus. The anterior interventricular vein, which lies in the anterior interventricular groove, is a commonly used vessel. The obtuse marginal cardiac vein, which lies along the posterolateral surface of the left ventricle, and small venous side branches may also be used.

■ IMPLANTABLE CARDIOVERTER-DEFIBRILLATORS

The first implantable cardioverter-defibrillators (ICDs) consisted of electrodes that were surgically placed along the surface of the heart after thoracotomy was performed. Modern ICDs consist of a defibrillator unit and one or more leads. The defibrillator unit comprises a titanium shell enclosing a computer, a capacitor that stores the charge, and a battery. Most current ICDs do not require thoracotomy for placement and are thus referred to as nonthoracotomy lead systems.

Nonthoracotomy systems have traditionally included combinations of intravenous, intracardiac, and subcutaneous leads, which are characterized by multiple metal coils. Today, placement of ICDs is completely transvenous and involves the implantation of a lead containing multiple exposed coils into the right ventricle. The current passes through the myocardium from the coil to the casing of the defibrillator unit implanted within the subcutaneous tissues of the chest wall. ICDs may be bundled with a pacemaker in patients as a treatment for cardiac arrhythmias and as a secondary system in the case of ventricular fibrillation or ventricular tachycardia.

Complications of Pacemaker and Implantable Cardioverter-Defibrillator Placement

Lead migration has been reported to occur in approximately 5% to 10% of patients with pacemakers and ICDs and may result in displacement of a lead into another section of a cardiac chamber or into another cardiac chamber altogether. This phenomenon typically occurs within a few weeks of lead placement because the formation of fibrous tissue at the sites of contact between the lead and the cardiovascular structures decreases the likelihood of migration after this time. Although first described in patients with pacemakers, Twiddler syndrome may also be encountered in defibrillators. This phenomenon is characterized by conscious or unconscious rotation (twiddling) of the pulse generator at the site of percutaneous implantation. If one or more of the electrodes become dislodged, then the device may fail to defibrillate appropriately.

Pacemaker and ICD leads may be inadvertently positioned into the coronary sinus at the time of implantation. This malpositioned lead may appear to be properly positioned within the right atrium on the frontal radiograph, but it is directed posteriorly on the lateral radiograph. Rare cases of inadvertent lead insertion into the left ventricle have been reported and are typically the result of a congenital cardiac anomaly such as PFO or ASD. Potential complications of such lead positioning include perforation of the left ventricle, injury to the mitral valve, endocarditis, and thromboembolism.

Another common complication that can occur is a fracture of one or more of the leads, which typically have a life span of approximately 20 to 30 years. The incidence of lead fracture has been reported to be approximately 2.6%. This phenomenon typically occurs at positions subjected to mechanical stresses and compression, such as along the costal margin or between the clavicle and the first rib. Leads may also fracture at the point of connection to the pulse generator, at venous entry points, and at sharp turns. Fractured leads may result in failure of the device to defibrillate properly, but they may be surgically removed and replaced. Chest radiographs may be normal or may demonstrate irregularity of the normal lead contour, typically at one of the common sites of stress and compression.

The incidence of pneumothorax on the side of placement has been estimated at approximately 1.6% to 2.6%. Pneumothorax development has been described on the contralateral side secondary to unsuccessful attempts at device placement.

The incidence of infection following pacemaker and ICD placement is approximately 2% to 5%, and infection usually occurs at the site of implantation within the chest wall. The most common causative organisms are *Staphylococcus* and *Streptococcus epidermidis*. Attempts at surgical removal of an infected lead can result in fragmentation, the residua of which may be present on subsequent chest radiographs.

Perforation of the right ventricular myocardium by screws at the electrode tip has been reported. Myocardial perforation can be identified on chest radiography when the lead extends beyond the normal cardiac border. Pericardial effusion or tamponade may also be present. Surgical removal of pacemaker leads may be difficult because fibrous tissue may form at points of contact between the leads and the subclavian vein, superior vena cava, right atrium, tricuspid valve, and right ventricle. In such cases, the existing leads are cut and embedded. Subsequent chest radiographs may demonstrate the remaining lead fragments.

Traditionally, the presence of a cardiac pacemaker or ICD has been an absolute contraindication to MRI. However, an initial study evaluating patients with pacemakers scanned with 0.5 T MRI demonstrated no evidence of device dysfunction when specific strategies were used, such as using asynchronous modes, adequate monitoring, and limited radiofrequency exposure. Other studies showed no evidence of pacemaker or ICD dysfunction when MRI of the extremities was performed. However, more research is needed to determine the safety of routinely performing MRI examinations in patients with cardiac pacemakers and ICDs, and such circumstances remain absolute contraindications in most institutions.

■ PULMONARY ARTERY CATHETERS

Background and Indications

The first use of pulmonary artery catheters was detailed by H.J.C. Swan, Willard Ganz, and colleagues in 1970. Today, the term Swan-Ganz usually refers to any multilumen catheter used primarily for measuring hemodynamic pressures and cardiac output, and it is a registered trademark of Edwards Lifesciences.

Pulmonary artery catheters are percutaneously inserted through the internal jugular vein, subclavian vein, or femoral vein and are then advanced through the right atrium, right ventricle, and across the pulmonic valve into the pulmonary artery. A balloon, measuring approximately 1.5 cm when inflated, is located proximal to the tip of the catheter and can be inflated to determine pulmonary capillary wedge pressure, which estimates left atrial pressure and left end-diastolic volume. The balloon is inflated only when measurements are recorded. When the balloon is deflated, the catheter

should terminate within the left or right pulmonary artery approximately 2 to 3 cm from the hilum. The catheter travels distally into smaller pulmonary arterial branches when the balloon is inflated.

Other features of the pulmonary artery catheter include a thermistor used to measure temperature changes and to calculate cardiac output. It is located 4 cm proximal to the balloon. The catheter may demonstrate multiple lumina with their individual openings, the most distal of which is present at the catheter tip. Additional lumina with fenestrations may be used for the delivery of medications to the right atrium. A fiberoptic probe has been developed that can be inserted into the ventricular wall and provide information on oxygen saturation of the ventricular myocardium.

Although pulmonary artery catheters have been widely used in intensive care settings since their introduction to clinical medicine in the 1970s, the clinical value of the data obtained from such devices remains uncertain. Results of studies evaluating the impact of these catheters on morbidity and mortality have been mixed, with some investigators demonstrating no impact and others suggesting an increase in morbidity and mortality. One prospective cohort study including medical and surgical patients in intensive care units observed increased mortality, length of hospital stay, and overall cost when pulmonary artery catheters were used.

Complications

One of the most common complications of pulmonary artery catheter placement is malposition of the device. The catheter may coil or loop within the right atrium or the right ventricle and result in arrhythmias, right bundle branch block, or complete heart block. The catheter may be advanced distally into a small pulmonary arterial branch of the lower lobes or placed into a tributary vessel such as the internal jugular vein, azygos arch, and internal mammary vein.

Pulmonary hemorrhage is more commonly seen in those patients with pulmonary arterial hypertension, and it may be encountered in isolation or as a complication of pseudoaneurysm formation. Pseudoaneurysms may form in patients with indwelling pulmonary artery catheters that have been advanced into the peripheral arterial system, with erosion and weakening of the vessel wall. The most common clinical symptoms encountered in pseudoaneurysm formation are hemoptysis and unexplained cardiopulmonary distress. Small pseudoaneurysms may not be detected on chest radiography. When visible on chest radiographs, pseudoaneurysms appear as nodular opacities distal to the position of the pulmonary artery catheter. Multidetector CT (MDCT) is the modality of choice in evaluating for the presence and number of pseudoaneurysms. On MDCT, pseudoaneurysms appear as nodular opacities that demonstrate contrast enhancement in phase with the pulmonary arteries. Surrounding ground glass opacities representing pulmonary hemorrhage may be seen.

The most serious complication of pulmonary artery catheter placement is pulmonary infarction, which may result from advancement of the catheter distally into a small arterial branch or protracted inflation of the balloon in a more proximal segment. In these situations, distal blood flow becomes impaired or obstructed, or both. The most common findings on chest radiography include patchy opacities or consolidation within the lung parenchyma distal to the position of the pulmonary artery catheter. On MDCT, pulmonary infarction typically appears as solid, ground glass, or mixed density within the lung parenchyma. Additional complications such as pulmonary artery rupture and bronchial-arterial fistula are uncommon.

Bibliography

Acker MA. Surgical therapies for heart failure. *J Card Fail.* 2004;10:S220-S224.

Attili A, Kazerooni E. Postoperative cardiopulmonary thoracic imaging. *Radiol Clin North Am.* 2004;42:543-564.

Baskett RJ, Ghali WA, Maitland A, Hirsch GM. The intraaortic balloon pump in cardiac surgery. *Ann Thorac Surg.* 2002;74:1276-1287.

Ben-Dor I, Waksman R, Hanna NN, et al. Utility of radiologic review for noncardiac findings on multislice computed tomography in patients with severe aortic stenosis evaluated for transcatheter aortic valve implantation. *Am J Cardiol.* 2010;105:1461-1464.

Burney K, Burchard F, Papouchado M, et al. Cardiac pacing systems and implantable cardiac defibrillators (ICDs): a radiological perspective of equipment, anatomy and complications. *Clin Radiol.* 2004;59:699-708.

Connors Jr AF, Speroff T, Dawson NV, et al. The effectiveness of right heart catheterization in the initial care of critically ill patients. *JAMA.* 1996;276:889-897.

Esmore D, Rosenfeldt FL. Mechanical circulatory support for the failing heart: past, present and future. *Heart Lung Circ.* 2005;14:163-166.

Farrar DJ, Bourque K, Dague CP, Cotter CJ, Poirier VL. Design features, developmental status, and experimental results with the HeartMate III centrifugal left ventricular assist system with a magnetically levitated rotor. *ASAIO J.* 2007;53:310-315.

Fowler RA, Cook DJ. The arc of the pulmonary artery catheter. *JAMA.* 2003;290:2732-2734.

Fuchs S, Stabile E, Kinnaird TD, et al. Stroke complicating percutaneous coronary interventions: incidence, predictors, and prognostic implications. *Circulation.* 2002;106:86-91.

Gregoric ID, Jacob LP, La Francesca S, et al. The TandemHeart as a bridge to a long-term axial flow left ventricular assist device (bridge to bridge). *Tex Heart Inst J.* 2008;35:125-129.

Hunter TB, Taljanovic MS, Tsau PH, et al. Medical devices of the chest. *Radiographics.* 2004;24:1725-1746.

Jauhar S. The artificial heart. *N Engl J Med.* 2004;350:542-544.

Jain VR, White CS, Pierson 3rd RN, Griffith BP, Sorensen EN. Imaging of left ventricular assist devices. *J Thorac Imaging.* 2005;20:32-40.

Klodell CT, McGiffin DC, Rayburn BK, et al. Initial United States experience with the Paracor HeartNet myocardial constraint device for heart failure. *J Thorac Cardiovasc Surg.* 2007;133:204-209.

Krahn AD, Klein GJ, Skanes AC, Yee R. Insertable loop recorder use for detection of intermittent arrhythmias. *Pacing Clin Electrophysiol.* 2004;27:657-664.

Kherani AR, Maybaum S, Oz MC. Ventricular assist devices as a bridge to transplant or recovery. *Cardiology.* 2004;101:93-103.

Leipsic J, Wood D, Manders D, et al. The evolving role of MDCT in transcatheter aortic valve replacement: a radiologists' perspective. *AJR Am J Roentgenol.* 2009;193:W214-W219.

Lembcke A, Wiese TH, Dushe S, et al. Effects of passive cardiac containment on left ventricular structure and function: verification by volume and flow measurements. *J Heart Lung Transplant.* 2004;23:11-19.

Mand'ak J, Lonsky V, Dominik J, Zacek P. Vascular complications of the intra-aortic balloon counterpulsation. *Angiology.* 2005;56:69-74.

Mandell VS, Nimkin K, Hoffer FA, Bridges ND. Devices for transcatheter closure of intracardiac defects. *AJR Am J Roentgenol.* 1993;160:179-184.

Mancini D, Burkhoff D. Mechanical device-based methods of managing and treating heart failure. *Circulation.* 2005;112:438-448.

Papaioannou TG, Stefanadis C. Basic principles of the intraaortic balloon pump and mechanisms affecting its performance. *ASAIO J.* 2005;51:296-300.

Rose EA, Gelijns AC, Moskowitz AJ, et al. Long-term mechanical left ventricular assistance for end-stage heart failure. *N Engl J Med.* 2001;345:1435-1443.

Sales V, McCarthy P. Understanding the C-Pulse device and its potential to treat heart failure. *Curr Heart Fail Rep.* 2010;7:27-34.

Sandham JD, Hull RD, Brant RF. A randomized, controlled trial of the use of pulmonary-artery catheters in high-risk surgical patients. *N Engl J Med.* 2003;348:5-14.

Schoenhagen P, Kapadia SR, Halliburton SS, et al. Computed tomography evaluation for transcatheter aortic valve implantation (TAVI): imaging of the aortic root and iliac arteries. *J Cardiovasc Comput Tomogr.* 2011;5:293-300.

Schulze MR, Ostermaier R, Franke Y, et al. Aortic endocarditis caused by inadvertent left ventricular pacemaker lead placement. *Circulation.* 2005;112:e361-e363.

Seki H, Fukui T, Shimokawa T, et al. Malpositioning of a pacemaker lead to the left ventricle accompanied by posterior mitral leaflet injury. *Interact Cardiovasc Thorac Surg.* 2009;8:235-237.

Sharifi M, Sorkin R, Sharifi V, et al. Inadvertent malposition of a transvenous-inserted pacing lead in the left ventricular chamber. *Am J Cardiol.* 1995;76:92-95.

Shellock FG, O'Neill M, Ivans V, et al. Cardiac pacemakers and implantable cardioverter defibrillators are unaffected by operation of an extremity MR imaging system. *AJR Am J Roentgenol.* 1999;172:165-170.

Sommer T, Vahlhaus C, Lauk G, et al. MR imaging and cardiac pacemakers: in vitro evaluation and in vivo studies in 51 patients at 0.5 T. *Radiology.* 2000;215:869-879.

Steiner RM, Tegtmeyer CJ, Morse D. The radiology of cardiac pacemakers. *Radiographics.* 1986;6:373-399.

Takasugi JE, Godwin JD, Bardy GH. The implantable pacemaker-cardioverter-defibrillator: radiographic aspects. *Radiographics.* 1994;14:1275-1290.

Trost JC, Hillis LD. Intra-aortic balloon counterpulsation. *Am J Cardiol.* 2006;97:1391-1398.

Trotman-Dickenson B. Radiology in the intensive care unit: part I. *J Intensive Care Med.* 2003;18:198-210.

Trotman-Dickenson B. Radiology in the intensive care unit: part 2. *J Intensive Care Med.* 2003;18:239-252.

Wong SC, Minutello R, Hong MK. Neurological complications following percutaneous coronary interventions (a report from the 2000-2001 NY State Angioplasty Registry). *Am J Cardiol.* 2005;96:1248-1250.

CHAPTER 19

Vascular Devices

Anil Kumar Pillai, Alexander Oscar Quiroz Casian, and Sanjeeva P. Kalva

■ STENT GRAFTS

Zenith Endograft

The Zenith endograft (Cook Medical, Inc., Bloomington, Ind) was released in 2003 (Fig. 19-1). This Food and Drug Administration (FDA)–approved woven polyester device, which consists of a stainless steel main body with a diameter of 22 to 36 mm and a length of 11.2 to 17.9 cm, allows suprarenal fixation. It is suitable for an abdominal aortic aneurysm (AAA) with a neck diameter of 18 to 28 mm, a length of 15 mm or more, and a neck angle of less than 60 degrees. The device is delivered through an integrated 20- to 26-Fr sheath. The Zenith endograft is unique in that it offers multiple combinations of lengths and diameters. Although it has a more complex delivery system, its newest design adds more flexibility with less kinking of limbs. This device is MRI conditional (Box 19-1).

Talent Endograft

The Talent endograft (Medtronic, Minneapolis, Minn) was FDA approved in 2008 (Fig. 19-2). This polyester graft sewn to a nickel titanium (nitinol) frame is characterized by a main body diameter of 22 to 36 mm and a main body length of 14 to 17 cm. The primary indication is for AAA with a neck length of at least 10 mm, a neck diameter of 18 to 32 mm, and a neck angle of less than 60 degrees. Its flexibility and suprarenal fixation make Talent a good choice for aortic aneurysms that are an anatomic challenge because of a short neck and large diameter. One of the main disadvantages of this endovascular device is its large delivery profile with an integrated sheath of 22 to 24 Fr. This device is MRI conditional (see Box 19-1). It can be identified on x-ray film by the uncovered suprarenal fixation spikes.

Endurant Endograft

The Endurant endograft (Medtronic) was FDA approved in 2010 (Fig. 19-3). This polyester graft sewn to a nitinol frame has a main body diameter of 23 to 36 mm and a length of 12.4 to 16.6 cm. This endograft is suitable for an AAA with a neck diameter of 19 to 32 mm, a neck length of at least 10 mm, and a neck angle of

less than 60 degrees. This graft has a suprarenal fixation and is delivered through an 18- to 20-Fr delivery sheath. It a good option for AAA with short necks and challenging anatomy. This device is MRI conditional (see Box 19-1). It can be identified on x-ray film by the uncovered suprarenal fixation spikes.

AneuRx Stent Graft

The AneuRx device (Medtronic) is an FDA-approved polyester-woven nitinol endograft with an infrarenal fixation and consists of a main body diameter of 20 to 28 cm and a main body length of 13.5 or 16.5 cm. It was approved for an AAA of 18 to 25 mm neck diameter and a neck length of 10 mm or more (Fig. 19-4). This device was released in 1999 for its use, but in 2003, a revision of the instruction for use changed the neck length to greater than 15 mm. This device has a delivery profile that consists of an integrated sheath of 21 Fr. One of the main disadvantages of the AneuRx is its high incidence of migration. This device is MRI conditional (see Box 19-1).

Excluder Endograft

The Excluder endograft (Gore Medical, Flagstaff, Ariz) was FDA approved and released in 2002 (Fig. 19-5). Its fabric material consists of expanded polytetrafluoroethylene (ePTFE). The main body has a diameter of 23 to 31 mm and a length of 12 to 18 cm. This device is suitable for an AAA with a neck length of at least 15 mm, a neck diameter of 19 to 26 mm, and a neck angle of less than 60 degrees. In contrast to other stent grafts, the Excluder is delivered through a separate sheath of 18 to 20 Fr and has a limited infrarenal fixation. The main advantage of this graft is its small profile, which makes it easy to deploy. This device is MRI conditional (see Box 19-1).

Anaconda Stent Graft

The Anaconda device (Vascutek, Renfrewshire, Scotland) is a trimodular stent graft and consists of a woven Dacron prosthesis supported by self-expanding nitinol ring stents (Fig. 19-6). The main body is available in diameters between 19.5 and 34 mm and lengths between 6 and 6.5 cm. This endograft has an active

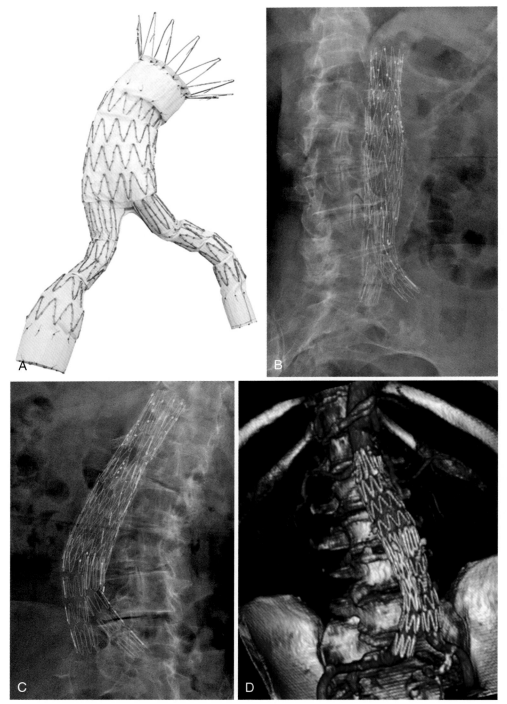

Figure 19-1 Zenith abdominal aortic aneurysm (AAA) endograft (Cook Medical, Inc.).**A,** Zenith device. **B** and **C,** Oblique radiographs of the abdomen showing the Zenith AAA device. **D,** Three-dimensional computed tomography of the Zenith AAA device in the aortoiliac arteries. (**A,** Courtesy of Medical, Inc., Bloomington, Ind.)

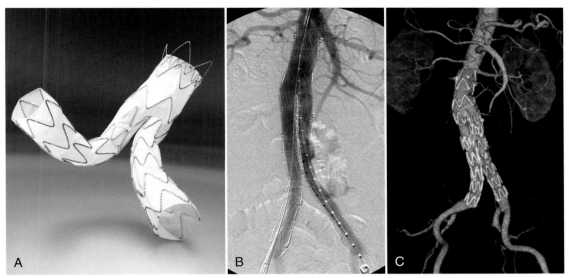

Figure 19-2 Talent abdominal aortic aneurysm (AAA) endograft (Medtronic). **A,** Talent device. **B,** Digital subtraction angiography of the aortoiliac arteries following Talent AAA endograft placement for an AAA. **C,** Three-dimensional computed tomography of the Talent AAA device in the aortoiliac arteries. (**A,** Courtesy of Medtronic, Minneapolis, Minn.)

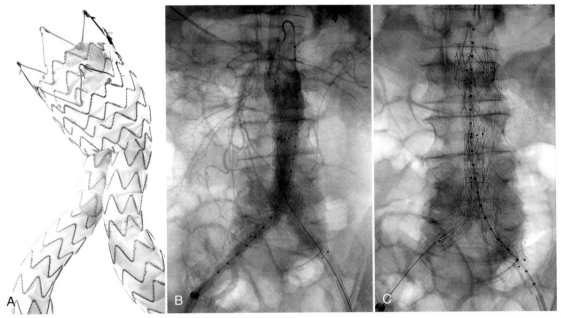

Figure 19-3 Endurant abdominal aortic aneurysm (AAA) endograft (Medtronic). **A,** Endurant device. **B,** Catheter angiography of aortoiliac arteries following Endurant AAA endograft placement. Note the most proximal bare metallic segment of the body of the graft placed across the renal artery ostia. **C,** Plain radiograph of the abdomen showing the Endurant AAA device. (**A,** Courtesy of Medtronic, Minneapolis, Minn.)

fixation system consisting of four pairs of hooks. The endograft is delivered through a 20.4 to 22.5 Fr sheath. This device is MRI conditional (see Box 19-1).

Endologix Endograft

The Endologix device (Endologix, Irvine, Calif) is an FDA-approved endograft that was released in 2004 (Fig. 19-7). This ePTFE device has a main body diameter of 22 to 28 mm and a length of 10 to 15.5 cm. It is approved for treatment of an AAA with an aortic neck diameter of 18 to 26 mm and a length of at least 15 mm, with an angle of less than 60 degrees. This graft is delivered through an integrated sheath of 21 Fr and has a fixation that sits on the aortic bifurcation with infrarenal or suprarenal extensions. Its unibody design with a unique support at the aortic bifurcation and a one side percutaneous make this device an attractive choice. The main disadvantages are the lack of sizing versatility and the minimal radial force that increases the risk of migration. This device is MRI conditional (see Box 19-1).

Vanguard Stent Graft

The Vanguard device (Boston Scientific, Natick, Mass) is a second-generation modular stent graft consisting of a nitinol metal framework covered with polyester graft material (Fig. 19-8). This graft was first implemented in 1994. Vanguard comes with a main body diameter of 22 to 30 mm and iliac components of 10 to 12 mm. It is delivered through an 18-Fr sheath. The contralateral limb is delivered through a 10-Fr sheath by a percutaneous approach. The indication for this device is an infrarenal AAA with a neck of 20 to 25 diameter, a length of at least 15 mm, and neck angulation less than 60 degrees. This device is MRI safe (see Box 19-1).

Ancure Endograft

The Ancure device is a unibody nonsupported woven polyester endograft (Guidant Corp., St. Paul, Minn) with a main body diameter of 26 mm (Fig. 19-9). This endograft is suitable for an aneurysm with an aortic neck diameter of 18 to 26 mm and a neck length greater than 15 mm. It is delivered through a 24-Fr introducer sheath. Although it was approved in 1999 by the FDA for the repair of AAA, Guidant suspended production of this device and announced a recall of all existing inventory in 2001. This

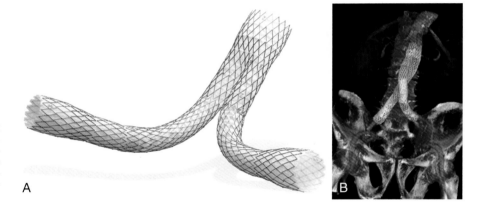

Figure 19-4 AneuRx abdominal aortic aneurysm (AAA) endograft (Medtronic). **A,** AneuRx AAA endograft device. **B,** Three-dimensional computed tomography of the AneuRx AAA device in the aortoiliac arteries. (**A,** Courtesy of Medtronic, Minneapolis, Minn.)

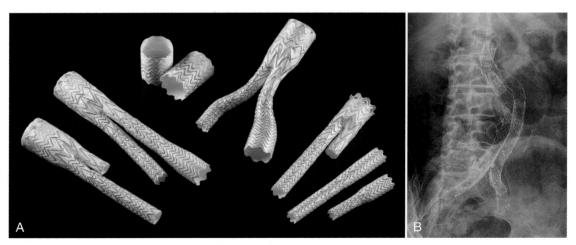

Figure 19-5 Excluder abdominal aortic aneurysm (AAA) endograft (Gore Medical). **A,** Gore Excluder AAA device. **B,** Oblique radiograph of the abdomen showing the Gore Excluder device. (**A,** Courtesy of Gore Medical, Flagstaff, Ariz.)

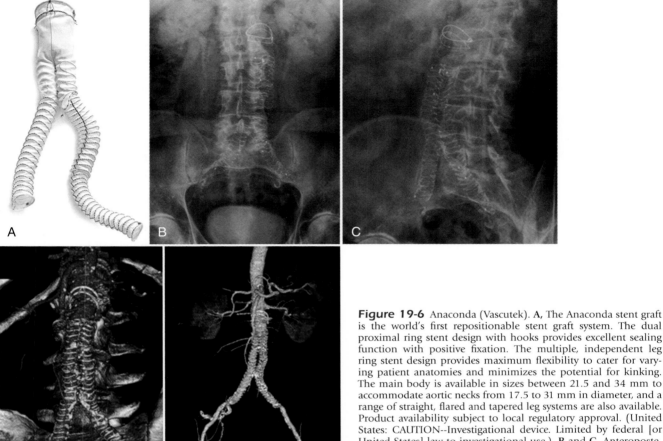

Figure 19-6 Anaconda (Vascutek). **A,** The Anaconda stent graft is the world's first repositionable stent graft system. The dual proximal ring stent design with hooks provides excellent sealing function with positive fixation. The multiple, independent leg ring stent design provides maximum flexibility to cater for varying patient anatomies and minimizes the potential for kinking. The main body is available in sizes between 21.5 and 34 mm to accommodate aortic necks from 17.5 to 31 mm in diameter, and a range of straight, flared and tapered leg systems are also available. Product availability subject to local regulatory approval. (United States: CAUTION--Investigational device. Limited by federal [or United States] law to investigational use.). **B** and **C,** Anteroposterior and oblique radiographs showing the Anaconda device. **D** and **E,** Three-dimensional computed tomography showing the Anaconda device in the aortoiliac arteries. (**A,** Courtesy of Vascutek, Renfrewshire, Scotland.)

device is MRI safe (see Box 19-1). It is easily identified by the absence of metalwork within the main body.

Talent Thoracic Endograft

The Talent thoracic endograft (Medtronic) is made of thin woven polyester fabric sewn to a self-expanding nitinol wire frame (Fig. 19-10). This device comes in four different configurations: proximal main, proximal extension, distal main, and distal extension. It has numerous device diameters, ranging from 22 to 46 mm, and lengths of 11.2 to 11.6 cm. The device profile requires 20- to 24-Fr introducer sheaths. A minimum aortic neck diameter of 20 mm is required at the sealing zone. This device is MRI conditional (see Box 19-1).

Conformable GORE TAG Thoracic Endoprosthesis

The Conformable GORE TAG thoracic endoprosthesis (Gore Medica; Fig. 19-11) is made of an expanded ePTFE tube that is reinforced with an ePTFE and fluorinated ethylene propylene (FEP) film and an external nitinol

self-expanded stent affixed to the graft. This device is available in a diameter of 26 to 40 mm and a length of 10 to 20 cm. The device profile requires 20- to 24-Fr introducer sheaths. A minimum aortic diameter of 20 mm is required at the sealing zones on either end. This device deploys from the middle of the graft toward each end, a design characteristic intended to prevent windsocking at the proximal fixation zone. This device is MRI conditional (see Box 19-1).

Zenith Thoracic Stent Graft

The Zenith thoracic endograft (Cook Medical, Inc.) has a stainless steel body frame and a polyester covering (Fig. 19-12). It has proximal and distal components and extension elements of varying sizes. It is MRI conditional (see Box 19-1).

Fluency Stent Graft

The Fluency device is a nitinol stent (Bard, Inc., Tempe, Ariz) covered with ePTFE. It is FDA approved for tracheobronchial use (Fig. 19-13). This device has

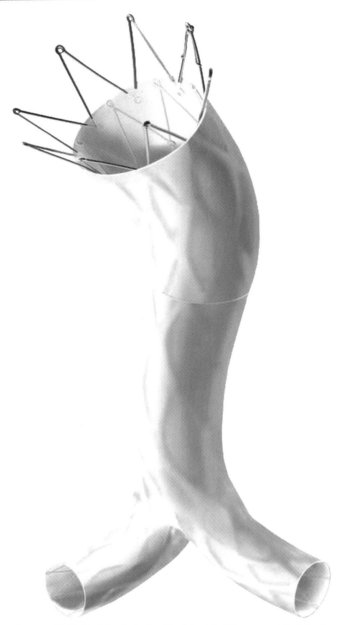

Figure 19-7 Endologix device (Endologix). (Courtesy of Endologix, Irvine, Calif.)

diameters of 6 to 10 mm and lengths of 40 to 80 cm. This stent graft requires an introducer sheath of 8 to 9 Fr and can be implanted over a 0.035-inch guidewire. The delivery system is 80 or 117 cm long. The stent can be identified on x-ray film by its characteristic four tantalum markers at each ends. The ends of the stent have a 2-mm uncovered portion. This device is MRI safe (see Box 19-1).

Flair Stent Graft

Similar to the Fluency device, the Flair (Bard, Inc.) stent graft is a nitinol stent covered with ePTFE (Fig. 19-14). It is FDA approved for treating venous anastomotic narrowing in synthetic arteriovenous grafts. The stent is

characterized by a diameter of 6 to 9 mm and a length of 30 to 50 mm. It comes in two configurations: one has straight ends, whereas the other has flared ends. The device is delivered through a 9-Fr introducer sheath and over a 0.035-inch guidewire. The delivery system is 80 cm long. This stent has no radiopaque markers at the ends. This device is MRI conditional (see Box 19-1).

Viabahn Endovascular Device

The Viabahn (Gore Medical) is an FDA-approved endovascular device made of nitinol and ePTFE (Fig. 19-15). The main indication for its use is for superficial femoral artery disease. This endovascular device is characterized by a diameter of 5 to 13 mm and a length of 25 to 150 mm. The device can be delivered over a 0.035- to 0.018-inch guidewire and requires an introducer of 6 to 12 Fr. The length of the delivery system is 75 to 120 cm. The newer devices are heparin coated to prevent thrombus formation. This stent has no radiopaque markers. This device is MRI conditional (see Box 19-1).

Viatorr Stent Graft

Viatorr (Gore Medical) is an FDA-approved stent graft indicated for transjugular intrahepatic portosystemic shunt (TIPS) (Fig. 19-16). This device is made of nitinol and ePTFE. The stent graft is available at a diameter of 8 to 12 mm and a length of 40 to 80 mm. The device can be delivered over a 0.038-inch guidewire and requires an introducer of 10 Fr. The delivery system is of 75 cm long. The stent graft has a 2-cm uncovered segment, which is positioned in the portal vein. The covered segment of the graft is positioned across the parenchymal tract and into the hepatic vein. A radiopaque ring separates the covered and uncovered segments of the stent. This device is MRI safe (see Box 19-1).

Viabil Stent Graft

The Viabil (Gore Medical) is an FDA-approved stent graft indicated for malignant biliary strictures (Fig. 19-17). This device is contraindicated for all cardiovascular applications. This device is made of nitinol and ePTFE. The Viabil is available at a diameter of 8 to 10 mm and a length of 40 to 100 mm. The device is delivered through a 10-Fr sheath and over a 0.035-inch guidewire. The delivery system is 40 cm long. A radiopaque ring at either end of the stent helps in identifying this device. The stent also has anchoring fins that prevent it from migrating. This device is MRI conditional (see Box 19-1).

WallFlex Stent

The WallFlex stent (Boston Scientific) is FDA approved for the biliary tract and is composed of Platinol (platinum core and nitinol encasing) wire mesh (Fig. 19-18). The device is available as a fully covered, partially covered, or uncovered stent. The covering material is made of Permalume. The ends of the stent have a retrieval loop for endoscopic removal. This device has a diameter

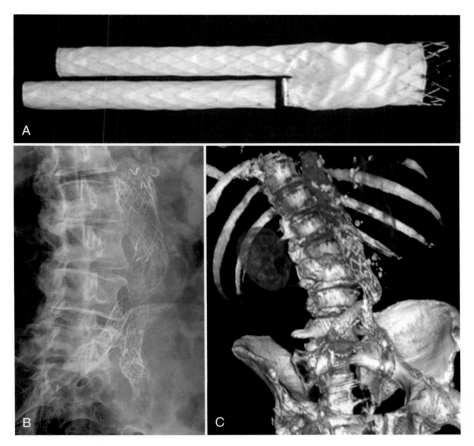

Figure 19-8 Vanguard abdominal aortic aneurysm endograft (Boston Scientific, Natick, Mass.). **A,** Vanguard device. **B,** Oblique radiograph of the abdomen showing the Vanguard device in the aortoiliac arteries. **C,** Three-dimensional computed tomography of the Vanguard device in the aortoiliac arteries. (**A,** From Diethrich EB. AAA stent grafts: current developments. *J Invasive Cardiol.* 2001;13. <http://www.medscape.com/viewarticle/407496_4>; Accessed 10.07.12.)

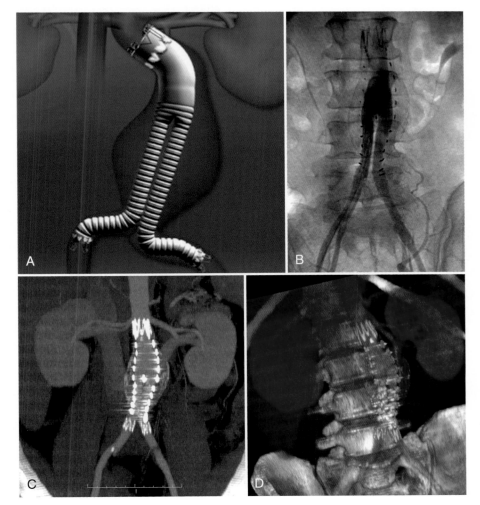

Figure 19-9 Ancure abdominal aortic aneurysm endograft (Guidant Corp.). **A,** Ancure device. **B,** Catheter angiography after deploying the Ancure device in the aortoiliac arteries. Three-dimensional maximum intensity projection (**C**) and three-dimensional volume-rendered (**D**) images show the Ancure device in the aortoiliac arteries. (**A,** Courtesy of Guidant Corp., St. Paul, Minn.)

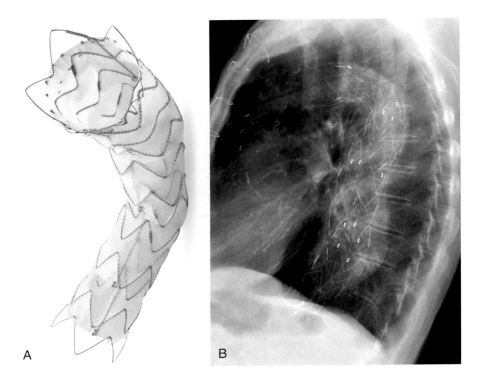

Figure 19-10 Talent thoracic endograft (Medtronic). **A,** Talent thoracic endograft device. **B,** Lateral thoracic radiograph demonstrating Talent thoracic endograft. (**A,** Courtesy of Medtronic, Minneapolis, Minn.)

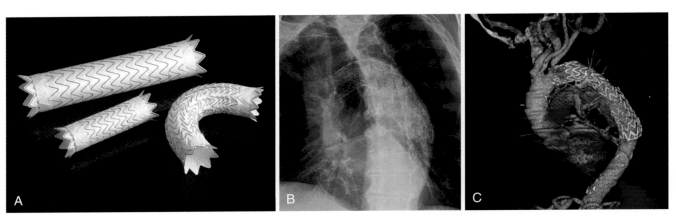

Figure 19-11 Comfortable GORE TAG thoracic endoprosthesis (Gore Medical). **A,** Gore TAG device. **B,** Oblique chest radiograph showing the Comfortable GORE TAG endoprosthesis. **C,** Three-dimensional computed tomography showing the Gore TAG device in the thoracic aorta. (**A,** Courtesy of Gore Medical, Flagstaff, Ariz.)

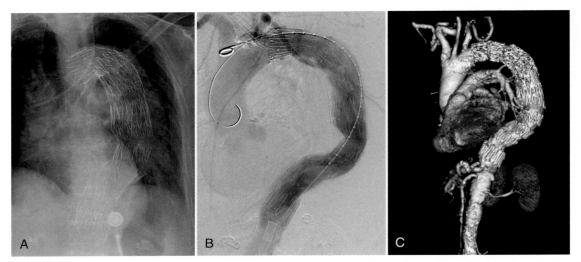

Figure 19-12 Zenith thoracic stent graft (Cook Medical, Inc., Bloomington, Ind.). **A,** Oblique plain radiograph of the chest showing the Zenith thoracic stent graft. **B,** Digital subtraction angiography of the aorta after placing a Zenith thoracic stent graft. **C,** Three-dimensional computed tomography of the thoracic aorta showing a Zenith thoracic stent graft.

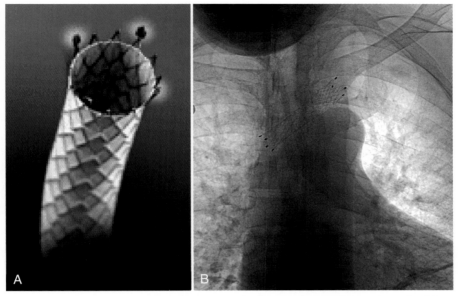

Figure 19-13 Fluency stent graft (Bard, Inc.). **A,** Fluency device: Note the four titanium markers at the ends of the graft. **B,** Anteroposterior chest radiography demonstrating a Fluency stent graft in the left innominate vein. (**A,** Courtesy of Bard, Inc., Tempe, Ariz.)

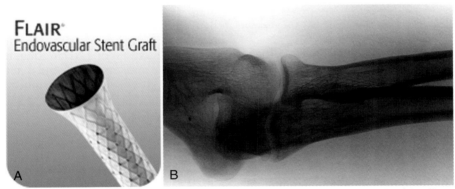

Figure 19-14 Flair stent graft (Bard, Inc.). **A,** Flair stent graft device with flared ends. **B,** Plain radiograph of the elbow showing the Flair graft in a dialysis graft venous outflow. (**A,** Courtesy of Bard, Inc., Tempe, Ariz.)

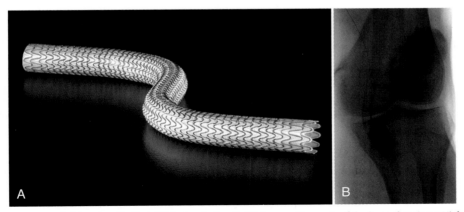

Figure 19-15 Viabahn stent graft (Gore Medical). **A,** Viabahn device. **B,** Oblique radiograph of the knee showing a Viabahn graft in the popliteal artery. (**A,** Courtesy of Gore Medical, Flagstaff, Ariz.)

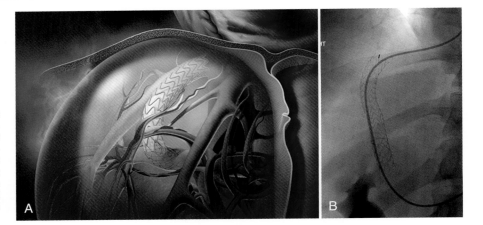

Figure 19-16 Viatorr stent graft (Gore Medical). **A,** Viatorr device. **B,** Plain radiograph of the abdomen showing the Viatorr graft in a patient who underwent a transjugular intrahepatic portosystemic shunt procedure. Note the radiopaque ring that separates the uncovered segment (2 cm long and positioned in the portal vein) and the covered segment. (**A,** Courtesy of Gore Medical, Flagstaff, Ariz.)

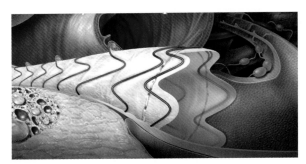

Figure 19-17 Viabil stent graft device (Gore Medical). (Courtesy of Gore Medical, Flagstaff, Ariz.)

of 8 to 10 mm and a stent length of 40 to 100 mm. The device is delivered through an 8- to 8.5-Fr introducer and over a 0.035-inch guidewire. This device is MRI conditional (see Box 19-1).

iCAST Stent Graft

The iCAST (Atrium Medical, Hudson, NH) is an FDA-approved balloon-expandable stent graft indicated for tracheobronchial use (Fig. 19-19). This 316L stainless steel device covered with thin film of PTFE has a diameter of 5 to 12 mm and a length of 16 to 59 mm. The device is delivered over a 0.035-inch guidewire and through an introducer of 6 to 7 Fr. The delivery system is 80 or 120 cm long. This device has no radiopaque markers. This device is MRI conditional (see Box 19-1).

HeRO Graft (Hemodialysis Reliable Outflow)

The HeRO graft (Hemosphere, Inc., Eden Prairie, Minn) consists of a venous outflow component and a proprietary ePTFE arterial graft component (Fig. 19-20). This device has a 5-mm inner diameter and a 19-Fr outer diameter and is 40 cm long. It consists of a radiopaque silicone catheter with braided nitinol reinforcement and a radiopaque marker band at the distal tip. This graft can be identified by the radiopaque marker and the titanium connector, which can be easily identified on x-ray film. This graft is intended for use in maintaining long-term vascular access in patients undergoing long-term

hemodialysis who have exhausted peripheral venous access. This device is MRI conditional (see Box 19-1).

■ STENTS

Protegé Stent

The Protegé stent is a self-expanding nitinol stent (ev3 Endovascular, Inc., Plymouth, Minn) approved for biliary use (Fig. 19-21). It is available in various sizes: diameter of 5 to 8 mm and length of 20 to 150 mm. It is delivered through a 6-Fr or larger introducer sheath and over a 0.035-inch guidewire. This device comes with a delivery system 80 or 120 cm long. It has four tantalum radiopaque markers at each end that can be identified on x-ray film. This device is MRI conditional (see Box 19-1).

Zilver Stent

The Zilver device (Cook Medical, Inc.) is a self-expanding nitinol endovascular stent (Fig. 19-22). This stent is available at a diameter of 6 to 10 mm and a stent length of 20 to 80 mm. The FDA indication is for iliac arteries. The stent is delivered over a 0.018-inch guidewire and requires an introducer of 5 Fr or larger. This device comes with a delivery system 125 cm long. The device has four radiopaque markers at each end that can be seen on x-ray film. This device is MRI conditional (see Box 19-1).

Absolute Stent

The Absolute stent is a self-expanding nitinol stent (Abbott Vascular, Abbott Park, Ill) approved for biliary use (Fig. 19-23). It is available in various sizes: diameter of 5 to 9 mm and stent length of 20 to 80 m. The stent is delivered over a 0.035-inch guidewire and requires an introducer of 6 Fr or larger. This device comes with a delivery system 80 cm long. The device has 6 radiopaque markers at each end which can be seen on x-ray film. This device is MRI safe (see Box 19-1).

LifeStent

The LifeStent is a self-expanding nitinol stent (Bard, Inc.) approved for use in the superficial femoral artery

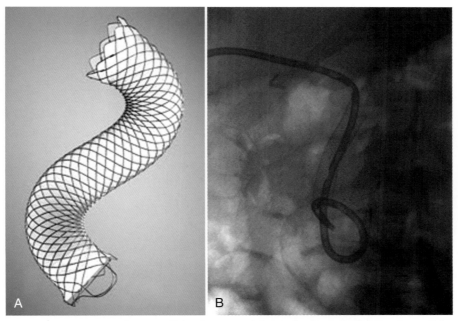

Figure 19-18 WallFlex device (Boston Scientific). **A,** WallFlex device. **B,** Abdominal radiograph showing the WallFlex device in the common bile duct. Also note the Simon nitinol filter in the inferior vena cava. (**A,** Courtesy of Boston Scientific, Natick, Mass.)

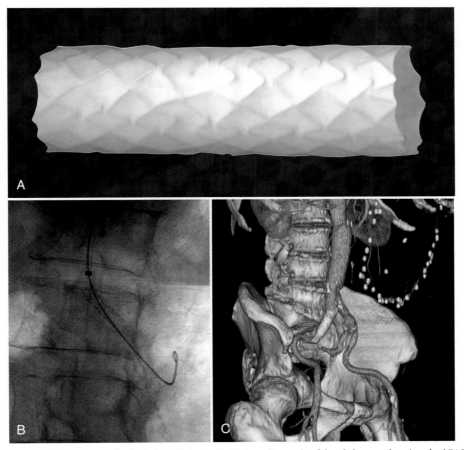

Figure 19-19 iCAST stent graft (Atrium Medical). **A,** iCAST device. **B,** Plain radiograph of the abdomen showing the iCAST stent graft in the left renal artery. **C,** Three-dimensional computed tomography showing the iCAST stent graft in the right common iliac artery. (**A,** Courtesy of Atrium Medical, Hudson, NH.)

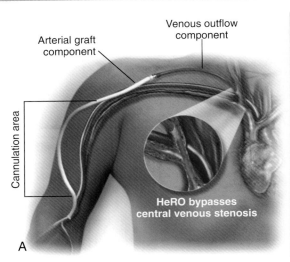

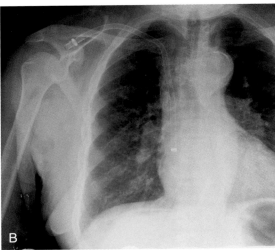

Figure 19-20 HeRO graft (Hemosphere, Inc.). **A,** HeRO device. **B,** Chest radiograph showing the HeRO device. Also note a Fluency graft in the right arm in an earlier dialysis access venous outflow. (A, Courtesy of Hemosphere, Inc., Eden Prairie, Minn.)

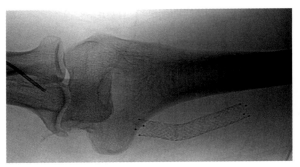

Figure 19-21 Plain radiograph of the arm with a Protegé stent (ev3 Endovascular, Inc., Plymouth, Minn) in a dialysis access venous outflow.

and proximal popliteal artery (Fig. 19-24). It is available in various sizes: diameter of 6 to 7 mm and stent length of 20 to 80 mm. The stent is delivered over a 0.035-inch guidewire and requires an introducer of 6 Fr or larger. This device comes with a delivery system 80 or 130 cm long. The device has 6 radiopaque markers at each end that can be seen on x-ray film. This device is MRI conditional (see Box 19-1).

S.M.A.R.T. Stent

The S.M.A.R.T. stent is a self-expanding nitinol stent (Cordis Corp., Warren, NJ) that is FDA approved for use in the iliac arteries (Fig. 19-25). It is available in various sizes: diameter of 6 to 8 mm and stent length of 20 to 100 mm. The stent is delivered over a 0.035-inch guidewire and requires an introducer of 6 Fr or larger. This device comes with a delivery system 80 or 120 cm long. The stent has 12 tantalum micromarkers at its end to increase radiopacity. This device is MRI conditional (see Box 19-1).

Wallstent

The Wallstent is a self-expanding stainless steel stent (Boston Scientific) approved for use in the biliary tract

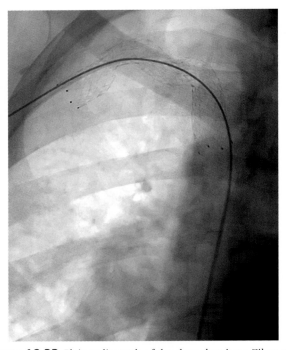

Figure 19-22 Plain radiograph of the chest showing a Zilver stent (Cook Medical, Inc., Bloomington, Ind) in the subclavian vein in a patient with dialysis access in the right arm.

(Fig. 19-26). It is available in various sizes: diameter of 6 to 10 mm and stent length of 27 to 100 mm. The stent is delivered over a 0.035-inch guidewire and requires an introducer of 6 Fr or larger. This device comes with a delivery system 75, 100, or 160 cm long. This device does not have radiopaque markers. This device is MRI conditional (see Box 19-1).

Carotid Wallstent

The carotid Wallstent endoprosthesis (Boston Scientific; Fig. 19-27) is indicated for the treatment of patients at high risk for adverse events from endarterectomy

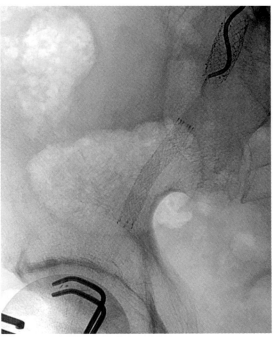

Figure 19-23 Plain radiograph of the pelvis showing an Absolute stent (Abbott Vascular, Abbott Park, Ill) in the right external iliac artery. Note the radiopaque markers at the ends of the stent.

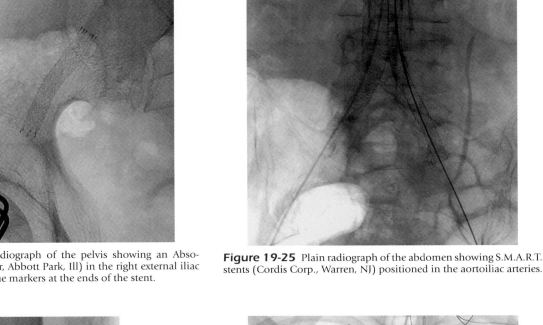

Figure 19-25 Plain radiograph of the abdomen showing S.M.A.R.T. stents (Cordis Corp., Warren, NJ) positioned in the aortoiliac arteries.

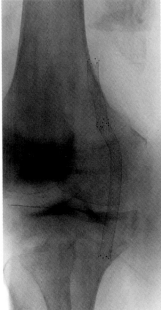

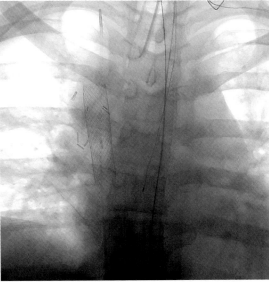

Figure 19-26 Chest radiograph showing a Wallstent (Boston Scientific, Natick, Mass) in the superior vena cava.

Figure 19-24 Plain radiograph of the knee showing a LifeStent (Bard, Inc., Tempe, Ariz) in the popliteal artery. Note the radiopaque markers at the ends of the stent.

resulting from anatomic or comorbid conditions who require carotid revascularization and who meet specific criteria. This device is available in various sizes: diameter of 6 to 10 mm and stent length of 21 to 37 mm. The stent is delivered over a 0.014-inch guidewire and requires an introducer of 5 Fr or larger. This device comes with a 135-cm delivery system. This device does

not have radiopaque markers. This device is MRI safe (see Box 19-1).

Express Stent

The Express balloon-expandable stent (Boston Scientific) is an FDA-approved device indicated for biliary use (Fig. 19-28). It is made of 316L stainless steel. The stent is available in different diameters of 6 to 10 mm and lengths of 17 to 57 mm. It comes with an introducer

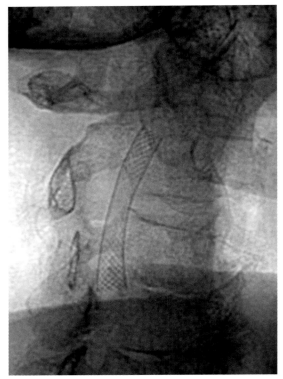

Figure 19-27 Lateral neck radiograph showing a carotid Wallstent (Boston Scientific). (Courtesy of Boston Scientific, Natick, Mass.)

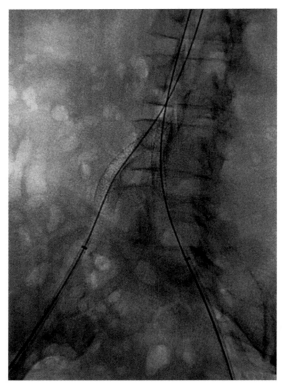

Figure 19-28 Abdominal radiograph showing bilateral kissing iliac Express stents (Boston Scientific, Natick, Mass).

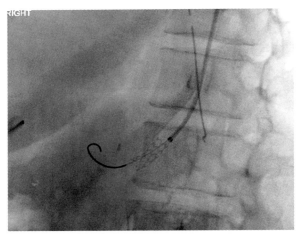

Figure 19-29 Oblique abdominal radiograph showing a Palmaz stent (Cordis Corp., Warren, NJ) in the celiac artery.

of 6 to 7 Fr, depending on length of the stent. The delivery system has a length of 75 to 135 cm. This device does not have radiopaque markers. This device is MRI conditional (see Box 19-1).

Palmaz Stent

The Palmaz balloon-expandable stainless steel stent (Cordis Corp.) is approved for iliac artery and renal artery disease (Fig. 19-29). It is made of 316L stainless steel. The stent is available in different diameters of 4 to 8 mm and lengths of 10 to 29 mm. It comes unmounted and is deployed through an introducer of 10 Fr or larger. This device does not have radiopaque markers. This device is MRI conditional (see Box 19-1).

■ INFERIOR VENA CAVA FILTERS

Greenfield Filter

The original Greenfield filter (Boston Scientific) is a stainless steel conical device (apex pointed toward the heart) with six legs. It is delivered through a 28-Fr introducer through a femoral or jugular venous access. This device is MRI conditional (see Box 19-1). The titanium Greenfield filter (Fig. 19-30, *A*) and the over-the-wire stainless steel Greenfield filter (see Fig. 19-30, *B*) are delivered through a 12-Fr introducer. These are permanent devices and are recommended for use in an infrarenal inferior vena cava 28 mm or less in diameter. The titanium Greenfield filter is MRI safe (see Box 19-1).

Bird's Nest Filter

As the name Bird's Nest suggests, this permanent filter (Cook Medical, Inc.) has a unique design with two V-shaped stainless steel barbs that point in opposite directions and a mesh of stainless steel wire (Fig. 19-31). The device is delivered through a 12-Fr introducer through the jugular or femoral vein. The filter is approved for use in an infrarenal vena cava 40 mm or less in diameter. This device is MRI conditional (see Box 19-1).

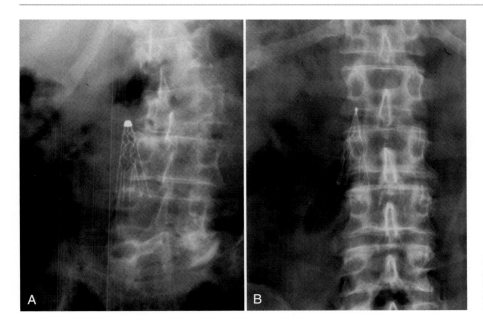

Figure 19-30 Plain radiographs of the abdomen showing titanium (**A**) and stainless steel (**B**) Greenfield filters (Boston Scientific, Natick, Mass). (**B,** Courtesy of Boston Scientific, Natick, Mass.)

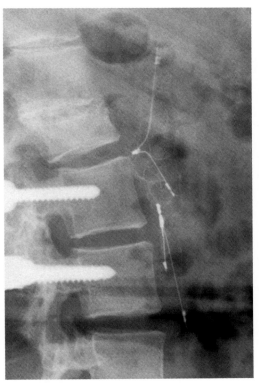

Figure 19-31 Lateral radiograph of the abdomen showing a Bird's Nest filter (Cook Medical, Inc., Bloomington, Ind).

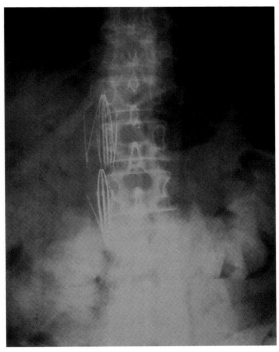

Figure 19-32 Vena Tech filter (B. Braun Medical, Inc., Bethlehem, Pa). The caudally located filter failed to open during deployment, and another Vena Tech filter was deployed superiorly.

Vena Tech Filter

The Vena Tech filter (B. Braun Medical, Inc., Bethlehem, Pa) is a permanent filter made of Phynox wire. It has a W-shaped configuration in which the peripheral struts provide anchoring and prevent tilting of the device (Fig. 19-32). The filtration system is conical and single level. This device is approved for use in an infrarenal vena cava 28 mm or less in diameter. This device is MRI conditional (see Box 19-1).

Simon Nitinol Filter

The Simon nitinol filter (Bard, Inc.) is a permanent filter made of nitinol and delivered through a 7-Fr introducer through the jugular, femoral, or other veins (Fig. 19-33). It provides two levels of filtration through flower-like superior and conical inferior filtration levels. This device is approved for use in an infrarenal vena cava 28 mm or less in diameter. This device is MRI conditional (see Box 19-1).

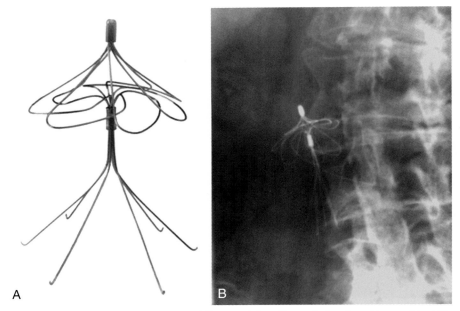

Figure 19-33 Simon nitinol filter (Bard, Inc.). **A,** Simon nitinol filter. **B,** Plain radiograph showing a Simon nitinol filter. (**A,** Courtesy of Bard, Inc., Tempe, Ariz.)

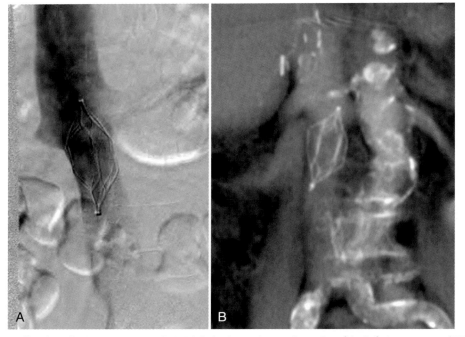

Figure 19-34 TrapEase filter (Cordis Corp., Warren, NJ). **A,** Digital substraction angiography of the inferior vena cava (IVC) following TrapEase filter placement. **B,** Muliformatted computed tomography of the abdomen showing the TrapEase filter in the infrarenal IVC.

TrapEase and OptEase Filters

TrapEase is a permanent filter (Cordis Corp.) made of nitinol that has a self-centering basket design (Fig. 19-34). It can be delivered through a 6-Fr introducer. It is recommended for a vena cava 30 mm or less in diameter. This device is MRI conditional (see Box 19-1).

The design of OptEase filter is similar to that of TrapEase but with an added hook in the caudal portion for retrieval through the femoral vein. The device is approved for permanent use and for retrieval. This device is MRI conditional (see Box 19-1).

Gunther Tulip Filter

The Gunther Tulip filter is a conical filter (Cook Medical, Inc.) made of Egiloy (nickel, chromium, and cobalt) (Fig. 19-35). It has four legs and petal-like barbed wire around the legs. It has an apical hook for retrieval through the jugular veins. It is delivered through a 7-Fr

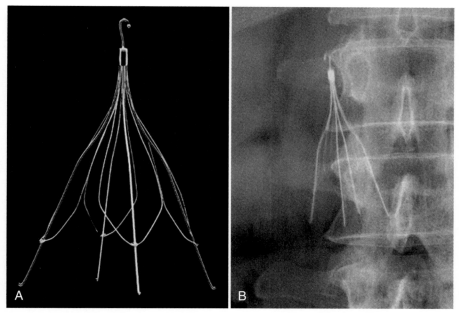

Figure 19-35 Gunther Tulip filter (Cook Medical, Inc.). **A,** Gunther Tulip filter device. **B,** Plain radiograph of the abdomen showing a Gunther Tulip filter. Note the apical hook for retrieval. (**A,** Courtesy of Cook Medical, Inc., Bloomington, Ind.)

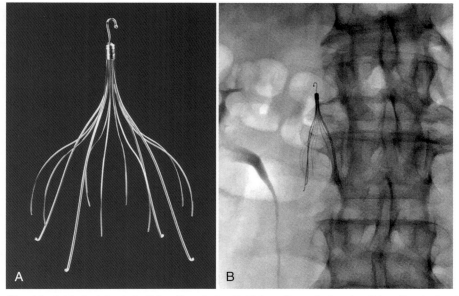

Figure 19-36 Celect filter (Cook Medical, Inc.). **A,** Celect filter device. **B,** Plain radiograph showing Celect filter in the abdomen. Note the apical hook for retrieval. (**A,** Courtesy of Cook Medical, Inc., Bloomington, Ind.)

femoral or an 8.5-Fr jugular introducer. This filter is approved for permanent use and for retrieval. It is recommended for an infrarenal vena cava 30 mm or less in diameter. This device is MRI conditional (see Box 19-1).

Celect Filter

The Celect filter (Cook Medical, Inc.) is a modification of the Gunther Tulip filter. It has four legs and eight arms that intersperse the legs (Fig. 19-36). It has an apical hook for jugular retrieval. It is delivered through a 7-Fr femoral or an 8.5-Fr jugular introducer. This filter is approved for permanent use and for retrieval. It is

recommended for an infrarenal vena cava 30 mm or less in diameter. This device is MRI conditional (see Box 19-1).

G2, G2 Express, and Eclipse Filters

The Recovery G2 (or simply G2), G2 X (Fig. 19-37), and Eclipse filters (Bard, Inc.) are modifications of the original Recovery filter. These optional filters are made of nitinol. These are delivered through a 7-Fr introducer by a femoral vein approach and a 10-Fr introducer by a jugular vein approach. These filters are recommended for an infrarenal vena cava 28 mm or less in diameter. The G2 X filter has a hook at the apex and is therefore retrievable

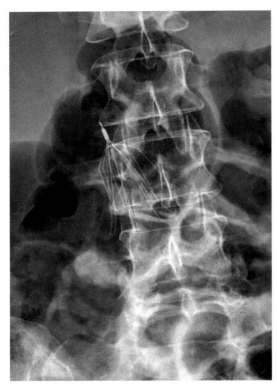

Figure 19-37 Recovery G2 X filter (Bard, Inc., Tempe, Ariz). Plain radiograph showing a Recovery G2 X filter. It has an apical hook for retrieval.

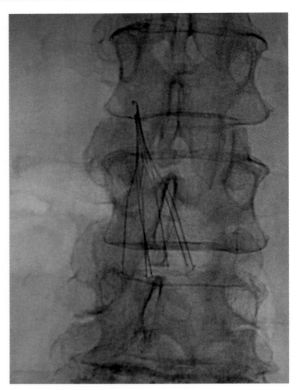

Figure 19-38 Option filter (Rex Medical, Conshohocken, Pa). Plain radiograph showing the Option filter in the abdomen. Note the apical hook of the filter for retrieval.

by the snare technique or with the cone retrieval kit that is supplied for G2 filter. The Eclipse filter is similar to the G2 X filter but has special coating on the nitinol frame. These devices are MRI conditional (see Box 19-1).

Option Filter

The Option filter (Rex Medical, Conshohocken, Pa) is an optional filter made of nitinol. It can be delivered through a 5-Fr introducer by the femoral or jugular approach (Fig. 19-38). It is recommended for an infrarenal vena cava 30 mm or less in diameter. This device is MRI conditional (see Box 19-1).

ALN Filter

The ALN filter (ALN International, Ghisonaccia, Corsica, France) is an optional filter made of stainless steel (Fig. 19-39). It can be delivered through a 7-Fr introducer through the femoral, jugular, or brachial veins. It is recommended for an infrarenal vena cava of 28 mm or less in diameter. This device is MRI conditional (see Box 19-1).

■ EMBOLIZATION DEVICES

Amplatzer Vascular Plug

The Amplatzer vascular plug (St. Jude Medical, St. Paul, Minn) is a self-expanding cylindrical device made of nitinol wires (Fig. 19-40). This device is available with

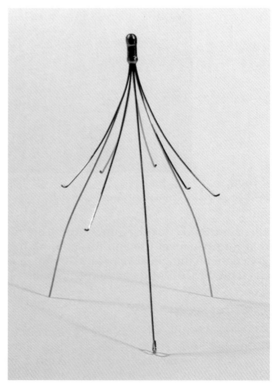

Figure 19-39 ALN filter device (ALN International). (Courtesy of ALN International, Ghisonaccia, Corsica, France.)

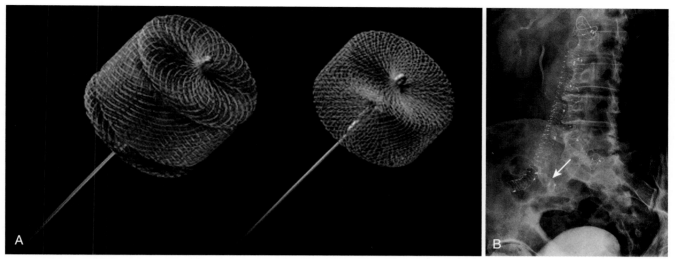

Figure 19-40 Amplatzer vascular plug (St. Jude Medical). **A,** Amplatzer vascular plug. **B,** Oblique radiograph of the abdomen showing the Amplatzer plug *(arrow)* in the right internal iliac vein. Note the Anaconda abdominal aortic aneurysm endograft. (**A,** Courtesy of St. Jude Medical, St. Paul, Minn.)

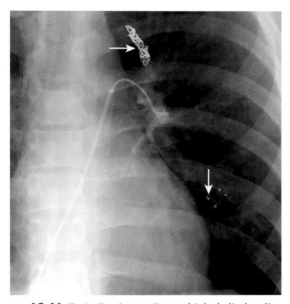

Figure 19-41 Embolization coils. Multiple helical radiopaque embolization coils *(horizontal arrow)* are used to treat a pulmonary arteriovenous malformation in this patient. Note the atrial septal occluders *(vertical arrow)* in the left lower lobe. These were used to embolize a large pulmonary arteriovenous malformation.

different diameters of 4 to 16 mm and length of 7 to 8 mm. The size of the introducer required to deliver the device varies with the diameter of the plug. The maximal length of the delivery system is 100 cm. This device is MRI conditional (see Box 19-1).

Embolization Coils

Embolization coils are mainly divided into pushable and detachable (Fig. 19-41). They are constructed of different types of materials: platinum, tungsten, gold, tantalum, and stainless steel. They are all radiopaque. They are available in various shapes: helical, spiral, and more complex. They are also available as standard coils (0.035 or 0.038 inch) or microcoils (0.014 or 0.018 inch).

Bibliography

Binkert C. Inferior vena cava filters. In: Mauro M, Murphy K, Thomson K, et al, eds. *Image-Guided Interventions.* 2nd ed. Philadelphia: Saunders; 2012.

Matsumura JS. Aortic stents and grafts. In: Cronenwett JL, Johnston W, eds. *Rutherford's Vascular Surgery.* 7th ed. Philadelphia: Saunders; 2010.

Pearce B, Jordan Jr WD. Nonaortic stents and stent-grafts. In: Cronenwett JL, Johnston W, eds. *Rutherford's Vascular Surgery.* 7th ed. Philadelphia: Saunders; 2010.

SPECIAL SITUATIONS

CHAPTER **20**

Imaging for Congenital Cardiovascular Disease

Kristopher W. Cummings, Ferenc Czeyda-Pommersheim, and Sanjeev Bhalla

Imaging of congenital heart disease is a complex and challenging topic that until recently was almost exclusively the domain of pediatric radiologists and cardiologists. With advances in surgical and percutaneous techniques since the 1990s, most patients with congenital heart disease now survive into adulthood and are imaged with increasing frequency. Adults with corrected congenital heart disease often come to attention decades after initial surgical repair when they become symptomatic from long-term complications arising from failure of their postoperative anatomy or from secondary complications. Most of these patients underwent surgical procedures long before the development of electronic medical record keeping, and they are often imaged at different institutions with little information available on the underlying lesion or surgical repair. The role of the imager in these situations is to recognize the lesion and the corrective measures, as well as the complications that bring the patient to clinical attention. Cross-sectional imaging now complements, and has sometimes come to replace, echocardiography and angiography because of technical advances in CT and magnetic resonance imaging (MRI), as well as the widespread availability of these modalities both in the emergency and outpatient settings. Therefore, every radiologist must be familiar with the cross-sectional imaging appearance of the most common congenital heart lesions, the basic operations used to correct them, and the long-term complications of surgical correction.

Providing a detailed account of every congenital heart defect and every conceivable corrective surgical procedure or complication is beyond the scope of this chapter. Instead, the focus is on the most common heart defects survived into adulthood and the most common operations, with the hope of giving the reader a basic framework for pattern recognition and problem solving when faced with an adult patient presenting with unknown, corrected congenital heart disease.

◼ TECHNIQUES

CT and MRI have few standard protocols for cardiac imaging of congenital heart disease. The modality and technique must be tailored to the patient and the clinical question. CT angiography (CTA) before and after the administration of intravenous nonionic contrast material with thin collimation on a 64-slice or newer-generation scanner is the preferred CT method of evaluation. Low-dose precontrast imaging may be important because it allows identification of calcified or high-density conduits and repair changes and lessens the risk of confusing these normal changes with postoperative complications such as vascular leaks. In most cases, automated bolus tracking or test bolus techniques to optimize contrast opacification to the aorta or vascular bed of interest are used, although this approach can certainly be altered depending on the congenital disease and the desired information. Splitting the contrast bolus with two different rates of injection, similar to performing triple rule out CTA, can be done to obtain adequate opacification of both the pulmonary and systemic arterial systems. One must be prepared to obtain delayed phase imaging because altered anatomy, such as secondary to Fontan procedures or cavopulmonary shunts, may not opacify on the initial phase as a result of upper extremity contrast injection. A fixed delay may be required when the clinical question centers on the right heart or superior vena cava (SVC). Generally, a 15- to 20-second delay allows for the evaluation of these structures and can be quite useful when the clinical issue concerns a Glenn shunt or the superior limb of a baffle.

Because coronary artery anomalies are common in many types of congenital heart disease, electrocardiogram (ECG) gating can also be performed for dedicated coronary analysis. Although dose reduction techniques are making inroads to lessen the issue of radiation exposure even with retrospective gating, coronary anomalies in origin and course are generally readily apparent on thin collimation examinations in the absence of gating. As a rule, multiphase imaging of the thorax is preferred to the added radiation of gating. Gated studies are usually used as problem-solving techniques or when ventricular parameters are required. If gating is to be performed, care must be taken with the use of beta-blockers in patients who are in right-sided heart failure because the use of these drugs can exacerbate heart failure. CTA also provides excellent multiplanar and three-dimensional postprocessing capability, as well as potentially functional information (if retrospective ECG-gating has been used). The advantages of CT compared with MRI are faster imaging time and more widespread availability.

A basic cardiac MRI protocol often includes noncine fast black-blood scout images in axial, sagittal, and coronal views throughout the chest (single shot half-Fourier fast spin echo sequences) to evaluate mediastinal and great vessel anatomy. These images are often followed by transaxial bright-blood images, which are usually gated, noncine single shot steady-state free precession (SSFP) images. Intravenous gadolinium-based contrast agents are often not required for congenital heart disease analysis, although angiographic postcontrast sequences can help clarify vascular anomalies or stenoses when information is unclear on noncontrast sequences. Breath-hold noncontrast SSFP cine images are obtained along both the short and long axis of the heart to assess the anatomy and function of the cardiac chambers. On these cine images, laminar flow appears as high signal because of flow-related enhancement. A low-signal jet appears on the high-signal background in areas of turbulence as a result of dephasing of protons in areas of nonlaminar flow. Close attention must therefore be paid to dephasing artifact, especially on the cine images, because this artifact occurs in areas of vascular or valvular stenosis, in regurgitation, and across shunt defects. If mural thrombus in a surgical conduit or in the left atrial appendage is of clinical concern, a spoiled gradient echo or fast low-angle shot sequence may be used. This sequence does not have the chemical shift artifact inherent in the SSFP and is less likely to obscure subtle thrombus.

In patients with an intracardiac or extracardiac shunt, cross-sectional flow quantification of the proximal aorta and pulmonary artery by using a phase-encoded inversion recovery sequence can be performed to calculate the ratio of pulmonic flow to systemic flow (Qp/Qs). The same sequence when positioned perpendicular to a dephasing jet can be used to calculate the maximum velocity of flow across areas of stenosis, with the gradient across the stenotic segment calculated using the modified Bernoulli equation [gradient in mm Hg = 4 × (peak velocity in m/second)^2]. When the slice position is placed in cross section above the aortic or pulmonic valve, a regurgitant volume and fraction can be calculated. Limitations of MRI include claustrophobia and the inability to image patients with non–MRI-compatible cardiac pacemakers, which represent most currently available devices.

■ BICUSPID AORTIC VALVE

Bicuspid aortic valve, the most common type of congenital heart disease, with an incidence of 0.9% to 2% in the general population, is the result of incomplete separation of the valve leaflets during embryogenesis. Morphologically, the incompletely separated leaflet usually contains a midline cleft or raphe, which is readily detected by echocardiography and cross-sectional imaging. In the most common form of this condition, the right and left leaflets comprise the "fused" leaflet, and the noncoronary leaflet is normal. This anomaly has a male predominance, with a male-to-female ratio of 4:1. Patients with a bicuspid valve are at risk of developing infectious endocarditis and require antibiotic prophylaxis before invasive procedures. Coarctation of the aorta and interrupted aortic arch are frequently associated

with a bicuspid aortic valve. Because of this association, the diagnosis of any of these conditions warrants interrogation for the others on initial imaging.

Although patients may be initially asymptomatic and a few may never become symptomatic, the natural history of bicuspid valve is progressive, premature calcification and degeneration of the valve leaflets resulting in aortic stenosis and, sometimes, concomitant regurgitation. Because of coexisting aortopathy, dilation of the aortic root or ascending aorta may be seen, the presence and degree of which are independent of the patient's age or the degree of valve stenosis. If aortic regurgitation is present, left ventricular dilation may develop, and aortic dilation can accelerate. Patients with a bicuspid aortic valve are predisposed to aortic dissection, also a function of the concomitant aortopathy, independent of the functional impairment of the valve. Therefore, in patients less than 40 years old who present with aortic dissection, bicuspid aortopathy, as well as heritable diseases such as Marfan syndrome, should be considered.

Echocardiography is the primary imaging modality in the evaluation of the aortic valve because of its ease of performance, widespread availability, relatively low cost, excellent spatial and temporal resolution, ability to estimate gradients and valve areas, and lack of need for nephrotoxic contrast agents and radiation. Because many of these patients are regularly followed up, the benefits of echocardiography make it an ideal choice for repetitive imaging, especially when patients are young. However, the use of CT and MRI for preoperative and postoperative imaging of a bicuspid aortic valve is becoming more common, usually to evaluate and follow aortic size. Both CT and MRI can provide high-resolution images of the aortic valve en face to characterize the morphology of the valve and allow for valve planimetry. CT is superior at demonstrating calcification, which is common in stenotic valves, as well as allowing for simultaneous evaluation of the coronary arteries and complete thoracic aortic assessment before surgical intervention (Fig. 20-1, *A* to *D*).

On MRI, phase contrast flow quantification sequences allow pressure gradient estimation from peak velocities across the aortic valve. After an oblique coronal view of the aortic root is obtained with a cine SSFP sequence, the flow quantification series is run with the imaging plane perpendicular to the dephasing jet of stenosis that occurs above the aortic valve and contains the maximum velocities (see Fig. 20-1, *E* and *F*). When the series is run perpendicular to the axis of flow within the aorta itself approximately 1 cm above the valve plane, estimates of stroke volume, cardiac index, and regurgitant volume and fraction can be obtained. MRI can also evaluate the thoracic aorta to exclude aneurysm or coarctation at the time of evaluation, as well as provide left ventricular chamber size and functional assessment. Although cine MRI and retrospectively gated cine CT are not as readily used in clinical practice, both techniques can provide estimates of valve opening area that have been shown to correlate well with similar data derived with transthoracic and transesophageal echocardiography.

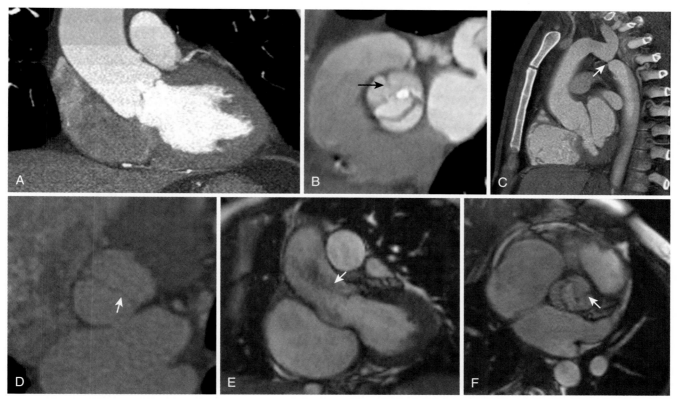

Figure 20-1 Bicuspid aortic valve. A and **B,** Aneurysmal dilatation of the ascending aorta effacing the sinotubular junction on oblique coronal computed tomography (CT) (**A**) can be seen with en face valve reconstruction demonstrating a bicuspid valve with raphe (*arrow* in **B**). **C,** Juxtaductal coarctation *(arrow)* can be seen on oblique sagittal volume-rendered CT image with enlargement of intercostal collateral arteries. **D,** This patient had a bicuspid aortic valve with a single commissure *(arrow).* Oblique coronal (**E**) and oblique axial (**F**) steady-state free precession images in systole of the aortic root and valve demonstrate a dephasing jet of stenosis above the aortic valve (*arrow* in **E**) and bicuspid morphology of the valve with a "fish-mouth" opening and a raphe (*arrow* in **F**) from fusion of the left and right leaflets.

Surgical intervention is necessary in patients with symptomatic aortic stenosis, if the valve area is less than 0.6 cm² or if moderate aortic regurgitation develops. The choice of mechanical versus bioprosthetic valve takes into account the risk from the required lifelong anticoagulation with mechanical valves, balanced against the risk from the anticipated need for reoperation with bioprosthetic valves 10 to 15 years after implantation. Traditional nonsurgical approaches to treatment of trileaflet aortic stenosis are often inadequate for patients with bicuspid valves. Balloon valvuloplasty is generally not optimal in the setting of the heavy valvular calcification that is frequently seen in bicuspid disease, and the procedure is complicated by recurrent stenosis or the development of progressive valvular regurgitation. Percutaneous valve replacement is becoming more readily available in those patients who are not surgical candidates, but patients with a bicuspid valve are not considered optimal candidates because of the abnormal morphology of the valve orifice, as well as frequent underlying coexisting aortic root dilatation.

Surgical correction in *symptomatic* pediatric and young adolescent patients with a bicuspid aortic valve is often accomplished through the Ross procedure, named after the British surgeon Donald Ross. The operation consists of replacement of the aortic valve using an autologous pulmonary homograft, reimplantation of the coronary arteries into the homograft, and reconstruction of the right ventricular outflow tract with a cadaveric cryopreserved allograft. This procedure is ideal for developing children and adolescents because the allograft has been shown to grow proportional to the growth of the patient and obviates the need for anticoagulation. Investigators have also suggested that this procedure may be associated with a relatively decreased long-term incidence of neoaortic stenosis. The most common long-term complications of the Ross procedure requiring reoperation are homograft stenosis, neoaortic valve regurgitation, and aneurysm formation, as well as stenosis or regurgitation of the pulmonary allograft. Neoaortic root dilatation may be observed postoperatively; however, this condition usually stabilizes during the first postoperative year.

In cases of ascending aortic or root aneurysm and bicuspid aortic valve stenosis, concomitant aortic root replacement is performed at the time of valve replacement if the maximum diameter is 4.5 cm or greater. In the setting of bicuspid aortic valve stenosis and ascending aortic dissection, valve replacement and ascending aortic and root replacement (Bentall or modified Bentall procedure) are performed. In patients with normally functioning bicuspid aortic valves and ascending aortic dissection, valve-sparing aortic root replacement may be considered.

ATRIAL SEPTAL DEFECTS

A congenital opening in the interatrial septum is one of the most common types of congenital heart disease, occurring in approximately 1 of 1000 live births. Most patients are asymptomatic, and this explains why young adults may present with a previously undiagnosed atrial septal defect (ASD). Other patients are identified by a detectable cardiac murmur, systemic embolic events, or, in the setting of long-standing shunting, pulmonary hypertension and right-sided heart failure. ASD results from abnormalities in the complex embryogenesis of the interatrial septum, with the normal septum developing through the apposition of the septum primum, a thin membrane originating in the roof of the primordial atrium, and the septum secundum, a crescentic membrane growing from the ventrocranial wall of the primitive atrium. A large defect in the central portion of the septum secundum, the foramen ovale, is normally sealed by the thin membrane of the septum primum to create an oval indentation in the atrial septal wall referred to as the fossa ovalis. This anatomy is important to understand because the septum primum, forming the floor of the fossa ovalis, may be imperceptibly thin on CT and MRI images and can be easily misinterpreted as a septal defect when slice thickness exceeds 2 mm.

In approximately 25% of the population, the foramen ovale remains probe patent, meaning that the membranes of the fossa ovalis can be separated. In this situation, the higher left atrial pressures keep the membranes apposed, but in certain situations, such as during the Valsalva maneuver, the right atrial pressures can increase enough to open the fossa ovalis transiently. Therefore, these patients are at risk for systemic embolic events. For unclear reasons, patent foramen ovale also has an association with migraine headaches.

A probe-patent foramen ovale (a potential risk factor for stroke) or ASD may be seen as contrast material extending across the atrial septum from the right atrium to the left atrium, on power injection of intravenous contrast, or as a dephasing jet across the interatrial septum on bright-blood gradient echo MRI images (Fig. 20-2, A and B).

The three main types of ASD are ostium secundum, ostium primum, and sinus venous defects. The fourth type of ASD is the unroofed coronary sinus, which is the rarest type, although it is not really a defect within the atrial septum (but has the same physiologic consequences). Failure of the septum primum to seal the foramen ovale completely results in an open communication between the atria at the level of the fossa ovalis known as an ostium secundum–type ASD (see Fig. 20-2, C and D). This type of ASD is the most common in the general population, and it comprises approximately 70% of lesions. Although secundum ASD is usually an isolated lesion, it can coexist with many other forms of congenital heart disease and has an association with mitral valve prolapse. Two of the more common associations are with mitral stenosis (Lutembacher syndrome) and with radial ray shortening (Holt-Oram syndrome).

Accounting for approximately 20% of ASDs, the ostium primum lesion occurs inferiorly between the fossa ovalis and the atrioventricular (AV) valve plane (see Fig. 20-2, E). Ostium primum ASDs are frequently encountered as part of the AV canal or endocardial cushion defects (ECDs). Seen most commonly in patients with trisomy 21 and heterotaxy syndromes, ECDs are made up of an ostium primum ASD, an inlet ventricular septal defect (VSD), and a variety of AV valve abnormalities. As a result of this frequent association with more complex congenital heart disease, ostium primum lesions tend to come to clinical attention during childhood.

The sinus venosus ASD (see Fig. 20-2, F and G) comprises most of the remaining ASDs. Although a few of these defects occur at the junction of the inferior vena cava (IVC) and right atrium (inferior type), most lesions are superior in location, found at the junction between the SVC and the right atrium. Superior sinus venosus ASD has a high association with partial anomalous pulmonary venous return (PAPVR), usually of the right upper lobe, to the SVC. In conjunction with this associated lesion, patients with sinus venosus ASD have a higher likelihood of developing pulmonary hypertension. A rare lesion, often referred to as an unroofed coronary sinus, may be encountered that results from a failure of separation of the superior wall of the coronary sinus with the left atrium. This lesion is challenging to identify on imaging studies and is frequently associated with a persistent left SVC. Because most of the shunting is from left to right, the coronary sinus tends to be larger than expected, with a left-sided SVC alone, a useful clue to this rare entity.

Another malformation of the interatrial septum is the atrial septal aneurysm, which results from excessive mobility of the septum with ballooning toward either the right or left atrial chamber. Atrial septal bowing is referred to as an aneurysm when it extends more than 1 cm beyond the plane of the fossa ovalis or when the overall excursion during the cardiac cycle is greater than 1.5 cm. Patients with atrial septal aneurysm have a significantly increased incidence of embolic stroke, especially if the septal aneurysm is associated with a patent foramen ovale. The reason for this is unknown and may be related to thrombus formation in the saclike segment, paradoxical embolization through the patent foramen ovale, or atrial arrhythmia. Septal aneurysm may be associated with patent foramen ovale, ASDs, and mitral valve prolapse.

Echocardiography (either transthoracic or transesophageal) is the study of choice for evaluation of suspected ASDs. Given the high spatial resolution and ability to assess blood flow with color Doppler imaging, echocardiography is ideal for the evaluation of most types of ASD. Normally filtered by the pulmonary circulation, intravenously injected agitated saline contrast can be employed with and without the Valsalva maneuver to assess for transeptal transit of saline bubbles, which are abnormally detected within the left atrium in patients with patent foramen ovale or ASD. Estimates of pulmonary arterial pressure and right-sided heart function can also be obtained with echocardiography. Because of the proximity of the transducer to the atrial septum, transesophageal echocardiography is sensitive for detection

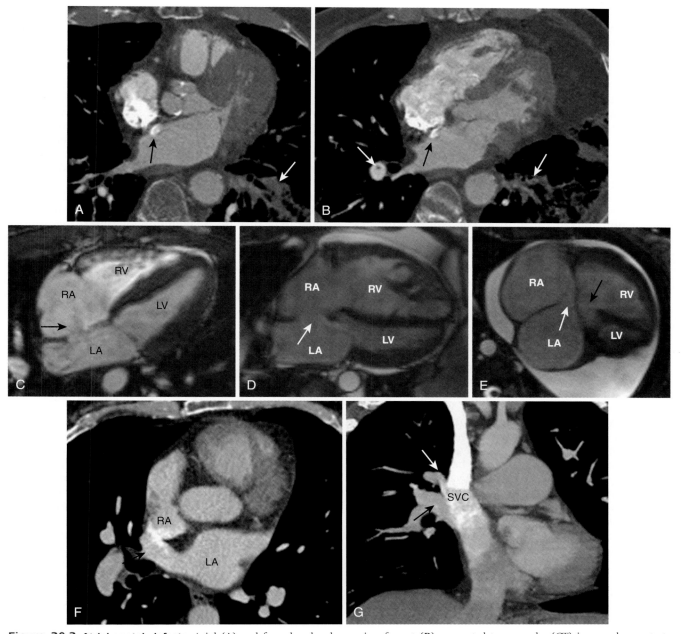

Figure 20-2 Atrial septal defects. Axial (**A**) and four-chamber long-axis reformat (**B**) computed tomography (CT) images demonstrate right-to-left high-density contrast shunting *(black arrows)* along the left atrial side of a patent foramen ovale in a patient with extensive acute pulmonary emboli *(white arrows)*. **C** and **D,** Four-chamber long-axis steady-state free precession(SSFP) magnetic resonance imaging (MRI) scans in two different patients demonstrate ostium secundum atrial septal defects *(arrows)* with subtle left-to-right dephasing across the defect (**C**) and right ventricular enlargement and hypertrophy (**D**). **E,** SSFP MRI scan in a patient with heterotaxy syndrome demonstrates an atrioventricular canal defect, consisting of an ostium primum atrial septal defect *(white arrow)*, an inlet ventricular septal defect *(black arrow)*, and a common atrioventricular valve. Axial (**F**) and oblique coronal reformat (**G**) CT images in another patient demonstrate a sinus venosus atrial septal defect *(arrow* in **F**) located high in the atrial septum near the junction with the superior vena cava (SVC), as well as right upper lobe partial anomalous pulmonary venous return of several branches into the superior vena cava–right atrial junction *(arrows* in **G**). *LA,* Left atrium; *LV,* left ventricle; *RA,* right atrium; *RV,* right ventricle.

of ASD. However, detection of sinus venosus ASD can be difficult, given the superior location of most lesions. Unroofed coronary sinus ASDs are frequently occult on echocardiography.

Cardiac MRI can serve as a method of primary detection or secondary evaluation of patients with suspected or known ASD. A dephasing jet can be detected on cine steady-state bright-blood imaging sequences. In patients without coexistent pulmonary hypertension, the dephasing jet is directed toward the right atrium as a result of higher left atrial pressures. However, in patients with a patent foramen ovale or elevated right-sided heart pressures, the dephasing jet may be bidirectional or even directed toward the left atrium. Large ASDs are usually readily apparent as a result of the lack of septal tissue, but they may not display a focal dephasing jet because of the unrestricted flow. In these cases, only mild low-velocity turbulence may be seen. An estimate of the diameter of the defect should be reported, as well as the presence or absence and minimal width of the circumferential rim of atrial septum, because this information is useful in evaluating transcatheter occluder device appropriateness and size.

In all patients with suspected ASD, flow quantification of the aorta and pulmonary arteries is required to assess the degree of shunting by comparing the forward flow across the pulmonic valve with the forward flow across the aortic valve (Qp/Qs). Care should be taken when setting the cross-sectional flow quantification sequences that the plane of imaging is truly orthogonal to the long axis of flow in each vessel, because off-axis imaging in one or both vessels can lead to false shunt estimates. Unlike echocardiography, during which assessment of right ventricular function can be restricted by retrosternal location and limited acoustic window, MRI can qualitatively and quantitatively assess right heart chamber size and function. Intravenous contrast material is not required for evaluation. If pulmonary hypertension is present, pulmonary arterial enlargement, right ventricular and atrial dilatation, right ventricular hypertrophy, tricuspid regurgitation, and interventricular septal dyskinesis may be seen. Care should be taken to identify all pulmonary veins and their course to the left atrium, best accomplished on multiplanar noncine SSFP brightblood sequences, to exclude partial anomalous venous return, which is frequently seen in patients with superior sinus venosus defects. Given that right upper lobe partial anomalous venous return can be challenging to identify, intravenous contrast may be used to assist in the detection of all right upper lobe veins.

Although CT is not a primary method of evaluation of ASD, these lesions can be seen on contrast-enhanced imaging studies performed for noncardiac reasons or during the evaluation of other cardiac diseases. Detection depends on the lack of septal tissue, which can be seen in large defects, or the presence of transeptal contrast flow, which requires differential degrees of opacification of the right and left atrium. Patent foramen ovale can be seen when high-density contrast material crosses the fossa ovale, frequently directed at a slight angle or parallel to the interatrial septum as it courses between the separated membranes at the fossa ovalis. Morphologic changes in keeping with pulmonary hypertension, including pulmonary arterial enlargement and right heart chamber size and ventricular hypertrophy, can be seen. Multidetector CT (MDCT) is also highly sensitive for detection of anomalous pulmonary venous drainage because of its superior isovolumetric spatial resolution.

In the adult patient, ASD and symptomatic patent foramen ovale are most commonly treated with percutaneous septal occluder devices, and open surgical procedures are reserved for patients with very large defects, unsuitable margins of a defect, or associated lesions requiring corrective intervention. In young children, surgical patch repair or primary closure is typically required. Sinus venosus defects are not amenable to occluder device placement and require surgical correction, which often includes baffling of associated anomalous pulmonary venous drainage back to the left atrium.

■ ATRIOVENTRICULAR SEPTAL DEFECTS

Fusion of the dorsal and ventral endocardial cushions gives rise to the ostium primum portion of the interatrial septum, the inlet portion of the interventricular septum, and the septal portions of the AV valve leaflets during the sixth week of embryologic development. Abnormal fusion or lack of fusion of the endocardial cushions results in a range of abnormalities known as ECDs, which include ostium primum ASD, inlet VSD, and AV valve abnormalities. A wide range of valvular abnormalities can be seen from a common AV valve to deformities of tricuspid or mitral septal leaflets. The relative position of the defects and the type of valve abnormality leads to various presentations, depending on the resulting direction of systemic and pulmonic blood flow.

Echocardiography readily identifies this defect in infants and even prenatally. In addition to shunting identified on color Doppler flow and an absence of portions of the interatrial and interventricular septa, the tricuspid and mitral valve planes are abnormally located along the same axis in ECDs. Normally, the tricuspid valve is slightly more apical in location with respect to the mitral valve. The types of valvular abnormalities can also be characterized.

MRI is often used in older patients with ECDs (adolescents and young adults) before and after surgical intervention (see Fig. 20-2, E). In addition to identifying the abnormalities described on echocardiography, MRI allows for flow quantification of the aorta and pulmonary artery to assess the direction and degree of shunting (Qp/Qs). Quantitative biventricular functional analysis is also performed, and the anatomic relationships of the defects to other cardiac structures such as the left ventricular outflow tract are noted. MDCT can play a complementary role, with its strength lying in multiplanar demonstration of the anatomic defects and relationships at the cost of radiation exposure.

Because shunting is often predominantly from left to right, increased pulmonary arterial flow, if left untreated, eventually may lead to Eisenmenger syndrome. Surgical correction is usually performed at 4 to 6 months of age or earlier if the patient is symptomatic in spite of medical therapy. Temporizing measures before definitive surgical correction are banding of the pulmonary artery to decrease pulmonary flow and ASD closure using a pericardial patch. If a complete AV canal exists, the double patch technique is often used. In this operation, the atrial defect is again closed with a pericardial patch, the VSD is closed with a synthetic patch, and the malformed AV valve leaflets are reconstructed and sandwiched between the atrial and ventricular septal patches.

Given that the AV node and bundles of His are in close proximity to the surgical field, conduction anomalies including AV block are common complications of repair. This can complicate ECG-gated MRI cine bright-blood sequences or even preclude MRI altogether if a non–MRI compatible implantable pacer device is required. On follow-up imaging, attention to residual ASDs or VSDs is necessary, including flow quantification of the aorta and pulmonary artery. Qualitative tricuspid and mitral valve evaluation for regurgitation should be performed. Aortic outflow tract obstruction can also occur.

■ VENTRICULAR SEPTAL DEFECTS

After the bicuspid aortic valve, VSD is one of the most common forms of congenital heart disease. VSDs can be isolated as a result of deficiency in septal tissue, part of a more complex congenital heart disease, or even acquired through penetrating injuries or myocardial infarction. VSDs are categorized according to their physiologic consequence and anatomic location. Physiologically, VSDs are classified as restrictive if they are flow limited and result in a significant pressure gradient between the left and right ventricles. Because these lesions are small and restrictive to flow, they do not result in significant shunting, but they do predispose patients to endocarditis, for which antibiotic prophylaxis before invasive procedures is required. Nonrestrictive VSDs are larger lesions that permit hemodynamically significant shunting and as a result are symptomatic, initially from right ventricular overload and over time from the development of irreversible pulmonary hypertension (Eisenmenger syndrome).

VSDs are also classified according to anatomic location. Accounting for the overwhelming majority of defects in adults, perimembranous VSDs occur in and extend from the membranous portion of the interventricular septum, which lies immediately beneath the aortic valve and is in continuity with the base of the septal leaflet of the tricuspid valve (Fig. 20-3, A to C). The most common defect in children and the second most common defect in the adult population, muscular VSDs are bordered entirely by myocardium and occur along the muscular interventricular septum (see Fig. 20-3, D and E). Many muscular VSDs spontaneously close in early childhood, a characteristic accounting for the finding that VSDs are more common than ASDs in this age group, yet ASDs are more commonly encountered in young adults. Most acquired VSDs are muscular.

Outlet VSDs occur above the level of the crista supraventricularis in the right ventricular infundibulum, are the most superior in location, are in proximity to the aortic and pulmonic valves, and are most frequently seen in the setting of conotruncal abnormalities such as tetralogy of Fallot (TOF), truncus arteriosus, and transposition of the great arteries (TGA) (see Fig. 20-3, F to H). Inlet VSDs occur immediately beneath the AV valve plane and are most commonly encountered in the setting of ECDs (see Fig. 20-3, I).

Echocardiography is the mainstay of evaluation of VSDs and, similar to ASD assessment, involves the use of color Doppler analysis and agitated saline contrast injection to detect shunting across the interventricular septum. Pulmonary artery pressure estimates can be made, as well as biventricular functional assessment.

As in evaluation of ASD, MRI can provide complementary information on VDSs, specifically, quantification of the Qp/Qs and biventricular function. Because of their close anatomic relationship with the undersurface of the aortic annulus, perimembranous and outlet VSDs can lead to eccentric aortic regurgitation and valvular degeneration resulting from high-velocity flow across the septum that exerts a pulling effect on what is typically the right or noncoronary aortic cusp. This phenomenon is referred to as the Venturi effect. If present or progressive, aortic insufficiency in the setting of an otherwise restrictive VSD may require surgical intervention to prevent damage to the aortic valve. MDCT can provide excellent anatomic localization and can demonstrate secondary effects of pulmonary hypertension, but it is not a primary method of evaluation in VSD. Unless the CT scan is ECG gated, detection of a perimembranous VSD can be quite challenging on CT because of pulsation artifact.

The goal of corrective therapy in VSD is closure of defects that cause a significant shunt (Qp/Qs >1.5:1), before irreversible pulmonary hypertension develops. In children, most muscular VSDs close spontaneously by muscular ingrowth before the age of 2 years, and, if they do not, these defects are surgically corrected. With the increasing use of MDCT and MRI, small, incomplete tubular invaginations within the interventricular septum can be seen, presumably small VSDs that have spontaneously healed. Perimembranous VSDs can also spontaneously heal because of the development of redundant tissue from the septal leaflet of the tricuspid valve that seals over the defect, thus leaving a wind sock type of deformity that extends toward the right ventricle from the interventricular septum.

Closure may be accomplished surgically with patch repair through median sternotomy and right or left ventriculotomy. Dyskinesia of the left or right ventricular wall, depending on the site of ventriculotomy, and conduction abnormalities are potential risks of the surgical approach; these complications can be seen on cine MRI and echocardiography. On CT, a felt pledget or fatty metaplasia often can be seen in an earlier ventriculotomy site.

A less invasive approach is transcatheter placement of a septal occluder device. This procedure carries a slightly higher risk of typically small residual defects. MRI and echocardiography may be used in the postrepair setting to detect residual shunting manifested by dephasing jets or in flow quantification measurements.

■ TETRALOGY OF FALLOT

This lesion, named after the French physician Etienne Fallot, who first described it in three cyanotic patients, represents approximately 10% of all congenital heart disease and is the most common cyanotic congenital heart disease manifesting after infancy. The lesion consists of right ventricular outflow stenosis, VSD (most commonly outlet type), rightward displacement of the aortic root (which overrides the VSD), and right ventricular hypertrophy. TOF results from anomalous migration of neural crest cells during embryonic development that results in abnormal truncal septation and abnormal position of the infundibular septum. TOF is often associated with other anomalies of vascular

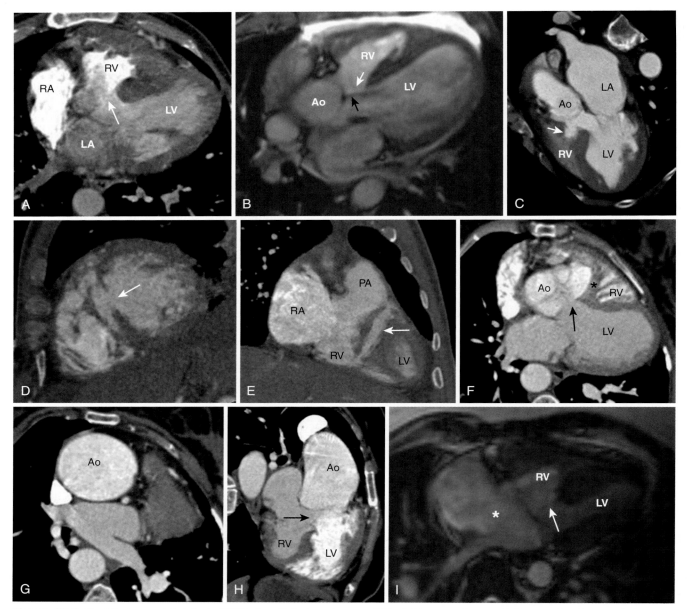

Figure 20-3 Ventricular septal defects (VSD). A to C, Perimembranous VSDs (*white arrows* in A to C) lie immediately beneath the aortic valve. Note pulmonary hypertension and right ventricular hypertrophy (A) and aortic insufficiency (*black arrow* in B). C, Spontaneously healed defect with wind sock deformity of the membranous septum *(arrow)*. Short-axis (D) and oblique coronal reformat (E) computed tomography images of a muscular VSD in an adult patient who was stabbed in the chest demonstrate a defect *(arrows)* coursing obliquely through the muscular septum from superior to inferior. F to H, Outlet VSDs in the setting of conotruncal abnormalities with pulmonary atresia. Axial (F and G) and four-chamber long-axis reformat (H) images demonstrate a high-outlet VSD *(arrows)* extending above the crista supraventricularis *(asterisk in F)*. Absence of the main pulmonary artery (G) is noted, as well as overriding of the aorta (Ao in H) above the defect. I, steady-state free precession four-chamber image shows inlet VSDs *(arrow)* in the setting of an atrioventricular canal defect resulting from trisomy 21. A large ostium primum atrial septal defect *(asterisk in I)* and a common atrioventricular valve are also seen. *Ao,* Aorta; *LA,* left atrium; *LV,* left ventricle; *PA,* pulmonary artery; *RA,* right atrium; *RV,* right ventricle.

development including right-sided aortic arch, (~25% of patients), coronary artery anomalies (including anomalous coronary origin and coronary fistulas in ~5% of patients), and progressive dilation of the aortic root and ascending aorta. Patent ductus arteriosus (PDA) is present in two thirds of patients with TOF; severe pulmonic stenosis or atresia and major aortico-pulmonary collateral arteries occur in one third. Associated tracheal anomalies have also been described in 11% of patients with TOF.

Although TOF is classically a cyanotic defect, the degree of cyanosis and the clinical presentation depend on the degree of right ventricular outflow stenosis. Right ventricular outflow obstruction results from a combination of septal deviation, rightward displacement of the overriding aortic root, hypoplasia of the pulmonic valve annulus, and muscular bands in the region of the pulmonic infundibulum. The stenosis may be subvalvular, valvular, or supravalvular and often occurs at multiple levels. If the obstruction is severe, the direction of flow across the VSD reverses and becomes a right-to-left shunt that causes the patient to be severely cyanotic. In relatively mild pulmonic stenosis, the degree of right-to-left shunting and cyanosis are less severe, and patients with minimal stenosis may have no significant shunting and thus no cyanosis ("pink tetralogy"). Patients with pink tetralogy may come to attention later in life as a result of a cardiac murmur or right-sided heart failure. Most patients, however, are cyanotic and present in the first year of life with cyanotic spells that may, in severe cases, lead to arrhythmias, ischemic strokes, and death.

Adults typically present with less drastic symptoms including chronic cyanosis, decreased exercise tolerance, and other symptoms and signs related to right-sided heart failure and hypoxemia. A variant of TOF consists of a large VSD and severe atresia or an absence of the main pulmonary arteries, with the lungs supplied by systemic aortopulmonary collateral vessels that reconstitute the pulmonary arteries at the segmental level. Depending on the degree of collateralization, these patients may be relatively asymptomatic early on and develop congestive heart failure later in infancy.

The current standard of care for patients with TOF is definitive repair in the first year of life. Very few patients survive to adulthood without early intervention. In the past, the goal of surgery was palliation by increasing pulmonary arterial flow through the creation of systemic pulmonary shunts, which were also used in other congenital heart diseases, in the hope of improving exercise tolerance and decreasing cyanosis (Fig. 20-4). Various approaches existed, including creation of a direct communication between the ascending aorta and the right pulmonary artery (Waterston shunt) or between the descending aorta and the left pulmonary artery (Pott shunt) and anastomosis of the subclavian artery to the pulmonary artery (Blalock-Taussig shunt). These approaches are no longer used because of the high incidence of postoperative complications, most importantly pulmonary hypertension and congestive heart failure. Other complications include stenosis of the pulmonary artery at the anastomotic site and preferential increase of flow to the lung ipsilateral to the shunt that leads to pulmonary artery hypertrophy. Although these procedures are no longer performed, the examiner should be familiar with them because many of these patients (≤85% at 36 years of postoperative follow-up) are now adults and may present for imaging.

Currently, the favored operative approach is primary definitive repair. The goals of repair are to relieve pulmonary outflow obstruction and patch the VSD. The older surgical technique involved repair of the septal defect through an incision in the right ventricular free wall (infundibulotomy) and relief of obstruction by valvectomy, but this technique was abandoned because of the frequent subsequent development of free pulmonic regurgitation and right ventricular dysfunction, which in many cases required reoperation for valve replacement. Valvotomy and transatrial repair of the VSD are currently favored. In patients with hypoplastic pulmonary arteries and collateral pulmonary supply, staged surgical repair through a modified (synthetic conduit) Blalock-Taussig shunt or reimplantation of the collateral vessels into a reconstructed pulmonary artery (known as unifocalization) is usually undertaken. The VSD repair may be accomplished at a later stage in these patients, who often need several repeat operations because of recurrent stenosis at the vessel reimplantation sites.

The most frequent long-term complication in patients who have undergone primary repair of TOF remains pulmonary regurgitation (Fig. 20-5, *A* to *C*), which may result in right ventricular dilation and failure and potentially life-threatening arrhythmias or sudden death. Patients with this complication have a significantly increased risk of mortality in the third postoperative decade. Other complications after repair are residual right ventricular outflow tract obstruction resulting from infundibular muscular bands, pulmonic stenosis or peripheral pulmonic arterial stenosis, and tricuspid regurgitation. The most important long-term factor associated with poor clinical status in the postoperative patient is decreased left ventricular systolic function, which may develop as a result of severe right heart failure.

Although most patients undergo serial echocardiography, imaging evaluation of patients with TOF is optimally performed with noncontrast MRI, which depicts valvular regurgitation, vascular stenoses, and clearly delineates postsurgical anatomy. All patients with TOF who are undergoing MRI should have quantification of right and left ventricular function, flow quantification of the pulmonic valve to assess for regurgitation and stenosis, and flow quantification of the aorta and Qp/Qs ratio to allow for assessment of residual shunting. In patients with pulmonic regurgitation, the most important parameter is the right ventricular end-diastolic volume, which should be normalized to body surface area. This value is often used to determine the severity of the situation and to assess whether surgery is warranted.

The central pulmonary arteries should be interrogated because peripheral pulmonic stenoses can develop (see Fig. 20-5, *D* and *E*), and the VSD patch repair should be evaluated for dephasing jets to exclude residual shunts. Patients who have undergone right ventricular infundibulotomy can develop aneurysmal outpouching along the anterior aspect of the outflow tract below the pulmonic valve (see Fig. 20-5, *F* to *H*). If the outpouching is large enough, preferential flow of blood into the aneurysm sac, as opposed to forward flow across the pulmonic valve, can lead to worsening clinical status. Although progressive right ventricular fibrosis can develop and be detected on delayed postcontrast-enhanced MRI, this is not routinely performed because of the added expense and contrast agent exposure.

In the setting of pulmonic atresia and aorticopulmonary collateral formation, dynamic postcontrast MRI may be required to delineate the number and size of feeding systemic arteries. MDCT can also be used in this setting and is equally well suited for detection of aorticopulmonary collateral vessels because of its high spatial resolution. CT may detect stenoses in central and peripheral pulmonic arterial branches and is superior for evaluation of any abnormalities in origin or course

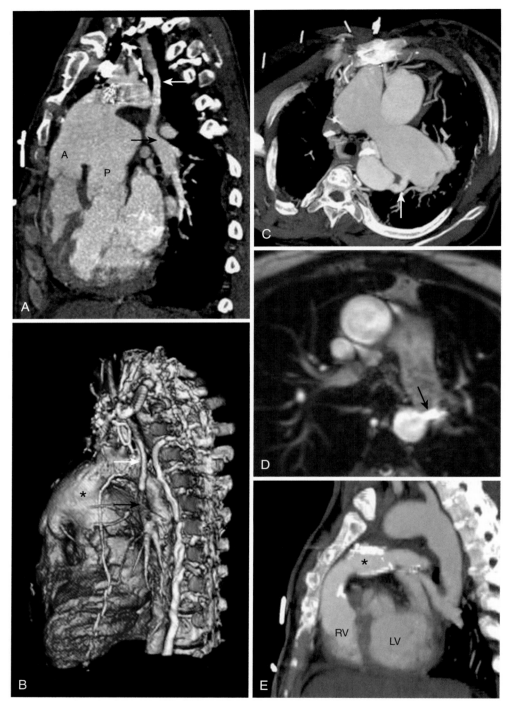

Figure 20-4 Surgical conduits for providing pulmonary blood flow. A and **B,** A modified Blalock-Taussig shunt *(white arrows)* provides blood flow to the left pulmonary artery *(black arrows)* in a patient with tricuspid atresia and D-transposition of the great arteries (D-TGA). This patient has undergone a Damus-Kaye-Stansel procedure *(asterisk* in **B)** with surgical anastomosis of the proximal aorta to the main pulmonary artery, which is used in some cases of D-TGA with aortic outflow obstruction to provide systemic arterial perfusion. **C,** A modified Potts shunt *(arrow)* connects the descending thoracic aorta to the left pulmonary artery in a patient with complex congenital heart disease. **D,** A classic Potts shunt *(arrow)* involves direct communication between the anterior aspect of the descending thoracic aorta and the posterior wall of the left pulmonary artery. Note the bright signal of flow from the aorta into the left pulmonary artery on steady-state free precession magnetic resonance imaging. **E,** In a different patient with pulmonary atresia and a ventricular septal defect, a Rastelli conduit *(asterisk)* connecting the right ventricle (RV) to the confluence of the pulmonary arteries is in place with calcification of conduit material, a common finding. *A,* Aorta; *LV,* left ventricle; *P,* pulmonary artery; *RV,* right ventricle.

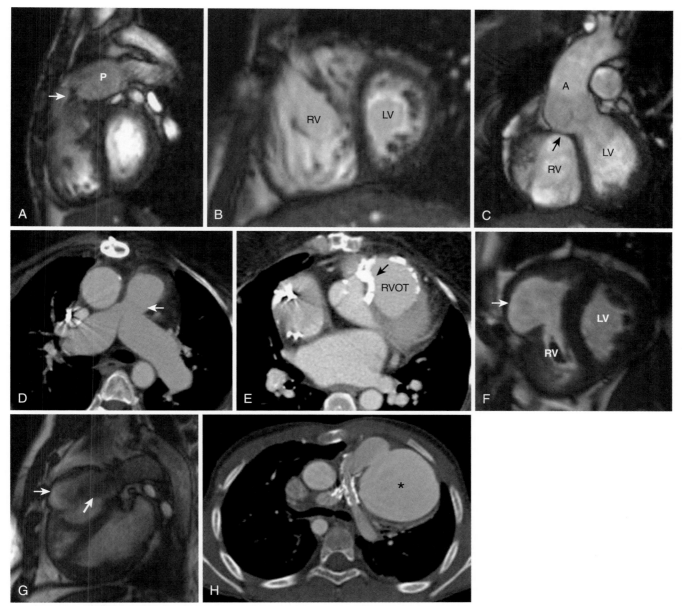

Figure 20-5 Tetralogy of Fallot (TOF) after surgical repair. A to C, Pulmonary outflow tract (A), midventricular two-chamber short-axis (B), and oblique coronal aortic outflow tract (C) steady-state free precession (SSFP) magnetic resonance imaging scans demonstrate a dephasing jet (*arrow* in **A**) of pulmonic insufficiency with diltation and hypertrophy of the right ventricle (RV in **B**) and patch repair (*arrow* in **C**) of a ventricular septal defect underneath a previously overriding aorta. Also note flattening of the interventricular septum (**B**) from increased volume and pressure in the RV. **D** and **E,** Narrowing of the main pulmonary artery (*arrow* in **D**) in a different patient with repaired TOF is demonstrated on axial computed tomography (CT) images, as well as calcification of the ventricular septal defect patch repair (*arrow* in **E**) and the right ventricular homograft. Note the aneurysmal dilatation of the right and left pulmonary arteries beyond the level of stenosis (**D**). **F** and **G,** Midventricular two-chamber short-axis (**F**) and oblique sagittal pulmonary outflow tract (**G**) SSFP MRI scans in a different patient show aneurysmal dilatation (*thin white arrows* in **F** and **G**) at the site of prior infundibulotomy with severe pulmonic insufficiency (*thick white arrow* in **G**). **H,** Axial CT image of a different patient demonstrates a large saccular aneursym *(asterisk)* arising from the right ventricular outflow homograft. Note the bilateral central pulmonary artery stents, which had been placed for treatment of stenoses. *A,* Aorta; *LV,* left ventricle; *P,* pulmonary artery; *RVOT,* right ventricular outflow tract.

of the coronaries. Retrosternal vessels may be at risk of injury if subsequent repeat sternotomy is performed, and reporting the presence of these vessels is required. The presence of anomalous vessels coursing anterior to the right ventricular infundibulum may require adjustment of the surgical approach. Right and left ventricular volumes and function can be assessed with retrospectively gated CT, which may be used if contraindications to MRI exist.

■ TRANSPOSITION OF THE GREAT ARTERIES

General Approach

Evaluation of TGA can be challenging because these lesions comprise a complex combination of abnormal vascular connections and cardiac anatomic anomalies and require a systematic approach for analysis. To ensure that all facets of the abnormality are included in the radiology report, an eight-step approach has been adopted for the analysis of patients with complex congenital heart disease, although not all components are relevant for TGA. The steps are the following:

1. Surgical repair. The most common types are patches, shunts, baffles, and valve replacements. Understanding the path of communication and potential complications is very important when evaluating the postsurgical patient. The most common forms of surgical correction are described later in this section.

2. Arch analysis, consisting of assessment of aortic arch side (left or right) and branching pattern. The two most common abnormal types of branching are mirror image branching (a left brachiocephalic artery, right common carotid artery, and right subclavian artery from proximal to distal) and right arch with aberrant left subclavian artery (left common carotid, right common carotid, right subclavian, and left subclavian artery arising from the proximal descending aorta). Aortic caliber should also be assessed. Focal narrowing of the aorta may be seen at the isthmus in patients with pseudocoarctation and coarctation. In patients with a double aortic arch, one of the two arch components may be narrowed, hypoplastic, or even atretic with a cord remnant.

3. Venous analysis. The most common types of systemic venous anomalies are left SVC, azygous continuation of an interrupted IVC, and aberrant retroaortic brachiocephalic vein. Left SVC runs to the left of the pulmonary artery and aortic arch through the ligament of Marshall to empty into the coronary sinus, which is commonly enlarged. Occasionally, a left SVC may empty into the left atrium, thus causing a right-to-left shunt. In the case of an interrupted IVC, the IVC is essentially absent (although an infrarenal portion of the IVC may be present), and venous return from the lower extremities and body is carried to the SVC by an enlarged azygous or hemiazygous vein, with the hepatic veins draining directly into the right atrium (sometimes through an extremely short IVC-like common vein). The aberrant retroaortic brachiocephalic vein travels posterior to the aorta underneath the arch and should not be confused with other mediastinal vascular anomalies.

4. Evaluation of the circuit of blood flow. Mapping out the direction of flow helps clarify the underlying lesion and also helps identify any potential sites of vascular shunting. When intravenous contrast is used in MRI or CT, following the flow of contrast material through the venous system and cardiac chambers helps detect not only the anatomic relationships but often also significant information on underlying physiology.

5. Chamber and septal analysis. Increased afterload results in hypertrophy of cardiac chamber walls. Increased volume causes chamber enlargement, which should prompt a search for the source (e.g., septal defect, regurgitant valve, or anomalous pulmonary venous return). Differentiation of the morphologic right and left cardiac chambers is important, especially in patients with complex congenital heart disease and

TGA, because a morphologic right ventricle in the systemic position will fail over time. The right atrium is defined by acceptance of the IVC blood return, and the right atrial appendage has a broad base and extends anteriorly in a horizontal orientation. The left atrium normally accepts drainage of the pulmonary veins, and the left atrial appendage has a narrower base and extends superiorly in a vertical orientation. The hallmarks of the morphologic right ventricle are as follows: the infundibulum, which separates the tricuspid and pulmonic valve planes; the crista supraventricularis, which is a marker of the beginning of the infundibulum; and the moderate band, although this can be difficult to identify in the setting of ventricular hypertrophy. The morphologic left ventricle does not have an infundibulum and has two papillary muscles. In patients with complex congenital heart disease, the best approach is often to refer to chambers as systemic or pulmonic and define the morphologic characteristics of the underlying chambers. A common pitfall of septal analysis is that a very thin, barely perceptible septal membrane may be mistaken for an ostium secundum ASD at the fossa ovalis or a membranous VSD, especially if slice thickness is significantly greater than the thickness of the membrane (usually >1 mm). A septal defect is confidently diagnosed by noting a jet of dephasing artifact on the cine SSFP MRI images or a thin thread of contrast material or nonopacified blood across the septum on CT.

6. Great vessel analysis. This is especially important in patients with TGA.

7. Pulmonary venous analysis. Normally, two left and two right pulmonary veins drain into the left atrium. Occasionally, all the pulmonary veins drain into the systemic circulation, a condition termed total anomalous pulmonary venous return. If only some of the main pulmonary veins drain systemically, PAPVR is present. PAPVR of the right upper lobe is commonly associated with sinus venosus–type ASD.

8. Mediastinal collateral vessels. These vessels may be arterial or venous. Arterial collateral vessels, also known as aorticopulmonary collateral arteries (Fig. 20-6), arise in situations characterized by obstruction to pulmonary arterial flow and provide arterial blood flow to the lungs that eventually drains through the pulmonary veins. Venovenous collateral vessels can result from alterations in transpulmonary pressure gradients between the upper and lower body, a complication of univentricular heart repair, and can drain directly into pulmonary veins or the left atrium, with resulting right-to-left shunt and cyanosis.

Dextrotransposition

Dextro-TGA (D-TGA) is the result of abnormal conotruncal rotation, with the aortic root positioned to the right and anterior to the pulmonary trunk. The great arteries migrate in parallel and do not cross, as they would in normal embryonic development. The morphologic ventricles are in their normal anatomic position and connect to the atria normally (AV concordance). The aorta arises from the right ventricle, and the pulmonary artery

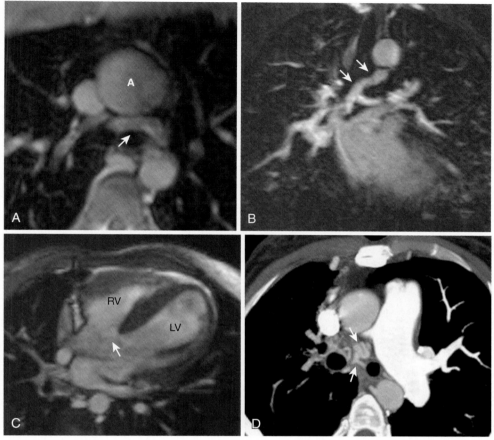

Figure 20-6 Aortopulmonary collateral arteries. A to C, Presenting in early adulthood with worsening dyspnea on exertion, a patient was found to have pulmonary atresia with a ventricular septal defect. Steady-state free precession (SSFP) axial image (**A**) and postcontrast coronal magnetic resonance angiography (**B**) demonstrate absence of the pulmonary arteries with a large branching aorticopulmonary collateral vessel (*arrows*) supplying the lungs. Four-chamber SSFP image (**C**) reveals a perimembranous ventricular septal defect (*arrow*) immediately inferior to the aortic valve. **D,** A different patient with congenital pulmonic and tricuspid valve stenoses who had initially been treated with a Waterston shunt from the ascending aorta to the right pulmonary artery presented for evaluation with computed tomography, which demonstrated chronic occlusion of the right pulmonary artery with collateral aorticopulmonary arteries (*arrows*) arising from the descending thoracic aorta. *A,* Aorta; *LV,* left ventricle; *RV,* right ventricle.

arises from the left ventricle (ventriculoarterial discordance). The direction of blood flow is vena cava to right atrium to right ventricle to aorta, parallel to the pulmonary circulation, which runs from pulmonary veins to left atrium to left ventricle to pulmonary artery. For the infant to survive the first few days of life without intervention, a shunt lesion such as an ASD, VSD, or PDA must be present to connect the systemic and pulmonary circulations. The incidence of D-TGA is approximately 1 in 3000 live births, with an increased incidence in infants of diabetic mothers reported.

Associated cardiac anomalies are present in approximately one-third of D-TGA patients. The most common associated cardiovascular anomalies are VSD (usually perimembranous or outlet types), coarctation, pulmonary outflow obstruction, and mitral and tricuspid stenosis and atresia. Anomalies of the coronary arteries frequently occur with the most common being the result of an anteriorly located noncoronary cusp.

Clinical presentation depends on the size of the VSD. If the VSD is large, cyanosis may be mild or initially absent. These patients present later with right (systemic) ventricular failure resulting from shunting

across the VSD and the systemic afterload for which the right ventricle is not adapted; pulmonary hypertension can develop from increased pulmonary blood flow from shunting across the VSD. More commonly, D-TGA patients are severely cyanotic in the early postnatal period. In patients with a small VSD, in which systemic to pulmonic shunting is through a PDA in the first few days of life, significant cyanosis develops after closure of the PDA. Immediate management is most critical in this patient group, with the goal of maintaining or increasing systemic-to-pulmonic shunting, to provide an opportunity for pulmonary oxygenation of blood. This goal can be accomplished with prostaglandin infusion, in an attempt to keep the PDA open. In patients with an intact ventricular septum, palliative atrial balloon septostomy is performed to create a systemic-to-pulmonic shunt, with later definitive surgical therapy. Few patients survive without early intervention, and the 6-month nonsurgical mortality rate is 90%.

Definitive correction may be accomplished by physiologic (atrial switch) or anatomic (arterial switch) repair. Physiologic repair was first developed, in the 1960s, by Canadian surgeon William Mustard and

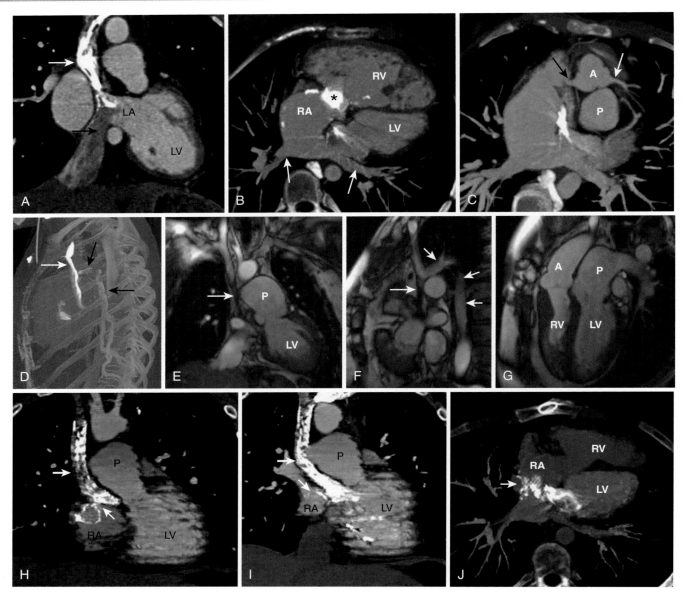

Figure 20-7 D-transposition of the great arteries (D-TGA) with atrial switch surgical correction. **A** and **B,** Oblique coronal computed tomography (CT) image (**A**) demonstrates superior (*white arrow* in **A**) and inferior (*black arrow* in **B**) limbs of a systemic baffle directing venous blood to the left atrium (LA) and subsequently left ventricle (LV). Axial thin maximum intensity projection (MIP) image (**B**) displays the pulmonic venous baffle directing pulmonary venous (*white arrows* in **B**) blood to the right atrium (RA) and subsequently the right ventricle (RV). Note the hypertrophy and dilatation of the morphologic RV, which is the systemic ventricle and surgical replacement of the tricuspid valve (*asterisk* in **B**). **C,** Axial MIP image shows that the aorta (A) lies anterior and to the right of the pulmonary artery (P) and the right (*black arrow*) and left (*white arrow*) coronary artery ostea and cusps are posterior, resulting in the unusual anterior position of the noncoronary cusp. **D,** Note reflux of injected contrast material into the azygous arch *(black arrows)* secondary to stenosis of the superior limb of the systemic baffle *(white arrow).* Oblique coronal (**E**) and sagittal (**F** and **G**) steady-state free precession magnetic resonance images from a different patient with D-TGA, after atrial switch, demonstrate stenosis of the superior limb of a systemic baffle *(long arrows* in **E** and **F**), with resultant dilatation of the azygous arch *(short arrows* in **F**). The aorta can be seen arising from the anterior RV with the pulmonary artery arising from the posterior LV (**G**). Oblique coronal reformats (**H** and **I**) and thin MIP (**J**) CT images of a different patient with the same condition and surgical correction demonstrate leakage of high-density intravenous contrast material (*thin arrows* in **H** and **I**) from the superior limb of the systemic baffle (*thick arrows* in **H** and **I**) into the RA, which should receive only pulmonary venous blood. This patient had also required previous stenting (*arrow* in **J**) of the pulmonic venous baffle anastomosis because of stenosis.

Swedish surgeon Ake Senning, and it involved creation of a pathway through the right atrium that redirects systemic venous blood through conduits (baffles) across the mitral valve to the left (pulmonic) ventricle. The atrial septum is removed, leaving the pulmonary veins to drain into a common (systemic) atrium across the tricuspid valve into the right (systemic) ventricle. The two methods differ in the way the baffle is created. The Senning procedure uses the atrial septum, and the Mustard procedure uses bovine pericardium for creation of the conduits. Even though baffle procedures are no longer performed, adult patients with surgically corrected D-TGA who present for treatment today are often postoperative from this type of repair (Fig. 20-7, *A* to *G*).

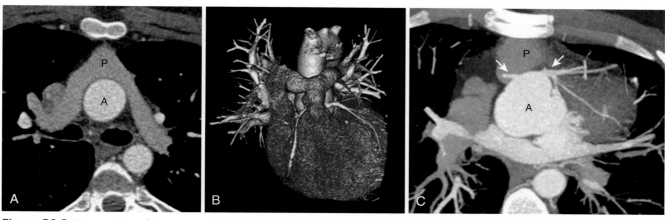

Figure 20-8 Transposition of the great arteries with arterial switch surgical correction. Axial (**A**), three-dimensional volume-rendered (**B**), and axial maximum intensity projection (**C**) computed tomography images demonstrate draping of the right and left pulmonary arteries (P) around the ascending aorta (A), with the pulmonary artery now anastomosed to the anterior right ventricle (**A** and **B**). The coronary arteries (*white arrows* in **C**) have been anastomosed to the anterior cusp of the aorta.

Overall, long-term outcomes after the Mustard and Senning procedures have been favorable. In a European study of 339 patients who underwent baffle operations, survival at 10, 20, and 30 years after surgery was 91.7%, 88.6%, and 79.3%, respectively, not including the 16.5% of patients who died within 30 days of the procedure. The most frequent complications are baffle leaks or stenoses (treated with stent placement and transcatheter occluder devices), tricuspid insufficiency, and right (systemic) ventricular failure. Arrhythmias also often develop and may result in sudden death, which, together with heart failure, is the most important cause of long-term mortality.

Atrial switch has been replaced by the arterial switch (Jatene) procedure (Fig. 20-8), which was developed in the late 1970s and early 1980s. The pulmonary artery is transected above the pulmonic valve, the aorta is transected above the coronary arteries, and the two vessels are switched and reanastomosed. To prevent stenosis of the pulmonary artery at the reimplantation site, augmentation of the pulmonary artery root is performed using a pericardial patch. The coronary arteries are excised from the aorta with a small cuff of surrounding vessel wall and are reimplanted into the neoaorta, after creation of small holes in the vessel wall just above its origin. The Lecompte maneuver, in which the pulmonary artery is placed anterior to the aortic root, was added in the 1980s, with the goal of elongating the neoaortic root to reduce kinking of the coronary arteries in the postsurgical patient. Any VSD is also repaired at the time of operation.

When patients present late (several months of life), reconditioning the left ventricle to handle systemic pressures may be necessary. This is accomplished by placing a synthetic or homograft band around the main pulmonary artery to increase left ventricular afterload before the Jatene switch is performed. The Jatene procedure, however, is ideally performed in the first or second week of life.

Some patients with D-TGA and a large VSD also have left ventricular outflow tract obstruction resulting from valvular stenosis. Initially, surgical repair in these patients

was done by arterial switch and concurrent repair of the stenotic valve. This approach was abandoned, however, because of frequent problems from recurrent left ventricular outflow tract obstruction. These defects are now repaired with the Rastelli procedure. In this operation, the pulmonary artery is divided from the left ventricle, and the site of stenosis in the left ventricular outflow tract is oversewn. A patch is then created to connect the left ventricle across the VSD and right ventricle to the aorta. The right ventricle is anastomosed through an extracardiac conduit to the pulmonary artery.

The Jatene arterial switch procedure has a more favorable outcome compared with the atrial switch operations because the morphologic ventricles are correctly paired with their respective workloads. The most common complication of the Jatene operation is pulmonic stenosis at the anastomotic site, which is often correctable by balloon angioplasty. Complications related to coronary artery kinking or stenosis at the reimplantation site are rare, occurring in less than 3% of patients. Left ventricular failure occurs but is also rare. Dilation of the neoaortic root has been described in approximately 50% of patients on long-term follow-up, but the cause of this complication is unclear. Dilation of the neoaortic annulus may lead to aortic regurgitation in a significant proportion of patients (~15% at a mean follow-up of 76 months and ≤30% by 15 years according to a study of 1156 of patients with D-TGA), although the degree of regurgitation is rarely significant. Most important, compared with baffle procedures, arrhythmias following Jatene switch are much less common.

Even though early complications of the Rastelli operation occur in less than 5% of patients, serious long-term complications are not uncommon. The incidence of late arrhythmia and sudden death is relatively high. Another common complication, frequently necessitating reintervention, is stenosis or obstruction of the right ventricle–to–pulmonary artery conduit, which, in a study of 94 survivors of the Rastelli procedure, occurred in 64 patients over a median follow-up of 8.7 years.

Imaging of patients with D-TGA can be performed with CT or MRI. CT is used more frequently in D-TGA because of the frequent presence of pacemakers. In patients who have undergone atrial switch correction, MDCT angiography (MDCTA) can be performed without gating, if no information about the coronary arteries or ventricular function is required. A noncontrast sequence should be performed to identify high-density or calcified baffles and patches, followed by an arterial phase timed to the systemic ventricle. A delayed phase is required to assess the inferior baffle limb connecting the IVC to the pulmonic ventricle. Multiplanar reconstructions on a three-dimensional workstation can display the course of the superior and inferior limbs of the baffle, to identify any areas of stenosis or leakage. Although the coronary artery origins and proximal courses may be visualized without gating, ECG-gated acquisition should be performed if detailed coronary analysis is desired. In patients who have undergone the arterial switch procedure, MDCTA including a low-dose precontrast sequence can be performed, timed to the aorta to assess for root dilatation or stenoses. A delayed phase in this case is not required.

In patients without contraindication who have undergone repair for D-TGA, quantitative assessment of pulmonic and systemic ventricular function can be performed using noncontrast MRI. Inversion recovery and SSFP sequences in oblique coronal and oblique sagittal planes are prescribed along the course of baffle limbs in patients after atrial switch. Dephasing jets and areas of focal narrowing indicate areas of baffle limb stenosis. Flow quantification with velocity encoded phase contrast imaging of the aorta and pulmonary artery is needed to exclude the presence of shunts. In cases of arterial switch, evaluation of aortic size and flow quantification to identify residual shunts and valvular regurgitation is required. Focal areas of narrowing and dephasing jets can be seen when pulmonary artery stenosis has developed, and flow quantification across these dephasing jets can provide pressure gradient estimates.

Levotransposition

Levo-TGA (L-TGA) is also an abnormality of conotruncal rotation, with the aortic root positioned to the left and anterior to the pulmonary trunk. The great vessels run parallel in their sagittal course, as they do in D-TGA. In contrast to D-TGA, however, the normal anatomic orientation of the ventricles is also reversed (ventricular inversion with AV discordance). The left atrium opens to the morphologic right ventricle, which is in the levo-position normally occupied by the left ventricle. As the AV valve follows its respective ventricle, the tricuspid valve separates the left atrium from the right (systemic) ventricle, which then gives rise to the aorta. The right atrium opens through the mitral valve to the morphologic left (pulmonic) ventricle, which is in dextroposition and gives rise to the pulmonary artery. Therefore, L-TGA is said to be congenitally corrected because both ventriculoarterial discordance and AV discordance are present (Fig. 20-9). In other words, two wrongs make it right. The direction of blood flow is cava to right atrium to (morphologic) left ventricle to pulmonary artery to pulmonary vein to left atrium to (morphologic) right ventricle to aorta. The coronary arteries tend to follow their respective ventricles.

Associated cardiac anomalies have been described. The most common are VSD, usually perimembranous and outlet types (incidence is ~70%), pulmonic stenosis (most commonly subvalvular affecting ~40% of patients), pulmonary atresia, and abnormalities of the tricuspid (systemic) AV valve that include displacement of the valve toward the apex (~32% of patients with L-TGA). Anomalies of the conduction system, which may predispose to arrhythmias, have also been reported, as has ventricular noncompaction.

Because the pulmonary and systemic circulations in L-TGA are not isolated, patients are mildly symptomatic or asymptomatic in infancy unless other cardiac anomalies are present. These patients may only come to attention, and may present for imaging for the first time, in adulthood. Long-term complications in patients who did not undergo surgical correction are most often the result of tricuspid valve failure and congestive heart failure as the right ventricle progressively fails against systemic vascular resistance. Clinical presentation in the adult patient may also be related to arrhythmia.

Historically, surgical correction, even in patients who were correctly diagnosed early on, focused on repair of any associated anomaly and left the underlying L-TGA intact. As complications in the adult with uncorrected L-TGA have become more widely recognized, surgical correction in early childhood is now advocated. Correction is accomplished by a combination of the atrial switch and arterial switch surgical procedures previously described in the discussion of D-TGA. This correction is accomplished by a Mustard or Senning operation, followed by either a Jatene switch or a Rastelli-type procedure (double switch procedure) (Fig. 20-10). The early operative morbidity is low, and results on intermediate follow-up have been encouraging. The double switch approach, however, is subject to the complications of its component surgical procedures, as described in the section on D-TGA.

■ HYPOPLASTIC LEFT HEART AND OTHER FUNCTIONALLY UNIVENTRICULAR CONDITIONS

Various conditions can result in cardiac circulation with a functionally single ventricle. Although a detailed discussion of each complex entity is beyond the scope of this chapter, the more commonly encountered lesions and their often shared surgical treatment are discussed briefly.

More commonly seen in boys, hypoplastic left heart syndrome is one of the most common reasons for cyanosis and congestive heart failure in the newborn. Encompassing hypoplasia of the left ventricle and varying degrees of hypoplasia or atresia of the aortic valve and ascending aorta, this syndrome is thought to arise from abnormalities in embryologic separation of the ventricles and conditions that limit left ventricular blood flow, believed to be required to form the left ventricle and proximal aorta. At birth, the infant derives systemic blood flow through a PDA, which is required for survival.

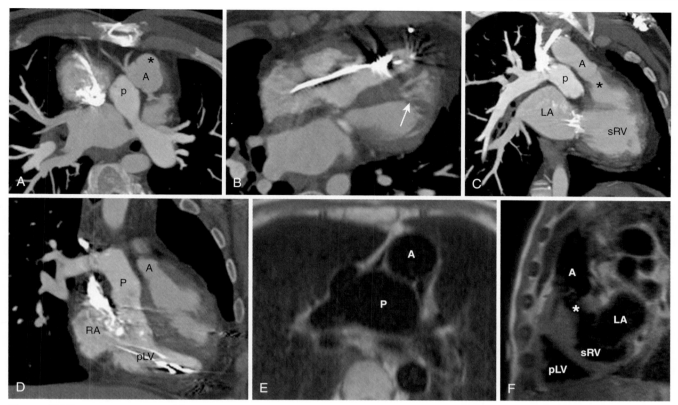

Figure 20-9 Levotransposition of the great arteries (L-TGA). **A to C,** Computed tomography images in a patient with uncorrected L-TGA show the aorta (A) arising anterior and left of the pulmonary artery (P) with the noncoronary cusp abnormally located in the anterior position (*asterisk* in **A**). The moderator band (*arrow* in **B**) and infundibulum (*asterisk* in **C**) are markers of the morphologic right ventricle (RV), which is in systemic position (sRV), giving rise to the aorta. Also visible is atrioventricular discordance with the pulmonary veins draining into the left atrium (LA) (**C**) that, in turn, feeds the sRV across a morphologic tricuspid valve that has been replaced (the atrioventricular valve generally follows its respective ventricle). **D,** The right atrium (RA) empties into the pulmonic left ventricle (pLV), thus giving rise to the pulmonary artery. **E** and **F,** Magnetic resonance imaging in a different patient with uncorrected L-TGA demonstrates similar findings on dark-blood images with the aorta lying anterior and to the left of the pulmonary artery (**E**) and the RV in systemic position (sRV in **F**) receiving blood from the LA and pumping across an infundibulum (asterisk in **F**) into the aorta.

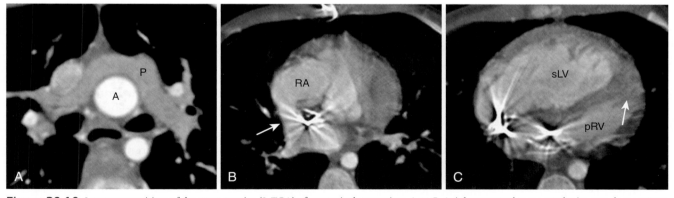

Figure 20-10 Levotransposition of the great arteries (L-TGA) after surgical correction. **A to C,** Axial computed tomography images demonstrate postsurgical changes of both atrial and arterial switch procedures in this pediatric patient who had undergone L-TGA repair with the double switch procedure. The pulmonary arteries are draped around the ascending aorta (A), with the main pulmonary artery (P) having been placed anterior to the aorta. The atrial inflow has also been switched, with the pulmonic venous return having been directed through a baffle (*arrow* in **B**) to the right atrium (RA). The right ventricle (RV), as identified by the moderator band (*arrow* in **C**) remains in an abnormal posterior location, but because of the atrial inflow and arterial outflow switches, is in pulmonic position (pRV). *sLV,* Systemic left ventricle.

Retrograde flow in the proximal aorta occurs during diastole to fill the great vessels and coronary arteries. Varying degrees of mitral stenosis or atresia may be present, and a patent foramen ovale or ASD allows pulmonary venous return to enter the right atrium. The severity of pulmonary venous congestion depends on the size of the ASD. In the era of staged surgical reconstruction that allows dedication of the morphologic single right ventricle to the systemic circulation and pulmonary blood flow through nonventricular conduits, patients now routinely survive into adulthood, although they are at risk for complications related to the surgical repair.

Univentricular AV connection syndromes, although rare, also result in single ventricle systems. Identification of the morphologic characteristics of the single ventricle as right or left is important. The characteristic features of the right ventricle are course trabeculations, separation of the inflow and outflow valves, and the presence of an infundibulum, whereas the left ventricle lacks separation of inflow and outflow valves and typically has fewer trabeculations. Double inlet, single inlet, and common inlet conditions exist.

Double inlet AV conditions have a single ventricle receiving inflow from both the tricuspid and mitral valves, with a variety of AV valvular malformations and the potential for unbalanced alignments of the valves with the ventricle. Most patients with double inlet ventricle have a morphologic left ventricle. Common inlet AV conditions are most frequently seen in patients with trisomy 21 or heterotaxy, who have AV canal defects, as discussed earlier in this chapter.

Single inlet ventricle occurs from atresia of the mitral or tricuspid valve that results in either a single right or left ventricle, respectively, that receives inflow from one atrial chamber. Patients with tricuspid atresia have varying degrees of hypoplasia of the right ventricle caused by lack of forward blood flow (preload) into the chamber during development. In many cases, the trabecular portion of the right ventricle is underdeveloped, whereas an infundibular component remains. In this disorder, an ASD, usually a patent foramen ovale or an ostium secundum type, allows venous blood to mix with systemic oxygenated blood in the left atrium. If a VSD is present, the systemic left ventricle provides pulmonary blood flow across the defect into the pulmonary artery. In the absence of a VSD, which is quite rare, pulmonary blood flow is through a PDA, and the patient usually has more severe atresia of the right ventricle and pulmonary artery.

Although countless different combinations of lesions and disorders leading to a functionally single ventricular system exist, the surgical treatment is often similar. The goal is to separate the systemic and pulmonic circulations by creating a systemic-to–pulmonary artery connection without an intervening ventricular chamber, thus allowing dedication of the single ventricle to the systemic circulation. In other words, the pulmonary arteries fill passively through vena cava–to–pulmonary artery shunts, and the single ventricle is used to pump against the aorta. Done in stages to protect the pulmonary circulation and avoid ventricular volume overload, the Norwood procedure, including the Fontan and modified Fontan procedures, was initially devised for treatment of patients with hypoplastic left heart syndrome, but its use has expanded for treatment of other univentricular conditions (Fig. 20-11).

The first stage is centered on establishment of reliable pulmonary blood flow. Initially, a Blalock-Taussig shunt was used. This shunt involved takedown of the subclavian artery and anastomosis to the ipsilateral pulmonary artery. Today, a modified Blalock-Taussig shunt, made of synthetic graft material, is used. It has fewer anastomotic complications and avoids sacrifice of the subclavian artery. A newer modification of this first stage is the Sano procedure, which involves creation of a right ventricle–to–pulmonary artery conduit that theoretically would avoid the potential for aorticopulmonary runoff by providing simultaneous perfusion of the systemic and pulmonic systems. In the past, anastomosis of the descending thoracic aorta to the distal left pulmonary artery (Potts shunt) or anastomosis of the ascending aorta to the proximal right pulmonary artery (Waterston shunt) was used to provide pulmonary artery blood flow in situations where this flow was compromised, but these procedures frequently resulted in the development of pulmonary arterial hypertension, pulmonary vascular bed injury, and distortion of the pulmonary artery at the anastomosis. In the case of hypoplastic left heart syndrome, the stage I procedure also includes creation of a neoaorta by using the main pulmonary artery. The hypoplastic ascending aorta is kept as a conduit for the coronary arteries. A nonrestrictive ASD may also be created to prevent pulmonary venous hypertension. In some patients, pulmonary artery banding may also be used to guard against pulmonary overcirculation and ensuing pulmonary hypertension.

In the second stage, a superior cavopulmonary connection is established, and the systemic-to–pulmonary arterial shunt is removed. Although no longer widely used, a classic Glenn connection involved isolation of the right pulmonary artery from the main pulmonary artery and right atrium and anastomosis to the SVC. In this situation, upper body venous return was completely to the right lung, and lower body venous return admixed with oxygenated blood in the now common systemic atrium. Today, a bidirectional Glenn anastomosis to the right pulmonary artery is used, with the main pulmonary artery isolated from the right atrium, thus leaving the branch pulmonary arteries in continuity. An alternative procedure, the hemi-Fontan operation, leaves the pulmonary arteries in continuity with the right atrium but creates an anastomosis from the SVC to the confluent pulmonary arteries by using a patch to close the normal SVC-to–right atrial communication. A bidirectional Glenn anastomosis is technically easier to perform, whereas the hemi-Fontan procedure allows for a faster stage 3 completion Fontan surgery.

In the third stage, the systemic and pulmonary circulations are completely isolated. In a classic Fontan repair, the IVC blood is directed to the pulmonary circulation through anastomosis of the right atrial appendage to the confluence of the pulmonary arteries, the stage 1 ASD is repaired, and the stage 2 classic Glenn anastomosis connecting the SVC to the isolated right pulmonary

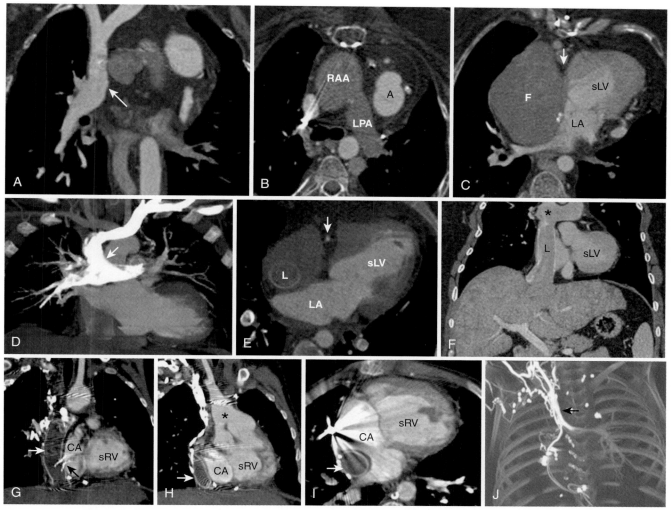

Figure 20-11 Cavopulmonary surgical treatments for univentricular heart conditions. A to **C,** Computed tomography (CT) images from a patient with tricuspid atresia who underwent a classic Fontan surgical correction demonstrate a unilateral Glenn anastomosis (*arrow* in **A**) that connects the superior vena cava to the isolated right pulmonary artery and a Fontan correction (F) formed by connecting the right atrial appendage (RAA) to the left pulmonary artery (LPA) directing blood flow from the lower body to the left pulmonary circulation. Note the fat bar (*arrow* in **C**) in the right atrioventricular groove indicating atresia of the tricuspid valve with resultant near complete atresia of the right ventricle in this patient with a functionally univentricular systemic left ventricle (sLV). **D** to **F,** In a different patient with tricuspid atresia, a modified surgical technique, commonly referred to as a hemi-Fontan procedure, was used for correction. A bidirectional Glenn anastomosis (*arrow* in **D**) connecting the superior vena cava to the confluence of the pulmonary arteries has been created, and an intracardiac lateral tunnel (L) has been created directing inferior vena caval blood to the confluence of the pulmonary arteries (*asterisk* in **F**). Differential enhancement of the blood pool outside the lateral tunnel (**E**) in the right atrium with respect to the left atrium (LA) results from the phase of contrast from an upper extremity injection because the atrial chambers are in free communication as part of the surgical correction. Note the heterogeneity of the liver (**F**) secondary to sluggish flow in the lateral tunnel and resulting in chronic passive hepatic congestion. The classic fat bar (*arrow* in **E**) is again noted, as a result of tricuspid atresia. **G** to **J,** A patient who underwent total cavopulmonary correction using an extracardiac lateral tunnel for underlying hypoplastic left heart syndrome is seen on CT to have a conduit (*white arrows* in **G** to **I**) lying outside the now common atrium (CA) directing inferior vena caval blood to the confluence of the pulmonary arteries. A bidirectional Glenn anastomosis (*arrow* in **J**) of the superior vena cava to the pulmonary arteries which have been left in continuity is present. This patient has had a stent placed within a fenestration of the conduit (*black arrow* in **G**) to allow a small degree of communication between the systemic venous system and the pulmonary venous chamber. Because of hypoplasia of the ascending aorta, in stage I of the Norwood procedure, a neoaorta was constructed, which in this case involved anastomosis (*asterisk* in **H**) of the main pulmonary artery and ascending aorta to create a systemic arterial feeding vessel arising from the functionally univentricular systemic right ventricle (sRV). *A,* Aorta.

artery is left in place. Today, two modified Fontan procedures are widely performed. In patients who have had a stage 2 bidirectional Glenn anastomosis, an extracardiac prosthetic conduit is placed connecting the IVC to the confluence of the pulmonary arteries. Those patients treated with a stage 2 hemi-Fontan procedure undergo creation of an intracardiac lateral tunnel that uses part of the atrial wall and prosthetic conduit to direct inferior caval blood to the confluence of the pulmonary arteries. In either modification, a fenestration allowing communication between either the lateral tunnel or the extracardiac prosthetic conduit and the systemic atrium is frequently created to allow a small portion of blood to bypass the pulmonary circulation when pulmonary vascular resistance is elevated. Although this technique preserves adequate filling of the systemic ventricle, it does

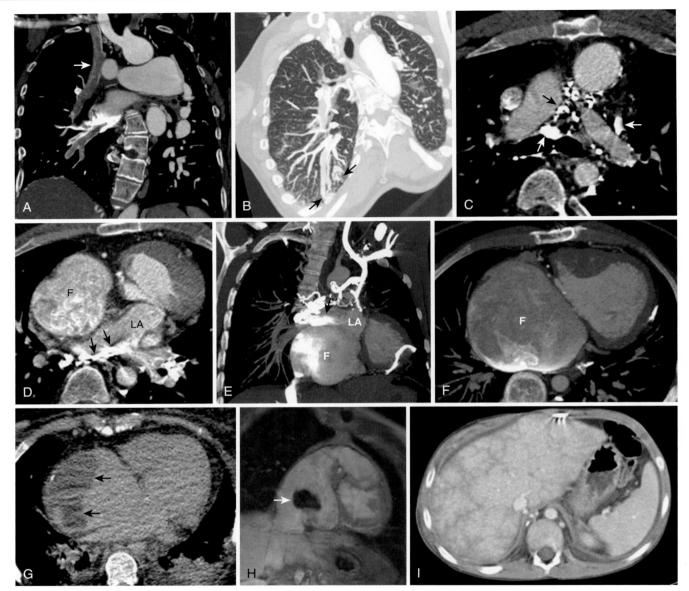

Figure 20-12 Complications of cavopulmonary surgical corrections. A and B, A patient with a unidirectional Glenn anastomosis to the right pulmonary artery (*arrow* in **A**) was found to have numerous right pulmonary arteriovenous malformations (*arrows* in **B**), a commonly reported complication of unidirectional or bidirectional Glenn anastomoses. **C** to **F**, Computed tomography (CT) images with contrast injected through the left upper extremity in a patient with tricuspid atresia treated with the classic Fontan (F) procedure demonstrates filling with high-density contrast material of numerous venovenous collateral channels (*arrows* in **C** to **F**) that drain directly into the left atrium (LA; *arrows* in **D** and **E**) and create a right-to-left shunt. Note the dilated Fontan baffle and absent tricuspid valve plane (*asterisk* in **F**) resulting from underlying tricuspid atresia and leaving a functionally univentricular left ventricle. Because of sluggish forward flow, Fontan baffles frequently dilate over time, and this can lead to atrial arryhthmias and stasis of blood flow. As demonstrated on axial CT (**G**) and oblique coronal postcontrast magnetic resonance imaging (**H**) scans in two different patients, thrombus (*arrows*) can form in this setting. **I**, A different patient who underwent total cavopulmonary anastomosis for hypoplastic left heart syndrome was found to have chronic passive congestion of the liver leading to the classic "nutmeg" appearance of the hepatic parenchyma on CT secondary to sluggish forward flow of inferior vena caval blood. This can lead to cardiac cirrhosis and is also thought to play a role in the development of protein-losing enteropathy.

allow for low-level right-to-left shunting that can exacerbate cyanosis. However, the fenestration can be closed if necessary by surgical or percutaneous transcatheter techniques.

In addition to knowledge of postsurgical anatomy, imagers must also be aware of complications associated with univentricular repair that can be seen on CT and MRI. Low levels of hypoxia are not uncommon following repair, although hypoxia can be exacerbated by

certain complications. A well-known complication of superior cavopulmonary anastomosis is the development of pulmonary arteriovenous malformations, estimated to occur in up to 25% of patients (Fig. 20-12, *A* and *B*). Although the exact mechanism remains unclear, lack of admixture with hepatic venous blood is thought to play a role because arteriovenous malformations have been reported to resolve with reestablishment of exposure to IVC blood flow. These complications are best seen on contrast-enhanced magnetic resonance angiography (MRA) or CTA, but given the inherent contrast difference between blood vessels and lung parenchyma, thin collimation noncontrast CT can also be used for evaluation.

Venovenous collateral vessels often develop after stage 2 correction and result from differences in upper body and lower body systemic venous pressures. This situation creates a gradient for collateral flow either through the azygos or hemiazygos system to the lower-pressure IVC system or by reopening of embryonic venous connections draining directly into the pulmonary veins and left atrium (see Fig. 20-12, C to F). The results are right-to-left shunting and exacerbation of cyanosis. Because most intravenous contrast injections are administered through the upper extremities, early phase imaging (at 15 seconds after injection) demonstrates filling of these collateral venous channels, with high-density contrast material shunting into the pulmonary veins and left atrium. Bilateral simultaneous upper extremity injections may be used to improve detection of venovenous collateral vessels. If evaluation is with MRI, close attention for residual ASD and VSD should be paid, as evidenced by dephasing jets, and flow quantification for Qp/Qs assessment should be performed.

Aortopulmonary collateral vessels (see Fig. 20-6), often from the bronchial or internal mammary circulation, can develop in the setting of chronic hypoxia as a way of increasing blood flow to the lungs. These vessels are best seen in systemic arterial phase, although often they can also be identified on noncontrast MRI SSFP sequences. In addition to increasing the workload of the systemic ventricle, these vessels can increase the risk of bleeding if reoperation is required. Percutaneous coil embolization of either venovenous or aortopulmonary collateral vessels can be performed.

Thrombus can develop within conduits or cardiac chambers from sluggish flow or exposure to thrombogenic suture material and can result in systemic or pulmonary thromboembolic events (see Fig. 20-12, G and H). Care must be taken when imaging patients with complicated postsurgical anatomy and shunts not to confuse nonopacification of a vessel or conduit with thrombus. Delayed phase CT sequences are often required to allow time for opacification of vessels not in direct communication with the site of contrast injection.

Systemic ventricular dysfunction can develop as a result of complications mentioned earlier, as well as inherent morphologic characteristics in the setting of a systemic right ventricle. MRI can accurately quantify ventricular volume and ejection fraction in addition to identifying AV valve insufficiency.

Arrhythmias are frequent in this patient population and are often atrial. This complication can result from surgical manipulation of the right atrium with suture lines, sinus node dysfunction, or, in the case of classic Fontan corrections, dilatation of the right atrium. Protein-losing enteropathy is another rare complication with high mortality that is thought to result from increased hepatic and portal venous pressures that lead to mucosal bowel injury and dysfunction (see Fig. 20-12, I).

■ CONCLUSION

As surgical advances continue to be made, many patients born with even complex forms of congenital heart disease are surviving into adulthood. Therefore, imagers will encounter these patients either as a result of cardiac complications or during routine evaluation of non--cardiac-related disease. Although imaging the patient with congenital heart disease can seem like a daunting task, familiarity with the more commonly used surgical procedures in conjunction with a systematic approach to evaluation can lead to accurate interpretation.

Bibliography

Abbara S, Soni AV, Cury RC. Evaluation of cardiac function and valves by multidetector row computed tomography. *Semin Roentgenol.* 2008;43:145-153.

Banerji D, Martinez F, Abbara S, Truong QA. Turner syndrome with aberrant right subclavian artery and partial anomalous pulmonary venous return. *J Cardiovasc Comput Tomogr.* 2011;5:189-191.

Bardo DM, Frankel DG, Applegate KE, Murphy DJ, Saneto RP. Hypoplastic left heart syndrome. *Radiographics.* 2001;21:705-717.

Braverman AC, Guven H, Beardslee MD, et al. The bicuspid aortic valve. *Curr Prob Cardiol.* 2005;30:470-522.

Brickner ME, Hillis LD, Lange RA. Congenital heart disease in adults. First of two parts. *N Engl J Med.* 2000;342:256-263.

Brickner ME, Hillis LD, Lange RA. Congenital heart disease in adults. Second of two parts. *N Engl J Med.* 2000;342:334-342.

Devaney E, Charpie J, Ohye RG, Bove EL. Combined arterial switch and Senning operation for congenitally corrected transposition of the great arteries: patient selection and intermediate results. *J Thorac Cardiovasc Surg.* 2003;125:500-507.

Dos L, Teruel L, Ferreira IJ, et al. Late outcome of Senning and Mustard procedures for correction of transposition of the great arteries. *Heart.* 2005;91:652-656.

Duerinckx A, Atkinson D, Klitzner TS, Perloff J, Drinkwater D, Laks H. MR imaging of surgical complications of systemic-to-pulmonary artery shunts. *Magn Reson Imaging.* 1996;14:1099-1105.

Duncan BW, Mee RB, Mesia CL, et al. Results of the double switch operation for congenitally corrected transposition of the great arteries. *Eur J Cardiothorac Surg.* 2003;24:11-19:discussion 19-20.

Fallot E. Contribution à l'anatomie pathologique de la maladie bleu (cyanose cardiaque). *Mars Med.* 1888:25.

Gaca AM, Jaggers JJ, Dudley LT, Bisset 3rd GS. Repair of congenital heart disease: a primer. Part 1. *Radiology.* 2008;247:617-631.

Geva T, Sandweiss BM, Gauvreau K, Lock JE, Powell AJ. Factors associated with impaired clinical status in long-term survivors of tetralogy of Fallot repair evaluated by magnetic resonance imaging. *J Am Coll Cardiol.* 2004;43:1068-1074.

Graham TP, Bernard YD, Mellen BG, et al. Long-term outcome in congenitally corrected transposition of the great arteries: a multi-institutional study. *J Am Coll Cardiol.* 2000;36:255-261.

Halliburton SS, Abbara S, Chen MY, et al. SCCT guidelines on radiation dose and dose-optimization strategies in cardiovascular CT. *J Cardiovasc Comput Tomogr.* 2011;5:198-224.

Hoffman JI, Kaplan S. The incidence of congenital heart disease. *J Am Coll Cardiol.* 2002;39:1890-1900.

Hornung TS, Derrick GP, Deanfield JE, Redington AN. Transposition complexes in the adult: a changing perspective. *Cardiol Clin.* 2002;20:405-420.

Hutter PA, Kreb DL, Mantel SF, Hitchcock JF, Meijboom EJ, Bennink GB. Twenty-five years' experience with the arterial switch operation. *J Thorac Cardiovasc Surg.* 2002;124:790-797.

Jacobs JP, Burke RP, Quintessenza JA, Mavroudis C. Congenital heart surgery nomenclature and database project: ventricular septal defect. *Ann Thorac Surg.* 2000;69(Suppl):S25-S35.

Karamlou T, McCrindle BW, Williams WG. Surgery insight: late complications following repair of tetralogy of Fallot and related surgical strategies for management. *Nat Clin Pract Cardiovasc Med.* 2006;3:611-622.

Knauth AL, Gauvreau K, Powell AJ, et al. Ventricular size and function assessed by cardiac MRI predict major adverse clinical outcomes late after tetralogy of Fallot repair. *Heart.* 2008;94:211-216.

Kouchoukos NT, Masetti P, Nickerson NJ, Castner CF, Shannon WD, Davila-Roman VG. The Ross procedure: long-term clinical and echocardiographic follow-up. *Ann Thorac Surg.* 2004;78:773-781.

Levin D, Fellows K, Sos T. Angiographic demonstration of complications resulting from the Waterston procedure. *AJR Am J Roentgenol.* 1978;131:431-437.

Liebman J, Cullum L, Belloc NB. Natural history of transposition of the great arteries: anatomy and birth and death characteristics. *Circulation.* 1969;40:237-262.

Nollert G, Fischlein T, Bouterwek S, Bohmer C, Klinner W, Reichart B. Long-term survival in patients with repair of tetralogy of Fallot: 36-year follow-up of 490 survivors of the first year after surgical repair. *J Am Coll Cardiol.* 1997;30:1374-1383.

Norgaard MA, Lauridsen P, Helvind M, Patterson G. Twenty-to-thirty-seven-year follow-up after repair for tetralogy of Fallot. *Eur J Cardiothorac Surg.* 1999;16:125-130.

Pasquali SK, Hasselblad V, Li JS, Kong DF, Sanders SP. Coronary artery pattern and outcome of arterial switch operation for transposition of the great arteries: a meta-analysis. *Circulation.* 2002;106:2575-2580.

Pouler AC, le Polain de Waroux JB, Pasquet A, Vanoverschelde JL, Gerber BL. Aortic valve area assessment: multidetector CT compared with cine MR imaging and transthoracic and transesophageal echocardiography. *Radiology.* 2007;244:745-754.

Rojas CA, El-Sherief A, Medina HM, et al. Embryology and developmental defects of the interatrial septum. *AJR Am J Roentgenol.* 2010;195:1100-1104.

Rojas CA, Jaimes CE, El-Sherief AH, et al. Cardiac CT of non-shunt pathology of the interatrial septum. *J Cardiovasc Comput Tomogr.* 2011;5:93-100.

Sideris EB, Walsh KP, Haddad JL, Chen CR, Ren SG, Kulkarni H. Occlusion of congenital ventricular septal defects: "buttoned device" clinical trials international register. *Heart.* 1997;77:276-279.

Thakrar A, Shapiro MD, Jassal DS, Neilan TG, King ME, Abbara S. Cor triatriatum: the utility of cardiovascular imaging. *Can J Cardiol.* 2007;23:143-145.

Wiant A, Nyberg E, Gilkeson RC. CT evaluation of congenital heart disease in adults. *AJR Am J Roentgenol.* 2009;193:388-396.

CHAPTER **21**

Role of Magnetic Resonance Imaging in Cardiomyopathies

Stephan Danik and Jeremy Ruskin

The use of magnetic resonance imaging (MRI) in cardiac diseases has been advancing rapidly, and this technique has become the gold standard for diagnosing many of the pathologic conditions encountered in clinical practice. MRI is an indispensable tool to aid in clinical decision making. Although traditional modalities such as single photon emission computed tomography (SPECT) and echocardiography continue to be the mainstays of cardiac imaging, MRI can provide data that are both complementary and uniquely distinct, thus allowing for insights into the disease process that until recently were not possible.

This chapter focuses on the ability of cardiac magnetic resonance (CMR) to aid in the management of both ischemic and nonischemic cardiomyopathies. Although much of this discussion highlights the ability of CMR to diagnose various myopathies, it also reviews the role of CMR as an important tool in various decision-making processes encountered on a daily basis by the clinician. Such instances include deciding whether to pursue revascularization in ischemic cardiomyopathies and determining when it is appropriate to recommend implantation of an implantable cardioverter-defibrillator (ICD) in the myopathic heart.

A clinical vignette is offered as an introduction to each topic discussed. The hope is that such a format will highlight the practical implications of the current data available on the use of CMR in a particular pathologic process. Although the amount and quality of supportive data may vary for each clinical instance, the data reflect the "real world" challenges that clinicians face when treating patients.

■ ISCHEMIC CARDIOMYOPATHY: WHEN TO REVASCULARIZE?

Case 1

A 70-year-old male patient with a history of diabetes, hypertension, and elevated cholesterol and a prior history of a distant myocardial infarction undergoes an evaluation for gradually progressive dyspnea on exertion. An echocardiogram shows a mildly dilated left ventricle and an ejection fraction of 38% with regional wall motion abnormalities. Exercise treadmill testing with SPECT imaging is performed, and the patient is able to exercise for 5 minutes of Bruce protocol (see Chapter 5 for details of Bruce protocol). No changes are noted on the electrocardiogram (ECG), and the patient has mostly fixed defects in the anterior and lateral walls with "mild reversibility." He is already taking a beta-blocker, a statin, aspirin, and an angiotensin-converting enzyme (ACE) inhibitor as part of his medical regimen.

Should the patient undergo cardiac catheterization even though the clinician knows that this patient will have significant coronary disease, given that noninvasive imaging seems to indicate mostly scarred myocardium? Would any benefit result from revascularization with the present data from the stress test and echocardiogram? Would an invasive strategy provide any benefit, given that the patient is already following a good medical regimen?

Importance of Viable Myocardium

The clinician should establish whether any chance exists that the patient has viable myocardium that will benefit from restoration of blood flow. In patients with an area of previously infarcted myocardium, the tissue is often a heterogeneous mixture of both scar and noncontractile but still surviving myofibers. Although the tissue has reduced perfusion from the ischemic substrate, residual metabolic function is present. This dysfunctional but viable tissue in the setting of chronic coronary disease has been classified as hibernating myocardium. In patients with viable myocardium, restoration of blood flow through revascularization improves survival as compared with patients who are treated medically (Fig. 21-1).

This mortality benefit occurs even without an improvement in left ventricular (LV) function. Studies also have shown that attempts to revascularize nonviable tissue provide no survival benefit and stress the need to be sure that the diagnostic imaging has high sensitivity and specificity. However, patients with severely dilated hearts tend to fare worse than do patients with smaller LV volumes. This finding may reflect the chronicity of the ischemia or the extent of adverse remodeling. Even in patients with demonstrable viable tissue, revascularization may not be possible, especially in those with prior coronary artery bypass grafting or diabetic patients with poor target vessels. Despite areas of viable myocardium, these patients are treated medically, with the subsequent risk of higher mortality. Not surprisingly, in small, nonrandomized studies, sudden cardiac death was the leading cause of mortality in patients with hibernating myocardium who were treated medically.

Role of Cardiac Magnetic Resonance in the Search for Viable Tissue

Is a superior method available to assess whether any of the tissue is viable? Most clinicians agree that all the traditional methods (dobutamine MRI, contrast-enhanced MRI, SPECT with thallium-201, SPECT with technetium-99m tracers, positron emission tomography/SPECT with fluorodeoxyglucose) provide the data necessary to assess whether and to what extent viable tissue is present. Few data are available that compare noninvasive methods "head to head" to determine which is superior. CMR is able to detect viable tissue by measuring end-diastolic wall thickness, evaluate contractile reserve, and detect the degree of transmurality of scar tissue. The ability to identify the presence of transmural scar (involving the entire thickness of myocardium) is important because this finding suggests that functional recovery will not improve even with restoration of blood flow. Earlier studies validated the use of MRI in the assessment of viable myocardium, and MRI can distinguish infarcts with variable degrees of nontransmural scar from transmural scars. Generally speaking, myocardium with a scar (delayed hyperenhancement) that occupies less than 50% of the wall thickness is likely to improve in function after revascularization.

Data suggest that the sensitivity and specificity of regional wall improvement as predicted by CMR are 82% and 67%, respectively. Studies suggest that CMR carries important prognostic information for general cardiovascular outcomes. An additional benefit of CMR is the absence of radiation, although caution must be taken if gadolinium is used in patients with severe renal insufficiency. In general, most clinicians agree that at least 25% of the left ventricle should be "viable" to pursue revascularization.

Case 1 Continued

The patient has diabetes and a depressed ejection fraction. If the patient has significant coronary disease (especially left anterior descending coronary artery disease) that can be revascularized, the patient's life can be prolonged. The use of CMR may be beneficial in this situation if the actual amount of viable tissue is near this cutoff, as may be suggested by the initial SPECT imaging (although it was not a viability study). Cardiac catheterization would be reasonable to establish coronary disease as the cause. Revascularization can then be performed if viable tissue is indeed present.

■ ISCHEMIC CARDIOMYOPATHY AND THE RISK OF SUDDEN CARDIAC DEATH

Case 2

A 69-year-old male patient with a history of coronary artery disease with prior coronary artery bypass grafting 10 years earlier and known ischemic cardiomyopathy presents to his cardiologist for a yearly checkup. The patient feels well and walks regularly 5 days a week for 20 minutes at a time. He has been closely followed by his cardiologist, and his last echocardiogram a year ago was remarkable for a mildly dilated left ventricle with an ejection fraction of 40% without significant valvular abnormalities. The patient's medication regimen includes aspirin, a beta-blocker, an ACE inhibitor, a statin, and a low-dose diuretic. His ECG shows sinus rhythm at 64 beats/minute with occasional premature ventricular contractions (PVCs), an old anterior wall myocardial infarction, and a QRS complex duration of 96 msec. He has New York Heart Association (NYHA) class II congestive heart failure (CHF), and a 24-hour Holter monitor shows occasional PVCs with couplets, but no triplets. A repeat echocardiogram shows an ejection fraction of 34%. Repeat stress testing with perfusion imaging results in his exercising for 9 minutes of Bruce protocol (10 metabolic equivalents [METS]) without ECG abnormalities. Perfusion imaging shows scar in the anterior apical region without reversible ischemia with a calculated ejection fraction of 38%. After the data are obtained, the patient's cardiologist opens the conversation about the role of an ICD. The patient feels well and desires more information and data about whether he really needs one. The patient's internist suggests cardiac MRI to obtain a "true" ejection fraction.

Sudden Cardiac Death: Can Cardiac Magnetic Resonance Provide Useful Prognostic Information?

Sudden cardiac death, the leading cause of cardiovascular mortality in the United States, claims approximately 400,000 lives each year. Patients with a history of coronary artery disease, previous myocardial infarction, and depressed LV function are at increased risk for ventricular

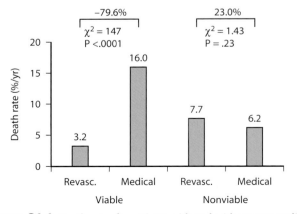

Figure 21-1 Death rates for patients with and without myocardial viability treated by revascularization or medical therapy. The reduction in mortality for patients with viability treated by revascularization is 79.6% ($P < .0001$). In patients without myocardial viability, no significant difference in mortality with revascularization (Revasc.) versus medical therapy is noted.

arrhythmias, which are responsible for most cases of this syndrome.

Based on data from the Sudden Cardiac Death from Heart Failure Trial (SCD-HeFT) and the Multicenter Automatic Defibrillator Implantation Trial (MADIT II), the current standard of care supports the implantation of an ICD in the patient in this case study. The SCD-HeFT enrolled patients with ischemic or nonischemic cardiomyopathy with an ejection fraction of up to 35% and class II or III NYHA, whereas the MADIT II enrolled patients with ischemic cardiomyopathy with an ejection fraction of up to 30% and NHYA class I, II, and III CHF. Further examination of the two trials found that approximately 20% of implanted ICDs had fired appropriately during 4 years of follow-up, thus subjecting most patients to the morbidity of having implanted hardware without receiving benefit. Although ejection fraction is a strong predictor of ventricular tachyarrhythmias, it is relatively nonspecific, and other clinical characteristics are needed to help stratify risk in these patients appropriately.

Because of the lack of a satisfactory way to stratify these patients, the search for a diagnostic test that could serve as a noninvasive means of identifying patients at risk for sudden cardiac death has rapidly evolved. Exercise treadmill testing and myocardial perfusion imaging have provided important prognostic information for patients at risk for cardiovascular morbidity and mortality, but not specifically for arrhythmogenic death.

Mechanism of Ventricular Tachycardia

To help identify patients at risk for sudden death, an understanding of the basic mechanism of ventricular tachycardia (VT) in the patient with coronary artery disease is critical. Earlier work in animal and human pathologic specimens showed that both a substrate and a trigger are required for the initiation and propagation of the reentry circuit. The trigger that initiates the arrhythmia may result from multiple factors such as ischemia, changes in autonomic tone, and neurohormonal and metabolic influences. The anatomic substrate is scar tissue around which propagation exhibits slow conduction and thus allows for maintenance of reentry circuits. The surviving myocardial fibers surrounding and interspersed within the infarcted region provide the electrical heterogeneity that is required for differences in conduction velocity, functional block, and alterations in cell-to-cell coupling.

The elucidation of this mechanism was demonstrated elegantly in explanted human hearts studied with high-resolution mapping (Fig. 21-2). In these hearts that had sustained VT, mapping localized slow conduction that

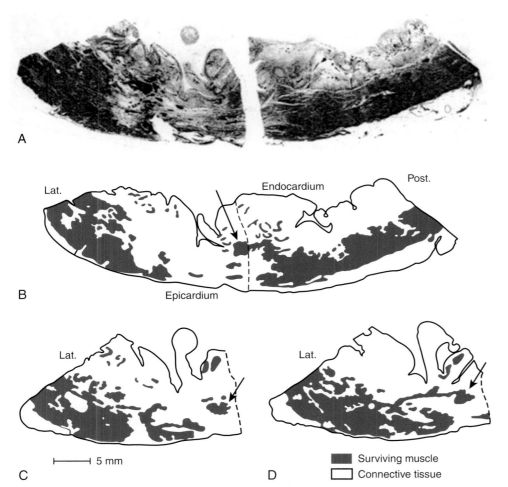

Figure 21-2 A, Photomicrograph of sections of Langendorff-perfused human heart. The patient had a history of myocardial infarction, coronary artery disease, and ventricular tachycardia. *Dark areas* mark surviving cardiac tissue; *light areas* point to fibrotic and fatty tissue. B, Schematic drawings of the section. C and D, Schematic drawings of sections beneath B. The *arrow* denotes a continuous patch of viable tissue coursing through the lateral and posterior wall.

is critical for reentry along a complex network of surviving myocytes interspersed in and around the scar. These findings helped to complement earlier work in animal models that demonstrated the presence of a circuit in the "border zone" of tissue made of scar and surviving myocardium.

Detecting Scar and Ventricular Tachyarrhythmias: Is Quantification of Scar Enough?

Knowing that the presence of scar or fibrosis could represent a potential substrate for ventricular tachyarrhythmias, investigators have sought to determine whether prognostic information can be obtained using CMR in various myopathic processes, including hypertrophic cardiomyopathy (HCM) and ischemic and nonischemic cardiomyopathies.

Earlier data suggested that total cardiac enzyme released during a myocardial infarction is a predictor of future cardiovascular outcomes. The absolute quantity of necrosed tissue may therefore be reflected by the extent of scarred myocardium. The extent of scar tissue, as determined by stress testing with myocardial perfusion (technetium) imaging, has been demonstrated to be an important predictor of death and ventricular arrhythmias. In 349 patients with ischemic cardiomyopathy and a depressed ejection fraction, the degree of quantifiable scar as determined by CMR was a predictor of death or the need for cardiac transplantation. In addition, this study found that female gender with scar was also a positive predictor of cardiac events. Similarly, delayed enhanced MRI (DE-MRI) performed in 231 patients with prior healed myocardial infarctions demonstrated that infarct size was a better predictor of long-term mortality than was LV ejection fraction.

Although the ability to quantify scar accurately in patients with coronary artery disease may be useful to reflect the size of a prior myocardial infarction accurately, whether this information will be useful to predict who is likely to develop ventricular tachyarrhythmias, as opposed to mortality resulting from CHF or myocardial infarction, is not clear. One small study found that infarct mass, as determined by DE-MRI, was shown to be a better predictor than LV ejection fraction of inducible monomorphic VT at electrophysiology study in patients ($n = 48$) with a history of coronary artery disease.

Investigators had hoped that the DETERMINE study would determine whether infarct mass alone could appropriately stratify risk in patients. This study was to test the hypothesis that patients with an infarct size of at least 10% randomized to ICD and medical therapy would have improved survival as compared with those randomized to medical therapy alone. Patients with coronary disease and an ejection fraction between 35% and 50% (or patients with an ejection fraction of 30% to 35% and NYHA class I heart failure without a history of ventricular tachyarrhythmias) would have undergone CMR imaging to determine the infarct size. Unfortunately, the trial was stopped by the sponsor. As of now, the investigators have no future plans to move

forward, and so the answer to this question remains unknown.

Characterizing the Border Zone: The Intersection of Scar and Viable Tissue

Although the presence of scar is critical in forming the basis of the substrate for ventricular tachyarrhythmias, a considerable effort has been made to try to "visualize" the interface between scar and surviving tissue. Attempts to characterize scar and the surrounding border zone in patients with a prior myocardial infarction have been made using CMR. Furthermore, initial reports seem to yield promising results regarding prognostic information in potentially high-risk patients.

An initial report characterized the mechanical properties of LV wall segments containing different degrees of scar tissue and the location of these segments from the interface between infarcted and noninfarcted myocardial tissue. A total of 46 patients underwent electrophysiologic testing before subsequent implantation of an ICD for primary prevention of sudden cardiac death. Patients with inducible monomorphic VT during electrophysiology study were more likely to have more infracted and border zone segments as compared with patients whose VT was noninducible. Furthermore, patients with inducible monomorphic VT were more likely to have border zones segments with greater systolic contractility as compared with patients with noninducible VT. These findings suggested that "enhanced" border zone function as determined by DE-MRI may be a marker of inducible monomorphic VT. This characterization of the mixture of viable and nonviable tissue (tissue heterogeneity) and how it relates to arrhythmogenesis further strengthened the potential prognostic capabilities of DE-MRI.

More recently, Roes et al examined whether infarct tissue heterogeneity could serve as a predictor of spontaneous ventricular tachyarrhythmias. Ninety-one patients with a prior myocardial infarction underwent DE-MRI before implantation of an ICD. After a median follow-up period of 8.5 months, 18 patients had received appropriate ICD therapy. Infarct tissue heterogeneity was a better predictor of appropriate ICD therapy as compared with LV function, LV volume, and total infarct size.

Specific characteristics of the interface between scar and surviving tissue are likely crucial determinants of whether a substrate exists. Although the hope is that CMR can identify and characterize the extent of this "gray" zone, several limitations must first be overcome. Certain technical considerations are important when assessing the characteristics of the periinfarct territory known as the border zone. This mixture of viable and nonviable tissue alters signal intensity because partial volume effects produce intermediate signal intensities along the border zone. The quality of the study is critical; proper adjustment of the inversion time is crucial in interpreting the images. Manually adjusting the inversion time to null signal from normal myocardium is necessary in each patient to optimize contrast between normal myocardium (black) and scar (white).

Case 2 Continued

CMR could provide the clinician and the patient with several pieces of relevant data. It could provide an ejection fraction that is likely to be the most accurate. In addition, it could quantify the extent and characteristics of scar that is present, and this could also help predict the likelihood of cardiovascular morbidity and mortality for this patient given the earlier (albeit limited) studies.

■ HYPERTROPHIC CARDIOMYOPATHY

Case 3

A 24-year-old white male patient without any significant medical history presents after a syncopal episode while food shopping. He lost consciousness, fell on his forehead, and required eight stitches to close a laceration. The patient has no recollection of the event. He has never had syncope or near syncope in the past and was active in high school sports. He has had "a few" palpitations once in a while that have lasted for seconds but has not thought anything of it. This patient is not taking any medications and has never used illegal drugs. He has no family history of sudden cardiac death. Physical examination is unremarkable, without any murmurs; laboratory study results are normal. An ECG shows sinus rhythm with nonspecific T-wave abnormalities. An echocardiogram shows normal biventricular size and function without significant valvular abnormalities. The interventricular septum is measured at 12 mm, as compared with 9 mm in other parts of the left ventricle. An exercise stress test is unremarkable; the patient exercises for 12 minutes of Bruce protocol with a normal blood pressure response and no ECG changes. A 24-hour Holter monitor shows rare PVCs.

The patient's cardiologist is concerned about the mild septal hypertrophy and brings up the possibility of HCM. The patient himself wonders whether this could have been his first episode of vasovagal syncope. The cardiologist refers him to an electrophysiologist and asks whether an electrophysiology study would help. The electrophysiologist decides to order a cardiac MRI. Is this reasonable?

Traditional Methods for Risk Stratification of Sudden Cardiac Death

The diagnosis of HCM can sometimes be challenging, especially in patients who are high-endurance athletes. Once the diagnosis is entertained, the concern for sudden cardiac death must be considered, and the patient must be assessed appropriately. The mechanism of sudden cardiac death in these patients has been shown to be mainly VT or ventricular fibrillation. Many patients present with sudden cardiac death, especially during an episode of exertion. At present, risk stratification of sudden cardiac death includes a family history of sudden death, a history of syncope, nonsustained VT (NSVT) on

Holter monitoring, abnormal blood pressure response during exercise stress testing, and LV hypertrophy of 30 mm or greater. However, data suggest that many patients experience an event with only one risk factor. Long-term follow-up in a large cohort suggested that appropriate ICD discharges are just as likely in patients with one risk factor as they are in those with three or more risk factors. As a result, recommendations about prophylactic implantation of a defibrillator are difficult in patients who may have only one such risk factor. A careful assessment must be made on an individual basis.

Cardiac Magnetic Resonance and Delayed Enhancement in Hypertrophic Obstructive Cardiomyopathy

The pattern of scarring in HCM that has been detected with CMR usually does not occur in the territory of the epicardial coronary arteries. Instead, typical patterns of fibrosis are seen on CMR. Unlike ischemic scars, which are always subendocardial with varying degrees of transmurality, the fibrosis in HCM is typically midmyocardial and shows sparing of the subendocardial myocardium. The patches of fibrosis are not confined to a coronary artery territory. Several studies have reported that fibrosis of the myocardium at the insertion sites of the right ventricle into the ventricular septum is characteristic of HCM (Fig. 21-3). Studies have also shown that the presence of scar and fibrosis in patients can be reliably detected using CMR, with good histologic correlation of the scar with areas of delayed enhancement. More important, the use of this imaging modality may have prognostic significance in these patients.

Several studies have attempted to demonstrate a correlation between scar and fibrosis detected by CMR and the presence of NSVT shown on Holter monitoring. One report found that delayed enhancement was present in 41% of 177 patients with HCM. Although this finding was an independent predictor of NSVT on Holter monitoring, no difference was noted in the extent of tissue with delayed enhancement in patients with or without NSVT. A smaller study ($N = 47$) also reported that delayed enhancement was present in nearly all patients with NSVT on Holter, but it was also present in 60% of patients without NSVT. Similarly, the degree of tissue with delayed enhancement was not different in patients with or without NSVT.

However, although patients with delayed enhancement may be more likely to have NSVT, the lack of delayed enhancement as seen on MRI does not preclude the presence of NSVT on Holter monitoring. As a result, whether MRI will prove to have a negative predictive value that is clinically acceptable during risk stratification of patients has yet to be determined.

A large, comprehensive study reported on the CMR findings of 424 patients with HCM. Although 56% of these patients had delayed enhancement, no relationship was found between delayed enhancement and symptoms or functional class. Patients with delayed enhancement were 3 times as likely to have NSVT on

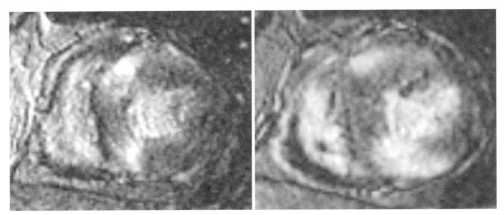

Figure 21-3 Short-axis cardiac magnetic resonance (CMR) images after contrast administration. Images from CMR in a 52-year-old male patient with a known history of hypertrophic cardiomyopathy. Delayed enhancement is seen in the anterior and inferior walls of the basal aspects of the left ventricle. This patient had one "high-risk factor" for sudden death; given these findings of significant amounts of scar, the electrophysiologist recommended an implantable cardioverter-defibrillator.

Holter monitoring compared with those without it (27% versus 8.5%). Many patients had undergone genotyping as well. "Gene-positive" patients were more likely to have areas of delayed enhancement. Sudden cardiac death occurred in 4 patients, and an additional 4 patients received appropriate ICD therapy; all 8 patients had tissue with delayed enhancement.

The absence of NSVT on Holter monitoring in children and younger adults is by no means reassuring. Indeed, certain genotypes have been shown to have higher rates of sudden death, but with extensive myocardial disarray and less myocardial hypertrophy and fibrosis at autopsy. In addition, these patients tend to be much younger. Myocardial disarray may serve as a substrate for ventricular arrhythmias resulting from the alteration of the location and the extent of gap junctions that are critical for cell coupling and impulse propagation. Fibrosis and scar may not be the substrate in these patients; microfoci of scar possibly may be responsible.

This concern is supported by earlier data showing that sudden death can occur in patients without significant LV hypertrophy. Whether these patients would demonstrate a significant amount of scarring on CMR that would warrant concern is still not known. Although the substrate is believed to be caused by myocardial disarray as well as by fibrosis, which of the two is the more important component in the maintenance of ventricular tachyarrhythmias is not clear. Patients can have significant amounts of disorganized myocardial architecture in myocardial tissue that is not hypertrophied. In addition, the relationship between myocardial disarray and fibrosis that is detected during imaging is uncertain.

Present Use of Cardiac Magnetic Resonance in Hypertrophic Obstructive Cardiomyopathy

Although no general consensus exists on how to use these data, many clinicians use CMR as a "tie breaker" in risk stratification for patients who have one or more of the established features in the original guidelines.

Other clinicians, however, suggest that the finding of scar alone is enough to warrant concern.

Case 3 Continued

The patient undergoes CMR, which measures part of his septum to be up to 15 mm in thickness. In addition, areas of delayed hyperenhancement are found at the right ventricular (RV) insertion site of the septum. A diagnosis of obstructive HCM (HOCM) is made, and the patient undergoes insertion of a single chamber ICD. Subsequent follow-up shows several detections of NSVT, although the patient has not yet had any sustained episodes.

■ ARRHYTHMOGENIC RIGHT VENTRICULAR CARDIOMYOPATHY AND DYSPLASIA

Case 4

A 48-year-old male patient is referred for a cardiovascular workup after a visit to his primary physician's office for palpitations. An ECG was unremarkable (without T-wave inversions in the precordial leads or epsilon waves), but a 24-hour Holter monitor showed moderate PVCs and two runs of NSVT lasting 4 beats at 190 beats/minute. An echocardiogram is unremarkable except for a concern of a right ventricle that seems to be at the upper limit of normal size. An exercise treadmill test is performed. The patient exercises for 10 minutes and reaches a peak heart rate of 175 beats/minute; no ECG changes and no episodes of VT are noted. The 12-lead ECG at rest just before exercise was initiated shows PVCs of outflow tract morphology. The PVCs are suppressed with exercise. The patient has never had syncope. The family history is remarkable for sudden cardiac death in his father at the age of 40 years. However, his father was a heavy smoker and had diabetes; no autopsy was performed. Because of a concern for arrhythmogenic RV cardiomyopathy/dysplasia (ARVC/D), a referral is made to a cardiac electrophysiologist, who performs a signal averaged ECG, which has 1 of 3 abnormal components that are associated with ARVC/D.

Does Cardiac Magnetic Resonance Have a Role in the Diagnosis?

Present Understanding

ARVC/D is a type of cardiomyopathy characterized by a progressive replacement of RV myocytes with adipose and fibrous tissue. Involvement of the left ventricle is not uncommon. The incidence has been estimated at 1 in 5000. ARVC/D can occur sporadically, or it can be inherited, most commonly in an autosomal dominant fashion. Data suggest that genetic mutations of desmosomal proteins located at the intercalated disk are responsible. The resultant alteration in structure leads to susceptibility to stress and damage and, ultimately, to myocyte death. The disease is progressive, and RV dilatation and dysfunction can occur over time. Sudden cardiac death is common, and up to half of these patients die before the age of 35 years. The diagnosis can be difficult to make, and criteria established by the task force on cardiomyopathies (the task force of the Working Group Myocardial and Pericardial Disease of the European Society of Cardiology and of the Scientific Council on Cardiomyopathies of the International Society and Federation of Cardiology) serve as an important guide. The task force updated the criteria to reflect important developments in the understanding of this disease entity.

Impact of Imaging in the Diagnosis

The use of MRI to aid in the diagnosis of ARVC/D has been widely adopted. Although the original task force recommendations included the diagnosis of fibrofatty replacement of myocardium on endomyocardial biopsy (a major criterion), this determination has been largely replaced by noninvasive imaging, either by CMR or computed tomography (CT). This practice has become more acceptable not only because of the potential complications of biopsy of the right ventricle, but also because of the patchy nature of the fibrofatty replacement that may result in sampling error and relatively low sensitivity. The updated task force recommendations recognize the practical utility of CMR in characterizing the myocardium, as opposed to relying on biopsy.

Case 4 Continued

CMR is performed, and the image shows normal biventricular size and function without any areas of delayed enhancement. However, a mild to moderate amount of fat is present in the right ventricle. What is the significance of these MRI findings? Before the MRI findings, the patient had two minor criteria (NSVT of outflow tract morphology and one of three abnormal parameters on signal averaged ECG), thus classifying him as "possible" based on the updated task force criteria.

Given the CMR findings, does the patient now have ARVC/D?

Which Findings on Cardiac Magnetic Resonance Are Important?

The concern for many clinicians is the difficulty in making a noninvasive diagnosis of this disease in the early stages, when life-threatening ventricular arrhythmias can occur before obvious structural abnormalities (e.g., dilatation, aneurysms, or wall motion abnormalities) of the right ventricle can be detected.

Although assessing the accuracy of CMR in the diagnosis of ARVC/D is difficult, data suggest that structural abnormalities detected by this imaging modality do correlate with areas of electrically abnormal tissue as determined by invasive electroanatomic mapping. Convincing data are not yet available to show whether CMR can be used to determine which patients are at risk for malignant tachyarrhythmias. Whereas several studies have attempted to determine whether the presence of scar in patients with HOCM may help stratify those at risk for VT, a thorough evaluation has not yet been undertaken in patients with ARVC/D.

One small study reported that 6 of 8 patients suspected of having ARVC/D who had delayed enhancement were found to have inducible sustained monomorphic VT during electrophysiologic testing. The presence of scar in the right ventricle, regardless of origin, has been found to be an ominous finding. This was demonstrated in a cohort of 64 patients with or without ARVC/D, all of whom presented with nonischemic scar-related VT of RV origin. The diagnosis of ARVC/D was made based on the task force criteria. Scar was determined either by CMR or contrast echocardiography. No difference was noted in the recurrence of VT in patients diagnosed with or without ARVC/D based on the task force criteria. With the updated task force criteria, more of these patients possibly would have been diagnosed with ARVC/D.

The potential for overdiagnosis of this disease entity exists if only fat is present on CMR images. Although the presence of fibrosis should raise concern, fat replacement of the right ventricle has been found to be present in patients without ARVC/D, and it likely represents a distinct entity of uncertain significance. The presence of fat replacement in the anterior wall of the apex is probably not an abnormal finding. Earlier data suggested that the presence of significant fat infiltration of the right ventricle occurs in more than half of normal hearts in older patients. The importance of this concern has been recognized by the fields of cardiac electrophysiology and cardiovascular imaging. For example, CMR has been used to show that patients with marked fat deposition without other morphologic features of ARVC/D have a distinct clinical entity that must be treated as such to avoid unnecessary referral for ICD implantation. The presence of fibrosis in the form of delayed enhancement appears to improve the diagnostic accuracy of CMR for ARVC/D. Based on these findings, the updated task force specifically commented on this concern by confirming that the ability of CMR to detect fat without concomitant fibrosis is of limited value in the diagnosis of ARVC/D. In addition, other findings that may represent normal variants can easily be misinterpreted as abnormal.

Case 4 Continued

The presence of fat without fibrosis does not constitute a major or minor criterion, according to the updated task force guidelines for the diagnosis of ARVC/D. This patient has two minor criteria and should be classified as "possible" regarding the diagnosis. He should have close follow-up with a reasonable strategy consisting of a repeat CMR to ensure that no structural abnormalities of the right ventricle have developed. Given that the patient has had NSVT of outflow tract morphology, a voltage map would be reasonable to see whether any abnormal areas of low voltage are present. These areas could represent areas of scar that may not have been adequately detected by CMR.

■ SARCOIDOSIS

Case 5

A 46-year-old male patient is referred to a cardiologist after he is diagnosed with pulmonary sarcoidosis. He had been well until he was deployed overseas for military duty. Toward the end of his tour, the patient "got sick" with a bad cold and was run down. When he returned, he found that his exercise tolerance was markedly diminished, and his main symptom was dyspnea on exertion. Because of an abnormal chest radiograph, the patient had a pulmonary workup that included a CT scan. A biopsy of mediastinal lymph nodes demonstrated noncaseating granulomas. An ECG showed sinus rhythm with bifascicular block and a prolonged PR interval; this ECG was markedly different from one performed by the military 3 years previously. An echocardiogram showed normal biventricular size and function. The patient exercised for 7 minutes of Bruce protocol and reached a peak heart rate of 153 beats/minute; no ECG changes occurred, but he stopped because of fatigue and dyspnea. Perfusion imaging was normal. The patient was treated with immunosuppressive agents and improved subjectively, as well as objectively (CT imaging of the chest revealed improvement of ground glass opacities).

Over the course of the next 6 months, the patient had been gradually resuming his very active lifestyle, but he developed an episode of near syncope while jogging that was preceded by palpitations and dizziness. A repeat ECG showed (Fig. 21-4, *A*) bifascicular block with a normal PR interval. A repeat exercise tolerance test showed that his exercise capacity had improved such that he was able to exercise for 11 minutes of Bruce protocol and reached a peak heart rate of 160 beats/minute. No ECG changes were noted. A Holter monitor showed occasional multiform PVCs and one 6-beat NSVT at 210 beats/minute. The patient was asymptomatic. A repeat echocardiogram was unchanged.

His cardiologist is concerned about cardiac involvement of his sarcoidosis. Would CMR help?

Background

Sarcoidosis is a multisystemic disease characterized by noncaseating granulomas most commonly affecting the lungs and lymph nodes. However, other organs and tissue, including the heart, liver, eyes, skin, and spleen, can be involved as well. The exact cause of the disease is not known; the granulomas may be an immunologic response to an antigenic trigger. In the United States, the annual incidence of sarcoidosis has been estimated at 10.9 per 100,000 in whites and up to 35.5 per 100,000 in African Americans.

Based on autopsy studies, cardiac involvement is present in at least 25% of patients with sarcoidosis in the United States and is responsible for up to 25% of the deaths. Noncaseating granulomas can be found anywhere in the heart, especially in the LV free wall and basal aspect of the interventricular septum. Conduction abnormalities are common, including complete heart block. Ventricular arrhythmias are not uncommon, and sudden cardiac death is responsible for up to 65% of cases of death resulting from cardiac sarcoid. CMR has been shown to correlate with cardiac involvement; findings of delayed enhancement suggest fibrogranulomatous replacement and inflammation.

Imaging and Prognostic Implications

Data on the prognostic utility of CMR in predicting future cardiac events in the setting of sarcoidosis are limited. One prospective study used CMR to evaluate 81 consecutive patients with biopsy-proven extracardiac sarcoidosis for cardiac involvement, and these patients were followed for approximately 2 years. Delayed enhancement was present in 26% of patients. This finding represented a twofold higher identification than the consensus criteria for the diagnosis of cardiac sarcoidosis developed by the Japanese Ministry of Health and Welfare. Coronary angiography was performed in all patients with hyperenhancement to exclude the presence of obstructive coronary disease. Although no difference in LV volumes was noted, patients with hyperenhancement had significantly lower ejection fractions (median, 45% versus 57%, respectively) as compared with patients without evidence of delayed enhancement. The finding of delayed enhancement was 9 times more likely to reach a combined end point of death, defibrillator therapy, or requirement of pacemaker implantation as compared with the absence of this finding. In addition, 4 patients with delayed enhancement reached the end point of cardiac death, as opposed to 1 patient without it.

Case 5 Continued

The patient undergoes CMR (see Fig. 21-4, *B*) imaging, which reveals extensive areas of fibrosis and scarring in a pattern not consistent with coronary disease but consistent with his known diagnosis of sarcoidosis. The present Heart Rhythm Society Guidelines lists as class IIa the implantation of a defibrillator for primary prevention of sudden cardiac death in patients with cardiac sarcoidosis. Given the patient's near syncope, palpitations during the episode, and findings of significant fibrosis on

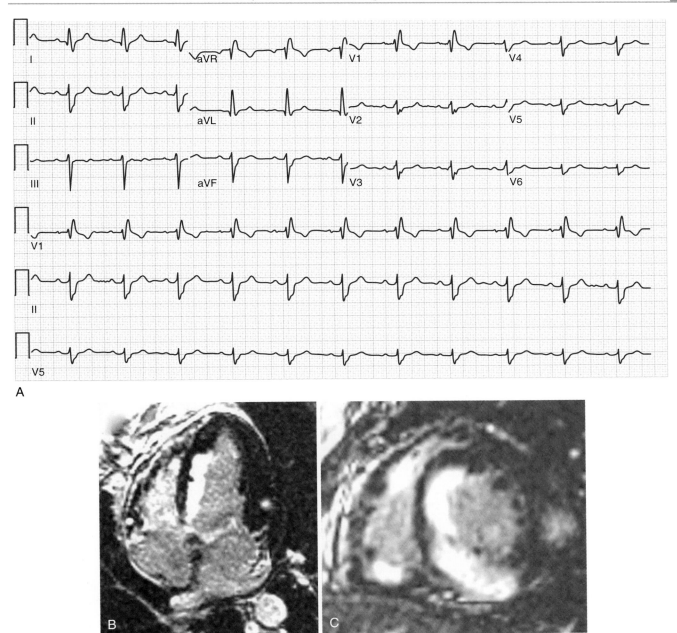

Figure 21-4 A, The electrocardiogram from case 5 shows bifascicular block (right bundle branch block with left anterior hemiblock). **B and C,** These images were obtained from cardiac magnetic resonance imaging of the patient in case 5. The delayed enhancement seen in the septal and inferior walls of the left ventricle likely accounts for the significant conduction disease seen on this patient's his electrocardiogram in **A.**

CMR, offering this patient a defibrillator is a reasonable approach.

■ LEFT VENTRICULAR NONCOMPACTION

Case 6

A 30-year-old male patient without any prior medical history presents with fatigue and dyspnea on exertion. He has been active all his life and played competitive soccer in high school and college. He notes a 6-month-long functional decline. His ECG (Fig. 21-5, *A*) shows sinus rhythm with biatrial enlargement. This finding leads to

an echocardiogram, which confirms the biatrial enlargement, as well as severe LV dilatation and severe dysfunction (ejection fraction of 18%). The patient undergoes left and right heart catheterization, which shows normal coronary arteries with mild elevation in central venous pressure, pulmonary pressures, and pulmonary capillary wedge pressures; the cardiac output is 4.3 L/minute. His physicians consult a cardiologist and raise the question of the need for a biopsy to determine the cause.

The cardiologist first decides to obtain a CMR (see Fig. 21-5, *B*) image, which shows a severely dilated left ventricle and findings consistent with LV noncompaction (LVNC). These results obviate the need for a biopsy.

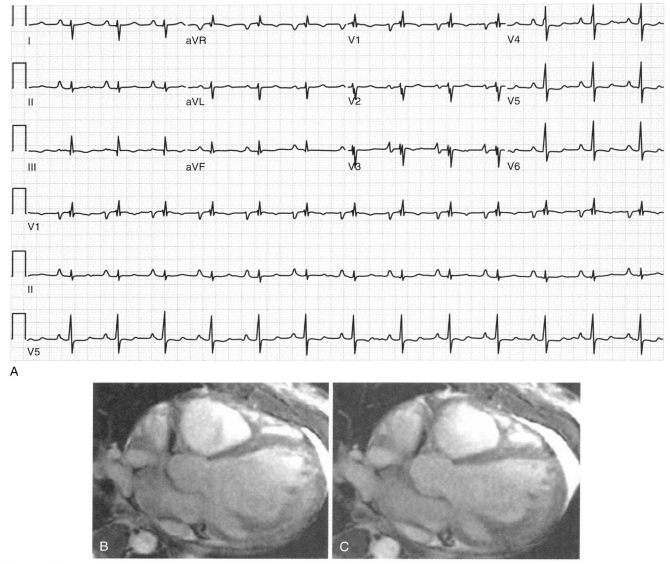

Figure 21-5 **A,** The electrocardiogram from the patient in case 6 shows biatrial enlargement and a narrow QRS complex. **B and C,** The corresponding oblique long-axis cardiac magnetic resonance image demonstrates left ventricular noncompaction in the lateral wall (noncompacted-to-compacted ratio >2.3).

Background and Available Data

Isolated LVNC is a type of cardiomyopathy characterized by persistent prominent ventricular trabeculations with deep intertrabecular recesses resulting from a defect in embryogenesis. Because of the relatively sparse data available, the natural course of this myopathy is not well known. It is considered to be a rare cause of cardiomyopathy, with an incidence of 0.06% to 0.3%; LVNC is especially important in the pediatric population. A genetic component appears to exist in some patients.

Reports vary on the prognosis of these patients. Initially, investigators thought that the outlook was poor, although more recent data suggested otherwise. In addition, most reports described patients who presented with symptoms. A registry of 105 adult patients in France whose condition was diagnosed by echocardiography

found that, over 2.3 years of follow-up, severe heart failure occurred in a third of these patients, ventricular arrhythmias occurred in 7, embolic events occurred in 9, and 12 patients died.

MRI is now considered to be the reference standard for the diagnosis of this entity, although cardiac-gated CT is a reasonable alternative. Diagnosis with CMR is based on measurement (in end-diastole) of the ratio of noncompacted versus compacted LV myocardial thickness in long-axis views. A ratio greater than 2.3: 1 is highly suggestive of this disease entity. One study examined 763 patients referred for CMR for further characterization of cardiomyopathy. Forty-two patients were diagnosed with LVNC, whereas echocardiography had made the diagnosis in only 10% of these patients. Half of the patients with LVNC had presented with dyspnea, and a further 14% had evidence of thromboembolic phenomenon (pulmonary embolism, stroke, and brachial artery embolism). The understanding of this disease is still in its infancy, and long-term data with prognostic indicators are lacking.

■ CONCLUSION

The use of CMR has proven to be an important tool in the diagnosis and characterization of various cardiomyopathies. It has helped to continue to advance the field in seeking to image the substrate for sudden cardiac death. Further progress continues to be made to quantify and characterize scar in various myopathic substrates. The hope is that the unique capabilities of CMR can ultimately provide the clinician with important prognostic information in identifying which myopathic substrates are more likely to give rise to ventricular arrhythmias that result in sudden cardiac death.

Bibliography

Adabag AS, Maron BJ, Appelbaum E, et al. Occurrence and frequency of arrhythmias in hypertrophic cardiomyopathy in relation to delayed enhancement on cardiovascular magnetic resonance. *J Am Coll Cardiol.* 2008;51:1369-1374.

Akhtar M, Garan H, Lehmann MH, Troup PJ. Sudden cardiac death: management of high-risk patients. *Ann Intern Med.* 1991;114:499-512.

Allman KC, Shaw LJ, Hachamovitch R, Udelson JE. Myocardial viability testing and impact of revascularization on prognosis in patients with coronary artery disease and left ventricular dysfunction: a meta-analysis. *J Am Coll Cardiol.* 2002;39:1151-1158.

Assomull RG, Prasad SK, Lyne J, et al. Cardiovascular magnetic resonance, fibrosis, and prognosis in dilated cardiomyopathy. *J Am Coll Cardiol.* 2006;48:1977-1985.

Bell MR, Gersh BJ, Schaff HV, et al. Effect of completeness of revascularization on long-term outcome of patients with three-vessel disease undergoing coronary artery bypass surgery: a report from the Coronary Artery Surgery Study (CASS) Registry. *Circulation.* 1992;86:446-457.

Bello D, Fieno DS, Kim RJ, et al. Infarct morphology identifies patients with substrate for sustained ventricular tachycardia. *J Am Coll Cardiol.* 2005;45:1104-1108.

Bogun F, Desjardins B, Good E, et al. Delayed-enhanced magnetic resonance imaging in nonischemic cardiomyopathy utility for identifying the ventricular arrhythmia substrate. *J Am Coll Cardiol.* 2009;53:1138-1145.

Bardy G, Lee KL, Mark DB, et al. Amiodarone or an implantable cardioverter-defibrillator for congestive heart failure. *N Engl J Med.* 2005;352:225-237.

Burke AP, Farb A, Tashko G, Virmani R. Arrhythmogenic right ventricular cardiomyopathy and fatty replacement of the right ventricular myocardium: are they different diseases? *Circulation.* 1998;97:1571-1580.

Chaudhry FA, Tauke JT, Alessandrini RS, et al. Prognostic implications of myocardial contractile reserve in patients with coronary artery disease and left ventricular dysfunction. *J Am Coll Cardiol.* 1999;34:730-738.

Cheong BY, Muthupillai R, Nemeth M, et al. The utility of delayed-enhancement magnetic resonance imaging for identifying nonischemic myocardial fibrosis in asymptomatic patients with biopsy-proven systemic sarcoidosis. *Sarcoidosis Vasc Diffuse Lung Dis.* 2009;26:39-46.

Cheong BY, Muthupillai R, Wilson JM, et al. Prognostic significance of delayed-enhancement magnetic resonance imaging: survival of 857 patients with and without left ventricular dysfunction. *Circulation.* 2009;120:2069-2076.

de Bakker JM, Coronel R, Tasseron S, et al. Ventricular tachycardia in the infracted, Langendoff-perfused human heart: role of the arrangement of surviving cardiac fibers. *J Am Coll Cardiol.* 1990;15:1594-1607.

de Bakker JM, van Capelle FJ, Janse MJ, et al. Slow conduction in the infracted human heart: "zigzag" course of activation. *Circulation.* 1993;88:915-926.

de Bakker JM, van Capelle FJ, Janse MJ, et al. Reentry as a cause of ventricular tachycardia in patients with chronic ischemic heart disease: electrophysiologic and anatomic correlation. *Circulation.* 1988;77:589-606.

de Leeuw N, Ruiter DJ, Balk AH. Histopathologic findings in explanted heart tissue from patients with end-stage idiopathic dilated cardiomyopathy. *Transpl Int.* 2001;14:299-306.

Dillon SM, Allessie AM, Ursell PC, Wit AL. Influences of anisotropic tissue structure on reentrant circuits in the epicardial border zone of subacute canine infarcts. *Circ Res.* 1988;63:182-206.

Dimitrow PP, Klimeczek P, Vliegenthart R, et al. Late hyperenhancement in gadolinium magnetic resonance imaging: comparison of hypertrophic cardiomyopathy patients with and without nonsustained ventricular tachycardia. *Int J Cardiovasc Imaging.* 2008;24:85-87.

Dumont C, Monserrat L, Soler R, et al. Clinical significance of late gadolinium enhancement on cardiovascular magnetic resonance in patients with hypertrophic cardiomyopathy. *Rev Esp Cardiol.* 2007;60:15-23.

El Sherif N, Scherlag BJ, Lazzara R. Electrode catheter recording during malignant ventricular arrhythmia following experimental acute myocardial ischemia: evidence for re-entry due to conduction delay and block in ischemic myocardium. *Circulation.* 1975;51:1003-1014.

Fahmy TS, Wazni OM, Jaber WA, et al. Integration of positron emission tomography/computed tomography with electroanatomical mapping: a novel approach for ablation of scar-related ventricular tachycardia. *Heart Rhythm.* 2008;5:1538-1545.

Fazio G, Corrado G, Zachara E, et al. Ventricular tachycardia in non-compaction of the left ventricle: is this a frequent complication? *Pacing Clin Electrophysiol.* 2007;30:544-546.

Fenoglio Jr JJ, Pham TD, Harken AH, Horowitz LN, Josephson ME, Wit AL. Recurrent sustained ventricular tachycardia: structure and ultrastructure of subendocardial regions in which tachycardia originates. *Circulation.* 1983;68:518-533.

Fernandes VR, Wu KC, Rosen BD, et al. Enhanced infarct border zone function and altered mechanical activation predict inducibility of monomorphic ventricular tachycardia in patients with ischemic cardiomyopathy. *Radiology.* 2007;245:712-719.

Fleming HA, Bailey SA. The prognosis of sarcoid heart disease in the United Kingdom. *Ann N Y Acad Sci.* 1986;465:543-550.

Fleming HA, Bailey SM. Sarcoid heart disease. *J R Coll Physicians Lond.* 1981;15:245-246:249-253.

Fontaliran F, Fontaine G, Fillette F, Aouate P, Chomette G, Grosgogeat Y. Nosologic frontiers of arrhythmogenic dysplasia: quantitative variations of normal adipose tissue of the right heart ventricle. *Arch Mal Coeur Vaiss.* 1991;84:33-38.

Frances RJ. Arrhythmogenic right ventricular dysplasia/cardiomyopathy: a review and update. *Int J Cardiol.* 2006;110:279-287.

Frenneaux MP, Counihan PJ, Caforio AL, et al. Abnormal blood pressure response during exercise in hypertrophic cardiomyopathy. *Circulation.* 1990;82:1995-2002.

Garan H, Fallon JT, Rosenthal S, Ruskin JN. Endocardial, intramural, and epicardial activation patterns during sustained monomorphic ventricular tachycardia in late canine myocardial infarction. *Circ Res.* 1987;60:879-896.

Gehi A, Haas D, Fuster V. Primary prophylaxis with the implantable cardioverter-defibrillator: the need for improved risk stratification. *JAMA.* 2005;294:958-960.

Gupta A, Lee VS, Chung YC, Babb JS, Simonetti OP. Myocardial infarction: optimization of inversion times at delayed contrast-enhanced MR imaging. *Radiology.* 2004;233:921-926.

Habib G, Charron P, Eicher JC, et al. Isolated left ventricular compaction in adults: clinical and echocardiographic features in 105 patients. Results from a French registry. *Eur J Heart Fail.* 2011;13:177-185.

Hamilton R. Arrhythmogenic right ventricular cardiomyopathy. *PACE.* 2009;32:S44-S51.

Hiraga H, Yuwa K, Hiroe M. *Guideline for the Diagnosis of Cardiac Sarcoidosis: Study Report on Diffuse Pulmonary Disease [in Japanese]* Tokyo: Japanese Ministry of Health and Welfare; 199323–24.

Iwai K, Sekiguti M, Hosoda Y, et al. Racial difference in cardiac sarcoidosis incidence observed at autopsy. *Sarcoidosis.* 1994;11:26-31.

Jain A, Tandri H, Calkins H, Bluemke DA. Role of cardiovascular magnetic resonance imaging in arrhythmogenic right ventricular dysplasia. *J Cardiovasc Magn Reson.* 2008;10:1-14.

Josephson ME, Almendral JM, Buxton AE, Marchlinski FE. Mechanisms of ventricular tachycardia. *Circulation.* 1987;75:III41-III47.

Josephson ME, Horowitz LN, Farshidi A, Kastor JA. Recurrent sustained ventricular tachycardia: mechanisms. *Circulation.* 1978;57:431-440.

Jones EL, Craver JM, Guyton RA, et al. Importance of complete revascularization in performance of the coronary bypass operation. *Am J Cardiol.* 1983;51:7-12.

Judd RM, Wagner A, Rehwald WG, Albert T, Kim RJ. Technology insight: assessment of myocardial viability by delayed-enhancement magnetic resonance imaging. *Nat Clin Pract Cardiovasc Med.* 2005;2:150-158.

Kadish A, Bello D, Finn JP, et al. Rationale and design for the Defibrillators to Reduce Risk by Magnetic Resonance Imaging Evaluation (DETERMINE) trial. *J Cardiovasc Electrophysiol.* 2009;20:982-987.

Kim JS, Judson MA, Donnino R, et al. Cardiac sarcoidosis. *Am Heart J.* 2009;157:9-21.

Kim RJ, Fieno DS, Parrish TB, et al. Relationship of MRI delayed contrast enhancement to irreversible injury, infarct age, and contractile function. *Circulation.* 1999;100:1992-2002.

Klocke FJ, Wu E, Lee DC. "Shades of gray" in cardiac magnetic resonance images of infarcted myocardium: can they tell us what we'd like to them? *Circulation.* 2006;114:8-10.

Kim RJ, Wu E, Rafael A, et al. The use of contrast-enhanced MRI to identify reversible myocardial dysfunction. *N Engl J Med.* 2006;343:1445-1453.

Kwon DH, Halley CM, Carrigan TP, et al. Extent of left ventricular scar predicts outcomes in ischemic cardiomyopathy patients with significantly reduced systolic function: a delayed hyperenhancement cardiac magnetic resonance study. *JACC Cardiovasc Imaging.* 2009;2:34-44.

Kwon DH, Smedira NG, Rodriguez ER, et al. Cardiac magnetic resonance detection of myocardial scarring in hypertrophic cardiomyopathy: correlation with histopathology and prevalence of ventricular tachycardia. *J Am Coll Cardiol.* 2009;54:242-249.

Kwong RY, Chan AK, Brown KA, et al. Impact of unrecognized myocardial scar detected by cardiac magnetic resonance imaging on event-free survival in patients with signs and symptoms of coronary artery disease. *Circulation.* 2006;113:2733-2743.

Macedo R, Prakasa K, Tichnell C, et al. Marked lipomatous infiltration of the right ventricle: MRI findings in relation to arrhythmogenic right ventricular dysplasia. *AJR Am J Roentgenol.* 2007;188:W423-W427.

Marcus FI, McKenna WJ, Sherrill D, et al. Diagnosis of arrhythmogenic right ventricular cardiomyopathy/dysplasia: proposed modification of the task force criteria. *Circulation.* 2010;121:1533-1541.

Maron BJ. Hypertrophic cardiomyopathy: a systematic review. *JAMA.* 2002;287:1308-1320.

Maron BJ, Kragel AH, Roberts WC. Sudden death in hypertrophic cardiomyopathy with normal left ventricular mass. *Br Heart J.* 1990;63:308-310.

Maron BJ, Shen WK, Link MS, et al. Efficacy of implantable cardioverter-defibrillators for the prevention of sudden death in patients with hypertrophic cardiomyopathy. *N Engl J Med.* 2000;342:365-373.

Maron B, Spirito P, Shen WK, et al. Implantable cardioverter-defibrillators and prevention of sudden cardiac death in hypertrophic cardiomyopathy. *JAMA.* 2007;298:405-412.

Maron BJ, Wolfson JK, Roberts WC. Relation between extent of cardiac muscle cell disorganization and left ventricular wall thickness in hypertrophic cardiomyopathy. *Am J Cardiol.* 1992;70:785-790.

McClellan MB, Tunis SR. Medicare coverage of ICDs. *N Engl J Med.* 2005;352: 222–224.

McCrohon J, Moon J, Prasad S, et al. Differentiation of heart failure related to dilated cardiomyopathy and coronary artery disease using gadolinium-enhanced cardiovascular magnetic resonance. *Circulation.* 2003;108:54-59.

McKenna WJ, Thiene G, Nava A, et al. Diagnosis of arrhythmogenic right ventricular dysplasia/cardiomyopathy: task force of the Working Group Myocardial and Pericardial Disease of the European Society of Cardiology and of the Scientific Council on Cardiomyopathies of the International Society and Federation of Cardiology. *Br Heart J.* 1994;71:215-218.

Moon JC, Reed E, Sheppard MN, et al. The histologic basis of late gadolinium enhancement cardiovascular magnetic resonance in hypertrophic cardiomyopathy. *J Am Coll Cardiol.* 2004;43:2260-2264.

Moss AJ, Zareba W, Jackson Hall W, et al. Prophylactic implantation of a defibrillator in patients with myocardial infarction and reduced ejection fraction. *N Engl J Med.* 2002;346:877-883.

Murphy RT, Thaman R, Blanes JG, et al. Natural history and familial characteristics of isolated left ventricular non-compaction. *Eur Heart J.* 2005;26:187-192.

Nazarian S, Bluemke DA, Lardo AC, et al. Magnetic resonance assessment of the substrate for inducible ventricular tachycardia in nonischemic cardiomyopathy. *Circulation.* 2005;112:2821-2825.

Norman M, Simpson M, Mogensen J, et al. Novel mutation in desmoplakin causes arrhythmogenic left ventricular cardiomyopathy. *Circulation.* 2005;112:636-642.

Pagano D, Lewis ME, Townend JN, et al. Coronary revascularization for postischemic heart failure: how myocardial viability affects survival. *Heart.* 1990;82:684-688.

Patel MR, Cawley PJ, Heitner JF, et al. Detection of myocardial damage in patients with sarcoidosis. *Circulation.* 2009;120:1969-1977.

Paya E, Marin F, Gonzalez J, et al. Variables associated with contrast-enhanced cardiovascular magnetic resonance in hypertrophic cardiomyopathy: clinical implications. *J Cardiac Fail.* 2008;14:414-419.

Pearlman JD, Laham RJ, Simons M. Coronary angiogenesis: detection in vivo with MR imaging sensitive to collateral neocirculation—preliminary study in pigs. *Radiology.* 2000;214:801-807.

Peters NS, Coromilas J, Severs NJ, Wit AL. Disturbed connexin43 gap junction distribution correlates with the location of reentrant circuits in the epicardial border zone of healing canine infarcts that cause ventricular tachycardia. *Circulation.* 1997;95:988-996.

Pfluger HB, Phrommintikul A, Mariani JA, Cherayath JG, Taylor AJ. Utility of myocardial fibrosis and fatty infiltration detected by cardiac magnetic resonance imaging in the diagnosis of arrhythmogenic right ventricular dysplasia: a single centre experience. *Heart Lung Circ.* 2008;17:478-483.

Podio V, Spinnler MT, Bertuccio G, et al. Prognosis of hibernating myocardium is independent of recovery of function: evidence from a routine based follow up study. *Nucl Med Commun.* 2002;23:933-942.

Poon M, Fuster V, Fayad Z. Cardiac magnetic resonance imaging: a "one-stop-shop" evaluation of myocardial dysfunction. *Curr Opin Cardiol.* 2002;17:663-670.

Rahimtoola SH. The hibernating myocardium. *Am Heart J.* 1989;117:211-221.

Ramani K, Judd RM, Holly TA, et al. Contrast magnetic resonance imaging in the assessment of myocardial viability in patients with stable coronary artery disease and left ventricular dysfunction. *Circulation.* 1998;98:268-294.

Reddy VY, Malchano ZJ, Holmvang G, et al. Integration of cardiac magnetic resonance imaging with three-dimensional electroanatomic mapping to guide left ventricular catheter manipulation: feasibility in a porcine model of healed myocardial infarction. *J Am Coll Cardiol.* 2004;44:2202-2213.

Roberts WC, McAllister HA, Ferrans VJ. Sarcoidosis of the heart: a clinicopathologic study of 35 necropsy patients and review of 78 previously described necropsy patients. *Am J Med.* 1977;63:86-108.

Roes SD, Borleffs CJ, van der Geest RJ, et al. Infarct tissue heterogeneity assessed with contrast-enhanced MRI predicts spontaneous ventricular arrhythmia in patients with ischemic cardiomyopathy and implantable cardioverter-defibrillator. *Circ Cardiovasc Imaging.* 2009;2:183-190.

Roes SD, Kelle S, Kaandorp TA, et al. Comparison of myocardial infarct size assessed with contrast-enhanced magnetic resonance imaging and left ventricular function and volumes to predict mortality in patients with healed myocardial infarction. *Am J Cardiol.* 2007;100:930-936.

Rubinshtein R, Glockner JF, Ommen SR, et al. Characteristics and clinical significance of late gadolinium enhancement by contrast-enhanced magnetic resonance imaging in patients with hypertrophic cardiomyopathy. *Circ Heart Fail.* 2010;3:51-58.

Rybicki BA, Major M, Popovich Jr J, et al. Racial differences in sarcoidosis incidence: a 5-year study in a health maintenance organization. *Am J Epidemiol.* 1997;145:234-241.

Sadoul N, Prasad K, Elliott PM, et al. Prospective prognostic assessment of blood pressure response during exercise in patients with hypertrophic cardiomyopathy. *Circulation.* 1997;96:2987-2991.

Samady H, Elefteriades JA, Abbott BG, et al. Failure to improve left ventricular function after coronary revascularization for ischemic cardiomyopathy is not associated with worse outcome. *Circulation.* 1999;100:1298-1304.

Santangeli P, Pieroni M, Dello Russo A, et al. Noninvasive diagnosis of electroanatomic abnormalities in arrhythmogenic right ventricular cardiomyopathy. *Circ Arrhythm Electrophysiol.* 2010;3:632-638.

Schinkel AF, Bax JJ, Delgado V, Poldermans D, Rhaimtoola SH. Clinical relevance of hibernating myocardium in ischemic left ventricular dysfunction. *Am J Med.* 2010;123:978-986.

Schinkel AF, Bax JJ, Poldermans D. Clinical assessment of myocardial hibernation. *Heart.* 2005;91:111-117.

Schmidt A, Azevedo CF, Cheng A, et al. Infarct tissue heterogeneity by magnetic resonance imaging identifies enhanced cardiac arrhythmia susceptibility in patients with left ventricular dysfunction. *Circulation.* 2007;115:2006-2014.

Shirani J, Berezowski K, Roberts WC. Quantitative measurement of normal and excessive (cor adiposum) subepicardial adipose tissue, its clinical significance, and its effect on electrocardiographic QRS voltage. *Am J Cardiol.* 1995;76:414-418.

Silverman KJ, Hutchins GM, Bulkley BH. Cardiac sarcoid: a clinicopathologic study of 84 unselected patients with systemic sarcoidosis. *Circulation.* 1978;58:1204-1211.

Simonetti OP, Kim RJ, Fieno DS, et al. An improved MR imaging technique for the visualization of myocardial infarction. *Radiology.* 2001;218:215-223.

Smedema JP, Snoep G, Van Kroonenburgh MP, et al. Evaluation of the accuracy of gadolinium-enhanced cardiovascular magnetic resonance in the diagnosis of cardiac sarcoidosis. *J Am Coll Cardiol.* 2005;45:1683-1690.

Soejima K, Suzuki M, Maisel WH, et al. Catheter ablation in patients with multiple and unstable ventricular tachycardias after myocardial infarction: short ablation lines guided by reentry circuit isthmuses and sinus rhythm mapping. *Circulation.* 2001;104:664-669.

Spirito P, Bellone P, Harris KM, et al. Magnitude of left ventricular hypertrophy and risk of sudden death in hypertrophic cardiomyopathy. *N Engl J Med.* 2000;342:1778-1785.

Spirito P, Seidman CE, McKenna WJ, Maron BJ. The management of hypertrophic cardiomyopathy. *N Engl J Med.* 1997;336:775-785.

Stevenson WG, Friedman PL, Sager PT, et al. Exploring postinfarction reentrant ventricular tachycardia with entrainment mapping. *J Am Coll Cardiol.* 1997;29:1180-1189.

Suk T, Edwards C, Hart H, Christiansen JP. Myocardial scar detected by contrast-enhanced cardiac magnetic resonance imaging is associated with ventricular tachycardia in hypertrophic cardiomyopathy patients. *Heart Lung Circ.* 2008;17:370-374.

Tandri H, Bomma C, Calkins H, Bluemke DA. Magnetic resonance and computed tomography imaging of arrhythmogenic right ventricular dysplasia. *J Magn Reson Imaging.* 2004;19:848-858.

Tandri H, Saranathan M, Rodriguez ER, et al. Noninvasive detection of myocardial fibrosis in arrhythmogenic right ventricular cardiomyopathy using delayed-enhancement magnetic resonance imaging. *J Am Coll Cardiol.* 2005;45:98-103.

Teraoka K, Hirano M, Ookubo H, et al. Delayed contrast enhancement of MRI in hypertrophic cardiomyopathy. *Magn Reson Imaging.* 2004;22:901.

Tian J, Smith MF, Chinnadurai P, et al. Clinical application of PET/CT fusion imaging for three-dimensional myocardial scar and left ventricular anatomy during ventricular tachycardia ablation. *J Cardiovasc Electrophysiol.* 2009;20:597-604.

Thompson PL, Fletcher EE, Katavatis V. Enzymatic indices of myocardial necrosis: influence on short- and long-term prognosis after myocardial infarction. *Circulation.* 1979;59:113-119.

Toda K, Mackenzie K, Mehra MR, et al. Revascularization in severe ventricular dysfunction (15% < OR = LVEF < OR = 30%): a comparison of bypass grafting and percutaneous intervention. *Ann Thorac Surg.* 2002;74:2082-2087.

van der Burg AE, Bax JJ, Boersma E, Pauwels EK, van der Wall EE, Schalij MJ. Impact of viability, ischemia, scar tissue, and revascularization on outcome after aborted sudden death. *Circulation.* 2003;108:1954-1959.

Varnava AM, Elliott PM, Baboonian C, Davison F, Davies MJ, McKenna WJ. Hypertrophic cardiomyopathy: histopathological features of sudden death in cardiac troponin T disease. *Circulation.* 2001;104:1380-1384.

Vignaux O, Dhôte R, Duboc D, et al. Clinical significance of myocardial magnetic resonance abnormalities in patients with sarcoidosis: a 1-year follow-up study. *Chest.* 2002;122:1895-1901.

Yousef ZR, Foley PW, Kadjooi K, et al. Left ventricular non-compaction: clinical features and cardiovascular magnetic resonance imaging. *BMC Cardiovasc Disord*. 2009;9:37.

Wagner A, Mahrholdt H, Thomson L, et al. Effects of time, dose and inversion time for acute myocardial infarct size measurements based on magnetic resonance imaging: delayed contrast enhancement. *J Am Coll Cardiol*. 2006;47:2027-2033.

Weinmann HJ, Laniado M, Mutzel W. Pharmacokinetics of Gd-DTPA/dimeglumine after intravenous injection into healthy volunteers. *Physiol Chem Phys Med NMR*. 1984;16:167-172.

Wijnmaalen AP, Schalij MJ, Bootsma M, et al. Patients with scar-related right ventricular tachycardia: determinants of long-term outcome. *J Cardiovasc Electrophysiol*. 2009;20:1119-1127.

Wit AL, Allessie MA, Bonke FI, et al. Electrophysiologic mapping to determine the mechanism of experimental ventricular tachycardia initiated by premature impulses: experimental approach and initial results demonstrating reentrant excitation. *Am J Cardiol*. 1982;49:166-185.

Wit AL, Dillon SM, Coromilas J, Saltman AE, Waldecker B. Anisotropic reentry in the epicardial border zone of myocardial infarcts. *Ann N Y Acad Sci*. 1990;591:86-108.

Wu E, Judd RM, Vargas JD, et al. Visualisation of presence, location, and transmural extent of healed Q-wave and non–Q-wave myocardial infarction. *Lancet*. 2001;357:21-28.

Wu E, Ortiz JT, Tejedor P, et al. Infarct size by contrast enhanced cardiac magnetic resonance is a stronger predictor of outcomes than left ventricular ejection fraction or end-systolic volume index: prospective cohort study. *Heart*. 2008;94:730-736.

Wu KC, Weiss RG, Thiemann DR, et al. Late gadolinium enhancement by cardiovascular magnetic resonance heralds an adverse prognosis in nonischemic cardiomyopathy. *J Am Coll Cardiol*. 2008;51:2414-2421.

Yan AT, Shayne AJ, Brown KA, et al. Characterization of the peri-infarct zone by contrast-enhanced cardiac magnetic resonance imaging is a powerful predictor of post-myocardial infarction mortality. *Circulation*. 2006;114:32-39.

Yao JA, Hussain W, Patel P, Peters NS, Boyden PA, Wit AL. Remodeling of gap junctional channel function in epicardial border zone of healing canine infarcts. *Circ Res*. 2003;92:437-443.

Zheng ZJ, Croft JB, Giles WH, Mensah GA. Sudden cardiac death in the United States, 1989 to 1998. *Circulation*. 2001;104:2158-2163.

Zipes DP, Wellens HJ. Sudden cardiac death. *Circulation*. 1998;98:2334-2351.

CHAPTER 22

Atherosclerosis: Role of Calcium Scoring

Sion K. Roy and Matthew J. Budoff

Six hundred fifty thousand asymptomatic patients with no known coronary artery disease (CAD) present with acute coronary events annually. These patients represent a grand failure of the current risk assessment system for CAD, which consists primarily of conventional cardiac risk factor assessment. Substantial evidence indicates that coronary artery calcium (CAC) scoring is the most powerful predictor of subclinical atherosclerosis today, and it is underused clinically in the United States. CAC scoring may be the key to preventing asymptomatic patients with subclinical CAD from experiencing coronary events.

■ PATHOPHYSIOLOGY

CAC is pathognomonic for coronary artery atherosclerosis because atherosclerosis is the only vascular disease that causes calcification of coronary arteries. Atherogenesis begins with lipid accumulation, cell proliferation, and extracellular matrix synthesis. These atherosclerotic plaques are also associated with circulating proteins normally associated with bone remodeling, and the proteins are believed to regulate the accumulation of the hydroxyapatite form of calcium phosphate in these lesions.

Whether coronary arterial calcification is a result of the ongoing inflammation associated with plaque formation or an attempt to repair damage to the vascular wall is not known. Whether coronary artery calcification is a dynamic phenomenon, like the ongoing formation and degradation of bone tissue, is also unknown.

Rumberger et al demonstrated that the total area of CAC highly correlates in a linear fashion with the total area of coronary artery plaque on a segmental, individual, and whole coronary artery system basis (Figs. 22-1 and 22-2). These investigators also demonstrated that CAC generally comprises approximately 20% of total plaque size.

■ METHODOLOGY

Technical Considerations

Until relatively recently, electron beam tomography (EBT) was the principal method for acquiring the images used for calcium scoring. In fact, most of the data substantiating the importance of calcium scoring were acquired through EBT. Multidetector computed tomography (MDCT) is a more recent, widely used development that will likely completely replace EBT for calcium scoring in the near future.

EBT uses a rotating electron beam (current, 630 mA; voltage, 130 kV) to acquire 50-ms x-ray images at 3-mm intervals by using prospective triggering in the space of a 30- to 40-second breath hold. The volume mode on EBT allows acquisition of a single image with each preselected movement of the patient table. Up to 40 continuous slices can be obtained by scanning 12 to 32 cm of anatomy, thus allowing adequate images for CAC scoring to be obtained.

MDCT uses a rotating gantry with a special x-ray tube and a variable number of detectors to acquire images while a patient advances through the machine on a moving table. MDCT is able to acquire 73- to 375-msec temporal resolution images in 0.5- to 3.0-mm intervals by using prospective triggering if the heart is steady and the rate is less than 60 beats/minute. To avoid coronary motion artifacts, image acquisition with temporal resolutions of less than 50 msec is needed because the right coronary artery exhibits translational motion of up to 60 mm/second. The left anterior descending and left circumflex arteries exhibit 20 to 40 mm/second of translational motion. Single source MDCT is therefore plagued by more motion artifacts than is EBT.

Radiation

The radiation exposure for each patient undergoing a calcium scan is approximately 1 mSv with either EBT or MDCT. Comparatively, mammograms, which are recommended annually for breast cancer screening in all women after the age of 40 years, cause approximately 0.6 mSv of radiation exposure.

Scoring

Multiple methods of calcium scoring are used. On EBT, CAC is defined as a lesion of at least two to three adjacent pixels in any of the three dimensions (effective pixel size, 0.68 to 1.02 mm^2 for a 512 × 512 reconstruction matrix and field of view size of 30 cm) greater than 130 Hounsfield units (HU) anywhere in the epicardial coronary system. On MDCT, calcified lesions are similarly defined, although the effective pixel size is 0.26 mm^2 with a typical field of view of approximately 26 cm.

Agatston et al originally determined a calcium score by the summation of the product of the calcified plaque area and a factor for maximum calcium density (1 for lesions with maximal density of 130 to 199 HU, 2 for 200 to 299 HU, 3 for 300 to 399 HU, 4 for >400 HU) in each lesion. Calcium scores are generally classified in as follows: 1 to 10, minimal; 11 to 100, mild; 101 to 400, moderate; and greater than 400, severe. The major weakness of the Agatston score is that it is reproducible only at approximately 20%. One reason for this limitation is that the calcium density score based on HU does not increase in a linear pattern, and small incremental differences in HU can result in nonlinear scoring differences.

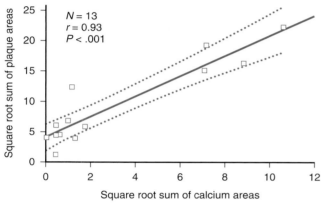

Figure 22-1 Correlation of whole heart coronary calcium and plaque areas. The figure shows the square root sum of coronary calcium areas (mm) by electron beam tomography versus the square root sum of atherosclerotic plaque areas (mm) for 13 autopsied hearts. The linear regression line and the 95% confidence limits are featured. (From Rumberger JA , Simons DB , Fitzpatrick LA , et al. Coronary artery calcium areas by electron beam computed tomography and coronary atherosclerotic plaque area: a histopathologic correlative study. *Circulation*. 1995;92:2157-2162.)

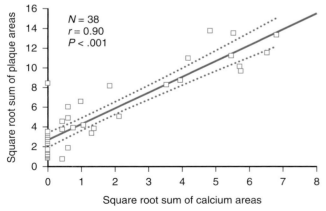

Figure 22-2 Correlation of individual coronary artery calcium and plaque areas. The figure shows the square root sum of coronary calcium areas (mm) by electron beam tomography versus the square root sum of atherosclerotic plaque areas (mm) for 38 individual coronary arteries. The linear regression line and the 95% confidence limits are featured. (From Rumberger JA , Simons DB , Fitzpatrick LA , et al. Coronary artery calcium areas by electron beam computed tomography and coronary atherosclerotic plaque area: a histopathologic correlative study. *Circulation*. 1995;92:2157-2162.)

The calcium volume score is a more reproducible measure of CAC score. The volume score is derived using an isotropic interpolation principle, and it represents a direct measurement of calcium volume in an atherosclerotic plaque (measured in picoliters). Unlike the Agatston score, the volume score accounts for pathophysiologic changes that are likely in a healing plaque. As volumetric contraction and loss of noncalcified contents on plaque occur, the Agatston score, with its dependence on density, could conceivably overestimate CAC in this situation. The volume score is not susceptible to this problem.

Two newer types of CAC scores are still being validated. The calcium mass score is calculated as the summation of the product of the volume and density of each voxel of each lesion. The calcium coverage score measures CAC score as a percentage of coronary artery segments that contain calcium.

The comparability of MDCT- and EBT-derived CAC scores has been well validated by several studies involving more than 400 patients. The most recent study between EBT and 64-slice MDCT demonstrated 99% interscan agreement for the presence of CAC. The linear relationship between the scores from the 2 scanners was significant, and the interscanner variability was not significantly different. Multiple studies further confirmed that 64-slice MDCT and EBT were comparable for both Agatston and volumetric CAC scanning.

■ EXAMPLES AND PITFALLS

Sample images of CAC scans on 64-slice MDCT scanner are shown in Figures 22-3 to 22-5.

The following common pitfalls can make CAC scoring challenging:

1. Mitral annular calcification can often complicate CAC scoring in the left circumflex artery territory (Fig. 22-6).
2. A beam hardening artifact causes the edges of an object to appear brighter than the center. Calcium

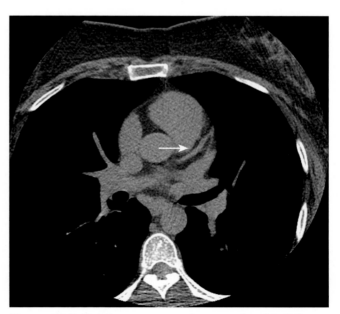

Figure 22-3 Multidetector computed tomography of the left anterior descending coronary artery with no calcium *(arrow)*.

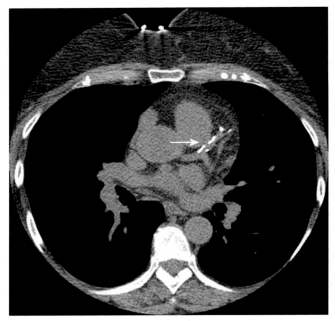

Figure 22-4 Multidetector computed tomography of moderate calcium in the left anterior descending coronary artery *(arrow)*.

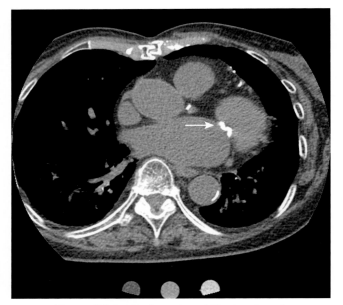

Figure 22-6 Mitral annular calcification *(arrow)*.

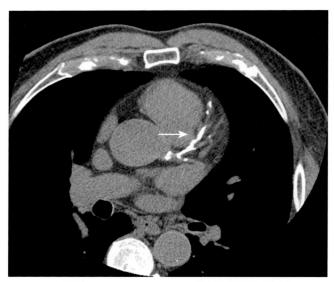

Figure 22-5 Multidetector computed tomography of severe calcium in the left anterior descending coronary artery *(arrow)*.

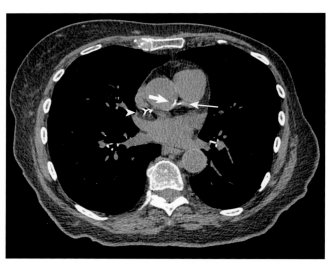

Figure 22-7 Beam hardening artifact *(arrowhead)*. The *thick arrow* points to aortic root calcium, and the *thin arrow* points to left main coronary artery calcium.

is particularly susceptible to this artifact, which can make CAC scoring difficult (Fig. 22-7).
3. Aortic root calcium can be mistaken for left main coronary artery calcium (see Fig. 22-7).
4. Refusal to compute a CAC score on segments that include a stent is appropriate because the presence of a stent falsely increases the CAC score.

■ EPIDEMIOLOGY

Figure 22-8 shows CAC score percentiles based on the age and gender of asymptomatic patients. These data are based on large databases of asymptomatic patients.

This nomogram, albeit useful, does not take into account race.

The Multi-Ethnic Study of Atherosclerosis (MESA), a study of 6814 asymptomatic patients with 53% women and an average age of 62 years, revealed more specific data on CAC scores according to race. As expected, the MESA showed that men have greater CAC scores on average than women. Additionally, among men, whites and Hispanics were first and second, respectively, in terms of average CAC score. Black men had the lowest CAC scores at younger ages, whereas Chinese men had the lowest CAC scores at older ages (Figs. 22-9 and 22-10).

In women, whites had the highest CAC scores. As in men, Chinese women had the lowest CAC scores in the oldest age groups.

Asymptomatic Women (*N* = 6,027)

	<*I* = 40	41–45	46–50	51–55	56–60	61–65	66–70	721–75	>75
Number	331	407	885	1,213	1,091	770	626	437	297
10%	0	0	0	0	0	0	0	0	0
20%	0	0	0	0	0	0	0	0	6
25%	0	0	0	0	0	0	0	4	25
30%	0	0	0	0	0	0	0	10	40
40%	0	0	0	0	0	0	3	29	86
50%	0	0	0	0	0	2	17	67	157
60%	0	0	0	0	2	17	48	120	314
70%	0	0	0	3	12	55	114	217	403
75%	0	0	2	7	29	81	163	310	577
80%	0	0	3	16	56	114	215	398	775
90%	2	5	35	79	166	273	481	738	1,193

Asymptomatic Men (*N* = 15,238)

	<*I* = 35	35–40	41–45	46–50	51–55	56–60	61–65	66–70	71–75	>75
Number	446	1,011	1,873	2,503	2,915	2,385	1,765	1,212	679	429
10%	0	0	0	0	0	0	0	1	8	17
20%	0	0	0	0	0	0	5	23	51	91
25%	0	0	0	0	0	1	12	41	81	148
30%	0	0	0	0	0	4	25	66	121	233
40%	0	0	0	0	4	15	59	128	216	358
50%	0	0	0	2	14	42	114	211	328	562
60%	0	0	1	8	36	89	206	351	493	816
70%	0	1	4	26	80	166	335	554	749	1,223
75%	0	3	8	41	116	227	421	709	918	1,409
80%	2	5	14	67	161	314	543	888	1,119	1,658
90%	12	23	56	174	379	654	996	1,484	1,667	2,396

Figure 22-8 Coronary artery calcium score percentiles based on the age and gender of asymptomatic patients. (From Wong ND, Budoff MJ, Pio J, et al. Coronary calcium and cardiovascular event risk: evaluation by age-and sex-specific quartiles. *Heart J.* 2002;143:456-459.)

The MESA demonstrated very strong CAC predictive value for all gender and ethnic groups. Additionally, younger patients with a family history of CAD had significantly higher CAC scores than did age-matched patients without this risk factor.

■ REVIEW OF THE LITERATURE

Guidelines

The main purpose of obtaining a CAC score is to detect subclinical atherosclerosis. In the 2010 American College of Cardiology/American Heart Association (ACC/AHA) guidelines for assessment of cardiovascular risk in asymptomatic patients, measurement of CAC score in asymptomatic patients at intermediate (10% to 20% 10-year risk based on Framingham risk score) risk to assess cardiovascular risk is a IIa recommendation (benefits substantially outweigh the potential risk; generally accepted as reasonable to perform the procedure or test). Measurement of CAC score in asymptomatic patients at low risk (<6% 10-year risk) is not recommended.

In the ACC/Society of Cardiovascular Computed Tomography/American College of Radiology/AHA/American Society of Nuclear Cardiology/Society for Cardiovascular Angiography and Interventions/Society for Cardiovascular Magnetic Resonance (ACC/SCCT/ACR/AHA/ASE/ASNC/SCAI/SCMR) 2010 appropriate use criteria for cardiac computed tomography, CAC scoring was deemed appropriate in asymptomatic patients with no known CAD who are at low risk if they have a family history of premature CAD. CAC scoring in asymptomatic patients with no history of CAD with intermediate risk was also deemed appropriate.

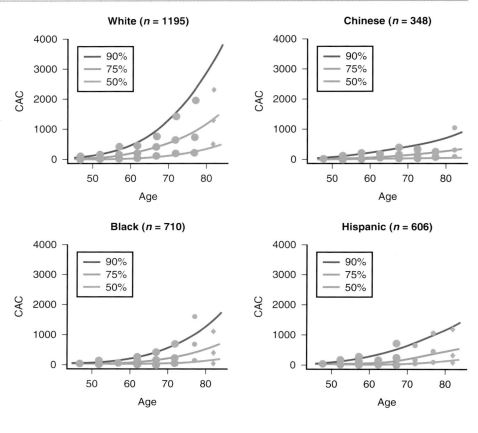

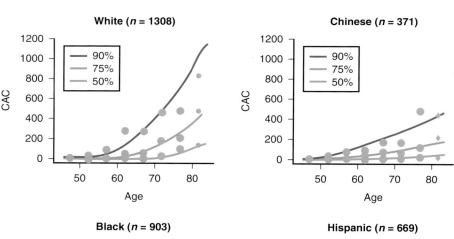

Figure 22-9 Estimated coronary artery calcium (CAC) score percentiles by age and race or ethnicity for men. Each plot shows the estimated curves for the 50th, 75th, and 90th percentiles across age. The observed empirical percentiles for each 5-year age interval also appear as *dots* for reference. (From McClelland RL, Chung H, Detrano R, et al: Epidemiology: distribution of coronary artery calcium by race, gender, and age results from the Multi-Ethnic Study of Atherosclerosis [MESA]. *Circulation.* 2006;113:30-37.

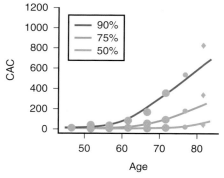

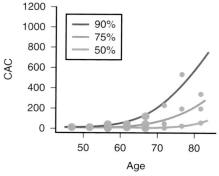

Figure 22-10 Estimated coronary artery calcium (CAC) score percentiles by age and race or ethnicity for women. Each plot shows the estimated curves for the 50th, 75th, and 90th percentiles across age. The observed empirical percentiles for each 5-year age interval also appear as *dots* for reference. (From McClelland RL, Chung H, Detrano R, et al: Epidemiology: distribution of coronary artery calcium by race, gender, and age results from the Multi-Ethnic Study of Atherosclerosis [MESA]. *Circulation.* 2006;113:30-37.

In the future, CAC scoring may be recommended in even low-risk patients. In a cohort of 222 young patients presenting with myocardial infarction (MI) as the first sign of CAD, Akosah et al showed that 70% were in lesser-risk categories. Schmermund et al and Pohle et al indicated that 95% of patients with acute MI would have been identified with a positive CAC score irrespective of age. Perhaps, in the future, as data accumulate on lower-risk patients, these patients will also be deemed appropriate for CAC scoring. In fact, the 2006 Screening for Heart Attack Prevention and Education (SHAPE) guidelines recommended CAC scoring (or carotid intima-media thickness [IMT]) in all but the very lowest-risk asymptomatic men more than 45 years old and women more than 55 years old, with treatment based on CAC score.

Finally, the 2010 American College of Cardiology Foundation (ACCF)/AHA guideline for assessment of cardiovascular risk in asymptomatic adults states that CAC scoring is reasonable for asymptomatic diabetic patients 40 years old and older (IIa recommendation). It further states that stress myocardial perfusion imaging may be considered in asymptomatic diabetic patients who are considered to be at high risk for CAD, including when the CAC score is greater than 400 (IIb recommendation).

Prognostic Value

The prognostic value of CAC scoring has been shown to be excellent in multiple, large studies. In 2000, Raggi et al elegantly demonstrated a graded annualized event rate in a cohort of 632 asymptomatic patients followed up for 32 months. Patients with 0 scores had an annualized event rate of 0.1%. Patients with scores of 1 to 99 had an event rate of 2.1%, those with scores of 100 to 400 had an event rate of 4.1%, and patients with scores higher than 400 had an annualized event rate of 4.8%. With all positive CAC scores having an annualized event rate of more than 2.0%, the risk associated with any positive CAC score exceeds the 2% annual event risk required for secondary prevention using the Framingham risk score.

Shaw et al subsequently showed that all-cause mortality increased proportionally to CAC score, even after adjustment for Framingham risk factors. In this retrospective study of 10,377 patients, Shaw et al also found that CAC scoring had superior area under the receiving operator characteristic (ROC) curves compared with Framingham risk assessment (0.73 versus 0.67; $P < .001$). Even more impressive, after patients were stratified according to their Framingham risk, CAC scores were able to further stratify risk in these patients accurately. This additional risk stratification was particularly strong in the group of patients with intermediate Framingham risk scores. Finally, Shaw et al also showed that the relative risk of death in patients with a CAC score of just 10 is comparable to the relative mortality risk of patients with diabetes, smoking, and hypertension (see Fig. 22-8).

In an asymptomatic cohort of 5635 patients Kondos et al showed that the relative risk for cardiac events with a positive CAC score is 10.5, compared with only 1.98 for diabetes and 1.4 for smoking. This finding is quite striking, especially considering that diabetes is considered a CAD equivalent.

The St. Francis Heart Study, a prospective study of 5585 predominantly moderate-risk to moderately high-risk asymptomatic patients, confirmed these various study results and showed an increasing event rate with increasing CAC scores. Additionally, CAC scores higher than 100 were associated with relative risks from 12 to 32 and were a secondary prevention equivalent with an event rate of more than 2% per year. Of the patients in this study who were classified as intermediate risk by Framingham risk scores, 67% were appropriately reclassified by using CAC tertiles, with outcomes confirmed by monitoring cardiac events in the study.

Prognostic Significance of Very High Scores

Extensive evidence confirms the prognostic significance of very high CAC scores. In a retrospective analysis of 25,203 patients, Budoff et al found that a CAC score higher than 400 was associated with a hazard ratio of 9.2. Additionally, Becker et al conducted a prospective study of 1724 patients and found that a CAC percentile of more than 75% versus 0% was associated with a hazard ratio of 6.8 in men and 7.9 in women. Becker et al also found that 82% of the patients in their cohort who developed MI or cardiac death were classified as high risk by their CAC percentile, compared with only 30% by Framingham risk scores. The area under the ROC curve for the CAC percentile (0.81) in this group was also significantly superior to that of Framingham scoring.

In the MESA, the National Heart, Lung, and Blood Institute sponsored a prospective trial of 6814 patients who were followed up for almost 4 years, and similar results were found. Patients with CAC scores of 101 to 300 had a hazard score of 7.73, whereas patients with CAC scores higher than 300 had a hazard score of 9.67 when compared with patients with no CAC ($P < .001$). Among the 4 racial or ethnic groups (white, Chinese, Hispanic, black), doubling of the CAC score increased the risk of a coronary event by 18% to 39%. ROC curve areas were significantly higher when the CAC score was added to the Framingham risk score ($P < .001$).

Prognostic Significance of Very Low Scores

Patients with 0 CAC scores may still have atherosclerosis in the form of noncalcified plaque, but their coronary event rates are very low. Raggi et al showed only a 0.11% annual event rate with a 1.1% 10-year risk in asymptomatic patients with 0 CAC scores. The MESA also showed a 0.11% annual event rate in asymptomatic patients without CAC, and the St. Francis Heart Study showed a 0.12% rate. A meta-analysis of 64,873 patients followed up over 4.2 years similarly showed a 0.13% annual event rate for patients with 0 CAC scores. In a cohort of more than 44,000 asymptomatic patients who were followed up for 5.6 years, Blaha et al showed that deaths per 1000 patient-years were 7.48 for patients with CAC scores higher than 10, 1.92 for those with CAC scores between 1 and 10, and 0.87 for those with a CAC score of 0.

Multiple studies have shown that only 5% of acute ischemic syndromes occur in patients with 0 CAC scores and exclusively noncalcified plaque. In their meta-analysis, Sarwar et al showed that only 2 of 183 (1.1%) patients with 0 CAC scores were ultimately diagnosed with acute coronary syndrome after they presented with acute chest pain, normal troponin values, and equivocal electrocardiographic findings. A CAC score higher than 0 had a 99% sensitivity, 57% specificity, 24% positive predictive value, and 99% negative predictive value for acute coronary syndrome.

Correlation with Obstructive Disease and Symptomatic Patients

The presence of CAC is essentially 100% specific for atherosclerosis. Pathologic specimens have shown that the amount of CAC only weakly correlates with the degree of luminal narrowing in the coronary arteries, but the likelihood of obstructive disease certainly increases with increasing CAC scores.

Clinically, Shavelle et al showed that a positive CAC score is 96% sensitive but only 47% specific for an obstructive lesion. This finding was compared with a 76% sensitivity and 60% specificity of treadmill testing for obstructive disease. Rumberger et al showed that higher calcium scores are more specific for obstructive disease, although the sensitivity decreases. Budoff et al later showed that CAC scores facilitated prediction of obstructive CAD when these scores were used collaboratively with age, gender, and risk factors. In the large meta-analysis by Sarwar et al, the cohort contained 10,355 symptomatic patients. This study found that positive CAC score was 98% sensitive and 40% specific for the presence of stenosis of more than 50% of luminal diameter. Additionally, the negative predictive value was 93%, whereas the positive predictive value was 68%.

Treatment

After CAC scoring, clinicians must make management decisions based on the results. According to prognostic data from the St. Francis Heart Study, a CAC score higher than 100 is a CAD equivalent. In this same study, CAC scores higher than 400 or higher than the 90th percentile were associated with a particularly high annual risk (4.8% and 6.5%), and these patients may be good candidates for more aggressive management.

Based on the AHA Prevention V Update and the most recent National Cholesterol Education Program recommendations, Hecht recommended that patients with 0 CAC scores should be treated as a low-risk Framingham equivalent. In addition, patients with CAC scores of 1 to 10 (as long as <75th percentile for age and gender) are at moderate risk, patients with CAC scores of 11 to 100 (as long as <75th percentile) are at moderately high risk, patients with CAC scores of 101 to 400 or higher than the 75th percentile are high risk and have a CAD equivalent, and those with CAC scores higher than 400 or higher than the 90th percentile are at the highest risk.

Numerous studies have reported that CAC scoring improves patient compliance with therapeutic interventions. In a study of 505 asymptomatic patients, Kalia et al showed that 3.6 years after visualizing their CAC scan, 90% of patients with CAC scores higher than 400 complied with their statin therapy, compared with 75% of patients with CAC scores of 100 to 399 and only 44% of patients with 0 CAC scores. Similarly, in a study of 980 asymptomatic patients, Orakzai et al showed that acetylsalicylic acid initiation, dietary changes, and exercise were much better in patients with CAC scores higher than 400 (61%, 67%, and 56%, respectively) than in patients with 0 CAC scores (29%, 34%, and 44%, respectively).

Symptomatic Patients

That symptomatic patients with CAC are also more likely to have events is well established. The National Institute for Health and Clinical Excellence (NICE) guidelines, developed by the National Clinical Guideline Centre for Acute and Chronic Conditions in the United Kingdom, recommended CAC scoring as the first diagnostic intervention in patients with chest pain without known CAD, who have a 10% to 29% likelihood of having CAD. The NICE guidelines further recommended finding noncardiac causes of chest pain in those patients whose CAC score is 0. If the CAC score is 1 to 400, computed tomography coronary angiography is recommended, and if the CAC score is higher than 400, then invasive angiography is recommended. In a meta-analysis of 3924 symptomatic patients with 3.5-year follow-up, patients with a positive CAC score had an event rate of 2.6% per year compared with only 0.5% per year in patients with no CAC.

In a cohort of 1031 patients who presented to the emergency department with chest pain and who had a nonischemic electrocardiogram, normal initial troponin values, and no history of CAD, Nabi et al showed that a CAC score of 0 predicted a normal nuclear stress test result and an excellent short-term outcome. In a cohort of 118 patients, La Mont et al showed that the absence of CAC in patients with false-positive treadmill stress test results had a negative predictive value of 90%. This finding suggests that CAC scoring could potentially be used to rule out CAD in low-probability patients with abnormal stress test results.

Despite these guidelines and studies, the practice of using calcium scoring in the workup of symptomatic patients is not part of the recommended algorithm in the United States.

Additional Applications

Raggi et al showed that diabetic patients with no CAC have the same prognosis as do patients without diabetes. Based on this finding, not treating these patients as having a CAD risk equivalent may be a reasonable approach.

Budoff et al showed that the presence of CAC in 120 patients with heart failure of unknown origin was 99% sensitive to the presence of ischemic cardiomyopathy.

Comparison With Other Biomarkers

CAC scoring has clearly been shown to be superior for predicting outcomes compared with conventional risk factors. Multiple studies in large groups of patients, however, have shown a clear association between CAC score and conventional risk factors, including premature family history of CAD, diabetes, and lipid values. Even so, Hecht et al showed that conventional risk factors do not always correlate with CAC score in individual patients. In a cohort of 930 patients, Hecht et al showed a significant correlation between increasing CAC scores with increasing low-density lipoprotein cholesterol (LDL-C) and decreasing high-density lipoprotein cholesterol (HDL-C), although a lack of correlation was noted in individual patients in this cohort between CAC percentile and levels of LDL-C, HDL-C, triglyceride, and homocysteine. Hecht et al showed that individual patients are certainly missed during screening for CAD with conventional risk factors and related biomarkers.

Individual groups of patients are particularly susceptible to inaccurate conventional risk analysis. Hecht and Superko showed that total cholesterol, LDL-C, and triglyceride levels were not higher in women more than 55 years old with positive CAC scores than in those with 0 CAC scores. This finding shows that risk in postmenopausal women is particularly difficult to stratify using conventional risk factors.

Taylor et al showed that conventional risk factors underestimated CAD in 630 active duty U.S. Army personnel 39 to 45 years old. This finding showed that conventional risk analysis is also a problem in this young, low-risk screening cohort.

Given the suboptimal relationship between lipid values and subclinical CAD, extensive efforts are being made to identify stronger markers for subclinical CAD. CAC scoring compares favorably with these other markers.

CAC scoring is superior to high-sensitivity C-reactive protein (hs-CRP) in predicting cardiac events. In 967 asymptomatic patients, Park et al showed that low to high CAC at any hs-CRP level increased the relative risk of MI or cardiac death fourfold to fivefold after adjustment for conventional risk factors. Low to high hs-CRP at any level of CAC, conversely, increased the relative risk by only 0.25-fold to 0.7-fold. After multivariate analysis, Park et al also showed that CAC score is significantly predictive of cardiac events ($P < .005$), whereas hs-CRP is not ($P = .09$), with or without adjustment for CAC score.

In the Study of Inherited Risk of Coronary Atherosclerosis, Reilly et al showed no significant relationship between hs-CRP and CAC score. The Dallas Heart Study had similar results. Additionally, in the St. Francis Heart Study, only the CAC score significantly predicted cardiac events ($P < .0001$) in a multivariate analysis including standard risk factors, hs-CRP, and baseline CAC score. The hs-CRP value did not predict events independent of CAC score ($P = .47$).

Additionally, CAC was more predictive of coronary disease than was carotid IMT because the hazard ratios per each standard deviation increment increased 2.5-fold for CAC (95% confidence interval [CI], 2.1 to 3.1), but only 1.1-fold for IMT (95% CI, 1.0 to 1.4).

Although atherosclerosis undeniably has metabolic and inflammatory components, thus making lipids and

hs-CRP worthy considerations for screening measurements, it also probably has a genetic component that is missed by today's screening blood tests. This is why screening with imaging is so important.

Coronary Artery Calcium Progression

Statins and Lipids

Researchers are currently exploring the utility of following CAC progression over time. They are also exploring CAC progression to help further understand the pathophysiology of CAD.

Numerous animal studies have analyzed CAC progression. In 2000, Stary published a study of 59 rhesus monkeys. These monkeys were fed high-cholesterol diets for several years, followed by a cholesterol-restricted diet. The monkeys were sacrificed at various time points in this experiment. Stary found that when these monkeys were fed cholesterol-rich diets, lipid-rich plaques developed with scattered calcific granules. As plaques expanded, more calcifications became visible. After 3 years of the cholesterol-restricted diet, however, the plaques became less lipid rich and more fibrotic, and the calcium burden remained unchanged.

In a study of 32 adult male cynomolgus monkeys initially fed an atherogenic diet, Williams et al further showed that pravastatin treatment led to a reduction in intimal neovascularization, diminished plaque macrophage infiltration, and a decrease in calcification of both early and advanced plaques. This study showed that statins not only may help lower LDL-C levels, but also may benefit existing plaques.

In similar studies, Daoud et al and Clarkson et al did not find a reduction in coronary artery plaque calcium deposition with intervention in either pigs or monkeys. These findings are a reminder that much more histologic work remains to be done in the field of CAC progression and CAC regression.

Studies have demonstrated that luminal stenosis improvements seen on quantitative invasive angiography result in cardiovascular event reduction, even with the minimal stenosis regression usually seen with medical therapy. Similar studies have been pursued to determine whether CAC regression or progression results in a predictable change in the cardiovascular event rate. Of course, these studies cannot strictly be compared with invasive angiography stenosis change because most of the patients undergoing invasive angiography are symptomatic, unlike most of the patients undergoing CAC scoring.

In 1998, Callister et al conducted an observational study of 149 asymptomatic patients with sequential CAC scans 12 to 15 months apart. The patients included in the cohort required a volume score higher than 30 to maximize reproducibility of the CAC scores. Forty-four of these patients did not receive statin therapy. These patients (mean LDL-C, 147 mg/dL, with standard deviation of 22 mg/dL) averaged CAC score progression of 52 ± 36% per year. Among the treated patients, 65 achieved an LDL-C level lower than 120 mg/dL. These patients showed a net regression of calcium volume score of −7 ± 22% per year. In those patients treated with statin therapy but with an LDL-C level higher than 120 mg/dL, the mean yearly calcium volume score progression was 25 ± 22%. All intergroup comparisons were statistically significant ($P < .0001$). This study suggested that the aggressiveness of LDL-C treatment correlates with atherosclerotic plaque change, which can be monitored with CAC scoring.

Budoff et al later showed that statin treatment in 299 asymptomatic patients followed up with sequential CAC scans for 1 to 6.5 years was beneficial. Statin therapy resulted in significant slowing of CAC progression when compared with untreated patients (15 ± 8% per year with treatment versus 39 ± 12% per year without treatment).

In a subsequent prospective study, Achenbach et al studied 66 asymptomatic patients. The patients had known CAC and LDL-C levels higher than 130 mg/dL at baseline. The patients were left untreated for 14 months and had repeat CAC scans. The patients were then started on statin therapy, and repeat CAC scans were obtained 12 months later. The median calcium volume score increase during the drug-free period was 25% during the untreated year, but it slowed to 8.8% during the treatment year ($P < .0001$). The 32 patients who achieved an average LDL-C level lower than 100 mg/dL actually achieved median calcium volume regression (−3.4%), whereas these same patients progressed 27% during the untreated year ($P = .0001$). This finding provided more evidence of the effectiveness of aggressive LDL-C reduction.

In a subanalysis of the Women's Health Initiative, Hsia et al studied 914 postmenopausal women. This group found that women with lower scores at baseline had smaller annual increases in CAC score; CAC scores increased 11, 31, and 79 units per year among women with baseline CAC scores in the lowest, middle, and highest tertiles, respectively. Hsia et al also found that age was not an independent predictor of CAC progression. Statin use at baseline was a negative predictor ($P = .015$), and baseline score was a strong positive predictor ($P < .0001$).

Despite all these favorable results, larger prospective studies failed to confirm an association between LDL-C reduction and CAC progression. The Beyond Endorsed Lipid Lowering with EBT Scanning trial was a randomized study of 615 postmenopausal, dyslipidemic women with sequential EBT CAC scans. The patients were randomized to either atorvastatin (80 mg/day) or pravastatin (40 mg/day). Although atorvastatin achieved better LDL-C levels (94 mg/dL) than pravastatin (129 mg/dL), no significant difference in CAC progression was noted between the 2 groups. The St. Francis Heart Study was also a prospective, randomized study of 1005 healthy patients with CAC scores higher than the 80th percentile for age and sex. The study compared atorvastatin (20 mg/day) with vitamin C and E supplementation versus placebo, and progression was similar (~20% per year) between the 2 treatment arms of the trial on follow-up (mean follow-up 4.3 years).

Other Studies of Coronary Artery Calcium Progression

Although the foregoing large studies did not show that lipid-lowering therapy slowed CAC progression, other interesting studies have been done on various therapies and their impact on CAC changes. In 109 patients with type 1 diabetes (22 to 50 years old) who had sequential EBT scans 2.7 years apart, Snell-Bergeon et al showed that CAC progression was associated with hyperglycemia (odds ratio, 7.11; 95% CI, 1.38 to 36.6; $P = .02$).

In the Women's Health Initiative, postmenopausal women in their 50s were randomized to treatment with estrogen or placebo. In a substudy of this group, 1064 of these patients underwent CAC scans after 8.7 years of being enrolled in the trial. Patients receiving estrogen had a significantly reduced CAC score compared with patients receiving placebo (83.1 versus 123.1; $P = .02$).

In a placebo-controlled, randomized, double-blind pilot study of 23 patients, Budoff et al showed that aged garlic extract slowed CAC progression. The 23 patients in this study were randomized to garlic or placebo and underwent sequential CAC scans 1 year apart. The group taking garlic had significantly lower CAC volume progression than did the group receiving placebo (7.5 versus 18.5; $P = .046$), with no significant differences in lipid values or CRP in the 2 groups.

Garlic has been shown to reduce cardiovascular risk factors by reducing blood pressure, cholesterol, and platelet function while stimulating endothelial cells to produce nitric oxide. In 2009, Budoff et al showed that aged garlic extract with supplements decreased total cholesterol, LDL-C, homocysteine, immunoglobulin G and immunoglobulin M autoantibodies to malondialdehyde-modified LDL-C, and apolipoprotein B–immune complexes. The group also showed that garlic increased HDL-C, lipoprotein (a), and temperature rebound (a marker of vascular function), as well as slowed calcium progression. All these findings were significant compared with placebo in this placebo-controlled, double-blind, randomized trial of 65 intermediate-risk patients. In this same trial, Budoff et al also showed that garlic significantly increased oxidized phospholipids on apolipoprotein B-100. In an interesting follow-up, Ahmadi et al showed that increased oxidized phospholipids on apolipoprotein B-100 correlated strongly with increases in vascular function and predicted a lack of CAC progression in the same cohort. In a more recent analysis of this cohort, Larijani et al showed a significant decrease in carotid-radial pulse wave velocity (marker correlating with decreased vascular stiffness) in the group taking aged garlic extract with supplement.

Nanobacteria have been implicated as a trigger for the initiation of CAC and atherosclerosis. In contrast, ethylenediaminetetraacetic acid (EDTA) disodium salt has been theorized to remove calcium from soft tissue deposits. Maniscalco et al conducted an interesting study in which 77 volunteers with stable CAD were given therapy composed of EDTA, tetracyclines, coenzyme Q10, and vitamins. This therapy reduced lipid levels in many of these patients, most of whom were already receiving statin therapy. Additionally, 44 of the patients showed CAC regression in CAC scans performed 4 months apart.

End-stage renal disease results in cardiovascular disease rates much higher than those in the general population. Calcium-based phosphate-binding therapy for hyperphosphatemia in these patients has been implicated in the development and progression of arterial and valvular calcification. In the Treat-to-Goal study, 200 patients who had received hemodialysis for at least 3 years before study entry were randomized to sevelamer, a calcium-free nonabsorbable polymer or the traditional calcium-based phosphate binders to control hyperphosphatemia. During the study period, serum phosphorus levels were maintained between 3 and 5 mg/dL, serum calcium levels were between 8.5 and 10.5 mg/dL, and serum parathyroid hormone levels were between 150 and 300 pg/mL. CAC scans were obtained at baseline and at 1-year follow-up. Both groups had CAC score progression, but no significant difference was noted between the groups. The group taking sevelamer had a significantly lower mean LDL-C level compared with the group taking calcium-based phosphate binders, even though the latter group received statins more frequently. CAC progression between the group taking sevelamer and the group taking calcium-based phosphate binders was similar when adjusted for LDL-C.

Block et al subsequently conducted a similar trial, but had very different results. At the end of 18 months follow-up, the group taking calcium-based phosphate binders had an 11-fold greater CAC progression than did the group taking sevelamer ($P < .002$). Additionally, after 4.5 years, the sevelamer group had significantly lower mortality (hazard ratio, 2.2; $P < .02$).

More recently, the Calcium Acetate Renagel Evaluation-2 (CARE-2) study failed to show a difference between sevelamer and the calcium-based phosphate binders. The investigators found that CAC progression was similar in both groups. This study was poor, however, because parathyroid hormone levels for the treated patients were double those of patients in earlier studies and suggested inadequate control of mineral metabolism.

Prognostic Value of Coronary Artery Calcium Progression

A few studies have investigated the clinical implications of CAC progression. Raggi et al followed 817 asymptomatic patients who were referred for sequential CAC scores at an average interval of 2.2 ± 1.3 years. The use of statin therapy in these patients was at the discretion of the treating physicians. Several years after the sequential CAC scans, telephone interviews were conducted to determine the occurrence of MI in these patients, among other end points. The mean yearly CAC volume score change for those patients who subsequently suffered an MI was $47 \pm 50\%$, but it was only $26 \pm 32\%$ for those who did not ($P < .001$). Both treatment of hyperlipidemia (likely secondary to greater baseline risk) and CAC progression were independent predictors of events.

Raggi et al did another observational study on 495 asymptomatic patients with sequential CAC scans followed for a median 3 years. The 41 patients in this group who had an MI had significantly higher CAC score progression compared with the event-free group (42 ± 23 versus $17 \pm 25\%$; $P < .001$). The subjects who had MIs also had an average relative CAC score increase of more than 15%, which has been identified as the cut-off for true score change, as opposed to a measurement

reproducibility error. Both groups had identical average LDL-C levels (~120 mg/dL). In a multivariable model, the best predictors of yearly CAC increase of more than 15% were smoking ($P = .032$), male gender ($P = .014$), and baseline CAC score ($P = .02$).

In the St. Francis Heart study, 4613 patients had CAC scores determined 2 years apart. The median absolute CAC score increase was 4 in patients who did not suffer from cardiac events during follow-up, but it was 247 for those with events ($P < .0001$). A 2-year change in CAC score was significantly associated with the risk of cardiovascular events ($P < .0001$).

More recently, in 4609 asymptomatic patients, Budoff et al showed that CAC progression added incremental value in predicting all-cause mortality over baseline score, time between scans, demographics, and cardiac risk factors.

The clinical implications of CAC progression have been demonstrated to be significant in observational studies, and standard therapies have shown variable utility in slowing CAC score progression. Whether sequential CAC scoring should be recommended in clinical practice remains controversial.

■ CONCLUSION

CAC scoring is a well-validated risk assessment tool that represents a major advance in screening for CAD. The evidence is sound, and cardiologists must be educated on the ways to incorporate this screening tool into clinical practice, as discussed in this chapter. Additionally, more research is needed on CAC progression and the impact of various treatments for CAD.

Bibliography

Achenbach S, Dieter R, Pohle K, et al. Influence of lipid-lowering therapy on the progression of coronary artery calcification. *Circulation.* 2002;106:1077-1082.

Agatston AS, Janowitz WR, Hildner FJ, et al. Quantification of coronary artery calcium using ultrafast computed tomography. *J Am Coll Cardiol.* 1990;15:827-832.

Ahmadi N, Tsimikas S, Hajsadeghi F, et al. Relation of oxidative biomarkers, vascular dysfunction, and progression of coronary artery calcium. *Am J Cardiol.* 2010;105:459-466.

Akosah K, Schaper A, Cogbill C, Schoenfeld P. Preventing myocardial infarction in the young adult in the first place: how do the National Cholesterol Education Panel III guidelines perform? *J Am Coll Cardiol.* 2003;41:1475-1479.

American Cancer Society. Recommendations for Early Breast Cancer Detection in Women Without Breast Symptoms. <http://www.cancer.org/cancer/breastcancer/moreinformation/breastcancerearlydetection/breast-cancer-early-detection-acs-recs; 2010> Accessed 03.02.11.

American Heart Association. *Heart and Stroke Statistical Update.* Dallas: American Heart Association; 2001.

Arad Y, Goodman KJ, Roth M, et al. Coronary calcification, coronary risk factors, and atherosclerotic cardiovascular disease events: the St. Francis Heart Study. *J Am Coll Cardiol.* 2005;46:158-165.

Arad Y, Spadaro LA, Roth M, Newstein D, Guerci A. Treatment of asymptomatic adults with elevated calcium scores with atorvastatin, vitamin C and vitamin E: the St. Francis Heart Study randomized clinical trial. *J Am Coll Cardiol.* 2005;46:166-172.

Becker A, Leber A, Becker C, Knez A. Predictive value of coronary calcifications for future cardiac events in asymptomatic individuals. *Am Heart J.* 2008;155:154-160.

Becker CR, Kleffel T, Crispin A, et al. Coronary artery calcium measurement: agreement of multirow detector and electron beam CT. *AJR Am J Roentgenol.* 2001;176:1295-1298.

Berber TC, Carr JJ, Arai AE, et al. Ionizing radiation in cardiac imaging: a science advisory from the American Heart Association Committee on Cardiac Imaging of the Council on Clinical Cardiology and Committee on Cardiovascular Imaging and Intervention of the Council on Cardiovascular Radiology and Intervention. *Circulation.* 2009;119:1056-1065.

Blaha M, Budoff MJ, Shaw LJ, et al. Absence of coronary artery calcification and all-cause mortality. *JACC Cardiovasc Imaging.* 2009;2:692-700.

Blankenhorn DH. Coronary arterial calcification: a review. *Am J Med Sci.* 1961;242:41-49.

Block GA, Spiegel DM, Ehrlich J, et al. Effects of sevelamer and calcium on coronary artery calcification in patients new to hemodialysis. *Kidney Int.* 2005;68:1815-1824.

Bostrom K, Watson KE, Horn S, et al. Bone morphogenetic protein expression in human atherosclerotic lesions. *J Clin Invest.* 1993;91:1800-1809.

Brown ER, Kronmal RA, Bluemke DA. Coronary calcium coverage score: determination, correlates, and predictive accuracy in the multi-ethnic study of atherosclerosis. *Radiology.* 2008;247:669-675.

Budoff MJ, Ahmadi N, Gul KM, et al. Aged garlic extract supplemented with B vitamins, folic acid and L-arginine retards the progression of subclinical atherosclerosis: a randomized clinical trial. *Prev Med.* 2009;49:101-107.

Budoff MJ, Georgiou D, Brody A, et al. Ultrafast computed tomography as a diagnostic modality in the detection of coronary artery disease: a multicenter study. *Circulation.* 1996;93:898-904.

Budoff MJ, Hokanson JE, Nasir K. Progression of coronary artery calcium predicts all-cause mortality. *JACC Cardiovasc Imaging.* 2010;3:1229-1236.

Budoff MJ, Lane KL, Bakheshi H, et al. Rates of progression of coronary calcium by electron beam tomography. *Am J Cardiol.* 2000;86:8-11.

Budoff MJ, Mao S, Zalace CP, Bakhsheshi H, Oudiz RJ. Comparison of spiral and electron beam tomography in the evaluation of coronary calcification in asymptomatic persons. *Int J Cardiol.* 2001;77:181-188.

Budoff MJ, Raggi P, Berman D, et al. Continuous probabilistic prediction of angiographically significant coronary artery disease using electron beam tomography. *Circulation.* 2002;105:1791-1796.

Budoff MJ, Shavelle DM, Lamont DH, et al. Usefulness of electron beam computed tomography scanning for distinguishing ischemic from non-ischemic cardiomyopathy. *J Am Coll Cardiol.* 1998;32:1173-1178.

Budoff MJ, Shaw LJ, Liu ST, et al. Long-term prognosis associated with coronary calcification: observations from a registry of 25,253 patients. *J Am Coll Cardiol.* 2007;29:1860-1870.

Budoff MJ, Takasu J, Flores FR, et al. Inhibiting progression of coronary calcification using aged garlic extract in patients receiving statin therapy: a preliminary study. *Prev Med.* 2004;39:985-991.

Callister TQ, Cooil B, Raya SP, et al. Coronary artery disease: improved reproducibility of calcium scoring with an electron-beam CT volumetric method. *Radiology.* 1998;208:807-814.

Callister TQ, Raggi P, Cooil B. Effects of HMG-CoA reductase inhibitors on coronary artery disease. *N Engl J Med.* 1998;399:1972-1977.

Chertow GM, Burke SK, Raggi P. Sevelamer attenuates the progression of coronary and aortic calcification in hemodialysis patients. *Kidney Int.* 2002;62:245-252.

Clarkson TB, Bond MG, Bullock BC, et al. A study of atherosclerosis regression in *Macaca mulatta.* IV. Changes in coronary arteries from animals with atherosclerosis induced for 19 months and then regressed for 24 months at plasma cholesterol concentrations of 300 or 200 mg/dl. *Exp Mol Pathol.* 1981;34:345-368.

Daoud AS, Jarmolych J, Augustyn JM, et al. Sequential morphologic studies of regression of advanced atherosclerosis. *Arch Pathol.* 1981;105:233-239.

Daviglus ML, Pirzada A, Liu K, et al. Comparison of low risk and higher risk profiles in middle age to frequency and quantity of coronary artery calcium years later. *Am J Cardiol.* 2004;94:367-369.

Detrano R, Guerci AD, Carr JJ, et al. Coronary calcium as a predictor of coronary events in four racial or ethnic groups. *N Engl J Med.* 2008;358:1336-1345.

Detrano R, Tang W, Kang X, et al. Accurate coronary calcium phosphate mass measurements from electron beam computed tomograms. *Am J Card Imaging.* 1995;9:167-173.

Folsom AR, Kronmal RA, Detrano RC, et al. Coronary artery calcification compared with carotid intima-media thickness in the prediction of cardiovascular disease incidence: the multi-ethnic study of atherosclerosis (MESA). *Arch Intern Med.* 2007;167:2437-2442.

Goodman WG, Goldin J, Kuizon BD, et al. Coronary-artery calcification in young adults with end-stage renal disease who are undergoing dialysis. *N Engl J Med.* 2000;342:1478-1483.

Greenland P, Alpert JS, Beller GA, et al. 2010 ACCF/AHA guideline for assessment of cardiovascular risk in asymptomatic adults: executive summary. *Circulation.* 2010;122:2748-2764.

Guerci AD, Spadaro LA, Popma JJ, et al. Electron beam tomography of the coronary arteries: relationship of coronary calcium score to arteriographic findings in asymptomatic and symptomatic adults. *Am J Cardiol.* 1997;79:128-133.

Guerin AP, London GM, Marchais SJ, et al. Arterial stiffening and vascular calcifications in end-stage renal disease. *Nephrol Dial Transplant.* 2000;15:1014-1021.

Hecht HS. Assessment of cardiovascular calcium: interpretation, prognostic value, and relationship to lipids and other cardiovascular risk factors. In: Budoff MJ, Shinbane JS, eds. *Cardiac CT Imaging: Diagnosis of Cardiovascular Disease.* 2nd ed. New York: Springer; 2010.

Hecht HS, Superko HR. Electron beam tomography and national cholesterol education program guidelines in asymptomatic women. *J Am Coll Cardiol.* 2001;37:1506-1511.

Hecht HS, Superko HR, Smith LK, et al. Relation of coronary artery calcium identified by electron beam tomography to serum lipoprotein levels and implications for treatment. *Am J Cardiol.* 2001;87:406-412.

Hideya Y, Budoff MJ, Lu B, et al. Reproducibility of three different scoring systems for measurement of coronary calcium. *Int J Cardiovasc Imaging.* 2002;18:391-397.

Hoff JA, Chomka EV, Krainik AJ, et al. Age and gender distributions of coronary artery calcium detected by electron beam tomography in 35,246 adults. *Am J Cardiol.* 2001;87:1335-1339.

Hsia J, Klouj A, Prasad A, Burt J, Adams-Campbell LL, Howard BV. Progression of coronary calcification in healthy postmenopausal women. *BMC Cardiovasc Disord.* 2004;4:21.

Ideda T, Shirasawa T, Esaki Y, et al. Osteopontin mRNA is expressed by smooth muscle–derived foam cells in human atherosclerotic lesions of the aorta. *J Clin Invest.* 1993;92:2814-2820.

Janowitz WR, Agatston AS, Kaplan G, Viamonte M. Differences in prevalence and extent of coronary artery calcium detected by ultrafast computed tomography in asymptomatic men and women. *Am J Cardiol.* 1993;72:247-254.

Kalia NK, Miller LG, Nasir K, et al. Visualizing coronary calcium is associated with improvements in adherence to statin therapy. *Atherosclerosis.* 2006;185:394-399.

Khera A, de Lemos JA, Peshock RM, et al. Relationship between C-reactive protein and subclinical atherosclerosis: the Dallas Heart Study. *Circulation.* 2006;113:38-43.

Knez A, Becker C, Becker A, et al. Determination of coronary calcium with multi-slice spiral computed tomography: a comparative study with electron-beam CT. *Int J Cardiovasc Imaging.* 2002;18:295-303.

Kondos GT, Hoff JA, Sevrukov A, et al. Electron-beam tomography coronary artery calcium and cardiac events: a 37-month follow-up of 5,635 initially asymptomatic low to intermediate risk adults. *Circulation.* 2003;107:2571-2576.

Kuller LH, Matthews KA, Sutton-Tyrrell K, et al. Coronary and aortic calcification among women 8 years after menopause and their premenopausal risk factors: the Healthy Women Study. *Arterioscler Thromb Vasc Biol.* 1999;19:2189-2198.

La Mont DH, Budoff MJ, Shavelle DM, et al. Coronary calcium screening identifies patients with false positive stress tests [abstract]. *Circulation.* 1997;96:306–I.

Larijani VN, Zed I, Flores F. Aged garlic extract and coenzyme Q10 decreases arterial stiffness and retards progression of coronary artery calcium in at risk fire fighters. J Am Coll Cardiol. 2011;57:E1487-E1487.

Levine GN, Keaney Jr JF, Vita JA. Cholesterol reduction in cardiovascular disease: clinical benefits and possible mechanisms. *N Engl J Med.* 1995;332:512-521.

Lockwood D, Einstein D, Davros W. Diagnostic imaging: radiation dose and patient concerns. *Cleve Clin J Med.* 2006;736:583-586.

Lu B, Budoff MJ, Zhuang N, et al. Causes of interscan variability of coronary artery calcium measurements at electron-beam CT. *Acad Radiol.* 2002;9:654-661.

Maniscalco BS, Taylor KA. Calcification in coronary artery disease can be reversed by EDTA-tetracycline long-term chemotherapy. *Pathophysiology.* 2004;11:95-101.

Manson JE, Allison MA, Rossouw JE, et al. Estrogen therapy and coronary-artery calcification. *N Engl J Med.* 2007;356:2591-2602.

Mao SS, Pal RS, McKay CR, et al. Comparison of coronary artery calcium scores between electron beam computed tomography and 64-multidetector computed tomographic scanner. *J Comput Assist Tomogr.* 2009;33:175-178.

Mautner GC, Mautner SL, Froelich J, et al. Coronary artery calcification: assessment with electron beam CT and histomorphometric correlation. *Radiology.* 1994;192:619-623.

McClelland RL, Chung H, Detrano R, et al. Distribution of coronary artery calcium by race, gender, and age: results from the Multi-Ethnic Study of Atherosclerosis (MESA). *Circulation.* 2006;113:30-37.

McCullough CH, Ulzheimer S, Halliburton SS. Coronary artery calcium: a multi-institutional, multimanufacturer internation standard for quantification at cardiac CT. *Radiology.* 2007;243:527-538.

Nabi F, Chang SM, Pratt CM, et al. Coronary artery calcium scoring in the emergency department: identifying which patients with chest pain can be safely discharged home. *Ann Emerg Med.* 2010;56:220-229.

Naghavi M, Falk E, Hecht HS, et al. From vulnerable plaque to vulnerable patient. Part III. Executive summary of the Screening for Heart Attack Prevention and Education (SHAPE) task force report. *Am J Cardiol.* 2006;98(suppl):2H-15H.

Nasir K, Michos ED, Rumberger JA, et al. Coronary artery calcification and family history of premature coronary heart disease: sibling history is more strongly associated than parental history. *Circulation.* 2004;110:2150-2156.

National Cholesterol Education Program. Third Report of the National Cholesterol Education Program (NCEP) Expert Panel on Detection, Evaluation, and Treatment of High Blood Cholesterol in Adults (Adult Treatment Panel III). <http://www.nhlbi.nih.gov/guidelines/cholesterol/atp3xsum.pdf;> 2011. Accessed 07.02.11.

National Institute for Health and Clinical Excellence. Chest Pain of Recent Onset: Assessment and Diagnosis of Recent Onset Chest Pain or Discomfort of Suspected Cardiac Origin. NICE clinical guideline 95. < http://www.nice .org.uk/nicemedia/live/12947/47938/47938.pdf;> 2010. Accessed 08.02.11.

Orakzai RH, Nasir K, Orakzai SH, et al. Effect of patient visualization of coronary calcium by electron beam computed tomography on changes in beneficial lifestyle behaviors. *Am J Cardiol.* 2008;101:999-1002.

Park R, Detrano R, Xiang M, et al. Combined use of computed tomography coronary calcium scores and C-reactive protein levels in predicting cardiovascular events in nondiabetic individuals. *Circulation*. 2002;106: 2073-2077.

Pelburg R, Mazur W. *Cardiac CT Angiography Manual*. New York: Springer; 2007.

Peyser PA, Bielak LF, Chu J, et al. Heritability of coronary artery calcium quantity measures by electron beam computed tomography in asymptomatic adults. *Circulation*. 2002;106:304-308.

Pohle K, Ropers D, Maffert R, et al. Coronary calcifications in young patients with first, unheralded myocardial infarction: a risk factor matched analysis by electron beam tomography. *Heart*. 2003;89:625-628.

Qunibi W, Moustafa M, Muenz LR, et al. A 1-year randomized trial of calcium acetate versus sevelamer on progression of coronary artery calcification in hemodialysis patients with comparable lipid control: the Calcium Acetate Renagel Evaluation-2 (CARE-2) study. *Am J Kidney Dis*. 2008;5:952-965.

Raggi P. Natural history and impact of interventions on coronary calcium. In: Budoff MJ, Shinbane JS, eds. *Cardiac CT Imaging: Diagnosis of Cardiovascular Disease*. 2nd ed. New York: Springer; 2010.

Raggi P, Callister T, Budoff M, Shaw L. Progression of coronary artery calcium and risk of first myocardial infarction in patients receiving cholesterol-lowering therapy. *Arterioscler Thromb Vasc Biol*. 2004;24:1272-1277.

Raggi P, Callister TQ, Cooil B, et al. Identification of patients at increased risk of first unheralded acute myocardial infarction by electron beam computed tomography. *Circulation*. 2000;101:850-855.

Raggi P, Cooil B, Shaw LJ, et al. Progression of coronary calcification on serial electron beam tomography scanning is greater in patients with future myocardial infarction. *Am J Cardiol*. 2003;92:827-829.

Raggi P, Davidson M, Callister TQ, et al. Aggressive versus moderate lipid-lowering therapy in hypercholesterolemic post-menopausal women: Beyond Endorsed Lipid Lowering with EBT Scanning (BELLES). *Circulation*. 2005;112:563-571.

Raggi P, Shaw LJ, Berman DS, Callister TQ. Prognostic value of coronary artery calcium screening in subjects with and without diabetes. *J Am Coll Cardiol*. 2004;43:1663-1669.

Reilly MP, Wolfe ML, Localio AR, Rader DJ. C-reactive protein and coronary artery calcification: the Study of Inherited Risk of Coronary Atherosclerosis (SIRCA). *Arterioscler Thromb Vasc Biol*. 2003;23:1851-1856.

Rumberger JA, Sheedy PF, Breen JF, et al. Electron beam CT coronary calcium score cutpoints and severity of associated angiography luminal stenosis. *J Am Coll Cardiol*. 1997;29:1542-1548.

Rumberger JA, Simons DB, Fitzpatrick LA, et al. Coronary artery calcium areas by electron beam computed tomography and coronary atherosclerotic plaque area: a histopathologic correlative study. *Circulation*. 1995;92:2157-2162.

Sarwar A, Shaw LJ, Shapiro MD, et al. Diagnostic and prognostic value of coronary artery calcification. *JACC Cardiovasc Imaging*. 2009;2:675-688.

Schmermund A, Baumgart D, Gorge G, et al. Coronary artery calcium in acute coronary syndromes: a comparative study of electron beam CT, coronary angiography, and intracoronary ultrasound in survivors of acute myocardial infarction and unstable angina. *Circulation*. 1997;96:1461-1469.

Shanahan CM, Cary NR, Metcalfe JC, Weissberg PL. High expression of genes for calcification-regulating proteins in human atherosclerotic plaque. *J Clin Invest*. 1994;93:2393-2402.

Shavelle DM, Budoff MJ, LaMont DH, et al. Exercise testing and electron beam computed tomography in the evaluation of coronary artery disease. *J Am Coll Cardiol*. 2000;36:32-38.

Shaw LJ, Raggi P, Schisterman E, et al. Prognostic value of cardiac risk factors and coronary artery calcium screening for all-cause mortality. *Radiology*. 2003;28:826-833.

Simons DB, Schwartz RS, Edwards WD, et al. Noninvasive definition of anatomic coronary disease by ultrafast computed tomographic scanning: a quantitative pathologic comparison study. *J Am Coll Cardiol*. 1992;20:1118-1126.

Smith SC, Greenland P, Grundy SM. Prevention Conference V. Beyond secondary prevention: identifying the high-risk patient for primary prevention. Executive summary. *Circulation*. 2000;101:111-116.

Snell-Bergeon JK, Hokanson JE, Jensen L, et al. Progression of coronary artery calcification in type 1 diabetes: the importance of glycemic control. *Diabetes Care*. 2003;26:2923-2928.

Stary HC. Natural history of calcium deposits in atherosclerosis progression and regression. *Z Kardiol*. 2000;89(suppl 2):28-35.

Taylor AJ, Cerqueira M, Hodgson JM, et al. ACCF/SCCT/ACR/AHA/ASE/ASNC/SCAI/SCMR 2010 appropriate use criteria for cardiac computed tomography. *J Am Coll Cardiol*. 2010;56:1864-1894.

Taylor AJ, Feuerstein I, Wong H, Barko W, Brazaitis M, O'Malley PG. Do conventional risk factors predict subclinical coronary artery disease? Results from the Prospective Army Coronary Calcium Project. *Am Heart J*. 2001;141:463-468.

U.S. Renal Data System. *USRDS 2004 Annual Data Report: Atlas of End-Stage Renal Disease in the United States*. National Institute of Diabetes and Digestive and Kidney Diseases. Bethesda, Md: National Institutes of Health; 2004.

Wexler L, Brundage B, Crouse J, et al. Coronary artery calcification: pathophysiology, epidemiology, image methods and clinical implications. A scientific statement from the American Heart Association. *Circulation*. 1996;94:1175-1192.

Williams JK, Sukhova GK, Herrington DM, Libby P. Pravastatin has cholesterol-lowering independent effects on the artery wall of atherosclerotic monkeys. *J Am Coll Cardiol*. 1998;31:684-691.

CHAPTER 23

Cardiac Computed Tomography for the Evaluation of Acute Coronary Syndrome in the Emergency Department

Felix M. Gonzalez, Sampson K. Kyere, and Charles S. White

From 1999 through 2008, most visits to the emergency departments (EDs) in the United States by adult patients (≥15 years old) were mainly for chest and abdominal pain, according to the latest National Hospital Ambulatory Medical Care Survey released in September of 2010 by the Centers for Disease Control and Prevention. In 2007 and 2008, approximately 5.5 million visits were primarily attributed to chest pain. Among the visits for chest pain, a minority was caused by acute coronary syndrome (ACS), aortic dissection, or pulmonary embolism.

Besides the introduction of multiple medical advances in the evaluation of acute chest pain in the ED, differentiating patients who need to be admitted from those who can be safely discharged poses a difficult and complex challenge for emergency medicine clinicians. Most patients who present with chest pain and who are ultimately admitted are eventually discharged without a diagnosis or with a diagnosis of a noncardiac condition. This situation represents a significant financial burden, estimated to be approximately $8 billion in the United States each year. Moreover, patients who are inappropriately discharged and who ultimately prove to have ACS have an increased mortality rate (almost double) when compared with those who are admitted. In a typical ED in the United States, approximately 2% of patients with acute myocardial infarction and 2% of those with unstable angina are inappropriately discharged; this finding exemplifies that no model exists to identify successfully all patients with medically serious chest pain.

■ STANDARD APPROACH IN DIAGNOSING ACUTE CORONARY SYNDROME

ACS, which is usually caused by a ruptured atherosclerotic plaque, has different clinical presentations, ranging from unstable angina to subendocardial or transmural infarction. The most common clinical presentation of acute myocardial ischemia is chest pain, which is primarily the result of interrupted blood flow to the myocardium. Nevertheless, the clinical manifestations of chest pain are often ambiguous, and they present a major challenge in accurately differentiating ACS from other serious conditions such as pulmonary embolism and aortic dissection, as well as less serious noncardiac causes of chest pain such as pneumonia, gastroesophageal reflux, and musculoskeletal discomfort.

Since 2000, multidetector computed tomography (MDCT) has become the standard modality used to diagnose pulmonary embolism. MDCT allows routine visualization of the pulmonary arteries to the subsegmental level, with reported sensitivity and specificity ranging from 83% to 100% and 89% to 97%, respectively. MDCT has also become the gold standard for detection of suspected aortic dissection, with reported sensitivity and specificity greater than 95%. The urgent nature of arriving at a diagnosis of aortic dissection in the ED, the short time it takes for a scan to be performed, and the proximity of scanners to most EDs make MDCT highly attractive. The nonenhanced component of the scan is useful to detect the presence of intramural hematoma. Such a hematoma is apparent as a thickened aortic wall with increased radiodensity. In the absence of a dissection flap and a false lumen, an intramural hematoma may not be visible following the administration of contrast media.

In most cases, the diagnosis of ACS follows a standard approach that includes an initial evaluation phase, followed by a period of prolonged observation related to the diagnostic complexity of ACS. This observation period also prevents inappropriate discharge of patients with ACS. The initial assessment of ACS incorporates the clinical triad of symptoms, electrocardiogram (ECG), and cardiac enzyme levels (creatine kinase and troponin). The most common physical symptoms have classically been described as chest pain with exertion and pressure-like chest discomfort with radiation to the neck or arms. Nevertheless, the clinical presentation of ACS is often nonspecific, thus limiting the use of this clinical triad. As many as 20% of patients with myocardial infarction present with atypical chest pain, and another subset of patients presents with no pain at all. The second component of the initial assessment, the ECG, has limitations because approximately 20% of ECGs are normal in acute myocardial infarction, 37% in the setting of unstable angina. Classically, the ECG is diagnostic in the case of ST-segment elevation myocardial infarction and occasionally diagnostic for non–ST-segment elevation myocardial infarction, an inconsistency attributed to the sporadic nature of coronary ischemia.

Cardiac troponin has become the biomarker of choice for patients with ACS, especially in the ED; however, multiple limitations restrict biomarker application to acute myocardial infarction. The presence of biomarker elevation confirms only that myocardial injury has occurred, and myocardial injury can be seen in multiple conditions in addition to ACS, such as heart failure, myocarditis, pericarditis, pulmonary embolism, sepsis, or any other condition resulting in ischemia or inflammation of the myocardium. The sensitivity of biomarkers for acute myocardial infarction has been found to vary depending on when biomarker levels are measured; increases in sensitivity have been reported with serial measurements. The use of these biomarkers in patients with ACS is often inconclusive initially because it generally requires approximately 2 to 4 hours after the onset of symptoms for biomarker levels to be detectable.

The reported sensitivity of initial biomarkers for acute myocardial infarction is between 37% and 49%, with an increase to 79% to 93% when serial measurements are performed. Because of the initial limitations, the American College of Cardiology and the American Heart Association recommend repeat testing 8 to 12 hours after the initial levels are measured. This recommendation justifies the current period of observation used to improve diagnostic sensitivity and overall detection of ACS, although this approach comes at a high financial burden to society. These limitations highlight the need for approaches that can provide high diagnostic sensitivity while reducing the number of unnecessary admissions and the exposure of risky procedures to patients without ACS. The use of noninvasive cardiac imaging has the potential to achieve these goals.

■ PATIENT STRATIFICATION IN THE EVALUATION OF ACUTE CORONARY SYNDROME

The Thrombolysis in Myocardial Infarction (TIMI) risk score was introduced to stratify patients more accurately based on risk of cardiac events. Noninvasive imaging plays different roles depending on the likelihood of ACS. From this perspective, patients can be categorized into three groups.

The first group consists of patients who present with clear evidence of ACS by physical examination, ECG, and cardiac biomarkers. According to the guidelines of the American College of Cardiology and the American Heart Association, these patients are usually admitted for further interventions such as coronary angiography and, if necessary, reperfusion invasive therapies. Noninvasive imaging has no role in the immediate care of these patients.

The second group includes patients who present with clearly benign symptoms or other noncardiac conditions that do not require admission. These patients can usually be safely discharged from the ED without any further cardiac imaging assessment.

The third group, previously labeled the indeterminate group, is the most difficult group of patients to treat. These patients, usually in their fourth to sixth decades of life, present with an atypical clinical conglomeration of symptoms and laboratory results that do not fit any specific traditional risk factor criteria: atypical chest pain that deviates from the classic ischemic type, either normal or nonspecific ECG changes (nonspecific T-wave changes), and normal cardiac biomarker levels. These patients fall between the two previously described groups with risk factors that are low to intermediate for ACS, and they are at high risk of inappropriate discharge from the ED and possible future complications. In the ED, these patients are usually evaluated by a cardiologist. In many cases, they undergo noninvasive evaluation with conventional techniques including exercise treadmill testing and noninvasive cardiac imaging such as single photon emission computed tomography (SPECT) myocardial perfusion, and echocardiography. More recently, coronary computed tomography angiography (CTA) has been developed as a tool to help in the triage of these patients by providing a high negative predictive value for the exclusion of ACS.

■ ROLE OF NONINVASIVE IMAGING IN THE CONVENTIONAL ASSESSMENT OF ACUTE CORONARY SYNDROME

The pathophysiologic process from myocardial ischemia to infarction is dynamic and involves multiple phases at the vascular level. This process can be associated either with normal findings or with perfusion mismatches that lead to abnormalities of diastolic and systolic myocardial function. The goal of imaging is to identify processes that occur upstream to myocardial infarction, thus providing a mechanism for prompt intervention either by modification of the patient's dietary habits or by the use of pharmacologic agents. To date, the most frequent noninvasive imaging modalities used for the evaluation of possible ACS are chest radiography, exercise tolerance testing (ETT), transthoracic echocardiography, and radionuclide perfusion imaging, as discussed in the following subsections. Echocardiography and radionuclide perfusion play important roles as noninvasive imaging modalities currently used for the stratification of risk in patients subsequent to observation and a negative serial biomarker evaluation. These modalities are important adjuncts in the identification of high-risk patients with coronary disease because cardiac biomarker findings can be negative in the absence of myocardial death.

Chest Radiograph

In the ED, the chest radiograph is most commonly the first imaging modality used in the evaluation of patients presenting with chest pain. The attractiveness of this

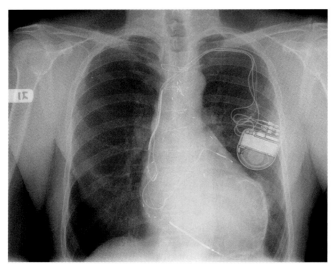

Figure 23-1 Chest radiograph of a 66-year-old male patient with chest pain. Frontal radiograph shows rimlike calcification along the left myocardial margin consistent with prior myocardial infarction. A defibrillator is present.

technique stems from its ability to exclude major noncardiac causes of chest pain (e.g., pneumonia, pneumothorax, or rib fracture) rapidly. The chest radiograph provides a global assessment of chest anatomy and any life-threatening conditions that require prompt intervention. The presence of myocardial calcification suggests prior myocardial infarction (Fig. 23-1). However, the detection of coronary artery calcification is neither sensitive nor specific for ACS.

Exercise Tolerance Testing

A sensitivity of 76% and a specificity of 60% have been described for ETT in the detection of myocardial ischemia. The reported high negative predictive value (98%) of ETT almost completely excludes ACS in the absence of inducible ischemia. One of the advantages of the ETT is its high negative predictive value; however, the test depends heavily on the physical ability of the patient to achieve the necessary heart rate. At least 33% of the patients are not suitable for ETT because of physical restrictions and many other factors.

Echocardiography and Radionuclide Perfusion Imaging

The use of resting echocardiography is limited in that ACS is a dynamic process. Therefore, in the absence of wall motion abnormalities, the examiner cannot exclude myocardial ischemia as a cause of the presenting chest pain episode if the pain is not present at the time of imaging. Conditions such as myocardial stunning can be appreciated on echocardiography because they can result in persistent wall motion abnormalities. Although studies have reported a high negative predictive value of resting echocardiography for the detection of myocardial infarction, conditions such as unstable angina have a considerably lower negative predictive

value. In the case of small regions of ischemia or infarction, a segmental wall motion abnormality may not be present.

Because of its prognostic value, stress echocardiography has been well established in the evaluation and triage of patients who present to the ED with acute chest pain. With a reported negative predictive value of 98%, a negative study result in most cases provides a reasonable basis for discharge from the ED and is associated with a very low adverse cardiac event rate. As compared with other techniques, stress echocardiography has many advantages, including portability, the capability to infer myocardial ischemia by demonstrating wall motion abnormalities and reduced ejection fractions, and physiologic information regarding baseline ventricular function, valvular function, and pericardial contour. Nevertheless, stress echocardiography has several disadvantages, including limited availability during off hours, the inability to exclude causes of chest pain outside the heart, limited use in patients with resolved symptoms and nontransmural infarcts, and the potential for a nondiagnostic test result when the necessary heart rate is not achieved. The use of newer technologies such as microbubble echocontrast that have shown to improve endomyocardial border definition and perfusion assessment may ultimately overcome some of the challenges with the use of echocardiography for the assessment of acute chest pain. Thus, stress and rest perfusion imaging has been promoted as an alternative modality.

Findings of multiple studies have shown sensitivity ranging from 90% to 100%, specificity from 60% to 78%, and a negative predictive value from 97% to 100% for radionuclide perfusion imaging for ACS if SPECT imaging is used. The addition of stress imaging in stable patients may improve diagnostic accuracy. In addition, radionuclide perfusion imaging has been shown to have prognostic value and permits risk stratification of patients for future cardiac events.

SPECT myocardial perfusion imaging has an important role both in patients at risk for coronary artery disease in the outpatient setting and in those who present with acute chest pain, as demonstrated in Figure 23-2. SPECT is performed after injection of technetium-99m–based perfusion tracer, with imaging obtained 45 to 60 minutes later, so that stress testing permits assessment of myocardial blood flow at the time of injection. In the ED setting, among low- to intermediate-risk patients with chest pain and nonspecific ECG changes, myocardial perfusion SPECT is effective in excluding ACS. In a series of observational studies, the negative predictive value for ruling out ACS was approximately 99%. Thus, a normal myocardial perfusion study result predicts a very small risk of ACS in this setting.

Myocardial perfusion imaging also provides greater risk stratification and prognostic value compared with clinical data for predicting adverse cardiac events. Patients who exhibit abnormal regional perfusion have a higher risk of cardiac events during hospitalization and subsequent to discharge. However, myocardial perfusion imaging has several disadvantages, both

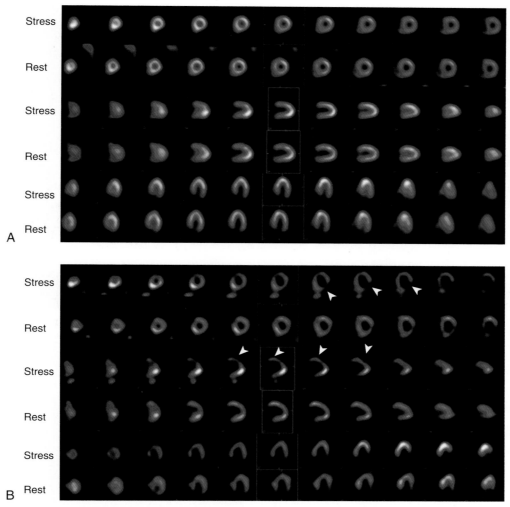

Figure 23-2 Normal and abnormal myocardial perfusion tests. **A,** A 16-year-old male patient with chest pain. Following treadmill exercise testing, thallium-201 was given intravenously, and stress tomographic imaging was performed. The patient returned to the department 2 hours later, and rest redistribution tomographic imaging was performed. Exercise stress myocardial perfusion single photon emission computed tomography (SPECT) shows no evidence of myocardial ischemia or prior infarction. The patient has normal left ventricular size, wall motion, and systolic function with a left ventricular ejection fraction (LVEF) of 61%. **B,** A 56-year-old female patient with a history of known coronary artery disease and an abnormal electrocardiogram. Following regadenoson pharmacologic stress testing, thallium-201 was given intravenously, and stress tomographic imaging was performed. The patient returned to the department 2 hours later, and rest redistribution tomographic imaging was performed. Myocardial perfusion SPECT scan demonstrated myocardial ischemia in the anterior and anteroseptal regions (left anterior descending vascular territory) and the middle to basal inferolateral region (circumflex vascular territory) of the left ventricle *(arrowheads)*. Globally, hypokinesis, dilated left ventricle with abnormal systolic function, and an LVEF of 24% were noted. (Courtesy of Dr. Qi Cao, MD, PhD, University of Maryland Medical Center, Baltimore.)

practical and intrinsic to the study. Because the test is generally not available during off hours, a patient with potential ACS who presents in the evening must wait until the following morning to be imaged. The nuclear medicine department is often not in the immediate vicinity of the ED suite, thus necessitating removal of the patient to a relatively unmonitored environment. Additionally, myocardial perfusion imaging is prone to artifacts that lead to false-positive results in certain populations. Finally, whereas a negative perfusion imaging study result largely excludes ACS, it does not address the potential for serious noncardiac causes of chest pain such as pulmonary embolism.

■ COMPUTED TOMOGRAPHIC CALCIUM SCORING FOR THE EVALUATION OF ACUTE CHEST PAIN

The progression of coronary atherosclerosis is marked by calcification of atherosclerotic plaque. With rapid advances in the technology of MDCT, ECG-gated coronary computed tomography (CT) allows for the detection of the extent and quantification of the calcification, properties that correlate with the presence of obstructive stenosis. In the Agatston method, software highlights pixels with Hounsfield units (HU) greater than 130, and the density and extent of these pixels

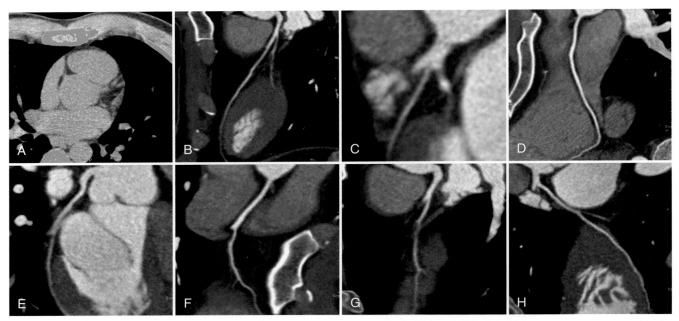

Figure 23-3 A 44-year-old male patient who presented with chest pain and shortness of breath. **A,** Computed calcium score by the Agatston method was zero, thus placing the patient below the 25th percentile for risk adjusted for age and gender. **B to H,** Curved multiplanar reconstruction views of the coronary vessels demonstrate no evidence of calcified or noncalcified plaque in the left main coronary artery (**B**), left anterior descending artery, ramus intermedius (**C**), right coronary artery (**D**), left circumflex artery (**E**), acute marginal artery (**F**), diagonal artery (**G**), or obtuse marginal artery (**H**), respectively. The patient had no pulmonary emboli or acute aortic disease.

are combined to create the Agatston score. Although this method was originally developed for the now abandoned electron beam CT, correlation of calcium scores is achieved by using volumetric or mass scoring methods. In symptomatic patients, the sensitivity of the presence of any coronary calcium for a stenosis greater than 50% is 95% to 99%. Calcium detected by coronary CT in symptomatic and asymptomatic patients is predictive of nonfatal myocardial infarction, cardiovascular death, and all-cause mortality. This score is then used to determine the calcium percentile, which compares the calcified plaque burden with that of other asymptomatic men and women of the same age.

The calcium score, in combination with the percentile, enables the physician to determine the patient's risk of developing symptomatic coronary artery disease and to measure the progression of disease and the effectiveness of treatment. A score of 0 indicates that the patient has no calcified plaque burden. This finding implies an absence of significant coronary artery narrowing and a very low likelihood of a cardiac event over at least the next 3 years, as illustrated in Figures 23-3 and 23-4. A score of 0 does not absolutely rule out the presence of soft, noncalcified plaque or totally eliminate the possibility of a cardiac event. A score that is greater than 0 indicates at least some coronary artery disease. As the score increases, so does the likelihood of a significant coronary narrowing and the likelihood of a coronary event over the next 3 years, compared with patients with lower scores. Similarly, the likelihood of a coronary event increases with increasing calcium percentiles, as seen in Figure 23-5.

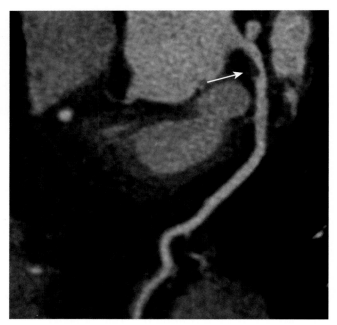

Figure 23-4 A 56-year-old male patient who presented with chest pain. Computed calcium score by the Agatston method was zero. Curved multiplanar reconstruction of the left anterior descending coronary artery shows at least 50% proximal stenosis resulting from a noncalcified plaque *(arrow)*.

In the setting of acute chest pain, the use of calcium scoring is limited in that it cannot identify noncalcified plaque or acute myocardial ischemia or infarction. In addition, because patients with a history of coronary artery disease are expected to have calcified

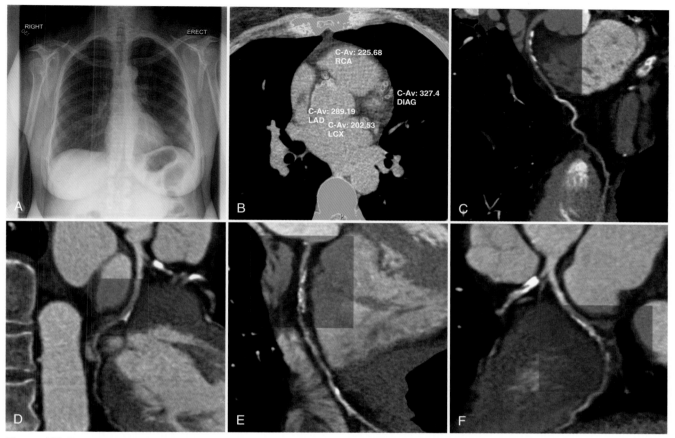

Figure 23-5 A 56-year-old female patient who presented with chest pain. **A,** Normal chest radiograph. **B,** Computed calcium score by the Agatston method was 1217, thus placing her at the 100th percentile for risk, adjusted for age and gender. *C-Av,* Calcium average; *DIAG,* diagonal artery; *LAD,* left anterior descending artery; *LCX,* left circumflex artery. **C** to **F,** Curved multiplanar reconstruction views of the coronary vessels demonstrate widespread atherosclerotic disease in the left anterior descending artery (**C**), left circumflex artery (**D**), right coronary artery (**E**), and obtuse marginal artery (**F**). There was no evidence of pulmonary emboli or acute aortic disease. Subsequent regadenoson pharmacologic stress thallium myocardial perfusion study revealed a reversible perfusion defect in the anteroseptal and inferolateral walls. The patient underwent a cardiac catheterization with a bare metal stent placed in the obtuse marginal.

atherosclerotic plaque whether or not they have ACS, the calcium score is less valuable in these patients. However, the ability to identify the presence of atherosclerotic plaque in patients at minimal risk for ACS who would not typically have coronary calcification gives calcium scoring the potential to serve as a screening tool in the ED. In fact, to date, four single center studies evaluated the use of coronary CT calcium scoring in patients with acute chest pain with minimal risk. Despite using different reference standards for the determination of the presence of ACS, these studies all demonstrated relatively high sensitivity, with values ranging from 82% to 100%. Specificities ranged from 37% to 63%, findings reflecting that the presence of calcium on coronary CT is not highly specific for underlying ACS. The low specificity of coronary CT calcium scoring for ACS translates into very low positive predictive values.

With its high sensitivity and low specificity, coronary CT calcium scoring could potentially be best used as a screening tool in the ED for quick discharge of patients who are at minimal risk for ACS and have coronary calcium scores of 0. This approach could possibly help relieve a large financial and resource burden by obviating the unnecessary diagnostic workup in this

group of patients. In using calcium scoring in this role, patient selection will be important because younger patients with obstructive coronary disease may have no or minimal calcium and therefore could possibly have false-negative results. As illustrated in a study by Schmermund et al of 118 patients with ACS, 12 patients without calcification were on average 12 years younger than those with calcification but had similar cardiac risk factors. Furthermore, in a retrospective study, Rubinshtein et al demonstrated that of 668 patients with chest pain who underwent coronary 64-slice CTA, 7% with an acute presentation of obstructive coronary disease had a calcium score of 0. These patients were younger and more likely to be women. These investigators also noted that obstructive coronary disease with no or minor calcification tended to be more frequent in acute chest pain presentations compared with stable chest pain presentations. This finding is consistent with a report of 64-slice coronary CTA results from 40 patients with ACS in whom only 14% of observed plaques were calcified, whereas 86% were mixed or noncalcified.

Screening based on CT calcium score may also have value in determination of long-term prognosis. Georgiou et al followed 192 patients who were admitted to

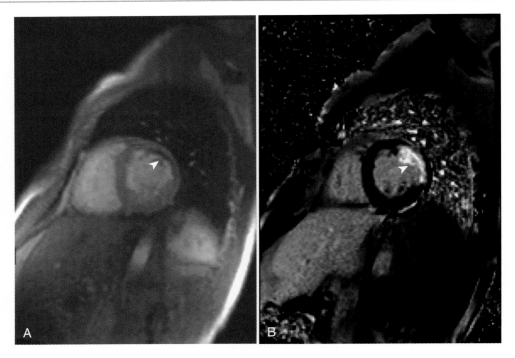

Figure 23-6 Abnormal cardiac magnetic resonance perfusion. A, Short-axis view of first-pass perfusion imaging after administration of intravenous gadolinium demonstrates a focal perfusion defect involving the subendocardial anterolateral left ventricular wall *(arrowhead).* **B,** Short-axis view of images obtained 10 minutes after the administration of gadolinium demonstrates marked delayed subendocardial enhancement in the same region of the anterolateral left ventricular wall *(arrowhead).* The region of delayed myocardial enhancement exceeds 50% of the myocardial thickness, with portions that appear transmural in extent. Cine clips (not shown) revealed marked focal hypokinesis involving the anterolateral left ventricular wall.

the ED with chest pain and who did not experience a cardiac event during the admission. Over an average follow-up of 50 months, the absence of coronary artery calcium was associated with a very low annualized event rate of less than 1%. In a multivariate analysis, including traditional risk factors, coronary calcium was a strong independent predictor of cardiac events.

The use of coronary CT calcium scoring for acute chest pain will require validation in larger, multicenter trials before it can be implemented clinically. The high negative predictive value of screening based on CT calcium score for acute chest pain could allow diagnostic performance equivalent to current standard approaches. To achieve such results, however, examiners perhaps would have to select patients older than a certain age and possibly according to gender. A potential problem with such a strategy is that the increase in coronary calcification seen with age will likely minimize the number of patients who have no calcification and thus decrease the benefit of coronary CT calcium scoring in this patient population.

■ COMPUTED TOMOGRAPHIC CORONARY ANGIOGRAPHY AND ITS ROLE IN THE EVALUATION OF ACUTE CHEST PAIN

A more comprehensive approach to the evaluation of acute chest pain caused by ACS is necessary, given the limitation of coronary CT calcium imaging in detecting noncalcified coronary plaques. The ideal imaging approach for the evaluation of ACS should include the ability to assess for the degree of coronary stenosis resulting from in situ thrombus formation on an underlying ruptured atherosclerotic plaque. Invasive coronary angiography meets this requirement and has traditionally been used in patients with ACS. Although

invasive coronary angiography remains the standard reference technique and is necessary for intervention, this approach carries serious risks to patients, high costs, and high resource requirements. With the advances in MDCT technology, coronary CTA now offers a noninvasive alternative to conventional coronary angiography that overcomes the limitations of the invasive approach. The most exciting application is the direct visualization of the coronary arteries, which formerly required invasive cardiac catheterization. Not only can MDCT determine the severity of stenosis, but also it directly permits assessment of the atherosclerotic plaque deposited in the vessel wall. It can identify the early stages of noncalcified (fatty and fibrous) plaque formation even before the plaque can be visualized on x-ray angiography images. MDCT also visualizes calcified plaque, which occurs in a later stage of atheroma development. As a comparison, perfusion cardiac magnetic resonance is depicted in Figure 23-6.

In the 1970s, the early CT technology was able to detect only large pathologic lesions in the heart. This limitation was largely the result of cardiac motion on the background of relatively long acquisition time (>10 seconds per slice). During the late 1980s, subsecond scanning became possible with helical scanners, which used a continuously rotating array of detectors and an x-ray fan beam around the patient. For the first time, examiners could visualize the coronary arteries, although the ability to diagnose obstruction was very limited. The first generation of helical CT scanners used a single row of x-ray detectors, but during the late 1990s, ECG-gated four-detector row MDCT scanners provided a noninvasive alternative to coronary angiography and became the standard choice for the noninvasive detection of coronary artery disease.

Substantial advances have been made in the capability of MDCT, with 16 rows, and then 64 rows, with the speed of image acquisition and volume coverage continuing to increase rapidly with each next generation of CT. The 64-slice CT scanners (which acquire 64 slices per rotation of the gantry around the patient) rotate around the patient in less than 400 msec (half a second). Because the coronary arteries and other cardiac structures move rapidly during the cardiac cycle, data are acquired during cardiac ECG monitoring, which allows retrospective reconstruction of slices acquired at different small segments of the cardiac cycle and thereby reduces motion artifact in the coronary arteries.

The current generation of MDCT scanners has 64 to 320 detector rows and 1 or 2 x-ray sources capable of imaging with spatial resolution of approximately 0.4 mm and temporal resolutions as low as 72 msec, which remain inferior to those of invasive coronary angiography (spatial resolution of approximately 0.2 mm and temporal resolution of approximately 5 msec). Despite these differences, coronary CTA is highly accurate for the detection of coronary stenosis. In a meta-analysis of published diagnostic accuracy studies using invasive angiography as a reference standard, Abdulla et al found the sensitivity and specificity of coronary CTA to be 97.5% and 91%, respectively, in a per-patient analysis. Most of the studies included in this meta-analysis were performed in populations of patients with stable angina who had an intermediate to high risk of coronary artery disease. Furthermore, similar findings were reported in studies including patients with non–ST-segment elevation ACS.

The second advantage of coronary CTA is the ability to identify intraluminal thrombi. In a sample of patients with ACS, Dorgelo et al noted thrombus in 53% by using certain criteria, including the recognition of a filling defect with an intraluminal position, irregular borders, and low density (19.3 ± 7.3 HU). Third, coronary CTA allows visualization of the vessel walls in addition to the lumen and hence has been used to characterize plaques based on morphology and MDCT density. With the ability to identify coronary stenoses and intraluminal thrombus and to characterize plaques, coronary CTA can identify the upstream event in the ischemic region, thus potentially making it a highly sensitive test for the detection of ACS, even compared with resting echocardiography or SPECT.

In the ED, coronary CTA can be used as an alternative diagnostic modality to serial ECGs, cardiac biomarkers, and even stress ECG, with or without the inclusion of echocardiographic or SPECT imaging. Coronary CTA has been demonstrated to be superior to exercise treadmill ECG testing in the setting of acute chest pain, as exemplified in a study by Rubinshtein et al. In this study, the investigators found evidence of obstructive coronary disease in 22% of patients with acute chest pain who had a negative treadmill result and in 39% of those with a nondiagnostic exercise treadmill test result. This study was a retrospective analysis of 103 patients who had undergone coronary CTA in addition to a standard evaluation including serial ECGs, serial biomarkers, and exercise treadmill testing for the evaluation of ACS.

The use of MDCT has been extrapolated to the ED, given that most of these sophisticated scanners are increasing positioned in or near the ED suite. One of the most attractive properties of MDCT is the ability to assess rapidly many nonthoracic emergency indications, such as abdominal pain, headache, and trauma, as well as critical noncardiac chest pain such as pulmonary embolism and aortic dissection. Two imaging protocols have been developed based on the need to perform dedicated coronary CTA or to scan the entire thorax. A dedicated coronary CTA examination affords the best possible visualization of the coronary arteries, including limited visualization of other structures such as the central pulmonary arteries. The other approach provides a comprehensive evaluation of the entire chest, to investigate both cardiac and noncardiac causes. This alternative method of scanning has been simplistically termed the triple rule-out approach to denote the triad of coronary artery disease, pulmonary embolism, and aortic dissection.

The triple rule-out protocol combines features the characteristics of a dedicated coronary CTA approach and a chest CT protocol used to evaluate for pulmonary emboli. The use of the triple rule-out protocol has been associated with challenges that require some compromises. With conventional single source 64-slice scanners, a breath hold may require as long as 15 to 20 seconds because of the longer caudocranial scan range (z-axis coverage). Because this examination typically excludes the abdominal aorta, it potentially limits the evaluation of suspected new aortic dissection, which may propagate inferiorly into the abdominal aorta. Moreover, a larger than usual contrast bolus is required to opacify the pulmonary artery optimally in addition to the coronary arteries, thus increasing the risk of renal toxicity.

An additional concern is that slightly greater radiation doses are delivered because of the larger coverage area included in these studies; the average exposure is 20 to 30 mSv, as opposed to 10 to 15 mSv for a dedicated coronary scan using the standard retrospective ECG-gated technique. These compromises may limit the quality of coronary artery visualization because of the longer scan time and, in some cases, the need to use a lower-quality scan for the larger field of view. Despite these challenges, studies have demonstrated no difference in imaging quality of the coronary arterial circulation between a dedicated coronary CTA and a triple rule-out CT study. By including a larger field of view compared with a dedicated coronary CT scan, the triple rule-out protocol has the potential to detect pulmonary emboli, as illustrated in Figure 23-7. One reasonable proposal may be to use the triple rule-out protocol in patients with suspected ACS who also are at risk of pulmonary embolism based on clinical history or serum markers.

Some technical aspects are shared among the CT protocols for the ED that are discussed in this chapter, including the use of intravenous contrast bolus injection facilitated by either an automatic triggering mechanism or an injection testing approach. Beta-blockade, typically achieved with metoprolol, is recommended in patients with a heart rate greater than 60 to 65 beats/minute. Contraindications such as asthma and heart block exclude the use of a beta-blocker. Visualization of

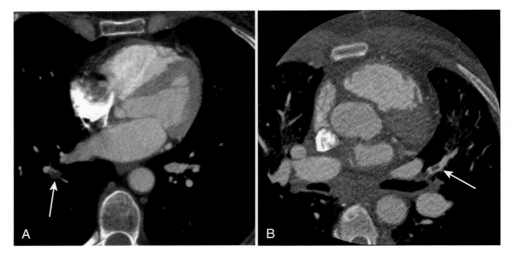

Figure 23-7 Two patients who presented with chest pain and computed calcium scores by the Agatston method of zero, with no noncalcified plaque identified. **A,** Right lower lobe acute pulmonary embolus *(arrow).* **B,** Lingula acute pulmonary embolus *(arrow).*

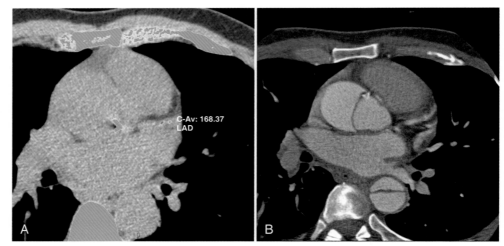

Figure 23-8 A 58-year-old male patient presenting with chest pain. **A,** Minimal calcified plaque was identified in the left anterior descending artery (LAD), and the computed calcium score by Agatston method was 6.6, thus placing the patient between the 50th and 75th percentile, adjusted for age and gender. *C-Av,* Calcium average. **B,** Contrast-enhanced computed tomography of the chest demonstrates a type A aortic dissection with the intimal flap visualized in the ascending and descending aorta *(arrows).*

the coronary arteries can be improved with indirect vascular vasodilation induced by sublingual nitroglycerin, which can be given in hemodynamically stable patients.

In patients undergoing CT evaluation for suspected coronary artery disease, vessel motion can result in blurred coronary outlines. ECG-gated data acquisition addresses this issue. This procedure was previously performed exclusively using retrospective gating but is now increasingly carried out with prospective triggering. For retrospective gating, 10 or 20 evenly spaced reconstructions or phases throughout the cardiac cycle, using a field of view restricted to the heart, may be reconstructed at 10% or 5% increments. Reconstruction of additional phases (e.g., defined as absolute values such as 350 msec after the R-peak or 300 msec before the following R-peak) can be acquired as needed. This approach allows selection of the phase with the least coronary artery motion, typically found in early or late diastole. Software permits in-plane reconstruction of the coronary arteries from their center lines, termed curved planar reconstructions, and additional reconstructions may be performed including maximum intensity projection and volumetric reformations. In the triple rule-out protocol, a separate full field of view data set encompassing

the entire chest is reconstructed and evaluated initially to exclude emboli, aortic dissection, and other noncardiac causes of chest pain, as depicted in Figure 23-8. The coronary arteries are then evaluated for the presence of calcified and noncalcified plaque and stenosis or obstruction of the coronary lumen.

Several single center trials assessed the value of CT in the ED for acute chest pain; these trials used both dedicated coronary CTA and the triple rule-out protocol. In the study by Hoffmann et al, the investigators reported a 100% negative predictive value of coronary CTA for subsequent diagnosis of ACS or major adverse cardiac events. The presence of atherosclerotic plaque and the severity of stenosis predicted ACS independent of coronary risk factors or the TIMI risk score used commonly for clinical risk stratification.

Goldstein et al performed a randomized dedicated coronary CTA trial in 197 patients with acute chest pain who were at low risk for ACS and who presented to the ED. These investigators compared the safety, diagnostic efficiency, and cost of 64-detector row CT with the standard of care diagnostic evaluation. Physicians using MDCT were able immediately to exclude or identify coronary disease as the source of chest pain in 75% of patients. The remaining 25% of patients required stress testing because of intermediate-severity lesions or nondiagnostic scans. The patients who underwent MDCT had a safety profile (no adverse coronary events for 6 months) equal to that of patients treated with the standard of care approach. Initial evaluation with MDCT reduced diagnostic time to an average of 3.4 hours compared with an average of 15 hours with a standard of care evaluation. Moreover, the average cost per patient was lowered from $1872 to $1586 when the MDCT algorithm was used. Patients in the MDCT arm of the study also required fewer subsequent evaluations for recurrent chest pain.

Takakuwa and Halpern demonstrated that triple rule-out coronary CTA in patients at low to moderate risk of having ACS who presented to the ED provided a noncoronary diagnosis that explained the presenting complaint in 11% of patients. This finding suggested the presence of significant moderate to severe coronary disease in 11% (22 of 197) of patients, and it precluded additional diagnostic cardiac testing in most of these patients, with no adverse outcomes at 30-day follow-up. However, the triple rule-out protocol differs from dedicated coronary CTA in several important aspects, such as the larger field of view with the triple rule-out protocol, imaging of the entire length of the thorax that results in increased radiation burden to the patient, and the delivery of additional contrast. High-pitch dual source acquisition is preferred for the triple rule-out protocol, if available, because it can be performed with a reasonably low overall contrast dose and at low radiation doses.

An approach to acute chest pain based on coronary CT has many theoretical advantages, and the results of small single center studies are promising, regardless of the imaging protocol used. However, future studies will need to address several important considerations in addition to diagnostic accuracy. In the past, most coronary CT used retrospective ECG gating, which resulted in substantial radiation exposure, even with the use of dose modulation. Radiation exposure from this type of coronary CT is comparable to that of a myocardial perfusion SPECT study; clinicians and patients will likely consider this acceptable if they are fully informed. However, newer technology results in substantially lower radiation doses that give coronary CT a clear advantage over radionuclide imaging with SPECT or positron emission tomography. The proportion of patients who may require nuclear stress testing and invasive cardiac catheterization in addition to coronary CT, with a resulting higher net radiation burden, is not clear. In the randomized trial by Goldstein et al, 24 of 99 patients in the coronary CT group required nuclear stress testing because of indeterminate coronary CT findings, and 11 required invasive angiography, compared with 3 patients in the standard of care group. Conversely, a strategy based on coronary CT may result in decreased exposure to medical radiation following discharge if it provides greater diagnostic certainty. In the same trial by Goldstein et al, no significant difference was reported in the overall number of invasive angiograms after 6-month follow-up.

In addition, prospective triggering is an important radiation-sparing technique that has been widely applied in the outpatient setting. Prospective triggering is an axial technique that involves a step and shoot approach in which the beam is turned on only during a limited part of the cardiac cycle, usually diastole, thus substantially lowering radiation dose. In outpatients, this approach has been found to decrease the radiation dose substantially. Shuman et al showed a dose reduction of 71% in the ED setting among patients who underwent coronary CTA with prospective gating. Unfortunately, large patients and individuals with high heart rates often cannot undergo prospective triggering. Moreover, functional imaging is not possible because images are obtained only during a limited portion of the cardiac cycle.

The potential of CT in the ED needs to be affirmed not only in single center trials but also in larger multicenter trials. The results of the Computed Tomographic Angiography for the Systematic Triage of Acute Chest Pain Patients to Treatment (CT-STAT) trial confirm those of early single center trials. In this large study, 699 low-risk patients with chest pain were randomized in 16 hospital sites to receive either CTA ($n = 361$) or standard of care and rest-test myocardial perfusion imaging ($n = 338$) with time to diagnosis as the primary end point. The investigators found that the use of CTA resulted in a mean diagnosis time of 2.9 hours, compared with 6.2 hours for the standard of care. CTA also significantly decreased overall radiation exposure: 12.8 mSv for the standard of care arm of the trial compared with 11.5 mSv for CTA. The overall costs for patients were less, with a mean of $3458 for standard of care and $2137 for CTA. The investigators concluded that CTA was safe, faster, and cheaper than the standard of care.

These findings encourage hospitals with EDs and cardiac CT technology to evaluate chest pain strategies based on cardiac CTA. However, they also caution that many factors must be considered with implementation, including the availability of CT (specifically technical staff and interpreting physicians) within the hospital (particularly beyond daytime hours), the development of protocols that highlight the indications and contraindications for the test, the importance of heart rate control, the administration of beta-blockers, and the recognition that not every patient is a suitable candidate for CTA. Other multicenter trials of CT in the ED are ongoing, including the second Rule Out Myocardial Infarction using Computer Assisted Tomography (ROMICAT2) trial and the American College of Radiology Imaging Network (ACRIN) trial. Both the ROMICAT2 and ACRIN trials are randomized controlled studies of a rapid rule-out strategy that aims to assess coronary CTA versus traditional care in the ED in low- to intermediate-risk patients with potential ACS. These trials are currently being conducted by principal investigators from Massachusetts General Hospital in Boston and the Hospital of the University of Pennsylvania in Philadelphia. The results of these multicenter trials will be important to know before a more formal assessment of the true value of CT in the ED can be made.

■ CONCLUSION

Although the triad of ACS, aortic dissection, and pulmonary embolism commonly manifests with the nonspecific complaint of chest pain, these conditions are associated with high morbidity and mortality. MDCT now has an established role in the evaluation of aortic dissection and pulmonary embolism. Growing numbers of small single and multicenter observational studies have demonstrated coronary CT to be a promising noninvasive alternative or adjunct modality to SPECT and echocardiography in the diagnosis of ACS. The combined triple rule-out CT protocol is well positioned as a noninvasive imaging approach to provide fast and highly accurate diagnostic information for patients with nonspecific chest pain symptoms. Notable concerns for its widespread adoption include the potential for overuse, the expense of the procedure, and subsequent radiation exposure. Therefore, ED physicians and cardiologists must set guidelines for appropriate triage and patient selection.

Based on study results, the ideal patient is one with a low to intermediate risk of ACS. With proper patient selection, evidence indicates that CT is less expensive than the standard of care. The potential cost of an additional diagnostic study was outweighed by savings from fewer admissions and from avoidance of unnecessary diagnostic studies. With the general proliferation of CT scans, increased concern exists for radiation exposure. Triple rule-out CT may result in a radiation dose as high as 20 to 30 mSv, depending on scanner technology, but it may be as low as 2 to 3 mSv with advanced scanners and scan algorithms. Concern regarding radiation exposure is mitigated by the overall longer-term reduction in number of tests, such as radionuclide imaging and invasive coronary angiography, which are also associated with substantial radiation exposure. As the use of cardiac CT becomes more widespread, longer-term follow-up of ongoing and published multicenter studies, determination of optimal protocols and patient-centered diagnostic algorithms, and cost-effectiveness analyses will be critical.

Bibliography

Abdulla J, Abildstrom SZ, Gotzsche O, Christensen E, Kober L, Torp-Pedersen C. 64-Multislice detector computed tomography coronary angiography as potential alternative to conventional coronary angiography: a systematic review and meta-analysis. *Eur Heart J.* 2007;28:3042-3050.

Achar SA, Kundu S, Norcross WA. Diagnosis of acute coronary syndrome. *Am Fam Physician.* 2005;72:119-126.

Achenbach S, Moselewski F, Ropers D, et al. Detection of calcified and noncalcified coronary atherosclerotic plaque by contrast-enhanced, submillimeter multidetector spiral computed tomography: a segment-based comparison with intravascular ultrasound. *Circulation.* 2004;109:14-17.

Achenbach S, Ropers D, Hoffmann U, et al. Assessment of coronary remodeling in stenotic and nonstenotic coronary atherosclerotic lesions by multidetector spiral computed tomography. *J Am Coll Cardiol.* 2004;43:842-847.

Amsterdsam EA, Kirk JD, Diercks DB, Lewis WR, Tunipseed SD. Early exercise testing in the management of low risk patients in chest pain centers. *Prog Cardiovasc Dis.* 2004;46:438-452.

Anderson JL, Adams CD, Antman EM, et al. ACC/AHA 2007 guidelines for the management of patients with unstable angina/non–ST-elevation myocardial infarction: executive summary. *J Am Coll Cardiol.* 2007;50:652-726.

Antman EM, Cohen M, Bernink PJ, et al. The TIMI risk score for unstable angina/non–ST elevation MI: a method for prognostication and therapeutic decision making. *JAMA.* 2000;284:835-842.

Balk EM, Ioannidis JP, Salem D, Chew PW, Lau J. Accuracy of biomarkers to diagnose acute cardiac ischemia in the emergency department: a meta-analysis. *Ann Emerg Med.* 2001;37:478-494.

Bastarrika G, Thilo C, Headden GF, et al. Cardiac CT in the assessment of acute chest pain in the emergency department. *AJR Am J Roentgenol.* 2009;193:397-409.

Bhuiya FA, Pitts SR, McCaig LF. Emergency department visits for chest pain and abdominal pain: United States, 1999-2008. *NCHS Data Brief.* 2010;43:1-8.

Bluemke DA, Achenbach S, Budoff M, et al. Noninvasive coronary artery imaging, magnetic resonance angiography and multidetector computed tomography angiography: a scientific statement from the American Heart Association Committee on Cardiovascular Imaging and Intervention of the Council on Cardiovascular Radiology and Intervention, and the Councils on Clinical Cardiology and Cardiovascular Disease in the Young. *Circulation.* 2008;118:586-606.

Braunwald E, Antman EM, Beasley JW, et al. ACC/AHA 2002 guideline update for the management of patients with unstable angina and non–ST-segment elevation myocardial infarction—summary article: a report of the American College of Cardiology/American Heart Association Task Force on Practice Guidelines. *J Am Coll Cardiol.* 2002;40:1366-1374.

Budoff MJ, Achenbach S, Blumenthal RS, et al. Assessment of coronary artery disease by cardiac computed tomography: a scientific statement from the American Heart Association Committee on Cardiovascular Imaging and Intervention, Council on Cardiovascular Radiology and Intervention, and Committee on Cardiac Imaging, Council on Clinical Cardiology. *Circulation.* 2006;114:1761-1791.

Budoff MJ, Diamond GA, Raggi P, et al. Continuous probabilistic prediction of angiographically significant coronary artery disease using electron beam tomography. *Circulation.* 2002;105:1791-1796.

Budoff MJ, Shaw LJ, Liu ST, et al. Long-term prognosis associated with coronary calcification: observations from a registry of 25,253 patients. *J Am Coll Cardiol.* 2007;49:1860-1870.

Camici PG, Prasad SK, Rimoldi OE. Stunning, hibernation, and assessment of myocardial viability. *Circulation.* 2008;117:103-114.

Detrano R, Hsiai T, Wang S, et al. Prognostic value of coronary calcification and angiographic stenoses in patients undergoing coronary angiography. *J Am Coll Cardiol.* 1996;27:285-290.

Dorgelo J, Willems TP, Geluk CA, van Ooijen PM, Zijlstra F, Oudkerk M. Multidetector computed tomography-guided treatment strategy in patients with non–ST elevation acute coronary syndromes: a pilot study. *Eur Radiol.* 2005;15:708-713.

Earls JP, Berman EL, Urban BA, et al. Prospectively gated transverse coronary CT angiography versus retrospectively gated helical technique: improved image quality and reduced radiation dose. *Radiology.* 2008;246:742-753.

Esteves FP, Sanyal R, Santana CA, Shaw L, Raggi P. Potential impact of noncontrast computed tomography as gatekeeper for myocardial perfusion positron emission tomography in patients admitted to the chest pain unit. *Am J Cardiol.* 2008;101:149-152.

Georgiou D, Budoff MJ, Kaufer E, Kennedy JM, Lu B, Brundage BH. Screening patients with chest pain in the emergency department using electron beam tomography: a follow-up study. *J Am Coll Cardiol.* 2001;38:105-110.

Georgiou D, Budoff MJ, Bleiweis MS, et al. A new approach for screening patients with chest pain in the emergency department using fast computed-tomography. *Circulation.* 1993;88:1-15.

Goldstein JA, Chinnaiyan KM, Abidov A, et al. The CT-STAT (Coronary Computed Tomographic Angiography for Systematic Triage of Acute Chest Pain Patients to Treatment) trial. *J Am Coll Cardiol.* 2011;58:1414-1422.

Goldstein JA, Gallagher MJ, O'Neill WW, Ross MA, O'Neil BJ, Raff GL. A randomized controlled trial of multi-slice coronary computed tomography for evaluation of acute chest pain. *J Am Coll Cardiol.* 2007;49:863-871.

Goodacre S, Locker T, Morris F, Campbell S. How useful are clinical features in the diagnosis of acute, undifferentiated chest pain? *Acad Emerg Med.* 2002;9:203-208.

Halpern EJ. Triple rule-out coronary angiography for evaluation of acute chest pain and possible acute coronary syndrome. *Radiology.* 2009;252:332-345.

Henneman MM, Schuijf JD, Pundziute G, et al. Noninvasive evaluation with multislice computed tomography in suspected acute coronary syndrome: plaque morphology on multislice computed tomography versus coronary calcium score. *J Am Coll Cardiol.* 2008;52:216-222.

Hlatky MA. Evaluating use of coronary computed tomography angiography in the emergency department. *J Am Coll Cardiol.* 2009;53:1651-1652.

Hoffmann U, Bamberg F, Chae CU, et al. Coronary computed tomography angiography for early triage of patients with acute chest pain: the ROMICAT (Rule Out Myocardial Infarction using Computer Assisted Tomography) trial. *J Am Coll Cardiol.* 2009;53:1642-1650.

Hoffmann U, Pena AJ, Cury RC, et al. Cardiac CT in emergency department patients with acute chest pain. *Radiographics.* 2006;26:963-978.

Jeremias A, Gibson CM. Narrative review: alternative causes for elevated cardiac troponin levels when acute coronary syndromes are excluded. *Ann Intern Med.* 2005;142:786-791.

Kontos MC, Arrowood JA, Jesse RL, et al. Comparison between 2-dimensional echocardiography and myocardial perfusion imaging in the emergency department in patients with possible myocardial ischemia. *Am Heart J.* 1998;136:724-733.

Lange RA, Hillis LD. Cardiovascular complications of cocaine use. *N Engl J Med.* 2001;345:351-358.

Laudon DA, Vukov LF, Breen JF, Rumberger JA, Wollan PC, Sheedy 2nd PF. Use of electron-beam computed tomography in the evaluation of chest pain patients in the emergency department. *Ann Emerg Med.* 1999;33:15-21.

Leber AW, Knez A, Becker A, et al. Accuracy of multidetector spiral computed tomography in identifying and differentiating the composition of coronary atherosclerotic plaques: a comparative study with intracoronary ultrasound. *J Am Coll Cardiol.* 2004;43:1241-1247.

Lewis WR. Echocardiography in the evaluation of patients in chest pain units. *Cardiol Clin.* 2005;23:531-539, vii.

Lieberman AN, Weiss JL, Jugdutt BI, et al. Two-dimensional echocardiography and infarct size: relationship of regional wall motion and thickening to the extent of myocardial infarction in the dog. *Circulation.* 1981;63:739-746.

Margolis JR, Chen JT, Kong Y, Peter RH, Behar VS, Kisslo JA. The diagnostic and prognostic significance of coronary artery calcification: a report of 800 cases. *Radiology.* 1980;137:609-616.

McLaughlin VV, Balogh T, Rich S. Utility of electron beam computed tomography to stratify patients presenting to the emergency room with chest pain. *Am J Cardiol.* 1999;84:327.

Min JK, Dunning A, Lin FY, et al. Age- and sex-related differences in all-cause mortality risk based on coronary computed tomography angiography findings: results from the International Multicenter CONFIRM (Coronary CT Angiography Evaluation for Clinical Outcomes: An International Multicenter Registry) of 23,854 patients without known coronary artery disease. *J Am Coll Cardiol.* 2011;58:849-860.

Mizuno K, Satomura K, Miyamoto A, et al. Angioscopic evaluation of coronary-artery thrombi in acute coronary syndromes. *N Engl J Med.* 1992;326:287-291.

Moselewski F, Ropers D, Pohle K, et al. Comparison of measurement of cross-sectional coronary atherosclerotic plaque and vessel areas by 16-slice multidetector computed tomography versus intravascular ultrasound. *Am J Cardiol.* 2004;94:1294-1297.

Pitts SR, Niska RW, Xu J, Burt CW. *National Hospital Ambulatory Medical Care Survey: 2006 Emergency Department Summary.* National Health Statistics reports no. 7. Hyattsville, Md: National Center for Health Statistics; 2008 <http://www.cdc.gov/nchs/data/nhsr/nhsr007.pdf> Accessed 10.05.12.

Pope JH, Aufderheide TP, Ruthazer R, et al. Missed diagnoses of acute cardiac ischemia in the emergency department. *N Engl J Med.* 2000;342:1163-1170.

Pope JH, Ruthazer R, Beshansky JR, Griffith JL, Selker HP. Clinical features of emergency department patients presenting with symptoms suggestive of acute cardiac ischemia: a multicenter study. *J Thromb Thrombolysis.* 1998;6:63-74.

Rahmani N, Jeudy J, White CS. Triple rule-out dedicated coronary artery CTA: comparison of coronary artery image quality. *Acad Radiol.* 2009;16:604-609.

Remy-Jardin M, Pistolesi M, Goodman LR, et al. Management of suspected acute pulmonary embolism in the era of CT angiography: a statement from the Fleischner Society. *Radiology.* 2007;245:315-329.

Ross R. The pathogenesis of atherosclerosis: a perspective for the 1990s. *Nature.* 1993;362:801-809.

Rubinshtein R, Gaspar T, Halon DA, Goldstein J, Peled N, Lewis BS. Prevalence and extent of obstructive coronary artery disease in patients with zero or low calcium score undergoing 64-slice cardiac multidetector computed tomography for evaluation of a chest pain syndrome. *Am J Cardiol.* 2007;99:472-475.

Rubinshtein R, Halon DA, Gaspar T, et al. Usefulness of 64-slice cardiac computed tomographic angiography for diagnosing acute coronary syndromes and predicting clinical outcome in emergency department patients with chest pain of uncertain origin. *Circulation.* 2007;115:1762-1768.

Rumberger JA, Sheedy PF, Breen JF, Schwartz RS. Electron beam computed tomographic coronary calcium score cutpoints and severity of associated angiographic lumen stenosis. *J Am Coll Cardiol.* 1997;29:1542-1548.

Rumberger JA, Simons DB, Fitzpatrick LA, Sheedy PF, Schwartz RS. Coronary artery calcium area by electron-beam computed tomography and coronary atherosclerotic plaque area: a histopathologic correlative study. *Circulation.* 1995;92:2157-2162.

Schlett CL, Banerji D, Siegel E, et al. Prognostic value of CT angiography for major adverse cardiac events in patients with acute chest pain from the emergency department: 2-year outcomes of the ROMICAT trial. *JACC Cardiovasc Imaging.* 2011;4:481-491.

Schmermund A, Baumgart D, Görge G, et al. Coronary artery calcium in acute coronary syndromes: a comparative study of electron-beam computed tomography, coronary angiography, and intracoronary ultrasound in survivors of acute myocardial infarction and unstable angina. *Circulation.* 1997;96:1461-1469.

Shiga T, Wajima Z, Apfel CC, Inoue T, Ohe Y. Diagnostic accuracy of transesophageal echocardiography, helical computed tomography, and magnetic resonance imaging for suspected thoracic aortic dissection: systematic review and meta-analysis. *Arch Intern Med.* 2006;166:1350-1356.

Shuman WP, Branch KR, May JM, et al. Whole-chest 64-MDCT of emergency department patients with nonspecific chest pain: radiation dose and coronary artery image quality with prospective ECG triggering versus retrospective ECG gating. *AJR Am J Roentgenol.* 2009;192:1662-1667.

Sosnouski D, Bonsall RP, Mayer FB, Ravenel JG. Extracardiac findings at cardiac CT: a practical approach. *J Thorac Imaging.* 2007;22:77-85.

Souza AS, Bream PR, Elliott LP. Chest film detection of coronary artery calcification: the value of the CAC triangle. *Radiology.* 1978;129:7-10.

Swap CJ, Nagurney JT. Value and limitations of chest pain history in the evaluation of patients with suspected acute coronary syndromes. *JAMA.* 2005;294:2623-2629.

Takakuwa KM, Halpern EJ. Evaluation of a "triple rule-out" coronary CT angiography protocol: use of 64-section CT in low-to-moderate risk emergency department patients suspected of having acute coronary syndrome. *Radiology.* 2008;248:438-446.

Walsh K, Chang AM, Perrone J, et al. Coronary computerized tomography angiography for rapid discharge of low-risk patients with cocaine-associated chest pain. *J Med Toxicol.* 2009;5:111-119.

White CS. Chest pain in the emergency department: potential role of multidetector CT. *J Thorac Imaging.* 2007;22:49-55.

White CS, Kuo D. Chest pain in the emergency department: role of multidetector CT. *Radiology.* 2007;245:672-681.

Zimetbaum PJ, Josephson ME. Use of the electrocardiogram in acute myocardial infarction. *N Engl J Med.* 2003;348:933-940.

CHAPTER 24

Imaging the Postoperative Thoracic Aorta

Santiago Martínez-Jiménez and Laura E. Heyneman

The thoracic aorta may be affected by various disorders including aneurysms, dissections, intramural hematomas, penetrating atherosclerotic ulcers, and acute aortic injury. Specific pathophysiologic details of these entities are beyond the scope of this chapter and are reviewed elsewhere in this book. This chapter focuses on the surgical and endovascular interventions used to treat the diseased thoracic aorta. The initial part of the chapter discusses the most common postoperative complications that may be seen after thoracic aortic repair, regardless of the surgical procedure. The chapter then details the different types of thoracic aortic surgical procedures, beginning with operations on the ascending aorta, followed by operations on the aortic arch, and finishing with endovascular procedures performed on the descending thoracic aorta. For each specific surgical procedure, the expected appearance of the postoperative aorta, as well as the appearance of common complications, will be described; the cardiovascular imager must be familiar with both normal and abnormal features, to interpret images of the postoperative aorta correctly.

■ INDICATIONS FOR TREATMENT

A consensus statement was published on the indications for open surgical and endovascular intervention in the thoracic aorta. The indications were based on data that demonstrated, in certain groups of patients, that the risk of mortality from untreated aortic disease outweighs the risk of intervention. Indications for intervention in the ascending thoracic aorta include the following: evidence of rupture; a diameter greater than 5.5 cm for the general population or greater than 5.0 cm in patients with Marfan syndrome, other connective tissue disorder, or a bicuspid aortic valve; aneurysm growth of more than 0.5 cm per year; or any aneurysm that is symptomatic. Indications for intervention in the descending thoracic aorta include a diameter of more than 6.5 cm in the general population or more than 6 cm in patients with Marfan syndrome and other connective tissue disorders.

■ OPEN SURGICAL PROCEDURES IN THE THORACIC AORTA, INCLUDING THEIR COMPLICATIONS

Most patients who have undergone open procedures of the thoracic aorta are often evaluated with computed tomography (CT), although magnetic resonance imaging (MRI) is an excellent alternative when necessary. Details on CT protocols are beyond the scope of this chapter; however, some fundamental and general concepts are described. Although no universally accepted protocol exists, in general, two CT acquisitions are recommended: an initial CT acquisition without intravenous contrast and a second CT acquisition after the administration of intravenous contrast material; imaging for the enhanced CT is most often obtained during the arterial phase. The purpose of the non-enhanced CT is to identify postoperative material that appears hyperdense and that could be misinterpreted as extraluminal contrast material on enhanced CT (e.g., anastomotic felt along the anastomosis). Moreover, nonenhanced CT can demonstrate a high-attenuation hematoma within the aortic wall; after the administration of intravenous contrast material, the high density of the hematoma may be obscured by the adjacent contrast. However, in the evaluation of the postoperative aorta, most of the information is obtained after the administration of intravenous contrast material. Acquiring images during the arterial phase is important because life-threatening complications such as pseudoaneurysm and dissection may be identifiable only during this phase. Cardiac gating can be helpful when precise assessment of the aortic valve, coronary arteries, and coronary bypass grafts is required. However, most assessments are currently performed without cardiac gating because most complications can be identified on nongated images.

When assessing the postsurgical aorta, radiologists and other clinicians must be aware of several components to avoid misinterpreting normal postoperative structures as pathologic. Synthetic grafts, often made from polyethylene, are smooth-walled, round structures that appear slightly hyperdense on unenhanced CT (Fig. 24-1) and are relatively hypodense to the enhanced blood pool on contrast-enhanced CT. Anastomoses of the graft to the native aorta are generally identified by a sharply demarcated change in caliber of the vessel; these changes in caliber are often most easily identified on multiplanar reformations, particularly reformations that demonstrate the vessel in its long axis. The anastomoses are also almost always marked by felt pledgets, strips, or rings that buttress the suture lines; these objects are hyperdense on both noncontrast and contrast-enhanced CT. Confirmation that the area of the felt objects is of high density on the noncontrast CT can prevent the misinterpretation of these foci as small pseudoaneurysms, a common pitfall. Furthermore, felt rings and strips tend to be located along the entire circumference of the anastomosis rather than being positioned along a single wall, as is often the case with pseudoaneurysms (Figs. 24-2 and 24-3).

Finally, aortic grafts generally fall into one of two types: inclusion grafts or interposition grafts. In an inclusion graft, a synthetic graft is positioned within the diseased aortic lumen, and the native aorta is wrapped around the graft; therefore, a potential space exists between the graft and the native aortic wall. An interposition graft replaces the diseased portion of the aorta; the diseased portion of the aorta is resected, and the graft is sewn from end to end to the remaining portion of the aorta. Most recent and current surgical procedures are interposition procedures. However, patients who have had remote surgical procedures may still present for CT with inclusion grafts. Therefore, radiologists must have an understanding of inclusion graft anatomy to interpret these examinations properly.

General Complications of Open Thoracic Aortic Operations

Radiologists must be familiar with the normal appearance of the aorta immediately after surgery, to differentiate normal postoperative findings from postoperative complications. Many of the normal postsurgical findings are described in the following subsections. Additionally, several general complications of open thoracic aortic procedures are also described.

Sterile and Infected Perigraft Fluid Collection

Sterile postoperative perigraft fluid collections may be seen as a result of evolving postoperative hematoma or as a result of an inflammatory reaction elicited by the synthetic graft material. Sterile perigraft fluid collections are common postoperative occurrences that can resolve or remain stable over time (Fig. 24-4). Data suggest that a large amount of perigraft hematoma (>1.5 cm in thickness) on initial postoperative imaging is associated with an increased risk of pseudoaneurysm formation at the anastomosis. Radiologic features that suggest superinfection of a perigraft collection include rim enhancement after contrast administration, increasing air within the collection, a fistulous connection to adjacent structures, and extension into other mediastinal compartments.

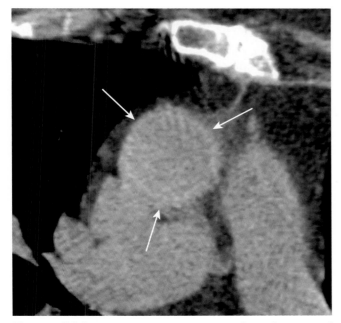

Figure 24-1 Supracoronary graft. Unenhanced computed tomography, axial image, demonstrates a polyethylene ascending aortic graft. The graft is slightly hyperdense *(arrows)* in comparison with the adjacent pulmonary artery.

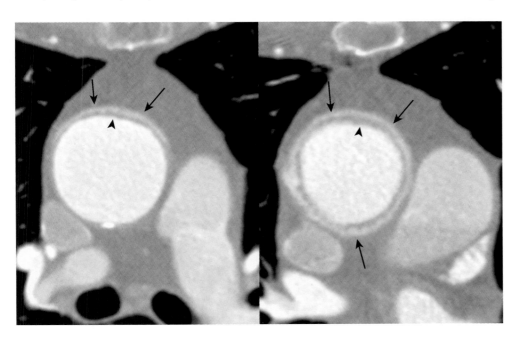

Figure 24-2 Normal graft anastomosis, axial view (left) and true cross-sectional reformation *(right)*. On the *left*, a felt ring appears hyperdense *(arrows)*, and the endograft is hypodense *(arrowhead)*. On the *right*, a true cross-sectional reformation of the entire anastomosis depicts the hyperdense felt ring *(arrows)* and the hypodense synthetic graft *(arrowhead)*.

Perigraft Gas Collections

The presence of mediastinal, perigraft air is an expected normal postsurgical finding that can persist for several weeks. However, the persistence of air for more than 8 weeks or an increasing amount of mediastinal air is highly suggestive of a developing infection or fistula (i.e., bronchial or esophageal) formation.

Sternal Osteomyelitis

Sternal osteomyelitis is a relatively common complication after median sternotomy. The infection can spread into the adjacent mediastinum and can result in mediastinitis. The radiologic findings of osteomyelitis include bone destruction, severe demineralization, change in orientation of the sternal wires, or frank sternal dehiscence. These findings are more conspicuous on CT than on radiography; furthermore, CT delineates other findings associated with osteomyelitis such as periosteal reaction, osseous sclerosis, and adjacent fluid collections (Fig. 24-5). When the CT appearance is nonspecific but osteomyelitis is of clinical concern, nuclear medicine studies with radiolabeled leukocytes may provide additional information.

■ SPECIFIC SURGICAL PROCEDURES INVOLVING THE ASCENDING AORTA

Supracoronary Grafts

Any repair that spares the aortic root (or sinuses of Valsalva) is generically called a supracoronary graft. If a repair involves both a supracoronary graft and an aortic valve replacement (thus sparing the sinuses of Valsalva), it is often referred to as the Wheat procedure (originally described by Wheat in 1964) (Fig. 24-6). Because the aortic root is spared, a supracoronary repair maintains the normal integrity of the coronary arteries. Therefore, a supracoronary repair is technically less complicated and avoids potential complications involving the coronary arteries (e.g., coronary pseudoaneurysm).

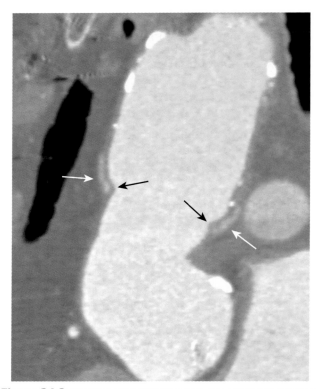

Figure 24-3 Normal graft anastomosis, long-axis reformation. Note the felt ring *(white arrows)* and the abrupt change in caliber, both of which help identify the anastomosis *(black arrows)*.

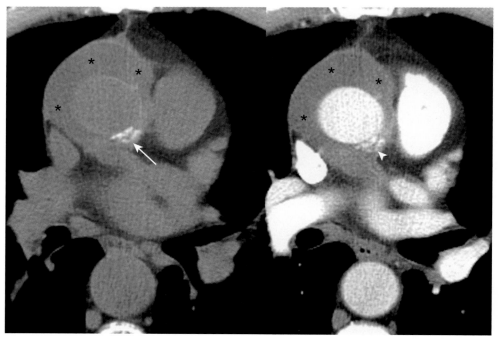

Figure 24-4 Supracoronary graft, Wheat procedure. Unenhanced and contrast-enhanced computed tomography (CT) axial views show a fluid collection *(asterisk)* surrounding the graft. Felt material is seen along the distal anastomosis *(arrow)*. The high density on the unenhanced CT scan is characteristic of felt pledgets and rings and is useful in differentiating the surgical material from a pseudoaneurysm on a contrast-enhanced CT scan. On the contrast-enhanced CT scan, the felt pledgets *(arrowhead)* may be misinterpreted as a pseudoaneurysm.

Potential complications of supracoronary reconstruction include the development of dissection or aneurysm involving the native aortic root. These complications occur most frequently in patients with connective tissue disorders or inflammatory processes such as aortitis. An additional possible complication is the development of a pseudoaneurysm at the anastomosis with the native aorta. The development of a pseudoaneurysm is the result of weakening of the surgical anastomosis; this may be caused by infection.

Complications of supracoronary repair are often identified in asymptomatic patients undergoing routine surveillance CT or MRI. Determining the possible presence of an aortic root aneurysm may be difficult because the normal size of the aortic root varies depending on gender and age. If, however, on serial examinations, the native aortic root changes in appearance or diameter, concern regarding a complication such as aneurysm formation should be raised. Aortic dissection involving the sinuses of Valsalva classically manifests with an intraluminal flap on cross-sectional imaging (Fig. 24-7). This is an emergency finding because dissection in this portion of the aorta may involve the coronary arteries and may place the patient at risk of myocardial infarction. Finally, a pseudoaneurysm at the anastomotic site usually appears as an extraluminal mass on noncontrast CT. After intravenous contrast administration, pseudoaneurysms usually enhance markedly, although they may have nonenhancing components related to the presence of peripheral thrombus (Fig. 24-8).

Composite Artificial Graft

When the aortic abnormality involves the sinuses of Valsalva, such as in patients with annuloaortic ectasia, the aortic reconstruction includes the aortic root. Two of the most common surgical techniques that involve the aortic root are the Bentall and Cabrol procedures (Figs. 24-9 and 24-10). In these operations, the aortic

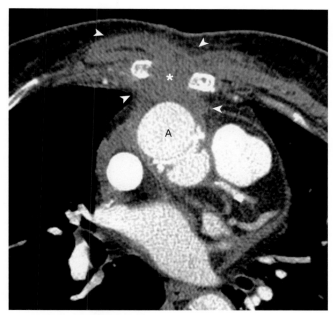

Figure 24-5 Supracoronary graft. Contrast-enhanced computed tomography axial views demonstrate a fluid collection in the anterior mediastinum that extends into the chest wall *(arrowheads)* through a sternal dehiscence *(asterisk)*. Needle aspiration confirmed the presence of infection. *A,* Aorta.

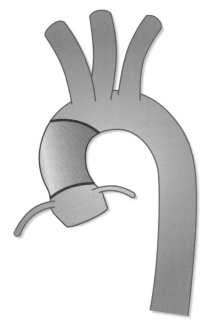

Figure 24-6 Supracoronary graft, Wheat procedure. Drawing depicts a tubular ascending aortic graft *(gray)* with preservation of the sinuses of Valsalva and replacement of the aortic valve *(blue).* The native aorta is shown in *red.*

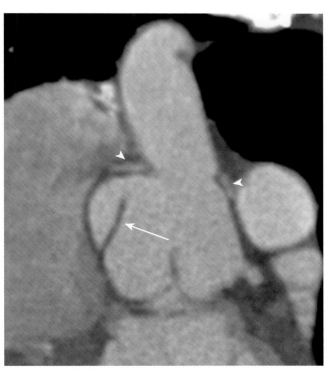

Figure 24-7 Supracoronary graft. Contrast-enhanced computed tomography, long-axis view, demonstrates an intimal flap *(arrow)* at the aortic root, proximal to the level of the proximal anastomosis *(arrowheads).*

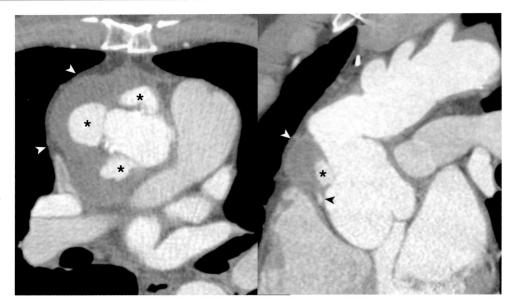

Figure 24-8 Supracoronary graft. Contrast-enhanced computed tomography axial image *(left)* and sagittal oblique reformation *(right)* depict a large pseudoaneurysm *(asterisks)* arising from the proximal anastomosis *(black arrowhead)*. Note the extensive surrounding thrombus *(white arrowheads)*.

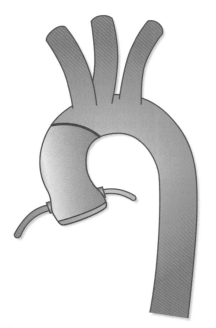
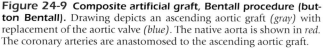

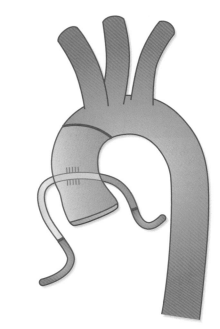

Figure 24-9 Composite artificial graft, Bentall procedure (button Bentall). Drawing depicts an ascending aortic graft *(gray)* with replacement of the aortic valve *(blue)*. The native aorta is shown in *red*. The coronary arteries are anastomosed to the ascending aortic graft.

Figure 24-10 Composite artificial graft, Cabrol procedure. Drawing shows an ascending aortic graft *(gray)* with replacement of the aortic valve *(blue)*. The native aorta is shown in red. The coronary arteries are anastomosed to the ascending aortic graft by a conduit.

valve is incorporated into the synthetic aortic graft; therefore, the aortic valve and the graft are implanted as a single unit. Because the sinuses of Valsalva are being replaced, the coronary arteries must be reimplanted onto the graft. The Bentall and Cabrol procedures differ from one another in the method by which the coronary arteries are reanastomosed to the aortic graft. In the Cabrol procedure, the coronary arteries are sewn onto a conduit that, in turn, is anastomosed to the ascending aorta. When the coronary conduit takes a retroaortic course, the wall of the conduit may mimic an intimal flap. Therefore, the radiologist must recognize the presence of the coronary conduit to

avoid misinterpreting this normal appearance as a dissection or a pseudoaneurysm.

In the Bentall procedure, the coronary arteries are directly implanted onto the ascending aortic graft. The original Bentall procedure had a high rate of complications involving the anastomoses of the coronary arteries onto the aortic graft. Therefore, the surgical procedure was revised; in the revised Bentall procedure, referred to as the button Bentall procedure, the coronary arteries are excised from the native aorta with a rind of native aortic wall, called a button. The button of native aortic tissue is then sewn to the ascending aortic graft. The button procedure has become the most common

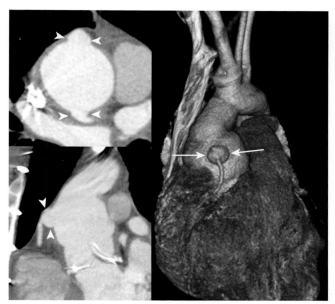

Figure 24-11 Composite artificial graft, Bentall procedure (button Bentall). Contrast-enhanced computed tomography axial view *(top left)*, sagittal oblique *(bottom left)*, and three-dimensional reformation *(right)* demonstrate the normal bulbous origin of the coronary buttons *(arrowheads and arrows)*.

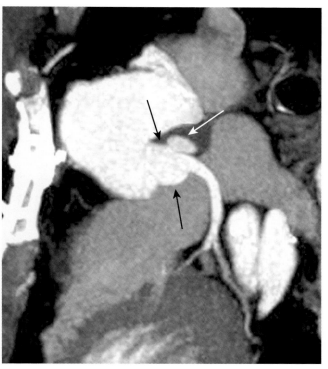

Figure 24-12 Composite artificial graft, Button Bentall procedure, with a pseudoaneurysm near the coronary anastomosis. Oblique axial reformation demonstrates a small focus of contrast extravasation *(white arrow)* from the left coronary artery button *(black arrows)*. This was a relatively common complication with the classic Bentall procedure, but it is less frequent in the setting of button Bentall modification.

method for attaching the coronary arteries onto an ascending aortic graft. The button may cause the origin of the coronary arteries to appear slightly dilated on CT (Fig. 24-11); the radiologist must be familiar with this normal appearance so as not to confuse the prominent button with an aneurysm or pseudoaneurysm, a common pitfall.

Postoperative complications of the Bentall procedure include pseudoaneurysms at the coronary anastomoses (Fig. 24-12) (which are much less common with the button Bentall modification) and at the aortic anastomoses (Fig. 24-13). Patients with Marfan syndrome are particularly prone to develop coronary pseudoaneurysms. In addition to pseudoaneurysm formation, patients who have undergone the Cabrol procedure are also at risk of complications related to the coronary conduit. On CT, thrombosis of the Cabrol coronary conduit may be diagnosed when contrast enhancement within the graft is lacking on contrast-enhanced CT (Fig. 24-14). Intimal hyperplasia of the conduit may appear on CT as low-density thickening of the conduit wall. Kinking of the conduit, with or without associated thrombosis, may also be seen. Because of the potential complications involving the coronary graft, the Cabrol procedure is now rarely performed; it is generally restricted to patients for whom a button Bentall is precluded, such as patients whose coronary arteries are difficult to mobilize.

Biologic Grafts

As an alternative to synthetic grafts, biologic grafts may be used in aortic reconstruction. Both cadaveric and autologous grafts have been used. The Ross procedure is an autograft that includes the pulmonic valve and

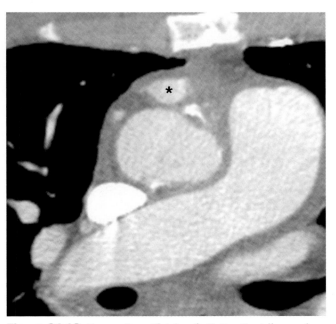

Figure 24-13 Composite artificial graft, Button Bentall procedure, with a pseudoaneurysm at the distal aortic anastomosis. Axial image depicts a small focus of contrast extravasation *(asterisk)* adjacent to the distal anastomosis.

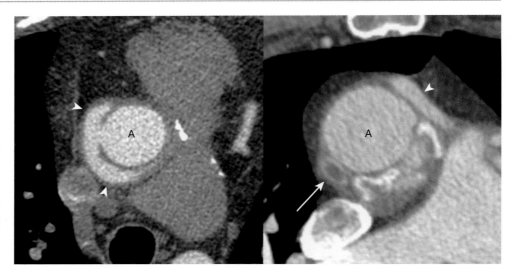

Figure 24-14 Composite artificial graft, Cabrol procedure. Contrast-enhanced computed tomography axial views of normal *(left)* and obstructed *(right)* coronary conduit grafts. Enhancing grafts *(arrowheads)* indicate normal flow. The lack of enhancement of the conduit to the left coronary artery *(arrow)* indicates obstruction. *A,* Aorta.

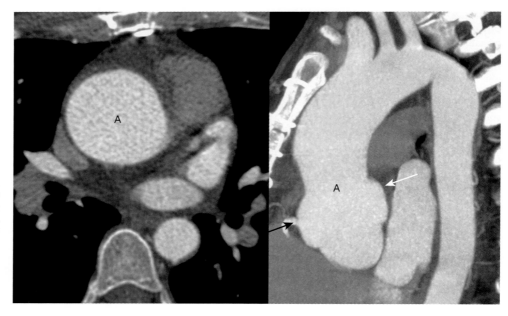

Figure 24-15 Biologic graft, Ross procedure. Contrast-enhanced computed tomography axial view *(left)* and sagittal oblique reformation *(right)* in a patient who underwent a Ross procedure several years earlier. Both the tubular and the sinus *(arrows)* portions of the ascending aorta are dilated. Aortic aneurysm formation is the most common complication of the Ross procedure. *A,* Aorta.

proximal pulmonary trunk; this pulmonary autograft is used to reconstruct the aortic root, with subsequent placement of a cadaveric or composite graft to reconstruct the pulmonary arterial trunk. This technique is most frequently used in children with aortic root disease because the autograft is thought to have favorable hemodynamics, a lower risk of endocarditis and thrombogenicity, and a higher growth potential.

Intrinsic complications of the Ross procedure include dilation of the aortic root (Fig. 24-15) with resultant valvular insufficiency, pseudoaneurysm formation, and ascending aortic dissection. All these complications are easily identified on CT or MRI, or both.

Aortic Valve-Sparing Procedures

Aortic valve-sparing procedures comprise a group of operations designed to preserve the aortic valve cusps in patients who have aortic root aneurysms with or without aortic insufficiency. This type of surgery is particularly useful in patients who have annuloaortic ectasia, in whom the aortic root is dilated but the aortic valve leaflets are normal. Several variations of this type of surgery are described in the literature, including the original supra-annular remodeling technique that was first performed by Yacoub and that keeps the aortic valve in situ. One of the most widely performed aortic valve-sparing surgical procedures was developed by David and Feindel. In this operation, the aneurysmal portion of the ascending aorta and sinuses of Valsalva are excised, but the aortic valve leaflets and some arterial wall are left attached to the left ventricular outflow tract. The aortic valve and the coronary arteries are then reimplanted inside a Dacron graft (Fig. 24-16). These aortic valve-sparing surgical procedures recreate the aortic sinuses and sinotubular junction, which is thought to improve hemodynamics; furthermore, the procedures allow for nearly normal cusp motion.

Total Arch Replacement

Elephant Trunk Procedure

Patients with extensive aortic aneurysms that involve the ascending, transverse, and descending aorta require complex surgical reconstruction, of which the "elephant trunk" (ET) technique is a commonly used example. The ET technique was originally described by Borst in 1983 and has undergone modifications since its introduction. The ET procedure is a two-stage operation that eventually results in total arch replacement. The first stage consists of an ascending aortic interposition graft that extends across the transverse aorta and has a free-floating distal end; the free-floating distal end of the graft dangles within the native descending aortic lumen. The "elephant trunk" designation is derived from the appearance of the unattached distal end of the graft as it floats within the lumen of the native descending aorta. During the first stage procedure, the arch vessels must be relocated. Frequently, the arch vessels are debranched from the native transverse aorta and are reattached to a trifurcated synthetic graft, which, in turn, is anastomosed to the ascending aortic graft. In the second stage of the ET procedure, the descending aorta is repaired by either an open or an endovascular approach, and the unattached distal end of the graft is anastomosed to a descending aortic graft (Fig. 24-17). When the second stage is performed by an endovascular approach, the combination of an open surgical first stage and an endovascular second stage is referred to as a hybrid ET procedure.

With the evolution of endovascular technology, a one-stage version of the ET procedure was introduced. This procedure is referred to as the frozen elephant trunk (FET). The initial portion of the FET surgery involves repairing the ascending and proximal transverse aorta, similar to the first stage of the traditional ET surgery. However, instead of terminating the operation after the proximal arch repair, in an FET procedure, the surgeon also repairs the distal arch and descending aorta by means of a composite graft that consists of a distal aortic stent graft that is sutured to a more proximal conventional tubular graft. The conventional synthetic graft is anastomosed to the proximal aortic arch repair, and the attached stent graft is deployed by an antegrade approach (i.e., from the arch).

Intrinsic complications of the conventional ET procedure after the first stage include aneurysm rupture, neurologic deficits, and stroke. After the second stage, spinal cord ischemia with resultant paraplegia is the most dreaded complication. Although the one-stage FET procedure prevents the patient from having to undergo a second surgical procedure with its associated morbidity and mortality, the risk of spinal cord ischemia may be higher with FET than with conventional ET surgery.

On CT after the first stage of the ET, the unattached free-floating graft within the descending aorta is well delineated within the descending aortic lumen. As intravenous contrast material fills the descending aorta, it surrounds the free ends of the graft (Fig. 24-18). The radiologist must recognize this normal postsurgical anatomy, to avoid misinterpreting the appearance of the free-floating

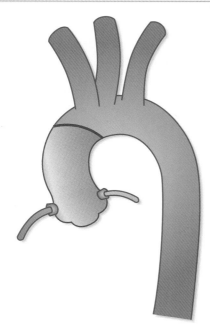

Figure 24-16 Aortic valve-sparing procedure. Drawing depicts an ascending aortic graft *(gray)* that includes the sinuses of Valsalva. The coronary arteries are anastomosed to the ascending aortic graft.

The most common intrinsic complication of aortic valve-sparing procedures is the development of aortic insufficiency. This complication can be assessed and quantified with echocardiography or cardiac MRI. Aortic dissection and pseudoaneurysm formation have also been reported.

■ SURGICAL PROCEDURES INVOLVING THE AORTIC ARCH

Any surgery involving the transverse aorta requires cerebral protection to prevent cerebral embolism or infarction. Many methods are used to maintain perfusion to the brain during aortic surgery, and these methods are beyond the scope of this chapter. In general, surgical procedures involving the aortic arch require the patient to undergo deep hypothermic circulatory arrest and either retrograde or antegrade cerebral perfusion.

Hemiarch Procedure

Disorders confined to the transverse aorta are exceedingly rare. Much more commonly, the aortic arch is involved in disease that extends from the ascending aorta into the descending aorta or that involves the entire thoracic aorta. When an ascending aortic aneurysm extends into just the proximal transverse aorta, thus sparing the arch vessels and distal transverse aorta, a hemiarch replacement may be performed. In this surgical procedure, the distal ascending aorta and proximal transverse aorta are removed; the remaining transverse aorta is beveled to leave the arch vessels intact. The graft that extends from the ascending aorta into proximal transverse aorta is then sewn onto the native aortic cuff.

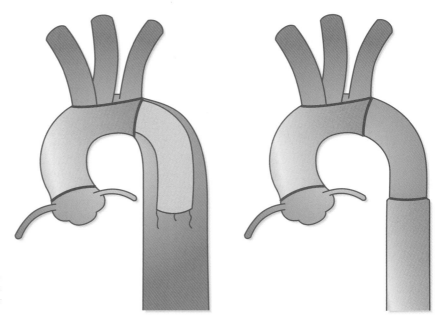

Figure 24-17 Elephant trunk procedure.
Drawings show stage I *(left)* and II *(right)* portions of the procedure. Typically, after stage I, the most distal portion of the graft remains unattached and is free floating within the descending aorta.

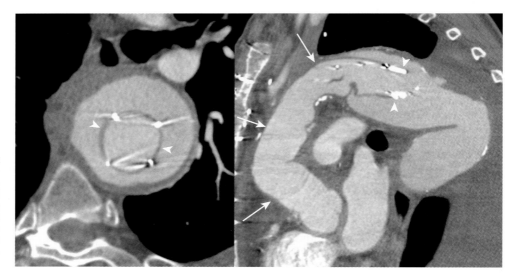

Figure 24-18 Elephant trunk procedure, stage I. Contrast-enhanced computed tomography, short-axis *(left)* and sagittal oblique reformations *(right)*. Note the ascending and aortic arch graft *(arrows)*. The distal portion *(arrowheads)* of the graft remains free floating within the descending aortic lumen.

distal graft as a dissection or pseudoaneurysm. Furthermore, the radiologist must recognize the appearance of the debranched arch vessels, which do not arise from the transverse aorta, but rather extend from a round conduit that courses from the ascending aortic graft.

Arch-First Technique
An alternative to the ET procedure is a one-stage surgical approach that replaces the entire diseased aorta in one setting through multiple incisions. To minimize cerebral ischemia, the one-stage surgical procedure requires early reanastomosis of the arch vessels; this is referred to as the arch-first technique. The arch vessels are removed from the native aortic arch and are attached to a curved, tubular graft that has branches onto which the arch vessels are anastomosed. This graft replaces the aortic arch. Antegrade perfusion of the arch vessels is established

through this branched graft. Attention is then turned to suturing the distal end of the branched graft onto a portion of the native descending aorta, which is normal in caliber. In this way, both the transverse aorta and descending aorta are repaired, and flow is reestablished both to the brain and the lower body. Finally, the proximal aspect of the branched graft is anastomosed to a normal-caliber aortic root, to a preexisting ascending aortic graft, or to a newly positioned ascending aortic interposition graft. The arch-first surgical procedure eliminates the risk of aneurysm rupture in the interval between staged procedures, eliminates the risks associated with a second thoracic aortic procedure, and is also associated with a low rate of reoperation on the remaining aorta. Compared with the ET procedure, the arch-first procedure has lower mortality and morbidity, especially regarding neurologic outcome.

■ SURGICAL PROCEDURES INVOLVING THE DESCENDING THORACIC AORTA

Disease that is limited to the descending thoracic aorta is often treated medically rather than surgically. In general, medical therapy for descending aortic disease carries a significantly lower morbidity and mortality as compared with surgical treatment. However, when descending aortic aneurysms exceed 5 to 6 cm, increase in size at a rate greater than 0.5 to 1.0 cm/year, or are symptomatic with refractory pain, surgical therapy is warranted. In the setting of descending aortic dissection, surgical treatment is initiated when the patient has symptoms of malperfusion. Aortic rupture from either aneurysm or dissection is a surgical emergency.

Some of the most common complications related to surgical repair of the thoracic descending aorta are left vocal cord paralysis, renal failure, paraplegia from spinal cord ischemia, stroke, and bleeding.

■ THORACIC AORTIC ENDOVASCULAR THERAPY AND ITS COMPLICATIONS

Since 1990, endovascular stent grafting of the thoracic aorta, often referred as thoracic endovascular aortic repair (TEVAR), has emerged as a viable option for treating aortic disease. The descending aorta is particularly suited to TEVAR because of its lack of curvature and the presence of few branch vessels. Thus, TEVAR is performed in the descending aorta more often than in the curved ascending and transverse aorta. A meta-analysis published in 2010 suggested that TEVAR may reduce early death, complications such as paraplegia and renal insufficiency, and length of hospitalization when compared with open surgery. However, sustained benefits on survival have yet to be proven. The meta-analysis concluded that, although the feasibility of TEVAR of the descending thoracic aneurysms had been widely established, indications for intervention remained to be fully defined.

In general, employment of a stent graft requires a 2-cm proximal and distal landing zone. In patients with descending aortic disease but an insufficient proximal landing zone, the left subclavian artery may be intentionally covered by the stent and thereby sacrificed. Perfusion to the left arm is restored by retrograde flow through the left vertebral artery or by a bypass graft. Sacrifice of the left subclavian artery may result in upper extremity ischemia or vertebrobasilar insufficiency, although these complications are uncommon. Occasionally, median sternotomy may be required to reroute the arch vessels and provide an adequate proximal landing zone. Alternatively, neck incision may be performed; the left subclavian artery is ligated proximally, and the distal end is anastomosed to the left common carotid artery, thus restoring flow to the arm and vertebral artery while allowing the ostium of the blind-ending subclavian artery to be covered by the stent graft. In general, TEVAR should be avoided in patients with Marfan syndrome or other connective tissue disorders because TEVAR in these patients may result in retrograde dissection, pseudoaneurysms, or endoleaks at the proximal and distal landing zones.

Imaging after aortic stent graft placement is performed shortly after the procedure to establish a baseline appearance of the graft and to detect early complications. Often, a 6-month follow-up scan is also obtained. Thereafter, imaging is generally performed annually, unless symptoms occur or an early complication must be monitored. Postprocedure imaging of TEVAR is mainly achieved with CT, although conventional angiography continues to have an important role. Most institutions obtain both noncontrast and arterial phased contrast-enhanced CT images in their evaluation of aortic stent grafts. Furthermore, data suggest that an additional set of images obtained approximately 60 seconds after intravenous contrast administration may also be useful in the evaluation of aortic stent grafts; approximately 10% of the complications called endoleaks (see the later discussion of endoleaks) are not visible on the arterial phase of contrast enhancement but may be seen on a delayed enhancement scan. Although it is generally considered optimal, a triphasic (noncontrast, arterial phase, delayed enhancement) CT is not used in every institution because most endoleaks are detected during the arterial phase of enhancement, and the performance of an additional delayed phase CT scan increases the patient's exposure to ionizing radiation. MRI angiography with gadolinium is an alternative to CT angiography but is less widely available; furthermore, the ability of MRI to evaluate the stent graft depends on the composition of the endograft, given that some grafts may cause a large amount of susceptibility artifact.

In addition to imaging, aortic stent grafts may be monitored by a wireless pressure sensor device (e.g., Endosure, CardioMEMS, Atlanta; Impressure, Remon Medical Technologies, Caesarea, Israel). This device, which is usually placed within the excluded portion of the aorta at the time the endograft is deployed, measures pressures within the excluded portion of the aorta. By sensing continued high pressures within the excluded aorta, the device may uncover a persistent communication between the systemic circulation and the excluded portion of the aorta, as seen in type I and III endoleaks (see the next section for a description of types of endoleaks).

Various different thoracic endografts are available on the market, including but not limited to the Gore TAG from Gore Medical (Flagstaff, Ariz), the Talent from Medtronic (Minneapolis), the Zenith TX2 from Cook Medical (Bloomington, Ind), the E Vita from Jotec (Muri, Switzerland), the TAArget from LeMaitre Vascular, Burlington, Mass), and the Relay from Bolton Medical (Sunrise, Fla). The specifics of the individual characteristics of each type of endograft are beyond the scope of this chapter. However, radiologists who frequently image aortic stent grafts are encouraged to become familiar with the different types of endografts because each type of graft has a characteristic appearance on imaging and may be prone to specific complications.

General complications specific to TEVAR include endoleaks, stent collapse, retrograde dissection, stent migration, and fistula formation. These complications are discussed in the following sections.

Table 24-1   Common Endoleaks After Thoracic Endovascular Aortic Repair

Endoleak		Description
I		Attachment site leaks
	A	Proximal
	B	Distal (outflow tract must be present)
II		Collateral vessel leaks
	A	Simple
	B	Two or more vessels
III		Graft failure
	A	Defect in the graft
	B	Junctional leak
Mixed		Combination

Endoleaks

The most common complication after TEVAR is an endoleak. An endoleak is defined as persistent perfusion of the excluded portion of the aorta after endoprosthesis deployment. Endoleaks are most often discovered on routine postprocedure contrast-enhanced CT, which is often performed when the patient is asymptomatic. The presence of contrast material within the excluded portion of the aorta, seen either on arterial phase or delayed phase postcontrast imaging, indicates the presence of an endoleak.

Five different types of endoleaks have been described in the setting of patients who have undergone TEVAR for aortic aneurysm repair. The different types of endoleak reflect different sources of persistent flow into the excluded portion of the aorta. Although five types of endoleaks have been described, only three types are commonly encountered; these are summarized in Table 24-1. A type I endoleak is caused by insufficient apposition of the endograft to the native aortic wall proximally or distally, thus allowing aortic flow around the attachment site into the excluded portion of the aorta. A type II endoleak results from perfusion of the excluded portion of the aorta through collateral vessels or retrograde flow from side branches. A type III endoleak is secondary to graft failure; most often, this is caused by a gap at the junction of two overlapping stent graft components. Each category of endoleak is divided into subtypes to define the source of persistent flow further.

Type IA endoleaks are more common than type IB endoleaks and are the result of insufficient apposition of the proximal aspect of the endograft to the aortic wall (Fig. 24-19). They may occur as an isolated complication, or they may be associated with endograft collapse (discussed later). In a type IA endoleak, the imperfect seal of the graft to the aortic wall allows aortic flow (and thus intravenous contrast material) to course around the edge of the graft into the aneurysm sac (Fig. 24-20). Therefore, contrast enhancement of the excluded portion of the aneurysm sac is seen, on either arterial phase or delayed phase imaging.

An entity that may mimic a type IA endoleak is "bird beaking." In bird beaking, the seal of the most proximal aspect of the endograft (the proximal landing zone) against the aortic wall is incomplete, but the remainder

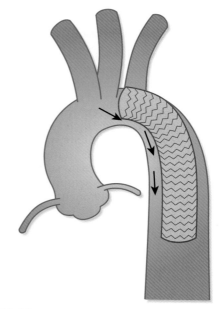

Figure 24-19 Endoleak type IA. Drawing shows an endograft deployed in the distal arch that extends into the descending aorta. *Arrows* demonstrate incomplete apposition of the stent to the aortic wall, thus allowing persistent flow around the edge of the graft into the aneurysm sac.

of the graft is sufficiently apposed to the aortic wall to prevent contrast material (and flow) from entering the excluded aneurysm sac (Fig. 24-21). The term bird beaking stems from the beaked appearance that the contrast forms when it undermines the proximal aspect of the stent graft. Bird beaking is not a true endoleak because flow and contrast material do not actually reach the excluded aneurysm sac. However, bird beaking requires close serial monitoring because it may progress to a true type IA endoleak.

Type II endoleaks are the most common type of endoleak and are caused by one or more collateral vessels feeding the excluded aneurysm sac. Frequently, the collateral vessel is small, such as an intercostal artery (Fig. 24-22). Perfusion of the excluded aorta from a small collateral vessel does not subject the excluded aorta to high pressure or high flow, and it may not result in growth of the aneurysm sac. However, occasionally, a type II endoleak is caused by perfusion from a large vessel such as the left subclavian artery (Fig. 24-23). When this occurs, flow to the excluded aorta may be sufficient to enlarge the aneurysm sac. These cases often warrant treatment. Measurement of the excluded sac diameter on serial follow-up CT scans is important because absence of sac shrinkage or sac growth may result from otherwise occult type II endoleaks.

Type III endoleaks are uncommon, and type IIIA (intrinsic graft defect) endoleaks are quite rare. Type IIIB endoleaks, also referred to as junctional endoleaks, are caused by an incomplete seal between two overlapping endografts or graft components. Although type IIIB endoleaks are usually isolated, they may occasionally result from endograft collapse (discussed later). On CT, a type IIIB junctional endoleak may be difficult to

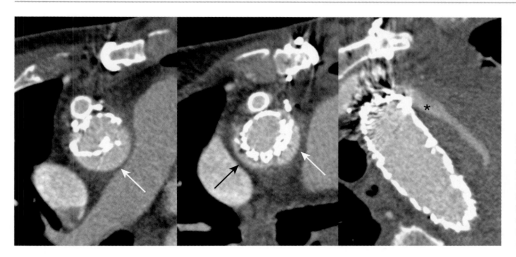

Figure 24-20 Endoleak type IA, proven at conventional angiography. Contrast-enhanced computed tomography axial oblique reformations. The proximal end of the stent is not apposed to the aortic wall. Contrast material extends around the edge of the graft *(arrows)* and forms a blush of enhancement *(asterisk)* within the aneurysm sac.

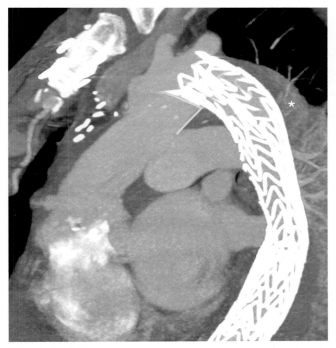

Figure 24-21 "Bird beaking" mimicking a type IA endoleak. Oblique sagittal reformat of contrast-enhanced computed tomography. The proximal stent graft is not completely sealed against the wall of the aortic lesser curvature. This allows contrast material to undermine the most proximal aspect of the stent *(yellow lines)*. However, contrast does not reach the excluded portion of the aorta *(asterisk)*. The angle formed by the stent relative to the lesser curvature *(yellow lines)* is referred to as bird beaking.

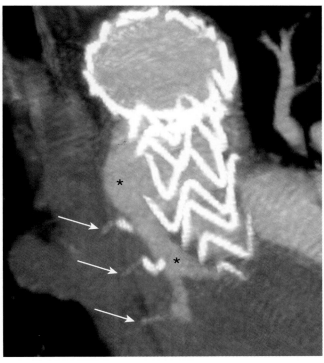

Figure 24-22 Endoleak type IIB. Contrast-enhanced computed tomography sagittal oblique maximum intensity projection reformation. Multiple small intercostal arteries *(arrows)* provide retrograde flow into the aneurysm sac that results in contrast enhancement *(asterisks)* outside the endograft.

differentiate from a type II endoleak arising from regional intercostal arteries.

Mixed types of endoleaks represent approximately 5% of all cases, and prospective diagnosis on imaging is extremely difficult. Martinez-Jimenez and Heyneman have seen two cases of a type IB endoleak that were associated with reopening of the ductus arteriosus (unpublished); the patent ductus, in turn, also fed the excluded portion of the aorta, a type IIA endoleak. This uncommon event was previously described in the setting of aortic dissection type B.

As mentioned previously, endoleak types I and III must be treated expeditiously because these endoleaks subject the excluded portion of the aorta to the high pressure of the native aorta and therefore place the aneurysm sac at risk of rupture. A type II endoleak typically does not subject the excluded aorta to very high pressures and therefore is usually treated conservatively. However, if the collateral vessels serving the excluded portion of the aorta are large (e.g., the left subclavian artery), the pressures within the excluded aorta may be elevated enough to enlarge the excluded portion.

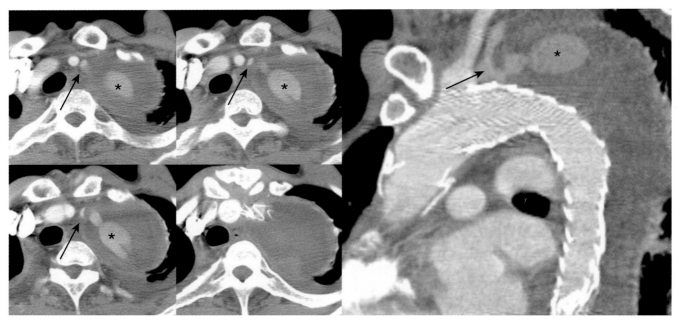

Figure 24-23 Endoleak type IIA, confirmed at conventional angiography. Contrast-enhanced computed tomography axial view montage *(left)* and sagittal oblique reformation *(right)*. The axial montage demonstrates the presence of an endoleak *(asterisk)* fed by retrograde flow from the left subclavian artery *(arrows)*. The sagittal oblique maximum intensity projection reformation more clearly delineates the extension of contrast material *(arrow)* from the left subclavian artery into the aneurysm sac.

In general, CT is excellent in detecting the presence of an endoleak (i.e., contrast material within the excluded aorta on either arterial or delayed phase imaging), but it may fail to identify the type of endoleak. The determination of the source of the endoleak may need to be made by conventional angiography. Decisions regarding management of the endoleak are made after consideration of multiple variables such as interval growth of the aneurysm sac on CT, measurement of aneurysmal sac pressures by a sensor such as the CardioMEMS device, or development of symptoms.

Persistent Flow Within False Lumen (Endoleak) After Thoracic Endovascular Aortic Repair for Aortic Dissection

Most of the literature on endoleaks stems from studies performed in patients who underwent TEVAR for aortic aneurysm repair. The data on TEVAR performed for aortic dissection are much more scarce. When an endograft is placed to repair an aortic dissection, the presence of persistent flow within the excluded false lumen likely constitutes an endoleak. However, the pathophysiology and the implications of an endoleak in the setting of dissection repair are currently not completely clear. The concern is that continued flow within the false lumen may expand the false lumen, thus placing it at risk of rupture. In general, persistent flow in the excluded false lumen requires at least two sites of communication between the true and false lumina: an entry point and an exit point. Often, multiple sites of communication (fenestrations) are present in a dissected aorta. After placement of an endograft,

continued communication between the true and false lumina may result from a type IA endoleak, in which lack of occlusive seal between the stent and the aortic wall allows flow to extend around the graft and into the false lumen. Additionally, type II endoleaks with retrograde flow through collateral vessels may permit continued perfusion of the false lumen. In one study, factors related to the presence of an endoleak after TEVAR for dissection were small radius of curvature of the transverse aorta and coverage of the left subclavian artery. Similar to the situation for stent grafts placed for aneurysm repair, endoleaks in the setting of aortic dissection may be complex and mixed (i.e., of more than one type).

Endograft Collapse

Endograft collapse is an uncommon complication that most often manifests after the initial deployment of the stent. Occasionally, however, the collapse occurs months after stent placement, usually as a result of a progressive type I (Fig. 24-24) or type III (Fig. 24-25) endoleak. The clinical presentation of stent collapse may be dramatic, with decreased or absent systemic perfusion distal to the graft. Stent collapse may be visualized on chest radiography, and it can be more apparent on bilateral oblique views than on a frontal or lateral radiograph. On CT, the deformed appearance of the stent and its lack of apposition to the aortic wall may be obvious. A collapsed stent is an emergency and requires immediate treatment. Treatment is often achieved by an endovascular approach with the deployment of a rigid stent inside the collapsed endograft. When the rigid stent (e.g., a Palmaz stent) is expanded, the collapsed endograft is opened, and distal flow is reestablished.

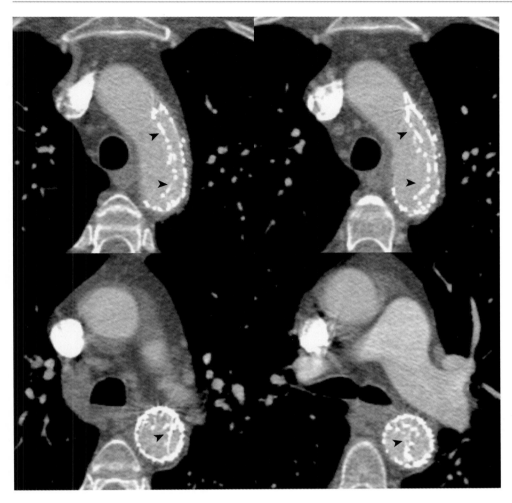

Figure 24-24 Endoleak type IA, confirmed at conventional angiography, with associated endograft collapse. Contrast-enhanced computed tomography axial view montage shows collapse and deformation of the endograft *(arrowheads).* This emergency complication of a type IA endoleak may result from undermining of the proximal graft by high-pressure aortic flow.

Dissection

The deployment of an endograft can injure the aortic intima and result in dissection that extends either in retrograde fashion (proximal to the stent) or in antegrade fashion (distal to the stent). The development and propagation of a dissection after endograft deployment are very uncommon. However, patients who have connective tissue disorders are more prone to dissection from endograft placement, and therefore TEVAR is not recommended in these patients. Dissection as a result of TEVAR usually manifests in the early postoperative period, although it has been reported several weeks after endograft placement. Treatment of the dissection is similar to that of a dissection involving the native aorta. A dissection that extends into the ascending aorta may be life-threatening, and open surgical repair may be performed. Imaging findings of dissection are identical to those of classic dissection (Fig. 24-26).

Migration

Stent migration is an uncommon complication that can result from type I endoleaks. In the setting of a type I endoleak, the systemic pressure around the edges of the endograft can displace the stent either cranially or caudally. The reported occurrence of proximal migration of

a Gore TAG thoracic endograft at 2-year follow-up is 4%. The change in position of the stent graft may be apparent on both radiography and CT. Therefore, the location of the stent relative to static anatomic landmarks should be assessed on all follow-up studies, and any change in stent location should be reported to the referring physician immediately.

Endograft Infection and Fistula Formation

Infection after TEVAR is uncommon, but if it occurs, it is often a devastating complication. The incidence is approximately 5%. The most commonly offending microorganisms are *Propionibacterium* species, *Staphylococcus aureus, Streptococcus* species, and *Enterobacter cloacae.* Infection often develops several months after stent placement. Although the pathogenesis is not clear, perioperative contamination, hematogenous seeding, and local bacterial translocation may play a role. Infection of the endograft carries an extremely poor prognosis, with a high mortality from sepsis.

CT findings that suggest endograft infection include air and fluid collections adjacent to the stent. A stent placed by an endovascular approach should never have air surrounding it (unless a concomitant open surgical

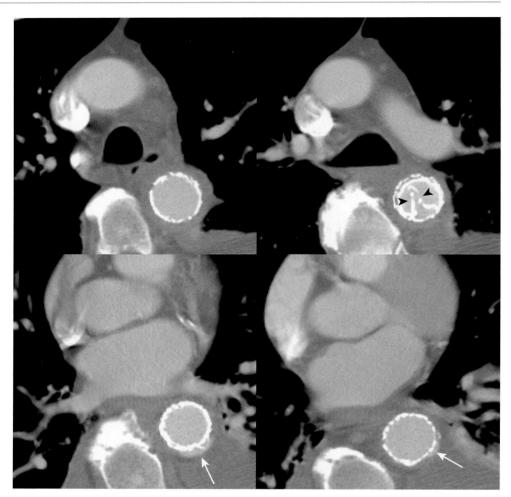

Figure 24-25 Endoleak type IIIB, confirmed at conventional angiography. Contrast-enhanced computed tomography axial view montage depicts collapse of a distal endograft *(arrowheads)*. This complication creates a junctional endoleak *(arrows)* and exposes the aorta to systemic pressure in this patient who had undergone thoracic endovascular aortic repair for type B aortic dissection.

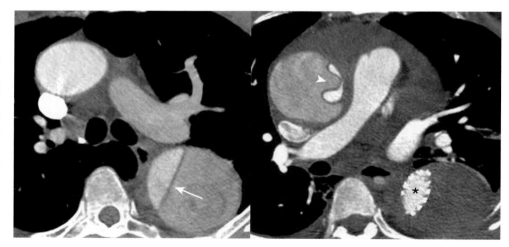

Figure 24-26 Retrograde aortic dissection after thoracic endovascular aortic repair. Axial contrast-enhanced computed tomography images performed before *(left)* and after *(right)* aortic endograft placement for descending aortic dissection in a patient with Marfan syndrome. Before the deployment of the aortic stent graft, the aortic dissection *(arrow)* is limited to the descending thoracic aorta. After placement of the descending aortic stent graft *(asterisk)*, a dissection flap is visible within the ascending aorta *(arrowhead)*.

procedure was also performed). In the setting of endograft infection, the amount of perigraft air is usually quite small.

Infection of the graft may lead to the formation of a fistula between the graft and the esophagus or the tracheobronchial tree. Alternatively, a fistula may develop primarily between the endograft and either the esophagus or the tracheobronchial tree if the stent's struts

perforate the aorta and its adjacent structures. When this occurs, secondary infection of the endograft invariably results.

A large amount of air in the perigraft space, the presence of air within the excluded portion of the aorta, or a perigraft air-fluid level should raise the possibility of a fistula between the endograft and the esophagus or tracheobronchial tree (Fig. 24-27). Obscuration of fat

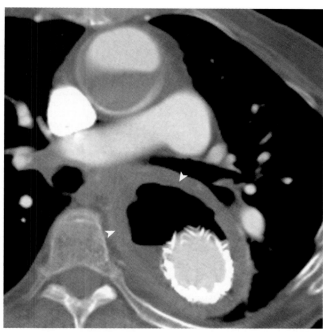

Figure 24-27 Fistula between the endograft and the esophagus after thoracic endovascular aortic repair. Contrast-enhanced computed tomography axial view depicts a large amount of air *(arrowheads)* within the aneurysm sac. The patient died as a result of sepsis.

planes between the aorta and the esophagus or the airways may also be seen in the setting of fistula formation. Visualization of the fistula itself is extremely rare.

Fistula between the endograft and either the esophagus or the tracheobronchial tree has a dismal prognosis. Patients often present with a sentinel episode of hematemesis or hemoptysis. Several hours after the initial presenting event, exsanguination may ensue. Treatment options are extremely limited. Definitive open surgical repair may be attempted, but perioperative mortality remains very high. Placement of an additional stent graft over the site of the fistula may be considered if the patient cannot tolerate the open surgical repair.

Transient Postimplantation Syndrome

Transient postimplantation syndrome (TPS) is a common inflammatory condition that occurs approximately 3 days after TEVAR. TPS consists of mild leukocytosis, elevated levels of C-reactive protein, and a moderately elevated body temperature. In addition to fever, patients may report mild to moderate back pain. Because of the presence of fever, the clinical presentation of TPS may be similar to that of stent infection. Therefore, in the setting of a febrile patient who recently underwent TEVAR, a normal CT scan that has no findings to suggest infection may be very reassuring.

■ CONCLUSION

Imaging the postsurgical aorta often requires a multidisciplinary and multimodality approach. Radiologists must understand various different aortic procedures so that they can recognize the expected postoperative appearances, as well as common postoperative complications.

Bibliography

Aronberg DJ, Glazer HS, Madsen K, Sagel SS. Normal thoracic aortic diameters by computed tomography. *J Comput Assist Tomogr.* 1984;8:247-250.

Azizzadeh A, Estrera AL, Porat EE, Madsen KR, Safi HJ. The hybrid elephant trunk procedure: a single-stage repair of an ascending arch and descending thoracic aortic aneurysm. *J Vasc Surg.* 2006;44:404-407.

Bavaria JE, Appoo JJ, Makaroun MS, et al. Endovascular stent grafting versus open surgical repair of descending thoracic aortic aneurysms in low-risk patients: a multicenter comparative trial. *J Thorac Cardiovasc Surg.* 2007;133:369-377.

Bentall H, De Bono A. A technique for complete replacement of the ascending aorta. *Thorax.* 1968;23:338-389.

Beregi JP, Haulon S, Otal P, et al. Endovascular treatment of acute complications associated with aortic dissection: midterm results from a multicenter study. *J Endovasc Ther.* 2003;10:486-493.

Borst HG, Walterbusch G, Schaps D. Extensive aortic replacement using "elephant trunk" prosthesis. *Thorac Cardiovasc Surg.* 1983;31:37-40.

Bortone AS, Schena S, D'Agostino D, et al. Immediate versus delayed endovascular treatment of post-traumatic aortic pseudoaneurysms and type B dissections: retrospective analysis and premises to the upcoming European trial. *Circulation.* 2002;106(suppl I):I234-I240.

Botta L, Buttazzi K, Russo V, et al. Endovascular repair for penetrating atherosclerotic ulcers of the descending thoracic aorta: early and mid-term results. *Ann Thorac Surg.* 2008;85:987-992.

Bozinovski J, Coselli JS. Outcomes and survival in surgical treatment of descending thoracic aorta with acute dissection. *Ann Thorac Surg.* 2008;85:965-970:discussion 970–971.

Brandt M, Hussel K, Walluscheck KP, et al. Stent-graft repair versus open surgery for the descending aorta: a case-control study. *J Endovasc Ther.* 2004;11:535-538.

Brinster DR, Wheatley 3rd GH, Williams J, et al. Are penetrating aortic ulcers best treated using an endovascular approach? *Ann Thorac Surg.* 2006;82:1688-1691.

Cabrol C, Pavie A, Gandjbakhch I, et al. Complete replacement of the ascending aorta with reimplantation of the coronary arteries: new surgical approach. *J Thorac Cardiovasc Surg.* 1981;81:309-315.

Cambria RP, Brewster DC, Lauterbach SR, et al. Evolving experience with thoracic aortic stent graft repair. *J Vasc Surg.* 2002;35:1129-1136.

Cao P, Verzini F, De Rango P, Maritati G, De Pasquale F, Parlani G. Different types of thoracic endografts. *J Cardiovasc Surg (Torino).* 2009;50:483-492.

Carroccio A, Spielvogel D, Ellozy SH, et al. Aortic arch and descending thoracic aortic aneurysms: experience with stent grafting for second-stage "elephant trunk" repair. *Vascular.* 2005;13:5-10.

Chen S, Yei F, Zhou L, et al. Endovascular stent-grafts treatment in acute aortic dissection (type B): clinical outcomes during early, late, or chronic phases. *Catheter Cardiovasc Interv.* 2006;68:319-325.

Cheng D, Martin J, Shennib H, et al. Endovascular aortic repair versus open surgical repair for descending thoracic aortic disease: a systematic review and meta-analysis of comparative studies. *J Am Coll Cardiol.* 2010;55:986-1001.

Cherry C, DeBord S, Hickey C. The modified Bentall procedure for aortic root replacement. *AORN J.* 2006;84:52-55:58-70; quiz 71–74.

Chiesa R, Melissano G, Marone EM, Marrocco-Trischitta MM, Kahlberg A. Aorto-oesophageal and aortobronchial fistulae following thoracic endovascular aortic repair: a national survey. *Eur J Vasc Endovasc Surg.* 2010;39:273-279.

Chiesa R, Tshomba Y, Kahlberg A, et al. Management of thoracic endograft infection. *J Cardiovasc Surg (Torino).* 2010;51:15-31.

Christensen JD, Heyneman LE. Case of the season: aortoesophageal fistula complicating thoracic aortic aneurysm stent graft repair. *Semin Roentgenol.* 2009;44:4-7.

Coady MA, Ikonomidis JS, Cheung AT, et al. Surgical management of descending thoracic aortic disease: open and endovascular approaches: a scientific statement from the American Heart Association. *Circulation.* 2010;121:2780-2804.

Coady MA, Rizzo JA, Hammond GL, et al. What is the appropriate size criterion for resection of thoracic aortic aneurysms? *J Thorac Cardiovasc Surg.* 1997;113:476-491:discussion 489–491.

Coselli JS, Plestis KA, La Francesca S, Cohen S, et al. Results of contemporary surgical treatment of descending thoracic aortic aneurysms: experience in 198 patients. *Ann Vasc Surg.* 1996;10:131-137.

Czerny M, Cejna M, Hutschala D, et al. Stent-graft placement in atherosclerotic descending thoracic aortic aneurysms: midterm results. *J Endovasc Ther.* 2004;11:26-32.

Czerny M, Grimm M, Zimpfer D, et al. Results after endovascular stent graft placement in atherosclerotic aneurysms involving the descending aorta. *Ann Thorac Surg.* 2007;83:450-455.

Dake MD, Kato N, Mitchell RS, et al. Endovascular stent-graft placement for the treatment of acute aortic dissection. *N Engl J Med.* 1999;340:1546-1552.

Dake MD, Miller DC, Semba CP, Mitchell RS, Walker PJ, Liddell RP. Transluminal placement of endovascular stent-grafts for the treatment of descending thoracic aortic aneurysms. *N Engl J Med.* 1994;331:1729-1734.

David TE, Armstrong S. Aortic cusp repair with Gore-Tex sutures during aortic valve-sparing operations. *J Thorac Cardiovasc Surg.* 2010;139:1340-1342.

David TE, Feindel CM, Webb GD, Colman JM, Armstrong S, Maganti M. Long-term results of aortic valve-sparing operations for aortic root aneurysm. *J Thorac Cardiovasc Surg.* 2006;132:347-354.

Davies RR, Goldstein LJ, Coady MA, et al. Yearly rupture or dissection rates for thoracic aortic aneurysms: simple prediction based on size. *Ann Thorac Surg.* 2002;73:17-27:discussion 27–28.

Demers P, Miller DC, Mitchell RS, Kee ST, Chagonjian L, Dake MD. Stent-graft repair of penetrating atherosclerotic ulcers in the descending thoracic aorta: mid-term results. *Ann Thorac Surg.* 2004;77:81-86.

Demers P, Miller DC, Mitchell RS, et al. Midterm results of endovascular repair of descending thoracic aortic aneurysms with first-generation stent grafts. *J Thorac Cardiovasc Surg.* 2004;127:664-673.

Eggebrecht H, Baumgart D, Schmermund A, et al. Endovascular stent-graft repair for penetrating atherosclerotic ulcer of the descending aorta. *Am J Cardiol.* 2003;91:1150-1153.

Eggebrecht H, Herold U, Kuhnt O, et al. Endovascular stent-graft treatment of aortic dissection: determinants of post-interventional outcome. *Eur Heart J.* 2005;26:489-497.

Eggebrecht H, Nienaber CA, Neuhäuser M, et al. Endovascular stent-graft placement in aortic dissection: a meta-analysis. *Eur Heart J.* 2006;27:489-498.

Erasmi A, Sievers HH, Scharfschwerdt M, Eckel T, Misfeld M. In vitro hydrodynamics, cusp-bending deformation, and root distensibility for different types of aortic valve-sparing operations: remodeling, sinus prosthesis, and reimplantation. *J Thorac Cardiovasc Surg.* 2005;130:1044-1049.

Erkut B, Ceviz M, Becit N, Gündogdu F, Unlü Y, Kantarci M. Pseudoaneurysm of the left coronary ostial anastomoses as a complication of the modified Bentall procedure diagnosed by echocardiography and multislice computed tomography. *Heart Surg Forum.* 2007;10:E191-E192.

Fann JI, Dake MD, Semba CP, Liddell RP, Pfeffer TA, Miller DC. Endovascular stent-grafting after arch aneurysm repair using the "elephant trunk." *Ann Thorac Surg.* 1995;60:1102-1105.

Fattori R, Napoli G, Lovato L, et al. Descending thoracic aortic diseases: stent-graft repair. *Radiology.* 2003;229:176-183.

Festic E, Steiner RM, Spatz E. Aortic dissection with extension to a patent ductus arteriosus. *Int J Cardiovasc Imaging.* 2005;21:459-462.

Garcia J, Ferreirós J, Santamaría M, Bustos A, Abades JL, Santamaría N. MR angiographic evaluation of complications in surgically treated type A aortic dissection. *Radiographics.* 2006;26:981-992.

Gelsomino S, Frassani R, Da Col P, et al. A long-term experience with the Cabrol root replacement technique for the management of ascending aortic aneurysms and dissections. *Ann Thorac Surg.* 2003;75:126-131.

Golzarian J, Dussaussois L, Abada HT, et al. Helical CT of aorta after endoluminal stent-graft therapy: value of biphasic acquisition. *AJR Am J Roentgenol.* 1998;171:329-331.

Golzarian J, Struyven J, Abada HT, et al. Endovascular aortic stent-grafts: transcatheter embolization of persistent perigraft leaks. *Radiology.* 1997;202:731-734.

Gorich J, Rilinger N, Krämer S, et al. Angiography of leaks after endovascular repair of infrarenal aortic aneurysms. *AJR Am J Roentgenol.* 2000;174:811-814.

Greenberg RK, Haddad F, Svensson L, et al. Hybrid approaches to thoracic aortic aneurysms: the role of endovascular elephant trunk completion. *Circulation.* 2005;112:2619-2626.

Grimm M, Loewe C, Gottardi R, et al. Novel insights into the mechanisms and treatment of intramural hematoma affecting the entire thoracic aorta. *Ann Thorac Surg.* 2008;86:453-456.

Hager A, Kaemmerer H, Rapp-Bernhardt U, et al. Diameters of the thoracic aorta throughout life as measured with helical computed tomography. *J Thorac Cardiovasc Surg.* 2002;123:1060-1066.

Heinemann MK, Buehner B, Jurmann MJ, Borst HG. Use of the "elephant trunk technique" in aortic surgery. *Ann Thorac Surg.* 1995;60:2-6:discussion 7.

Heyer KS, Modi P, Morasch MD, et al. Secondary infections of thoracic and abdominal aortic endografts. *J Vasc Interv Radiol.* 2009;20:173-179.

Hoang JK, Martinez S, Hurwitz LM. MDCT angiography after open thoracic aortic surgery: pearls and pitfalls. *AJR Am J Roentgenol.* 2009;192:W20-W27.

Idu MM, Reekers JA, Balm R, Ponsen KJ, de Mol BA, Legemate DA. Collapse of a stent-graft following treatment of a traumatic thoracic aortic rupture. *J Endovasc Ther.* 2005;12:503-507.

Ius F, Haql C, Haverich A, Pichlmaier M. Elephant trunk procedure 27 years after Borst: what remains and what is new? *Eur J Cardiothorac Surg.* 2011;40:1-11.

Kato N, Hirano T, Shimono T, et al. Treatment of chronic aortic dissection by transluminal endovascular stent-graft placement: preliminary results. *J Vasc Interv Radiol.* 2001;12:835-840.

Kidd JN, Ruel Jr GJ, Cooley DA, et al. Surgical treatment of aneurysms of the ascending aorta. *Circulation.* 1976;54(suppl III):III118-III122.

Klieverik LM, Takkenberg JJ, Elbers BC, Oei FB, van Herwerden LA, Bogers AJ. Dissection of a dilated autograft root. *J Thorac Cardiovasc Surg.* 2007;133:817-818.

Kouchoukos NT. One-stage repair of extensive thoracic aortic disease. *J Thorac Cardiovasc Surg.* 2010;140(suppl):S150-153:discussion S185–S190.

Kouchoukos NT. Complications and limitations of the elephant trunk procedure. *Ann Thorac Surg.* 2008;85:690-691:author reply 691-692.

Kouchoukos NT, Karp RB, Blackstone EH, Kirklin JW, Pacifico AD, Zorn GL. Replacement of the ascending aorta and aortic valve with a composite graft: results in 86 patients. *Ann Surg.* 1980;192:403-413.

Kouchoukos NT, Masetti P, Mauney MC, Murphy MC, Castner CF. One-stage repair of extensive chronic aortic dissection using the arch-first technique and bilateral anterior thoracotomy. *Ann Thorac Surg.* 2008;86:1502-1509.

Kouchoukos NT, Masetti P, Nickerson NJ, Castner CF, Shannon WD, Dávila-Román VG. The Ross procedure: long-term clinical and echocardiographic follow-up. *Ann Thorac Surg.* 2004;78:773-781:discussion 773-781.

Kouchoukos NT, Mauney MC, Masetti P, Castner CF. Single-stage repair of extensive thoracic aortic aneurysms: experience with the arch-first technique and bilateral anterior thoracotomy. *J Thorac Cardiovasc Surg.* 2004;128:669-676.

Kruser TJ, Osaki S, Kohmoto T, Chopra PS. Computed tomography finding mimicking aortic dissection after Cabrol procedure. *Asian Cardiovasc Thorac Ann.* 2009;17:108-109.

Lazar HL, Varma PK, Shapira OM, Soto J, Shaw P. Endograft collapse after thoracic stent-graft repair for traumatic rupture. *Ann Thorac Surg.* 2009;87:1582-1583.

LeMaire SA, Carter SA, Coselli JS. The elephant trunk technique for staged repair of complex aneurysms of the entire thoracic aorta*Ann Thorac Surg.* 2006;81:1561-1569:discussion 1569.

Leurs LJ, Bell R, Degrieck Y, et al. Endovascular treatment of thoracic aortic diseases: combined experience from the EUROSTAR and United Kingdom Thoracic Endograft registries. *J Vasc Surg.* 2004;40:670-679:discussion 679-680.

Leyh RG, Schmidtke C, Sievers HH, Yacoub MH. Opening and closing characteristics of the aortic valve after different types of valve-preserving surgery. *Circulation.* 1999;100:2153-2160.

Marcheix B, Dambrin C, Bolduc JP, et al. Midterm results of endovascular treatment of atherosclerotic aneurysms of the descending thoracic aorta. *J Thorac Cardiovasc Surg.* 2006;132:1030-1036.

Matsuda H, Tsuji Y, Sugimoto K, Okita Y. Secondary elephant trunk fixation with endovascular stent grafting for extensive/multiple thoracic aortic aneurysm. *Eur J Cardiothorac Surg.* 2005;28:335-336.

McCready RA, Pluth JR. Surgical treatment of ascending aortic aneurysms associated with aortic valve insufficiency. *Ann Thorac Surg.* 1979;28:307-316.

Midorikawa H, Ogawa T, Satou K, Hoshino S, Takase S, Yokoyama H. Long-term results of endoluminal grafting for descending thoracic aortic aneurysms. *Jpn J Thorac Cardiovasc Surg.* 2005;53:295-301.

Milano AD, Pratali S, Mecozzi G, et al. Fate of coronary ostial anastomoses after the modified Bentall procedure. *Ann Thorac Surg.* 2003;75:1797-1801:discussion 1802.

Miller DC, Stinson EB, Oyer PE, et al. Concomitant resection of ascending aortic aneurysm and replacement of the aortic valve: operative and long-term results with "conventional" techniques in ninety patients. *J Thorac Cardiovasc Surg.* 1980;79:388-401.

Minatoya K, Ogino H, Matsuda H, Sasaki H, Yagihara T, Kitamura S. Replacement of the descending aorta: recent outcomes of open surgery performed with partial cardiopulmonary bypass. *J Thorac Cardiovasc Surg.* 2008;136:431-435.

Mohan IV, Hitos K, White GH, et al. Improved outcomes with endovascular stent grafts for thoracic aorta transections. *Eur J Vasc Endovasc Surg.* 2008;36:152-157.

Monnin-Bares V, Thony F, Rodiere M, et al. Endovascular stent-graft management of aortic intramural hematomas. *J Vasc Interv Radiol.* 2009;20:713-721.

Murgo S, Dussaussois L, Golzarian J, et al. Penetrating atherosclerotic ulcer of the descending thoracic aorta: treatment by endovascular stent-graft. *Cardiovasc Intervent Radiol.* 1998;21:454-458.

Neschis DG, Moainie S, Flinn WR, Scalea TM, Bartlett ST, Griffith BP. Endograft repair of traumatic aortic injury—a technique in evolution: a single institution's experience. *Ann Surg.* 2009;250:377-382.

Neuhauser B, Greiner A, Jaschke W, Chemelli A, Fraedrich G. Serious complications following endovascular thoracic aortic stent-graft repair for type B dissection. *Eur J Cardiothorac Surg.* 2008;33:58-63.

Nienaber CA, Fattori R, Lund G, et al. Nonsurgical reconstruction of thoracic aortic dissection by stent-graft placement. *N Engl J Med.* 1999;340:1539-1545.

Okamoto K, Casselman FP, De Geest R, Vanermen H. Giant left coronary ostial aneurysm after modified Bentall procedure in a Marfan patient. *Interact Cardiovasc Thorac Surg.* 2008;7:1164-1166.

Parmer SS, Carpenter JP, Stavropoulos SW, et al. Endoleaks after endovascular repair of thoracic aortic aneurysms. *J Vasc Surg.* 2006;44:447-452.

Parsa CJ, Hughes GC. Surgical options to contend with thoracic aortic pathology. *Semin Roentgenol.* 2009;44:29-51.

Parsa CJ, Daneshmand MA, Lima B, Balsara K, McCann RL, Hughes GC. Utility of remote wireless pressure sensing for endovascular leak detection after endovascular thoracic aneurysm repair. *Ann Thorac Surg.* 2010;89:446-452.

Pauls S, Orend KH, Sunder-Plassmann L, Kick J, Schelzig H. Endovascular repair of symptomatic penetrating atherosclerotic ulcer of the thoracic aorta. *Eur J Vasc Endovasc Surg.* 2007;34:66-73.

Rabkin-Aikawa E, Aikawa M, Farber M, et al. Clinical pulmonary autograft valves: pathologic evidence of adaptive remodeling in the aortic site. *J Thorac Cardiovasc Surg.* 2004;128:552-561.

Restrepo CS, Martinez S, Lemos DF, et al. Imaging appearances of the sternum and sternoclavicular joints. *Radiographics.* 2009;29:839-859.

Rozenblit AM, Patlas M, Rosenbaum AT, et al. Detection of endoleaks after endovascular repair of abdominal aortic aneurysm: value of unenhanced and delayed helical CT acquisitions. *Radiology.* 2003;227:426-433.

Rubin S, Bayle A, Poncet A, Baehrel B. Retrograde aortic dissection after a stent graft repair of a type B dissection: how to improve the endovascular technique. *Interact Cardiovasc Thorac Surg.* 2006;5:746-748.

Safi HJ, Miller 3rd CC, Estrera AL, et al. Staged repair of extensive aortic aneurysms: morbidity and mortality in the elephant trunk technique. *Circulation.* 2001;104:2938-2942.

Sam 2nd A, Kibbe M, Matsumura J, Eskandari MK. Blunt traumatic aortic transection: endoluminal repair with commercially available aortic cuffs. *J Vasc Surg.* 2003;38:1132-1135.

Sasaki M, Usui A, Yoshikawa M, Akita T, Ueda Y. Arch-first technique performed under hypothermic circulatory arrest with retrograde cerebral perfusion improves neurological outcomes for total arch replacement. *Eur J Cardiothorac Surg.* 2005;27:821-825.

Schepens MA, Dossche KM, Morshuis WJ, van den Barselaar PJ, Heijmen RH, Vermeulen FE. The elephant trunk technique: operative results in 100 consecutive patients. *Eur J Cardiothorac Surg.* 2002;21:276-281.

Schoder M, Grabenwöger M, Hölzenbein T, et al. Endovascular stent-graft repair of complicated penetrating atherosclerotic ulcers of the descending thoracic aorta. *J Vasc Surg.* 2002;36:720-726.

Stavropoulos SW, Charagundla SR. Imaging techniques for detection and management of endoleaks after endovascular aortic aneurysm repair. *Radiology.* 2007;243:641-655.

Svensson LG, Kim KH, Blackstone EH, et al. Elephant trunk procedure: newer indications and uses. *Ann Thorac Surg.* 2004;78:109-116:discussion 109–116.

Svensson LG, Kouchoukos NT, Miller DC, et al. Expert consensus document on the treatment of descending thoracic aortic disease using endovascular stent-grafts. *Ann Thorac Surg.* 2008;85(suppl):S1-S41.

Symbas PN, Raizner AE, Tyras DH, et al. Aneurysms of all sinuses of Valsalva in patients with Marfan's syndrome: an unusual late complication following replacement of aortic valve and ascending aorta for aortic regurgitation and fusiform aneurysm of ascending aorta. *Ann Surg.* 1971;174:902-907.

Sze DY, van den Bosch MA, Dake MD, et al. Factors portending endoleak formation after thoracic aortic stent-graft repair of complicated aortic dissection. *Circ Cardiovasc Interv.* 2009;2:105-112.

Szeto WY, McGarvey M, Pochettino A, et al. Results of a new surgical paradigm: endovascular repair for acute complicated type B aortic dissection*Ann Thorac Surg.* 2008;86:87-93:discussion 93-94.

Tehrani HY, Peterson BG, Katariya K, et al. Endovascular repair of thoracic aortic tears*Ann Thorac Surg.* 2006;82:873-877:discussion 877-878.

Ueda T, Fleischmann D, Dake MD, et al. Incomplete endograft apposition to the aortic arch: bird-beak configuration increases risk of endoleak formation after thoracic endovascular aortic repair. *Radiology.* 2010;255:645-652.

Usui A, Ueda Y. Arch first technique under deep hypothermic circulatory arrest with retrograde cerebral perfusion. *MMCTS.* 2007;2007:1974.

Wellons ED, Milner R, Solis M, et al. Stent-graft repair of traumatic thoracic aortic disruptions. *J Vasc Surg.* 2004;40:1095-1100.

Wheat Jr MW, Wilson JR, Bartley TD. Successful replacement of the entire ascending aorta and aortic valve. *JAMA.* 1964;188:717-719.

Wolthuis AM, Houthoofd S, Deferm H, et al. Complex thoracic aortic aneurysm: a combined open and endovascular approach. *Acta Chir Belg.* 2005;105:400-402.

Wong CH, Wyatt MG, Jackson R, Hasan A. A dual strategic approach to mega-aortic aneurysms. *Eur J Cardiothorac Surg.* 2001;19:528-530.

Yoda M, Nonoyama M, Shimakura T, et al. Surgical case of aortic root and thoracic aortic aneurysm after the Wheat procedure. *Ann Thorac Cardiovasc Surg.* 2002;8:115-118.

Inflammatory and Infectious Vascular Disorders

Thorsten A. Bley and Christopher J. François

This chapter describes the role of noninvasive imaging modalities in the assessment of vascular manifestations of inflammatory and infectious disorders. Indications, limitations, technical aspects, and pitfalls and pearls of the following noninvasive imaging modalities are discussed: ultrasonography and color-coded Duplex sonography (CCDS), computed tomography (CT), magnetic resonance imaging (MRI) and MR angiography (MRA), fluorine-18 deoxyglucose positron emission tomography (FDG PET), and digital subtraction angiography (DSA). The chapter is subdivided in the two major parts: inflammatory disorders and infectious disorders.

■ INFLAMMATORY DISORDERS

Since the 1992 Chapel Hill, North Carolina consensus conference, primary systemic vasculitides have been subdivided according to the size of the affected vessel into large vessel vasculitis, medium vessel vasculitis, and small vessel vasculitis. Large vessel vasculitides include giant cell arteritis (GCA) and Takayasu arteritis (TA), whereas medium vessel vasculitides include polyarteritis nodosa (PAN) and Kawasaki disease. Small vessel vasculitides are further subdivided into those that demonstrate an association with antineutrophil cytoplasmic antibody (ANCA), such as granulomatosis with polyangitis formerly known as Wegener granulomatosis, Churg-Strauss vasculitis, and microscopic polyangiitis, and those small vessel vasculitides that are associated with immune complexes in the vessel. Inflammatory aortitis may also be present in other inflammatory diseases such as rheumatoid arthritis, (peri-)aortitis (Ormond), polychondritis, spondyloarthritis, sarcoidosis, Cogan syndrome, and Behçet disease.

This section focuses on the most common inflammatory disorders that affect the large and medium-sized arteries. Mural inflammatory changes in large and medium-sized arteries can be directly visualized by high-resolution imaging modalities. Vasculitic changes in small vessels can be visualized only indirectly. Inflammatory reactions of affected tissue, rather than the small vessel wall itself, can be demonstrated.

Imaging tools have been demonstrated to assess the extent and activity of vasculitic changes in a very sensitive way. The extent and distribution of vasculitic changes may help to narrow the potential differential diagnosis. However, inflammatory tissue reactions that can be demonstrated with noninvasive imaging may be similar in various vasculitides. For making a specific diagnosis, additional clinical or laboratory findings should be taken into account. For example, with noninvasive imaging, aortitis with subclavian stenoses caused by GCA may resemble aortitis with subclavian stenosis caused by TA. The patient's age is frequently very useful to distinguish between the two.

Large Vessel Vasculitides

Giant Cell Arteritis

GCA, also known as temporal arteritis, is the most common large vessel vasculitis. It has an incidence of up to 20 per 100,000 inhabitants. The prevalence is higher in northern urban populations as compared with southern rural populations. Female patients are more often affected than male patients. The typical age of initial presentation ranges from 60 to 80 years. Clinical presentations vary, and clinical signs may be nonspecific. Potential symptoms include scalp tenderness, new headaches, jaw claudication, and visual symptoms such as diplopia, amaurosis fugax, or even blindness. The following American College of Rheumatology criteria can be used for classification: age at onset of disease greater than 50 years, new onset or new type of localized pain of the head, temporal artery abnormality (tenderness, decreased pulsation), elevated erythrocyte sedimentation rate (>50 mm according to the Westergren method), and abnormal findings on biopsy of the temporal artery. Temporal artery biopsy demonstrating granulomatous mural inflammation with the presence of multinucleated giant cells or a disrupted internal elastic membrane is considered the diagnostic gold standard. Once GCA is suspected, immediate steroid treatment should be initiated. Typically, patients demonstrate rapid improvement of symptoms within a few days. However, long-term steroid treatment is mandatory to prevent relapsing disease. Alternative medications such as methotrexate or infliximab have been discussed, albeit controversially, to help reduce the amount of corticosteroid administered.

With more frequent use of noninvasive imaging modalities, the incidence of large vessel involvement has been found to be higher than previously believed. A study of 69 patients with GCA revealed presence of aortitis, for example, in 65% patients, and involvement of the subclavian arteries in 37%, followed by axillary, renal, carotid, and other large artery involvement. Non-invasive whole body vasculitis activity mapping would be desirable for assessment of vasculitis activity in therapeutic decision making.

CCDS can be considered the imaging modality of first choice for detection of mural inflammatory changes in GCA. In the hands of a well-trained observer, CCDS can be a powerful tool for identifying the typical halo, flow alterations, or stenoses of the superficial temporal artery (Fig. 25-1). With its high spatial resolution of approximately 100 mcm, clear depiction of the superficial cranial arteries and their mural anatomy is possible. A meta-analysis including more than 2000 patients revealed a weighted sensitivity and specificity of the halo sign of 69% and 82%, respectively, and a weighted sensitivity of stenosis or occlusion of 68% (compared with biopsy findings). CCDS is readily available, harmless, cost effective, and repeatable. However, it is observer dependent and can be rather time consuming, especially when the cranial involvement pattern and the supraaortic arteries are assessed at the same time. The thoracic aorta, which also can be involved, may not be clearly visible on CCDS because air in the lung may overlie the scan window.

FDG PET uses glucose metabolism for visualizing inflammatory tissue. The radioactive tracer FDG is metabolized in tumor cells and active inflammatory cells. Increased metabolic activity can be detected in areas of vascular inflammation (Fig. 25-2). Because of the small (picomolar) amount of tracer uptake necessary for visualization, FDG PET scanning is considered the most sensitive noninvasive imaging modality for detection of large vessel vasculitides. However, the increased metabolism is nonspecific, and FDG PET has low spatial resolution of approximately 4 mm. In addition, the underlying physiologic cerebral uptake of FDG precludes the ability of FDG PET to visualize the mural inflammatory changes of the superficial temporal arteries in GCA. Further, FDG PET is not everywhere available, it is costly, and it involves the use of ionizing radiation.

With its various tissue contrasts and the use of gadolinium-based contrast agents in imaging planes of any desired obliquity, MRI is a versatile tool for assessing inflammatory changes in many areas of the body. High-resolution MRI can noninvasively visualize mural inflammatory changes of arteries as small as the superficial temporal arteries. Typical MRI signs of vasculitic involvement include mural contrast enhancement and mural thickening (Figs. 25-3 and 25-4). To depict the occasionally subtle changes associated with GCA most clearly, a specific high-resolution protocol for visualization of the superficial temporal artery wall is necessary. This protocol includes a T1-weighted, contrast-enhanced multislice spin echo sequence with the following parameters: repetition time, 500 msec; time to echo, 22 msec; spectral fat saturation; field of view, 240 × 240 mm²; acquisition matrix, 1024 × 768; acquired in-plane resolution, 195 × 260 mcm; slice thickness, 3 mm; and acquisition time, 6:42 minutes at 1.5T and 4:52 minutes at 3T. Initial single center trials revealed a sensitivity and specificity of 80% and 97% and a positive and negative predictive value of 96% and

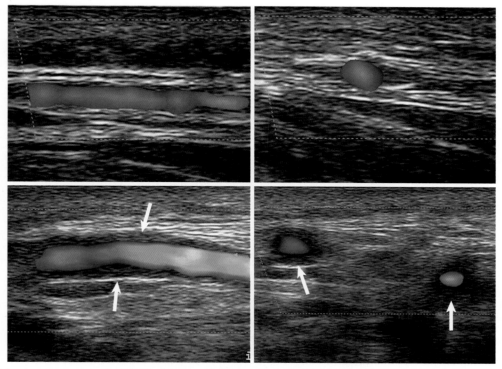

Figure 25-1 Color doppler sonography (CDS) of the superficial temporal arteries. *Upper row* demonstrates longitudinal and cross-sectional appearance of normal superficial temporal artery. The dark halo *(arrows in bottom row)* surrounding the superficial temporal artery represents a characteristic sign on CDS in patients with active giant cell arteritis. (Courtesy of Wolfgang Schmidt, MD, Vice Chair and Professor of Rheumatology, Medical Center for Rheumatology Berlin-Buch, Germany.)

84%, respectively. Sensitivity can be increased to 86% when imaging in the first few days of steroid treatment.

MRI follow-up studies of patients with biopsy proven GCA revealed that MRI signs were pronounced in active disease and decreased by steroid medication. This finding underlines the need for immediate scanning before steroid treatment effects diminish MRI-visible mural inflammatory changes. Relapsing disease has been visualized in individual cases in which repeated MRI scans have been performed.

High-resolution imaging of the superficial temporal arteries can be combined with MRA of the thoracic aorta

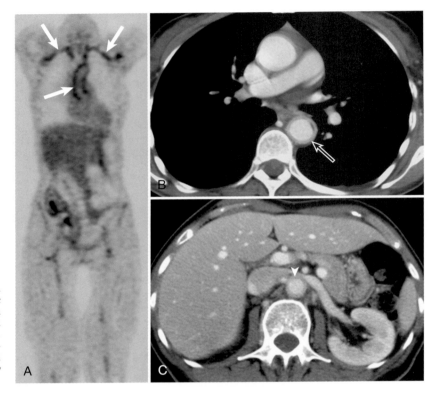

Figure 25-2 Fluorine-18 deoxyglucose positron emission tomography scan of a 56-year-old female patient with large vessel vasculitis affecting the aorta and supraaortic arteries demonstrates increased metabolic activity along the arterial walls *(arrows)*. The corresponding transversal computed tomography scans *(right)* readily reveal mural thickening and contrast enhancement of the descending aorta *(arrow in B)* and the abdominal aorta *(arrowhead in C)*.

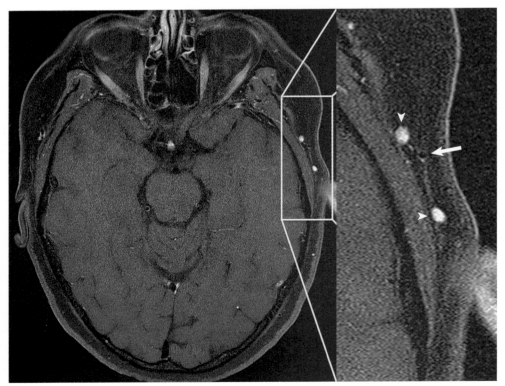

Figure 25-3 A 59-year-old female patient without giant cell arteritis. No mural thickening or increased contrast enhancement of the superficial temporal arteries is observed *(arrow)*. Please note the bright intraluminal signal in the superficial temporal veins *(arrowheads)* as compared with the flow-dependent signal void in the superficial temporal artery.

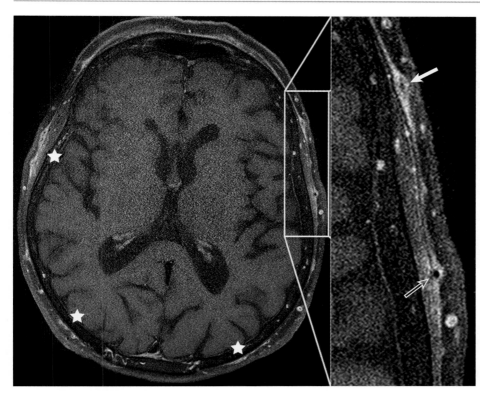

Figure 25-4 A 73-year-old female patient with giant cell arteritis. High-resolution magnetic resonance imaging reveals inflammatory mural thickening and contrast enhancement of the frontal *(solid arrow)* and parietal *(open arrow)* branches of the left superficial temporal artery. Please note inflammatory involvement of the frontal and parietal branches of the right superficial temporal artery and the superficial occipital arteries bilaterally *(stars)*.

and the supraaortic branches for assessment of large artery involvement within a single MRI or MRA study. This combined approach offers incremental value for the patient and the practitioner to understand the extent and activity of this systemic vasculitis.

An intraindividual head-to-head comparison of MRI and CCDS revealed that both imaging techniques had comparably high sensitivities and specificities in the detection of mural inflammatory changes in GCA. MRI demonstrated higher values for detection of disease, but differences did not reach the level of statistical significance. The intracranial and intradural arteries of the circle of Willis were not affected in a retrospective analysis of 50 patients with biopsy proven GCA and MRI signs of mural inflammation of the extracranial superficial temporal arteries. Increased contrast material enhancement of the intracranial and extradural medial meningeal artery was found in 32% of cases.

MRI images can be acquired by using a standard scanning protocol and are therefore observer independent. However, MRI is expensive and is not readily available everywhere. Published studies mainly report single center experiences. Higher levels of evidence from larger patient trials are warranted. Results from a multicenter trial based in Germany are expected soon.

Takayasu Arteritis

TA, also known as pulseless disease, is a chronic granulomatous form of vasculitis of unknown origin that affects the aorta and its major branches including the coronary and pulmonary arteries. Female patients less than 40 years old are predominantly affected. Inflammatory mononucleated infiltrates lead to mural thickening with multifocal stenosis and occlusion. Less than

10% of patients will also have dilatation and aneurysm formation of the affected arteries. Fatigue, mildly elevated body temperature, loss of weight, night sweats, myalgias, and arthralgias are typical presenting symptoms. Ischemic signs develop with progressive disease, predominantly claudication of the upper extremities and reduced cerebral perfusion, depending on the site of vasculitic manifestation. Aortic involvement is most common, followed by (in descending order) the subclavian, carotid, pulmonary, and abdominal arteries. The American College of Rheumatology criteria for classification of TA include age at onset of disease less than 40 years, ischemia of at least one extremity, reduced pulse of the radial or ulnar artery or both, systolic pressure gradient greater than 10 mm Hg between both arms, bruits over one or both subclavian arteries or abdominal aorta, and angiographic evidence of inflammatory changes of the aorta, its branches, or large extremity arteries.

Imaging in TA should ideally allow early diagnosis, including detailed assessment of the extent and severity of mural vasculitic changes and differentiation from atherosclerotic disease. Follow-up studies are used to monitor effectiveness of therapy and to identify relapsing disease. Ideally, therapy should be tailored according to disease activity, with the aims of reducing the amount of antiinflammatory medication necessary and therefore minimizing the risk of drug-induced side effects.

Similar advantages and limitations of the noninvasive imaging techniques CCDS, MRI or MRA, CT or CT angiography (CTA), and PET CT apply for imaging in TA and GCA. CCDS is readily available for assessment of mural thickening, luminal narrowing, and flow alterations in the carotid, subclavian, and axillary arteries. The thoracic aorta cannot be visualized

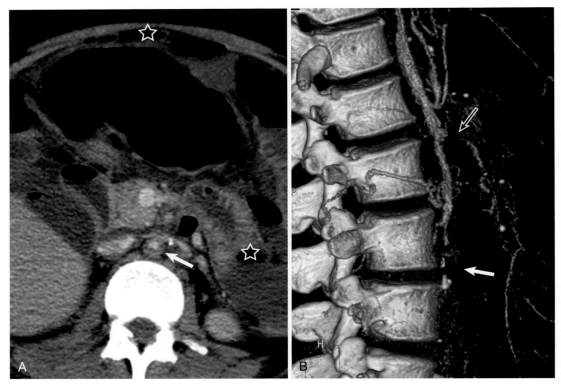

Figure 25-5 A 33-year-old female patient with fulminant Takayasu arteritis. **A** and **B**, Contrast-enhanced computed tomography reveals inflammatory obstruction of the infrarenal aorta (*solid arrows* in **A** and **B**) and the proximal mesenteric artery (*open arrow* in **B**). Ischemic complications include bowel perforation with free intraabdominal air (*stars* in **A**).

fully because of the overlying lung parenchyma. DSA displays the arterial lumen in very high resolution. However, mural inflammatory changes cannot be visualized directly. CTA and MRA do not have these limitations of CCDS and DSA (Figs. 25-5 and 25-6). Both CTA and MRA deliver angiographic images of the vessel lumen and can be combined with high-resolution imaging of the vessel wall in any desired orientation. Typical inflammatory changes include mural thickening and contrast enhancement. MRI, in particular, is useful for assessing the degree of vessel wall inflammation because of its various tissue contrasts (Fig. 25-7). High T2 signal intensity is considered consistent with mural inflammatory edema (Fig. 25-8). These mural changes may be present before the development of any vessel narrowing or dilatation. The role and diagnostic utility of increased mural T2 signal are controversial; different studies have reported varying levels of correlation between mural edema and inflammatory activity.

FDG PET is currently considered the most sensitive noninvasive imaging tool for assessing disease activity. The rationale for this recommendation is the very small amount (picomolar) of radioactive marked glucose necessary to produce positive PET findings. Furthermore, PET scanning covers the entire body and renders information about the distribution and extent of inflammatory changes. However, Arnaud et al reported no association between FDG uptake and clinical, biologic, and MRI signs of inflammatory activity in TA. FDG

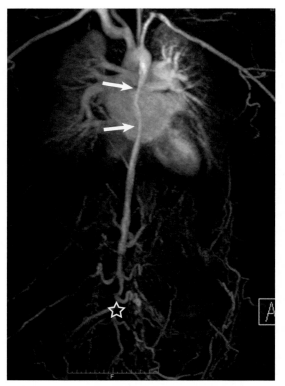

Figure 25-6 Magnetic resonance angiography of the same patient as in Figure 25-5 displays vasculitic stenoses *(arrows)* of the thoracic aorta and occlusion of the infrarenal aorta *(star)*. Please note the numerous lumbar and abdominal wall collateral arteries.

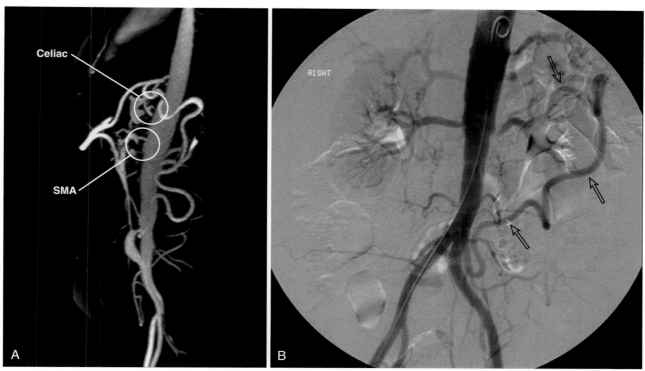

Figure 25-7 A, Contrast-enhanced magnetic resonance angiography in a 29-year-old man with Takayasu aortitis and occluded celiac and superior mesenteric (SMA) arteries. **B,** Digital subtraction angiography reveals collateral flow to the celiac and SMA branches through the arc of Riolan *(open arrows).*

uptake and increased T2 signal and mural thickening in MRI may persist despite clinical signs of remission. This persistence may result from vascular remodeling and may mimic inflammatory activity. Conversely, PET and MRI may be more sensitive than clinical and laboratory markers, and these changes may resemble persistent subclinical activity. This controversy is ongoing, and future studies may be necessary to resolve it. Because PET imaging does use ionizing radiation (~15 to 20 mSv), MRI and MRA are preferred over PET and CTA for repeated follow-up examinations. This is particularly true for patients with TA, who are younger than those with GCA.

Although noninvasive imaging modalities are promising for imaging TA, most studies reported thus far have been retrospective. Prospective multicenter trials assessing the sensitivity and specificity of MRI or MRA, CT or CTA, CCDS, and FDG PET are still needed. An ongoing U.S. multicenter cohort study evaluating the use of MRI or MRA and FDG PET for assessing disease activity in patients with TA is expected to help clarify this issue.

Medium Vessel Vasculitides

Kawasaki disease is a medium vessel vasculitis predominantly affecting young children less than 5 years of age. Skin, lymph nodes, and mucous membranes can be affected, as well as medium-sized arteries anywhere in the body. Coronary artery involvement is observed in 15% to 25% of patients with untreated cases. Approximately 20% of patients who present with coronary involvement in active disease will eventually develop coronary artery stenosis in the later course of the disease. Severe aneurysms can result if the disorder is untreated. Depending on the affected vascular territory, aneurysms of the coronary arteries or other large and medium-sized arteries can be assessed with ultrasound, CT or CTA, MRI or MRA, or DSA.

PAN is a form of necrotizing vasculitis characterized by segmental transmural infiltrates of medium or small arteries resulting in aneurysmal nodules, stenoses, or occlusions. Typically, the aneurysms seen in PAN are too small to be detected with noninvasive imaging and can be detected only with DSA, which is considered the diagnostic imaging gold standard. Occasionally, the aneurysms are large enough to be confidently identified with MRA (Fig. 25-9) or CTA. More frequently, MRA and CTA reveal multiple wedge-shaped cortical defects indicative of renal infarcts (see Fig. 25-9, *A*).

Small Vessel Vasculitides

Because of the small size of affected arteries in small vessel vasculitides such as granulomatous polyangiitis (formerly known as Wegener granulomatosis), microscopic polyangiitis, and Churg-Strauss syndrome, imaging focuses on inflammatory reactions in the affected tissues. For example, in granulomatosis with polyangitis granulomatous infiltrates can be seen in the nasopharynx, sphenoid bone, orbit, lungs, and trachea. Granulomatous inflammatory activity can be visualized most clearly by contrast enhancement in

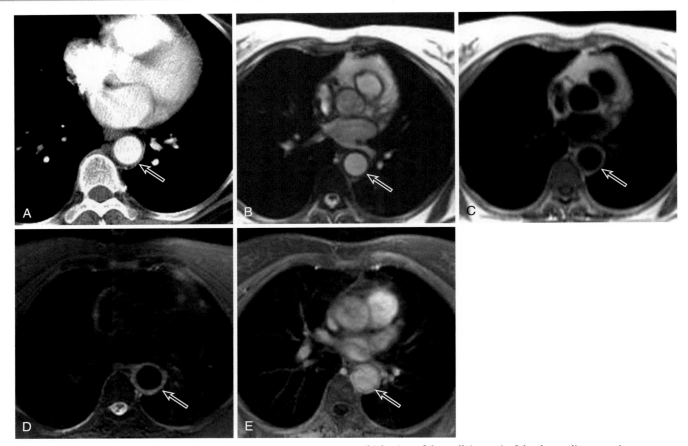

Figure 25-8 A 26-year-old female patient with Takayasu aortitis. **A** to **E,** Thickening of the wall *(arrows)* of the descending aorta is not as perceptible with computed tomography (**A**) as with magnetic resonance imaging (MRI) (**B** to **E**). With MRI, one can acquire multiple sequences with different T2 and T1 weighting to maximize tissue contrast. **B,** Balanced steady-state free precession. **C,** T1-weighted double inversion recovery. **D,** T2-weighted triple inversion recovery. **E,** Contrast-enhanced T1-weighted fast spoiled gradient echo.

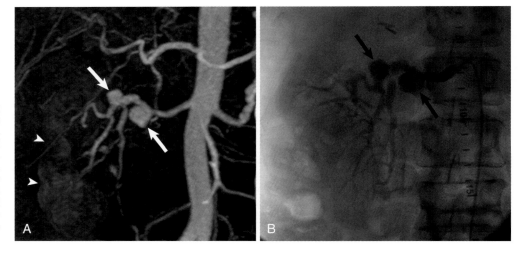

Figure 25-9 A 62-year-old female patient with hepatitis B virus infection and polyarteritis nodosa. Contrast-enhanced magnetic resonance angiography (**A**) and digital subtraction angiography (**B**) show relatively large aneurysms of the right renal artery *(arrows)*. Small peripheral perfusion defects in the right kidney are the result of infarction *(arrowheads in **A**).*

MRI. Bony destruction, however, is best depicted with CT. Direct imaging of mural inflammatory changes in the affected small vessels is not feasible with current imaging techniques. The inflammatory distribution, however, may indicate specific causes, such as granulomatous polyangiitis. Clinical presentation and serologic markers such as ANCA are typically used for differentiation of small vessel vasculitides.

■ INFECTIOUS DISORDERS

Mycotic Aneurysms

Mycotic aneurysms of the aorta are relatively uncommon, comprising less than 3% of abdominal aorta aneurysms. Unfortunately, mycotic aneurysms are associated with a relatively high rate of mortality and morbidity.

Factors associated with a poorer prognosis include rupture and suprarenal involvement, and the prognosis is even worse when the thoracic aorta is affected. Although the term mycotic would imply a fungal infection, fungi rarely cause infected aortic aneurysms, and bacteria are most often detected. Among the many different bacteria that can cause infected aortitis, *Staphylococcus*, *Streptococcus*, and *Salmonella* species are the most common. Less commonly associated organisms include *Escherichia coli*, *Listeria*, *Campylobacter*, *Acinetobacter*, and *Phialemonium* species.

Before the use of antibiotics, most patients were less than 40 years of age. In addition, in the preantibiotic era, mycotic aneurysms were almost always discovered in patients with infective endocarditis. Currently, the age at presentation of patients with mycotic aneurysms is older, with mean ages reported between 55 and 60 years. Comorbidities, such as diabetes mellitus, hypertension, intravenous drug use, and immune suppression, are frequently present as well. The association with infective endocarditis is less common now. Although the clinical presentation may be insidious, fever and back, chest, or abdominal pain are often present.

Patients with aortic aneurysms and bacteremia should be presumed to have infected aneurysms until proven otherwise. Negative blood culture results in patients with suspected infected aortic aneurysms are insufficient to exclude the diagnosis, and tissue culture may occasionally be necessary to establish the diagnosis. In patients with atherosclerosis, sepsis, and bacteremia, bacterial aortitis should be suspected, and cross-sectional imaging with CTA or MRA should be performed to confirm the diagnosis and locate the source of infection.

Angiographic findings suggestive of mycotic aortic aneurysm include a saccular aneurysm in an aorta without atherosclerotic disease (Fig. 25-10). In patients with infected aortic aneurysms, Macedo et al reported saccular aneurysms in 100% (13 of 13) of patients who underwent conventional angiography and in 93% (25 of 27) of patients who underwent CTA. Additional secondary criteria seen with CTA or MRA that assist in the diagnosis include periaortic soft tissue, stranding, and fluid (Figs. 25-11 and 25-12). Periaortic gas and adjacent vertebral body osteomyelitis are seen less commonly. FDG PET may be particularly useful in patients with potentially infected stent grafts to detect increased metabolic activity around the graft when it is infected (Fig. 25-13). Mycotic aneurysms usually occur adjacent to an atherosclerotic plaque. Another feature of mycotic aneurysms is their rapid growth when left untreated.

Whereas arteriosclerotic aortic aneurysms most frequently are infrarenal, only approximately one third of mycotic aortic aneurysms are infrarenal. Moreover, not all infected aortas are aneurysmal based on conventional criteria (aorta diameter >50% larger than normal).

Infectious Vasculitis

Various microorganisms can cause vasculitis that affects vessels of different sizes. Vasculitis associated with infectious agents is usually not ANCA positive.

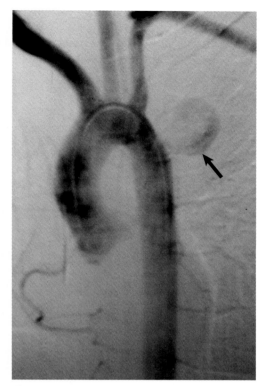

Figure 25-10 Digital subtraction angiography confirms a saccular aneurysm *(arrow)* in the proximal descending aorta in a patient with high-grade fever, bacteremia, and back pain from infectious aortitis. (Courtesy D. Yandow, MD, University of Wisconsin.)

Virus-associated vasculitis primarily mimics the small vessel vasculitides, especially PAN. The two main vasculitides associated with viral infections are hepatitis B virus (HBV PAN) and hepatitis C virus–associated cryoglobulinemic vasculitis (HCV CV). Other less frequently associated viruses include human immunodeficiency virus (HIV), cytomegalovirus (CMV), erythrovirus B19, varicella-zoster virus (VZV), and human T-cell lymphotrophic virus-1 (HTLV-1). In the 1970s, approximately one half of patients diagnosed with PAN were HBV positive. As a result of antiretroviral therapy and improved primary prevention, the frequency of HBV PAN has decreased substantially, and only approximately 5% of cases of PAN are related to HBV. HBV PAN usually manifests within 12 months of infection, generally before hepatitis is diagnosed clinically. Serum transaminase levels usually are less than double to triple normal levels. Clinical symptoms and imaging findings in HBV PAN are similar to those observed in noninfectious PAN (see also the earlier section on medium vessel vasculitides).

Although 30% to 50% of patients with HCV have evidence of mixed cryoglobulinemia, most remain asymptomatic. Symptoms present in patients with HCV CV include purpura, lower extremity ulcers, peripheral neuropathy, glomerulonephritis, arthritis, and sicca syndrome. Renal involvement in HCV CV is distinguished as membranoproliferative glomerulonephritis. Pauci-immune glomerulonephritis is not present. Additional complications reported in patients with HCV CV

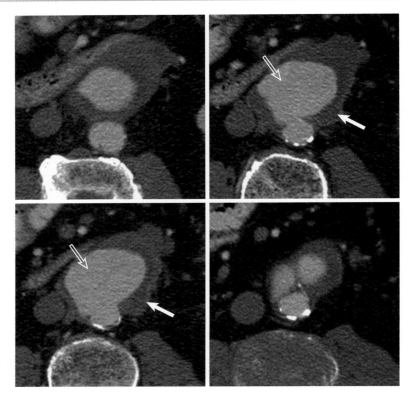

Figure 25-11 Mycotic saccular aneurysm *(open arrows)* with surrounding soft tissue inflammation *(solid arrows)* on contrast-enhanced computed tomography.

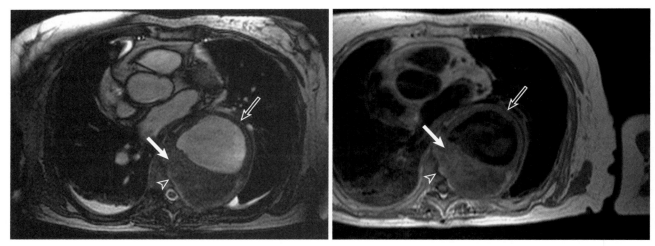

Figure 25-12 Balanced steady-state free precession *(left)* and double inversion recovery *(right)* magnetic resonance imaging images of a large descending aorta mycotic aneurysm. The wall of the aorta is diffusely thickened *(open arrows)*, and a large amount of inflammatory soft tissue *(solid arrows)* is present along the posteromedial wall of the aneurysm. This soft tissue component extends to and erodes the adjacent vertebral body *(arrowheads)*. (Courtesy of J. Kanne, MD, University of Wisconsin.)

include dilated cardiomyopathy, cerebral vasculitis, and mesenteric ischemia.

Less than 1% of patients with HIV infection will have vasculitis. Most of the cases are identified at autopsy or in large centers treating HIV-infected patients. HIV-related vasculitis can develop in children and adults at any stage of disease. Large, medium, and small vessel vasculitides, including necrotizing arteritis, nonnecrotizing arteritis, GCA, and eosinophilic arteritis, have all been described in patients with HIV infection. Although

the exact pathophysiology has not yet been determined, investigators believe the mechanism by which HIV causes vascular inflammation results from direct vessel wall injury or is secondary to an immune response to the virus.

These potential causative organisms should be recognized early because prolonged corticosteroid therapy should be avoided in these patients. Rather, the treatment of virus-related vasculitis is based on antiviral medications and plasma exchanges.

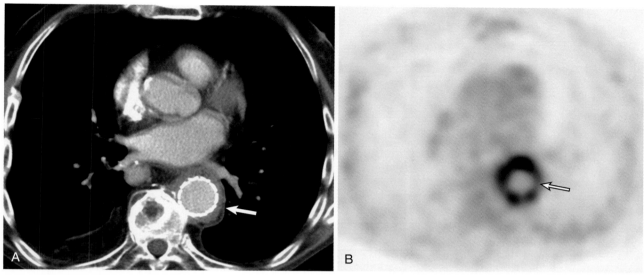

Figure 25-13 A 73-year-old male patient with an infected stent graft in the thoracic aorta. **A,** Contrast-enhanced computed tomography reveals a hypodense area around the thoracic stent graft *(solid arrow).* **B,** Fluorine-18 deoxyglucose positron emission tomography demonstrates increased periaortic glucose uptake *(open arrow)* consistent with stent graft infection.

Specific Infections

Tuberculous Aortitis

Tuberculous infections of the aorta are exceedingly rare, even when considering data from the preantibiotic era. Tubercle bacilli infect the aortic wall by direct implantation onto the intima, hematogenous dissemination through the vasa vasorum, or extension from adjacent tissues. Extension from adjacent infected lymph nodes, from paraspinal abscesses, or from other infected tissues is reported in most cases.

Tuberculous aortitis should be considered in patients with aortitis or atypical aortic aneurysms who have a history of pulmonary (Fig. 25-14) or extrapulmonary tuberculosis, patients with chronic immunosuppression, or patients who present with a cavitary lung lesion, pleural effusion, or lymphadenitis.

Thoracic and abdominal tuberculous aneurysms occur with relatively equal frequency, and thoracoabdominal aneurysms are much less common. The reason is thought to be related to the findings that atherosclerotic plaques are present less often in the thoracoabdominal aorta and that fewer lymph nodes are adjacent to the aorta in this region.

Most tuberculous aneurysms are saccular and false. Death in these patients is usually related to rupture and massive bleeding.

Syphilitic Aortitis

Syphilis was a disease that had a high degree of morbidity and mortality before the introduction of penicillin. After a marked decrease in incidence, a slight increase in the number of cases has occurred since 2000 as a result of changes in risk behavior, particular in persons at risk of acquiring HIV infection. Syphilitic aortitis occurs in tertiary syphilis, 10 to 30 years after the first stage of infection. Vascular findings in syphilitic aortitis include uncomplicated aortitis, aortic aneurysm (Fig. 25-15), aortic insufficiency, and coronary artery disease.

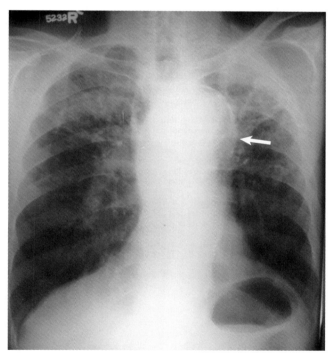

Figure 25-14 Aortic arch aneurysm *(arrow)* related to tuberculous aortitis in a patient with bilateral apical fibrosis secondary to chronic pulmonary tuberculosis. (Courtesy of D. Yandow, MD, University of Wisconsin, Madison.)

Most syphilitic aneurysms are solitary and saccular. Approximately 20% will have aortic calcifications. Histologically, syphilitic aortitis is characterized by arteritis obliterans of the vasa vasorum with perivascular plasma cell and lymphocytic infiltration, adventitial fibrosis, and intimal atherosclerosis. The ascending aorta is affected initially, with the aortic arch, descending aorta, and abdominal aorta affected in descending frequency.

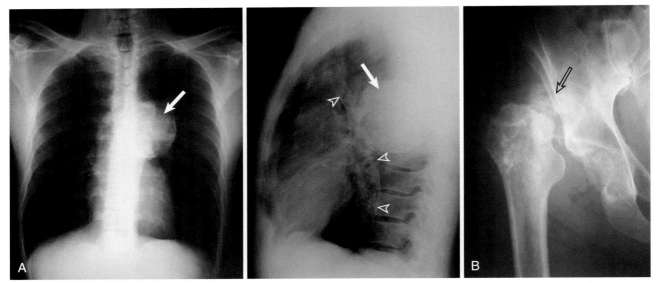

Figure 25-15 **A,** Posteroanterior and lateral chest radiographs in a patient with a calcified saccular aortic aneurysm related to syphilis *(solid arrows)*. Diffuse calcification is present in the thoracic aorta *(arrowheads)*. **B,** In addition, the patient had a Charcot joint in the right hip *(open arrow)*. (Courtesy D. Yandow, MD, University of Wisconsin, Madison.)

Bibliography

Andrews J, Al-Nahhas A, Pennell DJ, et al. Non-invasive imaging in the diagnosis and management of Takayasu's arteritis. *Ann Rheum Dis.* 2004;63:995-1000.

Arend WP, Michel BA, Bloch DA, et al. The American College of Rheumatology 1990 criteria for the classification of Takayasu arteritis. *Arthritis Rheum.* 1990;33:1129-1134.

Arnaud L, Haroche J, Malek Z, et al. Is (18)F-fluorodeoxyglucose positron emission tomography scanning a reliable way to assess disease activity in Takayasu arteritis? *Arthritis Rheum.* 2009;60:1193-1200.

Bley TA, Markl M, Schelp M, et al. Mural inflammatory hyperenhancement in MRI of giant cell (temporal) arteritis resolves under corticosteroid treatment. *Rheumatology (Oxford).* 2008;47:65-67.

Bley TA, Reinhard M, Hauenstein C, et al. Comparison of duplex sonography and high-resolution magnetic resonance imaging in the diagnosis of giant cell (temporal) arteritis. *Arthritis Rheum.* 2008;58:2574-2578.

Bley TA, Uhl M, Carew J, et al. Diagnostic value of high-resolution MR imaging in giant cell arteritis. *AJNR Am J Neuroradiol.* 2007;28:1722-1727.

Blockmans D, de Ceuninck L, Vanderschueren S, et al. Repetitive 18F-fluorodeoxyglucose positron emission tomography in giant cell arteritis: a prospective study of 35 patients. *Arthritis Rheum.* 2006;55:131-137.

Gornik HL, Creager MA. Aortitis. *Circulation.* 2008;117:3039-3051.

Heggtveit HA. Syphilitic aortitis: a clinicopathologic autopsy study of 100 cases, 1950-1960. *Circulation.* 1964;29:346-355.

Karassa FB, Matsagas MI, Schmidt WA, et al. Meta-analysis: test performance of ultrasonography for giant-cell arteritis. *Ann Intern Med.* 2005;142:359-369.

Leon Jr LR, Mills Sr JL. Diagnosis and management of aortic mycotic aneurysms. *Vasc Endovasc Surg.* 2010;44:5-13.

Long R, Guzman R, Greenberg H, et al. Tuberculous mycotic aneurysm of the aorta: review of published medical and surgical experience. *Chest.* 1999;115:522-531.

Lopes RJ, Almeida J, Dias PJ, et al. Infectious thoracic aortitis: a literature review. *Clin Cardiol.* 2009;32:488-490.

Macedo TA, Stanson AW, Oderich GS, et al. Infected aortic aneurysms: imaging findings. *Radiology.* 2004;231:250-257.

Maksimowicz-McKinnon K, Clark TM, Hoffman GS. Takayasu arteritis and giant cell arteritis: a spectrum within the same disease? *Medicine (Baltimore).* 2009;88:221-226.

Malouf JF, Chandrasekaran K, Orszulak TA. Mycotic aneurysms of the thoracic aorta: a diagnostic challenge. *Am J Med.* 2003;115:489-496.

Mason JC. Takayasu arteritis: advances in diagnosis and management. *Nat Rev Rheumatol.* 2010;6:406-415.

Meller J, Grabbe E, Becker W, et al. Value of F-18 FDG hybrid camera PET and MRI in early Takayasu aortitis. *Eur Radiol.* 2003;13:400-405.

Pagnoux C, Cohen P, Guillevin L. Vasculitides secondary to infections. *Clin Exp Rheumatol.* 2006;24(suppl 41):S71-S81.

Schmidt WA, Kraft HE, Vorpahl K, et al. Color duplex ultrasonography in the diagnosis of temporal arteritis. *N Engl J Med.* 1997;337:1336-1342.

Webb M, Chambers A, Al-Nahhas A, et al. The role of 18F-FDG PET in characterising disease activity in Takayasu arteritis. *Eur J Nucl Med Mol Imaging.* 2004;31:627-634.

CHAPTER 26

Current Role of Magnetic Resonance Imaging for Suspected Myocarditis

Emmanuelle Vermes and Matthias G. Friedrich

Myocarditis is an acute inflammatory process resulting from various infectious (mostly viral), immune, and nonimmune causes in the absence of ischemic injury. In many cases, myocarditis does not identify itself by specific cardiovascular symptoms or electrocardiogram (ECG) abnormalities, thus making diagnostic decisions difficult. Because many cases are not detected at the time of the acute illness, the true incidence and prevalence of myocarditis remain unknown. What is known, however, is that myocarditis is more prevalent in young men, who are also at greater risk of fatal myocarditis. Furthermore, myocarditis can be the underlying cause of dilated cardiomyopathy. Often, myocarditis causes nonspecific symptoms such as fatigue, dyspnea, palpitations, and fever. Occasionally, chest pain or ECG changes may mimic an acute coronary syndrome or may result in heart failure. The ECG may show ST-segment changes, arrhythmias, or atrioventricular block; laboratory tests may show elevation in the creatinine kinase or troponin, or both. However, these tests have limited sensitivity. Although endomyocardial biopsy is still considered the gold standard for diagnosing myocarditis, the value of myocardial biopsy is decreased by its low sensitivity, its high interosberver variability, and the invasive nature of this procedure. Cardiovascular magnetic resonance (CMR) offers the advantages of noninvasiveness and safety. It is also of special importance because of its ability to visualize tissue abnormalities associated with acute or severe remote inflammation.

■ SPECIFIC VALUE OF CARDIOVASCULAR MAGNETIC RESONANCE IN MYOCARDITIS

Since the late 1990s, CMR has emerged as a widely used tool for diagnosing myocarditis. In addition to the accuracy of functional and morphologic CMR data, this popularity mostly results from the value added by the ability of CMR to assess the activity of inflammatory changes including myocardial edema, hyperemia or capillary leak, and the degree of irreversible injury as defined by fibrosis.

Functional and Morphologic Ventricular Abnormalities

CMR is the noninvasive diagnostic tool of choice for assessing ventricular anatomy, structure, and function. This technique also allows the assessment of pericardial effusion.

High-resolution cine imaging with the best current steady-state free precession (SSFP) technique is widely considered the gold standard for the assessment of systolic function, ventricular volumes, and myocardial mass. Although nonspecific for myocarditis, cine CMR may reveal wall motion abnormalities that may be segmental or more diffuse, as well as transient increases of left ventricular (LV) volume. In severe forms of myocarditis, the LV ejection fraction can be severely depressed; however, LV dysfunction alone has a low sensitivity of 54% with a specificity of 76% and an overall accuracy of 64%.

Pericardial effusion is noted in 32% to 57% of patients with myocarditis. SSFP sequences are T1 or T2 weighted and therefore demonstrate pericardial effusion with bright signal intensity (SI) (Fig. 26-1). However, the differentiation from equally bright epicardial fat may be difficult. Epicardial fat is typically separated from pericardial effusion by a chemical shift artifact layer (see Fig. 26-1). Although nonspecific, pericardial effusion and LV dysfunction provide additional support for the presence of myocarditis.

Myocardial Edema

Because of interstitial edema and lymphocyte infiltrate with myocytolysis, free water content is increased in acute myocarditis. As a result, tissue T2 relaxation time is increased and causes hyperintense areas on T2-weighted images. In 1991, Gagliardi et al reported their preliminary results in 11 patients with clinically suspected myocarditis. These investigators demonstrated that, in patients with histologically confirmed myocarditis, abnormal SI of the myocardial walls was detected using T2-weighted spin echo sequences. In later years, T2-weighted imaging was optimized, leading to much better image quality. Today, detection of myocardial edema is typically performed by short tau inversion recovery (STIR) pulse sequences. This technique consists

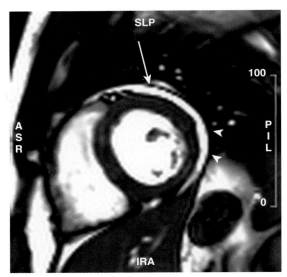

Figure 26-1 Small pericardial effusion on steady-state free precession sequences (short-axis images) in a patient with a severe acute myocarditis. Pericardial fluid demonstrates a high signal along the left side of the heart *(arrowheads)*. A chemical shift artifact (India ink) visible *(arrow on the top)* at fat-water interfaces reflects voxels that contain both epicardial fat and pericardial fluid. *A,* Anterior; *I,* inferior; *L,* left; *P,* posterior; *R,* right; *S,* superior.

of black-blood, T2-weighted triple inversion recovery with inversion pulses for fat and blood suppression. These pulse sequences are sensitive to the long T2 of water protons and provide excellent contrast between edematous myocardial tissue and normal myocardium. Edema in acute myocarditis may have a global (Fig. 26-2, *A*) or a regional (Fig. 26-3, *A*) distribution.

Because global edema is sometimes not recognizable to the eye, quantitative analysis is recommended (see the later discussion of global and regional edema assessment) by normalizing the SI of the myocardium to that of the skeletal muscle (T2 ratio). A T2 ratio of 2 or more is considered positive for myocardial edema (see Fig. 26-2, *B*). A high diagnostic accuracy of T2-weighted sequences (T2 ratio) has been shown in tissue edema detection in myocarditis. A group of experts proposed a set of criteria for the CMR diagnosis of myocarditis in which global edema (T2 ratio) and regional edema comprise one of three criteria for myocarditis. The other criteria are abnormal delayed hyperenhancement (fibrosis) and global relative enhancement (early enhancement) and are discussed in detail in the following sections.

The image quality of STIR may be limited by motion artifacts and its inherently low signal-to-noise ratio. Other T2-weighted sequences have been proposed. The value of T2 mapping for assessing myocardial inflammation appears promising, but it has yet to be established.

Myocardial Hyperemia (Myocardial Early Gadolinium Enhancement)

Tissue hyperemia, a component of the myocardial inflammatory reaction, can be detected by contrast-enhanced T1-weighted fast spin echo techniques with image acquisition during the first 3 minutes after gadolinium (Gd) injection. This technique visualizes reversible myocardial

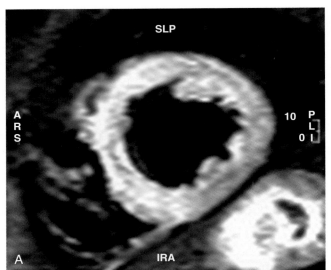

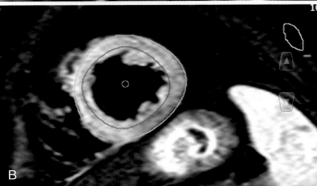

Figure 26-2 Global myocardial edema in a patient with acute myocarditis. **A,** T2-weighted cardiovascular magnetic resonance image in the midventricular short-axis view shows high signal intensity of the entire left ventricular myocardium, corresponding to global (diffuse) left ventricular edema. *A,* Anterior; *I,* inferior; *L,* left; *P,* posterior; *R,* right; *S,* superior. **B,** Quantitative assessment of global edema is performed by measuring signal intensity (SI) of the myocardium divided by SI of skeletal muscle. In this case, the T2 ratio of 2.7 is positive (normal is <2.0).

signal changes in acute myocarditis that showing Gd accumulation in regions of suspected myocardial inflammation. This Gd accumulation causes contrast enhancement compared with noninflamed myocardium. Increased volume of distribution from acute cell damage allows Gd enter into the intracellular space and could explain enhancement in the pathologic areas. Contrast-enhanced magnetic resonance imaging (MRI) was initially reported in 2 patients with myocarditis. Friedrich at al were the first to report an ECG-triggered T1-weighted contrast-enhanced technique in 44 patients with suspected acute myocarditis. These investigators measured the global relative signal enhancement of the LV myocardium related to skeletal muscle and found a focal myocardial enhancement pattern in the acute phase and a more diffuse pattern later. Other studies have confirmed the diagnostic value of this sequence in acute myocarditis.

Similar to the analysis of the T2-weighted images for edema, SI derived from regions of interest (ROIs) over the myocardium is compared with a reference ROI of skeletal muscle, and a normalized enhancement ratio (early Gd enhancement ratio [EGE ratio]) is calculated.

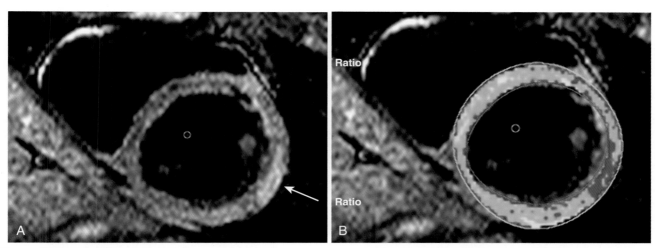

Figure 26-3 Regional myocardial edema in a patient with acute myocarditis. **A,** T2-weighted midventricular short-axis short time inversion recovery image shows a focus of high signal intensity within the lateral wall *(arrow)*, indicating regional edema. **B,** Computer-aided signal intensity analysis with color-coded display of relative signal intensity, normalized to skeletal muscle. *Blue* indicates a signal intensity ratio of myocardium to skeletal muscle of 2 or more, indicating edema; *green* indicates normal signal intensity.

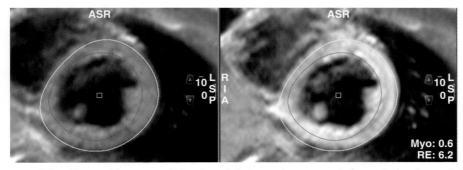

Figure 26-4 Acute myocarditis with a positive myocardial early gadolinium enhancement. Left ventricular short-axis T1-weighted spin echo images before *(left)* and shortly after *(right)* gadolinium administration show early gadolinium accumulation in the lateral and anterior walls. The global relative enhancement T1 ratio is positive (6.2) for myocardial inflammation, as is the absolute enhancement of 65% (normal is <45%). *A,* Anterior; *I,* inferior; *L,* left; *P,* posterior; *R,* right; *S,* superior.

An EGE ratio of 4 or more or an absolute increase of myocardium enhancement 45% or more is considered positive for myocardial inflammation (Fig. 26-4) and represents one of the three CMR criteria for myocarditis.

Fibrosis

Late Gd enhancement (LGE) imaging allows visualization of myocardial necrosis and fibrosis. This type of imaging, performed 10 to 20 minutes after contrast injection, uses inversion recovery gradient echo sequences with the inversion time set to null viable myocardium.

Gd, an extracellular agent, easily distributes in extracellular fluid space but not into intact myocyte cell membrane. In the acute stage of necrosis, cell membrane rupture allows Gd to enter into cells, and the volume of contrast distribution is increased. This process results in local accumulation of Gd with subsequently high SI values (hyperenhancement, LGE). In the chronic setting, necrotic myocytes are replaced by fibrous tissue, and the interstitial space is expanded. These changes lead to increased Gd concentration and hyperenhancement. This technique was initially developed for the noninvasive detection of myocardial scarring in coronary artery disease. The main

difference from infarcted regions is that areas of tissue damage within myocarditis generally do not involve the subendocardial layers in an isolated fashion; this characteristic distinguishes ischemic (which always has subendocardial involvement) from nonischemic injury. Moreover, areas of tissue damage in myocarditis are usually smaller and not as bright as infarct enhancement because inflammatory areas usually contain more living myocytes between the islands of necrosis than in myocardial infarction.

Several controlled studies investigated late contrast-enhanced CMR in patients with suspected myocarditis and confirmed a high specificity of LGE for the detection of irreversible injury. The pattern of myocardial fibrosis in myocarditis varies considerably, but it typically involves the subendocardial or midmyocardial wall focally without being confined to a coronary distribution. Usually, the inferolateral wall is involved (Fig. 26-5), and the anteroseptal segments are involved less frequently (see Fig. 26-5). In 2006, Mahrholdt et al suggested that in the setting of parvovirus B19 myocarditis, lateral subepicardial LGE was the most frequent distribution, and midwall interventricular septum LGE was the most common in human herpesvirus 6 myocarditis.

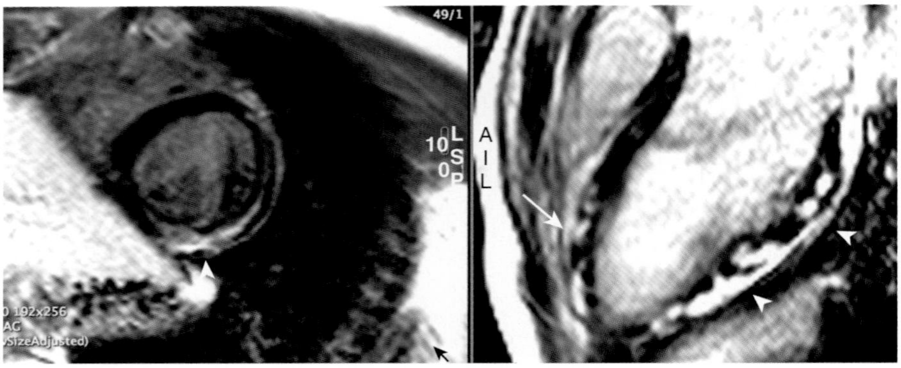

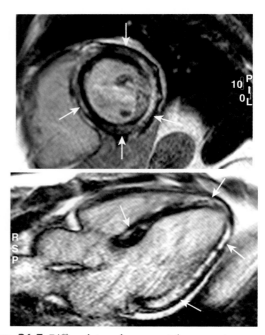

Figure 26-5 Late enhancement images in a young patient with acute myocarditis. Short-axis *(left)* and long-axis *(right)* images show regional midwall to subepicardial delayed hyperenhancement of the inferolateral *(arrowheads)* and anteroseptal wall *(arrows),* indicating fibrosis. *A,* Anterior; *I,* inferior; *L,* left; *P,* posterior; *S,* superior.

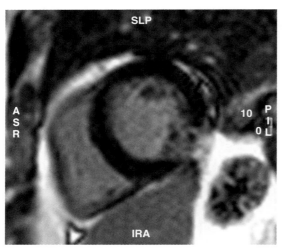

Figure 26-6 Focal late enhancement in a patient with acute myocarditis. Short-axis image shows necrosis as visualized by focal transmural late enhancement in the inferolateral wall. *A,* Anterior; *I,* inferior; *L,* left; *P,* posterior; *R,* right; *S,* superior.

Figure 26-7 Diffuse late enhancement in an acute myocarditis. Short-axis *(left)* and long-axis *(right)* images show extensive areas of high signal intensity *(arrows),* likely reflecting irreversible injury. *I,* Inferior; *L,* left; *P,* posterior; *R,* right; *S,* superior.

Areas of high SI in LGE images, however, may also appear focally transmural (Fig. 26-6) or diffuse (Fig. 26-7). The presence of myocardial fibrosis is more common in younger men compared with women, with an almost twofold greater frequency of myocardial fibrosis in men. LGE is one of the three criteria for the CMR diagnosis of myocarditis.

■ INTERNATIONAL CONSENSUS ON CARDIOVASCULAR MAGNETIC RESONANCE IN MYOCARDITIS: LAKE LOUISE CRITERIA

Several controlled trials evaluated the diagnostic accuracy of individual or combined CMR methods in patients with suspected acute myocarditis (Table 26-1). More recently, a group of CMR and myocarditis experts pooled these data and found that the combination of these methods was the most appropriate approach to achieve the highest diagnostic accuracy, sensitivity, and specificity. If two or more of the three criteria are positive, myocardial inflammation can be predicted or ruled out with a diagnostic accuracy of 78%; if only LGE imaging is performed, the diagnostic accuracy is 68% (Table 26-2). The international consensus group on

CMR in myocarditis proposed diagnostic CMR criteria for myocarditis that are known as the Lake Louise criteria (Table 26-3).

Indications for Lake Louise Criteria Assessment

The Lake Louise criteria for CMR are applicable only in patients with suspected myocarditis who have the following clinical presentation: recent onset or persisting symptoms (dyspnea, palpitations, chest discomfort, or fatigue); and evidence of significant myocardial injury (ventricular dysfunction or new ECG changes or elevated troponin) in the absence of coronary artery disease.

■ CARDIOVASCULAR MAGNETIC RESONANCE PROTOCOL

The international consensus group on CMR in myocarditis proposed a comprehensive CMR protocol including

Table 26-1   Diagnostic Accuracy of Individuals and Combined Cardiovascular Magnetic Resonance Criteria in Multiple Controlled Trials

CMR Parameters	Accuracy (%)	Sensitivity (%)	Specificity (%)
Single Approach			
T2 Signal Intensity Ratio			
Laissy	59	45	100
Rieker	76	100	50
Abdel-Aty	79	84	74
Gutberlet	67	67	69
Myocardial Early Gadolinium Enhancement			
Friedrich	86	84	89
Laissy	89	85	100
Abdel-Aty	74	80	68
Gutberlet	72	63	86
Late Enhancement			
Rieker	52	45	60
Abdel-Aty	71	44	100
Mahrholdt	96	95	96
Gutberlet	49	27	80
Yilmaz	51	35	83
Combined Approach			
Any 1 of 3			
Abdel-Aty	75	100	48
Gutberlet	67	81	49
Any 2 of 3			
Abdel-Aty	85	76	96
Gutberlet	73	63	89

CMR, Cardiovascular magnetic resonance.

Table 26-2   Diagnostic Accuracy of Individuals and Combined Cardiovascular Magnetic Resonance Criteria in Pooled Data

CMR Parameters	Accuracy (%)	Sensitivity (%)	Specificity (%)
Single Approach			
T2 signal intensity ratio (*n* = 178)	70	70	71
Myocardial early gadolinium enhancement (*n* = 19)	78	74	83
Late enhancement (*n* = 336)	68	59	86
Combined Approach			
Any 1 of 3 (*n* = 130)	70	88	48
Any 2 of 3 (*n* = 130)	78	67	91

CMR, Cardiovascular magnetic resonance.

Table 26-3   Lake Louise Consensus Criteria for Myocarditis

If clinical criteria for myocarditis are met, CMR findings are consistent with myocarditis if two of the following CMR criteria are present:

Criteria	Signal Intensity Threshold	CMR Sequences
Global myocardial edema or regional edema	T2 ratio ≥2	T2-weighted images (STIR)
Increased myocardial early gadolinium enhancement	EGE ratio ≥4	T1-weighted images (T1 FSE/TSE precontrast/postcontrast)
Presence of late enhancement	Visual assessment	Phase sensitive IR-GE

Modified from Friedrich MG, Sechtem U, Schulz-Menger J, et al. Cardiovascular magnetic resonance in myocarditis: A JACC White Paper. *J Am Coll Cardiol.* 2009;53:1475–1487.
CMR, Cardiovascular magnetic resonance; *EGE,* early gadolinium enhancement; *FSE,* fast spin echo; *GE,* gadolinium enhancement; *IR,* inversion recovery; *STIR,* short-tau-inversion recovery spin echo sequence; *TSE,* turbo spin echo.

assessment of global or regional myocardial edema, global relative enhancement, and LGE.

Global and Regional Edema Assessment

A STIR spin echo sequence is recommended with suppression pulses for blood and fat. Because of the required SI quantification, the body coil or an SI correction algorithm is recommended to avoid signal inhomogeneity. A slice thickness of 10 to 15 mm is required to maximize the signal-to-noise ratio. Short-axis slices covering the base, middle, and apex of the heart are recommended.

Myocardial edema appears as bright areas of high SI in T2-weighted images. In case of global myocardial edema, quantitative assessment is recommended by normalized SI quantification with manually traced endocardial and epicardial contours of the entire visible myocardium and skeletal muscle in the same slice

(T2 SI ratio; see Fig. 26-2, *B*). To identify skeletal muscle correctly, SSFP sequences or T1-weighted images are recommended to trace an ROI at the same slice position. Myocardial SI is related to that of the skeletal muscle by using the following equation:

$$\text{Relative myocardial T2 SI} = \frac{\text{SI myocardium}}{\text{SI skeletal muscle}}$$

A ratio of 2 or more is considered positive for global myocardial edema. Because skeletal muscle is used as a reference, this ratio is valid only in patients without clinical evidence of active myosis. No studies have addressed the diagnostic accuracy of T2 ratio in case of involvement of skeletal muscle in systemic inflammation.

Although regional edema can be identified visually, quantitative assessment of the signal abnormalities is

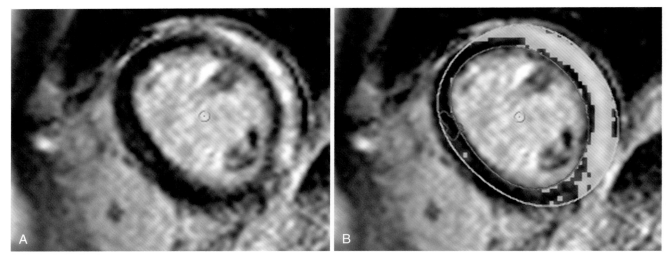

Figure 26-8 Quantitative assessment of late enhancement. A, Short-axis image shows late gadolinium hyperenhancement in the lateral and anterolateral walls. **B,** Quantitative assessment using 2 standard deviations above normal to define fibrosis: the late enhancement mass is calculated: at 6.1 g and 49% of all myocardium in this slice.

recommended. Regional edema is defined by a regional area (of ≥10 adjacent pixels) of SI of at least 2 standard deviations (SD) of remote myocardium in the absence of artifacts in any of these regions (see Fig. 26-3, *B*). Regions of increased SI that did not follow the contour of the myocardium or crossed endocardial or epicardial surfaces are usually considered image artifacts.

Myocardial Early Gadolinium Enhancement Assessment

T1-weighted turbo spin echo sequences should be applied in three short-axis slices (basal, middle, and apical region) before and during the first 3 minutes after an intravenous contrast bolus of 0.1 mmol/kg. Similar to T2-weighted imaging, the use of the body coil or SI correction software is required. The acquisition is performed during free breathing. If image quality is insufficient in short-axis views, axial slices can be acquired. Quantitative evaluation of an EGE ratio is required and calculated by using a similar T2 ratio approach. An ROI in the LV myocardium and in the skeletal muscle within the same section is drawn on the precontrast T1-weighted images and is copied to the postcontrast images (see Fig. 26-4). The EGE ratio is calculated by using the following equation:

$$\text{EGE ratio} = \frac{(\text{SI}[\text{myocardium post}] - \text{SI}[\text{myocardium pre}])/\ \text{SI}[\text{myocardium pre}]}{(\text{SI}[\text{sm post}] - \text{SI}[\text{sm pre}])/\ \text{SI}[\text{sm pre}]}$$

In this equation, sm denotes skeletal muscle.

A EGE ratio of 4 or more is considered positive for myocardial inflammation. An absolute increase of myocardial enhancement of 45% or more is also considered positive, especially in patients with evidence of skeletal muscle involvement, in whom the normalizing myocardial to muscular enhancement values may be invalid.

Fibrosis Assessment

Delayed enhancement imaging using inversion recovery prepared gradient echo sequences with individual determination of inversion time according to maximal suppression of normal myocardial signal is recommended. LGE images are assessed qualitatively for the presence, number, and transmurality of LGE areas by using complete short-axis coverage. The spatial extend of these lesions can also be assessed quantitatively. Although no consensus exists regarding the quantitative assessment of LGE in patients with myocarditis, most centers use the visual assessment or SD threshold method. In the SD threshold method, the endocardial and epicardial contours are traced, followed by placement of an ROI in a normal appearing area (low SI). An automated computer-aided threshold detection sets at either 2 or 5 SD above the mean SI of the normal myocardium ROI to define fibrosis (with at least five connecting pixels). This allows the clinician to quantify the amount of fibrosis in both volume or grams and the percentage of enhanced myocardium (Fig. 26-8).

■ FOLLOW-UP OF MYOCARDITIS: INSIGHTS FROM CARDIOVASCULAR MAGNETIC RESONANCE

In uncomplicated myocarditis, myocardial edema and inflammation, as well as functional abnormalities, if present, usually disappear within the first weeks. Zagrosek et al showed that ejection fraction significantly increased and both the T2 ratio and EGE ratio significantly decreased 18 months after acute myocarditis. In contrast, most of the time, LGE remains throughout the course of myocarditis but significantly decreases in size at follow-up. During healing, necrotic myocytes are replaced by fibrous tissue, and the result is persistent contrast enhancement. However, after healing, these scars remodel and shrink, and edema disappears, thus explaining the decrease of LGE (Fig. 26-9). Less

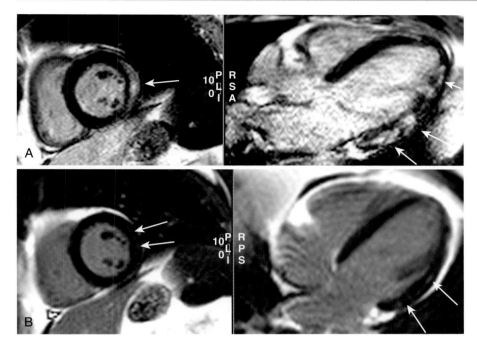

Figure 26-9 Late enhancement in the acute phase and at 1-year follow-up in a patient with myocarditis. **A,** Short-axis *(left)* and long-axis *(right)* images show extensive mesocardial late hyperenhancement in the lateral wall *(arrows)*. *A,* Anterior; *I,* inferior; *L,* left; *P,* posterior; *R,* right; *S,* superior. **B,** At 1 year later, late hyperenhancement has significantly decreased in the lateral wall *(arrows)*. *I,* Inferior; *L,* left; *P,* posterior; *R,* right; *S,* superior.

frequently, scars may become smaller than CMR pixels; this shrinkage explains the complete disappearance of LGE.

Although recovery may not leave sequelae, fibrosis may persist, or acute myocarditis may progress to chronic myocarditis or dilated cardiomyopathy. Pilot data indicate that EGE at 4 weeks after the onset of symptoms predicts the functional and clinical long-term outcome. More recently, another study indicated that, in patients with suspected chronic myocarditis, T2 ratio and EGE ratio could be helpful in identifying persistent myocardial inflammation. In a series of 83 patients with clinically suspected chronic myocarditis, Gutberlet et al found that the EGE ratio had the highest specificity and diagnostic accuracy for detection of immune histologic inflammation (86% and 72%, respectively), and the T2 ratio had the highest sensitivity (67%). CMR follow-up at least 4 weeks after the onset of disease is recommended using the same protocol as in the acute phase. Persistence of myocardial edema or a positive EGE ratio on the CMR follow-up examination suggests ongoing inflammation.

■ FUTURE CHALLENGES

Although T2-weighted CMR technology has improved in recent years, it suffers from several limitations including sensitivity to myocardial motion, high signal from stagnant blood that makes it difficult to differentiate edema from blood, and surface coil intensity variation. An alternative approach in the future could be quantitative T2 mapping, which offers the potential for improving identification of myocardial edema. T2 mapping could facilitate detection of global or diffuse changes in myocardium.

The LGE technique is not able to demonstrate diffuse myocardial changes in diffuse myocarditis. Indeed, this

technique is based on selecting an inversion time set to null the normal myocardium as defined by the absence of hyperenhancement. However, when the myocardial injury is diffuse, the signal generated by diffuse fibrosis is artificially suppressed. T1 mapping, which is able to visualize and quantify changes in T1, is an innovative approach that could offer the potential for visualizing diffuse myocardial fibrosis early in the disease.

■ CONCLUSION

CMR has become the diagnostic tool of choice for the noninvasive detection of myocardial tissue changes in acute myocarditis. Consensus CMR criteria have been published. Through the combined use of T2-weighted imaging of myocardial edema, T1-weighted EGE imaging of hyperemia and capillary leakage, and necrosis or fibrosis imaging using LGE, comprehensive CMR scans not only have improved our understanding of myocarditis, but also serve as safe and efficient tools for managing patients with suspected or known myocarditis.

Bibliography

Abdel-Aty H, Boye P, Zagrosek A, et al. Diagnostic performance of cardiovascular magnetic resonance in patients with suspected acute myocarditis: comparison of different approaches. *J Am Coll Cardiol.* 2005;45:1815-1822.

Aletras AH, Kellman P, Derbyshire JA, Arai AE. ACUT2E TSE-SSFP: a hybrid method for T2-weighted imaging of edema in the heart. *J Magn Reson Med.* 2008;59:229-235.

Ammann P, Naegeli B, Schuiki E, et al. Long-term outcome of acute myocarditis is independent of cardiac enzyme release. *Int J Cardiol.* 2003;89:217-222.

Assomull RG, Lyne JC, Keenan N, et al. The role of cardiovascular magnetic resonance in patients presenting with chest pain, raised troponin, and unobstructed coronary arteries. *Eur Heart J.* 2007;28:1242-1249.

Baccouche H, Mahrholdt H, Meinhardt G, et al. Diagnostic synergy of non-invasive cardiovascular magnetic resonance and invasive endomyocardial biopsy in troponin-positive patients without coronary artery disease. *Eur Heart J.* 2009;30:2869-2879.

Bruder O, Schneider S, Nothnagel D, et al. EuroCMR (European Cardiovascular Magnetic Resonance) registry: results of the German pilot phase. *J Am Coll Cardiol.* 2009;54:1457-1466.

Chow LH, Radio SJ, Sears TD, McManus BM. Insensitivity of right ventricular endomyocardial biopsy in the diagnosis of myocarditis. *J Am Coll Cardiol.* 1989;14:915-920.

Cocker MS, Abdel-Aty H, Strohm O, Friedrich MG. Age and gender effects on the extent of myocardial involvement in acute myocarditis: a cardiovascular magnetic resonance study. *Heart.* 2009;95:1925-1930.

Cocker MS, Shea SM, Strohm O, Green J, Abdel-Aty H, Friedrich MG. A new approach towards improved visualization of myocardial edema using T2-weighted imaging: a cardiovascular magnetic resonance (CMR) study. *J Magn Reson Imaging.* 2011;34:286-292.

Codreanu A, Djaballah W, Angioi M, et al. Detection of myocarditis by contrast-enhanced MRI in patients presenting with acute coronary syndrome but no coronary stenosis. *J Magn Reson Imaging.* 2007;25:957-964.

Cooper LT, Baughman KL, Feldman AM, et al. The role of endomyocardial biopsy in the management of cardiovascular disease: a scientific statement from the American Heart Association, the American College of Cardiology, and the European Society of Cardiology. Endorsed by the Heart Failure Society of America and the Heart Failure Association of the European Society of Cardiology. *J Am Coll Cardiol.* 2007;50:1914-1931.

Cooper Jr LT. Myocarditis. *N Engl J Med.* 2009;360:1526-1538.

Feldman AM, McNamara D. Myocarditis. *N Engl J Med.* 2000;343:1388-1398.

Felker GM, Hu W, Hare JM, Hruban RH, Baughman KL, Kasper EK. The spectrum of dilated cardiomyopathy: the Johns Hopkins experience with 1,278 patients. *Medicine (Baltimore).* 1999;78:270-283.

Friedrich MG, Sechtem U, Schulz-Menger J, et al. Cardiovascular magnetic resonance in myocarditis: A JACC White Paper. *J Am Coll Cardiol.* 2009;53:1475-1487.

Friedrich MG, Strohm O, Schulz-Menger J, Marciniak H, Luft FC, Dietz R. Contrast media–enhanced magnetic resonance imaging visualizes myocardial changes in the course of viral myocarditis. *Circulation.* 1998;97:1802-1809.

Gagliardi MG, Bevilacqua M, Di Renzi P, Picardo S, Passariello R, Marcelletti C. Usefulness of magnetic resonance imaging for diagnosis of acute myocarditis in infants and children, and comparison with endomyocardial biopsy. *Am J Cardiol.* 1991;68:1089-1091.

Garcia-Pavia P, Aguiar-Souto P, Silva-Melchor L, et al. Cardiac magnetic resonance imaging in the diagnosis of myocarditis mimicking myocardial infarction. *Int J Cardiol.* 2006;112:e27-e29.

Giri S, Chung YC, Merchant A, et al. T2 quantification for improved detection of myocardial edema. *J Cardiovasc Magn Reson.* 2009;11:56.

Gutberlet M, Spors B, Thoma T, et al. Suspected chronic myocarditis at cardiac MR: diagnostic accuracy and association with immunohistologically detected inflammation and viral persistence. *Radiology.* 2008;246:401-409.

Hauck AJ, Kearney DL, Edwards WD. Evaluation of postmortem endomyocardial biopsy specimens from 38 patients with lymphocytic myocarditis: implications for role of sampling error. *Mayo Clin Proc.* 1989;64:1235-1245.

Hendel RC, Patel MR, Kramer CM, et al. ACCF/ACR/SCCT/SCMR/ASNC/NASCI/SCAI/SIR 2006 appropriateness criteria for cardiac computed tomography and cardiac magnetic resonance imaging: a report of the American College of Cardiology Foundation Quality Strategic Directions Committee Appropriateness Criteria Working Group, American College of Radiology, Society of Cardiovascular Computed Tomography, Society for Cardiovascular Magnetic Resonance, American Society of Nuclear Cardiology, North American Society for Cardiac Imaging, Society for Cardiovascular Angiography and Interventions, and Society of Interventional Radiology. *J Am Coll Cardiol.* 2006;48:1475-1497.

Holzmann M, Nicko A, Kuhl U, et al. Complication rate of right ventricular endomyocardial biopsy via the femoral approach: a retrospective and prospective study analyzing 3048 diagnostic procedures over an 11-year period. *Circulation.* 2008;118:1722-1728.

Iles L, Pfluger H, Phrommintikul A, et al. Evaluation of diffuse myocardial fibrosis in heart failure with cardiac magnetic resonance contrast-enhanced T1 mapping. *J Am Coll Cardiol.* 2008;52:1574-1580.

Jeserich M, Olschewski M, Bley T, et al. Cardiac involvement after respiratory tract viral infection: detection by cardiac magnetic resonance. *J Comput Assist Tomogr.* 2009;33:15-19.

Karjalainen J, Heikkila J. "Acute pericarditis": myocardial enzyme release as evidence for myocarditis. *Am Heart J.* 1986;111:546-552.

Kawai C. From myocarditis to cardiomyopathy: mechanisms of inflammation and cell death: learning from the past for the future. *Circulation.* 1999;99:1091-1100.

Kim RJ, Fieno DS, Parrish TB, et al. Relationship of MRI delayed contrast enhancement to irreversible injury, infarct age, and contractile function. *Circulation.* 1999;100:1992-2002.

Korkusuz H, Esters P, Huebner F, Bug R, Ackermann H, Vogl TJ. Accuracy of cardiovascular magnetic resonance in myocarditis: comparison of MR and histological findings in an animal model. *J Cardiovasc Magn Reson.* 2010;12:49.

Kyto V, Saraste A, Voipio-Pulkki LM, Saukko P. Incidence of fatal myocarditis: a population-based study in Finland. *Am J Epidemiol.* 2007;165:570-574.

Laissy JP, Hyafil F, Feldman LJ, et al. Differentiating acute myocardial infarction from myocarditis: diagnostic value of early- and delayed-perfusion cardiac MR imaging. *Radiology.* 2005;237:75-82.

Laissy JP, Messin B, Varenne O, et al. MRI of acute myocarditis: a comprehensive approach based on various imaging sequences. *Chest.* 2002;122:1638-1648.

Lauer B, Niederau C, Kuhl U, et al. Cardiac troponin T in patients with clinically suspected myocarditis. *J Am Coll Cardiol.* 1997;30:1354-1359.

Mahrholdt H, Goedecke C, Wagner A, et al. Cardiovascular magnetic resonance assessment of human myocarditis: a comparison to histology and molecular pathology. *Circulation.* 2004;109:1250-1258.

Mahrholdt H, Wagner A, Deluigi CC, et al. Presentation, patterns of myocardial damage, and clinical course of viral myocarditis. *Circulation.* 2006;114:1581-1590.

Matsouka H, Hamada M, Honda T, et al. Evaluation of acute myocarditis and pericarditis by Gd-DTPA enhanced magnetic resonance imaging. *Eur Heart J.* 1994;15:283-284.

Morgera T, Di Lenarda A, Dreas L, et al. Electrocardiography of myocarditis revisited: clinical and prognostic significance of electrocardiographic changes. *Am Heart J.* 1992;124:455-467.

Rehwald WG, Fieno DS, Chen EL, Kim RJ, Judd RM. Myocardial magnetic resonance imaging contrast agent concentrations after reversible and irreversible ischemic injury. *Circulation.* 2002;105:224-229.

Rieker O, Mohrs O, Oberholzer K, Kreitner KF, Thelen M. Cardiac MRI in suspected myocarditis. *Rofo.* 2002;174:1530-1536:in German.

Roditi GH, Hartnell GG, Cohen MC. MRI changes in myocarditis: evaluation with spin echo, cine MR angiography and contrast enhanced spin echo imaging. *Clin Radiol.* 2000;55:752-758.

Simonetti OP, Kim RJ, Fieno DS, et al. An improved MR imaging technique for the visualization of myocardial infarction. *Radiology.* 2001;218:215-223.

Strohm O, Schulz-Menger J, Pilz B, Osterziel KJ, Dietz R, Friedrich MG. Measurement of left ventricular dimensions and function in patients with dilated cardiomyopathy. *J Magn Reson Imaging.* 2001;13:367-371.

Wagner A, Mahrholdt H, Holly TA, et al. Contrast-enhanced MRI and routine single photon emission computed tomography (SPECT) perfusion imaging for detection of subendocardial myocardial infarcts: an imaging study. *Lancet.* 2003;361:374-379.

Wagner A, Schulz-Menger J, Dietz R, Friedrich MG. Long-term follow-up of patients paragraph sign with acute myocarditis by magnetic resonance imaging. *MAGMA.* 2003;16:17-20.

Yilmaz A, Mahrholdt H, Athanasiadis A, et al. Coronary vasospasm as the underlying cause for chest pain in patients with PVB19 myocarditis. *Heart.* 2008;94:1456-1463.

Zagrosek A, Abdel-Aty H, Boye P, et al. Cardiac magnetic resonance monitors reversible and irreversible myocardial injury in myocarditis. *JACC Cardiovasc Imaging.* 2009;2:131-138.

Zagrosek A, Wassmuth R, Abdel-Aty H, Rudolph A, Dietz R, Schulz-Menger J. Relation between myocardial edema and myocardial mass during the acute and convalescent phase of myocarditis: a CMR study. *J Cardiovasc Magn Reson.* 2008;10:19.

CHAPTER 27
Radiation Issues
Jörg Hausleiter

Significant advances in modern radiology and cardiology have made noninvasive cardiac imaging more effective and appealing. With the introduction of 64-slice computed tomography (CT) scanners in 2004, the improved spatial and temporal resolution allowed for accurate almost motion-free image acquisition of the coronary arterial system in a single breath hold of approximately 10 to 15 seconds. The use of cardiac CT angiography (CTA) has escalated exponentially, and cardiac CTA has become a common noninvasive imaging modality for the evaluation of cardiac diseases, especially coronary artery disease. In a multisocietal approach, experts have defined clinical situations for which cardiac CTA is considered appropriate. Cardiac CTA requires the use of ionizing radiation, however, and the potential risk of developing cancer from radiation exposure is a public health concern. Several strategies have been recommended and implemented to reduce the radiation dose associated with multislice CTA in cardiac imaging.

The desire to achieve low radiation exposure must be balanced with the likelihood of obtaining a useful diagnostic image. A nondiagnostic study may lead to additional imaging with substantially higher net radiation or to inappropriate invasive testing, delayed or lack of targeted treatment, or nontreatment.

■ HOW IS RADIATION DOSE ESTIMATED IN CARDIOVASCULAR COMPUTED TOMOGRAPHY IMAGING?

The primary outcome parameters used to quantify radiation dose in cardiovascular CT imaging are the volume CT dose index ($CTDI_{vol}$) and the dose-length product (DLP). The physical details related to obtaining the $CDTI_{vol}$ are described by Morin et al. The $CTDI_{vol}$ is usually displayed on the CT console before and after CT data acquisition and allows the CT operator to compare the radiation doses that patients receive from different CT imaging protocols. The $CTDI_{vol}$ is unrelated to the length of the CT scan; in contrast, the DLP, which is the product of $CTDI_{vol}$ and the scan length, reflects the radiation exposure derived from a cardiovascular CT scan. The DLP, reported in milligray times centimeters (mGy × cm), is displayed after completion of the scan along with $CTDI_{vol}$ and can be used for

estimating effective radiation dose and risk from a cardiovascular CT scan.

The radiation risk from cardiovascular CT imaging is typically estimated and expressed by the concept of effective dose (E), which is used in radiation protection as an estimate of the stochastic effect of a nonuniform radiation dose on a human. E, expressed in millisievert (mSv), can be estimated from sophisticated Monte Carlo simulations in which absorbed doses to various organs are adjusted by a weighting factor that accounts for organ sensitivity, patient age, and patient sex. In clinical practice, a reasonable estimate of effective dose can be obtained by multiplying the DLP provided by the scanner with a weighting factor (k), in which k depends on the exposed body regions. A k value of 0.014 mSv/mGy × cm for the chest is currently used for estimating effective dose from cardiovascular CT imaging procedures for adult patients.

■ HOW HIGH IS THE RADIATION DOSE OF CARDIAC COMPUTED TOMOGRAPHY ANGIOGRAPHY?

Two large multicenter registries collected radiation dose data for coronary CTA. The Prospective Multicenter Study on Radiation Dose Estimates of Cardiac CT Angiography I (PROTECTION I), an international dose survey for cardiac CTA that included 50 study sites, collected representative radiation dose-relevant data for coronary CTA in 1960 patients. This study showed that cardiac CTA performed in 2007 was associated with a median DLP of 885 mGy × cm (value does not include radiation exposure from a localizer, coronary calcium scan, or contrast bolus timing scan). This DLP corresponded to an effective dose of approximately 12 mSv (interquartile range [IQR], 8 to 18 mSv). A second large registry included 4800 patients who underwent cardiac CTA in 2007 and 2008. Data were collected as part of a large multicenter interventional study by the Advanced Cardiovascular Imaging Consortium to investigate the effect of a formal program for lowering the radiation exposure from cardiac CTA. During a study period of 1 year, the investigators showed a 53% reduction in radiation exposure without impairment of diagnostic image quality. The median total DLP (including radiation exposure from

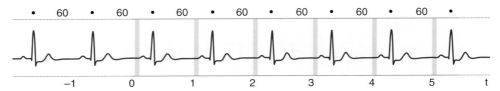

Figure 27-1 Electrocardiogram (ECG) tracing of a cardiac computed tomography scan acquired with the retrospective ECG-gated helical low-pitch scan mode at a heart rate of 60 beats/minute. The pink time interval represents the actual scan duration during which radiation exposure is administered. The narrow medium blue bars represent the time interval needed for image reconstruction, whereas the continuous light blue color represents a non–ECG-modulated tube current.

a localizer, coronary calcium scan, or contrast bolus timing scan, when performed) was reduced from 1493 mGy × cm (21 mSv; IQR, 12 to 26 mSv) in the initial control period to 697 mGy × cm (10 mSv; IQR, 6 to 16 mSv) in the final follow-up period.

In the years following the publication of these two large cardiac CTA dose registries, progressive refinements in CT technology have resulted in decreased cardiac CTA radiation exposures. The details of these technical developments are described in more detail later.

■ WHICH SCAN TECHNIQUES ARE AVAILABLE FOR CARDIAC COMPUTED TOMOGRAPHY ANGIOGRAPHY?

For many indications, correlation of raw CT data acquisition or reconstruction to the electrocardiogram (ECG) is required for obtaining images during a desired cardiac phase. This is accomplished using the ECG signal either to gate data acquisition retrospectively or to trigger data acquisition prospectively. These scan techniques encompass the retrospective ECG-gated helical low-pitch scan mode, as well as the prospective ECG-triggered axial and the prospective ECG-triggered helical high-pitch scan modes.

For those indications that do not require ECG synchronization, conventional helical scanning without ECG correlation is usually performed because it offers the advantage of shorter scan times compared with ECG-correlated scan modes on most CT systems. Such indications include pulmonary vein visualization before electrophysiologic ablation procedures or imaging of the descending aorta for stent planning. Non–ECG-correlated scan modes are often also associated with lower radiation exposures.

■ HOW DOES THE RETROSPECTIVE ELECTROCARDIOGRAM-GATED HELICAL LOW-PITCH SCAN MODE WORK IN CARDIAC COMPUTED TOMOGRAPHY ANGIOGRAPHY, AND HOW IS IT USED TO KEEP RADIATION EXPOSURE LOW?

The *retrospective ECG-gated helical low-pitch scan mode* is considered the conventional scan technique for ECG-correlated cardiovascular CT imaging because it is very robust and less prone to motion artifacts. With this scan mode, CT raw data are acquired during the entire cardiac cycle, with continuous rotation of the gantry and simultaneous table movement. By gating the simultaneously recorded ECG signal to the CT raw data and maintaining the tube current at a maximum throughout the cardiac cycle, image reconstruction can be performed at any time point during the cardiac cycle with identical image noise levels (Fig. 27-1). This technique also allows for manipulation of the ECG gating process in patients with arrhythmias, such as deletion of extra systolic beats, insertion of missed beats, or shifting of R peak locations to adjust for arrhythmia. However, the resulting radiation dose associated with a retrospective ECG-gated helical low-pitch coronary CT scan often ranges between 15 and 20 mSv.

The ability to reconstruct high-resolution images with low image noise at any time point in the cardiac cycle is rarely needed in cardiovascular CT. In fact, in patients with lower heart rates, diagnostic image quality is usually achieved when images are reconstructed in mid-diastole to late diastole when coronary artery motion is at its least. Accordingly, large amounts of acquired CT data during the remaining time of the cardiac cycle are not needed for image reconstruction and thus are not needed for coronary artery assessment. When applying *ECG-dependent tube current modulation* (EDTCM), the tube current is modulated according to the ECG, with the maximum tube current during the relevant phases of the cardiac cycle and downregulation of tube current to a lower level (e.g., 20%) during the remaining phases. When this technique was applied to evaluation of the coronary arteries, a 40% reduction in radiation dose values was reported for retrospective ECG-gated helical low-pitch scanning with EDTCM in clinical practice (Fig. 27-2).

Some CT scanners offer more "aggressive" downregulation of the tube current during the phases of cardiac cycle that are not necessary for image reconstruction. One of these algorithms, referred to as MinDose (Siemens Healthcare, Forchheim, Germany), reduces the tube current during phases not relevant for coronary diagnostic imaging down to a level of 4% (Fig. 27-3). Images acquired during phases of 4% tube current are of nondiagnostic quality for assessment of the coronary arteries, but they may still be sufficient for functional cardiac diagnostic purposes. With the use of this advanced EDTCM algorithm, an additional radiation dose reduction of 30% or more can be achieved when compared with standard EDTCM algorithms.

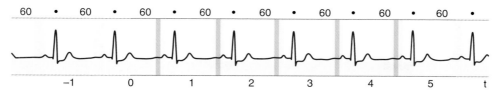

Figure 27-2 Electrocardiogram (ECG) tracing of a cardiac computed tomography scan acquired with the retrospective ECG-gated helical low-pitch scan mode and ECG-dependent tube current modulation at a heart rate of 60 beats/minute. The pink time interval represents the actual scan duration during which radiation exposure is administered. The narrow *medium blue bars* represent the time interval needed for image reconstruction, whereas the *light blue* color represents the ECG-modulated tube current, which is at 100% in the mid-diastolic phase used for image reconstruction and is downregulated to 20% in the remaining time of the R-R interval.

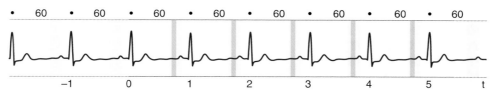

Figure 27-3 Electrocardiogram (ECG) tracing of a cardiac computed tomography scan acquired with the retrospective ECG-gated helical low-pitch scan mode and the MinDose ECG-dependent tube current modulation at a heart rate of 60 beats/minute. The *light blue* color represents the ECG-modulated tube current, which is at 100% in the mid-diastolic phase used for image reconstruction and is downregulated to only 4% in the remaining time of the R-R interval. The *medium blue bars* represent the time interval needed for image reconstruction.

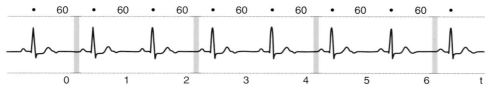

Figure 27-4 Electrocardiogram (ECG) tracing of a cardiac computed tomography scan acquired with the prospective ECG-triggered axial scan technique at a heart rate of 60 beats/minute. The four narrow *medium blue bars* represent the time interval needed for image reconstruction. The *pink* time intervals represent the short radiation exposures needed. After each acquisition, the table is incremented to the next position, so that every other beat is used for image acquisition.

■ HOW DOES THE PROSPECTIVE ELECTROCARDIOGRAM-TRIGGERED AXIAL SCAN MODE WORK IN CARDIAC COMPUTED TOMOGRAPHY ANGIOGRAPHY, AND HOW IS IT USED TO KEEP RADIATION EXPOSURE LOW?

When compared with retrospective ECG-gated helical low-pitch scanning, a considerable reduction of radiation dose can be achieved with the *prospective ECG-triggered axial scan technique*. In this axial mode, CT data acquisition is always prospectively triggered by the ECG signal during the desired cardiac phase while the examination table is stationary. Accordingly, radiation is applied only at a predefined time point of the cardiac cycle that is relevant for image reconstruction (i.e., the phase with greatest likelihood of minimal cardiac motion). Data acquisition is then suspended while the examination table is incremented to the next slice position, and the process is repeated until the entire scan range is covered (Fig. 27-4). Because images can be reconstructed only during the prespecified phase of data acquisition, functional analysis is limited. Some additional data beyond the minimum required for image reconstruction ("padding") can be acquired to permit minor retrospective adjustments of the reconstruction

window, thus potentially reducing cardiac motion artifacts. These adjustments are associated with higher radiation exposures, however. As a consequence, the CT data acquisition window should be kept as narrow as possible.

The total number of axial data acquisitions (steps) needed to cover the required scan length is inversely related to the CT detector array width. Wide detector arrays with up to 320 detector rows allow acquisition of a maximum of 16 cm along the z-axis per gantry rotation. Such wide coverage enables acquisition of data from the entire heart during two heartbeats with only one-step table movement or even at a single time point within one cardiac cycle without table movement.

A meta-analysis demonstrated that the diagnostic accuracy of prospective ECG-triggered axial coronary CTA is high when compared with invasive coronary angiography. Several other studies demonstrated that image quality of axial scanning is comparable to that of conventional retrospective ECG-gated helical low-pitch scanning, but the radiation exposure is reduced by 65% to 80%. As a consequence, the prospective ECG-triggered axial scan technique is currently considered the preferred cardiac CTA technique in patients with stable sinus rhythm and a well-controlled heart rate (preferably <60 to 65 beats/minute).

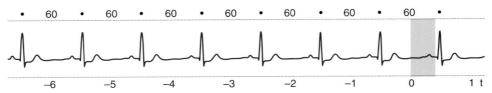

Figure 27-5 Electrocardiogram (ECG) tracing of a cardiac computed tomography (CT) scan acquired with the prospective ECG-triggered helical high-pitch scan mode at a heart rate of 60 beats/minute. The *medium blue bar* represents the time interval needed for cardiac CT scanning, which lasts approximately 300 msec. Radiation exposure is administered only in this single short phase of the cardiac cycle.

■ HOW DOES THE PROSPECTIVE ELECTROCARDIOGRAM-TRIGGERED HELICAL HIGH-PITCH SCAN MODE WORK IN CARDIAC COMPUTED TOMOGRAPHY ANGIOGRAPHY, AND HOW IS IT USED TO KEEP RADIATION EXPOSURE LOW?

The third scan technique available for cardiovascular CT imaging is the *prospective ECG-triggered helical high-pitch scan mode,* which is available on second-generation dual source CT systems. The pitch describes the movement of the examination table in relation to the nominal scan width (detector width) with helical CT data acquisition. The pitch equals 1 if the movement of the table during a single gantry rotation equals the detector width. With *low-pitch* helical scanning, the table movement is less than the detector width during one rotation, resulting in significant scan overlap with redundant CT data acquisition. Accordingly, the same region within the heart is exposed redundantly during several consecutive rotations, and this increases radiation dose. With conventional single-source CT systems, pitch is limited to a maximum value of 1.5 for gapless CT data acquisition in the z-direction. At higher pitch values, data gaps occur that may result in image artifacts and errors in image reconstruction. However, with second-generation dual source CT, the second tube or detector system is used to fill the data gaps, and the pitch can be increased to values greater than 3. This high pitch results in very short cardiac CTA data acquisition times of approximately 300 msec that allow scanning of the entire heart during a single diastolic phase (Fig. 27-5). Early studies showed the feasibility of the prospective ECG-triggered helical high-pitch scan mode for cardiac CTA in patients with a low and stable heart rate (<60 beats/minute) resulting in estimated effective doses consistently lower than 1 mSv when combined with tube potentials of 100 kV.

■ HOW DOES THE SCAN LENGTH AFFECT RADIATION EXPOSURE IN CARDIAC COMPUTED TOMOGRAPHY ANGIOGRAPHY?

Radiation exposure during CT imaging increases proportionally with every increase of the *scan length* in the z-direction. Therefore, accurate definition of the scan range to the volume of interest is an efficient means to reduce radiation exposure. For cardiovascular CT imaging, the scan should typically be started at the middle to lower level of the main pulmonary arteries and extended

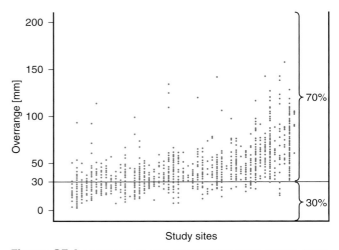

Figure 27-6 Variation in the noncardiac scan range (overrange) at different study sites of the PROTECTION I study. When applying a threshold of 30 mm as a maximum acceptable overrange (15 mm in the cranial and caudal directions), scan range was defined precisely in only 30% of patients. Although in some study sites overrange is less than 30 mm in nearly all patients, it is greater than 30 mm in more than 95% of patients at other study sites. Data from Bischoff B, Hein F, Meyer T, et al. Trends in radiation protection in CT: present and future status . *J Cardiovasc Comput Tomogr.* 2009; 3(suppl 2):S65–S73 .

through the apex of the heart. Other areas, such as the aortic arch, should be excluded unless imaging of these areas is specifically requested or otherwise indicated. The impact of setting the scan length to the lowest possible length on radiation exposure in daily practice is often underestimated; in fact, investigators showed that the scan length was well defined in only 30% of patients undergoing coronary CTA in the PROTECTION I study (Fig. 27-6).

■ HOW DOES THE X-RAY TUBE CURRENT AFFECT RADIATION EXPOSURE IN CARDIAC COMPUTED TOMOGRAPHY ANGIOGRAPHY?

The *x-ray tube current* is linearly related to radiation exposure such that a 20% reduction in tube current, for example, results in a 20% reduction in radiation exposure. Radiation dose reduction associated with lowering the tube current is achieved at the expense of increased image noise; image noise is proportional to $1/\sqrt{\text{tube}}$ current (mA) such that a 20% reduction in tube current results in a 12% increase in image noise. Patient size–adjusted settings of the tube current have been suggested to maintain comparable image noise levels while keeping the radiation exposure low. Furthermore, dose saving strategies exist for decreasing x-ray tube current and, subsequently, radiation exposure while achieving acceptable image noise. For cardiovascular CT imaging, these strategies include EDTCM with retrospective ECG-gated helical low-pitch scanning (discussed earlier).

■ HOW DOES THE TUBE POTENTIAL AFFECT RADIATION EXPOSURE IN CARDIAC COMPUTED TOMOGRAPHY ANGIOGRAPHY?

For cardiovascular CT imaging, *tube potentials* ranging from 80 to 140 kV are available in most CT systems; a tube potential of 120 kV is the most commonly used. The tube potential determines the energy of the x-ray beam. As with tube current, the tube potential can be adjusted according to a patient's size to avoid unnecessary exposure in slimmer patients. Assuming that no other changes to scan parameters are made, the radiation exposure is approximately proportional to the square of the tube potential such that a reduction in tube voltage from 120 to 100 kV results in a 31% reduction in radiation dose. The decreased radiation dose with lower tube potentials is achieved at the expense of increased image noise. Several smaller studies and one large randomized multicenter trial robustly showed comparable diagnostic image quality for the assessment of coronary arteries at 100 kV compared with 120 kV in nonobese patients. Accordingly, the use of 100 kV scan protocols has been recommended for patients weighing less than 90 kg or with a body mass index (BMI) lower than 30 kg/m^2. The use of tube potentials of 80 kV for very slim patients and of 135 or 140 kV for very obese patients has been studied in additional trials.

Adjustments in tube current or tube potential can be combined with other strategies for radiation dose reduction in cardiac CTA. Examples include EDTCM in retrospective ECG-gated helical low-pitch scan mode and the use of the prospective ECG-triggered axial or the prospective ECG-triggered helical high-pitch scan techniques.

■ HOW DO ITERATIVE IMAGE RECONSTRUCTION TECHNIQUES AFFECT RADIATION EXPOSURE IN CARDIAC COMPUTED TOMOGRAPHY ANGIOGRAPHY?

Compared with conventional image reconstruction using filtered back projection techniques, newer *iterative reconstruction techniques* are associated with lower image noise levels. Therefore, CT data can be acquired at lower tube parameter settings (tube current and potential) that result in lower radiation exposures. Iterative reconstruction techniques require more computational power and are more time consuming, but they may offer the additional advantages of improved low-contrast detectability and fewer streak artifacts. Although some experience with iterative reconstruction has been described in the literature, these iterative reconstruction algorithms are in their infancy; further development of and experience with these algorithms may expand their use in cardiovascular CT imaging.

■ WHICH VARIABLES ARE ASSOCIATED WITH RADIATION DOSE IN CARDIAC COMPUTED TOMOGRAPHY ANGIOGRAPHY?

Both previously described multicenter registries analyzed the independent predictors for estimated effective dose using multivariable linear regression models. The independent predictors can be grouped into patient-related, CT imaging center–related, and scan protocol-related factors.

Patient-Related Predictors

Increased *heart rates* and the *absence of regular sinus rhythm* have been found to be significantly associated with higher cardiac CTA radiation exposure. Most of the described techniques for radiation dose reduction in cardiac CTA depend on a low and regular heart rate (preferably <60 beats/minute). Thus, adequate patient preparation, usually with the administration of beta-blockers, is necessary in many patients for achieving such low heart rates. Accordingly, the administration of beta-blockers can be viewed as an additional strategy for radiation dose reduction.

Increased *body weight* (or BMI) was also identified as predictor for increased radiation exposure in cardiac CTA because heavier patients tend to require higher tube potential and current settings to achieve acceptable noise levels and to make diagnostic results possible. Furthermore, investigators showed that normal or reduced body weight (or BMI) allows for reducing tube potential and current settings without compromising diagnostic image quality.

Older patient *age* and *male sex* have also been associated with higher cardiac CTA radiation exposure. Although the causes are not entirely clear, one may hypothesize that the lowered risk of cancer development at higher age has led to the use of higher radiation scan protocols and the risk of breast cancer induction in female patients has resulted in an increased use of low-dose cardiac CTA scan strategies.

Computed Tomography Imaging Center–Related Predictors

Besides the imaging center *experience* and its *volume* in cardiac CTA, investigators showed that (1) *participation in special dose-reduction training* resulted in sustained lower median doses, and (2) considerable differences exist among CT scanner vendors and scanner models with regard to cardiac CTA radiation exposure. Besides some obvious differences in hardware characteristics, these differences among CT scanners and their vendors may also be explained by differences in the software realization of dose saving strategies, as well as the respective instructions on "how-to-use" dose-saving strategies in clinical practive by CT vendors and their acceptance by the CT user.

Scan Protocol-Related Predictors

As described earlier, selection of the most suitable scan technique for an individual patient and exact implementation of ECG-dependent tube current modulation (helical scan) or width of the data acquisition window (axial scan) typically have the greatest effects on radiation exposure, followed by selection of tube potential and tube current and planning of scan length.

■ COMPARING CARDIAC COMPUTED TOMOGRAPHY ANGIOGRAPHY AND ITS RADIATION DOSE WITH OTHER IMAGING MODALITIES

Modern cardiovascular imaging plays a central role in clinical cardiology and has contributed to the decrease in morbidity and mortality from coronary heart disease. The available diagnostic imaging technologies encompass several noninvasive and invasive imaging modalities. The most commonly used noninvasive techniques include chest radiography, stress ECG and stress echocardiography, cardiac magnetic resonance (CMR) imaging, single photon emission computed tomography (SPECT), positron emission tomography (PET), and cardiac CTA. These imaging modalities address different aspects of coronary artery disease, including cardiac and coronary anatomy, as well as myocardial function and its perfusion. Large comparative effectiveness trials are needed to demonstrate the superiority of one diagnostic technique over others. Superiority in this regard should focus not only on accuracy of the tests, but also on availability, cost effectiveness, reduction of unnecessary downstream testing and procedures, radiation exposure, and, finally, overall patient outcomes. Such trials are under way for establishing the role of cardiac CTA in clinical practice.

With the lack of current comparability trials, the radiation exposure of modern noninvasive and invasive imaging technologies can be summarized as follows. No radiation exposure is associated with stress echocardiography and CMR imaging. Representative effective radiation dose estimates for SPECT myocardial perfusion imaging range from 9 mSv (1-day stress-rest protocol with sestamibi) to 41 mSv (stress-rest protocol with thallium). The radiation exposure for PET myocardial perfusion imaging is also tracer dependent and ranges from 5 mSv (rubidium-82) to 14 mSv (fluorine-18 fluorodeoxyglucose). For a diagnostic invasive coronary angiogram, a representative effective dose of 7 mSv has been described. The radiation exposure of cardiac CTA is of comparable magnitude. In 2007, a median effective dose estimate of 10 to 12 mSv for cardiac CTA imaging was achieved in the previously mentioned Advanced Cardiovascular Imaging Consortium and PROTECTION I registries. Although newer data from large registries are lacking, it is perceivable that current cardiac CTA radiation exposure has been reduced to dose estimates lower than 5 mSv in daily practice with the introduction and consequent application of the previously described techniques for radiation dose reduction.

Bibliography

Achenbach S, Marwan M, Ropers D, et al. Coronary computed tomography angiography with a consistent dose below 1 mSv using prospectively electrocardiogram-triggered high-pitch spiral acquisition. *Eur Heart J.* 2010;31:340-346.

American Association of Medical Physicists (AAPM) Task Group 23. CT dosimetry: the measurement, reporting and management of radiation dose in CT. <http://www.aapm.org/pubs/reports/RPT_96.pdf.> Accessed 7.12.12.

Bischoff B, Hein F, Meyer T, et al. Comparison of sequential and helical scanning for radiation dose and image quality: results of the Prospective Multicenter Study on Radiation Dose Estimates of Cardiac CT Angiography (PROTECTION) I study. *AJR Am J Roentgenol.* 2010;194:1495-1499.

Bischoff B, Hein F, Meyer T, et al. Impact of a reduced tube voltage on CT angiography and radiation dose: results of the PROTECTION I study. *JACC Cardiovasc Imaging.* 2009;2:940-946.

Bischoff B, Hein F, Meyer T, et al. Trends in radiation protection in CT: present and future status. *J Cardiovasc Comput Tomogr.* 2009;3(suppl 2):S65-S73.

Bittencourt MS, Schmidt B, Seltmann M, et al. Iterative reconstruction in image space (IRIS) in cardiac computed tomography: initial experience. *Int J Cardiovasc Imaging.* 2011;27:1081-1087.

Blankstein R, Shah A, Pale R, et al. Radiation dose and image quality of prospective triggering with dual-source cardiac computed tomography. *Am J Cardiol.* 2009;103:1168-1173.

DeFrance T, Dubois E, Gebow D, Ramirez A, Wolf F, Feuchtner GM. Helical prospective ECG-gating in cardiac computed tomography: radiation dose and image quality. *Int J Cardiovasc Imaging.* 2010;26:99-107.

Earls JP, Berman EL, Urban BA, et al. Prospectively gated transverse coronary CT angiography versus retrospectively gated helical technique: improved image quality and reduced radiation dose. *Radiology.* 2008;246:742-753.

Einstein AJ, Henzlova MJ, Rajagopalan S. Estimating risk of cancer associated with radiation exposure from 64-slice computed tomography coronary angiography. *JAMA.* 2007;298:317-323.

Einstein AJ, Wolff SD, Manheimer ED, et al. Comparison of image quality and radiation dose of coronary computed tomographic angiography between conventional helical scanning and a strategy incorporating sequential scanning. *Am J Cardiol.* 2009;104:1343-1350.

Flohr TG, McCollough CH, Bruder H, et al. First performance evaluation of a dual-source CT (DSCT) system. *Eur Radiol.* 2006;16:256-268.

Gerber TC, Carr JJ, Arai AE, et al. Ionizing radiation in cardiac imaging: a science advisory from the American Heart Association Committee on Cardiac Imaging of the Council on Clinical Cardiology and Committee on Cardiovascular Imaging and Intervention of the Council on Cardiovascular Radiology and Intervention. *Circulation.* 2009;119:1056-1065.

Halliburton SS, Abbara S, Chen MY, et al. SCCT guidelines on radiation dose and dose-optimization strategies in cardiovascular CT. *J Cardiovasc Comput Tomogr.* 2011;5:198-224.

Hausleiter J, Bischoff B, Hein F, et al. Feasibility of dual-source cardiac CT angiography with high-pitch scan protocols. *J Cardiovasc Comput Tomogr.* 2009;3:236-242.

Hausleiter J, Martinoff S, Hadamitzky M, et al. Image quality and radiation exposure with a low tube voltage protocol for coronary CT angiography results of the PROTECTION II trial. *JACC Cardiovasc Imaging.* 2010;3:1113-1123.

Hausleiter J, Meyer T, Hermann F, et al. Estimated radiation dose associated with cardiac CT angiography. *JAMA.* 2009;301:500-507.

Hausleiter J, Meyer T, Hadamitzky M, et al. Radiation dose estimates from cardiac multislice computed tomography in daily practice: impact of different scanning protocols on effective dose estimates. *Circulation.* 2006;113:1305-1310.

Hendel RC, Patel MR, Kramer CM, et al. ACCF/ACR/SCCT/SCMR/ASNC/NASCI/SCAI/SIR 2006 appropriateness criteria for cardiac computed tomography and cardiac magnetic resonance imaging: a report of the American College of Cardiology Foundation Quality Strategic Directions Committee Appropriateness Criteria Working Group, American College of Radiology, Society of Cardiovascular Computed Tomography, Society for Cardiovascular Magnetic Resonance, American Society of Nuclear Cardiology, North American Society for Cardiac Imaging, Society for Cardiovascular Angiography and Interventions, and Society of Interventional Radiology. *J Am Coll Cardiol.* 2006;48:1475-1497.

Hou Y, Yue Y, Guo W, et al. Prospectively versus retrospectively ECG-gated 256-slice coronary CT angiography: image quality and radiation dose over expanded heart rates. *Int J Cardiovasc Imaging.* 2012;28:153-162.

Kalender WA, Deak P, Kellermeier M, van Straten M, Vollmar SV. Application- and patient size-dependent optimization of x-ray spectra for CT. *Med Phys.* 2009;36:993-1007.

Kitagawa K, Lardo A, Lima J, George R. Prospective ECG-gated 320 row detector computed tomography: implications for CT angiography and perfusion imaging. *Int J Cardiovasc Imaging.* 2009;25:201-208.

Leipsic J, Labounty TM, Heilbron B, et al. Estimated radiation dose reduction using adaptive statistical iterative reconstruction in coronary CT angiography: the ERASIR study. *AJR Am J Roentgenol.* 2010;195:655-660.

Leipsic J, Nguyen G, Brown J, Sin D, Mayo JR. A prospective evaluation of dose reduction and image quality in chest CT using adaptive statistical iterative reconstruction. *AJR Am J Roentgenol.* 2010;195:1095-1099.

Leschka S, Stolzmann P, Desbiolles L, et al. Diagnostic accuracy of high-pitch dual-source CT for the assessment of coronary stenoses: first experience. *Eur Radiol.* 2009;19:2896-2903.

Maruyama T, Takada M, Hasuike T, Yoshikawa A, Namimatsu E, Yoshizumi T. Radiation dose reduction and coronary assessability of prospective electrocardiogram-gated computed tomography coronary angiography: comparison with retrospective electrocardiogram-gated helical scan. *J Am Coll Cardiol.* 2008;52:1450-1455.

Morin RL, Gerber TC, McCollough CH. Radiation dose in computed tomography of the heart. *Circulation.* 2003;107:917-922.

PROspective Multicenter Imaging Study for Evaluation of Chest Pain (PROMISE). NCT01174550:< http://clinicaltrials.gov/ct2/show/NCT01174550.>; Accessed 13.01.12.

Qian Z, Joshi PH, Shaukat AF, et al. Relationship between chest lateral width, tube current, image noise, and radiation exposure associated with coronary artery calcium scanning on 320-detector row CT. *J Cardiovasc Comput Tomogr.* 2011;5:231-239.

Randomized Evaluation of Patients With Stable Angina Comparing Diagnostic Examinations (RESCUE). NCT01262625.< http://clinicaltrials.gov/ct2/show /NCT01262625:>. Accessed 13.01.12.

Raff GL, Chinnaiyan KM, Share DA, et al. Radiation dose from cardiac computed tomography before and after implementation of radiation dose-reduction techniques. *JAMA.* 2009;301:2340-2348.

Rybicki FJ, Otero HJ, Steigner ML, et al. Initial evaluation of coronary images from 320-detector row computed tomography. *Int J Cardiovasc Imaging.* 2008;24:535-546.

Stolzmann P, Scheffel H, Schertler T, et al. Radiation dose estimates in dual-source computed tomography coronary angiography. *Eur Radiol.* 2008;18:592-599.

von Ballmoos MW, Haring B, Juillerat P, Alkadhi H. Meta-analysis: diagnostic performance of low-radiation-dose coronary computed tomography angiography. *Ann Intern Med.* 2011;154:413-420.

Wang D, Hu XH, Zhang SZ, et al. Image quality and dose performance of 80 kV low dose scan protocol in high-pitch spiral coronary CT angiography: feasibility study. *Int J Cardiovasc Imaging.* 2012;28:415-423.

Weigold WG, Olszewski ME, Walker MJ. Low-dose prospectively gated 256-slice coronary computed tomographic angiography. *Int J Cardiovasc Imaging.* 2009;25:217-230.

DISEASE ENTITIES BY ANATOMIC REGION

Myocardial Ischemic Disease: Magnetic Resonance Imaging

John D. Grizzard, Christoph J. Jensen, and Raymond J. Kim

Ischemic heart disease is the leading cause of death in the United States and Europe. Advances in therapy have resulted in improved survival of patients suffering from acute myocardial infarction (MI). However, this improvement has led to an increase in the number of patients surviving with chronic coronary artery disease (CAD). Many of these patients require revascularization. Some may develop complications such as thrombus formation or ventricular aneurysm. Other patients present with chronic exercise-induced chest pain (angina) and may require revascularization, depending on their residual viable myocardium and coronary artery anatomy. Ischemic heart disease is a leading cause of heart failure, and differentiation from other cardiomyopathies that may cause heart failure is paramount to guide appropriate therapy.

Since 2000, substantial progress has been made in magnetic resonance imaging (MRI) hardware and software development such that cardiovascular MRI can now be considered a first-line modality in the evaluation of many facets of ischemic heart disease. For example, advances in coil design coupled with parallel acquisition techniques have resulted in significant shortening of examination time. A complete cardiac examination can now be performed in as little as 30 to 45 minutes. New pulse sequences provide improved visualization of irreversibly scarred myocardium in vivo with a precision that is unparalleled by any other modality. This chapter reviews the information MRI can provide that is useful in the evaluation of ischemic heart disease and its complications.

■ ISCHEMIC CASCADE

When considering the utility of cardiac magnetic resonance (CMR) imaging for the evaluation of ischemic heart disease, it may be useful first to consider the effects of ischemia on the myocardium at a tissue level because many of these events have MRI correlates. Myocardial ischemia reflects an imbalance between myocardial oxygen supply and demand, most often (but not exclusively) as a result of CAD. The initiating event in this ischemic cascade is the reduction of perfusion to less than the level needed to support myocardial metabolism. This process causes metabolic disorders at the tissue level, which then result in diastolic dysfunction, followed shortly by systolic dysfunction. If the imbalance persists, electrocardiogram (ECG) abnormalities may ensue, and symptomatic chest pain may develop. If the ischemic deficit is of sufficient severity and

duration, MI will result. This deficit occurs first in the subendocardium, but with prolonged ischemia, it may extend to involve the full thickness of the myocardium in a given segment. Indeed, if the ischemic injury persists for a period of time without restoration of normal epicardial coronary flow, not only myocytes supplied by the respective artery die, but also endothelial cells at the precapillary and capillary level in the region of infarction may undergo necrosis. In the acute phase, the infarcted myocardium is usually thickened and edematous, whereas chronic MIs typically show thinning of the affected segments, with diminished function.

Restoration of flow may not immediately result in restoration of function even in the absence of MI because the metabolic deficit may take some time to recover. *Myocardial stunning* describes reversible myocardial dysfunction resulting from an acute ischemic insult that resolves before myocardial necrosis in the affected tissue. In addition, a slowly developing, chronic reduction in myocardial blood flow has been postulated to result in myocardial "hibernation," a state of chronic myocardial dysfunction often accompanied by thinning of the affected segments. This state is believed to result from a downregulation of myocyte metabolism and ultrastructure to match its chronically impaired blood supply. This condition is also thought to be a reversible form of myocardial dysfunction.

The foregoing physiologic and anatomic abnormalities that are caused by ischemic injury can be well characterized using a variety of CMR techniques. For example, perfusion MRI allows detection of impaired perfusion occurring as a result of a significant coronary artery stenosis. Areas of segmental wall motion abnormality representing systolic and diastolic dysfunction can be clearly visualized using cine MRI. Global and regional myocardial function can be quantified accurately. MI can be visualized in both the acute and chronic phases by using the delayed enhancement MRI (DE-MRI) technique, which is widely recognized as the gold standard imaging test for the detection of MI and for the determination of myocardial viability (Table 28-1).

In the case of myocardial thinning and dysfunction, cases caused by potentially reversible hibernation can be clearly distinguished from those resulting from irreversible scar. These are important distinctions that in many cases can be made only with MRI.

Given the multiple techniques available, and the variety of clinical situations to which they can be applied, the difficulties in standardizing cardiac MRI protocols for the evaluation of ischemic heart disease are not surprising. However, the Society of Cardiovascular Magnetic Resonance developed suggestions for standard protocols, which are reviewed in the following sections. As an important modification of the standard examination, stress perfusion MRI is also discussed in some detail.

STANDARD CARDIOVASCULAR MAGNETIC RESONANCE EXAMINATION

Figure 28-1 illustrates many of the components, along with a timeline, of a typical multitechnique CMR protocol for cardiac imaging. Sequences are added

Table 28-1   Ischemic Cascade

Physiologic Abnormalities	CMR Imaging Correlates
Decreased perfusion	Focal deficit on perfusion imaging
Metabolic derangements	Spectroscopic abnormalities (research)
Wall motion abnormalities	Cine imaging abnormalities (regional or global)
Myocardial infarction	Delayed enhancement on DE-MRI
Microvascular injury	No-reflow zone on DE-MRI

CMR, Cardiovascular magnetic resonance; DE-MRI, delayed enhancement magnetic resonance imaging.

or excluded depending on the indication, patient considerations (e.g., the ability to breath hold), and even findings during the examination itself. Generally, all patients undergo *cine imaging* for the assessment of morphology, ventricular volumes, and contractile function. These images are typically acquired in 6- to 8-mm short-axis sections at contiguous 1-cm intervals from the mitral valve plane through the apex, as well as in the standard long-axis views (i.e., paraseptal long-axis, four-chamber, three-chamber views). DE-MRI after gadolinium administration is routinely performed with similar section thickness in locations spatially matched to the cine images. This technique allows the diagnosis and sizing of MI, assessment of viability, and other tissue characterization such as identification of thrombus and nonischemic scarring. Irregular heart rhythm or an inability to cooperate with breath holding may necessitate the use of single shot sequence variants to obtain diagnostic-quality images.

Optional elements include stress perfusion imaging to evaluate ischemia and velocity-encoded imaging for the assessment of hemodynamics and valvular function. Additionally, T2-weighted imaging has shown promise in assessing acute, inflammatory processes such as acute MI or myocarditis, and it may prove useful in distinguishing chronic lesions from those of recent onset. At experienced centers, coronary magnetic resonance angiography (MRA) may be performed to exclude left main or three-vessel CAD in selected patients or to evaluate coronary anomalies.

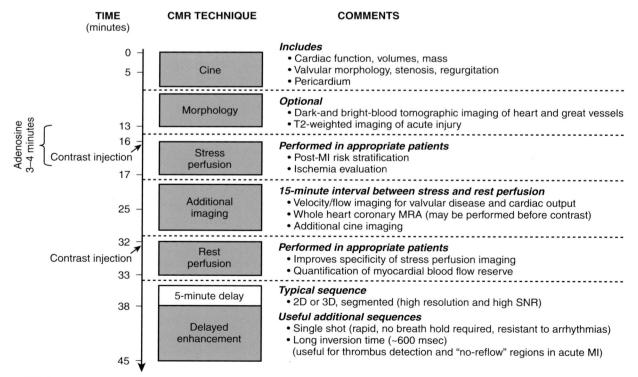

Figure 28-1 Timeline and potential components of a multitechnique cardiovascular magnetic resonance (CMR) examination for cardiac imaging. *2D*, Two-dimensional; *3D*, three-dimensional; *MI*, myocardial infarction; *MRA*, magnetic resonance angiography; *SNR*, signal-to-noise ratio. (Adapted from Kim HW, Farzaneh-Far A, and Kim RJ. Cardiovascular magnetic resonance in patients with myocardial infarction: current and emerging applications. *J Am Coll Cardiol.* 2010;55;1-16.).

Findings in Ischemic Heart Disease

Acute Ischemic Injury

CINE IMAGING

Acute ischemic injury of the myocardium usually results in myocardial dysfunction, with reduction of systolic wall thickening (not thickness) evident on cine images. This change may occur even in the absence of infarction, as expected from the discussion of the ischemic cascade. Acute infarctions may result in transient swelling of the affected segment, with increased signal often apparent on steady-state free precession (SSFP) cine imaging that reflects the presence of edema (Fig. 28-2).

DELAYED ENHANCEMENT MAGNETIC RESONANCE IMAGING

Acute ischemic injury that does not cause infarction does not result in hyperenhancement. Acute infarctions are recognized as focal areas of subendocardial

hyperenhancement on DE-MRI, and they may extend in a transmural fashion for a variable distance, depending on the duration and severity of the ischemia. More severe and long-standing ischemic episodes usually result in a greater transmural extent of infarction because necrosis proceeds in a "wavefront" fashion from the subendocardium toward the epicardium. If the injury is sufficiently severe, it may result in the development of a no-reflow zone, visible on DE-MRI as a dark, nonenhancing core at the center of an extensive infarction. These regions (discussed in more detail later in the chapter) are the DE-MRI correlates of microvascular occlusion from an ischemic injury that is sufficiently severe to cause endothelial damage in the core of the infarct (see the earlier section on the ischemic cascade).

T2 IMAGING

In the setting of acute myocardial injury, increased signal may be seen in areas of infarction, thus reflecting

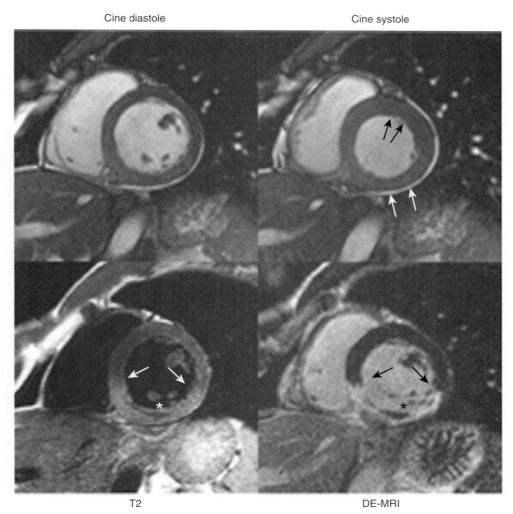

Cine diastole   Cine systole

T2   DE-MRI

Figure 28-2 Images from a patient with an acute inferior myocardial infarction (MI). The anterior wall demonstrates significant thickening in systole *(black arrows)*, but the inferior, inferoseptal, and inferolateral segments, although thicker at rest, do not show normal thickening *(white arrows)*. The T2-weighted image at the same location shows high signal consistent with edema. The hypointense core *(white asterisk)* within the edema likely represents myocardial hemorrhage. The delayed enhancement magnetic resonance imaging (DE-MRI) image shows transmural infarction of the inferior wall, as well as the inferoseptal and inferolateral segments, and matches the area of high signal on the precontrast T2-weighted image. The small dark area in the hyperenhanced inferior wall on the DE-MRI image is an area of microvascular damage, also known as a no-reflow zone *(black asterisk)*. The location and extent of the no-reflow zone are similar to the hemorrhagic region on the T2-weighted image.

the presence of edema (see Fig. 28-2). Investigators have proposed that the area at risk, but not infarcted, may be discerned by comparison of the edematous areas on T2-weighted images with the DE-MRI images, but this is controversial.

Chronic Ischemic Injury

CINE IMAGING

Chronic ischemic injury may result in impaired function, with regional or global hypokinesia, or even akinesia or dyskinesia. Wall thinning may also occur in the affected segments and may result from earlier infarction; however, it can also be seen with hibernation, a potentially reversible form of dysfunction. Cine imaging (without dobutamine stimulation) cannot differentiate between these possibilities.

DELAYED ENHANCEMENT MAGNETIC RESONANCE IMAGING

Similar to acute infarctions, chronic infarctions hyperenhance, whereas areas of hibernation do not. This finding allows differentiation between the two conditions, as discussed more fully later (Fig. 28-3).

T2 IMAGING

Chronic infarctions (>6 months' duration), lacking edema, do not show increased signal on T2-weighted

imaging, thus potentially allowing the distinction from acute MI. This distinction is often not possible with DE-MRI alone.

Clinical Reporting

For general clinical reporting, the 17-segment model recommended by the American Heart Association (AHA) is used. This model divides the basal and mid-cavity levels into 6 segments each, an apical level into 4 segments, and the true apex into 1 segment (see Fig. 14-4, *A* and *B*). For each segment, left ventricular (LV) systolic function is graded visually using a 5-point scale ranging from normal wall thickening to systolic thinning and dyskinesis. The LV ejection fraction is also provided and is estimated from visual inspection of all the short- and long-axis views. Occasionally, LV ejection fraction is quantitatively measured by planimetry, such as in patients undergoing chemotherapy with potentially cardiotoxic agents. DE-MRI images are also interpreted using a 5-point scale. For each segment, the area or transmural extent of hyperenhanced tissue is graded visually. Examples of myocardial segments with various transmural extents of hyperenhancement are shown in Figure 28-4.

DE-MRI images must be interpreted with the immediately adjacent cine images. The cine images can

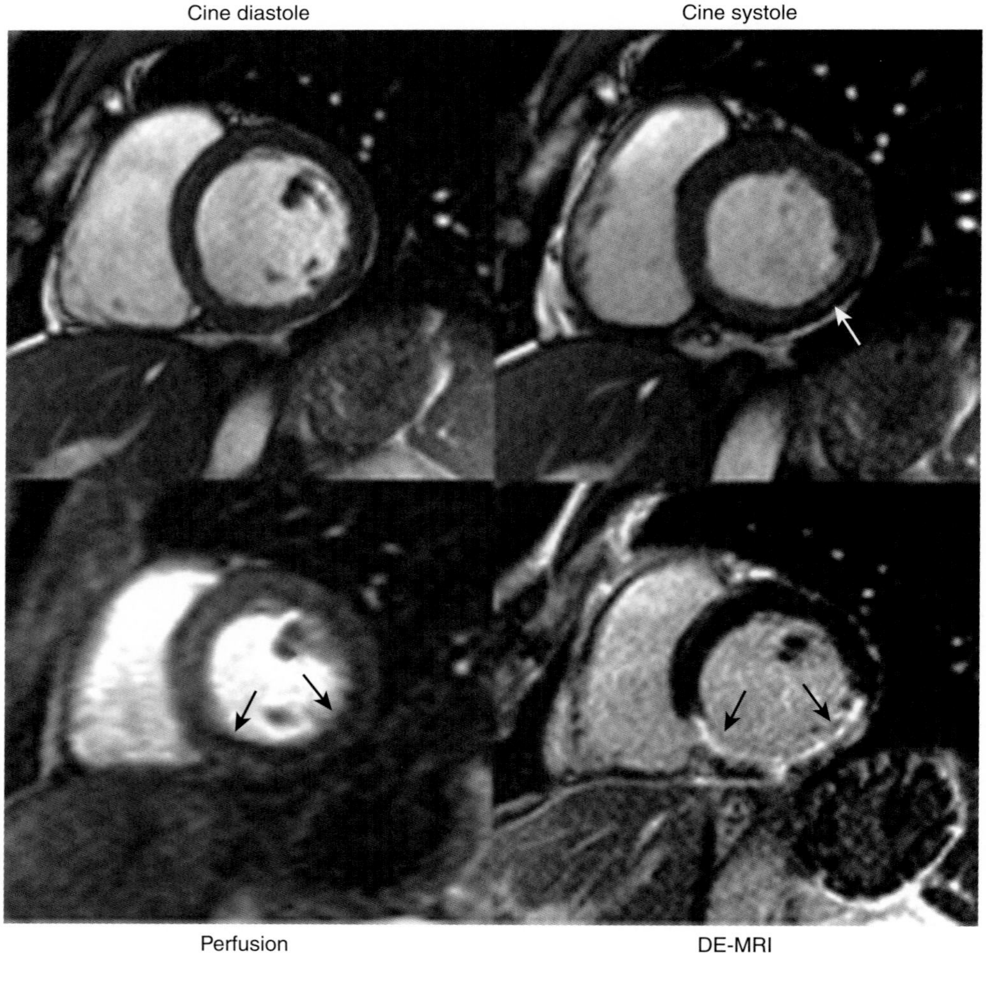

Cine diastole   Cine systole

Perfusion   DE-MRI

Figure 28-3 Images from the same patient as in Figure 28-2 obtained 4 months later. On the diastolic cine images, the swelling in the inferior, inferoseptal, and inferolateral segments has resolved. Now visible is thinning of the inferior and inferolateral segments, with akinesia noted on the systolic images as a failure to thicken *(white arrow)*. The perfusion image (obtained at rest) shows a residual perfusion deficit at the site of earlier infarction. The delayed enhancement magnetic resonance imaging (DE-MRI) image shows remodeling of the infarct.

provide a reference of the diastolic wall thickness of each region. This reference will be helpful if DE-MRI is performed before significant contrast washout from the LV cavity has occurred, and the examiner has difficulty in differentiating the bright signal from the LV cavity from hyperenhanced myocardium, as seen in Figure 28-5.

■ STANDARD EXAMINATION CLINICAL APPLICATIONS

Detection of Myocardial Infarction

In the usual clinical circumstance in which a patient presents with acute chest pain and testing shows elevated troponins as well as characteristic ECG changes (ST-segment elevation), the diagnosis of MI can be made with a high degree of certainty. However, many patients do not present during the acute phase and may not develop ECG changes diagnostic of earlier infarction. In these patients, significant myocardial injury may be missed. Troponin levels, although quite sensitive, may return to normal before the patient seeks medical attention. The ECG determination of infarction (postacute

phase) is based on the development of Q waves, but any non–Q-wave infarction will therefore be missed. A universal definition of MI has been developed. It indicates that a new regional wall motion abnormality or a loss of viable myocardium can be considered evidence of earlier MI. However, wall motion abnormalities may not occur unless the infarcted region exceeds 20% to 50% of the myocardial wall thickness. Similarly, scintigraphic defects may not be apparent until more than 10 g of tissue is infarcted.

Thus, because a sizable threshold of damage is required, echocardiography or single photon emission computed tomography (SPECT) may miss MI, particularly when it is small or subendocardial. In these instances, in which the diagnosis of MI by the universal definition is difficult, DE-MRI may prove helpful. In fact, DE-MRI is the only imaging technique used for the detection of MI that has been validated by an international multicenter trial. In that study, as well as in other studies, DE-MRI was shown to detect even small areas of infarction, regardless of the duration of the infarct or reperfusion status.

The DE-MRI technique has been demonstrated to be the most sensitive means of imaging small areas of

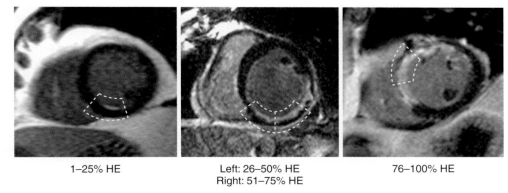

1–25% HE   Left: 26–50% HE   76–100% HE
                        Right: 51–75% HE

Figure 28-4 Typical delayed enhancement magnetic resonance imaging images showing myocardial segments *(dashed white lines)* with various degrees of hyperenhancement (HE). (From Kim RJ, Shah DJ, Judd RM. How we perform delayed enhancement imaging. *J Cardiovasc Magn Reson.* 2003;5:505-514.)

Cine frame   Delayed enhancement   Delayed enhancement
(before Gd)   (2 min after Gd)   (20 min after Gd)

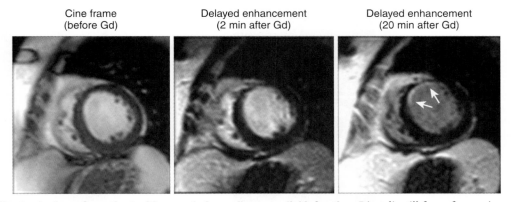

Figure 28-5 Short-axis view of a patient with an anterior wall myocardial infarction. Diastolic still-frame from a cine series is compared to the delayed enhancement images obtained early and late after gadolinium (Gd) administration. Differentiating the bright left ventricular cavity from the subendocardial infarction in the early (2-minute) delayed enhancement image is difficult. The cine frame, by showing the diastolic wall thickness of the anterior wall, provides evidence of subendocardial hyperenhancement in the anterior wall that is difficult to see on the early delayed enhancement image. The late (20-minute) delayed enhancement magnetic resonance imaging image confirms subendocardial hyperenhancement in the anterior wall *(arrows)*. (From Kim RJ, Shah DJ, Judd RM. How we perform delayed enhancement imaging. *J Cardiovasc Magn Reson.* 2003;5:505-514.)

myocardial necrosis in vivo, and experimental studies demonstrated a nearly perfect spatial correlation between areas of hyperenhancement noted on MRI and areas of tissue necrosis on histologic slides (Fig. 28-6). With standard imaging parameters, DE-MRI can detecting infarcts involving as little as one thousandth of total LV myocardial mass that may be undetectable by other techniques that assess myocardial perfusion or contractile function. DE-MRI is significantly more sensitive for the detection of infarction than is SPECT imaging. Although both modalities reliably detect *transmural* infarctions, MRI is superior for the detection of non-transmural *subendocardial* infarctions, more than 40% of which are missed by SPECT (Fig. 28-7). MRI has also been shown to be superior to positron emission tomography (PET) scanning in the detection of subendocardial infarcts.

Detection of Unrecognized Myocardial Infarction: Populations and Prognosis

Because of its exquisite sensitivity, DE-MRI has also been used in population studies to evaluate the prevalence of unrecognized MI. DE-MRI has been found to be significantly more sensitive than ECG testing, with a significant increase in lesion detection ranging from 76% to 390%. One could postulate that the MIs not recognized by standard criteria are likely small and of uncertain significance. However, in studies of patients not clinically known to have had an MI, the presence of unrecognized MI by DE-MRI has been shown to confer a greater than sevenfold increased risk of major adverse cardiac events. The information from DE-MRI is a stronger predictor of outcomes than are the standard clinical risk factors and even catheterization data.

Non–ST-Segment Elevation Myocardial Infarction

The improved sensitivity and spatial localization of infarction provided by MRI may also allow its use in the evaluation of patients with non–ST-segment elevation MI. Specifically, in many of these patients who go on to subsequent cardiac catheterization, multivessel disease is present. The culprit artery responsible for the infarction may not be apparent from the catheter angiogram, particularly if intervening clot dissolution has occurred or if the affected vessel is occluded at its origin. In this instance, performance of DE-MRI before catheterization may allow definitive localization of the culprit artery (Fig. 28-8).

Acute Chest Pain With Elevated Troponin: Myocardial Infarction or Not?

Other entities besides MI are known to cause acute chest pain syndromes, sometimes accompanied by troponin leak. Various studies evaluated the role of CMR in patients with chest pain, elevated troponins, and unobstructed coronary arteries. In this clinical setting, DE-MRI was reported to provide a new diagnosis in up to 65% of patients, and myocarditis was the most common identifiable cause. Similarly, in a large study of patients with ST-segment elevation MI (STEMI) who were undergoing coronary angiography, the investigators reported that 14% had no culprit artery detected, and 9.5% did not have significant CAD by invasive angiography. In the group without a clear culprit artery, MRI established that the most common diagnoses were myocarditis (31%), Takotsubo cardiomyopathy (31%), and STEMI without an angiographic lesion (28%)

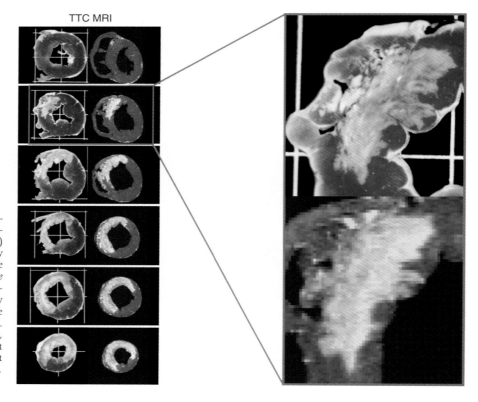

TTC   MRI

Figure 28-6 Comparison of high-resolution ex vivo delayed enhancement magnetic resonance imaging (DE-MRI) (right) with acute myocyte necrosis defined by histopathology (left). The size and shape of the infarcted region *(yellowish-white region)* defined histologically by triphenyltetrazolium chloride (TTC) stain are nearly exactly matched by the size and shape of the hyperenhanced *(bright)* region of DE-MRI. (Adapted from Kim RJ, Fieno DS, Parrish TB, et al. Relationship of MRI delayed contrast enhancement to irreversible injury, infarct age, and contractile function. *Circulation.* 1999;100:1996.)

(Fig. 28-9). These latter STEMIs may have been caused by coronary vasospasm, embolism, or occlusion with subsequent clot dissolution.

Potential causes responsible for acute coronary syndromes including MI in the absence of identifiable culprit artery include the absence of CAD, the absence of typical angiographic characteristics, or multivessel CAD in which more than one lesion is responsible.

Key Points

1. Current standard diagnostic criteria (and SPECT imaging) may miss many MIs.
2. The use of DE-MRI has been well validated as a means of detecting earlier infarction, and it may be useful in both population studies and prognostic studies.
3. The use of DE-MRI to evaluate for MI in acute chest pain syndromes may allow distinction between patients with acute coronary syndromes and those with other entities such as myocarditis or Takotsubo cardiomyopathy.
4. In those patients with MI and uncertainty regarding the culprit artery, MRI may provide additional helpful information.

Characterization of Myocardial Infarctions

Occasionally, circumstances arise in which the patient may have more than one MI, and the acuity of each is uncertain. As noted previously, DE-MRI demonstrates hyperenhancement in both acute and chronic MIs and thus cannot itself distinguish between these possibilities. However, findings suggesting that an area of hyperenhancement is likely chronic include wall thinning and lack of edema. Findings suggestive of acute MI include swelling of the affected segment, with edema noted as a bright signal abnormality on T2-weighted imaging.

The presence of a dark, nonenhancing central area contained within an area of hyperenhancement on DE-MRI is termed a no-reflow zone and is also indicative of acute MI. This zone reflects an area of markedly delayed diffusion of contrast material into the central core of what is usually an extensive MI (Fig. 28-10). The DE-MRI depiction of a no-reflow zone is thought to correspond to areas of profound microvascular obstruction indicative of an extensive ischemic injury resulting in microvascular destructive changes. These findings are often seen even after patency of the epicardial coronary artery

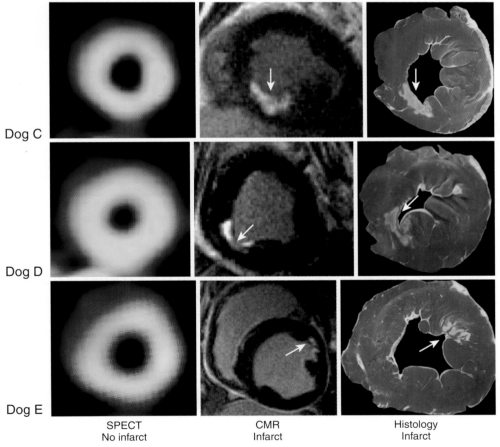

Dog C

Dog D

Dog E

SPECT
No infarct

CMR
Infarct

Histology
Infarct

Figure 28-7 Short-axis views from three dogs with subendocardial infarctions. Unlike single photon emission computed tomography (SPECT) images, delayed enhancement cardiovascular magnetic resonance (CMR) imaging readily demonstrates the infarcted regions *(arrows)*. (Adapted from Wagner A, Mahrholdt H, Holly TA, et al. Contrast-enhanced MRI and routine single photon emission computed tomography [SPECT] perfusion imaging for detection of subendocardial myocardial infarcts: an imaging study. *Lancet.* 2003;361:376.)

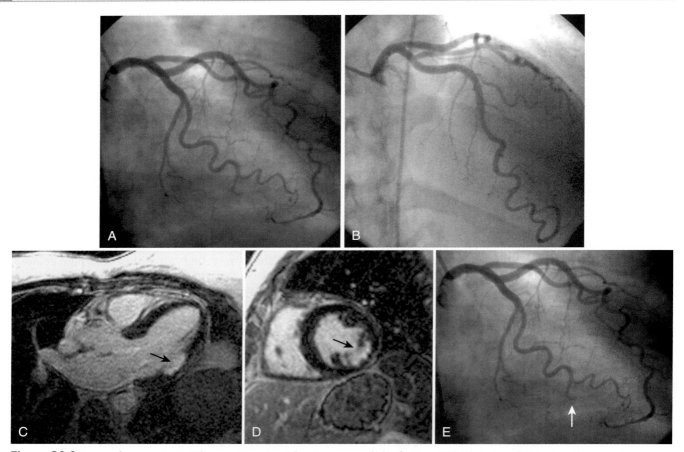

Figure 28-8 Images from a patient with non–ST-segment elevation myocardial infarction (MI). The initial diagnostic catheter angiogram was interpreted as negative (**A** and **B** are selected still frames), and the patient was referred for magnetic resonance imaging (MRI). Delayed enhancement MRI images (**C** and **D**) show a focus of hyperenhancement in the inferolateral wall *(arrows)*, consistent with a circumflex territory MI. Review of the angiogram confirmed a subtle occlusion of a small obtuse marginal branch *(arrow in E)*.

has been restored. They are seen in some acute MIs (usually transmural in extent) and are transient phenomena, given that they are usually not visualized after 4 to 6 weeks. Within a given examination, they are also transient phenomena, more apparent at earlier time points and diminishing over time as contrast material diffuses into the area of injury. These areas should probably be properly termed slow-reflow zones (Fig. 28-11). These areas of microvascular obstruction have been associated with worse outcomes, including adverse remodeling, an increased incidence of arrhythmia, and major adverse cardiac events and death.

Key Points

1. Both acute and chronic MIs demonstrate hyperenhancement on DE-MRI. As a corollary, nonhyperenhancing (nulled, black) myocardium is therefore viable, even if it is thinned (see later sections).
2. The area at risk that has suffered ischemic injury, but is not infarcted, does not demonstrate hyperenhancement. It may show diminished function, which is potentially reversible. Studies now suggest that it may be visualized on T2-weighted images up to 48 hours after injury, although this is somewhat controversial.

3. Although both acute and chronic MIs show hyperenhancement on DE-MRI, they can often be distinguished based on morphologic (myocardial thinning) and signal characteristics (T2-weighted sequences).
4. A no-reflow zone (as depicted on DE-MRI) is a manifestation of an acute infarction and is associated with an increased risk of adverse remodeling and diminished function.

■ VIABILITY STUDIES AND REVASCULARIZATION

Not all ischemic myocardial injury is irreversible. As noted in previous sections, areas of myocardium may be thinned and dysfunctional because of earlier infarction with scarring. However, they can also be thinned and dysfunctional from chronic ischemia in the *absence* of infarction. Revascularization of viable myocardium that is at ischemic risk is well known to be important. Therefore, the determination of viability versus nonviability in a given segment is of great importance in patients who have suffered earlier ischemic injury.

However, significant confusion often exists regarding what is meant by myocardial viability. Like the elephant described by the blind men, myocardial viability is

Patient 1

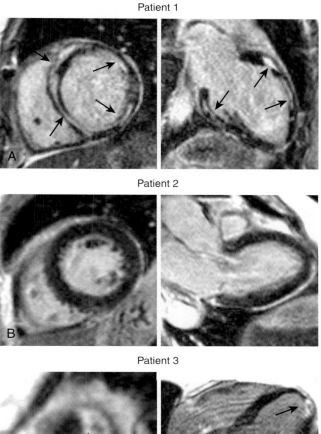

Patient 2

Patient 3

Figure 28-9 Typical delayed enhancement cardiovascular magnetic resonance (DE-CMR) images from 3 patients with chest discomfort, ST-segment elevation, positive troponins, and normal coronary arteries at angiography. **A,** Linear midmyocardial hyperenhancement *(arrows)* is present, particularly in the septum, and is indicative of myocarditis. **B,** In the setting of sudden emotional stress and apical ballooning, the absence of hyperenhancement is consistent with Takotsubo cardiomyopathy. **C,** Focal but transmural hyperenhancement *(arrow)* involving the lateral apex is present and indicative of myocardial infarction (MI) because of temporary occlusion of a small diagonal branch from the distal left anterior descending coronary artery *(top)*. DE-CMR with a long inversion time (600 msec) shows a thrombus *(arrowheads)* in the left atrial appendage *(bottom)*, a finding suggesting that an embolus is the cause of the MI. (Adapted from Kim HW, Farzaneh-Far A, Kim RJ. Cardiovascular magnetic resonance in patients with myocardial infarction: current and emerging applications. *J Am Coll Cardiol.* 2009;55:1-16.)

often defined incompletely by the information available through a given modality. For example, echocardiography may define it as myocardium exceeding 5.5 mm in thickness, below which is likely scar. Clearly, acute MIs, which often demonstrate swelling, do not meet this criterion. Nuclear imaging may define it as myocardium that shows perfusion and wall motion similar to other segments. However, hibernating, thinned myocardium may have reduced perfusion and wall motion but remain viable. Alternatively, acute MIs may have some preservation of perfusion despite significant loss of viability.

Rather than using these indirect measures of viability such as wall thickness or wall motion, the ultimate standard for viability should be the *presence of living myocytes*, and one characteristic of living cells is that they have intact cell membranes. As described earlier, loss of myocyte cell membrane integrity is thought to explain the presence of hyperenhancement in areas of acute infarction. A strong correlation exists between the presence of hyperenhancement and areas of cell death, whether acute or chronic. As a corollary, those myocytes that continue to exclude gadolinium are therefore alive and viable. This concept underlies the increasing acceptance of DE-MRI as the gold standard for the determination of myocardial viability.

Predictive Value of Delayed Enhancement Magnetic Resonance Viability Imaging

Acute Myocardial Injury

In the setting of acute MI, prompt restoration of coronary blood flow has been shown to result in salvage of viable myocardium, improvement in LV ejection fraction, and long-term improvement in survival. However, myocardial dysfunction may persist even after successful coronary reperfusion has been performed. The examiner should determine whether the dysfunction is caused by myocardial necrosis or stunning. DE-MRI has been shown to predict functional improvement after reperfused MI.

In the setting of acute MI, the transmural extent of infarction as measured on DE-MRI has been shown by multiple studies to be highly predictive of improvement in wall motion (Fig. 28-12). In other words, the greater the transmural extent of infarction is in a given segment, the lower will be the likelihood of recovery of function. For example, in one representative study, almost 80% of segments without infarction showed improvement, whereas only 5% of segments with greater than 75% transmural extent of infarction showed improvement. Areas of intermediate transmural extent of infarction demonstrated intermediate levels of recovery. In addition to predicting segmental functional recovery, DE-MRI also predicted improvement in global function; the presence of dysfunctional but viable myocardium with less than 25% transmural extent of infarction was directly related to change in mean wall thickening score and ejection fraction. Multiple other studies subsequently confirmed that the transmural extent of enhancement on DE-MRI predicts functional improvement following MI.

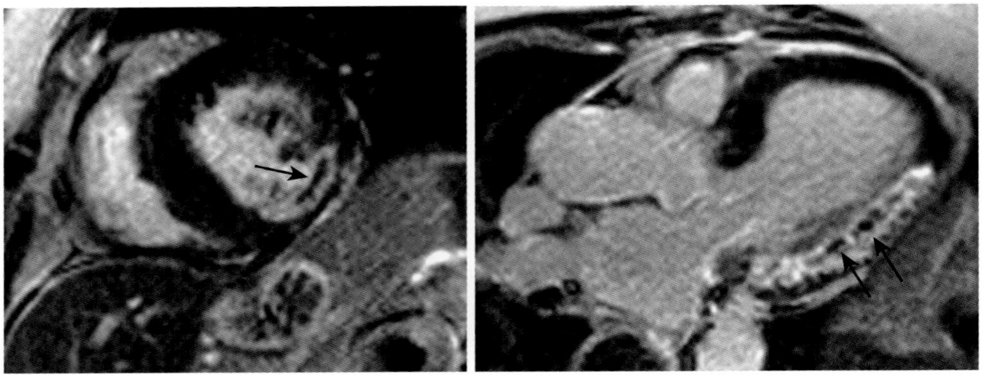

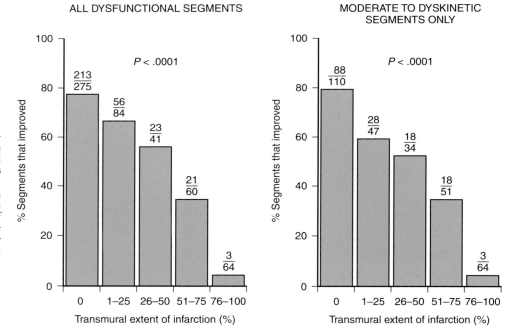

Figure 28-10 Short-axis **(A)** and three-chamber **(B)** delayed enhancement magnetic resonance imaging images from a patient with an acute inferolateral wall infarction. Note the presence of a no-reflow zone as seen as central dark nonenhanced areas *(arrows)* within the hyperenhanced infarcted myocardium.

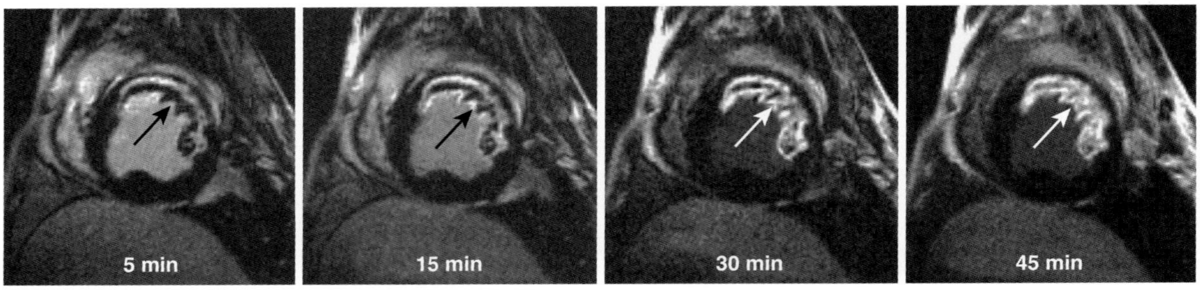

Figure 28-11 Sequential delayed enhancement magnetic resonance imaging images demonstrate a no-reflow zone *(arrows)* in an anterior infarction, manifested as a dark region surrounded by hyperenhancing myocardium. Labels refer to the time after administration of gadolinium. The no-reflow zone fills in and becomes smaller over time. (From Kim RJ, Choi KM, Judd RM. Assessment of myocardial viability by contrast enhancement. In: Higgins CB, de Roos A, eds. *Cardiovascular MRI & MRA.* Philadelphia: Lippincott Williams & Wilkins; 2003:209-237.)

Figure 28-12 Results of segmental analysis of patients with acute myocardial infarction. Of all dysfunctional segments on scans performed in the acute setting, the likelihood of improvement in contractile function decreases with increasing transmural extent of infarction (TEI). Numbers above each column refer to the number of segments. (Adapted from Choi KM, Kim RJ, Gubernikoff G, et al. Transmural extent of acute myocardial infarction predicts long-term improvement in contractile function. *Circulation.* 2001;104:1101-1107.)

Chronic Ischemic Heart Disease

In patients with known CAD and evidence of myocardial dysfunction, a common clinical question centers on the decision whether to proceed with revascularization. The clinical question is commonly phrased as follows: "Is sufficient residual viable myocardium sufficient to justify revascularization?" In this setting, DE-MRI has been shown to be extremely efficacious. Specifically, the transmural extent of infarction demonstrated on DE-MRI has been shown to predict response to myocardial revascularization in patients who have established CAD. Multiple studies demonstrated that, similar to findings in the acute setting, likelihood of functional improvement is inversely related in a progressive stepwise fashion to the transmural extent of infarction. In other words, the greater is the transmural extent of infarction, the lower

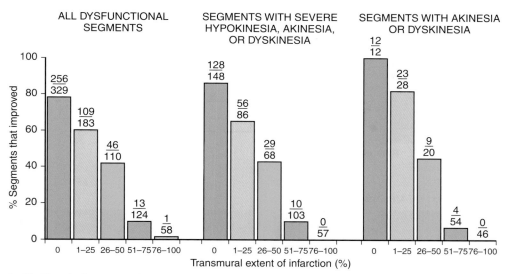

Figure 28-13 The likelihood of recovery of wall motion following revascularization is inversely related to the transmural extent of infarction (hyperenhancement) on delayed enhancement imaging, even in severely hypokinetic, akinetic, or dyskinetic segments. (From Kim RJ, Wu E, Rafael A, et al. The use of contrast-enhanced magnetic resonance imaging to identify reversible myocardial dysfunction. *N Engl J Med.* 2000;343:1445-1453.)

will be the likelihood of recovery of wall motion in any given segment. Alternatively, minimal or no enhancement is associated with a high probability of improvement following revascularization (Fig. 28-13). This is true even in segments that are akinetic or dyskinetic before revascularization. These data have led DE-MRI to be considered the current gold standard for the imaging of viability.

When interpreting the information that DE-MRI can provide in this setting, the examiner should take advantage of the technique's high spatial resolution. DE-MRI allows visualization of the transmural extent of viability or infarction, and thus it changes the assessment of viability from a binary yes/no characterization to that of a continuum, which better reflects reality. This ability to grade myocardial viability along a continuum is one of the great strengths of DE-MRI. As such, the use of a single cutoff value on which to base predictions of functional improvement would not have a physiologic basis and would be suboptimal.

Viability Imaging: Other Concepts

DE-MRI is recognized as a superior means of detecting small infarctions, particularly relative to the competing modality of SPECT imaging. The likely reason is the significantly better spatial resolution of DE-MRI. Specifically, the standard DE-MRI sequence demonstrates a greater than 40-fold improvement in spatial resolution relative to SPECT imaging. However, even if SPECT imaging had infinite spatial resolution, DE-MRI would still have a significant advantage because DE-MRI can show not only what is viable, but also what is infarcted, as well as their relative proportions. This information is particularly important in the differentiation of possibly hibernating myocardium from myocardium that is significantly thinned as a result of extensive scar.

To illustrate the importance of these additional parameters, Figure 28-14 is an example of a patient with

a 3.5-mm rim of viable but akinetic myocardium in the anterior wall. SPECT imaging or any other modality that shows only what is viable would see this patient as having poor tracer uptake and impaired wall motion. He would likely be assessed as having a scarred anterior wall with little viability. This is because modalities that only see what is viable use an *indirect* assessment of viability; that is, the thinned (but viable) rim is compared with the remote, normal segments (3.5 mm versus 9 mm = 39%). This would then be interpreted as showing no significant residual viable myocardium. In fact, by using DE-MRI, one can see (at most) only a 1.5-mm subendocardial infarction, and the 3.5-mm viable rim represents a wall that is 70% viable (3.5 mm out of 5 mm). As could be predicted by DE-MRI (but not by viability-only techniques or indirect assessment), this patient showed profound recovery of wall thickness and function following revascularization. Therefore, in the imaging evaluation of viability, it is extremely important to see not only what is alive, but also what is infarcted, and their relative proportions. This information is especially critical in differentiating thinned myocardium that is hibernating from irreversibly scarred myocardium, and only DE-MRI can provide this information.

Key Points

1. DE-MRI is the current gold standard for the detection of MI in vivo, and the absence of hyperenhancement is strong evidence of residual viability.

2. The transmural extent of infarction by DE-MRI correlates inversely with the likelihood of recovery of wall motion, in both acute and chronic settings.

3. When DE-MRI studies are interpreted for viability, myocardial regions are not interpreted in a binary fashion as viable or nonviable; rather, the transmural extent of viable and infarcted myocardium is directly visualized, and viability is assessed on a continuum.

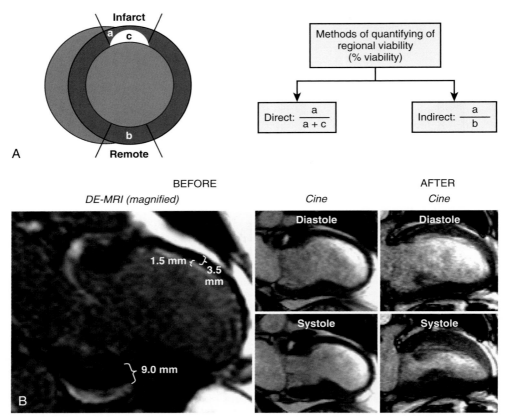

Figure 28-14 **A,** Illustration of the differences between direct and indirect methods of quantifying regional viability. Viable myocardium is displayed in *black;* infarcted myocardium is displayed in *white.* **B,** Long-axis magnetic resonance imaging (MRI) views of a patient before and 2 months after revascularization. Although the akinetic anterior wall is thinned (diastolic wall thickness = 5 mm; remote zone = 9 mm), delayed enhancement MRI demonstrates only a subendocardial infarction (1.5 mm thick). A direct assessment of viability would show that the anterior wall is predominantly viable (3.5 mm/5 mm = 70% viable), whereas an indirect assessment would show that the anterior wall is predominantly nonviable (3.5 mm/9 mm = 39% viable). Cine MRI images obtained following coronary revascularization demonstrate full recovery of wall motion and diastolic wall thickness. (Adapted from Kim RJ, Shah DJ. Fundamental concepts in myocardial viability assessment revisited: when knowing how much is "alive" is not enough. *Heart.* 2004;90:139.)

4. Modalities that demonstrate only what is viable are suboptimal in the evaluation of thinned, potentially hibernating myocardium. The examiner should evaluate not only what is viable, but also what is infarcted, and their relative proportions. Only DE-MRI can provide this information.

■ MODIFICATIONS OF THE STANDARD EXAMINATION

The preceding sections have described the use of the standard cardiac examination for the evaluation of acute and chronic ischemic heart disease. This section evaluates MRI techniques for the detection of CAD. Multiple MRI techniques are available, including coronary MRA, dobutamine stress MRI, and adenosine perfusion MRI.

Coronary Magnetic Resonance Angiography

As described in previous sections, coronary MRA is technically demanding for several reasons. The coronary arteries are small in caliber, usually measuring between 3 and 5 mm, and their course is complex compared with many other vascular beds that are imaged with MRA. More important, they are subject to nearly constant motion secondary to the cardiac cycle. Sequences that can be acquired during a breath hold usually have very limited coverage. Whole heart coverage takes several minutes to acquire and thus has a duration that far exceeds a single breath hold. In free-breathing examinations, compensation for respiratory motion with a diaphragm-tracking navigator adds an additional layer of complexity. In response to these complexities, several technical advances have been made to improve the robustness of coronary MRA, most particularly including the development of an ultrafast SSFP sequence that offers a superior signal-to-noise ratio and is used to provide whole heart imaging using the free-breathing technique. These sequences may be obtained with submillimeter in-plane spatial resolution (0.8 × 1.0 mm) and slice thickness of slightly more than 1 mm. With the use of modifications that can compensate for respiratory drift, imaging can usually be completed in 10 minutes or less.

Coronary MRA for the identification of native vessel coronary stenosis is not well established for routine clinical practice. Although some studies at specialized centers have reported high sensitivity and negative

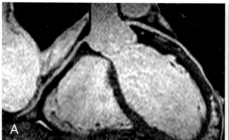 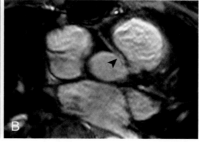 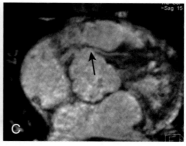

Figure 28-15 Coronary magnetic resonance angiography (MRA) images. **A,** Curved maximum intensity projection image from normal whole heart MRA. **B,** Coronary MRA showing an anomalous right coronary artery originating from the left coronary sinus *(arrowhead)*. **C,** Anomalous left anterior descending coronary artery arising from the right coronary sinus *(arrow)*. Both anomalous coronary arteries have a potentially dangerous interarterial course because they pass between the aorta and the pulmonary artery.

predictive value for the detection of left main coronary artery and triple vessel disease, other centers have reported less favorable results. Coronary MRA it is not a recommended first-line modality for the detection of CAD.

However, coronary MRA has been demonstrated to identify the proximal portion of the major epicardial coronary arteries reliably, and therefore this technique is believed to be a reasonable option for evaluating anomalous coronary artery origins. Although most coronary artery anomalies are benign, variants in which the anomalous coronary artery arises from the opposite cusp and transits between the great vessels are considered potentially dangerous, with a risk of sudden death. The right coronary artery originating from the left cusp and extending between the great vessels occurs more commonly than the left coronary artery originating from the right cusp with an interarterial course (Fig. 28-15). Studies have reported excellent accuracy for the CMR detection of these anomalies. Given the lack of ionizing radiation, consensus documents from the AHA indicated that coronary MRA may be a useful test for patients in whom an anomalous artery origin is suspected, or a known anomalous coronary artery origin requires further clarification. MRA may also be preferred over cardiac computed tomography angiography when concerns are heightened regarding the use of radiation or iodinated contrast material.

Dobutamine Stress Cardiovascular Magnetic Resonance

Similar in concept to dobutamine stress echocardiography, dobutamine stress CMR involves graded doses of dobutamine that are administered in a progressive stepwise fashion, with simultaneous cine CMR used to monitor for the development of ischemia-induced wall motion abnormalities. This technique has been shown to yield higher diagnostic accuracy than dobutamine stress echocardiography, and it can be effective in patients not suited for echocardiography because of poor acoustic windows. A meta-analysis of stress and functional CMR studies demonstrated an overall sensitivity of 83% and specificity of 86% for the demonstration of CAD on a per-patient level. However, the examination is technically complex, and logistic issues regarding patient safety and adequate monitoring are nontrivial matters that require planning and experienced personnel. This test is less widely performed than is adenosine stress perfusion.

Adenosine Stress Perfusion Cardiovascular Magnetic Resonance

In the ischemic cascade described previously, the earliest physiologic abnormality observed is abnormal perfusion. This change occurs before metabolic abnormalities and wall motion abnormalities. Thus, a technique that could reliably demonstrate impaired perfusion would seem to have a theoretical conceptual advantage over those techniques using the development of an ischemia-induced wall motion abnormality for the detection of a significant coronary artery lesion. Improvements in magnet hardware such as gradient and coil design, along with pulse sequence innovations, have resulted in increasingly robust stress perfusion MRI sequences capable of accurately depicting myocardial blood flow. Accordingly, adenosine stress MRI has become a competitive first-line test for the detection of CAD.

Modification of the Standard Examination for Perfusion Imaging

As seen in the CMR imaging timeline in Figure 28-16, stress perfusion can be seamlessly integrated into the standard examination. Following the acquisition of the standard short-axis cine images, stress perfusion imaging is performed, followed by completion of the cine imaging with the acquisition of long-axis images. Rest perfusion imaging is then performed, to aid in the differentiation of true perfusion defects from artifacts. After a short delay, DE-MRI images are obtained in the standard fashion. The entire examination can be performed in 35 to 40 minutes.

Magnetic Resonance Imaging Findings

Although research studies often emphasized analysis of the upslope curves and other complex postprocessing of the perfusion data, more recent reports using visual analysis demonstrated comparable sensitivity and specificity. Perfusion images, typically acquired in the short-axis plane, provide depiction of the sequential transit of the first pass of contrast agent, initially into the right ventricular (RV) cavity, then the LV cavity, and subsequently through the myocardium, thus causing its progressive enhancement (see Fig. 28-16). *True perfusion defects* are recognized as dark areas of contrast deficit extending from the subendocardium into the myocardium. They must be differentiation from artifacts, which are common on

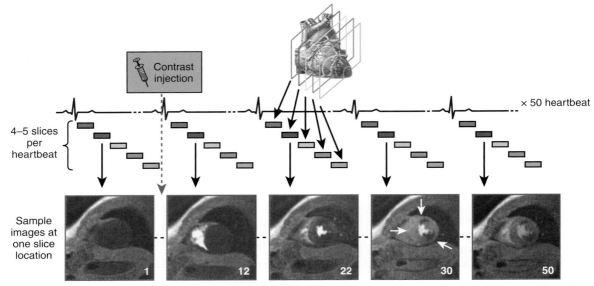

Figure 28-16 First-pass perfusion magnetic resonance imaging image acquisition. Images are acquired serially at multiple slice locations (usually four to five short-axis views for left ventricular [LV] coverage) every heartbeat to depict the passage of a compact contrast bolus as it transits the heart. Sample images of one slice location are shown at several representative time points: before arrival of contrast (frame 1); contrast in right ventricular (RV) cavity (frame 12); contrast in the LV cavity (frame 22); peak contrast in LV myocardium (frame 30), showing normal perfusion in the septum (*large arrow*) and abnormal perfusion in the inferolateral wall and anterior wall (*small arrows*); and the contrast washout phase (frame 50). (From Kim HW, Farzaneh-Far A, Klem I, et al. Magnetic resonance imaging of the heart. In: Fuster V, Walsh R, eds. *Hurst's The Heart*. New York: McGraw-Hill; 2010;631-666.

perfusion imaging and are most often seen as a thin dark rim at the interface of blood pool and the endocardium. Characteristics that may be useful in distinguishing between artifact and true perfusion defects include the following: (1) artifacts are more common in the phase encode direction; true perfusion defects should follow coronary artery distribution territories; (2) artifacts are transitory, varying in signal intensity in consecutive images during the transit of contrast media through the myocardium; true perfusion defects often linger for multiple image frames and should follow smooth image intensity trajectories; and (3) artifacts are often present at both stress and rest imaging; true perfusion defects generally appear only during vasodilator stress (Table 28-2).

Earlier infarctions can have several effects on perfusion images, and these effects can cause confusion if one thinks of CMR as similar to nuclear imaging, in which fixed or irreversible defects are evaluated. For example, if the infarct was sufficiently extensive to cause microvascular obstruction, they may show diminished perfusion on the initial stress images. On resting perfusion images, these defects may hyperenhance after the initial contrast bolus, and their enhancement may cause them to be less dark on perfusion images. This finding could lead to some confusion with true inducible ischemia, but correlation with the DE-MRI images allows identification of the correct diagnosis. Perfusion defects that significantly exceed the infarct size are then assessed as having perilesional ischemia.

Interpretation of the images follows the standard 17-segment AHA format described in the initial discussion of the standard examination. This interpretation is greatly facilitated by having side-by-side comparison of spatially matched cine, perfusion, and DE-MRI images, as seen in Figure 28-17.

Table 28-2 Differences Between Artifacts and True Perfusion Defects

Artifacts	True Perfusion Defects
Occur in the phase encode direction	Follow a coronary vascular territory
Transitory; vary from frame to frame	Persist over three or more heartbeats
Present on both stress and rest images	Present on stress images only

Comparison With Nuclear Imaging

MRI and SPECT perfusion imaging can both be performed with pharmacologic vasodilation, often using adenosine (or regadenoson, which does not require a second intravenous line). The underlying principle is similar in that a vasodilator is used to accentuate regional differences in myocardial blood flow. However, some important differences exist. As compared with nuclear perfusion imaging, perfusion MRI is a first-pass study that directly images the passage of contrast material and therefore is performed using an abbreviated adenosine protocol (approximately 3 minutes). Moreover, perfusion MRI has higher spatial resolution (>20 ×) than nuclear techniques, and it can depict a perfusion defect that is only subendocardial. Perfusion MRI has the additional advantage of providing a more linear depiction of myocardial blood flow in response to vasodilatation, without the plateau phenomenon seen with nuclear agents. The interpretation of the studies is also different in that regions of persistent contrast deficit present on both stress and rest perfusion MRI images are much more likely to represent artifact

BASAL ———————————————————→ APICAL

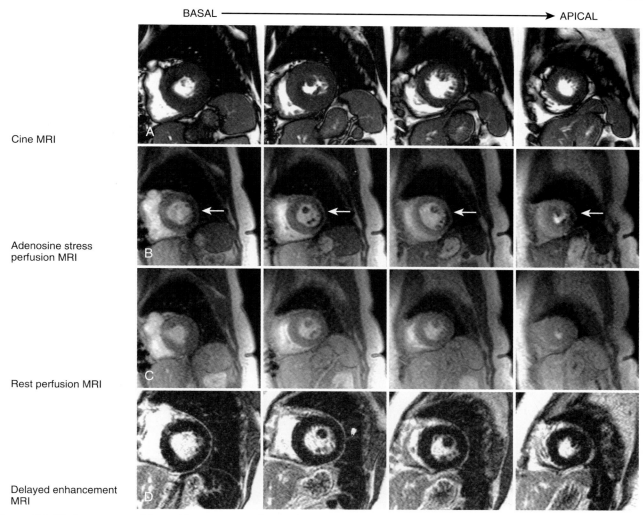

Cine MRI

Adenosine stress
perfusion MRI

Rest perfusion MRI

Delayed enhancement
MRI

Figure 28-17 Components of the multicomponent cardiovascular magnetic resonance stress test. Cine magnetic resonance imaging (MRI) (**A**), stress (**B**) and rest (**C**) perfusion MRI, and delayed-enhancement MRI (**D**) are performed at identical short-axis locations. During image interpretation, the different components are analyzed side by side to facilitate differentiation of perfusion defects resulting from infarction, ischemia, or artifact. *Arrows* point to perfusion defects seen during adenosine infusion, but not at rest, findings consistent with the presence of ischemic heart disease.

than earlier infarction. In rare instances, matched perfusion MRI defects may represent severe resting ischemia, but these regions may show abnormal wall motion or thinning on cine imaging and demonstrate absence of hyperenhancement on DE-MRI, findings indicating profoundly ischemic but viable myocardium.

Diagnostic Performance in Patients
The diagnostic performance of stress perfusion MRI has been evaluated in studies in humans. Analysis of the 20 published studies of perfusion imaging revealed that, on average, the sensitivity and specificity of perfusion MRI for detecting obstructive CAD were 83% (range, 44% to 93%) and 82% (range, 60% to 100%), respectively. However, the addition of DE-MRI information to the interpretation algorithm was shown to improve the specificity (to 87%) significantly while maintaining sensitivity of the examination for the detection of CAD (89%). Notably, evaluation of the DE-MRI images improved the specificity by correctly changing the

diagnosis from positive to negative for CAD. Studies in which infarction was not observed on DE-MRI even though perfusion MRI demonstrated matched stress-rest perfusion defects indicated that the findings were caused by artifact. Thus, these results likely reflect the actual real-world performance of a multicomponent CMR stress testing with appropriate image interpretation. Figure 28-18 demonstrates the interpretation algorithm with case examples.

Current Status
Perfusion MRI stress testing is emerging as an improved method for the detection of CAD. When it is combined with DE-MRI, the sensitivity, specificity, and diagnostic accuracy of the multicomponent stress CMR examination rival other currently available modalities for the evaluation of myocardial ischemia. In 2006, a consensus panel from the American College of Cardiology Foundation deemed the following indications as appropriate uses of stress perfusion CMR: (1) evaluating chest pain

syndromes in patients with intermediate probability of CAD and (2) ascertaining the physiologic significance of indeterminate coronary lesions. In the future, improvements in parallel imaging and pulse sequence technology, use of higher magnetic field strength, and protocol optimizations may continue the advance in image quality. Results of multicenter clinical trials, which are currently ongoing, will soon be available and will establish the diagnostic accuracy and prognostic value of MRI perfusion stress testing in a broad population of patients.

Key Points

1. Coronary MRA is an appropriate technique for the evaluation of coronary anomalies.
2. Dobutamine stress MRI has advantages over dobutamine stress echocardiography, but it requires experienced personnel.

3. Adenosine stress perfusion MRI is an increasingly well-validated technique for the detection of CAD.
4. Correct interpretation of CMR perfusion imaging is facilitated by simultaneous assessment of the spatially matched DE-MRI images, an approach that improves the recognition of artifact.

■ COMPLICATIONS OF ISCHEMIC HEART DISEASE

As noted earlier, patients are increasingly surviving an initial MI, and many go on to develop complications of ischemic heart disease, such as the development of intraventricular thrombi and aneurysm. With its comprehensive, multiplanar imaging capabilities, along with excellent soft tissue contrast, MRI is a superior means of evaluating these complications.

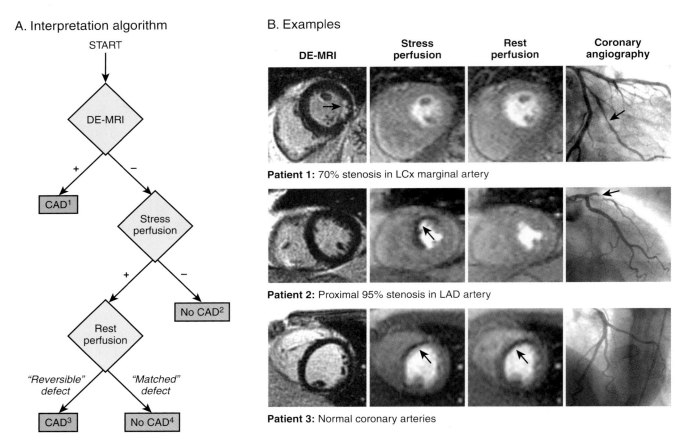

Figure 28-18 Interpretation algorithm for incorporating delayed-enhancement magnetic resonance imaging (MRI) with stress and rest perfusion MRI for the detection of coronary artery disease (CAD). **A,** Interpretation algorithm: (1) positive delayed enhancement magnetic resonance imaging (DE-MRI) study; hyperenhanced myocardium consistent with an earlier myocardial infarction (MI) is detected; does not include isolated midwall or epicardial hyperenhancement, which can occur in nonischemic disorders; (2) standard negative stress study; no evidence of earlier MI or inducible perfusion defects; (3) standard positive stress study; no evidence of earlier MI, but perfusion defects are present with adenosine that are absent or reduced at rest; and (4) artifactual perfusion defect; matched stress and rest perfusion defects without evidence of earlier MI on DE-MRI. **B,** Patient examples. *Top row,* Patient with a positive DE-MRI study demonstrating an infarct in the inferolateral wall *(arrow),* although perfusion MRI is negative. The interpretation algorithm (step 1) classified this patient as positive for CAD. Coronary angiography verified disease in a circumflex marginal artery. *LCx,* Left circumflex artery. Cine MRI demonstrated normal contractility. *Middle row,* Patient with a negative DE-MRI study but with a prominent reversible defect in the anteroseptal wall on perfusion MRI *(arrow).* The interpretation algorithm (step 3) classified this patient as positive for CAD. Coronary angiography demonstrated a proximal 95% left anterior descending coronary artery stenosis. *Bottom row,* Patient with a matched stress-rest perfusion defect *(arrows)* but without evidence of earlier MI on DE-MRI. The interpretation algorithm (step 4) classified the perfusion defects as artifactual. Coronary angiography demonstrated normal coronary arteries. (Adapted from Klem I, Heitner JF, Shah DJ, et al. Improved detection of coronary artery disease by stress perfusion cardiovascular magnetic resonance with the use of delayed enhancement infarction imaging. *Circulation.* 2006;47:1630-1638.)

Thrombus

Thrombus formation, a frequent complication of ischemic heart disease, occurs more often in patients with regional wall motion abnormalities, global systolic dysfunction, and ventricular aneurysms. MRI data suggest that patients with ischemic cardiomyopathy have an approximately fivefold increased risk relative to those with nonischemic systolic dysfunction of similar extent. Contrast-enhanced MRI is a sensitive imaging technique for the detection of thrombi and detects more than twice as many ventricular thrombi as does echocardiography. Clinically, investigators have frequently noted that ventricular thrombi are found adherent to sites of earlier infarction, where wall motion abnormalities and denudation of the endothelium produced by earlier infarction result in a nidus for thrombus formation. Studies have demonstrated that a greater than 50% transmural infarction is an additional risk factor for thrombus development (Fig. 28-19, *A* and *B*). In particular, thrombi are often noted along the endocavitary aspect of ventricular aneurysms (see Fig. 28-19, *C* and *D*).

Imaging Evaluation

Thrombus is recognized on cine imaging when it manifests as an intracavitary filling defect that is discernible from adjacent trabeculations and papillary muscles (see Fig. 28-19, *A* and *B*). Recognition of mural thrombus, however, can be quite difficult on noncontrast cine images, and it likely accounts for the lower sensitivity (40%) of cine CMR relative to contrast-enhanced CMR. The DE-MRI sequence is the most sensitive sequence for the depiction of thrombus. Thrombi usually appear as a dark intracavitary or mural filling defects, often attached to foci of hyperenhanced, infarcted myocardium (see Fig. 28-19, *B*). Although usually thrombi are low in signal intensity on DE-MRI obtained with an inversion time chosen to null normal myocardium, not infrequently they may show a black border with central higher signal, resulting in an etched appearance, particularly on DE-MRI images with SSFP readout. The likely reason is that thrombus has no contrast uptake; it has a long T1 value such that following an inversion pulse, it remains far below the zero baseline at the time point at

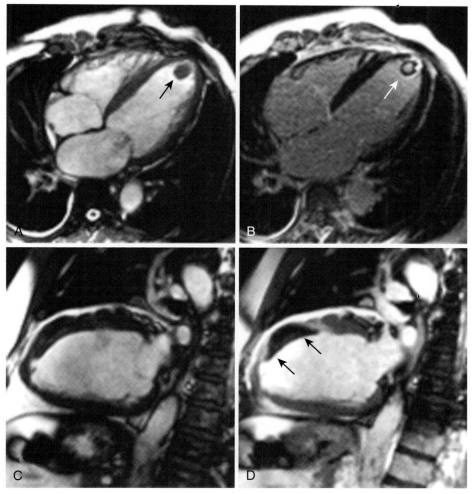

Figure 28-19 Intracavitary thrombus *(arrow)* is recognized as a filling defect separate from papillary muscles and trabeculae on the four-chamber cine view (**A**) and is noted on the delayed enhancement image (**B**) to be adherent to a site of previous apical infarction *(arrow)*. Mural thrombus can be difficult to detect in the absence of contrast, as in this two-chamber cine view (**C**). After the administration of contrast, the anterior mural thrombus *(arrows)* is readily detected (**D**).

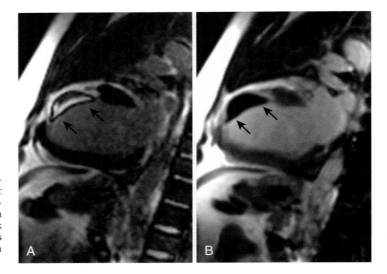

Figure 28-20 Two-chamber single shot delayed enhancement images with inversion times of 300 msec (**A**) and 600 msec (**B**) demonstrate a mural thrombus *(arrows)* adherent to an anterior wall infarct. In **A**, in which the inversion time was chosen to null the signal from myocardium, the thrombus has a dark rim surrounding a bright center, whereas in **B**, the thrombus is uniformly dark. See the accompanying text for an explanation of this finding.

which normal myocardium is at the zero-crossing point (Fig. 28-20, *A*).

Because the standard inversion recovery sequence is sensitive only to magnitude and not to phase, it appears to have a positive or bright signal. Acquiring the image at a later time point, such as an inversion time of 600 msec, allows the thrombus to recover longitudinal magnetization and arrive at or approach the zero-crossing point, whereas normal myocardium and infarct will have recovered above the zero-crossing point and will be light gray in signal intensity (see Fig. 28-20, *B*). Therefore, if any confusion exists regarding the signal characteristics of a suspected thrombus, repeating the inversion recovery DE-CMR sequence with a long inversion time (600 msec) is suggested. This same long inversion recovery variation of DE-CMR can be acquired using a single shot SSFP sequence in multiple planes to screen for thrombus rapidly, even in patients with arrhythmias or those who are uncooperative.

On occasion, diagnostic uncertainty may arise regarding whether a lesion is a thrombus or a no-reflow zone because both have very similar signal characteristics. The distinction can be made if it is possible to define the lesion as intracavitary (thrombus) rather than intramural and surrounded by hyperenhancing myocardium (no-reflow zone). When localization remains difficult, repeating the DE-MRI images 5 to 10 minutes later allows no-reflow zones to show progressive enhancement, whereas thrombi will not change in appearance.

Ventricular Aneurysms

The development of a ventricular aneurysm is estimated to occur in 5% to 7% of acute MIs. A ventricular aneurysm is best understood as an area of contour bulging in diastole that is dyskinetic in systole; that is, it bulges further outward in systole. In a true aneurysm, the myocardium is thinned and contains variable amounts of scar, but it remains intact. These findings are in contrast to the false aneurysm, which represents a contained

rupture of the myocardium. The pericardium serves to contain the rupture, resulting in a pseudoaneurysm.

Imaging Evaluation

Certain imaging characteristics have been noted to provide differentiation in most cases between true and false aneurysms. In general, true aneurysms tend to involve the anterior wall, whereas false aneurysms tend to involve the inferior wall. True aneurysms (Fig. 28-21) are known to have a wide neck that is similar or wider in diameter compared with the base of the aneurysm, whereas false aneurysms, representing a contained rupture, typically have a narrow neck (Fig. 28-22). Ultimately, however, the real distinction between the two is the presence of residual myocardium forming the boundary of the lesion in the case of a true aneurysm or the lack thereof in a false aneurysm. This distinction may be made with standard cine and DE-MRI. Visualization of the wall of the aneurysm as separate and distinct from the pericardium is usually possible with cine MRI. Conversely, if the pericardium appears to make up the boundary of the aneurysm without residual myocardium, the lesion should be deemed a false aneurysm. DE-MRI is also helpful in that pericardial enhancement has been described as occurring frequently in false aneurysms, with a lower incidence in true aneurysms. Both true and false aneurysms may have associated mural thrombus (see Fig. 28-22).

Key Points

1. Contrast-enhanced CMR using the DE-MRI technique is the most sensitive means of detecting thrombus and detects more than twice as many thrombi as does echocardiography.
2. Patients with ischemic cardiomyopathy are at significantly greater risk for the development of thrombi than are patients with nonischemic cardiomyopathy.
3. Thrombi are often found adherent to sites of earlier infarction, and infarcts greater than 50% in transmural extent are at increased risk.

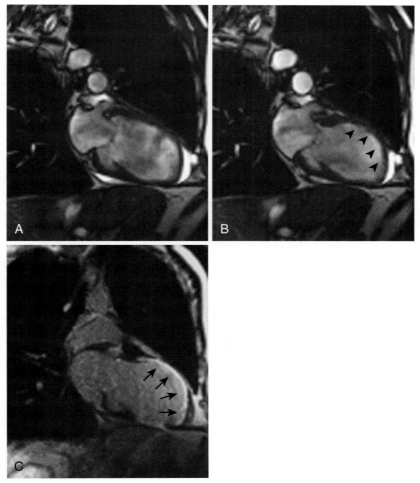

Figure 28-21 Images from a patient with a true aneurysm of the anterior wall and apex. Two-chamber cine images in diastole (**A**) and systole (**B**). The anterior wall and apex are aneurysmal and balloon out in systole *(arrowheads)*. Delayed enhancement magnetic resonance imaging in the two-chamber view (**C**) shows hyperenhancement of the anterior wall and apex consistent with scar *(arrows)*. Note the anterior wall location and the broad opening of the aneurysm.

4. Ventricular aneurysms are common, and true and false aneurysms can usually be accurately distinguished on CMR imaging.

■ DIFFERENTIATION BETWEEN ISCHEMIC AND NONISCHEMIC HEART DISEASE

With its exquisite sensitivity to small areas of scarring, DE-MRI has proven useful not only for the evaluation of ischemic heart disease, but also for the assessment of many nonischemic cardiomyopathies, as outlined in other chapters. DE-MRI also allows differentiation of ischemic from nonischemic cardiomyopathies, based on various patterns of hyperenhancement. Central to this use of DE-MRI is the concept of a CAD-type pattern of hyperenhancement. This pattern reflects the pathophysiology of ischemia, as described later.

Following coronary occlusion, myocardial contractility falls within seconds throughout the area at risk, which is the ischemic zone with reduced perfusion. Although blood begins to flow by way of preexisting collateral vessels (vascular channels that interconnect ordinary arteries), collateral flow is lowest and myocardial oxygen consumption is highest in the subendocardium. As a consequence, ischemia is most severe and necrosis begins first in the subendocardium, starting approximately 15 to 20 minutes after total occlusion. Necrosis then progresses as a wavefront toward the epicardium over the next few hours. During this period, the size of the area at risk remains the same, but the size of the infarcted region within the area at risk increases continuously toward a transmural infarction (Fig. 28-23).

Another facet of the wavefront phenomenon is that increasing the duration or severity of ischemic injury generally increases the transmurality of infarction, but the circumferential extent of infarction is not enlarged appreciably because the lateral margins are established relatively early in the ischemic period. Therefore, an ischemic-type or CAD-type pattern of hyperenhancement should always involve the subendocardium and should be located in a region that is consistent with the perfusion territory of an epicardial coronary artery. Figure 28-24 shows representative DE-MRI images of infarctions in the various coronary territories. DE-MRI

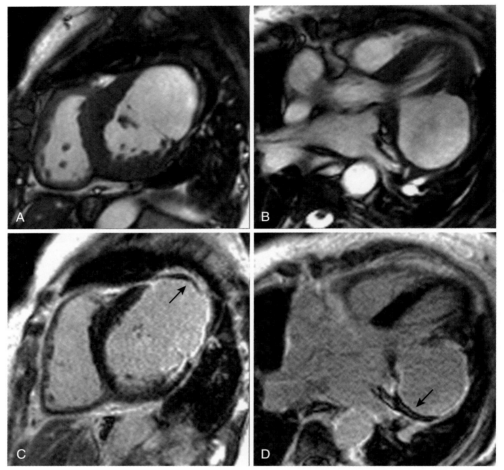

Figure 28-22 Images from a patient with a false aneurysm of the anterolateral wall at the base. Short-axis (**A**) and four-chamber cine (**B**) images and are compared with matched delayed enhancement magnetic resonance imaging images (**C** and **D**). Note the narrow opening of the false aneurysm compared with its base, a finding reflecting its nature as a contained rupture of the myocardium. In a false aneurysm, the retaining margin of the aneurysm is the pericardium. Note also the dark region along the margin of the lesion in **C** and **D** that represents a mural thrombus *(arrow)*.

studies that do not show such a pattern are likely the result of nonischemic cardiomyopathy. This information can be very useful in the stepwise assessment of cardiomyopathies.

Stepwise Approach to Differentiation of Cardiomyopathies

This approach is based on the following three steps:

Step 1. The presence or absence of hyperenhancement is determined. In the subset of patients with long-standing severe ischemic cardiomyopathy, the data indicate that virtually all patients had an earlier MI. The implication is that in patients with severe cardiomyopathy but without hyperenhancement, the diagnosis of idiopathic dilated cardiomyopathy should be strongly considered.

Step 2. If hyperenhancement is present, the location and distribution of hyperenhancement should be classified as a CAD or non-CAD pattern. For this determination, the concept that ischemic injury progresses as a wavefront from the subendocardium to the epicardium is crucial. Correspondingly, hyperenhancement patterns that spare the subendocardium and are limited to the middle or epicardial portion of the LV wall are clearly in a non-CAD pattern.

Step 3. If hyperenhancement is present in a non-CAD pattern, further classification should be considered. As described earlier, emerging data suggest certain nonischemic cardiomyopathies have predilection for specific scar patterns. For example, in the setting of LV hypertrophy, the presence of midwall hyperenhancement in one or both junctions of the interventricular septum with the RV free wall is highly suggestive of hypertrophic cardiomyopathy, whereas midwall or epicardial hyperenhancement in the inferolateral wall suggests Anderson-Fabry disease. Moreover, instead of an infinite variety of hyperenhancement patterns, it appears that broad stratification is possible into a limited number of common delayed enhancement phenotypes. Figure 28-25 provides a diagrammatic pattern recognition approach to the different common phenotypic patterns. Table 28-3 describes the diagnostic features of various cardiomyopathies.

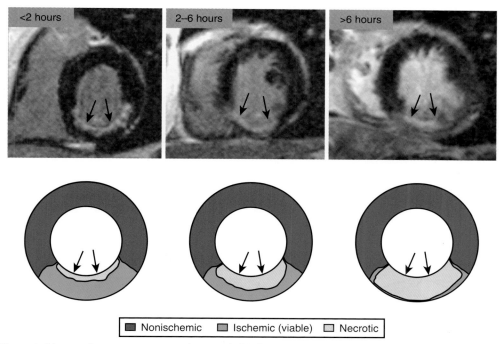

Figure 28-23 The typical hyperenhancement pattern of myocardial infarction can be explained by the pathophysiology of ischemia. Little or no cellular necrosis is found until about 15 minutes after occlusion. Over the next few hours, a wavefront of necrosis begins in the subendocardium and moves progressively toward the epicardium. During this period, the infarcted region *(arrows)* within the ischemic zone increases continuously and ultimately can become transmural. (From Mahrholdt H, Wagner A, Judd RM, et al. Delayed-enhancement cardiovascular magnetic resonance assessment of non-ischaemic cardiomyopathies. *Eur Heart J.* 2005;26:1464.)

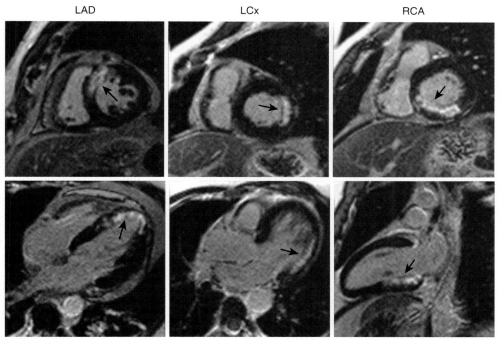

Figure 28-24 Delayed enhancement magnetic resonance imaging of infarctions *(arrows)* in the left anterior descending (LAD), left circumflex (LCx), and right coronary artery (RCA) territories. In each case, a subendocardial component is evident.

HYPERENHANCEMENT PATTERNS

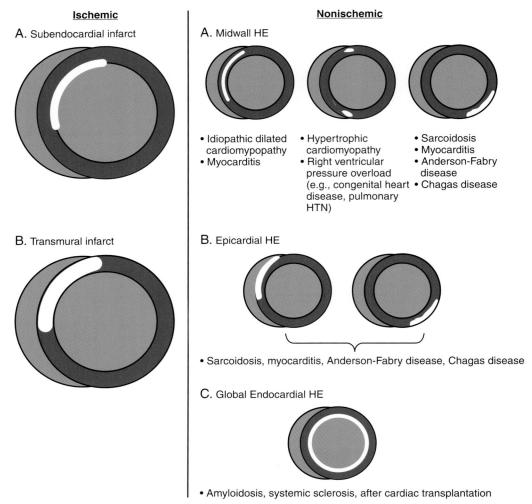

Figure 28-25 Representations of hyperenhancement patterns that are characteristic of ischemic and nonischemic disorders. Because myocardial necrosis resulting from coronary artery disease progresses as a wavefront from the subendocardium toward the epicardium, when hyperenhancement (HE) is present (white regions), the subendocardium should be involved in patients who have ischemic heart disease. Isolated midwall or epicardial hyperenhancement strongly suggests a nonischemic origin. *HTN,* Hypertension. (From Shah DJ, Judd RM, Kim RJ, et al. Magnetic resonance of myocardial viability. In: Edelman RR, Hesselink JR, Zlatkin MI, eds. *Clinical Magnetic Resonance Imaging.* 3rd ed. New York: Elsevier; 2005.)

Table 28-3   Diagnostic Features of Various Cardiomyopathies

Suspected Diagnosis	Cine Imaging	DE-MRI	Other
Amyloidosis	Thick ventricles, dilated atria	Diffuse subendocardial enhancement	Difficulty finding "null" point on inversion time scout sequence
ARVD	Large RV with poor function, microaneurysms	RV HE in two thirds	RV enhancement, fat
Fabry disease	Concentric hypertrophy	Midwall HE inferolateral wall at the base	Male predominance
HCM	Asymmetric, concentric or apical	Positive at RV insertion sites and in regions of thickening	
Myocarditis	Focal thickening, wall motion abnormality	Lateral epicardial or septal midwall HE common	T2-weighted imaging sometimes helpful
Sarcoidosis	Focal thickening, wall motion abnormality	Patchy uptake with slight basal or septal predominance	Mediastinal or hilar adenopathy often noted on morphologic images

ARVD, Arrhythmogenic right ventricular dysplasia; *DE-MRI,* delayed enhancement magnetic resonance imaging; *HCM,* hypertrophic cardiomyopathy; *HE,* hyperenhancement; *RV,* right ventricular.

Key Points

1. The DE-MRI hyperenhancement pattern seen with CAD reflects the pathophysiology of ischemia and proceeds in a wavefront from the subendocardium to involve a variably transmural portion of myocardium.
2. Myocardial dysfunction lacking this pattern is likely caused by nonischemic cardiomyopathy.
3. DE-MRI pattern recognition often allows a specific diagnosis of nonischemic disease.

Bibliography

Albert TS, Kim RJ, Judd RM. Assessment of no-reflow regions using cardiac MRI. *Basic Res Cardiol.* 2006;101:383-390.

Aletras AH, Tilak GS, Natanzon A, et al. Retrospective determination of the area at risk for reperfused acute myocardial infarction with T2-weighted cardiac magnetic resonance imaging: histopathological and displacement encoding with stimulated echoes (DENSE) functional validations. *Circulation.* 2006;113:1865-1870.

Arai AE. Using magnetic resonance imaging to characterize recent myocardial injury: utility in acute coronary syndrome and other clinical scenarios. *Circulation.* 2008;118:795-796.

Beek AM, Kuhl HP, Bondarenko O, et al. Delayed contrast-enhanced magnetic resonance imaging for the prediction of regional functional improvement after acute myocardial infarction. *J Am Coll Cardiol.* 2003;42:895-901.

Choi KM, Kim RJ, Gubernikoff G, Vargas JD, Parker M, Judd RM. Transmural extent of acute myocardial infarction predicts long-term improvement in contractile function. *Circulation.* 2001;104:1101-1107.

Eitel I, Desch S, Fuernau G, et al. Prognostic significance and determinants of myocardial salvage assessed by cardiovascular magnetic resonance in acute reperfused myocardial infarction. *J Am Coll Cardiol.* 2010;55:2470-2479.

Hundley WG, Bluemke DA, Finn JP, et al. ACCF/ACR/AHA/NASCI/SCMR 2010 expert consensus document on cardiovascular magnetic resonance: a report of the American College of Cardiology Foundation Task Force on Expert Consensus Documents. *Circulation.* 2010;121:2462-2508.

Ingkanisorn WP, Kwong RY, Bohme NS, et al. Prognosis of negative adenosine stress magnetic resonance in patients presenting to an emergency department with chest pain. *J Am Coll Cardiol.* 2006;47:1427-1432.

Jahnke C, Nagel E, Gebker R, et al. Prognostic value of cardiac magnetic resonance stress tests: adenosine stress perfusion and dobutamine stress wall motion imaging. *Circulation.* 2007;115:1769-1776.

Kim HW, Farzaneh-Far A, Kim RJ. Cardiovascular magnetic resonance in patients with myocardial infarction: current and emerging applications. *J Am Coll Cardiol.* 2009;55:1-16.

Kim HW, Klem I, Shah DJ, et al. Unrecognized non-Q-wave myocardial infarction: prevalence and prognostic significance in patients with suspected coronary disease. *PLoS Med.* 2009;6:e1000057.

Kim RJ, Fieno DS, Parrish TB, et al. Relationship of MRI delayed contrast enhancement to irreversible injury, infarct age, and contractile function. *Circulation.* 1999;100:1992-2002.

Kim RJ, Shah DJ. Fundamental concepts in myocardial viability assessment revisited: when knowing how much is "alive" is not enough. *Heart.* 2004;90:137-140.

Kim RJ, Shah DJ, Judd RM. How we perform delayed enhancement imaging. *J Cardiovasc Magn Reson.* 2003;5:505-514.

Kim RJ, Wu E, Rafael A, et al. The use of contrast-enhanced magnetic resonance imaging to identify reversible myocardial dysfunction. *N Engl J Med.* 2000;343:1445-1453.

Klem I, Heitner JF, Shah DJ, et al. Improved detection of coronary artery disease by stress perfusion cardiovascular magnetic resonance with the use of delayed enhancement infarction imaging. *J Am Coll Cardiol.* 2006;47:1630-1638.

Konen E, Merchant N, Gutierrez C, et al. True versus false left ventricular aneurysm: differentiation with MR imaging—initial experience. *Radiology.* 2005;236:65-70.

Kwong RY, Sattar H, Wu H, et al. Incidence and prognostic implication of unrecognized myocardial scar characterized by cardiac magnetic resonance in diabetic patients without clinical evidence of myocardial infarction. *Circulation.* 2008;118:1011-1020.

Kwong RY, Schussheim AE, Rekhraj S, et al. Detecting acute coronary syndrome in the emergency department with cardiac magnetic resonance imaging. *Circulation.* 2003;107:531-537.

Larose E, Rodes-Cabau J, Pibarot P, et al. Predicting late myocardial recovery and outcomes in the early hours of ST-segment elevation myocardial infarction traditional measures compared with microvascular obstruction, salvaged myocardium, and necrosis characteristics by cardiovascular magnetic resonance. *J Am Coll Cardiol.* 2010;55:2459-2469.

Mahrholdt H, Goedecke C, Wagner A, et al. Cardiovascular magnetic resonance assessment of human myocarditis: a comparison to histology and molecular pathology. *Circulation.* 2004;109:1250-1258.

Mahrholdt H, Wagner A, Judd RM, Sechtem U, Kim RJ. Delayed enhancement cardiovascular magnetic resonance assessment of non-ischaemic cardiomyopathies. *Eur Heart J.* 2005;26:1461-1474.

Nijveldt R, Beek AM, Hirsch A, et al. Functional recovery after acute myocardial infarction: comparison between angiography, electrocardiography, and cardiovascular magnetic resonance measures of microvascular injury. *J Am Coll Cardiol.* 2008;52:181-189.

Schvartzman PR, Srichai MB, Grimm RA, et al. Nonstress delayed-enhancement magnetic resonance imaging of the myocardium predicts improvement of function after revascularization for chronic ischemic heart disease with left ventricular dysfunction. *Am Heart J.* 2003;146:535-541.

Schwitter J, Nanz D, Kneifel S, et al. Assessment of myocardial perfusion in coronary artery disease by magnetic resonance: a comparison with positron emission tomography and coronary angiography. *Circulation.* 2001;103:2230-2235.

Schwitter J, Wacker CM, van Rossum AC, et al. MR-IMPACT: comparison of perfusion-cardiac magnetic resonance with single-photon emission computed tomography for the detection of coronary artery disease in a multicentre, multivendor, randomized trial. *Eur Heart J.* 2008;29:480-489.

Shah DJ, Kim HW, Kim RJ. Evaluation of ischemic heart disease. *Heart Fail Clin.* 2009;5:315-332:v.

Sievers B, Rehwald WG, Albert TS, et al. Respiratory motion and cardiac arrhythmia effects on diagnostic accuracy of myocardial delayed-enhanced MR imaging in canines. *Radiology.* 2008;247:106-114.

Simonetti OP, Kim RJ, Fieno DS, et al. An improved MR imaging technique for the visualization of myocardial infarction. *Radiology.* 2001;218:215-223.

Srichai MB, Junor C, Rodriguez LL, et al. Clinical, imaging, and pathological characteristics of left ventricular thrombus: a comparison of contrast-enhanced magnetic resonance imaging, transthoracic echocardiography, and transesophageal echocardiography with surgical or pathological validation. *Am Heart J.* 2006;152:75-84.

Stuber M, Weiss RG. Coronary magnetic resonance angiography. *J Magn Reson Imaging.* 2007;26:219-234.

Wagner A, Mahrholdt H, Holly TA, et al. Contrast-enhanced MRI and routine single photon emission computed tomography (SPECT) perfusion imaging for detection of subendocardial myocardial infarcts: an imaging study. *Lancet.* 2003;361:374-379.

Weinsaft JW, Kim HW, Shah DJ, et al. Detection of left ventricular thrombus by delayed-enhancement cardiovascular magnetic resonance prevalence and markers in patients with systolic dysfunction. *J Am Coll Cardiol.* 2008;52:148-157.

Weinsaft JW, Klem I, Judd RM. MRI for the assessment of myocardial viability *Cardiol Clin.* 2007;25:35-56.v.

Wince WB, Kim RJ. Molecular imaging: T2-weighted CMR of the area at risk: a risky business? *Nat Rev Cardiol.* 2010;7:547-549.

Wu KC, Kim RJ, Bluemke DA, et al. Quantification and time course of microvascular obstruction by contrast-enhanced echocardiography and magnetic resonance imaging following acute myocardial infarction and reperfusion. *J Am Coll Cardiol.* 1998;32:1756-1764.

CHAPTER 29

Myocardial Ischemic Disease: Nuclear

Sharmila Dorbala and Angela S. Koh

Myocardial perfusion imaging (MPI), using single photon emission computed tomography (SPECT) or positron emission tomography (PET) radionuclide techniques, is a commonly performed diagnostic imaging test to detect coronary artery disease (CAD) and determine risk of future events in patients with suspected or known CAD. The diagnostic and prognostic value of normal and abnormal MPI tests has been supported by many studies in the literature. This chapter explores the evaluation of patients with preclinical CAD, established chronic CAD, and acute chest pain evaluation, as well as postmyocardial infarction (MI) risk stratification and evaluation of myocardial viability.

■ PRECLINICAL CORONARY ATHEROSCLEROSIS

Key Questions

1. Does a role exist for radionuclide testing in asymptomatic patients for coronary atherosclerosis?
2. What are the modalities available for detection of preclinical coronary atherosclerosis?

Although robust medical literature supports the use of stress imaging for evaluation of symptomatic patients with known or suspected CAD, literature supporting testing in asymptomatic patients is not widely available. Various tests are available for the detection of subclinical atherosclerosis in asymptomatic patients with coronary risk factors (Box 29-1).

Practical Aspects

In patients with coronary risk factors, coronary atherosclerosis progresses gradually over the course of several decades. At the early stages, coronary risk factors can result in endothelial dysfunction with or without epicardial coronary artery narrowing. Subsequently, atherosclerosis can become evident initially as vessel wall abnormalities with preserved luminal diameter. With further progression of atherosclerosis, the outward remodeling process reaches a limit, and luminal encroachment ensues. Most results of tests of ischemia are positive at a stage in which atherosclerosis causes luminal narrowing and myocardial ischemia (Fig. 29-1). However, several studies have shown that nonobstructive coronary artery lesions can indeed lead to MI and associated complications from rupture of vulnerable albeit nonobstructive CAD. Thus, interest in identifying nonobstructive coronary plaque with imaging techniques is growing, but more evidence is needed to understand whether the identification of nonobstructive CAD in asymptomatic individuals is warranted. Although the idea is not without controversy, selected subsets of asymptomatic subjects may be considered appropriate for nuclear perfusion imaging, such as individuals with high coronary heart disease risk (Adult Treatment Panel III [ATP III] risk criteria) or high CAD risk with an Agatston score (coronary calcium score [CCS]) of 100 to 400 or persons with an Agatston score higher than 400.

Radionuclide imaging is widely used in research applications as a tool to identify preclinical atherosclerosis in asymptomatic individuals. Using quantitative PET, absolute myocardial blood flow can be quantified at rest and during peak stress. The coronary flow reserve (CFR; a unitless number) is computed as the ratio of hyperemic myocardial blood flow (after stress) to resting myocardial blood flow. Quantification of myocardial blood flow is better with radiotracers that are extracted linearly in relation to flow. Oxygen-15 (O-15) water is an ideal tracer for quantification of myocardial blood flow. Quantification of absolute myocardial blood flow is well validated with nitrogen-13 (N-13) ammonia, O-15 water, and rubidium-82 (Rb-82).

Abnormalities in myocardial blood flow have been reported in patients with coronary risk factors but without overt cardiovascular disease. The finding of abnormal CFR is the earliest abnormality associated with CAD and is an integrated parameter of endothelial function

---

BOX 29-1 Noninvasive Tools to Detect Subclinical Atherosclerosis in Asymptomatic Patients With Coronary Risk Factors

Treadmill exercise test
Single photon emission computed tomography or positron emission tomography myocardial perfusion imaging
Computed tomography coronary calcium scoring
Computed tomography coronary angiography
Endothelial or microvascular dysfunction
Carotid ultrasound
Ankle brachial index

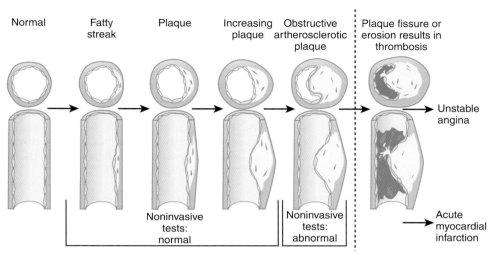

Normal Fatty streak Plaque Increasing plaque Obstructive artherosclerotic plaque Plaque fissure or erosion results in thrombosis

Noninvasive tests: normal

Noninvasive tests: abnormal

→ Unstable angina

→ Acute myocardial infarction

Figure 29-1 Progression of coronary atherosclerosis. Traditionally noninvasive tests become abnormal when atherosclerosis causes luminal narrowing and myocardial ischemia. However, coronary computed tomography angiography has the potential to detect early noncalcified or calcified plaque with positive remodeling before it causes luminal narrowing. (From Abrams J. Clinical practice. Chronic stable angina. *N Engl J Med.* 2005;352:2524-33.)

and endothelium-independent vascular smooth muscle relaxation. Changes in regional myocardial blood flow may also result from loss of myocytes, fibrosis, scar tissue formation, or high-grade stenosis of the epicardial coronary vessel. Measurement of flow responses to physiologic or pharmacologic challenges is done by PET and can be used to identify functional alterations of preclinical coronary atherosclerosis. Abnormal vasodilator response and reduced flow have been found in asymptomatic patients who are at high risk of CAD, with significant correlation between impairment of CFR and severity of lipid profile. Well-controlled studies of patients with isolated risk factors, such as diabetes, hypertension, smoking, postmenopausal state, and a family history of premature coronary atherosclerosis have been shown to demonstrate abnormalities in CFR in response to vasodilator stress agents (predominantly endothelium-independent flow abnormalities) or cold pressor testing (endothelium-dependent mechanisms). Furthermore, in one study, CFR was inversely related to the Framingham risk score (measuring a composite of risk factor burden), and patients with the highest tertile of Framingham risk score demonstrated the lowest CFR. Noninvasively estimated CFR measured using rest and vasodilator PET is also a very useful tool in assessing response to therapy after aggressive treatment of coronary risk factors.

■ ACUTE CORONARY SYNDROMES

Key Questions

1. In which groups of patients with acute chest pain can MPI be used for diagnosis?
2. What are the benefits of MPI testing beyond diagnosing CAD in patients with suspected or known acute coronary syndrome (ACS)?

Radionuclide MPI can be used in patients with acute chest pain and suspected ACS (low to intermediate risk), as well as for risk stratification and ischemia detection in a stable patient following a definite ACS diagnosis. For patients with acute chest pain and suspected ACS (low to intermediate risk), the role of radionuclide MPI is to

provide diagnostic and risk stratification information to direct management strategies.

In patients with acute and ongoing chest pain at rest, MPI may be performed using technetium-99m (Tc-99m) tracer injection during or soon after resolution of chest pain. Because of the minimal redistribution, the images reflect myocardial blood flow at the time of injection. This algorithm has been associated with a high negative predictive value for ruling out MI and was also useful for triage of patients presenting to the emergency department. An MPI-guided strategy was associated with reductions in unnecessary admission of patients, lower costs, and shorter lengths of stay. More recently, imaging of ischemic memory has been considered in patients with acute chest pain. Dilsizian et al demonstrated that using iodine-123 (I-123)–labeled 15-(p-iodo-phenyl)-3-R s-methylpentadecanoic acid (BMIPP), defects in fatty acid metabolism could be identified as long as 24 hours after an ischemic episode. More recently, BMIPP was used in the evaluation of patients with acute chest pain in the emergency department. The study demonstrated that in patients who presented to the emergency department with acute chest pain, compared with clinical variables alone, the addition of BMIPP SPECT scan was able to increase the sensitivity (from 43% to 81%) of diagnosing ACS, with higher negative (62% to 83%) and positive (41% to 58%) predictive values.

In patients with recent definite ACS (>48 hours and <3months), MPI may be used for risk stratification and management. The absence of reversible defects identifies a low-risk cohort, whereas the presence of reversible defects is a predictor of cardiac events for which coronary intervention may alter outcome. The Adenosine Sestamibi Post Infarction Evaluation (INSPIRE) trial was a large multicenter prospective randomized study that enrolled stable patients with ST-segment elevation MI or non–ST-segment elevation MI that used adenosine Tc-99m sestamibi SPECT as an initial noninvasive method for risk assessment and guidance for subsequent therapy. Expedited imaging was performed early (between 2 and 4 days from hospital admission), with no reported adverse events in these patients. The results of INSPIRE demonstrated that early SPECT MPI testing was able to stratify patients reliably into low-, intermediate-, and high-risk groups. Event rates at 1 year were lowest in patients with the smallest perfusion defects, but the event rates progressively increased when the defect size exceeded 20%. The rates of total cardiac events or death and reinfarction significantly increased within each INSPIRE risk group from low (5.4%, 1.8%), to intermediate (14%, 9.2%), to high (18.6%, 11.6%) ($P < .01$). The perfusion results significantly improved risk stratification beyond that provided by clinical and ejection fraction (EF) variables.

Practical Aspects

Patients With Suspected Acute Coronary Syndrome

- Patients at low to intermediate risk of ACS who are medically stable can be risk stratified by stress MPI, whereas patients with high-risk clinical characteristics in the setting of unstable angina or non–ST-segment elevation MI are recommended to undergo an early invasive strategy with cardiac catheterization. Patients with indeterminate clinical presentations are candidates for chest pain imaging with rest MPI.
- These subjects should be injected with radiotracer as soon as possible after chest pain resolution and preferably during chest pain.
- In this context, attenuation-corrected MPI can provide incremental value. Tc-99m tetrofosmin does not need preparation of the kit and may be better suited for this application. Thallium-201 (Tl-201) offers the advantage of having tracer available for use when needed (because of its 73-hour half-life), but it may be fraught with difficulties related to attenuation artifacts.
- The presence of a perfusion defect on a chest pain myocardial perfusion study does not differentiate between an earlier MI and a new perfusion defect from acute ischemia. Hence, patients with an earlier MI or Q waves on the electrocardiogram (ECG) are not optimal candidates for chest pain radionuclide study.
- Stress MPI in low- to intermediate-risk patients without infarct or ischemia in the presence of normal left ventricular (LV) function are at low risk of adverse outcome and can be managed conservatively, whereas patients found to have substantial inducible ischemia may be selected for cardiac catheterization.

Patients With Recently Diagnosed Acute Coronary Syndrome

- MPI may be used in the triage of patients who suffered unstable angina or an acute MI before hospital discharge; rest and vasodilator MPI may be considered for the risk stratification of patients without earlier coronary angiography or with coronary angiography but with incomplete coronary revascularization.
- In addition, sometimes viability assessment with SPECT or PET is performed in some of these patients (e.g., with late clinical presentation of ST-segment elevation MI) before consideration of coronary revascularization.

- Typically, because exercise increases myocardial oxygen demand, treadmill exercise testing is performed using a submaximal modified Bruce protocol (see Chapter 5). In contrast, vasodilator pharmacologic stress with adenosine or dipyridamole induces coronary hyperemia with minimal increase in oxygen demand. Hence, in the immediate post-MI phase, rest and vasodilator MPI is ideally suited for risk stratification and evaluation of ischemic burden even in patients who are able to exercise. Vasodilator stress testing has been demonstrated to be safe as early as 48 hours after an uncomplicated MI.

■ CHRONIC CORONARY ARTERY DISEASE

Key Questions

1. What is the diagnostic accuracy of radionuclide MPI?
2. What is the prognostic value of radionuclide MPI?
3. Is radionuclide MPI cost effective?

Diagnostic Accuracy, Sensitivity, and Specificity of Single Photon Emission Computed Tomography and Positron Emission Tomography Myocardial Perfusion Imaging

Extensive literature evaluating the sensitivity and specificity of SPECT MPI for detecting obstructive CAD has been published over the years. Pooled analysis of patients with known or suspected CAD demonstrated mean sensitivity and specificity of 87% and 73%, respectively, of exercise myocardial SPECT for detecting more than 50% stenosis. SPECT MPI provides incremental diagnostic value over exercise ECG testing in various patient cohorts. In patients with interpretable ECGs, the Duke treadmill score is able to separate patients into low-, intermediate-, and high-risk groups for future cardiac events. Within each of these Duke treadmill score risk categories, SPECT MPI is able to risk stratify patients further based on summed stress score (SSS) categories. Patients with low- and high-risk Duke treadmill scores may not require nuclear testing because the former group was found to have an extremely low event rate (0.9%), whereas the latter group usually proceeded with cardiac catheterization. In contrast, patients in the larger intermediate-risk category who had a cardiac event rate of 2.5% could be further stratified based on SSS. Those who had normal scans had an event rate of 0.4%, whereas those who had an SSS of 4 to 8 and an SSS of more than 8 had cardiac event rates of 6.4% and 8.9%, respectively.

The literature relating to the diagnostic value of PET MPI is more limited. One study directly comparing the diagnostic accuracy of Rb-82 myocardial perfusion PET and Tl-201 or Tc-99m SPECT showed higher sensitivity with PET than with SPECT (93% versus 76%) and similar specificity (78% versus 80%). However, Stewart et al observed a higher specificity for PET than with SPECT (83% versus 53%, respectively) without significant differences in sensitivity (86% versus 84%, respectively). The overall diagnostic accuracy is also higher for PET than for SPECT using either a 50% or a 70% angiographic threshold (87% versus 71% with a 50% threshold and 89% versus 79% with a 70% threshold), primarily driven by higher specificity. The average positive and negative predictive values of PET MPI for the diagnosis of obstructive CAD are 94% (range, 80% to 100%) and 73% (range, 36% to 100%), respectively.

Attenuation Artifacts Limit the Diagnostic Accuracy of Single Photon Emission Computed Tomography Myocardial Perfusion Imaging

Emitted photons undergo attenuation (absorption or deflection by soft tissues) when they traverse various soft tissue structures (muscle, adipose tissue, bone, breast, and diaphragm) before they reach the photo detectors of the gamma camera. This process of photon attenuation may result in lower sensitivity and specificity for the detection of CAD. Strategies to address attenuation include measurement and correction of soft tissue densities by using transmission scanning by external radioactive sources or cardiac computed tomography (CT). Attenuation correction improves the count uniformity of the image and helps distinguish attenuation artifacts from real defects. In stress-only imaging, if the stress images are normal, attenuation correction offers the possibility to skip the rest imaging and hence reduces time, cost, and radiation dose to the patient. In addition, quantitative estimation of myocardial blood flow in milliliters per gram per minute can be performed because accurate attenuation correction allows for precise measurements of absolute radiotracer concentration in the myocardium.

The disadvantages of using external radionuclide source transmission scans include additional radiation exposure (albeit small) associated with transmission scans that take longer to acquire and degradation of the radionuclide source over time that can diminish image quality. Conversely, CT attenuation correction is rapid (takes a few seconds) and of excellent quality, but it is also associated with additional radiation exposure (albeit small) and is more prone to misregistration with the emission images (as discussed later).

RADIONUCLIDE ATTENUATION CORRECTION
Studies showed that SPECT MPI with radionuclide attenuation correction compared with non–attenuation-corrected images is associated with better test specificity while maintaining sensitivity to detect obstructive CAD. Attenuation correction also increases the normalcy rate, a term used to define the percentage of normal studies in a low-risk cohort. Although publications have demonstrated the improved prognostic capability of attenuation-corrected SPECT MPI, widespread clinical adaptation of radionuclide attenuation correction with SPECT MPI has been slow. In contrast, PET MPI images without attenuation correction are significantly degraded by attenuation and are not interpreted clinically or for research purposes. As a result, PET MPI with radionuclide attenuation correction has been widely used clinically and for research applications.

Attenuation-corrected PET MPI has diagnostic and prognostic value. The sensitivity and specificity of attenuation-corrected PET MPI for the diagnosis of obstructive epicardial CAD are very high (a weighted sensitivity of 90% and specificity of 89% for the detection of a single coronary artery stenosis of >50%). Overall, when compared with the published data for SPECT imaging, current data suggest a higher diagnostic accuracy for PET MPI with a higher specificity for the diagnosis of CAD.

COMPUTED TOMOGRAPHY–BASED ATTENUATION CORRECTION
SPECT-CT and PET-CT use low-dose x-ray transmission CT for attenuation correction, rather than an external radiation source. As previously mentioned, misregistration of CT attenuation-corrected and SPECT or PET MPI images may result from inherent differences in image resolution between CT and SPECT or PET MPI. Accurate registration is critical for improving the diagnostic yield of CT attenuation-corrected MPI. SPECT-CT MPI has been validated in patients with and without underlying CAD. Compared with uncorrected images, attenuation-corrected SPECT-CT MPI had improvements in specificity and normalcy. Figure 29-2 demonstrates the effect of attenuation correction using a hybrid SPECT-CT system. In patients with CAD, Sampson et al showed, in an Rb-82 PET-CT MPI study, that the sensitivity, specificity, and normalcy rates of MPI in 64 consecutive patients with intermediate risk of CAD who underwent coronary angiography following stress testing were 93%, 83%, and 100%, respectively. In addition, in 1433 patients, gated Rb-82 PET-CT MPI was associated with an excellent outcome in patients with a normal scan, but the investigators found increased event rates in patients with mild, moderate, and severely abnormal scans.

Risk Stratification

Both PET and SPECT MPI provide important prognostic information. Risk assessment with radionuclide MPI is based on stress variables and MPI variables. The stress variables that predict high risk are listed in Box 29-2. Functional capacity is a very powerful predictor of adverse outcomes and should be carefully reviewed and reported.

Single Photon Emission Computed Tomography Myocardial Perfusion Imaging

The important MPI determinants of risk in patients with CAD are the extent of jeopardized myocardium, LV function, and other high-risk features. The extent and severity of perfusion defects are powerful predictors of outcome. Normal scans reflect a good prognosis, and abnormal scans reflect a poor prognosis. Further, the prognostic value of a given normal or abnormal scan result is modulated by patient-related factors, LVEF, and other high-risk scan features.

A meta-analysis that included 19 studies of more than 39,000 patients with an average 2.3-year follow-up found an event rate of 0.6% with a normal SPECT MPI result (64). The "warranty period" of a normal SPECT MPI study is considered to be approximately 2 years; however, patients with a history of CAD, pharmacologic stress, diabetes, and female gender appear to have higher

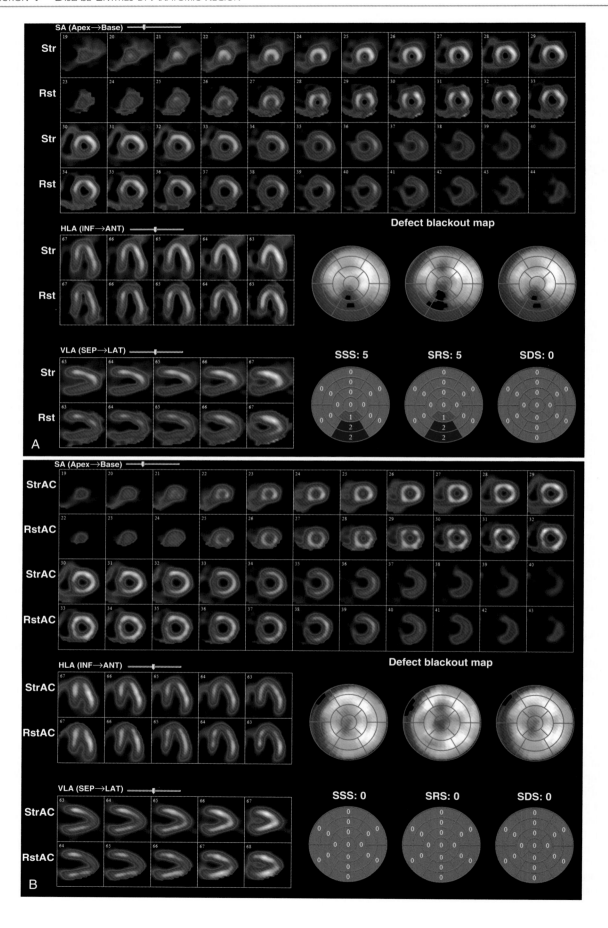

Figure 29-2 Attenuation correction with technetium-99m (Tc-99m)-sestamibi single photon emission computed tomography and computed tomography (SPECT) and computed tomography (CT). Tc-99m SPECT and CT images without attenuation correction (**A**) and with attenuation correction (**B**) are shown. The images without attenuation correction (**A**) demonstrate a medium-sized fixed perfusion defect in the entire inferior wall, likely caused by diaphragmatic attenuation, and this defect is corrected on the CT-based attenuation correction images (**B**). *ANT*, Anterior; *HLA*, horizontal long axis; *INF*, inferior; *LAT*, lateral; *Rst*, rest; *RstAC*, rest with attenuation correction; *SA*, short axis; *SEP*, septal; *Str*, stress; *StrAC*, stress with attenuation correction; *VLA*, vertical long axis.

In this figure, as well as in Figures 29-3, 29-6, 29-7, 29-8, and 29-13, paired stress *(top)* and rest *(bottom)* perfusion images are arranged in short-axis (apex to base), horizontal long-axis (inferior to anterior wall), and vertical long-axis (septum to lateral wall) views. Bull's eye plots *(middle panels, first row)* are created representing stress *(first plot from the left)*, rest *(middle plot)*, and reversibility *(third plot on the extreme right)*. The *bottom row* bull's eye plots display the summed stress score (SSS, fixed and reversible), summed rest score (SRS, fixed), and summed difference score (SDS, reversibility).

BOX 29-2   High-Risk Stress Variables

Duration of symptom limiting exercise <5 METs

Failure to increase SBP >120 mm Hg or a sustained decrease ≥10 mm Hg or lower than at rest during progressive exercise

ST-segment depression ≥2 mm, down sloping, at <5 METs, ≥5 leads, ≥5 minutes into recovery

Exercise-induced ST-segment elevation

Angina at low workloads

Sustained (>30 seconds) or symptomatic ventricular tachycardia

Poor heart rate recovery (<12 beats/minute)

Chronotropic incompetence

From Chaitman BR. Exercise stress testing. In: Libby P, Bonow RO, Mann DP, Zipes DP, editors. *Braunwald's Heart Disease: A Textbook of Cardiovascular Medicine.* Philadelphia: Saunders; 2008:195-226.

METs, Metabolic equivalents; *SBP,* systolic blood pressure.

---

event rates during year 2 after the index SPECT study. Patients with abnormal and high-risk MPI scans have much higher event rates (Figs. 29-3 and 29-4). The presence and extent of reversible defects on stress MPI reflect jeopardized myocardium at risk for future damage. The number of myocardial segments with reversible defects has been reported to be the best predictor of future cardiac events, over clinical and angiographic data.

LVEF is the most direct measure of LV systolic function, and measurement of resting EF has been shown to be a crucial predictor of future cardiac events. Sharir et al reported on the incremental prognostic value of poststress LVEF by gated SPECT MPI. In a study of 1680 patients, these investigators demonstrated that for any given degree of scan abnormality, patients with an EF of less than 45% had higher rates of cardiac death. Similarly, LV volumes (>70 mL) were also important for risk stratification. These variables were predictive of worse outcomes among patients undergoing exercise stress or adenosine stress.

Several other markers of high risk have been identified on MPI (Table 29-1). The presence of transient ischemic dilation of the LV cavity size with stress compared with rest on radionuclide MPI reflects global subendocardial hypoperfusion, as opposed to true cavity dilation from ischemia, as seen with exercise echocardiograms or dobutamine echocardiograms. Transient ischemic dilation is associated with severe and multivessel CAD. Increased lung uptake of radiotracer associated with elevated LV filling pressures also reflects LV dysfunction, extensive

angiographic disease, and risk of adverse cardiac events. This situation was more frequently seen with Tl-201 imaging, in which scanning was started 10 to 15 minutes after completion of stress. However, when increased lung uptake is seen with Tc-99m studies, the pathophysiologic implications are the same as with Tl-201 studies. These high-risk scan features are particularly helpful in risk assessment when the scan shows only mild perfusion defects. Finally, studies suggest that the use of multicategory reporting of scan results (normal, probably normal, equivocal, probably abnormal, and abnormal) that incorporates the image findings, the stress findings, and clinical information provides enhanced risk stratification compared with a dichotomous normal or abnormal categorization based solely on image scores.

Positron Emission Tomography Myocardial Perfusion Imaging

The prognostic value of PET MPI has been well documented. Both Rb-82 and N-13 ammonia PET MPI have been shown to have prognostic value in patients with known or suspected coronary disease (Table 29-2). In earlier studies, PET MPI was used in higher-risk patients with known CAD, whereas more contemporary studies confirmed the prognostic value of relative PET MPI in lower-risk patient cohorts. As with SPECT MPI, a normal relative PET MPI result is associated with excellent prognosis, and an increase in the extent and severity of stress perfusion defects is associated with worse outcomes. In a study of 685 patients with known CAD, Rb-82 dipyridamole stress demonstrated incremental prognostic value to clinical history and angiographic data. A normal study result was associated with a 0.9% annual event rate, whereas a positive study result was associated with a 4.3% annual event rate. Lertsburapa et al demonstrated that peak stress LVEF added significantly to clinical and MPI variables in predicting all-cause mortality. In addition, LVEF reserve (stress minus rest EF) provides significant independent and incremental value to Rb-82 PET MPI for predicting the risk of future adverse events. Annualized rates of cardiac events (2.1% versus 5.3%; $P < .001$) and all-cause death (4.3% versus 9.2%; $P < .001$) were significantly higher in patients who did not increase their LVEF from rest to peak stress. PET has also been found to be cost effective compared with angiography, exercise ECG, and SPECT in terms of quality-adjusted life-years.

The additional ability of PET to quantify absolute blood flow by dynamic imaging of tracer kinetics allows measurement of myocardial perfusion at rest and during

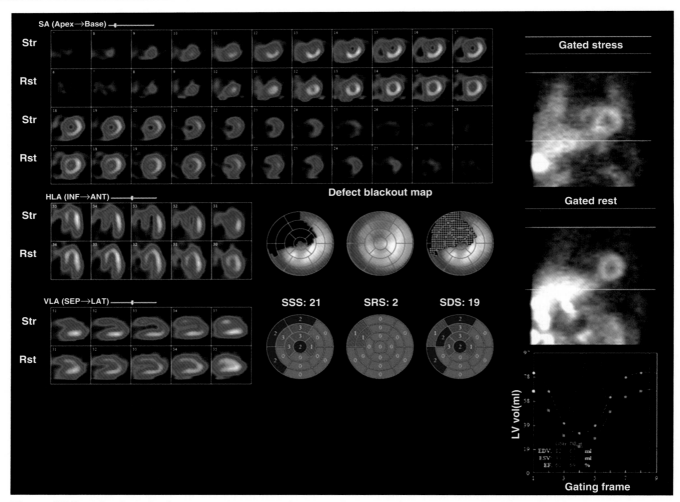

Figure 29-3 High-risk single photon emission computed tomography scan. Technetium-99m sestamibi images display a large and severe perfusion defect in the entire anterior and anteroseptal walls and apex showing complete reversibility. Transient ischemic dilation (TID) of the left ventricle is seen on the stress images. The scan demonstrates high-risk features of TID, transient increase in right ventricular tracer uptake, and increased lung uptake at stress compared with rest *(far right top and middle panels)*. *ANT*, Anterior; *HLA*, horizontal long axis; *INF*, inferior; *LAT*, lateral; *LV*, left ventricular; *Rst*, rest; *SA*, short axis; *SDS*, summed difference score; *SEP*, septal; *SRS*, summed rest score; *SSS*, summed stress score; *Str*, stress; *VLA*, vertical long axis.

stress, as well as CFR. CFR with vasodilators predominantly measures endothelium-independent coronary flow abnormalities and, to a lesser extent, endothelium-dependent flow abnormalities. In 51 patients with hypertrophic cardiomyopathy and 8-year follow-up, Cecchi et al showed that patients with the lowest tertile of dipyridamole-induced myocardial blood flow had worse outcomes compared with patients in the highest tertile. Furthermore, the degree of coronary microvascular dysfunction was an independent predictor of death and progressive heart failure in patients with dilated cardiomyopathy. Absolute myocardial perfusion may also be superior to quantitative coronary angiography in quantifying changes in myocardial blood flow in response to aggressive risk factor modification.

The prognostic value of vasodilator CFR when using N-13 ammonia or Rb-82 PET has also been investigated. In a study of 256 patients undergoing N-13 ammonia PET and a normal relative PET study, abnormal CFR was independently associated with a higher annual major adverse cardiac event rates over 3 years compared with normal CFR (1.4% versus 6.3%; $P < .05$). Despite the small number of patients, this was the first study to report the prognostic value of quantitative PET MPI in patients with known or suspected CAD. Similarly, another study that included 275 patients who underwent rest and dipyridamole stress Rb-82 PET MPI showed that a vasodilator CFR lower than the median value (2.11) was predictive of worse outcomes in the entire cohort, as well as in patients with normal relative PET MPI.

Endothelium-dependent flow abnormalities can be studied using cold pressor testing. In 72 subjects with chest pain and nonobstructive CAD, Schindler et al demonstrated that an impaired or decreased myocardial blood flow response to cold pressor test was associated with the highest incidence of cardiovascular events. Impaired cold pressor myocardial blood flow was independently associated with adverse cardiovascular events over and above coronary risk factors (smoking, hypercholesterolemia, hypertension, and increases in body mass index).

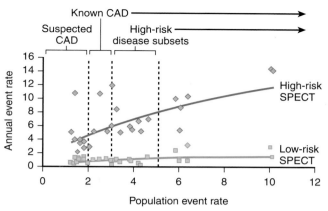

Figure 29-4 Relationship of population event rates with annual rates of cardiac death or nonfatal myocardial infarction in patients with low-risk and high-risk single photon emission computed tomography (SPECT) myocardial perfusion imaging (MPI) scans. High-risk SPECT MPI was defined as summed stress score higher than 8 and moderately to severely abnormal or multivessel disease perfusion patterns. Event rates were lower in populations with suspected coronary artery disease (CAD, defined as annual event rate <2%) as compared with patients with chronic CAD (defined as annual event rate ≥2%). Patients in the latter group with high-risk, severe, and extensive disease exhibited the highest overall event rates (defined as annual event rates ≥5%). (From Shaw LJ, Iskandrian AE. Prognostic value of gated myocardial perfusion SPECT. *J Nucl Cardiol.* 2004;11:171-185.)

Myocardial Perfusion Imaging to Guide Patient Management

Radionuclide MPI results are also used to guide patient management. Hachamovitch et al were the first to demonstrate that patients with a large ischemic burden (>10% ischemic myocardium) had a lower hazard of cardiac mortality in the revascularization group compared with the medical therapy group (Fig. 29-5). The nuclear substudy of the Clinical Outcomes Utilizing Revascularization and Aggressive Drug Evaluation (COURAGE) study also investigated this concept. The main COURAGE study was a randomized study that found no difference in major adverse cardiovascular events between patients who underwent percutaneous coronary revascularization and patients who received optimal medical therapy (OMT) alone. In the nuclear substudy of COURAGE, 314 patients underwent SPECT MPI at baseline and at 18 months. Percutaneous coronary intervention (PCI) plus OMT was found to reduce ischemic burden significantly compared with OMT alone, with the greatest benefit in patients with large ischemic burden, although this benefit was no longer evident on risk-adjusted analysis.

In response to therapeutic interventions, quantitative PET has been used in several research studies to evaluate progression or regression of atherosclerosis. In patients with dyslipidemia treated with aggressive risk factor modification (lifestyle changes and medications), quantitative PET is superior to quantitative coronary angiography in identifying response to therapy. This is because small changes in atherosclerosis that are not easily evident on coronary angiography may translate into much larger changes in myocardial blood flow that are readily imaged by quantitative PET imaging.

Table 29-1   High-Risk Myocardial Perfusion Imaging Variables

Features	Identification	Implication And Pathophysiology
Perfusion defect size, severity and location	Qualitative and semiquantitative analysis on reconstructed slices Correlation of location of defect with coronary distribution	Large defect size (reflecting extent of CAD) and severity (reflecting severity of CAD) implying worse prognosis More than one coronary distribution affected implying multivessel coronary disease
Increased lung uptake (particularly with Tl-201)	Increased lung uptake during cine review of raw projection data; software program can generate lung-to-heart ratios using region of interest	Lung-to-heart ratio >0.54 Tl-201, or >0.45 Tc-99m a poor prognostic indicator of extensive LV ischemia, earlier infarct, or LV dysfunction
Transient dilation of the left ventricle after stress (TID)	Increased stress-to-rest LV cavity ratio; software programs can generate TID ratio	TID ratio >1.22 abnormal; abnormal TID ratio based on the study protocol Marker of extensive and severe CAD Sensitivity 71% and specificity 95% Postulated to be related to diffuse subendocardial ischemia versus true LV dilation at stress
Increased right ventricular uptake	Qualitatively assessed on raw projection data and on reconstructed data; software programs can generate RV/LV tracer uptake ratios using region of interest	Increased in the presence of RV hypertrophy resulting from pulmonary hypertension *or* relatively "increased" in the setting of global LV uptake reduction during exercise stress
Decrease in left ventricular systolic function	Gated SPECT display on multiple ventricular slices and software-generated LVEF	Poor prognostic indicator related to high-risk coronary disease or cardiomyopathy
Poststress global stunning	Analyzed as stress LVEF – rest LVEF using commercial software programs; a decline of LVEF >5% considered abnormal	Related to severe ischemia and significant or multivessel CAD
Reversible regional wall motion abnormalities	Poststress regional dysfunction and regional wall motion abnormalities that are not present or less severe on rest; visual review of the rest and stress-gated images	53% sensitive and 100% specific for detection of severe CAD Presence of reversible regional wall motion abnormalities identifies >70% angiographic stenosis

CAD, Coronary artery disease; *LV,* left ventricular; *LVEF,* left ventricular ejection fraction; *RV,* right ventricular; *SPECT,* single photon emission computed tomography; *Tc-99m,* technetium-99m; *TID,* transient ischemic dilation; *Tl-201,* thallium-201.

Table 29-2   Summary of Studies Investigating the Prognostic Value of Positron Emission Tomography Myocardial Perfusion Imaging

First Author	Year	Stress Agent	Tracer	Patients (N)	Events (N)	Event Type	Prior CAD (%)	Normal Scans (%)	Event / Year In Normal MPI (%)	Event /Year In Abnormal MPI (%)
Marwick	1997	Dipyridamole	Rb-82	685	81	Cardiac death	Prior MI, 48%; prior revascularization, 37%	24	0.9	Mild, 2.6%; moderate, 5.1%; severe, 5.1%
Yoshinaga	2006	Dipyridamole	Rb-82	367	17	Cardiac death or MI	40.3	70.5	0.4	Mild, 2.3%; moderate to severe, 7.0%
Lertsburapa	2009	Dipyridamole	Rb-82	1,441	132	All-cause mortality	53.6	64.8	2.4	Mild, 4.1%; moderate to severe, 6.9%
Dorbala	2009	Dipyridamole Adenosine	Rb-82	1,432	140	Cardiac death or MI	30.6	54	0.7	Mild, 5.5%; moderate, 5%; severe, 11%
Herzog	2009	Adenosine	N-13	256	29	Cardiac death	66	45	0.5	3.1
Chow	2009	Exercise and dobutamine	Rb-82	124	16	Cardiac death, MI, revascularization	MI, 40%; PCI, 29%; CABG, 15%	37	1.7	13

From Al-Mallah MH, Sitek A, Moore SC, Di CM, Dorbala S. Assessment of myocardial perfusion and function with PET and PET/CT. *J Nucl Cardiol.* 2010; 17:498-513.
CABG, Coronary artery bypass graft; *MI,* myocardial infarction; *MPI,* myocardial perfusion imaging; *N-13,* nitrogen-13; *PCI,* percutaneous coronary intervention; *Rb-82,* rubidium-82.

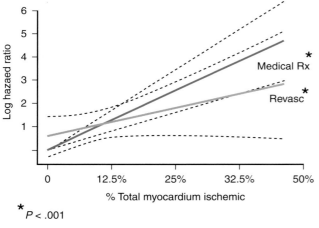

*P < .001

Figure 29-5 Relationship between the percentage of ischemic myocardium and survival advantage between revascularization (Revasc) and medical therapy (Rx). Based on this graph, medical therapy in patients with no or mild amounts of inducible ischemia conferred survival advantage over revascularization. The two lines intersect at 10% to 12.5% of ischemic myocardium, beyond which the survival benefit for revascularization over medical therapy increases as a function of increasing amounts of inducible ischemia. (From Hachamovitch R, Hayes SW, Friedman JD, et al. Comparison of the short-term survival benefit associated with revascularization compared with medical therapy in patients with no prior coronary artery disease undergoing stress myocardial perfusion single photon emission computed tomography. *Circulation.* 2003;107:2900-2907.)

Cost Effectiveness of Radionuclide Myocardial Perfusion Imaging

In patients with chronic stable angina, SPECT MPI has been shown to be cost effective. In the Economics of Noninvasive Diagnosis (END) study that looked at 11,249 consecutive patients with stable angina, a strategy of initial medical therapy with MPI-guided coronary angiography compared with a strategy of direct coronary angiography was associated with significantly lower diagnostic and follow-up evaluation costs with no differences in outcomes. The Economics of Myocardial Perfusion Imaging in Europe (EMPIRE) study was another study (retrospective case-controlled study) from four countries (France, Germany, Italy, and the United Kingdom) that found that when considering exercise ECG, MPI, and coronary angiography, a strategy including MPI was cheaper and at least as effective compared with strategies not including MPI. In one study, SPECT MPI had a lower cost-per-unit effectiveness compared with an exercise ECG test over a wide range of pretest probabilities of CAD, whereas PET MPI had the lowest cost-per-effectiveness or cost-per-utility unit in patients with intermediate pretest likelihood of CAD (pretest likelihood of 0.70). In a group of intermediate-risk subjects, Merhige et al also showed that the downstream costs of evaluation following PET MPI were lower than those of SPECT at their institution, and costs were lower than that reported with SPECT MPI from the END study. The results of the ongoing Study of Myocardial Perfusion and Coronary Anatomy Imaging Roles in CAD (SPARC) study will likely illustrate the utility of various imaging tests (SPECT, PET, CT angiography [CTA], or hybrid SPECT or PET with CTA) in evaluating patients with intermediate pretest likelihood of CAD.

Practical Aspects

The specificity of SPECT MPI is diminished when attenuation artifacts are interpreted as perfusion abnormalities resulting from CAD. ECG-gated SPECT improves specificity, as does attenuation-corrected SPECT. Attenuation correction algorithms are much more robust with PET MPI, and hence attenuation-corrected PET MPI has better specificity than non–attenuation-corrected SPECT MPI.

Stress perfusion defects reflect a combination of infarction (fixed) and viable but ischemic myocardium (reversible) (SSS). Specifically, although reversible defects predict MI and fixed defects predict cardiac death, the combination of reversible and fixed defects is a stronger predictor of overall events. Identification of reversible defects on stress MPI implies a modifiable risk that can be improved by therapeutic interventions, either revascularization by bypass surgery or PCI or medical therapy.

Routine stress imaging after successful PCI or coronary artery bypass graft (CABG) is not indicated, unless patients have symptoms. In selected asymptomatic patients, repeat MPI may be considered 5 or more years after CABG and 2 or more years after PCI. Repeat MPI should always be compared with a preintervention study, and the examiner should know the details of the PCI. In patients who have undergone CABG, abnormal perfusion may persist despite patent grafts because of residual disease in the native nongrafted vessels. A classic pattern of proximal defects with preserved perfusion in the distal portion of the left ventricle suggests a patent left internal mammary artery (LIMA) graft with progression of native left anterior descending coronary artery disease proximal to the LIMA insertion (Fig. 29-6). Moreover, in a patient with a pattern of perfusion defects in the apical segments with a patent LIMA graft on angiography, progression of vascular disease with subclavian artery stenosis should be considered. Septal wall motion abnormality is also common after CABG surgery, as is seen with any open heart surgery, left bundle branch block, or right ventricular pacing with left bundle branch block morphology.

Evaluation of Multivessel Coronary Artery Disease

Noninvasive diagnosis of underlying multivessel CAD is critical for proper patient management. The use of relative MPI in patients with underlying multivessel CAD can be problematic because of the potential for underestimation of the true extent of underlying CAD. In clinical practice, most commonly, exercise stress features of high risk (see Box 29-2) are useful to identify high-risk patients with an underlying large ischemic burden and or multivessel CAD. In addition, scan features of high risk (see Table 29-1), and low LVEF, although relatively insensitive, may help identify underlying severe multivessel CAD in the context of mild perfusion defects.

True balanced ischemia can result in completely normal MPI results and is a recognized pitfall, although this situation is uncommon. Normal MPI results in the setting of balanced ischemia may be occasionally seen in patients with left dominance and severe left main coronary artery disease. More commonly, three-vessel disease results in relative PET and SPECT MPI defects showing only the coronary territory supplied by the most severe stenosis (Fig. 29-7). This is because of the necessity to identify a reference segment for comparison of the defect territory; if all the segments are diseased, the most severely diseased segments may appear relatively worse than the less severely diseased segments. Absolute measurements of myocardial blood flow and vasodilator CFR by PET are inversely related to the severity of coronary artery stenosis and may identify more extensive underlying CAD. In a study of patients with three-vessel CAD, perfusion defect sizes were significantly larger using quantitative myocardial blood flow estimates as compared with circumferential profile methods. Quantitative PET may thus prove to be a useful tool to identify multivessel CAD.

How Are Discordant Stress Electrocardiogram and Perfusion Results Managed?

The presence of ischemic ECG changes in the context of the normal MPI portends worse outcomes compared with patients with normal scan results without ischemic ECG changes. Ischemic ECG changes during vasodilator imaging are very uncommon, but when present they are more likely to indicate ischemia from true coronary steal phenomenon. An abnormal perfusion scan remains an important indicator of ischemia with or without ECG changes, with powerful prognostic power for future cardiac events. Patients with normal perfusion but a positive ECG response have excellent outcomes with a low to intermediate Duke treadmill score, whereas clinical correlation is advised in patients with a high Duke treadmill score.

■ MYOCARDIAL VIABILITY AND HEART FAILURE

Key Questions

1. Is CAD the cause of heart failure?
2. Does the patient have myocardial ischemia?
3. Does the patient have myocardial viability?
4. Will regional and global function recover following successful revascularization?

Why Is Myocardial Viability Testing Important?

Heart failure is an enormous cause of cardiac morbidity and mortality. The aim of myocardial viability assessment in heart failure is to identify patients with potentially reversible LV dysfunction in whom the long-term prognosis may be improved with revascularization. The relationship between LV function and myocardial perfusion can be explained by the phenomenon of stunning and

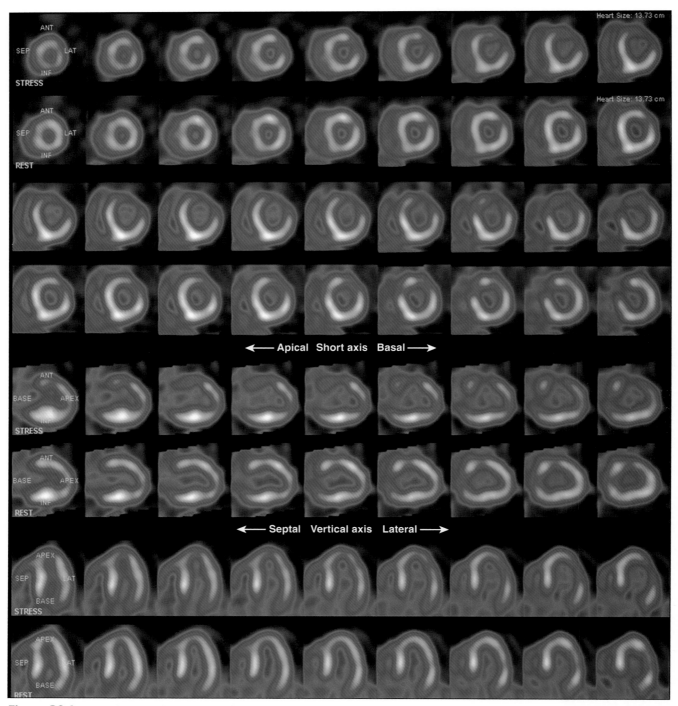

Figure 29-6 Rest and stress rubidium-82 perfusion images in a patient with earlier coronary artery bypass grafting. The medium-sized and severe perfusion defect in the middle and basal anterolateral walls spares the septum and apex. These findings suggest patent left internal mammary artery (LIMA) graft to the left anterior descending artery (LAD) with progression of native LAD and diagonal disease proximal to the LIMA graft insertion. *ANT,* Anterior; *INF,* inferior; *LAT,* lateral; *SEP,* septal.

hibernating myocardium. *Stunned myocardium* refers to the state of delayed recovery of regional LV dysfunction after a transient period of ischemia that has been followed by reperfusion. *Hibernating myocardium* refers to an adaptive response in which viable but dysfunctional myocardium arises from prolonged myocardial hypoperfusion at rest. In both stunned and hibernating myocardium, myocardial function is depressed at rest, but

myocytes remain viable. Prerequisites for cellular viability include the presence of adequate myocardial blood flow, cell membrane integrity, and preserved metabolic activity. Abnormalities in myocardial perfusion lead to cellular metabolic changes that result in contractile dysfunction. Therefore, to assess myocardial viability, several radionuclides can be used, such as myocardial perfusion tracers, tracers of myocardial metabolic activity, and low-dose dobutamine to assess contractile function (see Table 5-1, on SPECT and PET radionuclide characteristics in Chapter 5).

Nuclear Techniques for Viability Imaging

Several nuclear techniques can be used to image myocardial viability. Commonly used techniques include MPI (stress, rest, nitrate enhanced, dobutamine enhanced), Tl-201 redistribution imaging (with or without nitrate enhancement and reinjection), and imaging of myocardial metabolism (glucose metabolism or fatty acid metabolism).

Myocardial Perfusion Imaging

Radionuclides are taken up intracellularly, and normal myocardial perfusion indicates preserved cell membrane integrity (Tc-99m and Tl-201) and mitochondrial function (Tc-99m tracers) in the myocytes. A normal stress MPI study result in a patient with heart failure and LV dysfunction suggest a nonischemic origin of the cardiomyopathy with high sensitivity and high negative predictive value. In patients presenting with new-onset heart failure with LV dysfunction, SPECT MPI was able to exclude extensive CAD with a high negative predictive value of 96%.

Although no specific perfusion abnormality rules out CAD, extensive or severe perfusion defects are more likely to represent CAD, whereas smaller and milder defects are more likely to point to a nonischemic origin. Imaging of myocardial ischemia is a critical component in the management of patients with heart failure. Patients with normal resting myocardial perfusion can manifest extensive areas of stress-induced ischemia leading to global stunning and depressed LVEF (Fig. 29-8). The presence of ischemia and LV systolic dysfunction predicts a high likelihood of recovery of function following revascularization.

In regions with severe reduction of blood flow, absence of perfusion tracer alone can provide information about lack of viability. However, if reduction of blood flow is less severe, redistribution Tl-201 imaging or additional indices of metabolism may be required to determine viability. Compared with the detection of CAD, viability assessment has often incorporated quantitative techniques to report imaging patterns precisely. Investigators have demonstrated that with Tl-201 or Tc-99m MPI, regions of the myocardium with less than 40% peak activity on polar plots (non–attenuation-corrected SPECT MPI) are unlikely to be viable. The threshold for attenuation-corrected SPECT MPI is not well defined. The use of nitroglycerin infusion followed by injection of resting radiotracer has been advocated to improve collateral-related flow and identification of viable myocardium. More commonly, nitroglycerin is administered either in sublingual or spray form approximately 10 to 15 minutes before injection of the rest Tc-99m dose. Additionally, combined nitrate-enhanced perfusion and contractile reserve (nitroglycerin-enhanced rest SPECT followed by low-dose dobutamine-gated Tc-99m SPECT) have been shown to improve overall accuracy for the detection of viable myocardium.

Thallium-201 Redistribution Imaging

Stress or rest Tl-201 with redistribution imaging is another commonly used method for viability imaging. The initial Tl-201 perfusion images are acquired within 5 to 10 minutes after injection of 3 to 4 mCi of Tl-201. Normally perfused myocardial regions wash out Tl-201 rapidly, whereas hypoperfused but viable myocardium continues to accumulate Tl-201, resulting in redistribution of Tl-201. Redistribution images can be performed after 4 hours or 24 hours, with or without an additional reinjection of 1 to 1.5 mCi of Tl-201 before imaging. Redistribution of Tl-201 in regions with initially low Tl uptake is an insensitive but specific sign of myocardial hibernation. Enhanced Tl-201 uptake after redistribution or reinjection predicts improvement in regional LV function. The 24-hour redistribution images can be limited by radionuclide decay. Quantitative increase in the magnitude of Tl-201 uptake after reinjection has been found to be an important determinant of viability and potential recovery of function. Conversely, persistence of severe defects after reinjection identifies areas with a low likelihood of improvement. Similar results are found when Tc-based compounds such as sestamibi and tetrofosmin are used.

Myocardial Metabolism Imaging

Abnormalities in myocardial perfusion lead to changes in myocardial metabolism. Normal myocardium is a metabolic omnivore and uses glucose, fatty acids, lactic acid, and ketones for its metabolic needs, depending on the metabolic state. In the fasting state, fatty acids are the primary source of energy in the heart. In the fed state, high arterial glucose concentration results in increased insulin levels, thus stimulating glucose metabolism and inhibiting lipolysis. The step of beta oxidation in fatty acid metabolism is exquisitely sensitive to hypoxia, and therefore, ischemic myocardium preferentially relies on glucose for its metabolic needs in both fasting and fed states.

FLUORINE-18 FLUORODEOXYGLUCOSE POSITRON EMISSION TOMOGRAPHY IMAGING

Fluorine-18 (F-18) fluorodeoxyglucose (FDG), a glucose analogue, allows for imaging of myocardial glucose transport and uptake and is the most commonly used agent for the clinical imaging of myocardial metabolism. F-18 FDG enters into the myocytes through myocyte glucose transporter 4 receptors and is metabolized to FDG-6-phosphate by the enzyme hexokinase. FDG-6-phosphate remains in the myocyte without further metabolism. Because the myocytes switch their energy sources based on the metabolic state, the diagnostic accuracy of FDG imaging depends on substrate availability and hormonal conditions. In the fasting state, normal myocardium and scarred myocardium demonstrate no FDG uptake, and the only way to distinguish the two is based on MPI. Typical protocols involve imaging of myocardial perfusion using gated SPECT or PET MPI followed by F-18 FDG PET imaging (see Chapter 5). Given the heterogeneous myocardial uptake in the fasting state, FDG imaging is performed in a glucose-loaded state following 50 to 75 g of oral glucose loading to

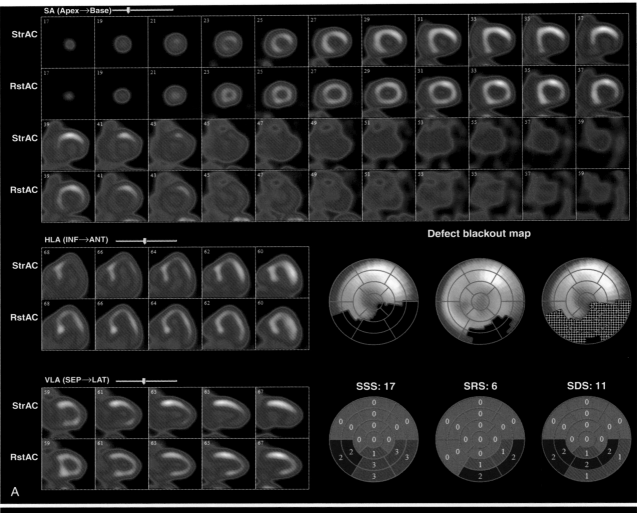

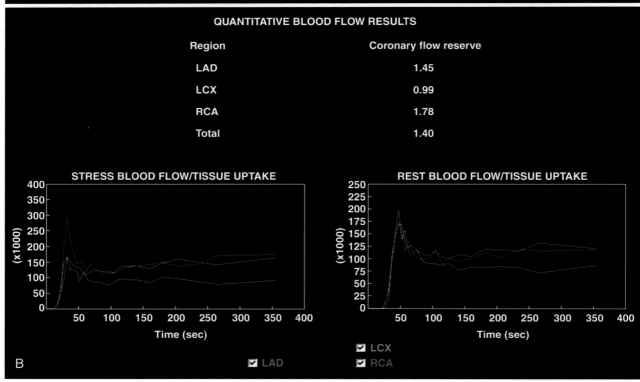

Figure 29-7 An example of balanced ischemia in a patient with relative positron emission tomography (PET) myocardial perfusion imaging (MPI) showing reduced perfusion in the most severe coronary distribution (A) but myocardial blood flow quantitation showing flow reduction in multiple coronary distributions (B). **A,** Rubidium-82 perfusion images demonstrate a large perfusion defect of severe intensity in the entire inferior wall, the middle and basal inferolateral walls, and the basal inferoseptal walls. The defect shows significant but not complete reversibility at rest. **B,** Stress and rest myocardial perfusion images with rubidium-82 as the flow tracer acquired in the same patient as in **A**. The quantitative data *(top panel)* demonstrate impaired coronary vasodilator reserve (stress flow and rest flow) in all three coronary territories and not only in the left circumflex (LCX) artery distribution as suggested by relative PET MPI images shown in **A**. From regions of interests assigned to the left ventricular myocardium on a polar map (corresponding to the territories of the left anterior descending artery [LAD], LCX artery, and right coronary artery [RCA]) on serially acquired images, time activity curves *(bottom left* and *right* panels) are derived that describe changes in radiotracer activity in arterial blood (counts/pixel/second) in all three coronary vessels as a function of time. Subsequent coronary angiogram demonstrated significant three-vessel coronary artery disease (CAD). This case illustrates the potential use of blood flow quantification to ascertain the extent of anatomic CAD more clearly. *ANT,* Anterior; *HLA,* horizontal long axis; *INF,* inferior; *LAT,* lateral; *RstAC,* rest with attenuation correction; *SA,* short axis; *SDS,* summed difference score; *SEP,* septal; *SRS,* summed rest score; *SSS,* summed stress score; *StrAC,* stress with attenuation correction; *VLA,* vertical long axis.

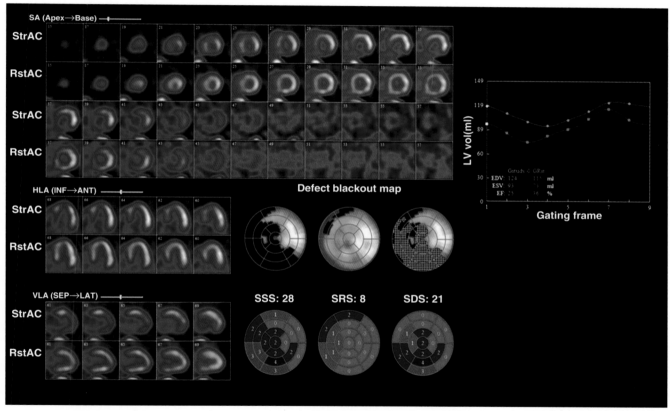

Figure 29-8 An example of a patient with normal resting myocardial perfusion and severe resting left ventricular dysfunction manifesting extensive areas of severe stress-induced ischemia. The images show a medium-sized and severe perfusion defect in the entire inferior wall and the basal inferoseptal wall that shows complete reversibility. In addition, a medium-sized perfusion defect of moderate intensity in the middle anteroseptal wall, the apical anterior and septal walls, and the apex showed nearly complete reversibility. Gated positron emission tomography images on the far right demonstrate enlarged left ventricular (LV) volumes with poststress ejection fraction (EF) of 25% compared with resting EF of 36%. These images suggest a high likelihood of functional recovery with successful revascularization. Depressed resting left ventricular EF is likely related to global stunning from severe ischemia. *ANT,* Anterior; *EDV,* end-diastolic volume; *ESV,* end-systolic volume; *HLA,* horizontal long axis; *INF,* inferior; *LAT,* lateral; *RstAC,* rest with attenuation correction; *SA,* short axis; *SDS,* summed difference score; *SEP,* septal; *SRS,* summed rest score; *SSS,* summed stress score; *StrAC,* stress with attenuation correction; *VLA,* vertical long axis.

increase glucose metabolism and stimulate FDG uptake. Forty-five minutes after the glucose load, serum glucose levels are checked. Intravenous insulin is then administered to reduce the glucose level to approximately 150 mg/dL before injection of FDG (see Tables 5-4 and 5-5 in Chapter 5). Imaging is performed approximately 60 to 90 minutes after FDG injection. In patients with limited FDG uptake by the myocardium (seen in insulin resistance), more insulin administration followed by repeated imaging can help. Possible myocardial perfusion and FDG patterns in a glucose-loaded study include the following:

I. Normal perfusion with normal FDG uptake
II. Reduced perfusion and correspondingly reduced FDG uptake (perfusion-metabolism match) signifying nonviable myocardium

III. Reduced perfusion with preserved or enhanced FDG uptake (perfusion-metabolism mismatch) signifying myocardial viability

IV. Nearly normal perfusion with reduced FDG uptake (reversed perfusion-metabolism mismatch) described in patients with repetitive myocardial stunning or left bundle branch block

The normal myocardium serves as a reference region for comparison of relative FDG uptake in the abnormal regions. A mismatch pattern of low perfusion but normal or enhanced FDG uptake identifies hypoperfused but viable myocardium with a potential for improvement in function after revascularization (Fig. 29-9). In contrast, myocardium with a match pattern of reduced flow and reduced FDG uptake is unlikely to recover function after revascularization (Fig. 29-10).

IMAGING MYOCARDIAL FATTY ACID AND OXIDATIVE METABOLISM

Carbon-11 (C-11)–labeled radiotracers to image myocardial fatty acid and oxidative metabolism are used in research applications. C-11 palmitate is a long-chain fatty acid. Uptake of C-11 palmitate in the myocardium depends on regional blood flow and acceptance in the cytosol by binding to C-11 acyl-coenzyme A (CoA), with resulting trapping of the tracer in the myocardium. In normally perfused myocardium, extraction fraction of C-11 palmitate is 40%. By using dynamic PET imaging, tracer inflow, peak accumulation, and tracer release can be quantified. C-11 acetate is a short-chain acid. Uptake of C-11 acetate in the myocardium is through first-pass extraction of approximately 63% at blood flows of 1 mL/g/minute. In the cytosol, C-11 acetate is converted to C-11 acetyl-CoA and is oxidized by the tricarboxylic acid cycle in the mitochondria. Hence myocardial turnover and clearance of C-11 acetate require oxidative metabolism and intact mitochondrial function of viable myocardium. A clearance rate of C-11 acetate within 2 standard deviations of the mean is associated with recovery of function after revascularization in patients after MI.

DIAGNOSTIC AND PROGNOSTIC VALUE OF FLUORODEOXYGLUCOSE POSITRON EMISSION TOMOGRAPHY

Techniques to assess myocardial perfusion abnormalities are very sensitive, whereas techniques to assess contractile reserve are highly specific for the diagnosis of viable myocardium. In pooled analysis, FDG PET demonstrated a high sensitivity (88%), good specificity (73%), and high positive (76%) and negative predictive values (82%) to identify viable myocardium. Imaging of contractile reserve using low-dose dobutamine echocardiography has a sensitivity of 84% and specificity of 81% to diagnose viable myocardium. Overall, FDG PET is slightly more accurate compared with other imaging techniques.

Extensive literature suggests that patients with viable myocardium have better outcomes, such as improvement in heart failure symptoms, reduced repeat hospitalizations, improvements in exercise capacity, improvements in EF, and a survival benefit following successful revascularization compared with patients without viable myocardium. In addition to good target vessels for revascularization and an optimal surgical risk, the magnitude of viable myocardium is important for improving the likelihood of recovery of function following revascularization. The threshold of viable myocardium to predict improved survival with revascularization compared with medical therapy varies from approximately 26% for PET to approximately 36% to 39% for echocardiography and SPECT imaging, respectively. Additionally, several other factors modulate the relationship between myocardial viability and patient outcomes (Table 29-3).

Furthermore, the role of demonstrating inducible ischemia by stress on top of demonstrating myocardial viability is important. Although most studies have focused on the analysis of resting tracer uptake (with Tl or Tc compounds) with metabolic activity at rest (by FDG or C-11 acetate), nontransmural infarction may occur in conjunction with some degree of viability in noncritically stenosed coronary vessels. The finding of stress-induced ischemia in such a setting is associated with a more favorable effect of revascularization predictive of future functional recovery than viability data alone. In addition, gated FDG PET provides LV volumes and function that correlate well with those obtained with magnetic resonance imaging (MRI). Measures of global LV function and remodeling can also be used to predict improvement in LV function after revascularization. Investigators have shown that increased LV volumes and cavity size predict poor outcome.

Randomized controlled trials assessing the utility of viability testing are limited. The PET and Recovery Following Revascularization-2 (PARR-2) study, a prospective randomized study of 428 patients with LVEF of up to 35% who were undergoing FDG PET imaging investigated whether FDG PET–assisted management of patients with suspected CAD and severe LV dysfunction altered outcomes compared with standard care. The study did not demonstrate a benefit for PET-guided management of patients with severe LV dysfunction (cumulative event rate 30% in the PET arm versus 36% in the standard arm; relative risk, 0.82; 95% confidence interval [CI], 0.59 to 1.14; $P = .16$). However, when patients who adhered to the PET recommendations for revascularization were considered, outcomes were better with a PET-guided strategy (hazard ratio for the composite outcome was 0.62; 95% CI, 0.42 to 0.93; $P = .019$).

More recently, the results of the prospective Surgical Treatment for Ischemic Heart Failure (STICH) trial were published. This study was a prospective study of 1212 patients with CAD amenable to CABG and an LVEF of up to 35% who were randomly assigned to medical therapy alone (602 patients) or medical therapy plus CABG (610 patients). In this study, no significant difference was noted in the primary outcome of all-cause death in the CABG arm (41%) compared with the medical therapy arm (36%) of the trial (hazard ratio with CABG, 0.86; 95% CI, 0.72 to 1.04; $P = .12$). Among the 1212 patients, 601 were enrolled in the STICH viability study, which included Tl-201, dobutamine, echocardiogram studies. Approximately 60% of the patients were

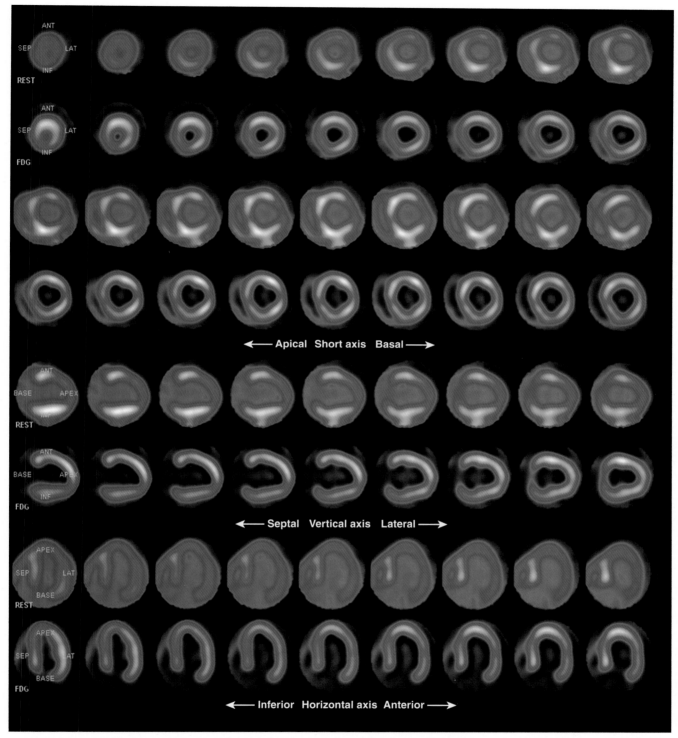

Figure 29-9 A pattern of perfusion-metabolism mismatch on rubidium-82 (Rb-82) and fluorine-18 (F-18) fluorodeoxyglucose (FDG) positron emission tomography. In Figures 29-9 and 29-10, paired Rb-82 resting perfusion images *(top)* and FDG *(bottom)* images are arranged in short-axis (first to fourth rows), vertical long-axis (fifth to sixth rows), and horizontal long axis (seventh to eighth rows) views. The perfusion images demonstrate a large perfusion defect of severe intensity in the middle to basal anterolateral walls, the midanterior wall, the apical four myocardial segments, and the left ventricular apex. The corresponding F-18 FDG images demonstrate preserved glucose metabolism and increased FDG activity in these regions, a mismatched perfusion-metabolism pattern consistent with hibernating myocardium. *ANT,* Anterior; *INF,* inferior; *LAT,* lateral; *SEP,* septal.

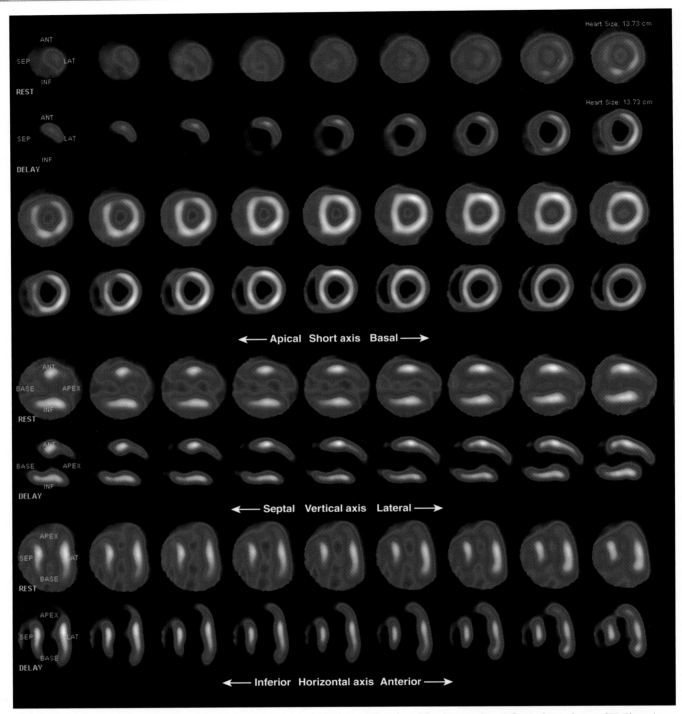

Figure 29-10 A pattern of perfusion-metabolism match on rubidium-82 (Rb-82) and fluorine-18 (F-18) fluorodeoxyglucose (FDG) positron emission tomography. Rb-82 resting perfusion images demonstrate a large perfusion defect of severe intensity in the middle anteroseptal wall, the midanterior wall, the apical four myocardial segments, and the left ventricular apex. The corresponding F-18 FDG images demonstrate lack of glucose use in these regions, a finding compatible with a matched perfusion-metabolism pattern consistent with scarred myocardium. *ANT,* Anterior; *INF,* inferior; *LAT,* lateral; *SEP,* septal.

symptomatic, and most had viable myocardium (81%). The presence of viable myocardium was associated with a greater likelihood of survival in patients with CAD and LV dysfunction (mortality, 37% viable myocardium versus 51% nonviable myocardium; hazard ratio for death among patients with viable myocardium, 0.64; 95% CI, 0.48 to 0.86; P = .003), but this relationship was not significant after adjustment for other baseline variables. The investigators concluded that the assessment of myocardial viability did not identify patients with a differential survival benefit from CABG, as compared with medical therapy alone. However, this study did not

Table 29-3   Factors That May Affect Outcomes During Assessment of Myocardial Viability

Factors Influencing Outcome	Reported Effects
Baseline LVEF	Accuracy of viability testing possibly lower in patients with LVEF <30%
Amount of myocardial viability	Varies widely based on type of test from 26% for PET, 36% for echocardiography, and 39% for SPECT imaging
Amount of myocardial scar	Extent of scar inversely related to recovery of LVEF following revascularization
Extent of LV remodeling	LVESVI >100 mL/m² on echocardiography a predictor of worse recovery of function despite presence of viability
Time to revascularization	Long waiting time for revascularization after detection of hibernating myocardium associated with no improvement of LVEF and a higher mortality rate compared with patients with early revascularization (<35 days)
Stress-induced ischemia	Presence of stress-induced ischemia associated with a more favorable outcome following revascularization

LV, Left ventricular; *LVEF,* left ventricular ejection fraction, *LVESVI,* left ventricular end-systolic volume index; *PET,* positron emission tomography; *SPECT,* single photon emission computed tomography.

include FDG PET or cardiac MRI, and separate analyses of the radionuclide versus dobutamine echocardiogram results will likely be limited by sample size. Further subgroup analyses of the STICH viability study are awaited.

■ ADDITIONAL AND NOVEL APPLICATIONS OF NUCLEAR CARDIOLOGY

Imaging of Inflammatory Heart Diseases and Infiltrative Heart Diseases

Radionuclide imaging has been used to evaluate cardiac involvement in patients with inflammatory heart diseases such as sarcoidosis (Tl-201, gallium-67, or F-18 FDG), cardiac amyloidosis (Tc-99m pyrophosphate), and myocarditis (indium-111 white blood cell scans). Investigators are considering multimodality hybrid imaging with SPECT-CT and PET-CT to identify sources of infection in patients with sepsis or artificial heart valves. Among these conditions, imaging of patients with known or suspected cardiac sarcoidosis is growing.

Cardiac sarcoidosis is frequently underdiagnosed. This may be because endomyocardial biopsy is typically performed from the right ventricle, whereas the disease frequently affects the LV myocardium; moreover, the disease is not diffuse, and foci of involvement may be missed by the blind biopsy procedure. Because a clinical diagnosis is made in 5% of patients, whereas autopsy series demonstrate cardiac involvement in 25% to 79% of patients, a need exists for imaging tests to diagnose

this disorder. The conventional diagnosis of cardiac sarcoidosis has been based on the Japanese Ministry of Health criteria. These criteria incorporate a histologic diagnosis based on endomyocardial biopsy; in addition, an extracardiac histologic diagnosis (extracardiac biopsy positive sarcoid) along with two or more major criteria and one major with two or more minor criteria (ECG, echocardiogram, EF, and imaging criteria) qualify for cardiac sarcoidosis. Gallium imaging (a major criterion) and perfusion defects on Tl-201 or Tc-99m imaging (minor criteria), but not FDG PET, are included in the Japanese Ministry of Health criteria.

FDG PET imaging is more sensitive (sensitivity of 91%, specificity of 96%, using the Japanese Ministry of Health criteria as the gold standard) than gallium-67, Tl-201, or Tc-99m imaging, but it is less widely available than SPECT techniques. The FDG PET protocol for cardiac sarcoid requires special dietary preparation with a low-carbohydrate, high-fat diet (with or without intravenous heparin to promote lipolysis). This dietary preparation allows for suppression or minimization of glucose use by normal myocytes, and areas of FDG uptake are considered abnormal. Perfusion imaging is also performed in conjunction with FDG images (see Fig. 5-2, J, in Chapter 5). Early stages of cardiac sarcoid demonstrate nearly normal myocardial perfusion with high FDG uptake, whereas later stages show declining perfusion with high FDG uptake (Fig. 29-11). End-stage sarcoid manifests as a severe perfusion defect with no FDG uptake (scar or inactive burnt-out stage). The various stages of sarcoid may coexist in any given patient. Because the pattern of perfusion and FDG may appear as a mismatch and may mimic hibernating myocardium, it is critical to exclude the presence of underlying epicardial CAD by using invasive or coronary CTA. The advantages of FDG PET for cardiac sarcoid imaging include its high sensitivity and its ability to stage disease activity and follow response to therapy. However, this technique may be challenging in diabetic patients, and the dietary preparation may not completely suppress normal myocardial FDG uptake, thus leading to false-positive results.

Hybrid Imaging

The development of CT technology with hybrid PET and SPECT scanners allows for attenuation correction, calcium scoring, and coronary CTA. Attenuation correction is possible with most hybrid devices and is discussed earlier. Select hybrid scanners combined with CT scanners with high temporal resolution can be used for calcium scoring and coronary CTA. The evaluation of subclinical coronary atherosclerosis in patients presenting for MPI is facilitated by combining MPI with calcium scoring or coronary CTA. The CCS derived from noncontrast CT assessment has become commonly used to assess coronary atherosclerotic burden in asymptomatic patients. In selected patients with normal perfusion scans (without known CAD and a regular rhythm) (Fig. 29-12), CCS may be used to evaluate the presence of atherosclerosis and to help guide management decisions. Results of studies that investigated patients with both MPI

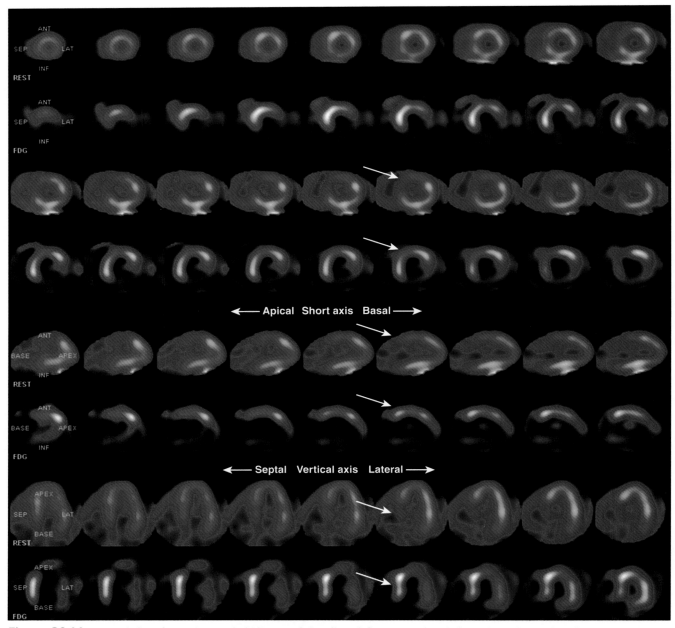

Figure 29-11 Myocardial perfusion images (rubidium-82 [Rb-82]) and fluorine-18 (F-18) fluorodeoxyglucose (FDG) positron emission tomography (PET) images in a patient with cardiac sarcoidosis. An example of Rb-82 and F-18 FDG PET for cardiac sarcoidosis. The rows 1, 3, and 5 represent Rb-82 perfusion images, whereas rows 2, 4 and 6 represent F-18 FDG images following a low-glucose, high-fat diet. On the resting perfusion images, one sees severely reduced blood flow in the anterior and anteroseptal regions in the middle and basal segments of the heart and preserved perfusion in the apical segments (in a noncoronary distribution of perfusion abnormality) with increased FDG uptake, a hallmark of active myocardial inflammation. In a patient with a histologic diagnosis of extracardiac sarcoid and without epicardial coronary artery disease, this pattern is consistent with active cardiac sarcoidosis. *ANT*, Anterior; *INF*, inferior; *LAT*, lateral; *SEP*, septal.

and CCS underscored the diagnostic value of the CCS in identifying the calcified atherosclerosis burden in patients with normal MPI results, although in the presence of extensive coronary artery calcification (Agatston score >400), as many as 45% of patients demonstrate ischemic MPI scans. Studies suggest that patients with normal myocardial perfusion SPECT MPI and a high CCS have a low short-term risk but an intermediate long-term risk compared with patients with normal MPI and no or minimal coronary artery calcium. Notably,

the presence of high coronary artery calcification may influence downstream patient behavior or physician practices that modify coronary risk factors. Calcium scoring is unlikely to provide much added utility in patients with known CAD, although this has not been specifically studied.

Contrast cardiac coronary CTA with a breath hold and prospective electrocardiographic triggering, if feasible (retrospective gating is less desirable if the heart rate is low and the rhythm is regular, because of the

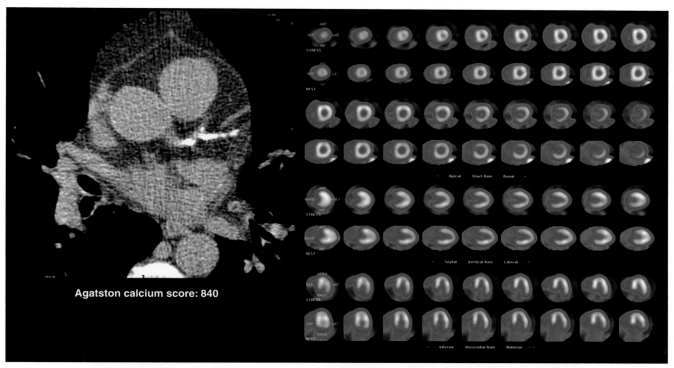

Figure 29-12 Hybrid positron emission tomography–computed tomography (CT) scanner showing both myocardial perfusion results and coronary calcium detected on noncontrast-gated cardiac CT. The rest and stress rubidium-82 myocardial perfusion images were normal. However, the gated noncontrast calcium score CT scan showed extensive calcification in the left anterior descending (LAD) artery with an Agatston score of 840 (high). In total, these images demonstrate extensive calcified LAD coronary atherosclerosis without flow limitation. *ANT,* Anterior; *INF,* inferior; *LAT,* lateral; *SEP,* septal.

higher radiation dose), can provide detailed information about coronary artery stenosis or coronary anomalies (Fig. 29-13). However, when used in conjunction with MPI, CTA provides an additional radiation burden. The radiation burden can be minimized if the CTA and MPI studies are performed by using dose reduction techniques (e.g., prospective triggering, low-kVP imaging, advanced iterative reconstruction, and high-pitch imaging). The use of stress-only MPI with coronary CTA has been accomplished with a low radiation dose and is an intriguing possibility. The utility of combined MPI and CTA is not well established. Several observational studies demonstrated that the information provided may be complementary, with CTA showing a high negative predictive value (>90%) but a low positive predictive value (45% to 67%) for the diagnosis of ischemia. In addition, investigators demonstrated in small studies that the information provided by SPECT MPI and CTA may be of prognostic value in risk stratification. In a study of 541 patients who were investigated with both CTA and MPI, CTA emerged as an independent predictor of events with an incremental prognostic value to MPI.

Volumetric representation of the left ventricle with three-dimensional color-coded perfusion quantification allows for identification of the extent of jeopardized myocardium in relation to the region of coronary stenosis, a technique that may be useful in patients with multivessel CAD for whom identification of flow-limiting coronary stenoses will provide important guidance

to revascularization. Hybrid imaging combining CT to localize structural abnormalities with radionuclide imaging to identify minute quantities of radionuclide uptake is playing an increasing role in molecular cardiology and translational research applications. Hybrid imaging is an evolving field, and readers are referred to extensive reviews on the topic for further information.

Ischemia Imaging

Direct imaging of myocardial ischemia can also be performed with F-18 FDG. Normal myocardium primarily uses fatty acids for energy metabolism during aerobic fasting conditions. During ischemia, anaerobic glycolysis is activated as myocardium metabolism switches to glucose use. This change results in increased glucose uptake by ischemic myocardium, which can persist for many hours after stress even when perfusion returns to baseline. Investigators showed that abnormal uptake of FDG on poststress images may show more abnormal coronary artery territories than seen with Tc MPI alone. SPECT imaging of BMIPP is also used in ischemia imaging. BMIPP is a fatty acid tracer that allows for imaging of regions of reduced fatty acid uptake in ischemic myocardium for as long as 30 hours after the ischemic event. This form of delayed imaging is referred to as ischemic memory imaging, and it has a reported sensitivity and specificity of 86% and 95%, respectively. BMIPP is a SPECT tracer that shows defects of fatty acid metabolism (compared with normal fatty acid metabolism

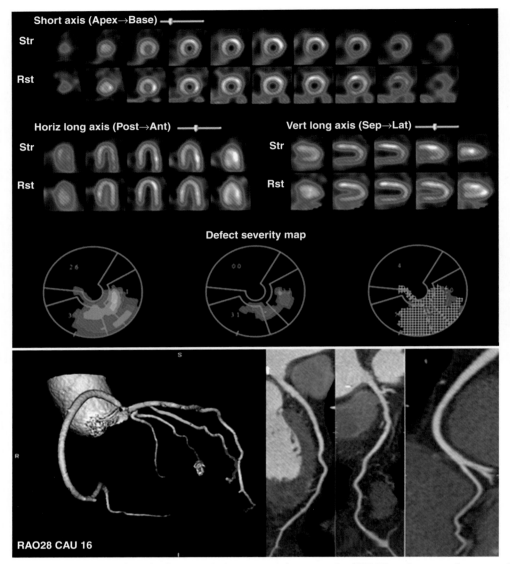

Figure 29-13 Technetium-99m (Tc-99m) single photon emission computed tomography (SPECT) and computed tomography (CT) coronary angiogram images. A 60-year-old woman underwent aortic valve replacement for bicuspid aortic valve 1 year earlier and presented with typical exertional angina. She exercised for 4:35 minutes of a standard Bruce protocol and attained a peak heart rate of 113 beats/minute (70% of age-predicted maximal heart rate). During exercise, she developed typical angina and 2 mm horizontal ST-segment segment depression in leads II, III, aVF, and V4 to V6. Because of her submaximal heart rate, she underwent an adenosine Tc-99m SPECT study, which demonstrated a medium-sized defect of moderate intensity throughout the inferior wall that was reversible. Because an invasive angiogram done 1 year earlier showed no evidence of atherosclerosis, a CT coronary angiogram was performed to identify possible anomalous coronary arteries. A gated contrast-enhanced CT coronary angiogram was performed (320 detector CT scanner) after using 10 mg of intravenous metoprolol, 0.4 mg of sublingual nitroglycerin, and 75 mL of iodinated contrast medium (Ultravist 370). The multidetector CT images demonstrate no evidence of atherosclerosis, but they do show an anomalous coronary artery with the right coronary arising from the left aortic sinus that likely accounts for her anginal symptoms. *Ant,* Anterior; *CAU,* caudal; *Horiz,* horizontal; *Lat,* lateral; *Post,* posterior; *RAO,* right anterior oblique; *Rst,* rest; *Sep,* septal; *Str,* stress; *Vert,* vertical.

in nonischemic myocardium), whereas FDG is a PET tracer, and ischemia is imaged as hot spot imaging (no reference segment because normal myocardium should not demonstrate any FDG uptake).

Imaging of Cardiac Innervation

Neuronal functional imaging of sympathetic innervation in the heart is performed by assessing for uptake and storage of radiolabeled neurotransmitters in presynaptic nerve terminals. I-123-Metaiodobenzylguanidine (MIBG) is a SPECT tracer that measures washout rate of the tracer over 3 to 5 hours by delayed imaging, as well as tracer uptake from the heart and mediastinum. An elevated washout rate indicates increased turnover of catecholamines and sympathetic activity. A washout rate of more than 27% has been shown to be associated with a higher incidence of sudden cardiac death in patients with chronic heart failure. The heart-to-mediastinum ratio of MIBG has been shown to predict clinical outcome in patients with dilated cardiomyopathy. A heart-to-mediastinum ratio of less than 1.2 was associated with a higher incidence of sudden death compared with patients with a normal heart-to-mediastinum ratio.

Molecular Imaging

Molecular imaging of atherosclerotic plaques is emerging as a research and potential clinical tool. Vulnerable plaque imaging will require a range of imaging techniques, as well as suitable agents that target plaque components such as macrophages, lipid pool, smooth muscle cells, adhesion molecules, extracellular matrix metalloproteinases, fibrous cap, and apoptotic cells. Studies have shown that FDG PET-CT can assess atherosclerosis because increased FDG uptake is seen in areas of plaque inflammation.

■ FUTURE OF CLINICAL POSITRON EMISSION TOMOGRAPHY AND SINGLE PHOTON EMISSION COMPUTED TOMOGRAPHY MYOCARDIAL PERFUSION IMAGING

Since 2000, enormous growth has occurred in new hardware and software techniques for SPECT and PET MPI. Improved quantification for SPECT MPI, with better attenuation and scatter correction algorithms, is anticipated to emerge, and low-dose and ultralow-dose protocols with reduced radiation dose to patients and staff will evolve, along with the possibility of quantitative myocardial blood flow evaluation with SPECT. SPECT-CT and PET-CT systems will likely evolve further with improved protocols for hybrid imaging. Fusion of coronary anatomy from CTA with perfusion patterns from SPECT is likely to grow over the years with better definition of its role in the diagnostic workup of the patient. Volumetric representation of the left ventricle with three-dimensional color-coded perfusion quantification is already available and allows identification and determination of the extent of jeopardized myocardium. An F-18 PET perfusion tracer (F-18 flurpiridaz) is currently under development. It targets the mitochondria and shows rapid and high myocardial uptake with better myocardial extraction fraction than Tc compounds. The longer half-life of F-18 also means that it would be suitable for exercise stress imaging. This agent may make unit dose radiotracers available and increase the use of clinical PET MPI and possibly encourage the development of dedicated cardiac PET scanners. Clinicians look forward to new radiotracer development for SPECT imaging over the next decade.

Bibliography

Abdelbaky A, Tawakol A. Noninvasive positron emission tomography imaging of coronary arterial inflammation. *Curr Cardiovasc Imaging Rep.* 2011;4:41-49.

Abidov A, Hachamovitch R, Hayes SW, et al. Are shades of gray prognostically useful in reporting myocardial perfusion single-photon emission computed tomography? *Circ Cardiovasc Imaging.* 2009;2:290-298.

Abrams J. Clinical practice. Chronic stable angina. *N Engl J Med.* 2005;352:2524-2533.

Alam M, Virani SS, Simpson L, Williams SB, Wilson JM. Cardiac sarcoidosis: a clinical entity uncommonly recognized. *Tex Heart Inst J.* 2009;36:501-503.

Alexanderson E, Slomka P, Cheng V, et al. Fusion of positron emission tomography and coronary computed tomographic angiography identifies fluorine 18 fluorodeoxyglucose uptake in the left main coronary artery soft plaque. *J Nucl Cardiol.* 2008;15:841-843.

Allman KC, Shaw LJ, Hachamovitch R, Udelson JE. Myocardial viability testing and impact of revascularization on prognosis in patients with coronary artery disease and left ventricular dysfunction: a meta-analysis. *J Am Coll Cardiol.* 2002;39:1151-1158.

Al-Mallah MH, Sitek A, Moore SC, Di CM, Dorbala S. Assessment of myocardial perfusion and function with PET and PET/CT. *J Nucl Cardiol.* 2010;17:498-513.

Amsterdam EA, Kirk JD, Bluemke DA, et al. Testing of low-risk patients presenting to the emergency department with chest pain: a scientific statement from the American Heart Association. *Circulation.* 2010;122:1756-1776.

Anand DV, Lim E, Hopkins D, et al. Risk stratification in uncomplicated type 2 diabetes: prospective evaluation of the combined use of coronary artery calcium imaging and selective myocardial perfusion scintigraphy. *Eur Heart J.* 2006;27:713-721.

Bacharach SL, Bax JJ, Case J, et al. PET myocardial glucose metabolism and perfusion imaging. Part 1. Guidelines for data acquisition and patient preparation. *J Nucl Cardiol.* 2003;10:543-556.

Baghdasarian SB, Noble GL, Ahlberg AW, Katten D, Heller GV. Risk stratification with attenuation corrected stress Tc-99m sestamibi SPECT myocardial perfusion imaging in the absence of ECG-gating due to arrhythmias. *J Nucl Cardiol.* 2009;16:533-539.

Baller D, Notohamiprodjo G, Gleichmann U, Holzinger J, Weise R, Lehmann J. Improvement in coronary flow reserve determined by positron emission tomography after 6 months of cholesterol-lowering therapy in patients with early stages of coronary atherosclerosis. *Circulation.* 1999;99:2871-2875.

Bateman TM, Heller GV, McGhie AI, et al. Diagnostic accuracy of rest/stress ECG-gated Rb-82 myocardial perfusion PET: comparison with ECG-gated Tc-99m sestamibi SPECT. *J Nucl Cardiol.* 2006;13:24-33.

Bax JJ, Poldermans D, Elhendy A, Boersma E, Rahimtoola SH. Sensitivity, specificity, and predictive accuracies of various noninvasive techniques for detecting hibernating myocardium. *Curr Probl Cardiol.* 2001;26:147-186.

Beanlands RS, Muzik O, Melon P, et al. Noninvasive quantification of regional myocardial flow reserve in patients with coronary atherosclerosis using nitrogen-13 ammonia positron emission tomography: determination of extent of altered vascular reactivity. *J Am Coll Cardiol.* 1995;26:1465-1475.

Beanlands RS, Nichol G, Huszti E, et al. F-18-fluorodeoxyglucose positron emission tomography imaging-assisted management of patients with severe left ventricular dysfunction and suspected coronary disease: a randomized, controlled trial (PARR-2). *J Am Coll Cardiol.* 2007;50:2002-2012.

Beanlands RS, Ruddy TD, deKemp RA, et al. Positron emission tomography and recovery following revascularization (PARR-1): the importance of scar and the development of a prediction rule for the degree of recovery of left ventricular function. *J Am Coll Cardiol.* 2002;40:1735-1743.

Beller GA. First annual Mario S. Verani, MD, Memorial lecture: clinical value of myocardial perfusion imaging in coronary artery disease. *J Nucl Cardiol.* 2003;10:529-542.

Berman DS, Hachamovitch R, Shaw LJ, et al. Roles of nuclear cardiology, cardiac computed tomography, and cardiac magnetic resonance: noninvasive risk stratification and a conceptual framework for the selection of noninvasive imaging tests in patients with known or suspected coronary artery disease. *J Nucl Med.* 2006;47:1107-1118.

Berman DS, Wong ND, Gransar H, et al. Relationship between stress-induced myocardial ischemia and atherosclerosis measured by coronary calcium tomography. *J Am Coll Cardiol.* 2004;44:923-930.

Bisi G, Sciagra R, Santoro GM, Fazzini PF. Rest technetium-99m sestamibi tomography in combination with short-term administration of nitrates: feasibility and reliability for prediction of postrevascularization outcome of asynergic territories. *J Am Coll Cardiol.* 1994;24:1282-1289.

Bisi G, Sciagra R, Santoro GM, Rossi V, Fazzini PF. Technetium-99m-sestamibi imaging with nitrate infusion to detect viable hibernating myocardium and predict postrevascularization recovery. *J Nucl Med.* 1995;36:1994-2000.

Bisi G, Sciagra R, Santoro GM, Zerauschek F, Fazzini PF. Sublingual isosorbide dinitrate to improve technetium-99m-teboroxime perfusion defect reversibility. *J Nucl Med.* 1994;35:1274-1278.

Blankstein R, Dorbala S. Adding calcium scoring to myocardial perfusion imaging: does it alter physicians' therapeutic decision making? *J Nucl Cardiol.* 2010;17:168-171.

Boden WE, O'Rourke RA, Teo KK, et al. Optimal medical therapy with or without PCI for stable coronary disease. *N Engl J Med.* 2007;356:1503-1516.

Bonow RO, Maurer G, Lee KL, et al. Myocardial viability and survival in ischemic left ventricular dysfunction. *N Engl J Med.* 2011;364:1617-1625.

Braunwald E, Antman EM, Beasley JW, et al. ACC/AHA 2002 guideline update for the management of patients with unstable angina and non-ST-segment elevation myocardial infarction: summary article: a report of the American College of Cardiology/American Heart Association task force on practice guidelines (Committee on the Management of Patients With Unstable Angina). *J Am Coll Cardiol.* 2002;40:1366-1374.

Braunwald E, Kloner RA. The stunned myocardium: prolonged, postischemic ventricular dysfunction. *Circulation.* 1982;66:1146-1149.

Brown KA. Prognostic value of thallium-201 myocardial perfusion imaging: a diagnostic tool comes of age. *Circulation.* 1991;83:363-381.

Brown KA, Boucher CA, Okada RD, et al. Prognostic value of exercise thallium-201 imaging in patients presenting for evaluation of chest pain. *J Am Coll Cardiol.* 1983;1:994-1001.

Brown KA, Heller GV, Landin RS, et al. Early dipyridamole (99m)Tc-sestamibi single photon emission computed tomographic imaging 2 to 4 days after acute myocardial infarction predicts in-hospital and postdischarge cardiac events: comparison with submaximal exercise imaging. *Circulation.* 1999;100:2060-2066.

Bureau JF, Gaillard JF, Granier R, Ollivier JP. Diagnostic and prognostic criteria of chronic left ventricular failure obtained during exercise-201Tl imaging. *Eur J Nucl Med.* 1987;12:613-616.

Bybee KA, Lee J, Markiewicz R, et al. Diagnostic and clinical benefit of combined coronary calcium and perfusion assessment in patients undergoing PET/CT myocardial perfusion stress imaging. *J Nucl Cardiol.* 2010;17:188-196.

Campisi R, Di Carli MF. Assessment of coronary flow reserve and microcirculation: a clinical perspective. *J Nucl Cardiol.* 2004;11:3-11.

Carrio I, Berna L, Ballester M, et al. Indium-111 antimyosin scintigraphy to assess myocardial damage in patients with suspected myocarditis and cardiac rejection. *J Nucl Med.* 1988;29:1893-1900.

Cecchi F, Olivotto I, Gistri R, Lorenzoni R, Chiriatti G, Camici PG. Coronary microvascular dysfunction and prognosis in hypertrophic cardiomyopathy. *N Engl J Med.* 2003;349:1027-1035.

Chaitman BR. Exercise stress testing. In: Libby P, Bonow RO, Mann DP, Zipes DP, eds. *Braunwald's Heart Disease: A Textbook of Cardiovascular Medicine.* 8th ed. Philadelphia: Saunders; 2008:195-226.

Chang SM, Nabi F, Xu J, et al. The coronary artery calcium score and stress myocardial perfusion imaging provide independent and complementary prediction of cardiac risk. *J Am Coll Cardiol.* 2009;54:1872-1882.

Chen W, Bural GG, Torigian DA, Rader DJ, Alavi A. Emerging role of FDG-PET/CT in assessing atherosclerosis in large arteries. *Eur J Nucl Med Mol Imaging.* 2009;36:144-151.

Chikamori T, Yamashina A, Hida S, Nishimura T. Diagnostic and prognostic value of BMIPP imaging. *J Nucl Cardiol.* 2007;14:111-125.

Chow BJ, Al Shammeri OM, Beanlands RS, et al. Prognostic value of treadmill exercise and dobutamine stress positron emission tomography. *Can J Cardiol.* 2009;25:e220-e224.

Cornel JH, Bax JJ, Elhendy A, et al. Biphasic response to dobutamine predicts improvement of global left ventricular function after surgical revascularization in patients with stable coronary artery disease: implications of time course of recovery on diagnostic accuracy. *J Am Coll Cardiol.* 1998;31:1002-1010.

Danias PG, Ahlberg AW, Clark III BA, et al. Combined assessment of myocardial perfusion and left ventricular function with exercise technetium-99m sestamibi gated single-photon emission computed tomography can differentiate between ischemic and nonischemic dilated cardiomyopathy. *Am J Cardiol.* 1998;82:1253-1258.

Dayanikli F, Grambow D, Muzik O, Mosca L, Rubenfire M, Schwaiger M. Early detection of abnormal coronary flow reserve in asymptomatic men at high risk for coronary artery disease using positron emission tomography. *Circulation.* 1994;90:808-817.

Depre C, Vanoverschelde JL, Taegtmeyer H. Glucose for the heart. *Circulation.* 1999;99:578-588.

DePuey EG, Rozanski A. Using gated technetium-99m-sestamibi SPECT to characterize fixed myocardial defects as infarct or artifact. *J Nucl Med.* 1995;36:952-955.

Di Carli MF. Myocardial viability assessment with PET and PET/CT. In: Di Carli MF, Lipton ML, eds. *Cardiac PET and PET/CT Imaging.* New York: Springer; 2007:250-269.

Di Carli MF. Predicting improved function after myocardial revascularization. *Curr Opin Cardiol.* 1998;13:415-424.

Di Carli MF, Asgarzadie F, Schelbert HR, et al. Quantitative relation between myocardial viability and improvement in heart failure symptoms after revascularization in patients with ischemic cardiomyopathy. *Circulation.* 1995;92:3436-3444.

Di Carli MF, Dorbala S, Meserve J, El FG, Sitek A, Moore SC. Clinical myocardial perfusion PET/CT. *J Nucl Med.* 2007;48:783-793.

Di Carli MF, Hachamovitch R. New technology for noninvasive evaluation of coronary artery disease. *Circulation.* 2007;115:1464-1480.

Di Carli MF, Janisse J, Grunberger G, Ager J. Role of chronic hyperglycemia in the pathogenesis of coronary microvascular dysfunction in diabetes. *J Am Coll Cardiol.* 2003;41:1387-1393.

Di Carli MF, Maddahi J, Rokhsar S, et al. Long-term survival of patients with coronary artery disease and left ventricular dysfunction: implications for the role of myocardial viability assessment in management decisions. *J Thorac Cardiovasc Surg.* 1998;116:997-1004.

Di Carli MF, Prcevski P, Singh TP, et al. Myocardial blood flow, function, and metabolism in repetitive stunning. *J Nucl Med.* 2000;41:1227-1234.

Dilsizian V, Bateman TM, Bergmann SR, et al. Metabolic imaging with beta-methyl-p-[(123)I]-iodophenyl-pentadecanoic acid identifies ischemic memory after demand ischemia. *Circulation.* 2005;112:2169-2174.

Dilsizian V, Bonow RO. Current diagnostic techniques of assessing myocardial viability in patients with hibernating and stunned myocardium. *Circulation.* 1993;87:1-20.

Dilsizian V, Freedman NM, Bacharach SL, Perrone-Filardi P, Bonow RO. Regional thallium uptake in irreversible defects: magnitude of change in thallium activity after reinjection distinguishes viable from nonviable myocardium. *Circulation.* 1992;85:627-634.

Dilsizian V, Rocco TP, Freedman NM, Leon MB, Bonow RO. Enhanced detection of ischemic but viable myocardium by the reinjection of thallium after stress-redistribution imaging. *N Engl J Med.* 1990;323:141-146.

Dorbala S, Hachamovitch R, Curillova Z, et al. Incremental prognostic value of gated Rb-82 positron emission tomography myocardial perfusion imaging over clinical variables and rest LVEF. *JACC Cardiovasc Imaging.* 2009;2:846-854.

Dorbala S, Hassan A, Heinonen T, Schelbert HR, Di Carli MF. Coronary vasodilator reserve and Framingham risk scores in subjects at risk for coronary artery disease. *J Nucl Cardiol.* 2006;13:761-767.

Dou KF, Yang MF, Yang YJ, Jain D, He ZX. Myocardial 18F-FDG uptake after exercise-induced myocardial ischemia in patients with coronary artery disease. *J Nucl Med.* 2008;49:1986-1991.

El FG, Kardan A, Sitek A, et al. Reproducibility and accuracy of quantitative myocardial blood flow assessment with (82)Rb PET: comparison with (13)N-ammonia PET. *J Nucl Med.* 2009;50:1062-1071.

El FG, Sitek A, Guerin B, Kijewski MF, Di Carli MF, Moore SC. Quantitative dynamic cardiac 82Rb PET using generalized factor and compartment analyses. *J Nucl Med.* 2005;46:1264-1271.

Elhendy A, Schinkel AF, van Domburg RT, et al. Prognostic value of exercise stress technetium-99m-tetrofosmin myocardial perfusion imaging in patients with normal baseline electrocardiograms. *Am J Cardiol.* 2006;98:585-590.

Eriksson P, Backman C, Bjerle P, Eriksson A, Holm S, Olofsson BO. Non-invasive assessment of the presence and severity of cardiac amyloidosis: a study in familial amyloidosis with polyneuropathy by cross sectional echocardiography and technetium-99m pyrophosphate scintigraphy. *Br Heart J.* 1984;52:321-326.

Fagan Jr LF, Shaw L, Kong BA, Caralis DG, Wiens RD, Chaitman BR. Prognostic value of exercise thallium scintigraphy in patients with good exercise tolerance and a normal or abnormal exercise electrocardiogram and suspected or confirmed coronary artery disease. *Am J Cardiol.* 1992;69:607-611.

Falk RH, Lee VW, Rubinow A, Hood Jr WB, Cohen AS. Sensitivity of technetium-99m-pyrophosphate scintigraphy in diagnosing cardiac amyloidosis. *Am J Cardiol.* 1983;51:826-830.

Ficaro EP, Fessler JA, Shreve PD, Kritzman JN, Rose PA, Corbett JR. Simultaneous transmission/emission myocardial perfusion tomography: diagnostic accuracy of attenuation-corrected 99mTc-sestamibi single-photon emission computed tomography. *Circulation.* 1996;93:463-473.

Fletcher GF, Balady GJ, Amsterdam EA, et al. Exercise standards for testing and training: a statement for healthcare professionals from the American Heart Association. *Circulation.* 2001;104:1694-1740.

Flotats A, Knuuti J, Gutberlet M, et al. Hybrid cardiac imaging: SPECT/CT and PET/CT: a joint position statement by the European Association of Nuclear Medicine (EANM), the European Society of Cardiac Radiology (ESCR), and the European Council of Nuclear Cardiology (ECNC). *Eur J Nucl Med Mol Imaging.* 2011;38:201-212.

Fricke E, Fricke H, Weise R, et al. Attenuation correction of myocardial SPECT perfusion images with low-dose CT: evaluation of the method by comparison with perfusion PET. *J Nucl Med.* 2005;46:736-744.

Fukushima K, Javadi MS, Higuchi T, et al. Prediction of short-term cardiovascular events using quantification of global myocardial flow reserve in patients referred for clinical 82Rb PET perfusion imaging. *J Nucl Med.* 2011;52:726-732.

Garcia EV, Esteves FP. Attenuation corrected myocardial perfusion SPECT provides powerful risk stratification in patients with coronary artery disease. *J Nucl Cardiol.* 2009;16:490-492.

Gibbons RJ, Balady GJ, Beasley JW, et al. ACC/AHA guidelines for exercise testing: a report of the American College of Cardiology/American Heart Association Task Force on Practice Guidelines (Committee on Exercise Testing). *J Am Coll Cardiol.* 1997;30:260-311.

Gibson RS, Watson DD, Taylor GJ, et al. Prospective assessment of regional myocardial perfusion before and after coronary revascularization surgery by quantitative thallium-201 scintigraphy. *J Am Coll Cardiol.* 1983;1:804-815.

Gill JB, Ruddy TD, Newell JB, Finkelstein DM, Strauss HW, Boucher CA. Prognostic importance of thallium uptake by the lungs during exercise in coronary artery disease. *N Engl J Med.* 1987;317:1486-1489.

Go RT, Marwick TH, MacIntyre WJ, et al. A prospective comparison of rubidium-82 PET and thallium-201 SPECT myocardial perfusion imaging utilizing a single dipyridamole stress in the diagnosis of coronary artery disease. *J Nucl Med.* 1990;31:1899-1905.

Goodwin GW, Taylor CS, Taegtmeyer H. Regulation of energy metabolism of the heart during acute increase in heart work. *J Biol Chem.* 1998;273:29530-29539.

Gould KL, Martucci JP, Goldberg DI, et al. Short-term cholesterol lowering decreases size and severity of perfusion abnormalities by positron emission tomography after dipyridamole in patients with coronary artery disease: a potential noninvasive marker of healing coronary endothelium. *Circulation.* 1994;89:1530-1538.

Gould KL, Ornish D, Scherwitz L, et al. Changes in myocardial perfusion abnormalities by positron emission tomography after long-term, intense risk factor modification. *JAMA.* 1995;274:894-901.

Gropler RJ, Geltman EM, Sampathkumaran K, et al. Functional recovery after coronary revascularization for chronic coronary artery disease is dependent on maintenance of oxidative metabolism. *J Am Coll Cardiol.* 1992;20:569-577.

Gropler RJ, Siegel BA, Sampathkumaran K, et al. Dependence of recovery of contractile function on maintenance of oxidative metabolism after myocardial infarction. *J Am Coll Cardiol.* 1992;19:989-997.

Guethlin M, Kasel AM, Coppenrath K, Ziegler S, Delius W, Schwaiger M. Delayed response of myocardial flow reserve to lipid-lowering therapy with fluvastatin. *Circulation.* 1999;99:475-481.

Hachamovitch R, Berman DS, Kiat H, et al. Exercise myocardial perfusion SPECT in patients without known coronary artery disease: incremental prognostic value and use in risk stratification. *Circulation*. 1996;93:905-914.

Hachamovitch R, Hayes S, Friedman JD, et al. Determinants of risk and its temporal variation in patients with normal stress myocardial perfusion scans: what is the warranty period of a normal scan? *J Am Coll Cardiol*. 2003;41:1329-1340.

Hachamovitch R, Hayes SW, Friedman JD, Cohen I, Berman DS. A prognostic score for prediction of cardiac mortality risk after adenosine stress myocardial perfusion scintigraphy. *J Am Coll Cardiol*. 2005;45:722-729.

Hachamovitch R, Hayes SW, Friedman JD, Cohen I, Berman DS. Comparison of the short-term survival benefit associated with revascularization compared with medical therapy in patients with no prior coronary artery disease undergoing stress myocardial perfusion single photon emission computed tomography. *Circulation*. 2003;107:2900-2907.

Hachamovitch R, Johnson JR, Hlatky MA, et al. The Study of Myocardial Perfusion and Coronary Anatomy Imaging Roles in CAD (SPARC): design, rationale, and baseline patient characteristics of a prospective, multicenter observational registry comparing PET, SPECT, and CTA for resource utilization and clinical outcomes. *J Nucl Cardiol*. 2009;16:935-948.

He ZX, Hedrick TD, Pratt CM, et al. Severity of coronary artery calcification by electron beam computed tomography predicts silent myocardial ischemia. *Circulation*. 2000;101:244-251.

He ZX, Shi RF, Wu YJ, et al. Direct imaging of exercise-induced myocardial ischemia with fluorine-18-labeled deoxyglucose and Tc-99m-sestamibi in coronary artery disease. *Circulation*. 2003;108:1208-1213.

Heller GV, Brown KA, Landin RJ, Haber SB. Safety of early intravenous dipyridamole technetium 99m sestamibi SPECT myocardial perfusion imaging after uncomplicated first myocardial infarction: Early Post MI IV Dipyridamole Study (EPIDS). *Am Heart J*. 1997;134:105-111.

Hendel RC, Berman DS, Cullom SJ, et al. Multicenter clinical trial to evaluate the efficacy of correction for photon attenuation and scatter in SPECT myocardial perfusion imaging. *Circulation*. 1999;99:2742-2749.

Hendel RC, Berman DS, Di Carli MF, et al. ACCF/ASNC/ACR/AHA/ASE/SCCT/ SCMR/SNM 2009 appropriate use criteria for cardiac radionuclide imaging: a report of the American College of Cardiology Foundation Appropriate Use Criteria Task Force, the American Society of Nuclear Cardiology, the American College of Radiology, the American Heart Association, the American Society of Echocardiography, the Society of Cardiovascular Computed Tomography, the Society for Cardiovascular Magnetic Resonance, and the Society of Nuclear Medicine. *J Am Coll Cardiol*. 2009;53:2201-2229.

Henneman MM, Bengel FM, van der Wall EE, Knuuti J, Bax JJ. Cardiac neuronal imaging: application in the evaluation of cardiac disease. *J Nucl Cardiol*. 2008;15:442-455.

Herzog BA, Husmann L, Valenta I, et al. Long-term prognostic value of 13N-ammonia myocardial perfusion positron emission tomography added value of coronary flow reserve. *J Am Coll Cardiol*. 2009;54:150-156.

Huggins GS, Pasternak RC, Alpert NM, Fischman AJ, Gewirtz H. Effects of short-term treatment of hyperlipidemia on coronary vasodilator function and myocardial perfusion in regions having substantial impairment of baseline dilator reverse. *Circulation*. 1998;98:1291-1296.

Hutchins GD, Schwaiger M, Rosenspire KC, Krivokapich J, Schelbert H, Kuhl DE. Noninvasive quantification of regional blood flow in the human heart using N-13 ammonia and dynamic positron emission tomographic imaging. *J Am Coll Cardiol*. 1990;15:1032-1042.

Inaba Y, Chen JA, Bergmann SR. Quantity of viable myocardium required to improve survival with revascularization in patients with ischemic cardiomyopathy: a meta-analysis. *J Nucl Cardiol*. 2010;17:646-654.

Iskandrian AE, Heo J. Myocardial perfusion imaging during adenosine-induced coronary hyperemia. *Am J Cardiol*. 1997;79:20-24.

Jaffer FA, Libby P, Weissleder R. Molecular imaging of cardiovascular disease. *Circulation*. 2007;116:1052-1061.

Jaffer FA, Libby P, Weissleder R. Molecular and cellular imaging of atherosclerosis: emerging applications. *J Am Coll Cardiol*. 2006;47:1328-1338.

Jain D, He ZX. Direct imaging of myocardial ischemia: a potential new paradigm in nuclear cardiovascular imaging. *J Nucl Cardiol*. 2008;15:617-630.

Kaiser KP, Feinendegen LE. [Planar scintigraphy versus PET in measuring fatty acid metabolism of the heart]. *Herz*. 1987;12:41-50:in German.

Kaufmann PA, Camici PG. Myocardial blood flow measurement by PET: technical aspects and clinical applications. *J Nucl Med*. 2005;46:75-88.

Kaufmann PA, Di Carli MF. Hybrid SPECT/CT and PET/CT imaging: the next step in noninvasive cardiac imaging. *Semin Nucl Med*. 2009;39:341-347.

Kioka H, Yamada T, Mine T, et al. Prediction of sudden death in patients with mild-to-moderate chronic heart failure by using cardiac iodine-123 metaiodobenzylguanidine imaging. *Heart*. 2007;93:1213-1218.

Kitsiou AN, Srinivasan G, Quyyumi AA, Summers RM, Bacharach SL, Dilsizian V. Stress-induced reversible and mild-to-moderate irreversible thallium defects: are they equally accurate for predicting recovery of regional left ventricular function after revascularization? *Circulation*. 1998;98:501-508.

Klocke FJ, Baird MG, Lorell BH, et al. ACC/AHA/ASNC guidelines for the clinical use of cardiac radionuclide imaging—executive summary: a report of the American College of Cardiology/American Heart Association Task Force on Practice Guidelines (ACC/AHA/ASNC Committee to Revise the 1995 Guidelines for the Clinical Use of Cardiac Radionuclide Imaging). *Circulation*. 2003;108:1404-1418.

Kluge R, Sattler B, Seese A, Knapp WH. Attenuation correction by simultaneous emission-transmission myocardial single-photon emission tomography using a technetium-99m-labelled radiotracer: impact on diagnostic accuracy. *Eur J Nucl Med*. 1997;24:1107-1114.

Knaapen P, de Haan S, Hoekstra OS, et al. Cardiac PET-CT: advanced hybrid imaging for the detection of coronary artery disease. *Neth J Med*. 2010;18:90-98.

Koh AS, Chia S. Update on clinical imaging of coronary plaque in acute coronary syndrome. *Ann Acad Med Singapore*. 2010;39:203-209.

Kontos MC, Dilsizian V, Weiland F, et al. Iodofiltic acid I 123 (BMIPP) fatty acid imaging improves initial diagnosis in emergency department patients with suspected acute coronary syndromes: a multicenter trial. *J Am Coll Cardiol*. 2010;56:290-299.

Krishnan R, Lu J, Dae MW, Botvinick EH. Does myocardial perfusion scintigraphy demonstrate clinical usefulness in patients with markedly positive exercise tests? An assessment of the method in a high-risk subset. *Am Heart J*. 1994;127:804-816.

Kuhle WG, Porenta G, Huang SC, et al. Quantification of regional myocardial blood flow using 13N-ammonia and reoriented dynamic positron emission tomographic imaging. *Circulation*. 1992;86:1004-1017.

Kumar SP, Brewington SD, O'Brien KF, Movahed A. Clinical correlation between increased lung to heart ratio of technetium-99m sestamibi and multivessel coronary artery disease. *Int J Cardiol*. 2005;101:219-222.

Kushner FG, Hand M, Smith Jr SC, et al. 2009 focused updates: ACC/AHA guidelines for the management of patients with ST-elevation myocardial infarction (updating the 2004 guideline and 2007 focused update) and ACC/ AHA/SCAI guidelines on percutaneous coronary intervention (updating the 2005 guideline and 2007 focused update): a report of the American College of Cardiology Foundation/American Heart Association Task Force on Practice Guidelines. *J Am Coll Cardiol*. 2009;54:2205-2241.

Kwok JM, Miller TD, Hodge DO, Gibbons RJ. Prognostic value of the Duke treadmill score in the elderly. *J Am Coll Cardiol*. 2002;39:1475-1481.

Ladenheim ML, Pollock BH, Rozanski A, et al. Extent and severity of myocardial hypoperfusion as predictors of prognosis in patients with suspected coronary artery disease. *J Am Coll Cardiol*. 1986;7:464-471.

Laine H, Raitakari OT, Niinikoski H, et al. Early impairment of coronary flow reserve in young men with borderline hypertension. *J Am Coll Cardiol*. 1998;32:147-153.

Lanza GA, Mustilli M, Sestito A, Infusino F, Sgueglia GA, Crea F. Diagnostic and prognostic value of ST segment depression limited to the recovery phase of exercise stress test. *Heart*. 2004;90:1417-1421.

Leoncini M, Marcucci G, Sciagra R, et al. Prediction of functional recovery in patients with chronic coronary artery disease and left ventricular dysfunction combining the evaluation of myocardial perfusion and of contractile reserve using nitrate-enhanced technetium-99m sestamibi gated single-photon emission computed tomography and dobutamine stress. *Am J Cardiol*. 2001;87:1346-1350.

Lertsburapa K, Ahlberg AW, Bateman TM, et al. Independent and incremental prognostic value of left ventricular ejection fraction determined by stress gated rubidium 82 PET imaging in patients with known or suspected coronary artery disease. *J Nucl Cardiol*. 2008;15:745-753.

Lette J, Lapointe J, Waters D, Cerino M, Picard M, Gagnon A. Transient left ventricular cavitary dilation during dipyridamole-thallium imaging as an indicator of severe coronary artery disease. *Am J Cardiol*. 1990;66:1163-1170.

Lin JW, Laine AF, Akinboboye O, Bergmann SR. Use of wavelet transforms in analysis of time-activity data from cardiac PET. *J Nucl Med*. 2001;42: 194-200.

Links JM, DePuey EG, Taillefer R, Becker LC. Attenuation correction and gating synergistically improve the diagnostic accuracy of myocardial perfusion SPECT. *J Nucl Cardiol*. 2002;9:183-187.

Litzler PY, Manrique A, Etienne M, et al. Leukocyte SPECT/CT for detecting infection of left-ventricular-assist devices: preliminary results. *J Nucl Med*. 2010;51:1044-1048.

Liu P, Kiess M, Okada RD, et al. Increased thallium lung uptake after exercise in isolated left anterior descending coronary artery disease. *Am J Cardiol*. 1985;55:1469-1473.

Lopaschuk GD, Stanley WC. Glucose metabolism in the ischemic heart. *Circulation*. 1997;95:313-315.

Maes AF, Borgers M, Flameng W, et al. Assessment of myocardial viability in chronic coronary artery disease using technetium-99m sestamibi SPECT: correlation with histologic and positron emission tomographic studies and functional follow-up. *J Am Coll Cardiol*. 1997;29:62-68.

Mahmarian JJ, Dakik HA, Filipchuk NG, et al. An initial strategy of intensive medical therapy is comparable to that of coronary revascularization for suppression of scintigraphic ischemia in high-risk but stable survivors of acute myocardial infarction. *J Am Coll Cardiol*. 2006;48:2458-2467.

Mahmarian JJ, Mahmarian AC, Marks GF, Pratt CM, Verani MS. Role of adenosine thallium-201 tomography for defining long-term risk in patients after acute myocardial infarction. *J Am Coll Cardiol*. 1995;25:1333-1340.

Mahmarian JJ, Shaw LJ, Filipchuk NG, et al. A multinational study to establish the value of early adenosine technetium-99m sestamibi myocardial perfusion imaging in identifying a low-risk group for early hospital discharge after acute myocardial infarction. *J Am Coll Cardiol*. 2006;48:2448-2457.

Mahmarian JJ, Shaw LJ, Olszewski GH, Pounds BK, Frias ME, Pratt CM. Adenosine sestamibi SPECT Post Infarction Evaluation (INSPIRE) trial: a randomized, prospective multicenter trial evaluating the role of adenosine

Tc-99m sestamibi SPECT for assessing risk and therapeutic outcomes in survivors of acute myocardial infarction. *J Nucl Cardiol.* 2004;11:458-469.

Malkerneker D, Brenner R, Martin WH, et al. CT-based attenuation correction versus prone imaging to decrease equivocal interpretations of rest/stress Tc-99m tetrofosmin SPECT MPI. *J Nucl Cardiol.* 2007;14:314-323.

Mannting F, Zabrodina YV, Dass C. Significance of increased right ventricular uptake on 99mTc-sestamibi SPECT in patients with coronary artery disease. *J Nucl Med.* 1999;40:889-894.

Manrique A, Bernard M, Hitzel A, et al. Prognostic value of sympathetic innervation and cardiac asynchrony in dilated cardiomyopathy. *Eur J Nucl Med Mol Imaging.* 2008;35:2074-2081.

Mark DB, Shaw L, Harrell Jr FE, et al. Prognostic value of a treadmill exercise score in outpatients with suspected coronary artery disease. *N Engl J Med.* 1991;325:849-853.

Marwick TH, Nemec JJ, Lafont A, Salcedo EE, MacIntyre WJ. Prediction by postexercise fluoro-18 deoxyglucose positron emission tomography of improvement in exercise capacity after revascularization. *Am J Cardiol.* 1992;69:854-859.

Marwick TH, Shan K, Patel S, Go RT, Lauer MS. Incremental value of rubidium-82 positron emission tomography for prognostic assessment of known or suspected coronary artery disease. *Am J Cardiol.* 1997;80:865-870.

Marwick TH, Zuchowski C, Lauer MS, Secknus MA, Williams J, Lytle BW. Functional status and quality of life in patients with heart failure undergoing coronary bypass surgery after assessment of myocardial viability. *J Am Coll Cardiol.* 1999;33:750-758.

Masood Y, Liu YH, DePuey G, et al. Clinical validation of SPECT attenuation correction using x-ray computed tomography-derived attenuation maps: multicenter clinical trial with angiographic correlation. *J Nucl Cardiol.* 2005;12:676-686.

Maurea S, Cuocolo A, Soricelli A, et al. Enhanced detection of viable myocardium by technetium-99m-MIBI imaging after nitrate administration in chronic coronary artery disease. *J Nucl Med.* 1995;36:1945-1952.

Mazzanti M, Germano G, Kiat H, et al. Identification of severe and extensive coronary artery disease by automatic measurement of transient ischemic dilation of the left ventricle in dual-isotope myocardial perfusion SPECT. *J Am Coll Cardiol.* 1996;27:1612-1620.

McLaughlin MG, Danias PG. Transient ischemic dilation: a powerful diagnostic and prognostic finding of stress myocardial perfusion imaging. *J Nucl Cardiol.* 2002;9:663-667.

Medrano R, Lowry RW, Young JB, et al. Assessment of myocardial viability with 99mTc sestamibi in patients undergoing cardiac transplantation: a scintigraphic/pathological study. *Circulation.* 1996;94:1010-1017.

Merhige ME, Breen WJ, Shelton V, Houston T, D'Arcy BJ, Perna AF. Impact of myocardial perfusion imaging with PET and (82)Rb on downstream invasive procedure utilization, costs, and outcomes in coronary disease management. *J Nucl Med.* 2007;48:1069-1076.

Merlet P, Benvenuti C, Moyse D, et al. Prognostic value of MIBG imaging in idiopathic dilated cardiomyopathy. *J Nucl Med.* 1999;40:917-923.

Min JK, Hachamovitch R, Rozanski A, Shaw LJ, Berman DS, Gibbons R. Clinical benefits of noninvasive testing: coronary computed tomography angiography as a test case. *JACC Cardiovasc Imaging.* 2010;3:305-315.

Morguet AJ, Munz DL, Kreuzer H, Emrich D. Scintigraphic detection of inflammatory heart disease. *Eur J Nucl Med.* 1994;21:666-674.

Muzik O, Beanlands RS, Hutchins GD, Mangner TJ, Nguyen N, Schwaiger M. Validation of nitrogen-13-ammonia tracer kinetic model for quantification of myocardial blood flow using PET. *J Nucl Med.* 1993;34:83-91.

Naya M, Tsukamoto T, Morita K, et al. Olmesartan, but not amlodipine, improves endothelium-dependent coronary dilation in hypertensive patients. *J Am Coll Cardiol.* 2007;50:1144-1149.

Neglia D, Michelassi C, Trivieri MG, et al. Prognostic role of myocardial blood flow impairment in idiopathic left ventricular dysfunction. *Circulation.* 2002;105:186-193.

Nishimura M, Tsukamoto K, Hasebe N, Tamaki N, Kikuchi K, Ono T. Prediction of cardiac death in hemodialysis patients by myocardial fatty acid imaging. *J Am Coll Cardiol.* 2008;51:139-145.

Nitzsche EU, Choi Y, Czernin J, Hoh CK, Huang SC, Schelbert HR. Noninvasive quantification of myocardial blood flow in humans: a direct comparison of the [13N]ammonia and the [15O]water techniques. *Circulation.* 1996;93:2000-2006.

Nowak B, Sinha AM, Schaefer WM, et al. Cardiac resynchronization therapy homogenizes myocardial glucose metabolism and perfusion in dilated cardiomyopathy and left bundle branch block. *J Am Coll Cardiol.* 2003;41:1523-1528.

Nunes H, Freynet O, Naggara N, et al. Cardiac sarcoidosis. *Semin Respir Crit Care Med.* 2010;31:428-441.

Ohira H, Tsujino I, Yoshinaga K. ^{18}F-Fluoro-2-deoxyglucose positron emission tomography in cardiac sarcoidosis. *Eur J Nucl Med Mol Imaging.* 2011;38:1773-1783.

Okayama K, Kurata C, Tawarahara K, Wakabayashi Y, Chida K, Sato A. Diagnostic and prognostic value of myocardial scintigraphy with thallium-201 and gallium-67 in cardiac sarcoidosis. *Chest.* 1995;107:330-334.

Ornish D, Scherwitz LW, Billings JH, et al. Intensive lifestyle changes for reversal of coronary heart disease. *JAMA.* 1998;280:2001-2007.

Osborn EA, Jaffer FA. The year in molecular imaging. *JACC Cardiovasc Imaging.* 2009;2:97-113.

Parkash R, deKemp RA, Ruddy TD, et al. Potential utility of rubidium 82 PET quantification in patients with 3-vessel coronary artery disease. *J Nucl Cardiol.* 2004;11:440-449.

Pasquet A, Robert A, D'Hondt AM, Dion R, Melin JA, Vanoverschelde JL. Prognostic value of myocardial ischemia and viability in patients with chronic left ventricular ischemic dysfunction. *Circulation.* 1999;100:141-148.

Patterson RE, Eisner RL, Horowitz SF. Comparison of cost-effectiveness and utility of exercise ECG, single photon emission computed tomography, positron emission tomography, and coronary angiography for diagnosis of coronary artery disease. *Circulation.* 1995;91:54-65.

Pazhenkottil AP, Herzog BA, Husmann L, et al. Non-invasive assessment of coronary artery disease with CT coronary angiography and SPECT: a novel dose-saving fast-track algorithm. *Eur J Nucl Med Mol Imaging.* 2010;37:522-527.

Pazhenkottil AP, Nkoulou RN, Ghadri JR, et al. Prognostic value of cardiac hybrid imaging integrating single-photon emission computed tomography with coronary computed tomography angiography. *Eur Heart J.* 2011;32:1465-1471.

Pena FJ, Banzo I, Quirce R, et al. Ga-67 SPECT to detect endocarditis after replacement of an aortic valve. *Clin Nucl Med.* 2002;27:401-404.

Perrone-Filardi P, Pace L, Prastaro M, et al. Dobutamine echocardiography predicts improvement of hypoperfused dysfunctional myocardium after revascularization in patients with coronary artery disease. *Circulation.* 1995;91:2556-2565.

Pitkanen OP, Raitakari OT, Niinikoski H, et al. Coronary flow reserve is impaired in young men with familial hypercholesterolemia. *J Am Coll Cardiol.* 1996;28:1705-1711.

Pollack Jr CV, Braunwald E. 2007 update to the ACC/AHA guidelines for the management of patients with unstable angina and non–ST-segment elevation myocardial infarction: implications for emergency department practice. *Ann Emerg Med.* 2008;51:591-606.

Risk stratification and survival after myocardial infarction. *N Engl J Med.* 1983;309:331-336.

Rohatgi R, Epstein S, Henriquez J, et al. Utility of positron emission tomography in predicting cardiac events and survival in patients with coronary artery disease and severe left ventricular dysfunction. *Am J Cardiol.* 2001;87:1096-1099:A6.

Roman CD, Habibian MR, Martin WH. Identification of an infected left ventricular assist device after cardiac transplant by indium-111 WBC scintigraphy. *Clin Nucl Med.* 2005;30:16-17.

Sampson UK, Dorbala S, Limaye A, Kwong R, Di Carli MF. Diagnostic accuracy of rubidium-82 myocardial perfusion imaging with hybrid positron emission tomography/computed tomography in the detection of coronary artery disease. *J Am Coll Cardiol.* 2007;49:1052-1058.

Schaefer WM, Lipke CS, Nowak B, et al. Validation of an evaluation routine for left ventricular volumes, ejection fraction and wall motion from gated cardiac FDG PET: a comparison with cardiac magnetic resonance imaging. *Eur J Nucl Med Mol Imaging.* 2003;30:545-553.

Schalet BD, Kegel JG, Heo J, Segal BL, Iskandrian AS. Prognostic implications of normal exercise SPECT thallium images in patients with strongly positive exercise electrocardiograms. *Am J Cardiol.* 1993;72:1201-1203.

Schelbert HR, Phelps ME, Hoffman E, Huang SC, Kuhl DE. Regional myocardial blood flow, metabolism and function assessed noninvasively with positron emission tomography. *Am J Cardiol.* 1980;46:1269-1277.

Schelbert HR, Phelps ME, Huang SC, et al. N-13 ammonia as an indicator of myocardial blood flow. *Circulation.* 1981;63:1259-1272.

Schepis T, Gaemperli O, Koepfli P, et al. Added value of coronary artery calcium score as an adjunct to gated SPECT for the evaluation of coronary artery disease in an intermediate-risk population. *J Nucl Med.* 2007;48:1424-1430.

Schindler TH, Nitzsche EU, Olschewski M, et al. Chronic inflammation and impaired coronary vasoreactivity in patients with coronary risk factors. *Circulation.* 2004;110:1069-1075.

Schindler TH, Nitzsche EU, Schelbert HR, et al. Positron emission tomography-measured abnormal responses of myocardial blood flow to sympathetic stimulation are associated with the risk of developing cardiovascular events. *J Am Coll Cardiol.* 2005;45:1505-1512.

Schindler TH, Zhang XL, Vincenti G, et al. Diagnostic value of PET-measured heterogeneity in myocardial blood flows during cold pressor testing for the identification of coronary vasomotor dysfunction. *J Nucl Cardiol.* 2007;14:688-697.

Sharir T, Germano G, Kang X, et al. Prediction of myocardial infarction versus cardiac death by gated myocardial perfusion SPECT: risk stratification by the amount of stress-induced ischemia and the poststress ejection fraction. *J Nucl Med.* 2001;42:831-837.

Sharir T, Germano G, Kavanagh PB, et al. Incremental prognostic value of post-stress left ventricular ejection fraction and volume by gated myocardial perfusion single photon emission computed tomography. *Circulation.* 1999;100:1035-1042.

Sharma S. Cardiac imaging in myocardial sarcoidosis and other cardiomyopathies. *Curr Opin Pulm Med.* 2009;15:507-512.

Shaw L, Chaitman BR, Hilton TC, et al. Prognostic value of dipyridamole thallium-201 imaging in elderly patients. *J Am Coll Cardiol.* 1992;19:1390-1398.

Shaw LJ, Berman DS, Maron DJ, et al. Optimal medical therapy with or without percutaneous coronary intervention to reduce ischemic burden: results from the Clinical Outcomes Utilizing Revascularization and Aggressive Drug Evaluation (COURAGE) trial nuclear substudy. *Circulation.* 2008;117:1283-1291.

Shaw LJ, Hachamovitch R, Berman DS, et al. The economic consequences of available diagnostic and prognostic strategies for the evaluation of stable angina patients: an observational assessment of the value of precatheterization ischemia. Economics of Noninvasive Diagnosis (END) Multicenter Study Group. *J Am Coll Cardiol*. 1999;33:661-669.

Shaw LJ, Iskandrian AE. Prognostic value of gated myocardial perfusion SPECT. *J Nucl Cardiol*. 2004;11:171-185.

Shaw LJ, Peterson ED, Shaw LK, et al. Use of a prognostic treadmill score in identifying diagnostic coronary disease subgroups. *Circulation*. 1998;98:1622-1630.

Shen YT, Depre C, Yan L, et al. Repetitive ischemia by coronary stenosis induces a novel window of ischemic preconditioning. *Circulation*. 2008;118:1961-1969.

Smanio PE, Watson DD, Segalla DL, Vinson EL, Smith WH, Beller GA. Value of gating of technetium-99m sestamibi single-photon emission computed tomographic imaging. *J Am Coll Cardiol*. 1997;30:1687-1692.

Smedema JP, van Kroonenburgh MJ, Snoep G, Bekkers SC, Gorgels AP. Diagnostic value of PET in cardiac sarcoidosis. *J Nucl Med*. 2004;45:1975.

Sobol SM, Brown JM, Bunker SR, Patel J, Lull RJ. Noninvasive diagnosis of cardiac amyloidosis by technetium-99m-pyrophosphate myocardial scintigraphy. *Am Heart J*. 1982;103:563-566.

Soman P, Lahiri A, Mieres JH, et al. Etiology and pathophysiology of new-onset heart failure: evaluation by myocardial perfusion imaging. *J Nucl Cardiol*. 2009;16:82-91.

Staniloff HM, Forrester JS, Berman DS, Swan HJ. Prediction of death, myocardial infarction, and worsening chest pain using thallium scintigraphy and exercise electrocardiography. *J Nucl Med*. 1986;27:1842-1848.

Stanley WC, Lopaschuk GD, Hall JL, McCormack JG. Regulation of myocardial carbohydrate metabolism under normal and ischaemic conditions: potential for pharmacological interventions. *Cardiovasc Res*. 1997;33:243-257.

Stewart RE, Schwaiger M, Molina E, et al. Comparison of rubidium-82 positron emission tomography and thallium-201 SPECT imaging for detection of coronary artery disease. *Am J Cardiol*. 1991;67:1303-1310.

Storch-Becker A, Kaiser KP, Feinendegen LE. Cardiac nuclear medicine: positron emission tomography in clinical medicine. *Eur J Nucl Med*. 1988;13:648-652.

Stowers SA, Eisenstein EL, Th Wackers FJ, et al. An economic analysis of an aggressive diagnostic strategy with single photon emission computed tomography myocardial perfusion imaging and early exercise stress testing in emergency department patients who present with chest pain but nondiagnostic electrocardiograms: results from a randomized trial. *Ann Emerg Med*. 2000;35:17-25.

Tadamura E, Mamede M, Kubo S, et al. The effect of nitroglycerin on myocardial blood flow in various segments characterized by rest-redistribution thallium SPECT. *J Nucl Med*. 2003;44:745-751.

Taegtmeyer H. Tracing cardiac metabolism in vivo: one substrate at a time. *J Nucl Med*. 2010;51(suppl 1):80S-87S.

Tahara N, Tahara A, Nitta Y, et al. Heterogeneous myocardial FDG uptake and the disease activity in cardiac sarcoidosis. *JACC Cardiovasc Imaging*. 2010;3:1219-1228.

Tarakji KG, Brunken R, McCarthy PM, et al. Myocardial viability testing and the effect of early intervention in patients with advanced left ventricular systolic dysfunction. *Circulation*. 2006;113:230-237.

Tauberg SG, Orie JE, Bartlett BE, Cottington EM, Flores AR. Usefulness of thallium-201 for distinction of ischemic from idiopathic dilated cardiomyopathy. *Am J Cardiol*. 1993;71:674-680.

Tawarahara K, Kurata C, Okayama K, Kobayashi A, Yamazaki N. Thallium-201 and gallium 67 single photon emission computed tomographic imaging in cardiac sarcoidosis. *Am Heart J*. 1992;124:1383-1384.

Thomson LE, Goodman MP, Naqvi TZ, et al. Aortic root infection in a prosthetic valve demonstrated by gallium-67 citrate SPECT. *Clin Nucl Med*. 2005;30:265-268.

Udelson JE, Beshansky JR, Ballin DS, et al. Myocardial perfusion imaging for evaluation and triage of patients with suspected acute cardiac ischemia: a randomized controlled trial. *JAMA*. 2002;288:2693-2700.

Udelson JE, Coleman PS, Metherall J, et al. Predicting recovery of severe regional ventricular dysfunction: comparison of resting scintigraphy with 201Tl and 99mTc-sestamibi. *Circulation*. 1994;89:2552-2561.

Udelson JE, Shafer CD, Carrio I. Radionuclide imaging in heart failure: assessing etiology and outcomes and implications for management. *J Nucl Cardiol*. 2002;9:40S-52S.

Uebleis C, Becker A, Griesshammer I, et al. Stable coronary artery disease: prognostic value of myocardial perfusion SPECT in relation to coronary calcium scoring—long-term follow-up. *Radiology*. 2009;252:682-690.

Underwood SR, Godman B, Salyani S, Ogle JR, Ell PJ. Economics of myocardial perfusion imaging in Europe: the EMPIRE Study. *Eur Heart J*. 1999;20:157-166.

Uren NG, Crake T, Lefroy DC, de Silva R, Davies GJ, Maseri A. Reduced coronary vasodilator function in infarcted and normal myocardium after myocardial infarction. *N Engl J Med*. 1994;331:222-227.

van Werkhoven JM, Schuijf JD, Gaemperli O, et al. Prognostic value of multislice computed tomography and gated single-photon emission computed tomography in patients with suspected coronary artery disease. *J Am Coll Cardiol*. 2009;53:623-632.

Velazquez EJ, Lee KL, Deja MA, et al. Coronary-artery bypass surgery in patients with left ventricular dysfunction. *N Engl J Med*. 2011;364:1607-1616.

Wackers FJ, Brown KA, Heller GV, et al. American Society of Nuclear Cardiology position statement on radionuclide imaging in patients with suspected acute ischemic syndromes in the emergency department or chest pain center. *J Nucl Cardiol*. 2002;9:246-250.

Wagner B, Anton M, Nekolla SG, et al. Noninvasive characterization of myocardial molecular interventions by integrated positron emission tomography and computed tomography. *J Am Coll Cardiol*. 2006;48:2107-2115.

Weiss AT, Berman DS, Lew AS, et al. Transient ischemic dilation of the left ventricle on stress thallium-201 scintigraphy: a marker of severe and extensive coronary artery disease. *J Am Coll Cardiol*. 1987;9:752-759.

Werner GS, Fritzenwanger M, Prochnau D, et al. Determinants of coronary steal in chronic total coronary occlusions donor artery, collateral, and microvascular resistance. *J Am Coll Cardiol*. 2006;48:51-58.

Williams KA, Schneider CM. Increased stress right ventricular activity on dual isotope perfusion SPECT: a sign of multivessel and/or left main coronary artery disease. *J Am Coll Cardiol*. 1999;34:420-427.

Wisenberg G, Schelbert HR, Hoffman EJ, et al. In vivo quantitation of regional myocardial blood flow by positron-emission computed tomography. *Circulation*. 1981;63:1248-1258.

Wong ND, Detrano RC, Diamond G, et al. Does coronary artery screening by electron beam computed tomography motivate potentially beneficial lifestyle behaviors? *Am J Cardiol*. 1996;78:1220-1223.

Yalamanchili P, Wexler E, Hayes M, et al. Mechanism of uptake and retention of F-18 BMS-747158-02 in cardiomyocytes: a novel PET myocardial imaging agent. *J Nucl Cardiol*. 2007;14:782-788.

Yamaguchi A, Ino T, Adachi H, et al. Left ventricular volume predicts postoperative course in patients with ischemic cardiomyopathy. *Ann Thorac Surg*. 1998;65:434-438.

Yamaguchi A, Ino T, Adachi H, Mizuhara A, Murata S, Kamio H. Left ventricular end-systolic volume index in patients with ischemic cardiomyopathy predicts postoperative ventricular function. *Ann Thorac Surg*. 1995;60:1059-1062.

Yamamoto N, Gotoh K, Yagi Y, et al. Thallium-201 myocardial SPECT findings at rest in sarcoidosis. *Ann Nucl Med*. 1993;7:97-103.

Yasuda T, Palacios IF, Dec GW, et al. Indium 111-monoclonal antimyosin antibody imaging in the diagnosis of acute myocarditis. *Circulation*. 1987;76:306-311.

Yoshinaga K, Katoh C, Noriyasu K, et al. Reduction of coronary flow reserve in areas with and without ischemia on stress perfusion imaging in patients with coronary artery disease: a study using oxygen 15–labeled water PET. *J Nucl Cardiol*. 2003;10:275-283.

Yu M, Guaraldi MT, Mistry M, et al. BMS-747158-02: a novel PET myocardial perfusion imaging agent. *J Nucl Cardiol*. 2007;14:789-798.

CHAPTER 30

Myocardial Ischemic Disease: Computed Tomography

John W. Nance Jr. and U. Joseph Schoepf

The scope of clinically relevant myocardial ischemic disease renders it one of the most important problems facing modern medicine. Risk stratification, diagnosis, management, and monitoring of patients with suspected or known ischemic disease heavily depend on imaging. Broadly speaking, the goals of imaging in ischemic heart disease can be categorized as anatomic or functional evaluation. Coronary computed tomography (CT) angiography has repeatedly been shown to have excellent diagnostic capabilities in the anatomic assessment of ischemic heart disease, specifically the detection of coronary artery atherosclerosis and stenosis. The physiologic relevance of coronary artery disease, however, is generally considered more important in establishing prognosis and management plans. Although myocardial morphology provides diagnostic clues in ischemic disease, dedicated myocardial evaluations generally focus on functional assessments, with specific goals depending on the clinical situation.

The diagnosis of acute and chronic ischemia can be made with myocardial functional imaging; more important, differentiation of viable from nonviable tissue is available and extremely important in guiding clinical management. Several strategies are used to determine tissue viability, depending on the clinical scenario; however, most of these rely on time-resolved imaging, myocardial perfusion imaging, delayed enhancement imaging, or a combination thereof. Therefore, CT has lagged behind other modalities in dedicated myocardial analyses. Temporal resolution and contrast resolution are inferior to those of other modalities, and the inevitable exposure to iodinated contrast material and ionizing radiation poses risks to the patient not associated with some techniques. However, the rapidly increasing rate of CT scans encompassing the heart, whether in a dedicated cardiac protocol or otherwise, necessitates knowledge of typical CT imaging findings in ischemic disease; furthermore, emerging techniques are showing progress in expanding the role of CT in physiologic assessments. Future refinement of these techniques could lead to a single-modality integrative evaluation of cardiac structure and function, the ultimate goal of cardiac imaging.

This chapter reviews the spectrum of imaging findings of myocardial ischemic disease in established CT applications, including routine thorax CT and dedicated cardiac CT angiography studies. In addition, technical considerations, imaging findings, and potential applications of experimental and emerging techniques are explored.

■ NONCARDIAC COMPUTED TOMOGRAPHY EXAMINATIONS

Although the value of non–electrocardiogram (ECG)-gated CT studies in assessing ischemic heart disease is limited, the sheer volume of such studies combined with the prevalence of the disease in current society necessitates knowledge of the possible imaging manifestations of acute and chronic ischemic disease. In addition, advances in scanner technology have decreased scan acquisition times sufficiently to allow assessment of the myocardium on some non–ECG-gated studies. All examinations that encompass the heart should be assessed for image quality and motion artifacts, and the myocardium should not be ignored when adequate assessment is possible.

Suggestions of acute myocardial infarction on non-gated CT studies are mainly found outside the myocardium itself. Pulmonary vascular congestion suggests acute left ventricular dysfunction. Assessment of cardiac chamber size is inaccurate, but a grossly enlarged left atrium in severe acute left ventricular failure may be apparent. Similarly, right ventricular failure from an isolated right ventricular myocardial infarction is rare, but a dilated right ventricular chamber, right atrial chamber, or systemic veins may be apparent, and contrast reflux deep into the hepatic or azygos veins may be present. Contrast-enhanced studies may display subendocardial attenuation deficits in normal-thickness myocardium, findings suggestive of acute infarction if the contrast medium bolus is timed correctly and motion artifacts are not severe; however, quantifying the size or severity of defects is difficult.

Major structural complications of myocardial infarction may also be apparent on non–ECG-gated scans. Left ventricular aneurysms or pseudoaneurysms may be seen as nonspecific morphologic abnormalities on unenhanced scans, whereas most contrast-enhanced studies should allow one to diagnose but not fully characterize wall deformities. Left ventricular free wall rupture or septal wall rupture may also be apparent on contrast-enhanced studies, but again this varies depending on image quality and the nature of the abnormality.

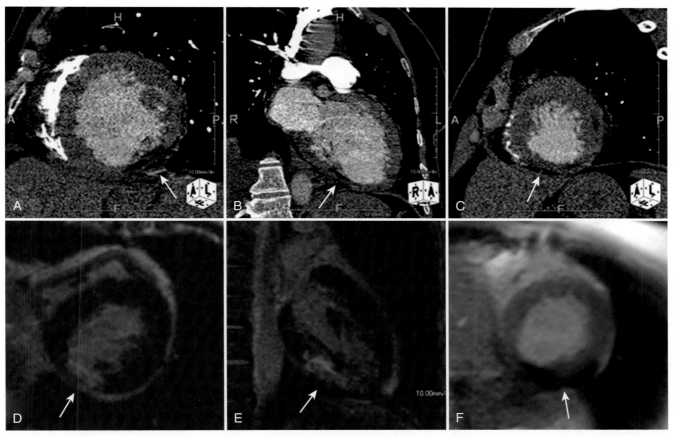

Figure 30-1 A 42-year-old male patient with no known coronary history presented to the emergency department with respiratory insufficiency and lower extremity edema. **A** to **C**, Non–electrocardiogram-gated pulmonary computed tomography angiography was performed, and it showed thinning, hypoattenuation, and fatty metaplasia of the inferior myocardium (*arrows* in **A** to **C**). **D** to **F**, Cardiac magnetic resonance imaging was subsequently performed and showed late enhancement on delayed phase imaging (*arrows* in **D** and **E**) and hypointensity on proton-density–weighted images (*arrow* in **F**), consistent with a chronic transmural inferior left ventricular wall infarct. *A*, Anterior; *L*, left; *R*, right.

Manifestations of chronic myocardial infarction are also apparent on many noncardiac CT protocols of the thorax. Left ventricular dilation should be noted, along with other signs of remodeling and functional inadequacy, such as an enlarged left atrial chamber, pulmonary venous hypertension, enlarged hilar lymph nodes, thickening of the pulmonary interlobular septa, bronchovascular bundle thickening, or ground glass opacities in dependent portions of the lungs. Again, depending on image quality, assessment of the myocardium itself may be possible. The interpreting physician should look for and comment on focal subendocardial fatty metaplasia, linear myocardial calcifications, and myocardial thinning, all of which are especially suggestive of remote infarction if they are present in a specific vascular territory (Fig. 30-1).

■ CARDIAC COMPUTED TOMOGRAPHY

The rapid rise of cardiac CT largely sprang from concomitant advances in the underlying technology, namely, decreased image acquisition times and increased detector coverage, the combination of which provided dramatic improvements in temporal resolution and isotropic submillimeter spatial resolution.

These advances allow robust assessment of the coronary arteries, with diagnostic accuracy for the detection of stenoses that approaches that of the gold standard, invasive coronary angiography. Furthermore, the technique has other inherent advantages that make it attractive in the diagnostic workup of cardiac disease. In contrast to invasive angiography, extraluminal coronary artery morphology, such as wall remodeling, is visualized. In addition, valuable information on the myocardium itself is available, both morphologic and, to a limited extent, functional.

Arterial Phase Imaging

Early researchers in CT recognized that contrast-enhanced scans were able to show areas of decreased myocardial attenuation that could be related to decreased blood flow to that area (Fig. 30-2). However, relatively poor temporal and spatial resolution limited the utility of CT for dedicated myocardial evaluation. Technical improvements combined with the increasing clinical use of coronary CT angiography revived interest in arterial phase myocardial imaging, especially given that routine coronary CT angiography scan protocols provide this information with no increase in radiation exposure, contrast dose, or study cost. The rationale

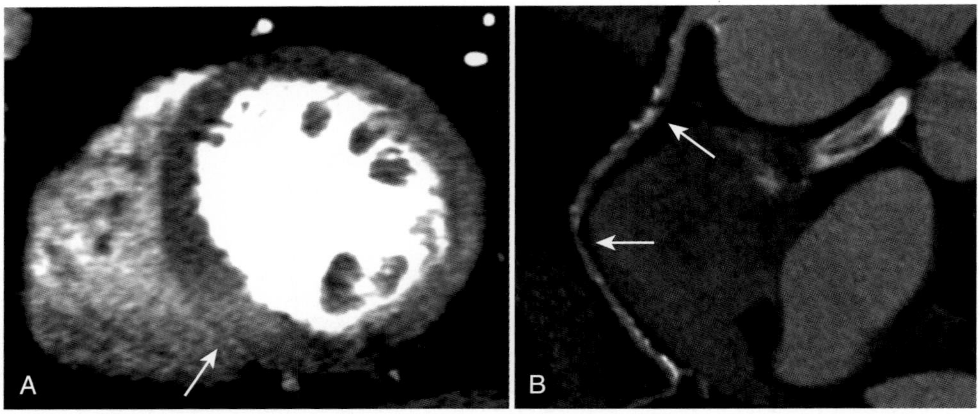

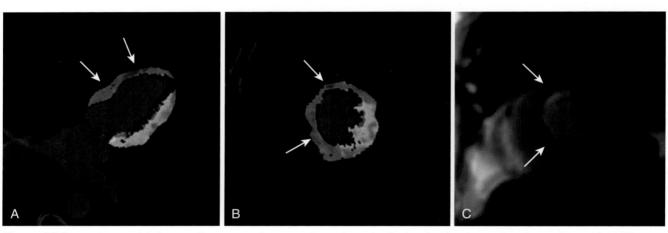

Figure 30-2 **A,** Electrocardiogram-gated coronary computed tomography angiography in a 59-year-old female patient with acute chest pain shows hypoattenuation in the posterior septal wall on short-axis imaging *(arrow)*. **B,** Coronary evaluation shows significant atherosclerotic disease of the right coronary artery *(arrows)*.

Figure 30-3 **A** and **B,** Arterial phase cardiac computed tomography angiography displayed with color overlays shows a large region of hypoattenuation in the anterior, interventricular septal, and inferior myocardial walls in a patient with known coronary artery disease *(arrows)*. **C,** Subsequent cardiac magnetic resonance imaging displayed subendocardial hypoperfusion compatible with ischemia *(arrows)*.

behind the technique is quite simple: contrast enhancement reflects myocardial blood volume, and both animal and human studies have shown that decreased contrast enhancement reflects decreased blood flow. This characteristic may allow the identification of hemodynamically significant coronary artery stenosis, acute infarction, or chronic scarring.

Arterial phase imaging, or first-pass perfusion, requires no modification of standard coronary CT angiography acquisition or reconstruction. Contrast material bolus timing is important, but both bolus tracking and test bolus techniques have been successfully applied. Some researchers have suggested the use of a lower energy setting (e.g., 100 kV), to increase contrast resolution. However, this should not be used unless it is in accordance with the intended coronary CT angiography protocol because myocardial evaluation is a secondary goal. Furthermore, although this technique has been shown to increase the specificity of identifying perfusion defects, it does not clearly enhance diagnostic accuracy and may decrease specificity compared with higher energy settings.

The evaluation of arterial phase myocardial CT images has not been standardized. Experienced researchers advocate starting with a narrow window and level (center, 100 to 150 Hounsfield units [HU], and width, 150

to 200 HU) and adjusting as desired. Individual diagnostic accuracy varies with the threshold used to call positive findings. In general, defects should occupy a known vascular territory. Attenuation values should be lower than 50% (in Hounsfield units) those of remote normal myocardium, although some researchers have used an attenuation difference of 20 HU to define a positive finding. Most studies have found normal myocardium to display attenuation values between 100 and 120 HU, whereas ischemic areas average 40 to 60 HU. As expected, the thickness of defects occupies a gradient between subendocardial and transmural, depending on the severity of the ischemia, and other patterns (e.g., subepicardial) should arise suspicion of nonischemic entities or artifact. Some examiners advocate comparison of end-systolic and end-diastolic images, with only those abnormalities seen on both regarded as true-positive results; this comparison is not possible in prospectively triggered studies. Finally, advanced visualization software, namely perfusion-weighted color mapping, is useful and has been shown to increase sensitivity (Fig. 30-3).

The ultimate goals of arterial phase CT are the same as other modalities used for myocardial analysis: risk stratification, prognostication, and better patient outcomes through improved clinical management decisions. These goals require appropriate characterization of defects regarded as true-positive results. Ideally, nonviable tissue should be distinguished from viable myocardium in the settings of acute and chronic disease. Unfortunately, no way exists to predict the recoverability of a given myocardial segment definitively based on arterial phase imaging alone because hibernating, stunned, vulnerable, and irreversibly damaged myocardium all may demonstrate areas of decreased attenuation. However, correlation with lesions seen on coronary artery analysis and wall motion abnormalities seen on time-resolved left ventricular functional analysis can add evidence of significant disease. In addition, the transmural extent of defects has been shown to correlate with functional recovery and should be reported. The volume of hypoperfused myocardium in relation to overall left ventricular volume may also provide useful information. Relative attenuation differences among defects can suggest acute versus chronic disease when fatty infiltration accompanies myocardial scarring. These areas may have negative attenuation values, whereas acute lesions should not display values lower than those found in unenhanced edematous myocardium. Chronic infarction is also suggested by relative thinning of the hypoattenuating segment.

Research on diagnostic accuracy is limited but has provided sensitivity values ranging from 67% to 100% and specificity values ranging from 57% to 97%. The technique has been evaluated in the setting of both acute and chronic infarction and compared with clinical, magnetic resonance imaging (MRI), and single photon emission CT (SPECT) reference standards, with similar results. Diagnostic accuracy figures highly depend on the methodology used for defining positive results by the gold standard. Several studies showed that the size of perfusion defects is underestimated in comparison with MRI and histopathologic examination; however, at least one study showed good correlation with SPECT in quantifying the volume of hypoperfused myocardium. Early work also suggested that the transmural extent of disease may be accurately assessed. Unfortunately, no currently available data suggest the appropriate integration of the technique into risk stratification or clinical management schemes; however, this integration should become possible as the clinical use of coronary CT angiography continues to expand.

Clear guidelines for the acquisition and evaluation of arterial phase myocardial CT imaging do not exist. However, the information is inherently available with any coronary CT angiography acquisition and should be considered when reporting findings. Although differentiation of viable from nonviable myocardium is often impossible without supplementary techniques (e.g., time-resolved, rest-stress, or delayed phase imaging; see later), clues to suggest acute versus chronic disease are often present, and correlation with angiographic and functional findings is useful. Future work should refine technical considerations and provide increased integration of findings into clinical decision making.

Stressed Arterial Phase Imaging

The rationale behind myocardial CT assessment under stress is equivalent to that in other modalities: to differentiate fixed from reversible myocardial perfusion defects, to guide management decisions. Technique and interpretation are identical to those of arterial phase imaging. Stress is most commonly achieved with 140 mcg/minute/kg of intravenous (IV) adenosine over 6 minutes, with rest imaging acquired 15 minutes following adenosine administration. A dose of up to 15 mg of IV metoprolol is usually given if the patient's heart rate does not decrease to 60 to 65 beats/minute or lower. The rest images are used for coronary CT angiography analysis and usually use collimator settings with the minimum detector width, whereas stress phase acquisitions require less fine anatomic detail and may be acquired with collimation using wider detector element configurations, such as 2 × 32 × 1.5 mm, which improves contrast-to-noise ratio values at the cost of lower spatial resolution.

Fixed defects are defined as those present on both rest and stress images, whereas reversible defects are present only under stress (Fig. 30-4). Combined assessments with coronary CT angiography and rest-stress CT myocardial perfusion imaging have shown good diagnostic accuracy in comparison with other combined assessments, namely, invasive angiography and nuclear medicine myocardial perfusion imaging. Prognostic and clinical value, however, has not been evaluated. Whether this technique is equivalent to dual energy CT (DECT), myocardial perfusion imaging, or time-resolved dynamic perfusion imaging (see later) is also unclear. As with all experimental techniques, institutional experience and additional radiation exposure should be strongly considered during patient selection.

Left Ventricular Function Analysis

The prognostic value of global left ventricular functional status is well established in patients with known ischemic myocardial disease, especially following myocardial infarction, in which global cardiac function is considered the strongest determinant of left ventricular pump failure and death. In addition, regional myocardial motion can be a valuable addition to coronary artery anatomy in routine coronary CT angiography examinations by providing clues to the hemodynamic significance of visualized stenoses. Information on global and regional function of the myocardium is available from all retrospectively ECG-gated examinations without any additional radiation or contrast dose. More recent prospective ECG-triggering techniques have been important in limiting ionizing radiation to the patient, but information across the entirety of the cardiac cycle is lost, thus disallowing left ventricular functional analysis. ECG gating with dose modulation, another trend in radiation dose reduction, may provide a compromise because it has been shown to provide adequate image quality to retain analytic capabilities while still decreasing radiation exposure by 30% to 50%.

The decision whether to perform left ventricular function analysis must take into consideration patient factors, institutional experience, and the clinical scenario. No guidelines currently exist to guide protocol decisions, but a reasonable approach is to place more

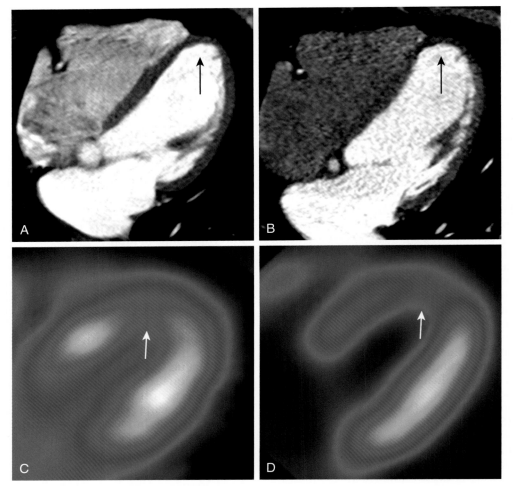

Figure 30-4 A 65-year-old male patient presented to his family physician with substernal chest pain on exertion. Rest (**A**) and stress (**B**) phase computed tomography (CT) myocardial imaging reveals an inducible attenuation defect in the apical anteroseptal left ventricular wall *(arrows)* that corresponds to an area of reversible ischemia seen on rest (**C**) and stress (**D**) single photon emission CT myocardial perfusion imaging *(arrows)*.

weight on the value of left ventricular function analysis in patients with a higher likelihood of disease, in those in whom radiation is less of a concern, and in institutions at which this analysis is integrated into routine cardiac CT protocol. In addition, CT may have some role as a primary test for cardiac functional evaluations in those patients with suboptimal examinations or contraindications to other, preferred modalities, such as echocardiography or MRI.

Few variations are required in the acquisition of cardiac CT data sets capable of functional analysis. The only prerequisite is a data set acquired across the entire cardiac cycle. However, several considerations optimize the value of subsequent interpretation. The most important technical parameter is temporal resolution, which must be approximately 100 msec or lower to provide adequate image quality for most heart rates. Some investigators argue that resolution of 30 to 50 msec is optimal, whereas temporal resolution as low as 19 msec may be necessary for true motion-free imaging. Temporal resolution has been improved by performing multisegment reformations (which can provide resolution down to 50 msec) and with the development of dual

source machines with increasingly fast gantry rotation speeds. These dual source machines can provide resolution to 75 msec with monosegment reconstructions that, in comparison with multisegment reformations, allow an increased pitch (lowering radiation burden) and provide greater spatial resolution (allowing better delineation of epicardial and endocardial borders) while suffering less image quality degradation from heart rate variability. Dual segment reconstructions with these newer scanners may provide even greater gains in temporal resolution in the future.

Patient-specific factors also weigh heavily in the final quality of functional examinations. High and irregular heart rates affect quantitative, time-resolved imaging disproportionately. Yet the administration of beta-blockers, routine in some institutions, alters hemodynamics and can confound results. In most cases, functional analysis should be considered a secondary goal of cardiac CT examinations, and beta-blockers should be administered as required, with the knowledge that functional parameters will be affected (see later). In addition, proper breath-hold technique is vital, and patients should be instructed accordingly.

Adequate image quality for functional assessment with dose modulation techniques has been shown with tube current reductions up to 80%, typically in the systolic portion of the cardiac cycle. However, the ability to perform functional analysis with reductions greater than this is not established. Otherwise, standard scan parameters may be used. Although routine contrast material delivery protocols have also shown adequacy, some evidence indicates that multiphase delivery may improve the accuracy of some quantitative measures, especially myocardial mass, by providing better delineation of the left ventricular septum from the right ventricular cavity.

Images are reconstructed across the cardiac cycle in a double oblique short-axis plane, from the level of the mitral annulus to the left ventricular apex. Although 20-phase reconstructions, at 5% intervals across the R-R cycle, have been proposed as possibly more accurate, especially in regional cine analyses, several studies showed that 10-phase reconstructions, at 10% intervals, provide equivalent results with advantages in processing time and system requirements.

Two main methods are used for global function analysis. Semiquantitative techniques using the Simpson method have been available for some time. This method uses two-dimensional planimetric measurements from contiguous 8-mm short-axis reformations along the length of the ventricular long axis that are summed to provide left ventricular volume. Software using this method is subject to problems in the reconstruction of the short-axis plane, delineation of endocardial and epicardial contours, and determination of the most basal and apical left ventricular segments; these errors often necessitate extensive and time-consuming manual intervention. This technique also fails to account for myocardial trabeculations and papillary muscles when blood volumes are quantified. Newer software systems use a three-dimensional segmentation technique based on attenuation differences between the contrast-filled left ventricular cavity and the myocardium (the region-growing approach). This method may provide several advantages over semiquantitative techniques, not the least of which is decreased postprocessing time, from 5 to 10 minutes to less than 3 minutes. In addition, trabeculations and papillary muscles are excluded from left ventricular volumes, and this may provide more accurate values. Software using this method is variable in the required amount of manual intervention; some systems provide automatic detection of basal and apical boundaries, whereas others do not. These techniques may also require adjustment of the attenuation threshold or endocardial contours to provide optimal results. However, even with these requirements, the three-dimensional region-growing approach is significantly faster than are semiquantitative techniques. Either method is used to quantify left ventricular myocardial mass, end-systolic and end-diastolic volumes, stroke volume, ejection fraction, and cardiac output.

Regional myocardial function is most commonly evaluated subjectively using multiphase cine reconstructions with 0.5- to 2-mm reconstruction width and increment. Left ventricular myocardial motion should be segmentally evaluated in accordance with the American Heart Association 17-segment model of the myocardium, excluding the apex. Regional wall motion is characterized, as with other modalities, as normal, akinetic, hypokinetic, or dyskinetic. Correlation with findings from coronary CT angiography analysis is vital to improving the predictive value of the cardiac CT examination as a whole.

The diagnostic value of CT left ventricular functional analysis has been well validated, with certain caveats. Both global assessment methods have excellent interobserver agreement and reproducibility, although the region-growing approach has slightly better values. The tendency has been for CT to overestimate end-systolic volume and subsequently underestimate ejection fraction in comparison with MRI. However, this tendency has been attributed in part to the use of beta-blockers and the inclusion of trabeculae and papillary muscles when chamber volumes are calculated. More recent studies using three-dimensional segmentation decreased this trend, and phantom studies suggested that CT may even be more accurate than MRI under ideal circumstances (i.e., slow and regular heart rates) because of its superior spatial resolution. Subjective regional wall motion analysis has also shown good correlation with echocardiography and MRI; in addition, more recent attempts to quantify regional motion with CT-based myocardial strain mapping have shown promise.

Future work should help guide optimal scan acquisition and postprocessing. The promise of greater radiation dose reductions with advanced acquisition and reconstruction methods also exists. The prognostic and clinical value of CT functional analysis has not been studied and will require validation. Furthermore, normalized sex- and gender-specific morphometric data should be established to aid interpretation of quantitative parameters.

Delayed Phase Imaging

The current gold standard for detecting myocardial viability is delayed phase MRI for the detection of late contrast enhancement. Late enhancement patterns are well established tools that provide clinically valuable information in the setting of acute and chronic ischemia. The same principles provide the rationale for delayed phase CT myocardial imaging. Both gadolinium-based and iodine-based contrast agents remain in the extracellular space. Acute ischemia causes membranous disruption in affected myocytes, which are normally tightly packed. This structural insult, along with accompanying edema, increases the volume of contrast agent distribution in infarcted areas and causes a relative increase in concentration and delayed washout compared with normal myocardium (Fig. 30-5).

Delayed phase imaging may also identify necrotic tissue in acute ischemia if it is accompanied by microvascular obstruction. Necrotic areas do not display late contrast enhancement, whereas adjacent ischemic myocardium demonstrates delayed hyperenhancement. The proposed mechanism of late enhancement in chronic ischemia is similar: scar tissue is formed with deposition

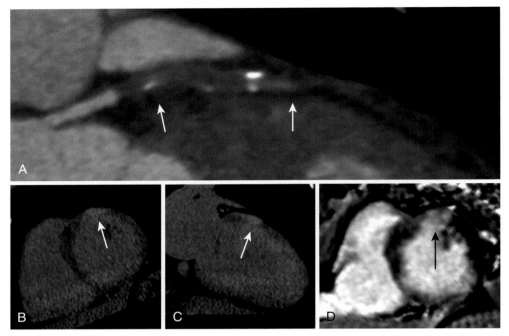

Figure 30-5 **A,** Coronary computed tomography (CT) angiography shows complete occlusion of the proximal left anterior descending artery *(arrows)* in a 57-year-old male patient being assessed for new-onset systolic heart failure. **B** and **C,** Delayed phase CT myocardial imaging performed 10 minutes later shows an area of increased attenuation in the anterior basal left ventricular myocardium *(arrows).* **D,** Delayed phase magnetic resonance imaging shows a corresponding area of hyperenhancement *(arrow)* indicative of infarcted myocardium.

of a collagenous matrix that increases the extracellular space, with a resulting increase in contrast concentration and delayed washout following delayed washin.

Late enhancement imaging provides independent information on myocardial viability, the likelihood of contractile recovery after revascularization, and clinical prognosis. Late enhancement MRI has been used in various clinical settings, usually in addition to sequences to evaluate myocardial perfusion, morphology, and function as a part of a comprehensive myocardial MRI protocol. The most common indication is in the setting of subacute myocardial infarction (>1 week after the initial insult). Late enhancing areas with greater than 50% transmural extent are considered by many examiners to represent nonviable tissue that does not warrant revascularization, especially if it is accompanied by significant contractile dysfunction. Less extensive areas are associated with a better prognosis and a greater chance of contractile recovery, and they may warrant surgical revascularization. In acute ischemia, late enhancement MRI can demonstrate the extent of infarct and somewhat differentiate necrotic tissue associated with microvascular obstruction from ischemic but potentially salvageable areas. In addition to aiding management decisions, the identification of microvascular obstruction and the evaluation of infarct size provide valuable prognostic information.

As with most emerging CT techniques used in the evaluation of myocardial ischemia, a combination of factors led to increasing interest in late phase CT imaging; namely, the increasing acceptance and application of coronary CT angiography combined with improved temporal and spatial resolution of newer-generation scanners. However, data are insufficient to provide

explicit recommendations for scan acquisition, reconstruction, interpretation, or clinical application. The technique must therefore be individually optimized for each clinical situation, by accounting for institution- and patient-specific factors.

Because delayed phase CT is currently an adjunct to routine coronary CT angiography, data sets are acquired following arterial phase scans. Protocols should be designed to maximize image quality while minimizing the patient's radiation dose. Although most studies have reported retrospective ECG-gated acquisitions, the ready availability of high-quality but low-dose prospectively ECG-triggered protocols should prompt clinicians to use prospective techniques whenever possible. Images often are acquired at end-systole if a prospective examination is used to maximize myocardial wall thickness. The examination is acquired similarly to a routine ECG-gated cardiac scan, with several modifications. Collimation may be increased to minimize the radiation dose. Slices of 1.5 mm are recommended as a compromise for z-axis spatial resolution and decreased dose. However, thinner cuts allowing isotropic resolution provide more detailed information, whereas slices as high as 5 mm have been reported to provide adequate image quality. No consensus exists on tube potential settings. Some investigators report increased contrast resolution with 80-kV settings, but this approach has also been associated with unacceptable increases in quantum noise and image artifacts. The exact setting should take the patient's body habitus into account. A setting of 80-kV may be appropriate in thin patients (body mass index [BMI] <25), but 100-kV or 120-kV settings should be employed in normal (BMI 25 to 30) or obese (BMI >30) patients, respectively. Optimum tube current is also debated, but several studies showed that low-current scans experience significant image quality degradation. Therefore, the same settings used in arterial phase scans are recommended.

Optimization of the contrast material protocol is also important in acquiring safe, high-quality scans. The speed of current-generation CT scanners has allowed a progressive decrease in required contrast material dose while maintaining good opacification of the coronary arteries. However, delayed phase imaging requires more contrast material to differentiate normal from abnormal myocardium. Animal studies showed that unacceptably high contrast volumes provide optimum diagnostic accuracy; therefore, human protocols should be individualized to provide adequate contrast material while minimizing the possibility of nephrotoxicity. In general, a dose of 120 to 150 mL (or ≥1.5 mL/kg) contrast material provides a sufficient gradient to allow washin to areas of infarct or scar. Studies showed success with simple delayed phase acquisitions following a standard cardiac CT contrast injection protocol, whereas some investigators advocated supplementing a routine high flow-rate coronary CT angiography infusion (e.g., 50 to 75 mL at 5 mL/second) with a slow infusion before delayed imaging (e.g., 70 to 100 mL at 0.1 mL/second). If this technique is used, a 5-minute washout period following the slow infusion should be undertaken before acquisition to allow contrast material clearance from the left ventricle. The optimum delay period is also not clearly established: studies showed the highest iodine concentration in diseased myocardium 5 to 15 minutes following contrast administration, although the highest ratio of iodine concentration between abnormal and normal myocardium was reported with a delay as high as 180 minutes. A 10-minute delay is recommended following a standard contrast delivery protocol, whereas a 5-minute washout period should be provided if a second, slow contrast infusion is performed.

Image reconstruction, postprocessing, and interpretation have several caveats. Maximum and minimum intensity projections have not been shown to be useful. Some investigators claimed that thin sections decrease sensitivity and recommended 1-cm reconstruction width, and others advocated 1.5-mm reconstructions; personal and institutional experience should guide the exact technique. As in arterial phase myocardial perfusion imaging, narrow window widths increase sensitivity. Window level and width of 100 and 200 HU, respectively, are reasonable starting points; alternatively, the level may be set to the attenuation value of hyperenhancing myocardium. Images are interpreted in the short-axis plane, similar to MRI or scintigraphic imaging. Supplemental orientations (cardiac or noncardiac) are available for further characterization.

Delayed phase CT shares the same considerations as MRI when findings are interpreted and reported. Because the absolute and relative attenuation values of normal and abnormal myocardium differ from scan to scan, the identification of "abnormal" myocardium is a largely subjective measure that should take into account the clinician's experience, the distribution of findings (i.e., in a coronary or noncoronary pattern), and the results of current and earlier diagnostic studies. Correlation with coronary artery morphology, myocardial perfusion, and left ventricular function can improve the characterization of abnormalities. Manual or software-assisted planimetry is used to quantify infarct size and extent. In the acute setting, particular attention should be paid to areas of hypoattenuation within an abnormal area of myocardium, findings that signify microvascular obstruction and portend a poor prognosis independent of infarct size. The transmural extent (quantified as a percentage of total wall thickness) and associated wall motion abnormalities are the most clinically important parameters in the assessment of subacute or chronic ischemia.

Delayed phase CT evaluation of the myocardium has been studied in various settings, with generally positive results. Animal models showed strong correlation with both MRI and histologic examination in quantifying acute and chronic infarct size, whereas most studies in humans had sensitivity and specificity values ranging from 70% to 98% for the overall detection of delayed enhancement (compared with SPECT, MRI, or clinical reference standards). CT was also shown to be robust in detecting microvascular obstruction, quantifying transmurality of infarcts, and characterizing delayed enhancement patterns seen in nonischemic myocardial diseases such as dilated cardiomyopathy, myocarditis, sarcoidosis, and amyloidosis. Outcome studies are emerging and indicate that delayed phase CT holds independent prognostic value in the setting of chronic ischemia.

Further studies are necessary to establish the clinical role of delayed phase CT imaging. Currently, this technique must be considered experimental, for use in research and special situations. However, signs indicate that the technique could enjoy more widespread adoption. Although MRI certainly has greater contrast resolution because of the ability to null normal myocardium, delayed phase MRI has known limitations, which include the increased costs, longer acquisition times, and infrastructure needs inherent in the technique. In addition, many patients have contraindications, such as implanted devices. MRI has been shown to overestimate the size of acute infarcts, and whether CT may be more accurate in this setting is not currently known. CT also provides greater spatial resolution and thinner image slices than does MRI, thus allowing more versatility in image reconstruction with CT. Finally, special applications of delayed phase CT have been described that warrant further evaluation, including the assessment of myocardial remodeling following postinfarction stem cell treatment and myocardial evaluation following percutaneous coronary angiography. The latter technique involves no additional contrast material administration; rather, a delayed phase data set is acquired shortly after coronary catheterization, by using the contrast material administered during that study. Future work is anticipated to provide additional potential indications as technology improves and clinicians move further in the quest for more comprehensive cardiovascular examinations.

Dynamic Perfusion Imaging

Although arterial phase imaging has shown promise in identifying regional areas of myocardium with decreased blood flow, it does not actually represent myocardial perfusion. Rather, it is a static representation of relative blood volume. In addition, inconsistencies in scan acquisition relative to the contrast bolus position decrease reproducibility. Time-resolved myocardial blood flow imaging has several advantages, including the ability to quantify myocardial perfusion. Modalities such as MRI have shown diagnostic and prognostic value for various quantitative parameters of time-resolved (dynamic) myocardial perfusion imaging. Formerly, the role of cardiac CT was limited by insufficient temporal resolution and narrow detector widths that prevented the simultaneous evaluation of the entire myocardium. Newer detectors, however, have overcome some of these limitations, largely through increased detector widths, and early investigations showed that quantitative whole heart CT myocardial imaging is feasible.

Various clinical applications have been suggested (see later), but dynamic perfusion imaging appears to be most suitable as a complement to routine coronary CT angiography, specifically, to determine the hemodynamic significance of coronary lesions seen on coronary angiography. The most commonly reported examination protocol includes a standard coronary CT scan followed by time-resolved cardiac acquisition under pharmacologically induced stress. Adenosine is the most frequently described agent, but dipyridamole has also been used, both in standard fashion. Myocardial blood flow is calculated from the perfusion scan, and findings are compared with coronary angiography results to evaluate the functional significance of coronary lesions. More comprehensive protocols have also been described that include additional rest-phase dynamic perfusion or delayed phase scans, either of which can be used to solve more specific diagnostic problems.

The technical basis behind the interest in dynamic perfusion imaging is largely a result of the increasing detector widths of current-generation CT scanners. The 256- and 320-slice scanners can provide volume coverage of the entire heart in most individuals, whereas the 128-slice machines employ a "shuttle mode," with rapid table movement (300 mm/second^2) between two positions and subsequent merging of the 2 simultaneously acquired data sets. The latter technique is most commonly described. Detector coverage is 38 mm, and with a 10% overlap between the 2 acquisitions; 73-mm coverage is available, enough to cover the entire left ventricular myocardium in most (>66%) individuals. The 128-slice dual source scanners should have both tubes set at 100 kV with 300 to 320 mAs. Gantry rotation time is 280 msec. A test bolus is used to determine delay time, followed by 50 mL iodinated contrast material and then 50 mL saline solution, all injected at 5 mL/second. Data are acquired at end-systole by using prospective ECG triggering. A complete data set is acquired for each heartbeat if the patient's heart rate is slower than 63 beats/minute, whereas every other heartbeat is acquired in patients with heart rates faster than 63 beats/minute.

The scan is generally performed over 30 seconds, thus providing 10 to 15 data sets for analysis. Proper breath-hold technique is very important because respiratory motion artifacts are a major source of nondiagnostic studies. Patients who are unable to complete the 30-second breath hold should be carefully instructed to release their breath slowly.

Examinations are reconstructed using a hybrid algorithm, which merges a low-frequency reconstruction from a full 360-degree data set with a high-frequency reconstruction from one-fourth rotation of the gantry. This approach eliminates the asymmetry inherent in partial data reconstructions from the myocardial enhancement (low-frequency) portion of the final images while maintaining the high temporal resolution necessary to evaluate sharp edges optimally. Slices are reconstructed with a 3-mm width every 2 mm, and a medium-soft convolution kernel (B25 or B30) is applied.

Postprocessing is performed using commercially available dedicated volume perfusion software. The most common method for quantifying myocardial perfusion uses a dedicated parametric deconvolution technique based on a two-compartment model of intravascular and extravascular space to fit time attenuation curves. Myocardial blood flow is calculated by dividing the maximum slope of tissue time attenuation curves by the maximum arterial input function. The maximum arterial input function is sampled from regions of interest in the descending aorta at each table position and then combined into one arterial input function that has double the sampling rate of tissue time attenuation curves (a technique that increases the precision of fit). Myocardial blood flow is calculated for each myocardial segment by sampling 2.5 cm^2 in each area and excluding 1 mm of subendocardium and 1 mm of subepicardium. Semiquantitative assessments may also be acquired by simply comparing the slopes of time attenuation curves in various myocardial segments.

The value of dynamic perfusion imaging lies in the ability to quantify and compare regional myocardial blood flow. Myocardial blood flow values for normal and hypoperfused myocardium have significant inter-individual variations, but studies uniformly report significant intraindividual differences between healthy and diseased tissue, with values ranging from 100 to 150 mL/mL/minute in normal myocardium to 55 to 100 mL/mL/minute in ischemic areas (Fig. 30-6). A rate of 75 mL/mL/minute was determined to be the optimal cutoff to identify disease in one study, but patient-specific comparisons between myocardial segments are likely more appropriate. CT-derived myocardial blood flow measurements have shown strong correlation with MRI and microsphere myocardial blood flow measurements, and identification of diseased tissue has compared favorably with histologic and scintigraphic findings. Compared with MRI, the overall diagnostic accuracy of CT has been shown to be as high as more than 90%, and one study showed incremental diagnostic performance compared with SPECT myocardial perfusion.

CT perfusion is not, however, a comprehensive assessment of myocardial ischemia. Myocardial blood flow measurements from stress phase protocols provide

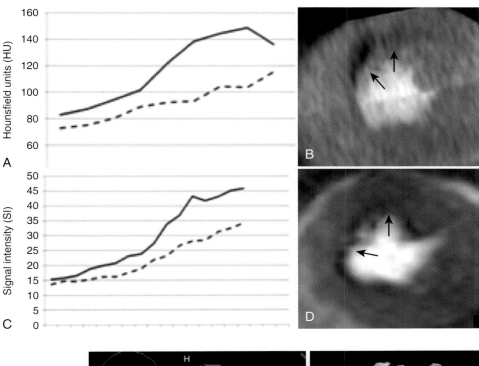

Figure 30-6 A 70-year-old male patient with angina equivalent underwent a contrast-enhanced time-resolved computed tomography (CT) myocardial perfusion study during adenosine-induced hyperemia (**A** and **B**), followed by myocardial perfusion magnetic resonance imaging (MRI) (**C** and **D**). Time-attenuation curves show hypoperfusion of the anteroseptal wall (*dashed lines* in **A** and **C**) relative to healthy myocardium (*solid lines* in **A** and **C**) that corresponds to an area of decreased attenuation and signal on CT and MRI, respectively (*arrows* in **B** and **D**).

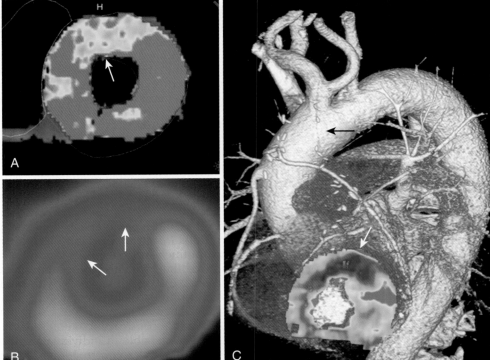

Figure 30-7 A 69-year-old female patient who had undergone coronary artery bypass grafting presented with worsening chest pain. **A,** Contrast-enhanced time-resolved computed tomography (CT) myocardial perfusion during adenosine-induced hyperemia showed relative hypoperfusion of the anterior left ventricular myocardium on color-overlay short-axis myocardial perfusion imaging *(arrow)*. **B,** This corresponded to an area of irreversible ischemia on single photon emission CT myocardial perfusion imaging *(arrows)*. **C,** A three-dimensional volume-rendered image with myocardial perfusion overlay shows complete occlusion of the left internal mammary artery bypass graft *(black arrow)* with patent grafts to the right and circumflex coronary arteries and the previously seen anterior wall infarction *(white arrow)*.

incremental value compared with coronary CT angiography alone in determining the physiologic significance of coronary artery stenoses but are unable to differentiate viable from nonviable myocardium or determine the acuity of ischemia. The addition of rest myocardial perfusion or delayed phase acquisitions may allow further characterization of disease, but this has not been well established. Interpretation of examinations should also include nonquantitative assessment of myocardial perfusion (Fig. 30-7), similar to arterial phase interpretations (see earlier). Specifically, the transmural extent and relative percentage of involved myocardium should be examined.

Dynamic CT myocardial perfusion is associated with several problems and unknown issues. Optimal scan acquisition, reconstruction, postprocessing, and interpretation techniques are uncertain. Prognostic and clinical value has not been examined. No trials have compared dynamic perfusion with static first-pass enhancement. When the additional ionizing radiation (~9 mSv) and iodinated contrast medium doses (50 mL) required for time-resolved scans are considered, strong validation will be required for widespread clinical adoption. Few studies have examined wide coverage scanners (i.e., 256- and 320-slice machines); however, the CORE 320 (Coronary Evaluation using 320 Detector CT) trial is ongoing and should provide more evidence on the efficacy of wide detector systems and dynamic CT myocardial perfusion in general. Several technical problems also require further study. Beam-hardening artifacts produce significant diagnostic limitations; beam-hardening correction algorithms have been developed that may partially mitigate the problem. Beta-blockers used to decrease cardiac motion related artifacts must be used with caution because they alter blood hemodynamics and may decrease sensitivity. Postprocessing is more involved than in routine studies and may limit clinical workflow. Finally, the large variations in individual myocardial blood flow make standardized interpretation guidelines difficult.

Dual Energy Computed Tomography

Traditional CT data sets rely on x-ray attenuation differences, largely a function of density, to provide contrast among tissues. However, substances have variable and unique x-ray absorption characteristics when different x-ray spectra are applied. This phenomenon can be exploited in CT imaging by reconstructing corresponding data sets acquired under different energies (tube kilovolt settings) that may then be postprocessed to isolate and map the distribution of specific materials. Theoretically, this approach can augment tissue characterization and contrast resolution. Early work in the 1970s and 1980s explored this technique, but data sets were necessarily acquired noncontemporaneously, thus limiting the ability to obtain exact spatial matches for postprocessing. The introduction of dual source CT in 2007 overcame this limitation because these machines provided two x-ray tubes mounted at 90-degree angles within the same gantry that allowed simultaneous acquisition of two data sets using different kilovolt settings. Other scanner vendors have developed alternatives that allow simultaneous acquisition of data sets at different tube current settings, including rapid tube current-switching technology.

Several groups of investigators have attempted to use dual energy techniques during cardiac CT examinations to map myocardial iodine distribution, which can serve as a surrogate for myocardial perfusion and blood volume. Early studies examined first-pass perfusion (Fig. 30-8), rest-stress perfusion (Fig. 30-9),

and delayed enhancement (Fig. 30-10) protocols, and results suggested that DECT can identify functionally relevant coronary artery disease and differentiate viable from nonviable myocardium. Because a DECT data set includes coronary CT angiography, this technique could feasibly be used as a stand-alone test for both anatomic and functional evaluation of acute and chronic myocardial ischemia (see Fig. 30-8, C), which traditionally requires a combination of tests.

Current data are insufficient to assert optimal scanner settings, contrast delivery, and reconstruction methods for DECT examinations definitively. The following represent the most commonly reported techniques for first- and second-generation dual source scanners; however, minor variations in tube settings and contrast delivery protocols have been described. Single phase examinations using first-generation scanners employ a 330-msec gantry rotation time, pitch of 0.2 to 0.43 (depending on heart rate), and $2 \times 32 \times 0.6$ mm collimation with z-flying focal spot technique. Tube A is set to 140 kV, 150 mAs, and tube B to is set to 80 kV, 165 mAs for slim (<140 lb) individuals or 100 kV, 165 mAs for larger subjects. Scans are retrospectively ECG gated, and tube current modulation may be employed to reduce dose without compromising necessary data. For individuals with slower (<65 beats/minute), regular heart rates, 60% to 70% pulse windows should be used; wider (35% to 75%) windows are used in patients with fast or irregular heartbeats. The dose is set to 20% outside the pulsing window. Triphasic contrast protocols adapted from standard coronary CT have provided acceptable results, and most studies have used a test bolus to determine delay time. Heart rate control with IV metoprolol has been variably used.

Coronary angiography analysis is performed in standard fashion by creating a merged reconstruction using 30% of the low-energy (tube B) spectrum with 70% of the high-energy (tube A) spectrum, thus providing a virtual 120-kV data set that combined the lower noise of the higher-energy data with the increased contrast resolution of the lower-energy data. Independent reconstructions from the low- and high-energy data sets are also routinely collected, but their use beyond the creation of the merged data set is not well established. The phase of the cardiac cycle with the least motion is used for reconstruction, with a 0.75-mm section width, 0.4-mm increment, and 165-msec temporal resolution. B26f reconstruction kernels are routinely used, with B46f available in individuals with stents. A series of merged serial reconstructions (1.5-mm reconstruction section width and 1.0-mm increment, B10f kernel, 165-msec temporal resolution) across the cardiac cycle at 10% increments is used to evaluate cardiac function. Postprocessing and analyses are performed as in routine coronary CT examinations.

Dual energy myocardial perfusion analysis requires reconstructions from both low-energy and high-energy spectra, each using a dedicated dual energy convolution kernel (D30f), 165-msec temporal resolution, 1.5-mm reconstruction section width, and 0.5-mm increment. Postprocessing requires a dedicated analysis platform and algorithm. Contrast material distribution is

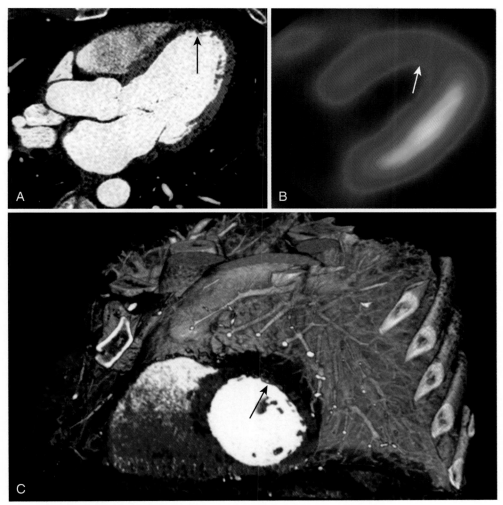

Figure 30-8 A 45-year-old male patient with a known history of coronary artery disease presented with new-onset angina at rest. Three-chamber view from a contrast-enhanced dual energy examination shows an iodine defect in the anteroapical myocardium (*arrow* in **A**) that corresponds to a fixed defect on single photon emission computed tomography myocardial perfusion imaging (*arrow* in **B**). Dual energy computed tomography has the ability to combine functional and anatomic evaluations during a single acquisition, as seen in this volume-rendered image with iodine map overlay (**C**) displaying a perfusion defect in the anterior myocardium *(arrow)*.

calculated by using the specific x-ray absorption characteristics of iodine at low and high energies; once identified, contrast material is subtracted from the images to create a virtual noncontrast series. The subtracted data are then used to create an iodine distribution map series that is overlaid onto the virtual noncontrast images. The result is a three-dimensional color-coded map of myocardial blood volume over a grayscale multiplanar data set. Although this process is fully automated, best results are obtained by individually adjusting the algorithm parameters and normalizing the iodine map to an area of myocardial perfusion (e.g., a well-attenuating segment of left ventricular wall). Reconstruction of the smallest field of view that fully encompasses the heart also improves spatial resolution and therefore image quality. Analysis is performed with the aid of routine postprocessing software. Short-axis and two-chamber views of the heart with 5-mm multiplanar reformations have been reported to work well for visualization of perfusion defects, which are seen as contiguous, circumscribed areas of absent or decreased iodine relative to the remainder of the myocardium. Results are reported according to the 17-segment American Heart Association and American College of Cardiology model.

Rest-stress and delayed enhancement acquisitions are similarly acquired. Stress imaging is performed first, with pharmacologic stressing achieved by 140 mcg/minute/kg IV adenosine over 6 minutes. Rest imaging is performed next, with up to 15 mg IV metoprolol given if the heart rate does not decrease to 65 beats/minute or lower after stressing. Finally, delayed enhancement images are acquired 6 minutes after the last contrast material was administered. Rest imaging uses an identical scan, reconstruction, and postprocessing protocol, as described earlier, whereas stress and delayed enhancement images are acquired with a 2 × 32 × 1.5 mm scanner collimation because only the dual energy heart perfusion blood volume series is acquired.

Second-generation dual source CT scanners have been introduced. These scanners have a wider detector array and faster gantry, thus providing increased temporal resolution

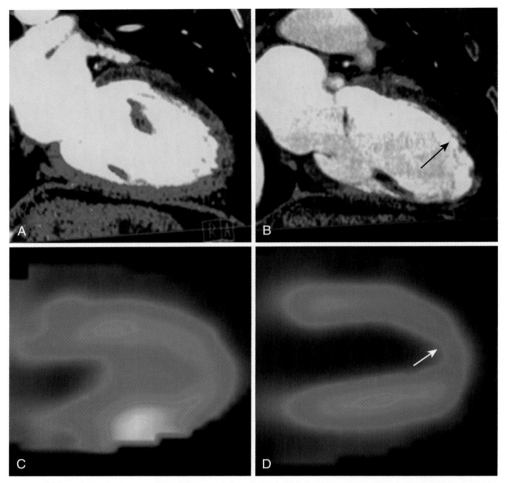

Figure 30-9 A 52-year-old female patient was referred for rest (**A**) and stress (**B**) dual energy cardiac computed tomography, which showed an area of decreased iodine in the anterior wall on stress but not rest images *(arrow* in **B**). Rest (**C**) and stress (**D**) single photon emission computed tomography myocardial perfusion imaging confirmed reversible anterior wall ischemia *(arrow* in **D**).

by faster acquisition times. In addition, a prepatient tin filter was added that improves material separation capabilities and signal-to-noise ratio without additional dose. Second-generation scanners may therefore provide increases in diagnostic capability with decreases in dose. Few protocol modifications are needed: scanner collimation is 2 × 64 × 0.6 mm in single phase and the rest phase of stress-rest protocols, and scanner collimation is 2 × 64 × 1.5 mm for stress and delayed enhancement acquisitions. The gantry rotation time is 280 msec; this time approximately corresponds to the temporal resolution of the heart perfusion blood volume series, whereas coronary angiography and functional reconstructions have temporal resolution that approaches 75 msec by a unique hybrid reconstruction algorithm. The pitch should be set to 0.17 to 0.2, depending on heart rate. Finally, suggested tube settings are 140 kV, 140 mAs for tube A and 100 kV, 165 mAs for tube B.

To date, DECT has been tested in the setting of known acute and chronic myocardial infarction, the assessment of known or suspected coronary artery disease (with or without acute symptoms), and the evaluation of coronary artery bypass or stent patency. Initial results have been generally positive. Single arterial phase DECT scans

(see Fig. 30-8) have shown sensitivities and specificities greater than 90% in detecting perfusion defects compared with SPECT in patients with known or suspected coronary artery disease and only slightly lower diagnostic accuracy compared with histopathologic examination in a canine model of acute myocardial infarction.

Arterial phase DECT scans can also identify areas of chronic infarction, with strong correlation with late enhancement MRI in patients with earlier coronary artery bypass grafting. However, the diagnostic accuracy of DECT images in this patient population has been shown to suffer from pronounced artifacts from median sternotomy wires, and grayscale reconstructions had slightly greater diagnostic accuracy than did DECT. Several studies found that single acquisition DECT examinations performed without a dedicated stress phase detected reversible defects seen only on SPECT stress series. Several theories have been postulated to account for this finding. The increased spatial resolution inherent in CT may allow visualization of more subtle defects. In addition, iodinated contrast material has a vasodilatory effect, which may produce a pharmacologic stress effect by a mechanism similar to that of adenosine. Finally, DECT may have a wider effective

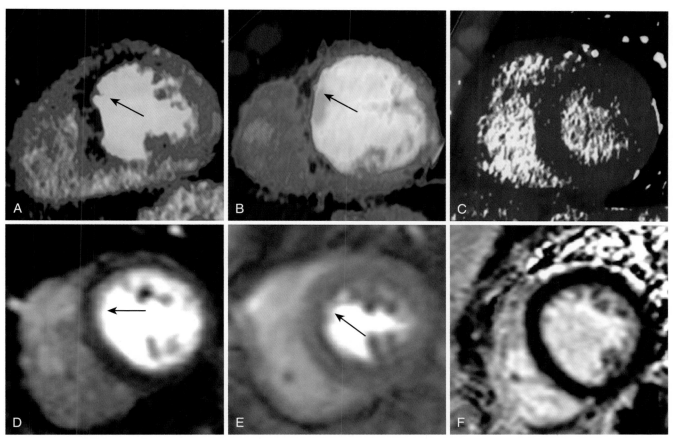

Figure 30-10 Stress, rest, and delayed phase contrast-enhanced dual energy computed tomography (DECT) (**A** to **C**) and magnetic resonance imaging (MRI) (**D** to **F**) in a 69-year-old female patient with acute chest pain display hypoperfusion of the interventricular septum during stress (*arrows* in **A** and **D**) that is not apparent at rest (*arrows* in **B** and **E**). Delayed phase DECT (**C**) and MRI (**F**) confirm that no late enhancement is present to suggest an irreversible infarct.

range to measure different rates of myocardial perfusion. Contrast attenuation has a linear relationship with myocardial perfusion, whereas in SPECT, signal intensity has a nonlinear relationship with perfusion and plateaus above a certain perfusion rate, thus limiting the ability to differentiate perfusion rates higher than a certain value and necessitating pharmacologic stressing to increase perfusion differences.

DECT examinations have also shown promise in differentiating viable from nonviable myocardium. Delayed enhancement DECT had a diagnostic accuracy comparable to that of delayed enhancement MRI in a pig model of reperfused chronic infarction; interreader agreement was very good, and infarct size correlated very well with histopathologic findings. Arterial phase DECT images with adenosine stress induction have also shown promise in correctly identifying reversible perfusion defects (see Fig. 30-9). DECT examinations with rest, stress, and delayed enhancement DECT phases (see Fig. 30-10) represent the most comprehensive uses of cardiac DECT, and early work suggested that DECT is able to detect fixed, reversible, and scarred myocardium.

DECT is currently in an early investigative phase; as such, no guidelines for appropriate clinical use are available. DECT should be considered a potential ancillary test to appropriately ordered coronary CT angiography studies. Acquiring a cardiac CT scan in the dual energy mode on first-generation dual source scanners decreases temporal resolution because a full data set necessitates a one-half, rather than a one-fourth, rotation of the gantry. Second-generation systems have shown some success in overcoming this limitation with advanced reconstruction techniques. Specific acquisition protocols should be individualized to the patient and clinical scenario. In particular, the increased radiation exposure associated with multiphase examinations should be considered.

Bibliography

Ali B, Hsiao E, Di Carli MF. Combined anatomic and perfusion imaging of the heart. *Curr Cardiol Rep.* 2010;12:90-97.

Bamberg F, Klotz E, Flohr T, et al. Dynamic myocardial stress perfusion imaging using fast dual-source CT with alternating table positions: initial experience. *Eur Radiol.* 2010;20:1168-1173.

Bastarrika G, Arraiza M, De Cecco CN, Mastrobuoni S, Ubilla M, Rábago G. Quantification of left ventricular function and mass in cardiac dual-source CT (DSCT) exams: comparison of manual and semiautomatic segmentation algorithms. *Eur Radiol.* 2008;18:939-946.

Bastarrika G, Ramos-Duran L, Rosenblum MA, Kang DK, Rowe GW, Schoepf UJ. Adenosine-stress dynamic myocardial CT perfusion imaging: initial clinical experience. *Invest Radiol.* 2010;45:306-313.

George RT, Arbab-Zadeh A, Miller JM, et al. Adenosine stress 64- and 256-row detector computed tomography angiography and perfusion imaging: a pilot study evaluating the transmural extent of perfusion abnormalities to predict atherosclerosis causing myocardial ischemia. *Circ Cardiovasc Imaging.* 2009;2:174-182.

Mahnken AH, Bruners P, Katoh M, Wildberger JE, Günther RW, Buecker A. Dynamic multi-section CT imaging in acute myocardial infarction: preliminary animal experience. *Eur Radiol.* 2006;16:746-752.

Mendoza DD, Joshi SB, Weissman G, Taylor AJ, Weigold WG. Viability imaging by cardiac computed tomography. *J Cardiovasc Comput Tomogr.* 2010;4:83-91.

Rocha-Filho JA, Blankstein R, Shturman LD, et al. Incremental value of adenosine-induced stress myocardial perfusion imaging with dual-source CT at cardiac CT angiography. *Radiology.* 2010;254:410-419.

Rodriguez-Granillo GA, Rosales MA, Baum S, et al. Early assessment of myocardial viability by the use of delayed enhancement computed tomography after primary percutaneous coronary intervention. *JACC Cardiovasc Imaging.* 2009;2:1072-1081.

Ruzsics B, Schwarz F, Schoepf UJ, et al. Comparison of dual-energy computed tomography of the heart with single photon emission computed tomography for assessment of coronary artery stenosis and of the myocardial blood supply. *Am J Cardiol.* 2009;104:318-326.

Sayyed SH, Cassidy MM, Hadi MA. Use of multidetector computed tomography for evaluation of global and regional left ventricular function. *J Cardiovasc Comput Tomogr.* 2009;3(Suppl):S23-S34.

Thilo C, Hanley M, Bastarrika G, Ruzsics B, Schoepf UJ. Integrative computed tomographic imaging of cardiac structure, function, perfusion, and viability. *Cardiol Rev.* 2010;18:219-229.

Weininger M, Schoepf UJ, Ramachandra A, et al. Adenosine-stress dynamic real-time myocardial perfusion CT and adenosine-stress first-pass dual-energy smyocardial perfusion CT for the assessment of acute chest pain: initial results. *Eur J Radiol.* 2010 Dec 29: [Epub ahead of print].

CHAPTER 31

Myocardial Nonischemic Cardiomyopathies

Travis S. Henry and Kristopher W. Cummings

The term nonischemic cardiomyopathy refers to a heterogeneous group of disorders that ultimately lead to impaired cardiac performance, either from decreased function or from abnormal conduction. Although the diseases are extremely diverse, they share important characteristics: the *absence of ischemic myocardial damage from atherosclerotic coronary artery disease (CAD) and the absence of other cardiac disorders such as valvular disease, systemic hypertension, or congenital heart disease that could otherwise explain the cardiac dysfunction.* Classification of cardiomyopathies has frequently changed over the past several decades as understanding of these diseases has improved, thus leading to confusion among clinicians about appropriate terminology. The current classification system of the American Heart Association (AHA) categorizes cardiomyopathies as either primary or secondary based on the most up-to-date understanding of the pathogenesis. Primary cardiomyopathies are those disorders that are confined to the heart muscle and are subdivided into genetic (e.g., hypertrophic cardiomyopathy [HCM]), acquired (e.g., myocarditis), or mixed (e.g., dilated cardiomyopathy [DCM]). Secondary cardiomyopathies represent cardiac involvement from systemic diseases (e.g., sarcoidosis, amyloidosis) (Table 31-1).

The role of the imager can be challenging when patients have potential nonischemic cardiomyopathy because these diseases often have overlapping appearances. The primary objective in many cases is to ensure that the cardiac dysfunction is not caused by CAD-related ischemia or infarction. Correlation with catheter angiography, the gold standard, is ideal; however, coronary computed tomography (CT) angiography (CTA) has been validated as an alternative noninvasive method for evaluation of the coronary arteries, especially in younger patients and those with a low pretest probability of atherosclerotic disease. Moreover, certain patterns of enhancement on delayed gadolinium–enhancement (DGE) magnetic resonance imaging (MRI), including subendocardial or transmural enhancement in a vascular distribution, are highly suggestive of ischemia, whereas other patterns of enhancement suggest nonischemic cardiomyopathy.

Although the AHA classification system of cardiomyopathies is a useful tool for clinical organization, its utility for an imager is limited because several cardiomyopathies (e.g., ion channelopathies and other conduction disorders) do not have specific imaging findings, or imaging features may be entirely normal. Characteristic imaging features of each disease are described where applicable.

■ APPROACH TO IMAGING NONISCHEMIC CARDIOMYOPATHIES

Common modalities in evaluation of nonischemic cardiomyopathy are as follows:

Chest radiograph. Findings in nonischemic cardiomyopathy on chest radiographs are often nonspecific and may be normal in spite of severe disease (e.g., HCM, infiltrative cardiomyopathies), or radiographs may show findings of congestive heart failure (e.g., DCM, myocarditis). Associated findings in the lungs (e.g., sarcoid) may be the best clue to the cause of underlying cardiomyopathy.

Echocardiography. This technique is typically the initial noninvasive test of choice in patients with nonischemic cardiomyopathy. Echocardiography is excellent at providing functional assessment of the heart including chamber size, wall thickness, ejection fraction, valvular dysfunction, pressure estimations, and wall motion abnormalities. Echocardiography is limited in patients with poor acoustic windows (e.g., obese patients), and visualization of the right ventricle (RV) or apex can sometimes be difficult or impossible. Furthermore, tissue characterization is limited, and echocardiography cannot evaluate the coronary circulation when wall motion abnormality may be caused by ischemia or nonischemic cardiomyopathy.

MRI. Cardiac MRI is a versatile examination that provides not only provides anatomic and functional imaging similar to echocardiography but also tissue characterization and assessment of myocardial perfusion and viability. The examination should be customized based on the clinical scenario, but any basic examination for evaluation of nonischemic cardiomyopathy should include the following:

■ Anatomic imaging: Black-blood imaging can be performed with either T1 or T2 weighting with blood suppression performed through a double inversion recovery pulse technique. These sequences are typically acquired in all three orthogonal planes (transaxial, sagittal, and coronal) to include the heart and great vessels.

Table 31-1   American Heart Association Classification of Cardiomyopathies (Excluding Ischemic, Vascular, Hypertensive, or Congenital Heart Disease)

	Primary		Secondary
Genetic	**Acquired**	**Mixed**	
Hypertrophic cardiomyopathy	Myocarditis	Dilated cardiomyopathy	Infiltrative (amyloid)
ARVC/D	Stress cardiomyopathy	Restrictive	Storage (hemochromatosis)
Ventricular noncompaction	Peripartum		Toxicity (drugs)
Glycogen storage diseases	Tachycardia-induced		Endomyocardial (Loeffler)
Ion channel disorders	Infants of mothers with insulin-dependent diabetes mellitus		Inflammatory (sarcoid)
Mitochondrial myopathies			Autoimmune
Conduction defects			

ARVC/D, Arrhythmogenic right ventricular cardiomyopathy and dysplasia.

Table 31-2   Patterns of Cardiac Magnetic Resonance Imaging Delayed Myocardial Enhancement

Subendocardial	**Mesocardial**	**Subepicardial**	**Transmural**
Infarct*	Hypertrophic cardiomyopathy	Myocarditis	Infarct*
Hypereosinophilic syndrome	Fabry disease	Sarcoid	Myocarditis
Amyloid	Dilated cardiomyopathy		Sarcoid
Cardiac transplantation	Right ventricular insertional fibrosis Sarcoid		

*Infarct usually confined to a coronary vascular territory.

- Functional imaging: Electrocardiogram (ECG)–gated cine imaging of the heart (images obtained throughout the cardiac cycle) is typically performed with a steady-state free precession (SSFP) sequence that takes advantage of the signal difference between flowing blood and myocardium. Stacks of cine sequences through the heart (6- to 10-mm slice thickness) in the two-chamber short-axis and four-chamber planes, with at least one image in the two-chamber long-axis plane, are usually sufficient.

Additional sequences and techniques used in assessment of nonischemic cardiomyopathy are as follows and are covered in more detail for specific diseases:

- Delayed contrast-enhanced imaging: Assessment of myocardial scar or viability, fibrosis, or infiltration is performed with DGE imaging, which can provide crucial information that differentiates among causes of nonischemic cardiomyopathy (Table 31-2). The contrast agent accumulates in regions of expanded extracellular space, either because of myocyte death and fibrosis or because of deposition of abnormal material (e.g., amyloid). The typical dose is 0.1 to 0.2 mmol/kg, and imaging is performed approximately 10 minutes after contrast administration. An inversion recovery gradient recalled echo (GRE) pulse is performed to null normal myocardial signal and increase the signal-to-noise ratio. This sequence requires acquisition of a series of scout images to determine the optimal myocardial nulling time (typically ~200 to 300 msec). Alternatively, a phase sensitive inversion recovery (PSIR) sequence can be performed that improves nulling of the normal myocardium over a wider range of inversion times. Imaging is usually performed in the two-chamber short-axis plane, but orthogonal views to confirm the presence of an abnormality and exclude artifact are often useful. At a minimum, mid–two-chamber long-axis or mid–four-chamber images should be obtained for assessment of the cardiac apex, which cannot be adequately evaluated on short-axis sequences.

- Long inversion time contrast-enhanced imaging for evaluation of thrombus: Intraluminal cardiac chamber filling defects are commonly encountered in the evaluation of nonischemic cardiomyopathy and usually represent clot. To confirm that a filling defect represents a thrombus (and not a mass such as a myxoma or metastasis), the inversion time can be lengthened to 600 msec; this will cause vascular tissue to appear gray and thrombus to be black.

- T2* for evaluation of iron deposition: Iron is a paramagnetic element that alters the local magnetic field and results in significant reduction in T2* for affected tissues. Myocardium with abnormally increased iron concentrations (i.e., hemochromatosis or siderotic cardiomyopathy) shows decreased signal on T2-weighted and T2*-weighted sequences, and measurement of T2* can help to quantify cardiac iron levels.

■ HYPERTROPHIC CARDIOMYOPATHY

HCM, the most common genetic cardiomyopathy, affects approximately 1 in 500 individuals. HCM is the result of

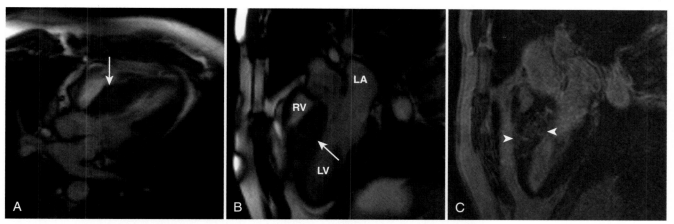

Figure 31-1 A 56-year-old man with the septal variant of hypertrophic cardiomyopathy (HCM). **A,** Static four-chamber steady-state free precession (SSFP) image at end-diastole shows asymmetric thickening of the basal septum *(arrow)*. **B,** Three-chamber static SSFP image shows the hypertrophic septum *(arrow)* in relation to the left ventricular outflow tract and is the ideal view to evaluate for outflow tract obstruction on cine images. LA, Left atrium; LV, left ventricle; RV, right ventricle. **C,** Delayed contrast-enhanced image in the same three-chamber view as **B** shows patchy mesocardial enhancement *(arrowheads)* confined to the region of hypertrophy, the typical pattern of contrast enhancement of HCM.

hundreds of different genetic mutations that result in myocyte disarray and variable amounts of hypertrophy and scar within the myocardium. The underlying genotypic variability results in a spectrum of phenotypes that vary in imaging appearance, clinical presentation, and severity of disease.

Most cases of HCM manifest in adolescence or early adulthood, although the disease has been seen across the spectrum of age range from infants to older adults. HCM is associated with a mortality rate of approximately 0.5% to 1.0% per year. Most patients are referred for imaging because of a positive family history of HCM, unexplained sudden cardiac death (SCD), or ECG abnormalities. Most symptomatic patients present with dizziness or syncope (from left ventricular outflow obstruction or arrhythmia) or dyspnea (from diastolic dysfunction).

Normal myocardium is less than 12 mm in thickness, and the following criteria indicate HCM:
1. Wall thickness greater than 15 mm
2. Normal-sized ventricular chambers
3. Normal afterload (i.e., absence of severe aortic stenosis or uncontrolled systemic hypertension)

The most common form of HCM involves the septum (asymmetric septal), but other variants exist, including apical, circumferential (diffuse), and midcavity.

Historically, the obstructive form of HCM received the most attention because of the well-known cases of SCD that result from lethal arrhythmia. Various names have been used as understanding of this entity has evolved, including idiopathic hypertrophic subaortic stenosis (IHSS), hypertrophic obstructive cardiomyopathy (HOCM), and muscular subaortic stenosis. These terms can be misleading because only 25% of cases cause left ventricular outflow tract (LVOT) obstruction, and many involve areas of myocardium other than the interventricular septum. HCM is now the preferred, all-inclusive term.

Because the overall size of the heart is normal in HCM, the chest radiograph is usually not helpful.

Imaging in HCM relies heavily on echocardiography and MRI for diagnosis, quantification of severity

of disease, and response to therapy. Echocardiography is typically the first modality used to evaluate HCM. In the setting of the septal variant of HCM, echocardiographers frequently use the estimate of interventricular septal thickness greater than 1.5 times that of the opposed posterior wall for diagnosis. Systolic function (left ventricular ejection fraction) is normal to increased (complete obliteration of the left ventricle [LV] lumen during systole), and diastolic function may be decreased. With increasing use of MRI, however, an estimated 6% to 12% of cases of HCM go undetected on echocardiography. MRI is quickly becoming the imaging modality of choice.

MRI for the evaluation of HCM should include a basic cardiac examination and delayed contrast-enhanced sequences. Additional sequences that may be helpful in HCM include a three-chamber cine sequence and phase contrast cine images across the LVOT. The three-chamber view offers an excellent look at the LVOT and is best for evaluating turbulent flow resulting from subaortic stenosis and systolic anterior motion of the anterior mitral valve leaflet that further exacerbates obstruction and causes mitral regurgitation (Fig. 31-1). The phase contrast sequence is used to measure peak velocities across the LVOT that can be translated into a pressure gradient using the modified Bernoulli equation (mm Hg = square of peak velocity in meter/second multiplied by 4).

Cine images show a normal to increased LV ejection fraction, and obliteration of the LV cavity may be observed during systole. Measurement of wall thickness and myocardial mass should be performed at end-diastole. MRI offers precise delineation of hypertrophied segments of myocardium, is highly accurate and reproducible, and offers a better evaluation of the LV apex and the RV than echocardiography; these areas can be affected by variants of HCM (Fig. 31-2). As previously mentioned, normal myocardium is less than 12 mm thick in end-diastole, and segments affected with HCM are usually at least 15 mm thick. Patients with wall thickness greater than 30 mm are at increased risk of SCD.

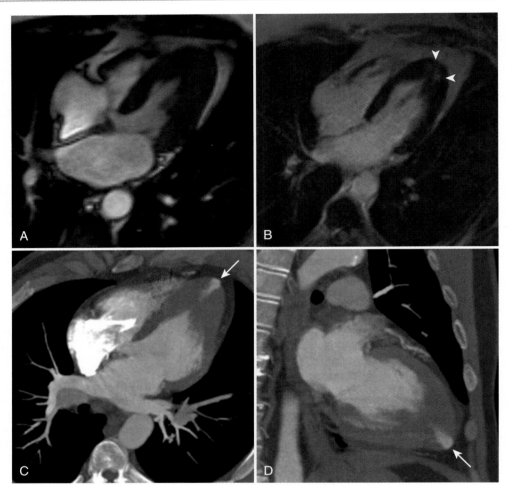

Figure 31-2 Apical variant of hypertrophic cardiomyopathy (HCM). Static four-chamber steady-state free precession image (**A**) and four-chamber delayed contrast-enhanced image (**B**) in a 58-year-old man with apical variant HCM. The left ventricle assumes a typical "spade" shape with obliteration of the apical lumen at end-systole. The hypertrophic myocardium also demonstrates patchy mesocardial enhancement (*arrowheads* in **B**). Oblique axial (**C**) and oblique sagittal (**D**) maximum intensity projection images from a contrast-enhanced computed tomography examination in a 53-year-old man with arrhythmia demonstrates the apical variant of HCM with a small area of apical thinning (*arrows*).

Abnormal delayed contrast enhancement is seen in up to 50% of cases of HCM. The hyperenhancement is typically patchy and usually mesocardial (midmyocardial); these findings help differentiate HCM from ischemic infarcts, which always are subendocardial with variable degree of transmurality. These areas of delayed hyperenhancement represent foci of fibrosis within the hypertrophic myocardium. Multiple studies have shown that more extensive areas of enhancement correlate with poorer prognosis because the areas of fibrosis serve as arrhythmogenic foci.

At institutions where alcohol ablation of the septum is performed, MRI may be used as a follow-up imaging modality to assess response to treatment (i.e., decrease in septal thickness and improved LVOT flow). Other MRI applications including myocardial tissue tagging and myocardial perfusion imaging are being investigated but are not currently used in routine clinical practice.

CT is not typically performed in the workup of HCM; however, because of the use of CT as a first-line imaging modality (particularly in emergency departments), cases may be incidentally detected by the imager (Fig. 31-3). The diagnosis is difficult on nongated CT examinations because motion artifact may simulate increased wall thickness, and the imager may be unaware of underlying systemic hypertension or other mimics of HCM. Cardiac-gated CT may be indicated in patients with

inconclusive echocardiographic evaluations and contraindications to MRI. Care should be taken to include functional data at end-diastole for wall thickness measurements. Delayed enhanced CT may detect areas of abnormal late enhancement, but the contrast-to-noise ratios are much inferior to those of MRI, and therefore the use of this technique is usually not recommended.

■ ARRHYTHMOGENIC RIGHT VENTRICULAR CARDIOMYOPATHY/ DYSPLASIA

Arrhythmogenic right ventricular cardiomyopathy/dysplasia (ARVC/D) is a primary genetic form of cardiomyopathy that, despite a low incidence of 1 in 5000 to 1 in 10,000 in the United States, accounts for 5% of cases of SCD in persons less than 35 years old. Because of this risk despite its relatively low incidence, ARVC/D is a common referral for cardiac MRI, either as part of an arrhythmia workup or for evaluation of patients with a positive family history.

ARVC/D is an autosomal dominant type of cardiomyopathy that results from one of several genetic mutations in the cardiac desmosome (responsible for cellular binding) and pathologically results in progressive fibrofatty infiltration of the myocardium. The disease almost always involves the RV and may progress

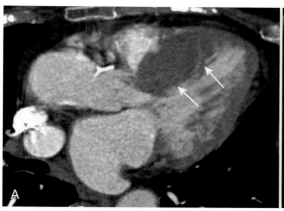
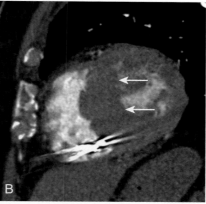

Figure 31-3 A 66-year-old woman with septal variant hypertrophic cardiomyopathy. Axial **(A)** and sagittal **(B)** reformation contrast-enhanced computed tomography images show marked asymmetric hypertrophy of the septum *(arrows)* relative to the normal thickness lateral and inferior walls of the left ventricle. Note the implantable cardioverter-defibrillator lead in the right ventricle that was placed to prevent arrhythmia.

to biventricular involvement. The earliest stages of the disease may not manifest on a macroscopic level, and imaging findings may be normal (although patients are still at risk for SCD). As the disease progresses, abnormalities in RV structure and function become visible on imaging, including fat infiltrating the myocardium of the RV free wall (seen on MRI), as well as chamber enlargement, decreased RV function, dyskinesis, and focal aneurysmal outpouchings (seen on MRI or echocardiography). End-stage ARVC/D may result in heart failure and a DCM pattern on imaging.

Diagnostic criteria for ARVC/D were established by the Arrhythmogenic Right Ventricular Dysplasia Task Force in 1994 and include major and minor criteria for structural, histologic, ECG, arrhythmic, and genetic features. Because of the high interobserver variability of the original imaging criteria for assessment of RV function and structural changes, revised criteria were proposed in 2010 to increase the sensitivity for the diagnosis of ARVC/D while maintaining specificity. These newer criteria include specific imaging criteria for two-dimensional echocardiography, MRI, and angiography (Table 31-3). Even though fat infiltration of the myocardium is a pathologic hallmark of ARVC/D, the presence of fat on imaging is not included in either set of criteria.

Echocardiography is often the initial imaging test of choice in suspected cases of ARVC/D. Structurally, right ventricular outflow tract (RVOT) dilation is the most common abnormality in patients who satisfy the Task Force Criteria, with an RVOT long axis greater than 30 mm in 89% of cases. Other structural abnormalities seen on echocardiography include trabecular derangement and a hyperreflective moderator band, present in 54% and 34% of cases, respectively. Functionally, regional wall motion abnormalities are present in 79% of cases, with the apex and anterior wall the most commonly affected (72% and 70%, respectively).

MRI has several advantages over echocardiography in the evaluation of ARVC/D, including better visualization of the RV, more accurate volume measurements, and the ability to characterize tissue composition (i.e., muscle versus fat). MRI examination for evaluation of ARVC/D should include a modified basic examination with breath-hold, high-resolution black-blood sequences through the RV free wall for evaluation of the presence of fat.

Table 31-3   Imaging Criteria for the Diagnosis of Arrhythmogenic Right Ventricular Dysplasia: Global or Regional Dysfunction and Structural Alterations

Major Criteria

Two-Dimensional Echocardiography

Regional RV akinesia, dyskinesia, or aneurysm and one of the following:

Parasternal long axis RVOT ≥32 mm (≥19 mm/m² corrected for BSA)

Parasternal short axis RVOT ≥36 mm (≥21 mm/m² corrected for BSA)

Fractional area change ≥33%

Cardiac MRI

Regional RV akinesia or dyskinesia, or dyssynchronous RV contraction and one of the following:

Ratio of RV EDV to BSA ≥110 mL/m² (male) or ≥100 mL/m² (female)

or RVEF ≥40%

Minor Criteria

Two-Dimensional Echocardiography

Regional RV akinesia or dyskinesia and one of the following:

Parasternal long axis RVOT ≥29 to <32 mm (≥16 to <19 mm/m² corrected for BSA)

or Parasternal short axis RVOT ≥32 to <36 mm (≥18 to <21 mm/m² corrected for BSA)

Cardiac MRI

Regional RV akinesia or dyskinesia or dyssynchronous RV contraction and one of the following:

Ratio of RV EDV to BSA ≥100 to <110 mL/m² (male) or ≥90 to <100 mL/m² (female)

or RVEF >40% to ≤45%

Modified from Marcus FI, McKenna WJ, Sherrill D, et al. Diagnosis of arrhythmogenic right ventricular cardiomyopathy/dysplasia: proposed modification of the task force criteria. *Circulation.* 2010;121:1533-1541; nonimaging criteria are not included in this table.

BSA, Body surface area; *EDV,* end-diastolic volume; *MRI* magnetic resonance imaging; *RV,* right ventricular; *RVEF,* right ventricular ejection fraction; *RVOT,* right ventricular outflow tract.

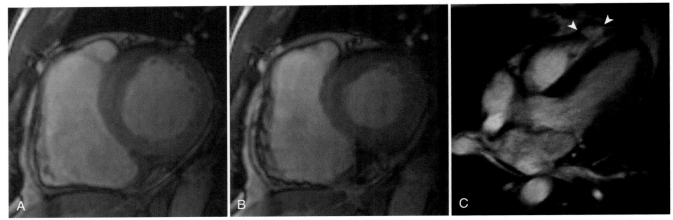

Figure 31-4 Two patients with a clinical diagnosis of arrhythmogenic right ventricular cardiomyopathy and dysplasia based on modified Task Force Criteria. Static two-chamber short-axis images at end-diastole (**A**) and end-systole (**B**) show a dyskinetic, enlarged right ventricle (RV) with decreased function. Measured RV ejection fraction was 31%. Steady-state free precession four-chamber image (**C**) in a 34-year-old woman shows a focal aneurysm of the RV free wall *(arrowheads)*. The RV was dyskinetic on cine images (not shown).

RV enlargement (defined as an RV larger than the LV at end-diastole on four-chamber cine views) was the most specific finding in a study of 40 patients imaged for suspected ARVC/D, with a specificity of 96% and a sensitivity of 68%. Enlargement of the RVOT (defined as larger than the LVOT) has 94% specificity and 78% sensitivity. Fat infiltration of the RV is the most sensitive finding (84%), but it is less specific (79%) and can easily be confused with epicardial or pericardial fat. Quantitative measurement of RV end-diastolic volume and RV ejection fraction were incorporated into the 2010 Task Force Criteria modifications (Fig. 31-4).

Delayed contrast-enhanced imaging can also be performed to look for areas of fibrous infiltration. Enhancement is seen in up to 70% of patients, but it is not a component of the Task Force Criteria.

■ LEFT VENTRICULAR NONCOMPACTION

Left ventricular noncompaction (LVNC) is a rare type of nonischemic cardiomyopathy characterized by spongy, hypertrabeculated myocardium. Familial and nonfamilial cases have been described, but the disease is classified as primary genetic cardiomyopathy by the AHA.

The exact pathogenesis is uncertain; however, LVNC is theorized to be caused by arrest of endomyocardial morphogenesis during embryonic development. The absence of compacted myocardium results in underdevelopment of capillary networks, decreased perfusion, and predisposition to ischemia, infarction, and fibrosis. During development, the myocardium compacts in a coordinated fashion that begins at the base and the septum and proceeds toward the apex and lateral wall; this pattern explains why the apex, midlateral wall, and midinferior wall are the most commonly involved regions.

The incidence of LVNC is estimated at 0.05%, and patients typically present with LV systolic dysfunction, thromboembolic disease, arrhythmias, or SCD. The prognosis of LVNC varies by inclusion criteria and length of follow-up, but in the largest study of 105

patients who were followed up over an approximately 2-year period, 30% experienced episodes of heart failure requiring hospitalization, 28% received implantable cardioverter-defibrillators, and 20% died or received a heart transplantation.

The major mimics of LVNC on imaging include hypertrabeculation from LV hypertrophy (e.g., long-standing systemic hypertension or aortic stenosis), DCM, and ischemic cardiomyopathy. In addition, up to 70% of anatomically normal individuals may also have areas of increased trabeculation that can lead to significant confusion for the imager and overdiagnosis if strict criteria are not used. In an effort to prevent overdiagnosis, many groups have published specific criteria for echocardiography and MRI, the preferred noninvasive tests in the diagnostic workup of LVNC.

The four major echocardiographic criteria for the diagnosis of LVNC are as follows: (1) the absence of coexisting cardiac abnormalities; (2) a ratio of noncompacted to compacted myocardium of more than 2:1 measured at *end-systole;* (3) segmental distribution predominantly involving the apex, midlateral wall, and/or midinferior wall; and (4) color Doppler evidence of flow within the deep trabecular recesses. The RV may also be involved in this disease; however, the RV is believed to be an unreliable marker because of its natural tendency to be much more trabeculated in anatomically normal individuals.

MRI offers better tissue characterization (delayed contrast imaging) and improved visualization of the apex in some patients. On cine MRI images, measurement of the noncompacted to compacted myocardium is performed at *end-diastole* (as opposed to end-systole for echocardiography), and a ratio of more than 2.3:1 is considered specific for LVNC. The apex, apical lateral wall, and inferolateral wall are most commonly involved, but involvement of the midventricular segments is associated with increased clinical severity of disease.

Abnormal delayed enhancement is seen in 17% of cases, predominantly in a subendocardial distribution. The hyperenhancement typically involves the areas

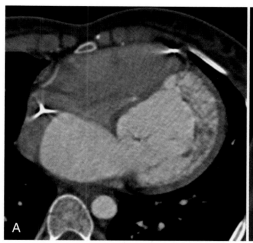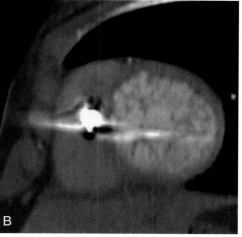

Figure 31-5 A 23-year-old woman with left ventricular non-compaction (LVNC). Axial (**A**) and sagittal (**B**) reformations from electrocardiogram-gated cardiac computed tomography angiography show markedly increased trabeculation of the apical and lateral walls of the left ventricle typical of LVNC. The ratio of noncompacted to compacted myocardium is at least 3:1 (normal is <2.3:1). The patient was unable to undergo magnetic resonance imaging because of the implanted defibrillator (tip visible in the right ventricle).

of noncompaction, but areas of apparently normal-thickness myocardium may also show enhancement. At times, distinguishing blood pool signal within deep trabecular recesses with true myocardial delayed enhancement can be difficult. Quantification of the amount of enhancement has been shown to correlate with clinical severity of disease.

Hypertrabeculation may be seen on ECG-gated contrast-enhanced CT examinations with a similar ratio of noncompacted to compacted myocardium, but specific CT criteria for the diagnosis of LVNC do not exist (Fig. 31-5).

■ DILATED CARDIOMYOPATHY

DCM is the most common type of nonischemic cardiomyopathy worldwide, with a prevalence of approximately 1 in 2500 individuals. DCM occurs across all age ranges (but is more common in adults) and can either be genetic or secondary. The familial (genetic) form of DCM may be responsible for up to 48% of cases, and similar to other inherited diseases such as HCM, numerous genetic mutations have been identified that result in identical imaging appearances. Common secondary causes of DCM include earlier myocarditis, substance use (i.e., alcohol, cocaine), anthracycline-based chemotherapeutic regimens, and systemic diseases (Box 31-1).

DCM is characterized by LV enlargement, decreased contractility (typically global hypokinesis), and depressed systolic function *out of proportion to CAD*, the major differential diagnostic consideration for this entity. Distinguishing a DCM pattern caused by CAD (ischemic DCM) from nonischemic DCM is one of the main objectives in imaging these patients because ischemic DCM has a poorer prognosis and a radically different treatment regimen, including possible coronary revascularization. In patients with DCM in whom ischemia has been excluded as a cause, the diagnostic workup centers on a search for either a genetic or a secondary cause.

Chest radiographic findings include an enlarged cardiac shadow with or without overt heart failure and pulmonary edema. On echocardiography, DCM appears as

---

BOX 31-1   Secondary Causes of Dilated Cardiomyopathy

Infections
  Viral (coxsackievirus, adenovirus, parvovirus, human immunodeficiency virus infections)
  Bacterial (rickettsial, mycobacterial, spirochetal infections)
  Fungal
  Parasitic (Chagas disease)
Toxins
  Chronic alcohol consumption
  Cocaine
  Anthracyclines (doxorubicin, daunorubicin)
  Heavy metals (lead, mercury, arsenic, cobalt)
Systemic disorders
  Autoimmune
  Collagen vascular disease (systemic lupus erythematosus, scleroderma)
  Sarcoidosis
  End-stage renal disease
Endocrine/metabolic conditions
  Thyroid dysfunction
  Pheochromocytoma
  Nutritional deficiencies
Peripartum conditions
Idiopathic causes

---

ventricular enlargement and decreased systolic function with global hypokinesis and decreased fractional shortening.

Historically, invasive coronary catheter angiography was performed to exclude CAD in patients with DCM. However, noninvasive imaging (coronary CTA and delayed enhancement MRI, in particular) is increasingly used as an alternative in evaluation.

Generalized findings of DCM including an enlarged heart, possibly with signs of heart failure, may be seen on a conventional chest CT scan for the workup of nonspecific symptoms such as shortness of breath or chest pain. Coronary CTA takes these findings a step further by providing a noninvasive evaluation of the coronary

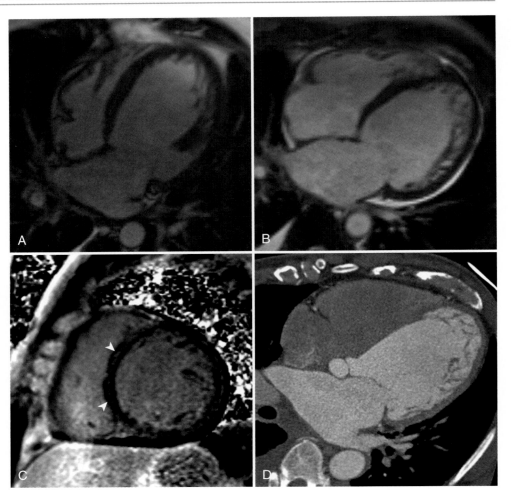

Figure 31-6 Dilated cardio-myopathy (DCM). A, Static four-chamber steady-state free precession (SSFP) image from a 36-year-old man with idiopathic DCM. The left ventricle is markedly enlarged, but the right ventricle and atria are not involved. No delayed enhancement was noted on postcontrast images (not shown). Static four-chamber SSFP image (B) and two-chamber delayed contrast-enhanced phase sensitive inversion recovery image (C) in a different patient, a 47-year-old man with DCM, demonstrate enlargement of both ventricles. Associated enlargement of the left atrium is attributable to mitral valve dysfunction secondary to dilation and incomplete coaptation of the leaflets. Linear meso-cardial enhancement is present in the interventricular septum (arrowheads). D, An oblique axial image from contrast-enhanced coronary computed tomography angiography in a 46-year-old man with DCM shows four-chamber enlargement and normal coronary arteries.

arteries in addition to anatomic and volumetric information. The high negative predictive value of coronary CTA is particularly useful in patients with a low index of suspicion for CAD, such as those with suspected nonischemic DCM. The negative predictive value and accuracy of 64-row coronary CTA approach 99% when compared with catheter angiography for the presence of stenosis greater than 50%. Furthermore, coronary CTA can provide useful data such as ventricular mass and chamber size and can also provide functional assessment if images are acquired throughout the cardiac cycle (i.e., retrospective ECG gating), albeit at an increase in radiation dose.

A cardiac MRI protocol for the evaluation of DCM should include a basic examination with delayed contrast-enhanced sequences. DCM results in increased myocardial mass (from an overall increase in size of the chamber, not increased wall thickness), increased ventricular volumes, and decreased ejection fraction (Fig. 31-6). Whereas ischemic disease usually causes wall motion abnormalities within a vascular territory, nonischemic DCM usually manifests as global hypokinesis. MRI offers a better functional evaluation of the RV than does echocardiography, particularly in patients with poor imaging windows. MRI is also useful for evaluating valvular dysfunction (i.e., mitral regurgitation) secondary to DCM.

Delayed enhancement sequences are essential components of MRI examination for confidently differentiating ischemic from nonischemic DCM. Ischemic disease manifests as either subendocardial or transmural delayed myocardial enhancement within a coronary vascular territory, whereas delayed enhancement in DCM is usually absent. A study of 63 patients with unobstructed coronary arteries demonstrated no delayed enhancement in 58% of patients and patchy or longitudinal mesocardial enhancement in 29% of patients. The presence of mesocardial enhancement has been associated with a greater risk of SCD, presumably resulting from fibrosis within conduction pathways predisposing to arrhythmia. The remaining 13% of patients showed an enhancement pattern indistinguishable from ischemic disease, and the investigators postulated that these patients may have suffered from infarction caused by coronary thrombus formation followed by lysis of the thrombus. Delayed enhancement imaging also offers the ability to assess for LV intraluminal thrombus that may form in a poorly functioning ventricle.

Finally, nuclear stress myocardial examinations are also used in the noninvasive evaluation of suspected DCM. Sensitivity of ECG-gated technetium-99m sestamibi single photon emission CT stress examinations ranges from 87% to 94%, but the test suffers from limited specificity (32% to 63%), often related to diaphragmatic attenuation of the dilated LV.

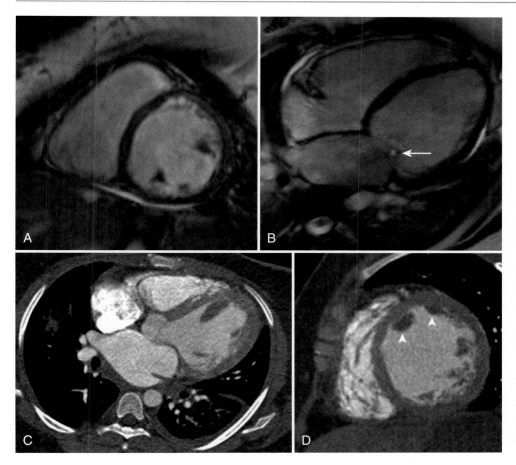

Figure 31-7 Peripartum cardiomyopathy (PPCM). Steady-state free precession (SSFP) two-chamber short-axis (**A**) and four-chamber (**B**) images in a 21-year-old woman who developed PPCM 1 week after a term delivery demonstrate marked biventricular enlargement. Note the turbulent flow jet of mitral regurgitation (*arrow* in **B**) secondary to chamber enlargement and incomplete coaptation of the valve leaflets. Axial (**C**) and sagittal reformat (**D**) contrast-enhanced computed tomography images in a different 26-year-old woman with PPCM demonstrate nonenhancing thrombus adherent to the anterior and apical walls of the left ventricle (*arrowheads* in **D**). Thrombus resolved and cardiac chamber size and function returned to normal on a follow-up echocardiogram 3 months later.

■ PERIPARTUM CARDIOMYOPATHY

Peripartum cardiomyopathy (PPCM) is defined as heart failure developing within the last month of pregnancy or up to 5 months after delivery in the absence of pre-existing heart disease. PPCM typically manifests with an imaging appearance similar to that of DCM. However, it deserves special consideration given the significantly improved survival rate and the complex issues of radiation (CT) and gadolinium (MRI) with respect to the fetus.

The incidence of PPCM is approximately 1 in 3000 to 1 in 4000 in the United States, with a higher incidence in African Americans. Historically, the survival rate was approximately 50%, but more recent data, in the United States in particular, report up to a 94% 5-year survival, with approximately half of all patients completely recovering cardiac function. Numerous causes of PPCM have been proposed, including viral infection (myocarditis), autoimmune disorders, abnormal response to altered hemodynamics of pregnancy, genetic factors, and abnormal metabolism of prolactin, but the exact cause is uncertain.

Patients with PPCM present with signs of heart failure. However, the diagnosis is often delayed because of the overlap with normal physiologic changes during the final months of pregnancy, including pedal edema, fatigue, and dyspnea. Less common presentations include emboli (either systemic or pulmonary) from ventricular thrombi, arrhythmia, and SCD. The differential diagnosis of PPCM includes underlying heart conditions that are either unmasked or exacerbated by the altered hemodynamics of pregnancy, such as previously unknown DCM, valvular heart disease, congenital heart disease, or acute myocardial infarction (AMI). Because the imaging appearances of PPCM and DCM are virtually indistinguishable at the time of presentation, the goals of imaging should be to quantify the severity of cardiac dysfunction and exclude the other aforementioned diseases in the differential diagnosis. Predictors of poor outcome include an LV end-diastolic diameter greater than 6.0 cm, LV ejection fraction of less than 30%, or the presence of thrombus in a cardiac chamber.

Echocardiography is most commonly used for functional assessment, but CT and MRI both have utility in the imaging of PPCM in the appropriate clinical context. Contrast-enhanced CT is frequently performed in the postpartum patient (radiation should be avoided before the patient delivers) who presents with acute onset of shortness of breath or chest pain, especially if pulmonary embolism is clinically suspected, and PPCM may be an incidental diagnosis (Fig. 31-7). In addition to evaluating the heart size, CT is more sensitive than radiography for detection of pulmonary edema or heart failure. The imager should interrogate the heart chambers carefully for the presence of thrombus because the combination of the peripartum state and cardiac dysfunction creates a hypercoagulable state. Patients with

PPCM may present with troponin elevation, and coronary CTA may be used to evaluate the coronary arteries (see the earlier discussion of CTA for DCM).

A basic noncontrast MRI scan can be performed in the pregnant patient for chamber function and valvular assessment. However, gadolinium is a class C drug in pregnancy and should be avoided. In the postpartum patient, gadolinium can be used, but data on its utility are limited. In one series of eight patients with PPCM, none of the patients exhibited delayed enhancement, although other case reports have shown areas of nonvascular, predominantly mesocardial enhancement that may resolve as cardiac function improves.

■ AMYLOIDOSIS

Cardiac amyloidosis is a type of secondary nonischemic cardiomyopathy that results from extracellular accumulation of insoluble fibrillary amyloid proteins. The proteins accumulate throughout the heart—including the ventricles, atria, atrial appendages, valves, perivascular tissues, and conduction system—and produce thickened, nondilated ventricles. Several different forms of cardiac amyloidosis are recognized, including light chain (also known as AL amyloidosis), familial, and senile amyloidosis, which can have widely varying clinical presentations.

AL amyloidosis is the most common form, associated with plasma cell dyscrasias and the production of light chain proteins. Approximately 2000 to 2500 new cases are diagnosed in the United States each year, and cardiac involvement is present in half of these patients. Cardiac involvement by AL amyloidosis has a particularly poor prognosis, with a median survival of less than 6 months in untreated patients with symptoms of heart failure. Arrhythmia and SCD from involvement of the conduction system are rare.

Echocardiography is usually the initial noninvasive imaging test performed. Features of amyloidosis include concentric hypertrophy of both ventricles (>12 mm thickness), prominent valves, and increased echogenicity of the myocardium from amyloid infiltration. Doppler echocardiography shows a restrictive pattern with progressive diastolic dysfunction over serial examinations. Ejection fraction is usually preserved until late in the disease.

Cardiac MRI in suspected amyloidosis should include a basic protocol and delayed contrast-enhanced sequences. Functional images show findings similar to those of echocardiography, including concentric ventricular hypertrophy, enlarged atria, restricted diastolic filling, and normal to decreased ejection fraction. Expansion of the extracellular space by the amyloid proteins results in gadolinium retention, which manifests as delayed contrast enhancement in 79% to 97% of patients (Fig. 31-8). Systemic expansion of the extracellular space is also believed to explain the absence of residual contrast material within the blood pool on delayed enhancement images that results in the characteristic dark blood pool. Four distinct patterns of delayed contrast enhancement have been described. The two most common patterns, global transmural and global subendocardial enhancement, correlate with the greatest amount of amyloid deposition (and the worst prognosis) and have been reported in 49% to 83% of cases. Focal patchy enhancement (in a nonvascular distribution) is present in 6% to 14% of cases. Incomplete nulling of the myocardial signal on the inversion recovery scout sequence (from elongation of the T1 signal time) is seen in 8% to 16% of cases. In general, if difficulty with myocardial suppression is noted, then cardiac amyloidosis should strongly be considered as the cause. Phase sensitive inversion recovery sequences, which are less sensitive to the selection of a specific inversion time for myocardial nulling, are often useful in this setting.

■ STRESS CARDIOMYOPATHY (TAKOTSUBO CARDIOMYOPATHY)

Stress cardiomyopathy is also known as broken heart syndrome, apical ballooning syndrome, or takotsubo cardiomyopathy (takotsubo is Japanese for "octopus trap"). It is an acquired, acutely reversible cause of left ventricular systolic dysfunction with a characteristic imaging appearance from which it receives its name. Takotsubo cardiomyopathy is usually precipitated by profound psychological or physical stress, and patients

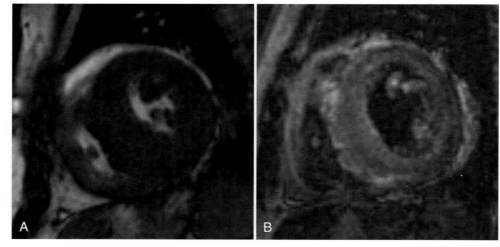

Figure 31-8 Amyloidosis. A, Steady-state free precession two-chamber image in a 47-year-old woman with familial amyloidosis demonstrates circumferential hypertrophy of the ventricles, the left affected more severely than the right. **B,** Delayed postcontrast image in the same patient shows diffuse subendocardial enhancement and a dark blood pool signal, both characteristic findings of amyloidosis. Also note enhancement of the papillary muscles

present with signs and symptoms that are difficult to distinguish from those of AMI, including elevated troponin levels and ST-segment elevations. This disease most commonly affects postmenopausal women and is estimated to represent 1% to 2% of patients presenting with symptoms of acute coronary syndrome. Proposed diagnostic criteria for the diagnosis of takotsubo cardiomyopathy are provided in Box 31-2.

BOX 31-2 Diagnostic Criteria for Stress Cardiomyopathy (Based on Modified Mayo Criteria)

1. Transient dysfunction (hypokinesis, akinesis, or dyskinesia) of the left ventricular midsegments, with or without apical involvement; wall motion abnormalities extending beyond a vascular territory, usually following a stressful trigger
2. Absence of obstructive coronary artery disease or angiographic evidence of acute plaque rupture
3. New electrocardiographic abnormalities (ST-segment elevation; T-wave inversion); possible cardiac troponin elevation
4. Absence of pheochromocytoma or myocarditis

Adapted from Akashi YJ, Goldstein DS, Barbaro G, et al. Takotsubo cardiomyopathy: a new form of acute, reversible heart failure. *Circulation.* 2008;118:2754-2762.

The pathogenesis of takotsubo cardiomyopathy is uncertain, but the disease may be caused by diffuse coronary artery spasm (from stress), catecholamine-induced myocyte damage, microvascular obstruction (without angiographic evidence of large vessel disease), or neurogenic myocardial stunning. Symptoms typically resolve on the order of weeks, and imaging is typically performed to exclude AMI or myocarditis and to evaluate for complications such as LV thrombus or, less commonly, LVOT obstruction.

Coronary angiography is the gold standard for diagnosis of takotsubo cardiomyopathy, with akinesis or dyskinesis of the mid-LV (with or without apical involvement) that results in dilation of the midchamber, without obstructing CAD. The basal LV wall either functions normally or is hyperdynamic, which results in the characteristic apical ballooning.

Echocardiographic findings correlate with angiography but better demonstrate akinetic or hypokinetic middle and apical portions of the LV and either a normal or hyperdynamic LV base. Complications such as LV thrombus or LVOT obstruction may also be seen.

The MRI protocol should include a basic examination and delayed enhancement sequences. Functional sequences show findings similar to those of echocardiography (Fig. 31-9). In the acute phase, takotsubo cardiomyopathy results in myocardial edema with

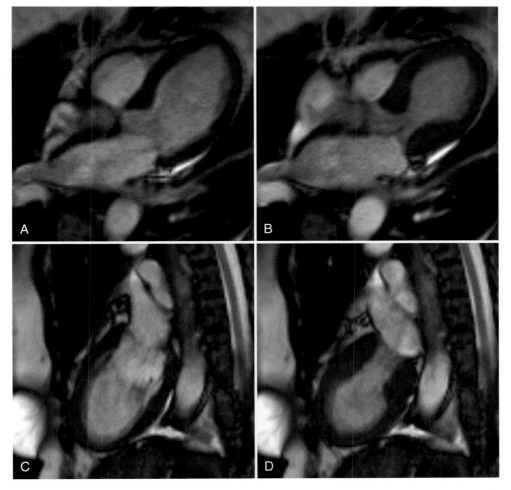

Figure 31-9 Stress cardiomyopathy (SCM). A 71-year-old woman with SCM that was diagnosed shortly after the death of her husband with a concomitant diagnosis of breast cancer. SSFP four-chamber images at end-diastole (**A**) and end-systole (**B**) demonstrate the characteristic appearance of the left ventricle with a contractile base and akinetic apex resulting in the characteristic apical ballooning or takotsubo appearance. The same findings are seen on the two-chamber long-axis images at end-diastole (**C**) and end-systole (**D**).

increased myocardial signal intensity on T2-weighted sequences. The edema may be transmural, although in a nonvascular distribution, and it typically resolves within approximately 2 weeks. Conversely, edema from AMI tends to be in a vascular distribution and does not resolve as rapidly. Findings of both first-pass perfusion and delayed enhancement imaging studies should be normal, thus allowing differentiation from ischemic or infiltrative cardiomyopathies.

CT perfusion and coronary CTA have also been described in takotsubo cardiomyopathy and may be particularly useful in patients with symptoms of acute chest syndrome but low pretest probability of CAD. As with other imaging modalities, CT in takotsubo cardiomyopathy should not show perfusion abnormalities or significant coronary artery stenoses, and the characteristic apical ballooning should be appreciated in the acute setting.

■ SARCOID CARDIOMYOPATHY

Sarcoidosis is a systemic inflammatory disorder of unknown origin that is characterized by the presence of noncaseating granulomas in affected organs. Pulmonary involvement is most common, and symptomatic cardiac involvement is seen in only 5% of cases. However, clinically silent cardiac involvement is present in up to 50% of cases at autopsy. Prevalence of sarcoidosis in the United States ranges from 10 to 35 per 100,000; African Americans are the most commonly affected ethnic group.

The origin of sarcoidosis is unknown and may be environmental or infectious, but some evidence indicates at least a partial genetic predisposition, with an increased incidence among identical twins. The clinical course varies widely, from asymptomatic to spontaneous regression to progressive organ failure and death. Cardiac involvement is a relatively poor prognostic factor and is responsible for 13% to 25% of sarcoid-related deaths, typically from left-sided heart failure or arrhythmia. Cardiac involvement may be difficult to detect, and, in addition to any patient with known sarcoidosis and new cardiac symptoms, the diagnosis should be considered in any young patient who presents with new complete heart block or heart failure. Cor pulmonale can also be seen with sarcoidosis; however, it is secondary to

end-stage sarcoid lung disease and is not directly caused by cardiac sarcoid involvement.

The imaging differential diagnosis for cardiac sarcoid includes ischemic cardiomyopathy, HCM, autoimmune diseases, and myocarditis. Progression of disease can result in a DCM-pattern in later stages.

The chest radiograph may show an enlarged cardiac silhouette but no specific signs of cardiac sarcoid. Characteristic right paratracheal and bilateral hilar lymphadenopathy or upper lung–predominant parenchymal disease may be present as a result of associated pulmonary sarcoid.

Echocardiographic findings are also nonspecific. In acute disease, thickening of the ventricular wall and increased echogenicity may be seen, as well as regional wall motion abnormalities that most commonly affect the basilar septum. In chronic disease, the ventricle may be enlarged with thinned myocardium, global hypokinesis, and a DCM pattern.

Cardiac MRI for sarcoidosis should include a basic protocol with delayed contrast sequences. The cine series may show regional wall motion abnormalities and normal or decreased function. Myocardial edema manifests as increased T2 signal intensity with or without increased wall thickness. Delayed enhancement is characteristically subepicardial or mesocardial, often with a patchy or nodular appearance (Fig. 31-10). In chronic stages, small focal areas of wall thinning and transmural enhancement can be seen. The nonvascular distribution distinguishes sarcoid from ischemic cardiomyopathy. Delayed enhancement is most commonly seen in the base of the interventricular septum, involving other ventricular walls, papillary muscles, or atria less commonly. If myocardial perfusion imaging is performed, sarcoid may show areas of hyperenhancement (rather than decreased enhancement seen in ischemia) resulting from inflammation. Edema and inflammation may decrease on follow-up studies in response to appropriate steroid or immunosuppressant therapy, and delayed contrast enhancement sometimes resolves. Noncardiac thoracic manifestations of sarcoidosis, such as mediastinal lymphadenopathy and pulmonary parenchymal changes, are typically present at the time of cardiac involvement diagnosis, so care should be taken to look for these supportive findings.

Figure 31-10 A 56-year-old man with cardiac sarcoidosis. **A,** Delayed contrast-enhanced two-chamber image through the midleft ventricle demonstrates patchy areas of mesocardial and transmural enhancement *(arrowheads)* not confined to a vascular territory, a finding typical of sarcoidosis. **B,** Black-blood axial T2-weighted image shows associated bilateral hilar lymphadenopathy and subtle reticular opacities in the lungs also typical of sarcoidosis *(arrows)*.

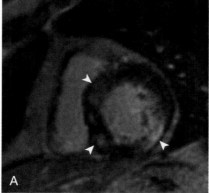
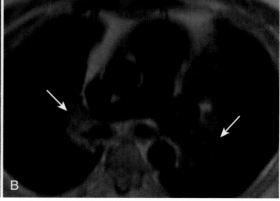

CT is not currently in routine use for evaluation of cardiac sarcoid. However, delayed enhancement images show patterns of enhancement similar to those of MRI and may be an adequate substitution in certain situations, such as in patients with pacemakers or other contraindications to MRI. CT offers superior evaluation of pulmonary sarcoid.

■ MYOCARDITIS (INFLAMMATORY CARDIOMYOPATHY)

Classified as an acquired form of nonischemic cardiomyopathy, myocarditis is acute or chronic myocardial inflammation and may have many causes, the most common being viral infection (Box 31-3). The incidence is likely underestimated because of the varying and often nonspecific presentations of this disease, but evidence of myocarditis has been identified in 1% to 9% of routine autopsies and in 5% to 12% of autopsies of patients with SCD. Clinically, myocarditis can be difficult to recognize because the symptoms range from chest pain and dyspnea to overt heart failure. Moreover, the clinical presentation can be nearly identical to that of AMI in that patients frequently have abnormal ECGs and cardiac enzyme elevation. Endomyocardial biopsy is extremely specific for the diagnosis but suffers from a sensitivity of only 10% to 22%, mostly resulting from

---

BOX 31-3   Causes of Inflammatory Cardiomyopathy

Viral infections (coxsackievirus, parvovirus, adenovirus, human immunodeficiency virus infections)
Bacterial infections (diphtheria, meningococcal infection, streptococcal infection, psittacosis)
Rickettsial (typhus, Rocky Mountain spotted fever)
Fungal (aspergillosis, candidiasis)
Parasitic (Chagas disease, toxoplasmosis)
Whipple disease
Giant cell myocarditis
Drug hypersensitivity reaction
Cocaine

---

sampling error. Most patients fully recover cardiac function, but up to one third may progress to DCM eventually requiring heart transplantation.

Accurate diagnosis of myocarditis (and differentiation from myocardial infarction in the acute setting or DCM in the chronic setting) is essential because the treatment and prognosis vary greatly. Noninvasive imaging, particularly MRI, is increasingly relied on to identify patients who may benefit from biopsy and to monitor response to treatment.

The chest radiographic findings are nonspecific in myocarditis and may be normal. Enlargement of the cardiac silhouette may be present, and distinguishing a large pericardial effusion (acute enlargement of the cardiac silhouette) from cardiomegaly caused by a DCM pattern is important. Patients may also present with signs of congestive heart failure and pulmonary edema.

The echocardiographic appearance of myocarditis is variable and nonspecific. Patterns similar to DCM, HCM, ischemic cardiomyopathy, and restrictive cardiomyopathy have all been described. Regional wall motion abnormalities of the LV are the most common finding, with normal to mildly increased LV volume. Other findings include transient increase in LV wall thickness secondary to edema and increased echogenicity of the myocardium. Echocardiography is helpful for identifying complications of myocarditis including LV thrombus, LV aneurysm, and pericardial effusion.

Cardiac MRI has become a very useful noninvasive imaging test for evaluation of myocarditis and differentiation from other nonischemic and ischemic conditions. The role of MRI in the setting of myocarditis is discussed in more detail in Chapter 26. Essentially, the evaluation of myocarditis should include a basic protocol and delayed contrast sequences, with perfusion sequences optional. Delayed contrast enhancement is seen in 90% of cases (most commonly in the inferior and inferolateral walls) and, if limited to the subepicardial region, is highly suggestive of myocarditis (Fig. 31-11). Mesocardial enhancement may also be present, but the subendocardium should appear to be spared, thus allowing differentiation from ischemic disease even when confined to a vascular territory. Perfusion MRI with early

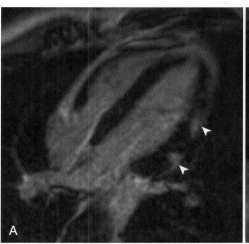
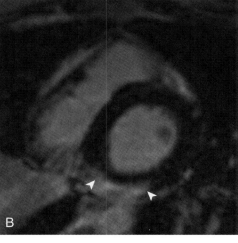

Figure 31-11 Myocarditis. Delayed contrast-enhanced four-chamber (**A**) and two-chamber short-axis (**B**) images in a 17-year-old male patient with myocarditis. Note the subepicardial enhancement along the inferior and inferolateral walls (*arrowheads*).

contrast-enhanced sequences is more time intensive but has been reported to increase the sensitivity and specificity of the diagnosis. The presence of any two of three criteria (increased T2 signal intensity, early hyperenhancement, and delayed enhancement in a distribution mentioned earlier) has a sensitivity and specificity of approximately 76% and 95.5%, respectively.

If the diagnosis is in doubt, or if tissue is required, then endomyocardial biopsy should be directed to any areas of delayed enhancement to increase sensitivity. In less straightforward cases with extensive involvement, excluding infiltrative disease such as sarcoidosis can be difficult. Because myocarditis typically shows improvement or resolution of delayed enhancement with conservative treatment, a follow-up examination in 6 to 8 weeks may be useful. More severely affected portions of the myocardium may demonstrate persistent enhancement resulting from the development of fibrous scar tissue.

CT is not routinely performed for the evaluation of myocarditis, but it may be used in acutely ill patients, those with confusing clinical presentations, or patients with contraindications to MRI. Coronary CTA shows an absence of CAD that would otherwise suggest ischemic cardiomyopathy. Delayed enhancement may be seen, but the data are limited to case reports. Complications of myocarditis including pericardial effusion and pericarditis can also be effectively imaged with CT.

■ HYPEREOSINOPHILIC SYNDROME AND ENDOMYOCARDIAL FIBROSIS

Hypereosinophilic syndrome (HES) is a systemic disorder characterized by increased peripheral eosinophils for more than 6 months with resultant end-organ damage. HES is seen in different clinical scenarios and may be secondary to neoplasm (i.e., eosinophilic leukemia), infections, or allergic agents, or it may be idiopathic. Cardiac involvement, also known as Loeffler endomyocarditis,

is a restrictive type of cardiomyopathy with progressive fibrosis of the endomyocardium. HES has significant overlap in the clinical, pathologic, and imaging appearances with endomyocardial fibrosis, and both entities are speculated to result from abnormal eosinophils.

Endomyocardial damage occurs in three pathologic stages:

1. Acute necrotic stage. Eosinophilic infiltration and degranulation result in damage to the endocardium and formation of microabscesses.
2. Thrombotic stage. The damaged endomyocardium creates a prothrombotic environment in which large mural thrombi can form.
3. Fibrotic stage. The end results of the endocardial damage are fibrosis and scar.

The chest radiograph may show atrial enlargement secondary to the restrictive physiology and atrioventricular valve dysfunction. LV failure may result in signs of pulmonary congestion.

The hallmark features of HES on echocardiography are obliteration of the ventricular apex and associated dilation of the atrium. These findings can resemble the apical variant of HCM; however, the restrictive pattern with associated atrial enlargement should suggest HES. Severe atrioventricular valve dysfunction may also be seen when the scar results in papillary muscle dysfunction. Complications such as mural thrombus and elevated pulmonary pressures (from left-sided heart dysfunction) may also be observed.

MRI evaluation of HES should include a basic protocol with delayed contrast imaging. Obliteration of the ventricular apex, atrial enlargement, and severe atrioventricular valve regurgitation appear similar to the echocardiographic findings. The most specific finding for HES is endocardial or subendocardial enhancement in a nonvascular distribution on delayed contrast images (Fig. 31-12). The major differential diagnosis of this pattern of enhancement is amyloid, and the two conditions can often be distinguished by the appearance of

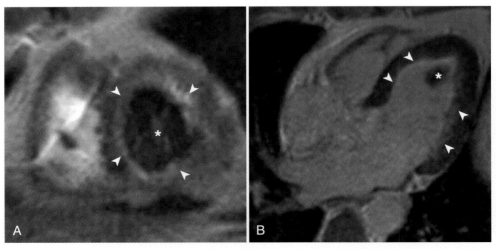

Figure 31-12 Two patients with hypereosinophilic syndrome. **A,** Delayed contrast-enhanced two-chamber short-axis image near the left ventricular apex in a 59-year-old man shows characteristic diffuse subendocardial enhancement in the left ventricle *(arrowheads)* and nonenhancing thrombus occupying the lumen *(asterisk)*. Contractility of the left ventricle on cine images (not shown) was normal. **B,** Delayed contrast-enhanced four-chamber image in a different patient, a 63-year-old man, shows more subtle diffuse subendocardial enhancement *(arrowheads)* and a smaller thrombus at the left ventricular apex *(asterisk)*.

the blood pool, which is usually dark in amyloidosis from loss of contrast but bright in HES. As previously discussed, infarction can also manifest with subendocardial enhancement, but it should be confined to a vascular territory. Mural thrombus may be seen in the thrombotic stage, and preserved LV contractility and wall thickness distinguish HES from thrombus because of infarct or aneurysm formation.

CT is not specifically indicated for evaluation of cardiac HES. However, thrombus should be visible on contrast-enhanced imaging if it is present. Pulmonary eosinophilia with typical peripheral areas of consolidation may be seen but are not necessary for the diagnosis of HES.

■ HEMOCHROMATOSIS AND SIDEROTIC CARDIOMYOPATHY

Abnormally high levels of iron are toxic to myocardium and, when untreated, can result in arrhythmia or restrictive cardiomyopathy that can ultimately progress to DCM. Iron overload may be caused by primary disorders of iron metabolism (i.e., hemochromatosis) or secondary iron overload (i.e., thalassemia major or other conditions requiring repeated blood transfusions), and types of both disorders have similar cardiac findings. Endomyocardial biopsy has traditionally been the method of choice for assessing myocardial iron content because most noninvasive tests are nonspecific; however, cardiac MRI can be used to assess myocardial iron deposition based on changes in the T2* signal characteristics of the tissue.

Primary hemochromatosis is an autosomal recessive disorder with a prevalence of approximately 5 to 8 per 1000. The disease has a variable presentation, partly determined by comorbidities, and cardiac involvement is seen clinically in approximately one third of patients. Hemochromatosis usually manifests in middle age, and initial clinical features include skin pigmentation changes or elevated liver function tests, or both. Siderotic cardiomyopathy (also known as secondary hemochromatosis) is most commonly associated with thalassemia major, and cardiac findings usually manifest at an earlier age (typically adolescence). Sickle cell anemia can also cause signs of secondary hemochromatosis in organs such as the liver and spleen, but the myocardium is usually spared.

Chest radiographic findings are nonspecific and may consist of an enlarged cardiac silhouette with or without signs of heart failure. Similarly, echocardiography is nonspecific for iron deposition and may show a restrictive pattern or DCM based on severity of disease. Patients with thalassemia major typically have increased cardiac output secondary to chronic anemia.

MRI is the imaging test of choice for evaluation of cardiac iron deposition. A routine protocol can suffice for diagnosis; however, optional T2*-weighted sequences and dedicated imaging through the liver, pancreas, and spleen can provide additional useful information. Iron causes local alterations in the magnetic field, with resultant shorter T2* relaxation time. In the setting of iron deposition, myocardium should appear darker than skeletal muscle on T2-weighted and T2*-weighted sequences, and if the disease is severe enough, it is also dark on T1-weighted sequences (Fig. 31-13). Primary hemochromatosis also causes signal loss in the liver and pancreas, but it spares the spleen. Siderotic cardiomyopathy causes decreased signal intensity in the liver and spleen (reticuloendothelial system) but spares the pancreas. Measurement of T2* values can also be performed, both as an indirect assessment of severity of disease (T2* <20 msec is usually associated with abnormal ventricular function) and for assessing response to appropriate therapy (T2* levels should increase with appropriate iron chelation therapy).

■ FABRY DISEASE

Fabry disease represents an example of infiltrative cardiomyopathy, a class of nonischemic cardiomyopathies caused by abnormal accumulation of a substance that results in myocardial dysfunction. Typically, infiltrative cardiomyopathies produce diastolic dysfunction in their early stages that progresses to overt systolic dysfunction and heart failure if the condition is not recognized and managed appropriately. Fabry disease, an autosomal recessive lysosome mutation, results in increased glycosphingolipid accumulation, LV hypertrophy, and increased myocardial mass in a pattern similar to that of the diffuse variant of HCM. In fact, 6% to 12% of patients who present with late-onset HCM (diagnosed in middle age or later) are subsequently found to have Fabry disease. The distinction is critical because Fabry

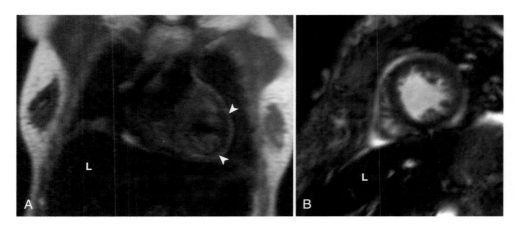

Figure 31-13 A 14-year-old female patient with siderotic cardiomyopathy. Coronal black-blood T2-weighted image (**A**) and two-chamber short-axis steady-state free precession image (**B**) demonstrate the typical low myocardial signal intensity (*arrowheads* in **A**) that is darker than skeletal muscle and liver (L).

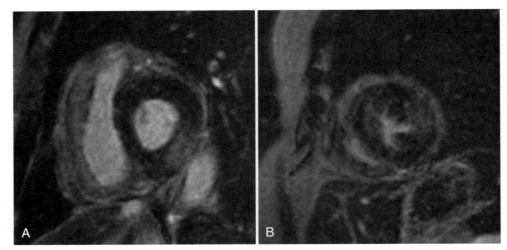

Figure 31-14 A 63-year-old woman with Fabry disease. Delayed contrast-enhanced images through the base (**A**) and apex (**B**) demonstrate diffuse left ventricular hypertrophy and areas of mesocardial enhancement typical of Fabry disease. Note the similarity of the enhancement pattern to that of hypertrophic cardiomyopathy.

disease can be managed with enzyme replacement therapy. The diagnosis of Fabry disease may be made during childhood or adolescence, but cardiac involvement is usually not seen until the third or fourth decade.

The chest radiographic appearance of Fabry disease is nonspecific and may be normal or consist of varying signs of left-sided heart failure based on the stage of disease.

Echocardiography typically shows diastolic dysfunction with a diffusely thickened LV wall (>12 mm in thickness at end-systole) and increased LV mass but preserved fractional shortening and ejection fraction. Glycosphingolipid deposition in the subendocardium may result in a characteristic binary appearance, defined as *hypo*echoic subendocardium that separates the *hyper*echoic endocardium from the myocardium.

A routine MRI protocol with delayed enhancement sequences should be performed for evaluation of suspected infiltrative cardiomyopathies. Results of functional imaging may resemble those in HCM, and an LVOT gradient may be seen. Delayed enhancement of Fabry disease involves the mesocardial layer, with sparing of the subendocardium, similar to HCM, but the enhancement is typically confined to the inferior and inferolateral walls (Fig. 31-14).

■ CONCLUSION

Nonischemic cardiomyopathy is a challenge for clinicians to diagnose and manage. Imaging, especially cardiac MRI, plays a key role that will likely continue to expand in the future. Therefore, imagers must be able to differentiate ischemic from nonischemic patterns of disease, as well as recognize patterns of disease that can help narrow the differential diagnosis in patients with nonischemic cardiomyopathy.

Bibliography

Akashi YJ, Goldstein DS, Barbaro G, et al. Takotsubo cardiomyopathy: a new form of acute, reversible heart failure. *Circulation.* 2008;118:2754-2762.

Anderson LJ, Westwood MA, Holden S, et al. Myocardial iron clearance during reversal of siderotic cardiomyopathy with intravenous desferrioxamine: a prospective study using T2* cardiovascular magnetic resonance. *Br J Haematol.* 2004;127:348-355.

Andreini D, Pontone G, Bartorelli AL, et al. Sixty-four-slice multidetector computed tomography: an accurate imaging modality for the evaluation of coronary arteries in dilated cardiomyopathy of unknown etiology. *Circ Cardiovasc Imaging.* 2009;2:199-205.

Andreini D, Pontone G, Pepi M, et al. Diagnostic accuracy of multidetector computed tomography coronary angiography in patients with dilated cardiomyopathy. *J Am Coll Cardiol.* 2007;49:2044-2050.

Belloni E, De Cobelli F, Esposito A, et al. MRI of cardiomyopathy. *AJR Am J Roentgenol.* 2008;191:1702-1710.

Bluemke DA. MRI of nonischemic cardiomyopathy. *AJR Am J Roentgenol.* 2010;195:935-940.

Bluemke DA, Achenbach S, Budoff M, et al. Noninvasive coronary artery imaging: magnetic resonance angiography and multidetector computed tomography angiography: a scientific statement from the American Heart Association Committee on Cardiovascular Imaging and Intervention of the Council on Cardiovascular Radiology and Intervention, and the Councils on Clinical Cardiology and Cardiovascular Disease in the Young. *Circulation.* 2008;118:586-606.

Bomma C, Rutberg J, Tandri H, et al. Misdiagnosis of arrhythmogenic right ventricular dysplasia/cardiomyopathy. *J Cardiovasc Electrophysiol.* 2004;15:300-306.

Brooks MA, Sane DC. CT findings in acute myocarditis: 2 cases. *J Thorac Imaging.* 2007;22:277-279.

Castillo E, Tandri H, Rodriguez ER, et al. Arrhythmogenic right ventricular dysplasia: ex vivo and in vivo fat detection with black-blood MR imaging. *Radiology.* 2004;232:38-48.

Chang SA, Kim HK, Park EA, et al. Images in cardiovascular medicine: Loeffler endocarditis mimicking apical hypertrophic cardiomyopathy. *Circulation.* 2009;120:82-85.

Cummings KW, Bhalla S, Javidan-Nejad C, et al. A pattern-based approach to assessment of delayed enhancement in nonischemic cardiomyopathy at MR imaging. *Radiographics.* 2009;29:89-103.

Danias PG, Papaioannou GI, Ahlberg AW, et al. Usefulness of electrocardiographic-gated stress technetium-99m sestamibi single-photon emission computed tomography to differentiate ischemic from nonischemic cardiomyopathy. *Am J Cardiol.* 2004;94:14-19.

De Cobelli F, Esposito A, Belloni E, et al. Delayed-enhanced cardiac MRI for differentiation of Fabry's disease from symmetric hypertrophic cardiomyopathy. *AJR Am J Roentgenol.* 2009;192:W97-W102.

Demant AW, Schmiedel A, Buttner R, et al. Heart failure and malignant ventricular tachyarrhythmias due to hereditary hemochromatosis with iron overload cardiomyopathy. *Clin Res Cardiol.* 2007;96:900-903.

Di Bella G, Minutoli F, Mazzeo A, et al. MRI of cardiac involvement in transthyretin familial amyloid polyneuropathy. *AJR Am J Roentgenol.* 2010;195:W394-W399.

Dimitrow PP, Chojnowska L, Rudzinski T, et al. Sudden death in hypertrophic cardiomyopathy: old risk factors re-assessed in a new model of maximalized follow-up. *Eur Heart J.* 2010;31:3084-3093.

Dodd JD, Holmvang G, Hoffmann U, et al. Quantification of left ventricular noncompaction and trabecular delayed hyperenhancement with cardiac MRI: correlation with clinical severity. *AJR Am J Roentgenol.* 2007;189:974-980.

Doughan AR, Williams BR. Cardiac sarcoidosis. *Heart.* 2006;92:282-288.

Falk RH. Diagnosis and management of the cardiac amyloidoses. *Circulation.* 2005;112:2047-2060.

Felker GM, Thompson RE, Hare JM, et al. Underlying causes and long-term survival in patients with initially unexplained cardiomyopathy. *N Engl J Med.* 2000;342:1077-1084.

Fernandez-Perez GC, Aguilar-Arjona JA, de la Fuente GT, et al. Takotsubo cardiomyopathy: assessment with cardiac MRI. *AJR Am J Roentgenol.* 2010;195:W139-W145.

Goitein O, Matetzky S, Beinart R, et al. Acute myocarditis: noninvasive evaluation with cardiac MRI and transthoracic echocardiography. *AJR Am J Roentgenol.* 2009;192:254-258.

Hansen MW, Merchant N. MRI of hypertrophic cardiomyopathy. Part I. MRI appearances. *AJR Am J Roentgenol.* 2007;189:1335-1343.

Hansen MW, Merchant N. MRI of hypertrophic cardiomyopathy. Part 2. Differential diagnosis, risk stratification, and posttreatment MRI appearances. *AJR Am J Roentgenol.* 2007;189:1344-1352.

Hundley WG, Bluemke DA, Finn JP, et al. ACCF/ACR/AHA/NASCI/SCMR 2010 expert consensus document on cardiovascular magnetic resonance: a report of the American College of Cardiology Foundation Task Force on Expert Consensus Documents. *J Am Coll Cardiol.* 2010;55:2614-2662.

Hussain J, Ghandforoush A, Virk Z, et al. Viability assessment by multidetector computed tomography in Takotsubo cardiomyopathy. *J Thorac Imaging.* 2011;26:W7-W8.

Ichinose A, Otani H, Oikawa M, et al. MRI of cardiac sarcoidosis: basal and subepicardial localization of myocardial lesions and their effect on left ventricular function. *AJR Am J Roentgenol.* 2008;191:862-869.

Inati A, Musallam KM, Wood JC, et al. Absence of cardiac siderosis by MRI T2* despite transfusion burden, hepatic and serum iron overload in Lebanese patients with sickle cell disease. *Eur J Haematol.* 2009;83:565-571.

Jacquier A, Thuny F, Jop B, et al. Measurement of trabeculated left ventricular mass using cardiac magnetic resonance imaging in the diagnosis of left ventricular non-compaction. *Eur Heart J.* 2010;31:1098-1104.

Jefferies JL, Towbin JA. Dilated cardiomyopathy. *Lancet.* 2010;375:752-762.

Kirsch J, Williamson EE, Araoz PA. Non-compaction visualization using ECG-gated dual-source CT. *Int J Cardiol.* 2007;118:e46-e47.

Lim RP, Srichai MB, Lee VS. Non-ischemic causes of delayed myocardial hyperenhancement on MRI. *AJR Am J Roentgenol.* 2007;188:1675-1681.

Marcus FI, McKenna WJ, Sherrill D, et al. Diagnosis of arrhythmogenic right ventricular cardiomyopathy/dysplasia: proposed modification of the task force criteria. *Circulation.* 2010;121:1533-1541.

Maron BJ. Hypertrophic cardiomyopathy: a systematic review. *JAMA.* 2002;287:1308-1320.

McCrohon JA, Moon JC, Prasad SK, et al. Differentiation of heart failure related to dilated cardiomyopathy and coronary artery disease using gadolinium-enhanced cardiovascular magnetic resonance. *Circulation.* 2003;108:54-59.

McKenna WJ, Thiene G, Nava A, et al. Diagnosis of arrhythmogenic right ventricular dysplasia/cardiomyopathy: Task Force of the Working Group Myocardial and Pericardial Disease of the European Society of Cardiology and of the Scientific Council on Cardiomyopathies of the International Society and Federation of Cardiology. *Br Heart J.* 1994;71:215-218.

Mouquet F, Lions C, de Groote P, et al. Characterisation of peripartum cardiomyopathy by cardiac magnetic resonance imaging. *Eur Radiol.* 2008;18:2765-2769.

Nance JW, Schoepf UJ, Ramos-Duran L. Tako-tsubo cardiomyopathy: findings on cardiac CT and coronary catheterization. *Heart.* 2010;96:406-407.

O'Hanlon R, Grasso A, Roughton M, et al. Prognostic significance of myocardial fibrosis in hypertrophic cardiomyopathy. *J Am Coll Cardiol.* 2010;56:867-874.

Pearson GD, Veille JC, Rahimtoola S, et al. Peripartum cardiomyopathy: National Heart, Lung, and Blood Institute and Office of Rare Diseases (National Institutes of Health) workshop recommendations and review. *JAMA.* 2000;283:1183-1188.

Pennell DJ. T2* magnetic resonance and myocardial iron in thalassemia. *Ann N Y Acad Sci.* 2005;1054:373-378.

Pieroni M, Chimenti C, De Cobelli F, et al. Fabry's disease cardiomyopathy: echocardiographic detection of endomyocardial glycosphingolipid compartmentalization. *J Am Coll Cardiol.* 2006;47:1663-1671.

Ptaszek LM, Price ET, Hu MY, et al. Early diagnosis of hemochromatosis-related cardiomyopathy with magnetic resonance imaging. *J Cardiovasc Magn Reson.* 2005;7:689-692.

Salanitri GC. Endomyocardial fibrosis and intracardiac thrombus occurring in idiopathic hypereosinophilic syndrome. *AJR Am J Roentgenol.* 2005;184:1432-1433.

Seward JB, Casaclang-Verzosa G. Infiltrative cardiovascular diseases: cardiomyopathies that look alike. *J Am Coll Cardiol.* 2010;55:1769-1779.

Skouri HN, Dec GW, Friedrich MG, et al. Noninvasive imaging in myocarditis. *J Am Coll Cardiol.* 2006;48:2085-2093.

Sliwa K, Hilfiker-Kleiner D, Petrie MC, et al. Current state of knowledge on aetiology, diagnosis, management, and therapy of peripartum cardiomyopathy: a position statement from the Heart Failure Association of the European Society of Cardiology Working Group on peripartum cardiomyopathy. *Eur J Heart Fail.* 2010;12:767-778.

Sparrow PJ, Merchant N, Provost YL, et al. CT and MR imaging findings in patients with acquired heart disease at risk for sudden cardiac death. *Radiographics.* 2009;29:805-823.

Tandri H, Bomma C, Calkins H, et al. Magnetic resonance and computed tomography imaging of arrhythmogenic right ventricular dysplasia. *J Magn Reson Imaging.* 2004;19:848-858.

Tandri H, Castillo E, Ferrari VA, et al. Magnetic resonance imaging of arrhythmogenic right ventricular dysplasia: sensitivity, specificity, and observer variability of fat detection versus functional analysis of the right ventricle. *J Am Coll Cardiol.* 2006;48:2277-2284.

van Spaendonck-Zwarts KY, van Tintelen JP, van Veldhuisen DJ, et al. Peripartum cardiomyopathy as a part of familial dilated cardiomyopathy. *Circulation.* 2010;121:2169-2175.

Vignaux O. Cardiac sarcoidosis: spectrum of MRI features. *AJR Am J Roentgenol.* 2005;184:249-254.

White JA, Patel MR. The role of cardiovascular MRI in heart failure and the cardiomyopathies. *Cardiol Clin.* 2007;25:71-95, vi.

Yoerger DM, Marcus F, Sherrill D, et al. Echocardiographic findings in patients meeting task force criteria for arrhythmogenic right ventricular dysplasia: new insights from the multidisciplinary study of right ventricular dysplasia. *J Am Coll Cardiol.* 2005;45:860-865.

CHAPTER 32

Cardiac Masses

John P. Lichtenberger III, Brett W. Carter, and Suhny Abbara

Advances in cardiac gated computed tomography (CT) and magnetic resonance imaging (MRI) have significantly expanded the role of imaging in the evaluation of cardiac lesions. Echocardiography is the most common imaging study performed, and incidentally discovered cardiac lesions on echocardiography account for a significant proportion of cardiac mass evaluations. Additionally, the increasing temporal resolution of conventional CT allows better visualization of the heart on dedicated chest or abdominal examinations that may, in turn, increase the detection of cardiac masses.

Once a cardiac lesion is detected, dedicated cardiac imaging provides detailed information crucial for patient management. Anatomic localization of the lesion is the first and most important step in evaluating a suspected cardiac mass. To begin, a lesion must be confirmed to be of or from the heart. Occasionally, lesions mimicking masses turn out to be normal structures. Masses originating within the pericardium, mediastinum, and lung may invade the heart or compress the heart sufficiently to suggest falsely that they are cardiac masses. The epicardial fat is helpful in discerning whether a mass is truly cardiac in origin. Masses external to the heart displace this thin layer of fat toward the heart, whereas masses of the myocardium often outwardly displace or infiltrate this layer. Similarly, the pericardium can help in distinguishing an anterior mediastinal mass from a myocardial mass. Tenting of pericardium away from the heart or draping of the pericardium over the mass suggests a myocardial origin.

The location of a mass within the heart provides important diagnostic information and is the next step in evaluating myocardial lesions. Lesions originating from the valves are most commonly vegetations or adherent thrombus, although rare primary cardiac tumors such as papillary fibroelastoma may originate from the valves.

After localization, tissue characterization of cardiac lesions is paramount to diagnosis. For instance, detecting fat within a lesion narrows the differential diagnosis of a cardiac lesion considerably to include lipomas, teratomas, and lipomatous hypertrophy of the interatrial septum. Calcifications are rare in malignant myocardial tumors, with the exception of metastases that calcify, such as osteosarcoma and the extremely rare primary cardiac osteosarcoma. Cystic components are less helpful in differentiating myocardial tumors, although the presence of cystic components makes lymphoma less likely.

When a lesion is detected in the heart on imaging, regardless of the modality, the first clinical question is typically whether the mass is a thrombus or a neoplasm. Imaging findings favoring a neoplastic cause include vascularity and infiltration of the mass into the myocardium. Behavior on repeat imaging such as resolution with anticoagulation (which would indicate thrombus) is an important clinical diagnostic factor. Although contrast enhancement of a lesion excludes acute thrombus, organized thrombus may exhibit low levels of enhancement.

Finally, an understanding of the epidemiology of myocardial disease is helpful in organizing a differential diagnosis for cardiac lesions. Primary cardiac masses are rare, occurring with a frequency of between 0.002% and 0.19%. Most primary cardiac masses are benign, and more than half of benign cardiac masses are myxomas. Among malignant cardiac masses, metastatic disease is by far the most common, followed distantly by angiosarcoma and lymphoma.

■ IMAGING OF CARDIAC MASSES

Multiple imaging tools are employed in the evaluation of cardiac masses. Because each modality has strengths and weaknesses, echocardiography, cardiac CT, and cardiac MRI are often used in concert. Although transthoracic echocardiography is accessible and is often the first imaging modality used to assess cardiac masses, cardiac MRI has improved resolution and soft tissue contrast. Cardiac-gated CT can provide detailed anatomic information, can evaluate extent of local invasion, and can better assess calcium. Detailed anatomic and functional evaluation of myocardial masses is often required for surgical or radiation therapy planning. Additionally, postsurgical or follow-up examinations may be required. Understanding the available imaging modalities and their complementary nature is important when diagnosing a suspected cardiac mass or when recommending subsequent studies.

Radiography

Myocardial masses are rarely detected or evaluated using radiography. Even when large, intracavitary masses may not significantly distort the cardiac silhouette. When arising from the myocardium, masses alter the normal cardiac contour or appear as cardiac enlargement. Calcifications may be localized to the heart when they are present in masses such as myxomas. Masses in the left atrium may result in pulmonary venous congestion and pulmonary edema by impeding pulmonary blood flow back to the heart or obstructing the mitral valve.

Echocardiography

Ultrasound is a safe and effective means of evaluating both the anatomy and function of the heart. Echocardiography is the most common imaging study, and imaging evaluation of heart disease most often begins with this modality. Cardiac masses are frequently first detected as an incidental finding on echocardiography. Multiple imaging planes are available, thus allowing targeted examination of the cardiac chambers, the cardiac valves, the pericardium, and the proximal aorta. Real-time imaging provides valuable information about myocardial global and regional wall motion. Doppler echocardiography allows estimation of important functional parameters such as ejection fraction, stroke volume, and cardiac output. Valvular dysfunction can also be quantified. Serial imaging with echocardiography provides important surveillance information for worsening cardiac dysfunction. Newer echocardiographic tools such as three-dimensional echocardiography have been developed.

Because ultrasound is so frequently used in the evaluation of heart disease, cardiac masses are often first discovered by this modality. Masses in the fetal heart such as rhabdomyoma are almost always first discovered during fetal ultrasound, and important mimics of cardiac masses such as thrombus or vegetations are often first characterized by echocardiography. Mass characterization on echocardiography often centers on vascularity, attachment site and morphology (e.g., stalklike or broad-based attachment site), and relationship with adjacent anatomy. Transesophageal echocardiography is the best modality to evaluate small masses arising from the cardiac valves. Real-time evaluation can depict valvular dysfunction associated with a cardiac mass, such as prolapse of a pedunculated atrial myxoma across the mitral or tricuspid valve.

Echocardiography is operator dependent and targeted, and certain regions of the heart and cardiac masses are challenging to detect. The left ventricular apex, inferior vena cava, and aortic arch may be difficult to image. Small masses centered in the myocardium may be visible only as focal thickening of the myocardium. Distinguishing myocardial from pericardial origin may be impossible with large and infiltrating masses. Additionally, the extent of extracardiac disease is not well evaluated with echocardiography, particularly into the pulmonary and systemic veins. Adjacent lungs, airways, and calcifications can be obstacles to detailed mass characterization when using echocardiography. Body habitus can limit transthoracic echocardiography.

Computed Tomography

Multidetector CT has established a role in imaging cardiac tumors, primarily secondary to its short imaging time, its high spatial resolution, and its unsurpassed ability to evaluate calcification. Depending on imaging parameters such as heart rate and mode of imaging, the entire heart can be imaged in as little as one heartbeat. Submillimeter detector arrays provide spatial resolution superior to that of MRI. Additionally, high spatial resolution in three planes (isovoxel) during image acquisition allows for post hoc multiplanar reconstructions. CT is the best imaging modality to demonstrate calcifications. The presence of calcification within a mass may provide important diagnostic information, and linear calcification in the myocardium indicative of earlier myocardial infarction can provide important information when thrombus is suspected. Fat can also be readily identified on CT as low attenuation regions (–30 to –100 Hounsfield units) within cardiac masses.

Fundamental to the use of CT to evaluate cardiac tumors is electrocardiogram (ECG) gating. Not only does it eliminate blurring secondary to cardiac motion, but also it can provide functional analysis. If scanned retrospectively such that the heart is effectively imaged throughout the entire cardiac cycle, an intracavitary mass can be depicted in both diastolic and systolic positions. This is perhaps most applicable when a mass is associated with or originating from a cardiac valve. Cardiac movement may reveal the pedunculated nature of the mass or assist in evaluating for the site of origin or attachment. Finally, high spatial resolution of cardiac CT when combined with ECG gating is an advantage of this modality over MRI.

Intravenous, nonionic contrast material is an important element of evaluating cardiac masses on CT. Opacification of the cardiac chamber helps to delineate the borders of an intracavitary mass. Contrast may also depict the differential enhancement of normal myocardium from an intramyocardial mass. The timing and composition of the contrast bolus are special considerations when performing cardiac CT. If the approximate anatomic location is known before imaging, the contrast bolus can be timed to opacify the involved or most adjacent cardiac chamber when the images are acquired. This typically involves bolus tracking or test bolus techniques, in which an anatomic site such as the ascending aorta is serially imaged in rapid succession after contrast injection to trigger the scan (bolus tracking technique) or to time the diagnostic contrast bolus (test bolus technique). Configuring the contrast bolus is particularly challenging when evaluating a right atrial mass. Inflow of nonopacified contrast material from the inferior vena cava and coronary sinus and concentrated contrast material inflowing from the superior vena cava and causing beam-hardening artifact may obscure the borders of a mass. Accurate imaging may require injecting a dilute mix of contrast material and saline solution after the typical concentrated contrast bolus, or early delayed scans (90 seconds) after injection of a large amount of contrast material to capture the second phase after systemic venous return. Injecting contrast material from a lower extremity vein may be considered when evaluating masses involving or near the inferior cavoatrial junction or when a mass has obstructed the superior vena cava.

When considering cardiac CT for the evaluation of myocardial masses, the examiner must be familiar with the limitations of this modality. Significant and persistent arrhythmias can make adequate ECG gating difficult or impossible. Similarly, high resting heart rates may limit the spatial resolution secondary to excessive motion artifact. Temporal resolution is lower in CT as compared with both echocardiography and MRI. With the exception of calcification, tissue characterization is inferior to that available with MRI. CT uses ionizing radiation, which is potentially hazardous. This factor is particularly important to consider when imaging young patients. Finally, cardiac CT almost always employs the use of intravenous contrast material, which is potentially nephrotoxic.

Magnetic Resonance Imaging

The high tissue contrast resolution, multiplanar imaging capability, and standardized and reproducible imaging planes make MRI the modality of choice for imaging most cardiac tumors. Unlike MRI examinations of other anatomic structures that may rely on standardized protocols and imaging planes, cardiac MRI for myocardial masses often requires real-time input from the cardiac imager to characterize a mass optimally and to delineate its anatomy more clearly. Anatomic definition and tissue characterization are evaluated using T1-weighted, proton density, and T2-weighted sequences. Cystic components and hemorrhage products can be distinguished using these sequences as elsewhere in the body. Gradient echo cine images provide wall motion and functional data and may demonstrate the dynamic interaction of a mass with cardiac valves. Early T1-based sequences and delayed enhancement sequences after gadolinium administration are usually employed both to evaluate enhancement and vascularity of the mass and to detect underlying myocardial scars when thrombus is suspected.

Imaging protocols for evaluating cardiac tumors on MRI usually begin with scout images and fast spin echo axial images, which provide early localization of the tumor. From this point, two-chamber steady-state free precession (SSFP) sequences are prescribed, depending on the location of the tumor (e.g., oriented along the tricuspid valve and right ventricular apex for tumors in the right side of the heart, oriented along the mitral valve and left ventricular apex for tumors in the left side of the heart). Four-chamber and short-axis SSFP sequences are then acquired, to provide an anatomic overview of the heart and functional information. T2-weighted triple-inversion recovery sequences are used to evaluate edema or necrosis in the mass and adjacent myocardium.

Gadolinium is an important component of the MRI evaluation of cardiac masses and should be used when possible. The principles of gadolinium enhancement were originally developed to evaluate myocardial infarction. T1-weighted fast spin echo sequences are acquired before and after the administration of intravenous gadolinium to detect abnormal enhancement of the mass or to highlight the differential enhancement compared with normal myocardium. Cardiac masses may enhance after the administration of intravenous gadolinium by one mechanism or by a combination of several mechanisms. Gadolinium accumulates in the extracellular space. When cellular damage has occurred, such as in necrotic or fibrotic portions of a mass, gadolinium may enter the intracellular space and result in enhancement. Another mechanism of gadolinium enhancement is its collection in a region of increased extracellular space, as in the case of myocardial edema. Local myocardial hyperemia incited by the presence of a mass may increase delivery of gadolinium to the mass.

Cardiac MRI has a role not only in tumor characterization but also in differentiating mass from thrombus, an important and common clinical question when a mass is discovered. MRI has superior soft tissue resolution and better reproducibility than echocardiography. MRI is a valuable tool for both the diagnosis and follow-up imaging of intracavitary thrombus. Intravenous gadolinium is also helpful in differentiating tumor from thrombus in that thrombus is typically avascular and therefore not expected to enhance. Large, chronic thrombus may demonstrate thin peripheral enhancement near the attachment site from neovascular ingrowth.

MRI is also useful for determination of the degree of myocardial infiltration and pericardial involvement. Differential enhancement of tumor and normal myocardium may provide important information about infiltrating tumors. Localized thickening of the pericardium in association with a cardiac mass may suggest involvement of the pericardium. An enhancing pericardial nodule or the presence of a hemopericardium in the setting of a cardiac tumor provides compelling evidence of the malignant nature of the cardiac tumor and indicates neoplastic pericardial involvement.

Limitations of MRI include long imaging times, the presence of contraindications such as claustrophobia or preexisting pacemakers, accessibility, and poor spatial resolution. Calcification is not well evaluated on MRI, an important component of tissue characterization best depicted on CT. Nephrogenic systemic fibrosis, previously known as nephrogenic fibrosing dermopathy, is a disease characterized by fibrosis of the skin and internal organs that has been associated with gadolinium. This association is derived from gadolinium found in biopsied fibrotic tissues in patients with this disease. All patients with nephrogenic systemic fibrosis have a history of renal insufficiency (except one report of two transplant recipients in which the donors' exposure to gadolinium was not reported). Relatively poor spatial resolution of cardiac MRI compared with echocardiography and CT limits its evaluation of very small masses, especially when associated with cardiac valves.

■ BENIGN CARDIAC MASSES

Myxoma

Background

Comprising approximately 50% of primary cardiac neoplasms, myxoma is the most common primary cardiac tumor. Histologically, myxomas are mesenchymal in origin, although they are distinct from noncardiac myxomas. Most sporadic myxomas occur in adults between 30 and 60 years old. Cardiac myxomas may also be seen in younger patients with Carney complex, an autosomal dominant syndrome of cardiac myxomas, hyperpigmented skin lesions, and extracardiac neoplasms such as breast fibroadenomas, pituitary adenomas, and psammomatous melanotic schwannomas. The myxomas in the setting of Carney complex may be uncharacteristically multifocal, extraatrial, and recurrent.

Most (>90%) cardiac myxomas are solitary, atrial, and intracavitary. They tend to arise from the interatrial septum (78%) near the fossa ovalis. From this site, they are more commonly within the left atrium (~80%) than the right atrium, and they may occasionally grow through the fossa ovalis to occupy both atria. Approximately 16% of these tumors contain calcification at surgical resection. Myxomas may be cystic, necrotic, or hemorrhagic. Although most are broad based, their occasional stalklike attachment to the cardiac chamber wall is a distinctive feature when present.

The clinical presentation of cardiac myxoma is attributable to embolization, functional obstruction, or idiopathic symptoms. Systemic and central nervous system embolization from these tumors may be from bland thrombus associated with the mass or from tumor embolization. Even embolization into the coronary arteries that causes small myocardial infarction has been described. When intracavitary and atrial, these masses may clinically mimic mitral or tricuspid stenosis.

Imaging

The imaging appearance of cardiac myxomas reflects the pathologic features, although internal structure characterization is nonspecific (Fig. 32-1). Although most myxomas are homogenous on echocardiography, they may show internal hypoechoic structures consistent with cysts or hyperechoic foci if calcifications are present. These masses are heterogeneously low attenuating on cardiac CT. CT is the optimal modality to evaluate for calcification and may show heterogeneity reflecting hemorrhage or necrosis. In the absence of calcification or hemorrhage, myxomas typically have high signal intensity on T2-weighted imaging because of their high water content, are isointense to myocardium on T1-weighted images, and demonstrate heterogeneous low-grade enhancement with gadolinium administration. Features that confer greater confidence in making the diagnosis of myxoma include stalklike attachment to the interatrial septum and mobility. In addition, prolapse of an atrial mass through the mitral or tricuspid valve is also frequently seen in myxomas and can be demonstrated on echocardiography, CT, and MRI. However, prolapse through the tricuspid valve is more frequently encountered when tumor thrombus extends from the IVC into the right atrium such as from renal, liver, adrenal, retroperitoneal, or uterine tumors. Tumor prolapse through the mitral valve may also occasionally be encountered by lung masses that invade the atrium through the pulmonary veins. Hence, if a prolapsing tumor is encountered, it is critical to identify the entire mass and its origin and attachment site.

Cardiac Papillary Fibroelastoma

Background

Cardiac papillary fibroelastoma is a connective tissue tumor (cardiac endothelial papilloma) lined by a single layer of endothelium. It is the second most common benign primary cardiac tumor based on large surgical and pathologic series, and it represents 10% of all primary cardiac tumors. Papillary fibroelastomas are by far the most common tumors to involve the cardiac valves,

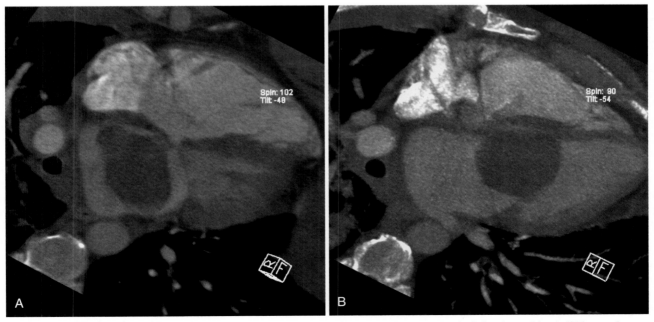

Figure 32-1 **A,** Retrospectively gated cardiac computed tomography angiography shows a mass in the left atrium with a stalklike attachment to the interatrial septum near the mitral valve. **B,** This mass prolapses through the mitral valve during diastolic filling.

with greater than 75% of these tumors occurring in this location. The aortic valve is the most common valve affected (29%), followed by the mitral and tricuspid valves. The mean age at diagnosis is approximately 60 years, with a slight male predominance.

Papillary fibroelastomas are typically less than 1 cm in size, although tumors ranging up to 7 cm have been reported. They often have a stalklike attachment to the avascular valvular endocardium. They tend to be on the aortic side of the aortic cusps and on the atrial side of the atrioventricular valves. That these tumors usually do not arise from the free leaflet edges or coaptation margins may help differentiate them from vegetations. The central portion and villous fronds of connective tissue are also avascular, and the overall appearance has been compared to a sea anemone on gross pathologic examination. Elastic fiber layers are the hallmark of these tumors when present in histologic samples.

Most patients with cardiac papillary fibroelastomas are asymptomatic, and most tumors are discovered incidentally. The friable nature of these tumors, the associated thrombus, and their predilection for the valves account for their clinical presentation in symptomatic patients. Stroke and transient ischemic attacks are the most frequent presenting symptoms, and peripheral embolization has also been reported. Despite the predilection of these tumors for the cardiac valves, valvular dysfunction is not typical.

Imaging

Cardiac papillary fibroelastomas are most frequently discovered on echocardiography (Fig. 32-2). Classic echocardiographic findings include a small, pedunculated mass with peripheral stippled edges, attributed to the echogenic interfaces of small papillary projections. Advances in CT and MRI have established a role for these modalities in the evaluation of this tumor.

Surgical excision is curative and is therefore the treatment of choice for symptomatic cardiac papillary fibroelastomas. Tumor mobility is an independent predictor of major morbidity and mortality. Surgery may also be considered in an asymptomatic patient if the mass is mobile.

Lipoma

Background

Cardiac lipomas are encapsulated tumors composed of adipose tissue, typically arising from a broad pedicle extending from the epicardium. These tumors are rare, although multiple intramyocardial cardiac lipomas have been associated with tuberous sclerosis. They may arise from the epicardium, myocardium, or interatrial septum.

Symptomatic, cardiac lipomas have been known to cause cardiac arrhythmias, obstruction when intracavitary, and symptoms such as shortness of breath secondary to local mass effect. Lipomatous hypertrophy of the interatrial septum is a distinct entity that is discussed separately later. Differentiating features are its absence of a capsule and the finding that this tumor is composed of immature brown fat.

Imaging

Cardiac lipomas are typically incidental findings, seen on chest radiographs as an abnormal contour of the cardiomediastinal silhouette or on echocardiography as a homogenous, hyperechoic mass when intracavitary. The echocardiographic appearance of lipomas in the pericardial space is more varied, and tumors in this location may be heterogeneous, hyperechoic, or hypoechoic. Necrosis and hemorrhage are uncommon. CT and MRI provide superior tissue characterization (Fig. 32-3). Lipomas on CT are homogeneous, fat attenuation, encapsulated masses without demonstrable enhancement. On MRI, these masses are T1 hyperintense and suppress with chemical fat saturation. These pliable masses may encase the coronary arteries without obstruction. Septations, if present, are thin and without nodularity or a nonfatty component.

Treatment of symptomatic cardiac lipomas is typically surgical. Infiltrating and unresectable tumors are the rare exception.

Fibroma

Background

Cardiac fibromas are rare, congenital tumors that are composed of fibroblasts and collagen and have no capsule. These tumors predominantly occur in children and infants, in whom they are the second most common tumor after rhabdomyomas, although up to 15% of fibromas occur in adolescents and young adults. These tumors occur with increased prevalence in patients with Gorlin syndrome (basal cell nevus syndrome), an autosomal dominant cancer syndrome characterized by basal cell carcinoma, odontogenic keratocysts of the mandible, plantar, and palmar pits, and other neoplasms. Patients may present with a murmur, arrhythmias, or heart failure. Cardiac fibromas are a recognized cause of sudden cardiac death, which may occur if the tumor extends into the conduction system.

Imaging

Cardiac fibromas are almost always solitary and without cystic features on imaging. Most of these tumors occur in the interventricular septum and left ventricular free wall (Fig. 32-4). Their size ranges between 2 and 5 cm. They are homogeneous, with the exception of dystrophic calcification, which is a common finding best identified on CT or echocardiography. On MRI, these tumors are typically discrete, focal myocardial masses or focal thickening isointense to hyperintense on T1-weighted images and slightly hypointense on T2-weighted images. Intense delayed enhancement is typical, indicating the expanded extracellular volume of distribution relative to the ventricular myocardium. Because this tumor is diagnosed predominantly in children and infants, the primary differential diagnosis is rhabdomyoma.

Rhabdomyoma

Cardiac rhabdomyomas are the most common primary cardiac tumors in infants (Fig. 32-5). They are histologically hamartomatous, and approximately half of the

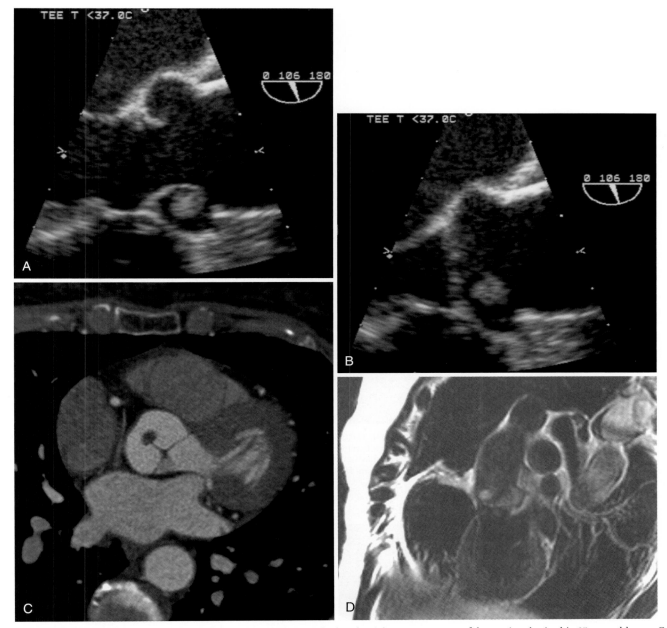

Figure 32-2 **A** and **B,** Echocardiographic images show a mass attached to the right coronary cusp of the aortic valve in this 65-year-old man. **C,** The mass was confirmed on computed tomography. **D,** Short-axis oblique black-blood technique magnetic resonance image shows a round mass attached to the right coronary cusp that was found to be a papillary fibroelastoma at surgical resection.

cases occur in patients with tuberous sclerosis. These tumors are often multiple, and they tend to occur in the ventricular myocardium. T2 hyperintensity can help to distinguish this tumor from cardiac fibroma, the next most common primary cardiac tumor in this age group. Cardiac rhabdomyomas spontaneously regress in most cases, and conservative management is often pursued unless the tumors demonstrate aggressive features.

Teratoma

Cardiac teratomas are rare cystic tumors of multiple germ cell layers, most frequently diagnosed in children. These tumors are most commonly found in the

pericardial space and are often accompanied by a pericardial effusion. CT may demonstrate the cysts, fat, and calcification comprising these tumors.

Hemangioma

Cardiac hemangiomas are rare tumors, accounting for less than 2% of all cardiac tumors. Symptoms are rarely attributed to cardiac hemangiomas, although arrhythmias, pericardial effusions, and chest pain have been reported. On imaging, these are well-defined, often lobular, broad-based but mobile masses that are typically heterogeneously low attenuating on CT. These tumors have high signal intensity on T1-weighted imaging, are

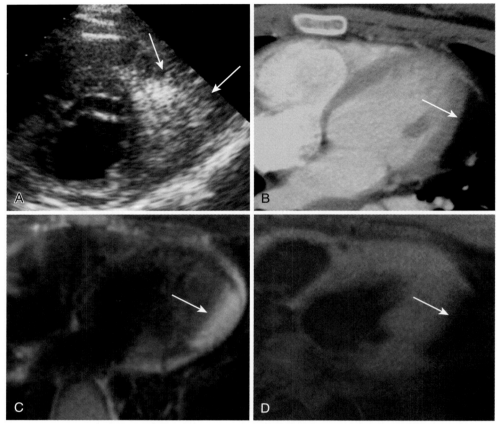

Figure 32-3 **A,** A 45-year-old man with a history of tuberous sclerosis and an incidental mass *(arrows)* on echocardiography. **B,** Computed tomography image shows a fat attenuation mass *(arrow)* in the left ventricular wall. **C** and **D,** This mass suppresses with chemical fat suppression on magnetic resonance imaging *(arrows),* thus confirming a cardiac lipoma. (From Lichtenberger JP, et al. Cardiac lipoma in a patient with tuberous sclerosis complex. In: Abbara S, Mamuya F. *Massachusetts General Hospital Cardiovascular Images.* <http://www.mgh-cardiovascimages.org/index .php?src=gendocs&ref=cv_september_2010>.)

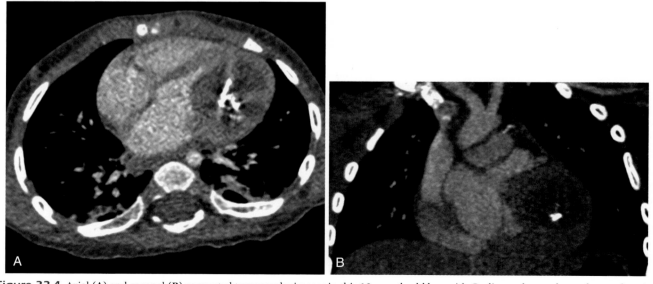

Figure 32-4 Axial (**A**) and coronal (**B**) computed tomography images in this 12-month-old boy with Gorlin syndrome show a hypoenhancing low attenuation cardiac mass centered in the left ventricular lateral wall with internal calcifications consistent with a cardiac fibroma.

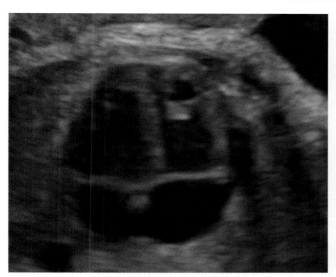

Figure 32-5 Transabdominal fetal ultrasound shows a right ventricular mass in this 34-week fetus that suggests a cardiac rhabdomyoma.

isointense on T1-weighted imaging, and are characterized by intense enhancement after iodinated contrast or gadolinium administration. They may contain fat and extend into the pericardial space. Cardiac hemangiomas may be distinguished from cardiac lipomas by their heterogeneity and intense enhancement.

Lymphangioma

Cardiac lymphangiomas are extremely rare, composed of thin-walled lymphatic cysts separate from the lymphatic system. They typically occur in the pericardial space and may be associated with chylous pericardial effusion. They are cystic on echocardiography, and the cysts follow fluid signal intensity on MRI. Portions of the tumor may be T1 hyperintense, a feature attributed to components of fatty stroma.

Paraganglioma

Background

Cardiac paragangliomas are very rare tumors composed of clusters of neuroendocrine cells. They most commonly occur in the posterior wall of the left atrium, although they have been reported in the interatrial septum and arising from paraganglia associated with the coronary arteries. They usually have a broad attachment to the myocardium. As with paragangliomas found elsewhere in the body, these tumors are highly vascular and tend to be necrotic.

Cardiac paragangliomas are usually benign and typically occur in the third and fourth decades. When symptomatic from a functioning paraganglioma, patients present with hypertension or symptoms attributable to catecholamine overproduction.

Imaging

When paragangliomas are suspected clinically, iodine-123 or iodine-131 metaiodobenzylguanidine (MIBG) scintigraphy is a highly specific imaging

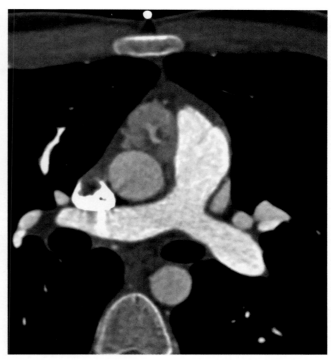

Figure 32-6 Axial contrast-enhanced computed tomography in a 16-year-old patient with a hypervascular mass along the right ventricular outflow tract that partially encompasses the right coronary artery. Pathologic examination revealed a paraganglioma.

modality. A norepinephrine analogue, MIBG is selectively taken up by extraadrenal paragangliomas. After localization to the heart or mediastinum on MIBG, further workup typically involves CT or MRI. The typical appearance on CT of cardiac paragangliomas is a homogeneous, well-circumscribed, hypoattenuating mass that avidly enhances (Fig. 32-6). These tumors are typically T2 hyperintense and avidly enhance on MRI.

Surgical resection of these tumors is often difficult secondary to their highly vascular nature and their tendency to involve the coronary arteries.

Hamartoma

Cardiac hamartomas are very rare, benign tumors that lack a true capsule and are characterized by hypertrophied, disorganized myocytes (Fig. 32-7). Patients described in case reports range in age from 6 months to 74 years and may be symptomatic or present with arrhythmia. Surgical resection can be curative.

■ MALIGNANT CARDIAC NEOPLASMS

Metastatic Disease

Background

Metastatic disease to the heart is approximately 20 to 40 times more common than are primary cardiac neoplasms, and it is associated with a poor prognosis. The most common primary malignant disease to metastasize to the heart is lung cancer, followed by lymphoma, leukemia, breast cancer, and esophageal cancer. The

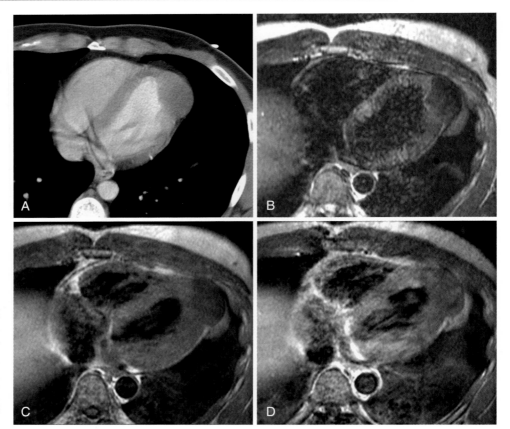

Figure 32-7 A, Axial computed tomography image shows a low attenuation mass in the left ventricle in this 33-year-old man with new-onset arrhythmia. Axial T2 (**B**), T1 pregadolinium (**C**) and post-gadolinium (**D**) images show a well-circumscribed mass of low signal intensity with central enhancement that was found to be a cardiac hamartoma at surgical resection.

pericardium is the most frequently involved site, with or without involvement of the underlying myocardium. The most common clinical presentation includes shortness of breath related to impaired cardiac function, which occurs in 30% of patients. Other symptoms include chest pain, cough, arrhythmias, and peripheral edema. Death from cardiac metastases is typically the result of heart failure, cardiac tamponade, coronary artery invasion, or sinoatrial node extension.

Noncardiac tumors may reach the heart by lymphatic spread, hematologic dissemination, direct extension, or transvenous spread. The most common route is retrograde extension through the lymphatic system, which results in implants along the epicardial surface of the heart and within the epicardial portion of the myocardium. Most of the lymphatic channels draining the pericardium coalesce at the level of the aortic root, and tumor involvement of this region can produce pericardial effusions. Melanoma and the sarcomas are the primary malignant diseases that have the highest propensity to spread hematogenously to the heart. These tumors spread to the epicardium and myocardium through the coronary arteries and venae cavae. Tumors of the lung, tracheobronchial tree, breast, and esophagus may directly invade the heart. Finally, transvenous extension may be encountered with renal cell carcinoma, hepatocellular carcinoma, adrenal cortical carcinoma, retroperitoneal tumors, and some lung cancers. These tumors access the right atrium through the superior or inferior vena cava or the left atrium through the pulmonary veins.

Imaging

The most common imaging manifestations of cardiac metastatic disease, as demonstrated by CT and MRI, are pericardial abnormalities and filling defects within vessels and cardiac chambers (Fig. 32-8). Pericardial nodularity and effusions are commonly encountered in cases of metastatic disease, especially primary malignant tumors of the lung or breast, lymphoma, and leukemia. Autopsy studies demonstrated that approximately one third of patients with lung cancer had pericardial metastatic disease. Malignant pericardial effusions are associated with a poor prognosis. Malignant pericardial disease may be suggested by thickening and enhancement of the pericardium on CT and MRI. Pericardiocentesis is necessary for definitive diagnosis, however, because the differential diagnosis of these findings includes sequelae of radiation therapy, drug-related pericarditis, infection, and idiopathic causes. If hemorrhagic and serosanguineous, pericardial effusions may appear hyperintense on T1-weighted images. In general, most metastatic lesions involving the heart and pericardium tend to be hypointense on T1-weighted images and hyperintense on T2-weighted images relative to myocardium. After the administration of gadolinium, enhancement is typically heterogeneous. However, in patients with metastatic melanoma, lesions may be hyperintense on both T1- and T2-weighted images secondary to the presence of paramagnetic melanin.

In the case of direct invasion by a primary malignant tumor such as lung cancer, obliteration of a superior pulmonary vein and, to a lesser extent, an inferior pulmonary

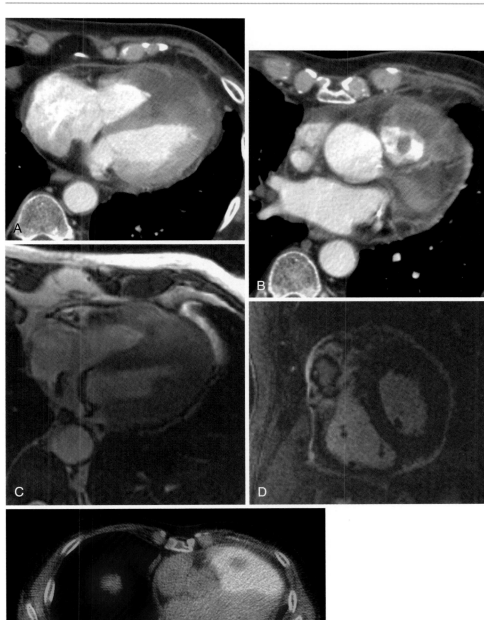

Figure 32-8 A 67-year-old man with history of non–small cell lung cancer and worsening fatigue. A and B, Axial computed tomography (CT) images show an infiltrative low attenuation mass centered on the right ventricular apex and extending to the right ventricular outflow tract to involve the tricuspid valve. Axial fast imaging employing steady state acquisition (FIESTA) (**C**) and delayed enhancement (**D**) images at short axis to the right ventricle confirm an enhancing mass consistent with metastatic disease to the heart. **E,** Positron emission tomography–CT fusion shows increased fluorodeoxyglucose avidity of the cardiac metastases relative to the remaining myocardium.

vein on CT or MRI suggests intrapericardial extension of tumor. In transvenous spread of tumor, most commonly from right-sided renal cell carcinomas and hepatocellular carcinomas, contrast-enhanced CT or multiphase MRI may demonstrate filling defects within an expanded inferior vena cava or filling defects within one or more cardiac chambers, typically the right atrium (Fig. 32-9). However, thrombus within these structures may be indistinguishable from metastatic disease. On MRI, recent thrombus may also be hyperintense on T2-weighed images. However, tumor is more likely to enhance following the

administration of gadolinium contrast, which may help in distinguishing between these two entities. An unusual and rather specific manifestation of osteosarcoma, a rare cause of cardiac metastatic disease, is the production of bone, which can aid in the diagnosis.

Sarcomas

Background
Sarcomas are the most common primary malignant tumors of the heart and pericardium and the second most

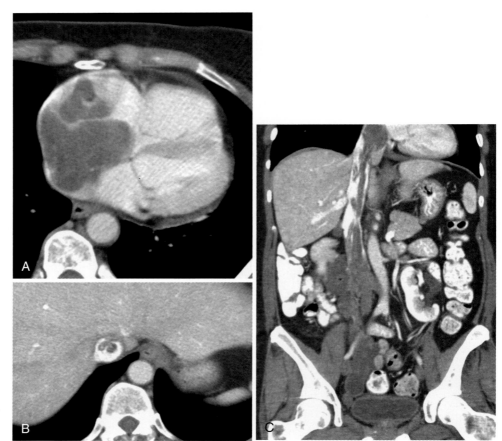

Figure 32-9 **A** and **B**, Axial computed tomography images show a lobulated mass filling the right atrium with extension into the inferior vena cava (IVC). **C**, Coronal reformatted image shows that the right atrial mass is the result of direct extension of a pelvic leiomyoma ascending the IVC.

common primary cardiac neoplasms overall, after myxoma. Primary cardiac sarcomas most commonly affect adults and are extremely rare in children and infants. The most common clinical symptom is dyspnea. Other presentations include chest pain, arrhythmias, peripheral edema, cardiac tamponade, and sudden death. Primary cardiac sarcomas are by definition restricted to the heart and pericardium, without evidence of extracardiac involvement. However, when metastatic, these tumors most frequently affect the lungs.

Angiosarcoma, the most common primary cardiac malignant tumor, accounts for approximately 37% of all cases. Additional types include undifferentiated sarcoma, malignant fibrous histiocytoma, leiomyosarcoma, myxofibrosarcoma, and osteosarcoma. Angiosarcoma, in contrast to the other sarcomas, usually occurs in the right atrium, and presenting symptoms are related to impaired right cardiac filling and pericardial tamponade. Undifferentiated sarcoma involves the left atrium approximately 80% of the time, but it can also originate from the cardiac valves. In contrast to metastatic osteosarcoma, primary cardiac osteosarcoma occurs predominantly in the left atrium. Leiomyosarcoma, a rare tumor arising from smooth muscle, usually involves the left atrium and results in symptoms related to mitral obstruction, such as dyspnea and cardiac obstruction. Although primary cardiac sarcomas are primarily tumors of adults, the most common childhood cardiac malignant tumor is rhabdomyosarcoma. This tumor does not have a chamber predilection, may involve multiple sites, and is the most common sarcoma to involve the cardiac valves.

Imaging

The most common radiographic abnormality in primary cardiac sarcomas is cardiomegaly. Additional findings include a discrete mass, consolidation, pleural effusion, pericardial effusion, and sequelae of heart failure. Contrast-enhanced CT can demonstrate pericardial and myocardial involvement, mediastinal invasion, involvement of the great vessels and airways, and pulmonary metastatic disease. Pericardial invasion manifests as pericardial thickening, effusion, and nodularity. Cardiac-gated MRI provides optimal imaging of primary cardiac sarcomas, thus allowing characterization of morphology and extent of disease. The most common imaging appearance is that of large, heterogeneous masses, often with irregular surface, occupying one or more cardiac chambers (Fig. 32-10). Disruption, thickening, and nodularity of the pericardium suggest invasion. Myocardial infiltration may appear as thickening and infiltration. Mediastinal invasion, valvular destruction, and metastatic disease may also be seen (Fig. 32-11). Sarcomas enhance heterogeneously following the administration of gadolinium, and nonenhancing regions usually represent tissue necrosis.

Two morphologic types of angiosarcoma have been described using CT. The first is a well-formed, hypodense mass protruding into a cardiac chamber, and the second is a diffusely infiltrating mass. Both types demonstrate

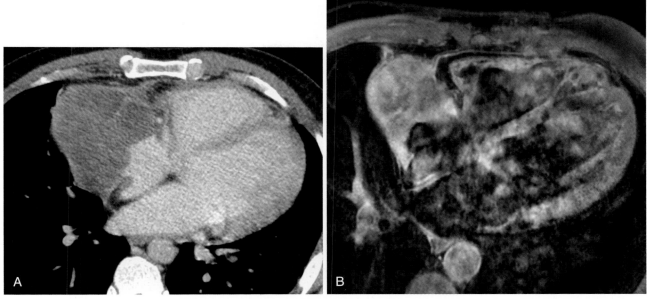

Figure 32-10 **A,** Axial computed tomography image shows a large mass extending into the anterior atrioventricular groove that invades the epicardial fat and displaces the right coronary artery. **B,** Axial delayed enhancement magnetic resonance imaging shows avid, heterogeneous enhancement of this proven angiosarcoma.

heterogeneous enhancement after the administration of intravenous contrast material. Angiosarcomas usually demonstrate pericardial invasion and hemorrhagic pericardial effusions on MRI. These tumors are heterogeneous in signal intensity on T1-weighted images, with areas of low, intermediate, and high signal intensity resulting from areas of necrosis, viable tumor, and methemoglobin, respectively. T2-weighted images show heterogeneous hyperintensity. Heterogeneous enhancement occurs after the administration of gadolinium, with marked surface enhancement and central necrosis.

Undifferentiated sarcomas may appear as discrete, hypodense myocardial masses protruding into the cardiac chamber on CT or as polypoid masses that are isointense to myocardium on MRI. These tumors have also been described as hemorrhagic masses replacing the pericardium and involving the cardiac valves. Leiomyosarcomas are usually depicted as lobulated, hypodense masses on CT that arise from the posterior wall of the left atrium, thus distinguishing them from myxomas. Contrast-enhanced CT may demonstrate filling defects within the pulmonary veins, consistent with invasion, a common phenomenon in these tumors. These tumors are nonspecific on MRI, and they appear intermediate in signal intensity on T1-weighted images and hyperintense on T2-weighted images. Osteosarcomas may be depicted as hypodense masses containing calcification on CT. However, calcification may be mistaken for dystrophic calcification or may not be present at all. Because of their origin from the left atrium, osteosarcomas may be mistaken for myxomas. Imaging features that suggest an osteosarcoma include a broad base of attachment, pulmonary venous extension, infiltrative growth along the epicardium, and invasion of the interatrial septum.

Lymphoma

Background
Although lymphoma metastasizing to the heart is common, primary cardiac lymphoma is rare. When it occurs, however, it is usually of the non-Hodgkin B-cell type. Primary cardiac lymphoma is confined to the heart and pericardium at the time of diagnosis. Although primary cardiac lymphoma is much more common in immunocompromised patients, particularly those with acquired immunodeficiency syndrome, immunocompetent individuals may also be affected. This entity much more commonly involves the right side of the heart, particularly the right atrium, with extension into the pericardium. The most common clinical presentations include chest pain, heart failure, arrhythmias, and cardiac tamponade. Primary cardiac lymphoma carries a poor prognosis, and most cases are diagnosed shortly before death or at autopsy.

Imaging
The most common findings on chest radiography include enlargement of the cardiac silhouette, pericardial effusion, and sequelae of heart failure. CT depicts primary cardiac lymphoma as isodense or hypodense masses relative to myocardium (Fig. 32-12). Following the administration of intravenous contrast material, these masses demonstrate heterogeneous enhancement. Echocardiography typically shows hypoechoic masses involving the right atrium or ventricle and pericardial effusion. On MRI, these lesions are isointense to hypointense relative to myocardium on T1-weighted images and isointense to hyperintense on T2-weighted images. Heterogeneous enhancement occurs following the administration of intravenous gadolinium contrast.

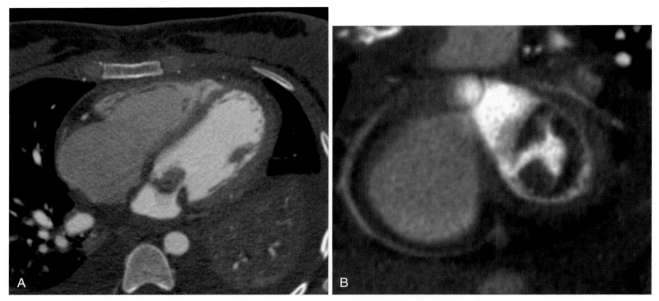

Figure 32-11 Axial computed tomography (**A**) and short-axis reformatted image (**B**) in this 28-year-old woman with shortness of breath show circumferential, irregular thickening of the mitral valve that was found to be a myxofibrosarcoma at surgical resection.

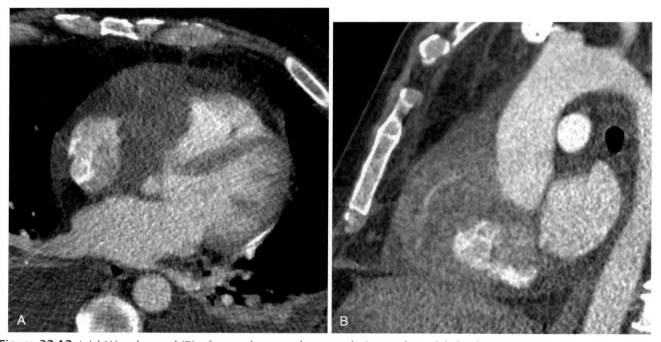

Figure 32-12 Axial (**A**) and coronal (**B**) reformatted computed tomography images show a lobulated mass centered in the anterior atrioventricular groove that infiltrates along the atrioventricular groove fat and encases the right coronary artery without obstructing it in this 55-year-old man with human immunodeficiency virus infection and non-Hodgkin lymphoma.

■ PSEUDOTUMORS

Normal Anatomic Variants

Several normal anatomic variants can be mistaken for a cardiac mass. Knowledge of both typical and atypical appearances of normal anatomic structures can help to avoid unnecessary imaging and intervention.

The crista terminalis is a muscular ridge within the right atrium that extends from the superior vena cava to the inferior vena cava at the point of fusion between the smooth posterior right atrial wall and the trabeculated anterior portion of the right atrium. This structure may be mistaken for a mass or for thrombus when it is viewed in a single imaging plane, particularly in echocardiography. It has a characteristic location and shape. Similarly, a ridge formed at the junction of the left superior pulmonary vein and the left atrial appendage may mimic a mass, particularly when it is bulbous or redundant.

A remnant of the fetal eustachian valve may occasionally be identified as a thin, mobile structure attached to the junction of the inferior vena cava and the right atrium. It may be thickened and mobile, appearing as an intracavitary mass. Similarly, fat may protrude into the inferior vena cava at the inferior cavoatrial junction and mimic a mass within the right atrium. Cardiac tumors do not typically involve this portion of the right atrium, and significant venous flow at this location also makes thrombus unlikely. Coronal and sagittal reconstructions are helpful in excluding a cardiac mass.

Thrombus

Clinical information, location, and imaging characteristics are important factors to consider when differentiating a cardiac tumor from an intracavitary thrombus. Peripheral embolization occurs in up to 10% of mural thrombi in the left ventricle and may be the presenting sign of left-sided heart thrombus. Pulmonary arterial emboli from right-sided heart thrombi may also occur. Atrial fibrillation, particularly in the setting of rheumatic heart disease, is an important predisposing clinical condition to the formation of thrombus in this location. Mitral stenosis and left atrial transvenous ablation procedures for atrial fibrillation also predispose to left atrial thrombus. In patients with a history of myocardial infarction, regional turbulence and slow flow of blood in the region of akinetic or dyskinetic scar may predispose to intraventricular thrombus formation. If not receiving anticoagulation, 40% to 60% of patients with anterior myocardial infarction may have left ventricular mural thrombus. Ventricular aneurysm similarly predisposes to thrombus formation. Finally, indwelling devices such as Swan-Ganz catheters and pacemaker wires may predispose to foreign body thrombus.

Intracavitary thrombus is the most frequent intracardiac mass, most commonly occurring in the left atrium and left atrial appendage. Thrombi are typically homogeneous on CT, and their MRI appearance depends on the evolution of red blood cells comprising the thrombus. Pedunculated thrombi may be mobile on echocardiography, retrospectively ECG-gated CT, and MRI. Delayed enhancement on cardiac MRI allows differentiation between enhancing myocardium and nonvascular acute thrombus. Low-grade enhancement at the attachment site may be demonstrated in large, chronic thrombi. Contrast-enhanced MRI has the additional benefit of detecting delayed enhancement in myocardial scars, an independent risk factor for the development of thrombus. Thrombus is best identified when using extremely long inversion times (e.g., ~600 msec).

Aneurysms

Vascular aneurysms in and about the heart may be mistaken for cardiac tumors when they are thrombosed or in the setting of slow, turbulent blood flow. Sinus of Valsalva aneurysms may be large and protrude onto the interatrial septum or into cardiac chambers. Coronary artery aneurysms and bypass graft aneurysms may also be large and exert a local mass effect simulating a cardiac mass.

Lipomatous Hypertrophy of the Interatrial Septum

An increase in the number of adipocytes in the interatrial septum may mimic a cardiac lipoma or other fat-containing mass. This hyperplasia of fat within the interatrial septum typically occurs in obese and older patients. The term lipomatous hypertrophy of the interatrial septum is typically applied when the fat in the atrial septum causes the transverse diameter near the fossa ovalis to exceed 2 cm. Histologically, this lesion is composed of adipose tissue and cells resembling brown fat. Although this condition is benign and usually asymptomatic, it is reported to cause atrial or ventricular arrhythmias. Rarely, inflow into the right atrium may be obstructed.

The involved atrial septum follows the tissue characteristics of fat on echocardiography, CT, and MRI. Fluorodeoxyglucose positron emission tomography may show increased uptake in this lesion correlating with the thickness of the septum (Fig. 32-13). This is not a true neoplasm, however, and it may be distinguished from the much rarer cardiac lipoma by the lack of a capsule and by the characteristic dumbbell appearance of this entity as it spares the fossa ovalis.

Vegetations

Pedunculated masses of the valve leaflets along the line of closure are characteristic of vegetations, particularly in the clinical setting of fever, heart murmur, and bacteremia (Fig. 32-14). Vegetations in nonbacterial thrombotic endocarditis are smaller and occur typically near the cusps of the valve leaflets. The clinical situation and multiplicity of vegetations usually differentiate this entity from cardiac tumors, although resolution with antibiotic treatment is confirmatory.

Caseous Mitral Annular Calcification

Although mitral annular calcification is a common and easily recognized degenerative abnormality in older patients, caseous calcification of the mitral valve annulus may be masslike and mimic a calcified cardiac tumor (Fig. 32-15). Caseous mitral annular calcification typically occurs in the posterior mitral annulus, following the contour of this structure in a semilunar shape. Echocardiography shows peripheral hyperechogenicity consistent with calcification and central hypoechogenicity. CT is the definitive imaging modality to evaluate this lesion, and it shows a peripheral rim or eggshell calcified lesion centered in the posterior mitral valve annulus with lower central homogeneous density that corresponds to liquefied calcium and tissue. These tumors are also known as toothpaste tumors because of the consistency of the material seen by surgeons and on gross pathologic examination.

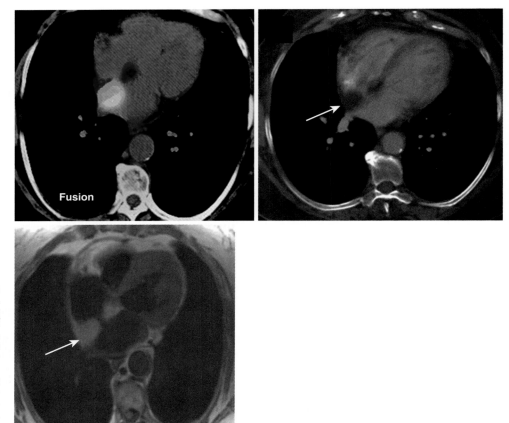

Figure 32-13 Axial *(top)* and coronal *(bottom)* reformatted images show thickening of the interatrial septum with sparing of the fossa ovalis. Fat attenuation and the classic dumbbell shape confirm lipomatous hypertrophy of the interatrial septum *(arrows)*. (From Fan CM, Fischman AJ, Kwek BH, Abbara S, Aquino SL. Lipomatous hypertrophy of the interatrial septum: increased uptake on FDG PET. AJR Am J Roentgenol. 2005;184:339-342.)

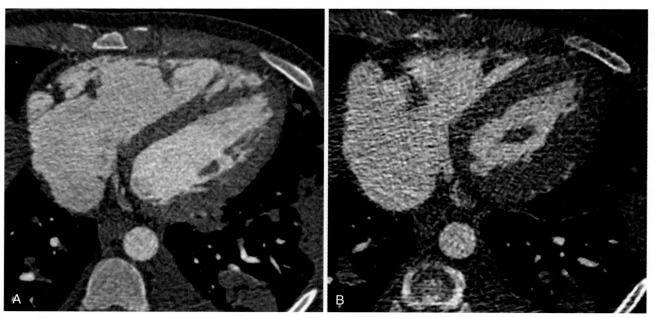

Figure 32-14 Axial computed tomography images in diastole (A) and systole (B) show small masses on the tricuspid valve and in the right ventricular trabeculations. Peripheral opacities representing septic emboli are important clues in this 32-year-old man with a history of intravenous drug abuse and cardiac vegetation.

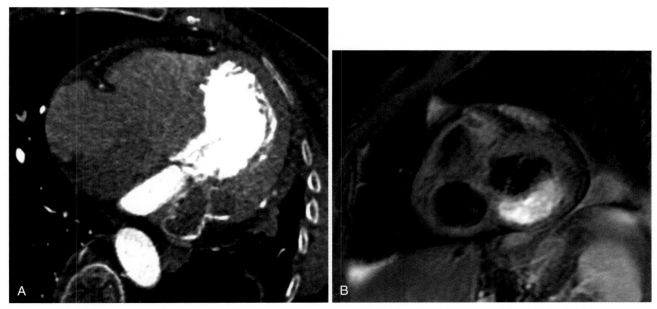

Figure 32-15 **A,** Axial computed tomography image shows extensive eggshell calcification in the region of the mitral valve that exerts a mass effect and mimics a calcified mass in this patient with caseous mitral annular calcification. **B,** Short-axis T2-weighted image shows high T2 signal intensity consistent with the myxoid component of central necrosis.

Cardiomyopathy

Focal and apical forms of hypertrophic cardiomyopathy may mimic a myocardial mass. Infiltrative cardiomyopathies may also mimic localized, space-occupying lesions on imaging. Myocardial contractility in these suspected masses may exclude a cardiac tumor. Contractility may be supported visually with special MRI techniques such as myocardial tagging, which employs desaturation bands across the myocardium that persist during cine acquisition.

Bibliography

Alkadhi H, Leschka S, Hurlimann D, Jenni R, Genoni M, Wildermuth S. Fibroelastoma of the aortic valve: evaluation with echocardiography and 64-slice CT. *Herz.* 2005;30:438.

Altinok D, Yildiz YT, Tacal T, Karapinar K, Eryilmaz M. MRI of intravascular leiomyomatosis extending to the heart. *Eur Radiol.* 2000;10:871.

Araoz PA, Mulvagh SL, Tazelaar HD, Julsrud PR, Breen JF. CT and MR imaging of benign primary cardiac neoplasms with echocardiographic correlation. *Radiographics.* 2000;20:1303-1319.

Beghetti M, Gow RM, Haney I, Mawson J, Williams WG, Freedom RM. Pediatric primary benign cardiac tumors: a 15-year review. *Am Heart J.* 1997;134:1107-1114.

Best AK, Dobson RL, Ahmad AR. Best cases from the AFIP: cardiac angiosarcoma. *Radiographics.* 2003;23:S141-S145.

Broderick LS, Brooks GN, Kuhlman JE. Anatomic pitfalls of the heart and pericardium. *Radiographics.* 2005;25:441-453.

Burke AP, Rosado-de-Christenson M, Templeton PA, Virmani R. Cardiac fibroma: clinicopathologic correlates and surgical treatment. *J Thorac Cardiovasc Surg.* 1994;108:862-870.

Butany J, Nair V, Naseemuddin A, Nair GM, Catton C, Yau T. Cardiac tumours: diagnosis and management. *Lancet Oncol.* 2005;6:219-228.

Can C, Arpaci F, Celasun B, Gunhan O, Finci R. Primary pericardial liposarcoma presenting with cardiac tamponade and multiple organ metastases. *Chest.* 1993;103:328.

Carney JA. The complex of myxomas, spotty pigmentation, and endocrine overactivity. *Arch Intern Med.* 1987;147:418-419.

Ceresoli GL, Ferreri AJ, Bucci E, Ripa C, Ponzoni M, Villa E. Primary cardiac lymphoma in immunocompetent patients: diagnostic and therapeutic management. *Cancer.* 1997;80:1497-1506.

Chiles C, Woodard PK, Gutierrez FR, Link KM. Metastatic involvement of the heart and pericardium: CT and MR imaging. *Radiographics.* 2001;21:439-449.

Clarke NR, Mohiaddin RH, Westaby S, Banning AP. Multifocal cardiac leiomyosarcoma: diagnosis and surveillance by transoesophageal echocardiography and contrast-enhanced cardiovascular magnetic resonance. *Postgrad Med J.* 2002;78:492-493.

Deluigi CC, Meinhardt G, Ursulescu A, Klem I, Fritz P, Mahrholdt H. Noninvasive characterization of left atrial mass. *Circulation.* 2006;113:e19-e20.

Donsbeck AV, Ranchere D, Coindre JM, Le Gall F, Cordier JF, Loire R. Primary cardiac sarcomas: an immunohistochemical and grading study with long-term follow-up of 24 cases. *Histopathology.* 1999;34:295-304.

Edwards FH, Hale D, Cohen A, Thompson L, Pezzella AT, Virmani R. Primary cardiac valve tumors. *Ann Thorac Surg.* 1991;52:1127-1131.

Elbardissi AW, Dearani JA, Daly RC, et al. Survival after resection of primary cardiac tumors: a 48-year experience. *Circulation.* 2008;118(suppl):S7-S15.

Georghiou GP, Vidne BA, Sahar G, Sharoni E, Fuks A, Porat E. Primary cardiac valve tumors. *Asian Cardiovasc Thorac Ann.* 2010;18:226-228.

Gowda RM, Khan IA, Nair CK, Mehta NJ, Vasavada BC, Sacchi TJ. Cardiac papillary fibroelastoma: a comprehensive analysis of 725 cases. *Am Heart J.* 2003;146:404-410.

Grebenc ML, Rosado-de-Christenson ML, Green CE, Burke AP, Galvin JR. Cardiac myxoma: imaging features in 83 patients. *Radiographics.* 2002;22:673-689.

Grebenc ML, Rosado de Christenson ML, Burke AP, Green CE, Galvin JR. Primary cardiac and pericardial neoplasms: radiologic-pathologic correlation. *Radiographics.* 2000;20:1073-1103:quiz 1110-1111, 1112.

Hunold P, Schlosser T, Vogt FM, et al. Myocardial late enhancement in contrast-enhanced cardiac MRI: distinction between infarction scar and non–infarction-related disease. *AJR Am J Roentgenol.* 2005;184:1420-1426.

Jain D, Maleszewski JJ, Halushka MK. Benign cardiac tumors and tumorlike conditions. *Ann Diagn Pathol.* 2010;14:215-230.

Kiaffas MG, Powell AJ, Geva T. Magnetic resonance imaging evaluation of cardiac tumor characteristics in infants and children. *Am J Cardiol.* 2002;89:1229-1233.

Kim RJ, Wu E, Rafael A, et al. The use of contrast-enhanced magnetic resonance imaging to identify reversible myocardial dysfunction. *N Engl J Med.* 2000;343:1445-1453.

Kimura F, Matsuo Y, Nakajima T, et al. Myocardial fat at cardiac imaging: how can we differentiate pathologic from physiologic fatty infiltration? *Radiographics.* 2010;30:1587-1602.

Lim RP, Srichai MB, Lee VS. Nonischemic causes of delayed myocardial hyperenhancement on MRI. *AJR Am J Roentgenol.* 2007;188:1675-1681.

Lo FL, Chou YH, Tiu CM, et al. Primary cardiac leiomyosarcoma: imaging with 2-D echocardiography, electron beam CT and 1.5-Tesla MR. *Eur J Radiol.* 1998;27:72-76.

Lotto AA, Earl UM, Owens WA. Right atrial mass: thrombus, myxoma, or cardiac papillary fibroelastoma? *J Thorac Cardiovasc Surg.* 2006;132:159-160.

Luna A, Ribes R, Caro P, Vida J, Erasmus JJ. Evaluation of cardiac tumors with magnetic resonance imaging. *Eur Radiol.* 2005;15:1446-1455.

Mandegar MH, Rayatzadeh H, Roshanali F. Left atrial myxoma: the role of multislice computed tomography. *J Thorac Cardiovasc Surg.* 2007;134:795.

Mollet NR, Dymarkowski S, Volders W, et al. Visualization of ventricular thrombi with contrast-enhanced magnetic resonance imaging in patients with ischemic heart disease. *Circulation.* 2002;106:2873-2876.

Morris MF, Maleszewski JJ, Suri RM, et al. CT and MR imaging of the mitral valve: radiologic-pathologic correlation. *Radiographics.* 2010;30:1603-1620.

O'Donnell DH, Abbara S, Chaithiraphan V, et al. Cardiac tumors: optimal cardiac MR sequences and spectrum of imaging appearances. *AJR Am J Roentgenol.* 2009;193:377-387.

Paydarfar D, Krieger D, Dib N, et al. In vivo magnetic resonance imaging and surgical histopathology of intracardiac masses: distinct features of subacute thrombi. *Cardiology.* 2001;95:40-47.

Perchinsky MJ, Lichtenstein SV, Tyers GF. Primary cardiac tumors: forty years' experience with 71 patients. *Cancer.* 1997;79:1809-1815.

Pugliatti P, Patane S, De Gregorio C, Recupero A, Carerj S, Coglitore S. Lipomatous hypertrophy of the interatrial septum. *Int J Cardiol.* 2008;130:294-295.

Putnam Jr JB, Sweeney MS, Colon R, Lanza LA, Frazier OH, Cooley DA. Primary cardiac sarcomas. *Ann Thorac Surg.* 1991;51:906-910.

Restrepo CS, Largoza A, Lemos DF, et al. CT and MR imaging findings of benign cardiac tumors. *Curr Probl Diagn Radiol.* 2005;34:12-21.

Sahdev A, Sohaib A, Monson JP, Grossman AB, Chew SL, Reznek RH. CT and MR imaging of unusual locations of extra-adrenal paragangliomas (pheochromocytomas). *Eur Radiol.* 2005;15:85-92.

Siripornpitak S, Higgins CB. MRI of primary malignant cardiovascular tumors. *J Comput Assist Tomogr.* 1997;21:462-466.

Stiller B, Hetzer R, Meyer R, et al. Primary cardiac tumours: when is surgery necessary? *Eur J Cardiothorac Surg.* 2001;20:1002-1006.

Sutsch G, Jenni R, von Segesser L, Schneider J. Heart tumors: incidence, distribution, diagnosis—exemplified by 20,305 echocardiographies. *Schweiz Med Wochenschr.* 1991;121:621-629;[in German].

Tesolin M, Lapierre C, Oligny L, Bigras JL, Champagne M. Cardiac metastases from melanoma. *Radiographics.* 2005;25:249-253.

Weinsaft JW, Kim HW, Shah DJ, et al. Detection of left ventricular thrombus by delayed-enhancement cardiovascular magnetic resonance prevalence and markers in patients with systolic dysfunction. *J Am Coll Cardiol.* 2008;52:148-157.

Xanthos T, Giannakopoulos N, Papadimitriou L. Lipomatous hypertrophy of the interatrial septum: a pathological and clinical approach. *Int J Cardiol.* 2007;121:4-8.

CHAPTER 33

Pericardial Disease

Nikhil Goyal, Carlos Andres Rojas, and Suhny Abbara

Pericardial disease is an important cause of morbidity and mortality. In general, diseases that affect the pericardium tend to affect it diffusely. Focal disease may be related to masses, cysts, or calcification. Imaging plays a key role in establishing a diagnosis of pericardial disease because the clinical manifestations of pericardial disease can be complex and range from incidental to life-threatening. As such, a working knowledge of pericardial anatomy and common pericardial diseases is essential for the cardiac imager to aid in proper diagnosis and potentially to guide treatment.

■ ANATOMY AND PHYSIOLOGY

The pericardium protects the heart, reduces friction between the heart and surrounding structures, supports atrial filling with negative systolic pericardial pressure, and limits acute cardiac distention. The pericardium is composed of two layers, the fibrous and the serous pericardium. The serous pericardium consists of the visceral and the parietal layers. The visceral pericardial layer covers the myocardium, epicardial fat, and epicardial vessels and is also referred to as the epicardium. It is continuous with the parietal pericardial layer at the pericardial recesses.

The space between the visceral and parietal pericardial layers is the pericardial space, which normally contains a small amount (15 to 50 mL) of pericardial fluid. The parietal serous pericardium is intimately adhered to the fibrous pericardium and cannot be separated from it. This portion of the pericardium is commonly referred to as the pericardium, as opposed to the epicardium. The epicardium and pericardium are normally inseparable to the eye on imaging, but in certain disease states, such as pericardial effusion, they become separated and visible (Fig. 33-1).

One useful way to recall the fat layers that surround the pericardium is that the *peri*cardial fat is around the *peri*meter of the pericardial membrane. Thus, it surrounds the pericardium (see Fig. 33-1). The epicardial fat is deep to the epicardium and is immediately adjacent to the myocardium.

In the craniocaudal direction, the pericardium extends all the way up to the proximal aortic arch and the pulmonary artery. This feature is, again, usually not evident, but when effusion or thickening is present, this becomes more apparent (Fig. 33-2).

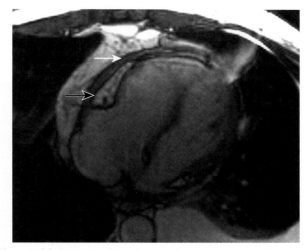

Figure 33-1 Balanced steady-state free precession axial magnetic resonance imaging showing the inner, serous, visceral layer (*black arrow;* epicardium) and the outer, fibrous, parietal (*white arrow;* often referred to simply as pericardium) layers of the pericardium in a 54-year-old patient with pericardial thickening. The epicardium and pericardium appear thicker than they are because of India ink artifact of voxels that border fat. Incidental note is made of left greater than right pleural effusions.

Reflections of the serous pericardium around the great vessels and the base of the heart are termed pericardial sinuses. The two main pericardial sinuses are the transverse and oblique sinuses (Fig. 33-3). The pericardial recesses arising from the transverse sinus are the superior aortic recess, inferior aortic recess, right pulmonic recess, and left pulmonic recesses. The recess originating from the oblique sinus is the posterior pericardial recess (see Fig. 33-3). The recesses originating from the pericardium proper are the pulmonic vein and the postcaval recesses.

Pitfall

Fluid accumulation in these recesses can be confused with lymphadenopathy.

■ PATHOLOGY

Pericardial Effusion

Pericardial effusion is defined as an excessive accumulation of pericardial fluid. Normally, only a small amount

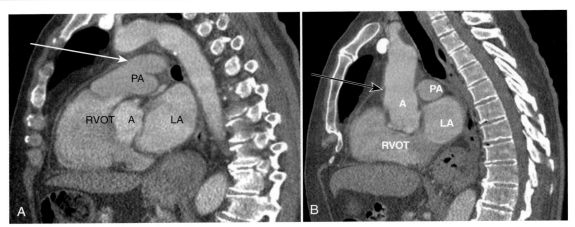

Figure 33-2 **A** and **B,** Sagittal contrast-enhanced computed tomography in a 67-year-old man demonstrates the cranial extent of the pericardium to envelope the proximal ascending aorta *(black arrow)* and the proximal pulmonary artery *(white arrow)* approximately 3 cm distal to their respective origins (pericardial reflection). *A,* Aorta; *LA,* left atrium; *PA,* pulmonary artery; *RVOT,* right ventricular outflow tract.

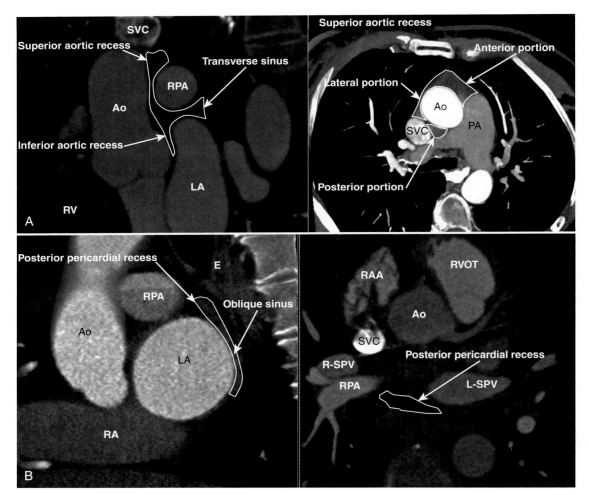

Figure 33-3 **A** and **B,** Sagittal and axial oblique cardiac computed tomography images demonstrate the location of the two major pericardial sinuses and their respective recesses. *Ao,* Aorta; *E,* esophagus; *L,* left; *LA,* left atrium; *PA,* pulmonary artery; *R,* right; *RA,* right atrium; *RAA;* right atrial appendage; *RPA,* right pulmonary artery; *RV,* right ventricle; *RVOT,* right ventricular outflow tract; *SPV,* superior pulmonary vein; *SVC,* superior vena cava.

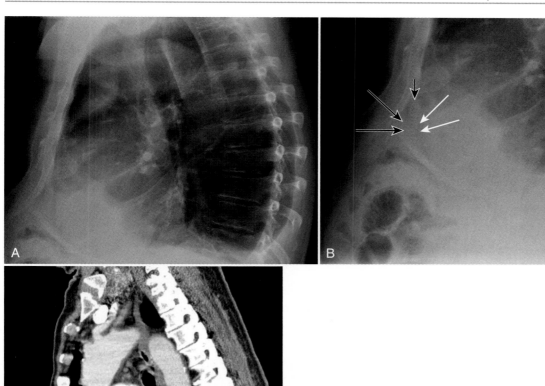

Figure 33-4 A, Lateral chest radiograph shows a small pericardial effusion with the classic "Oreo cookie" sign anteriorly. Small bilateral pleural effusions are also present. **B,** Magnified version demonstrates the composite layer: pericardial fat *(long black arrows),* pericardial fluid *(short black arrow),* and epicardial fat *(white arrows).* **C,** The corresponding layers are seen on sagittal computed tomography reconstruction.

of fluid is present between the visceral and parietal layers. This fluid serves to minimize friction between the two layers from cardiac motion. However, some disease states (heart or renal failure; infection, particularly viral infection or tuberculosis;, trauma; myocardial infarction; autoimmune disorders; malignant disease; and other systemic diseases) can lead to abnormal fluid pooling within the pericardial space.

Pericardial effusion can be a purely incidental finding in an asymptomatic patient. In a patient with symptoms, or in a patient with clinically suspected pericardial effusion, echocardiography is the first-line imaging that is performed. This technique can help delineate the size of the effusion and measure any hemodynamic consequences.

The fluid that accumulates can be simple, hemorrhagic, or infected. As such, it may be transudative, hemorrhagic, or exudative, respectively.

On conventional radiographs, the finding is classically described as a "water bottle" heart on the frontal view. On a properly performed lateral view, the classic "Oreo cookie sign" can be seen. The alternating dark-light-dark

appearance of the pericardial fat–effusion fluid–epicardial fat resembles an Oreo cookie when it is viewed in profile (Fig. 33-4).

On magnetic resonance imaging (MRI), the presence of pericardial effusion separates the two pericardial layers. The resulting appearance consists of two thin, dark lines separated by high signal fluid on T2-weighted spin echo or gradient recalled echo cine sequences. On echocardiography, pericardial effusion is seen as an echolucent space surrounding the heart. Swinging motion of the heart on multiphase imaging can be seen with massive pericardial effusion.

On echocardiography, pericardial fluid appears as a low-echo or anechoic space adjacent to the cardiac structures (Fig. 33-5). Pericardial fluid can be confused with pericardial fat and left-sided pleural effusion. The presence of fibrin strands, in the setting of an infectious inflammatory origin, can help differentiate pericardial fluid from pericardial fat. The circumferential involvement surrounding the heart and the separation between the descending aorta and the left atrium are most suggestive of pericardial effusion, rather than

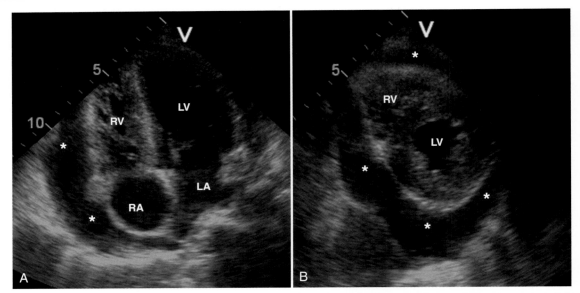

Figure 33-5 **A** and **B**, Four-chamber and short-axis two-dimensional echocardiography demonstrating anechoic or hypoechoic fluid surrounding the heart consistent with pericardial effusion *(asterisks)*. *LA,* Left atrium; *LV,* left ventricle; *RA,* right atrium; *RV,* right ventricle.

left-sided pleural effusion. Effusion size is assessed by measuring the distance between the two layers of the pericardium. A separation of less than 0.5 cm corresponds to a small effusion, a separation of 0.5 to 2.0 cm is moderate, and a separation greater than 2.0 cm is considered large.

Problem Solving: Deciphering Pericardial Thickening Versus Effusion

The maximum normal pericardial thickness is 2 mm on computed tomography (CT) images and 2.5 on echocardiography. Normal pericardium demonstrates low signal on T1- and T2-weighted spin echo and gradient recalled echo cine sequences, whereas pericardial effusion demonstrates high signal on fluid-sensitive sequences. On echocardiographic images, the pericardium is seen as a thin, echogenic, linear structure, and accumulated pericardial fluid is anechoic or hypoechoic.

On nongated chest CT, the pericardium appears as a thin membrane within the fat surrounding the heart. It is most easily detected anteriorly along the right ventricle (RV) free wall, and it can be followed peripherally around the cardiac chambers (Fig. 33-6). In physiologically normal individuals, the pericardium frequently cannot be clearly traced all the way around, perhaps because of a combination of cardiac motion and volume averaging. (Defects in the pericardial membrane can also cause it to not be seen, and these defects are discussed later.) Pericardial fluid, conversely, tends to layer posteriorly and inferiorly in the dependent portions of the pericardial space and in the anterior angle at the junction of inferior and anterior free walls of the RV.

The normal pericardium is not seen on conventional radiographs.

A special note should be made about hemopericardium. This condition can be seen in the setting of trauma, in cardiac malignant disease, after cardiac or aortic surgery, with improper line placement, or as a

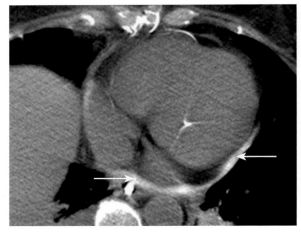

Figure 33-6 Noncontrast computed tomography in a 58-year-old patient after cardiac catheterization. During the catheterization procedure, focal laceration of a proximal coronary artery led to contrast extravasation into the pericardial space. The layering contrast material *(arrows)* is seen within the posterior pericardium.

complication of type A aortic dissection. On conventional radiographs, rapid change in the cardiac silhouette size, especially in the setting of falling hematocrit levels or known aortic dissection, should alert the physician to possible hemopericardium. Placing the Hounsfield unit (HU) cursor on *any* pericardial effusion should become automatic as part of the search pattern. Characteristically, a density of 30 to 70 HU is indicative of blood (Fig. 33-7). Type A aortic dissection should be excluded in any patient with hemopericardium. Conversely, *any* patient with type A dissection or intramural hematoma in the ascending aorta warrants a comment about the presence or absence of hemopericardium.

The volume of pericardial fluid is not all that should be reported. Comparison with prior examinations (especially recent ones) should involve an assessment of how

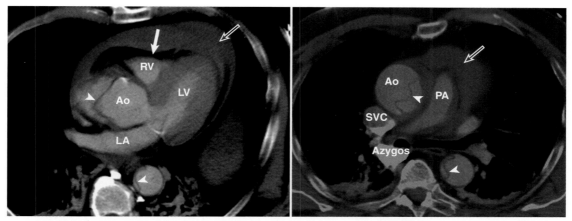

Figure 33-7 Axial images from an aortic computed tomography angiogram in a 55-year-old man demonstrate a large, dense (30 to 60 HU) pericardial effusion *(arrows)* consistent with hemopericardium secondary to ruptured type A aortic dissection *(arrowheads)*. Note the deformity of the right ventricle (RV) and contrast reflux into the azygos vein that suggest increased intrapericardial pressure. *Ao,* Aorta; *LA,* left atrium; *LV,* left ventricle; *PA,* pulmonary artery; *SVC,* superior vena cava.

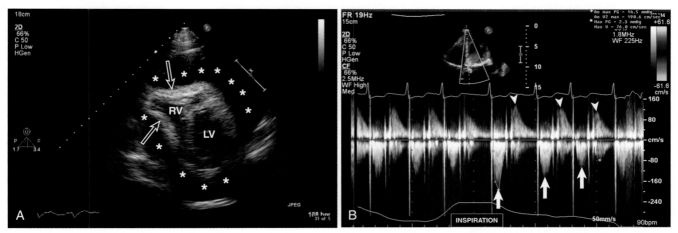

Figure 33-8 A, Parasternal short-axis view in a 72-year-old man with myelodysplastic syndrome demonstrates a large pericardial effusion *(asterisks)* associated with diastolic deformity of the inferior and anterior right ventricular free walls *(arrows)* consistent with cardiac tamponade. *LV,* Left ventricle; *RV,* right ventricle. **B,** Pulsed wave interrogation at the left ventricular outflow tract demonstrates inspiratory decrease in the time velocity integral size *(arrows)* representing inspiratory decrease in left ventricular cardiac output. This variation results from exaggerated interventricular interdependence. Incidentally noted is aortic insufficiency *(arrowheads)*.

rapidly the effusion has formed. Rapid accumulation of fluid or a large amount of fluid may lead to increased pressure within the pericardial space. Chamber filling and subsequently cardiac output can be impaired, and this condition can be life-threatening.

Cardiac Tamponade

Cardiac tamponade occurs when increased intrapericardial pressure, from accumulation of pericardial fluid, compromises both the systemic venous return and the effective cardiac output. The amount of volume necessary to cause pericardial tamponade depends on the velocity of fluid accumulation. Entities that result in rapid accumulation of fluid, such as ruptured aortic dissection (see Fig. 33-7), require a smaller amount of volume to cause cardiac tamponade. Conversely, chronic fluid accumulation, such as in patients with systemic lupus erythematosus, requires larger volumes to result in cardiac tamponade.

Two-dimensional echocardiography features of pericardial tamponade include pericardial effusion with early diastolic RV invagination, late diastolic right atrial invagination, and lack of inferior vena cava (IVC) collapse during deep inspiration resulting from increased intrapericardial pressure to more than the intracardiac pressures (see Fig. 33-5; Fig. 33-8). The main tool in the diagnosis of cardiac tamponade is Doppler echocardiography. Distinctive features include inspiratory decrease in mitral inflow and expiratory decrease in tricuspid inflow (noticed during pulsed wave interrogation). The changes in mitral inflow are analogous to pulsus paradoxus (blood pressure drop >10 mm Hg during inspiration).

Similar to echocardiography, CT and MRI can show deformity of cardiac chambers, in the presence of pericardial effusion, resulting from elevated intrapericardial pressures. Flattening of the interventricular septum, compression of the coronary sinus and intrathoracic IVC, and dilatation of the superior vena cava (SVC) and intraabdominal IVC can also be seen.

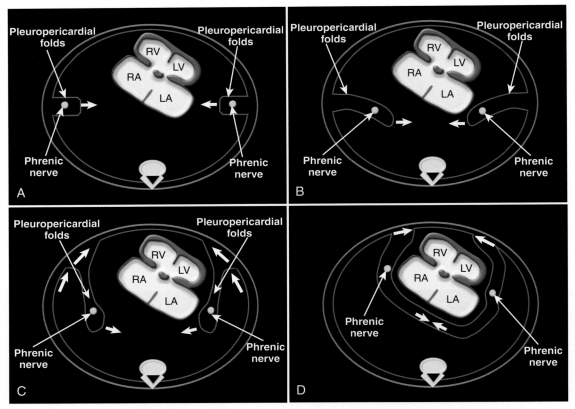

Figure 33-9 Diagram representing the normal development of the pericardium. **A,** The pericardium begins its development during the fifth week of fetal life from two infoldings of the coelomic layer called the pleuropericardial folds. **B,** These folds are located laterally and grow medially carrying the phrenic nerves with them. **C** and **D,** The base of the pleuropericardial folds moves ventrally until the folds reach their final position in the anterior chest. *LA,* Left atrium; *LV,* left ventricle; *RA,* right atrium; *RV,* right ventricle.

Development and Developmental Defects of the Pericardium

The pericardial sac originates from two mesoderm infoldings known as the pleuropericardial folds. The pleuropericardial folds eventually divide the thorax into a pericardial and two pleural cavities (Fig. 33-9). Up to one third of patients with congenital defects of the pericardium have associated malformations of the heart, aorta, lungs, chest wall, and diaphragm.

Congenital Absence of the Pericardium

Congenital absence of the pericardium results from decreased blood supply to the developing pericardium. Premature atrophy of the left common cardinal vein results in congenital absence of the left pericardium, either partial or complete. Most common is absence of the left pericardium (partial or complete); absence of the right pericardium and total absence of the pericardium are less common.

Complete absence of the left pericardium has characteristic imaging features that allow for its detection. On chest radiography, levorotation of the heart is noted, with apparent loss of the right heart border and prominence of the pulmonary artery contour on the frontal view that give the appearance of a "Snoopy dog" profile (Fig. 33-10).

On CT and MRI, interposition of lung parenchyma between the aortic knob and the main pulmonary artery is characteristic (see Fig. 33-10). On cine MRI, excessive motion of the cardiac apex can suggest this diagnosis. Although complete absence of the left pericardium is usually asymptomatic, partial absence of the left pericardium can result in intermittent herniation of the heart through the defect and compression of the left coronary arterial branches.

Other congenital anomalies can be associated with pericardial absence such as atrial septal defect, bicuspid aortic valve, and pulmonary malformations.

Problem Solving: Levocardia

Leftward shift of the heart on plain radiography carries a differential diagnosis: left lung volume loss, right heart enlargement resulting in levocardia, pectus excavatum, and absent pericardium. A few key points can help discern absent pericardium from the other diagnoses. In pericardial absence, lucency represents interpositioned lung between the aorta and the pulmonary artery. This finding is sometimes visible on chest radiographs, but it is more readily appreciated on CT. Right-sided heart enlargement resulting in levocardia is often caused by a left-to-right shunt. Therefore, the presence of shunt vascularity with levocardia should suggest this diagnosis. In absent pericardium, the lungs are normal, and no shunt vascularity is present. Pectus excavatum deformity can

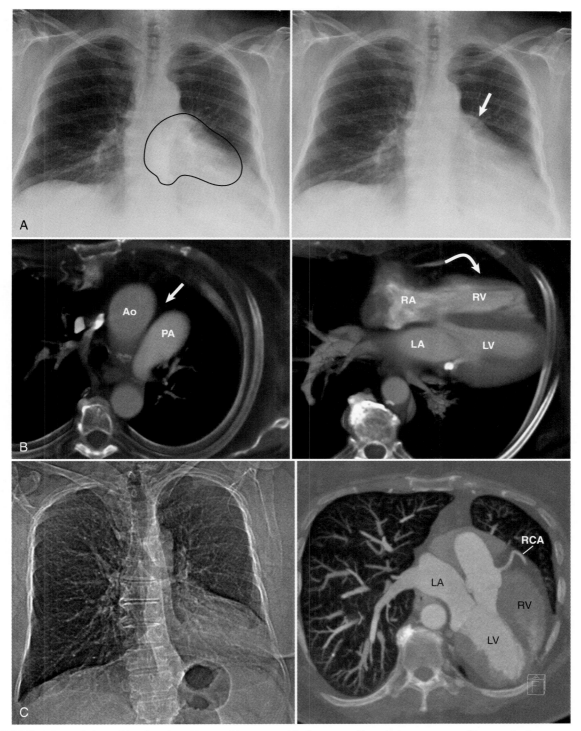

Figure 33-10 **A,** Frontal view of the chest in a 67-year-old woman with shortness of breath demonstrates a "Snoopy dog" appearance *(arrow)* of the cardiac silhouette secondary to prominence of the pulmonary artery and levorotation of the heart. **B,** Axial images of a computed tomography (CT) pulmonary angiogram in the same patient demonstrate complete absence of the left pericardium with interposition of lung between the aortic knob (Ao) and the main pulmonary artery (PA; *arrow, left image),* as well as levorotation of the heart *(arrow, right image).* **C,** Anteroposterior scout and axial cardiac CT images in a different patient with suspected coronary anomaly on invasive angiography. CT reveals absent left pericardium with marked rotation of the heart into the left hemothorax. The right ventricle (RV) is left lateral to the left ventricle (LV), and the right coronary artery (RCA) originates normally from the right coronary cusp, which is abnormally rotated toward the left. No coronary anomaly is present. *LA,* Left atrium; *RA,* right atrium.

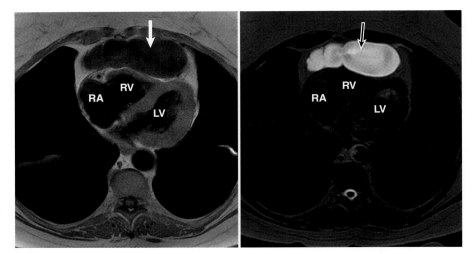

Figure 33-11 T1-weighted *(left)* and T2-weighted *(right)* images of the chest in a 44-year-old man demonstrate a large lobulated lesion anterior to the right ventricular (RV) free wall. The lesion demonstrates high T2 signal and low T1 signal compatible with a pericardial cyst *(arrows)*. The lack of related symptoms has prevented biopsy or drainage of this lesion. *RA,* Right atrium; *LV,* left ventricle.

be easily diagnosed with a lateral view demonstrating posterior sternal displacement, a feature not seen with congenitally absent pericardium.

Pericardial Cysts or Diverticula

A pericardial cyst is a rare anomalous mediastinal fluid collection arising from the parietal pericardium. These cysts are often congenital, but they can be acquired following cardiothoracic surgery or pericarditis. A pericardial diverticulum is a cyst that communicates with the pericardial sac. Clinically, pericardial cysts are asymptomatic; however, a few rare complications have been reported: cyst torsion, intracyst hemorrhage with resultant right-sided heart failure, cardiac tamponade from cyst rupture or intracyst hemorrhage, cyst infection, and obstruction of the right main stem bronchus from mass effect. Pericardial cysts have been reported to resolve spontaneously, possibly secondary to rupture into the adjacent pleural space.

Pericardial cysts are most often located in the right cardiophrenic angle (approximately two thirds of cases), followed by the left cardiophrenic angle (10% to 40% of cases); pericardial cysts may rarely be found in the anterior, superior, or posterior mediastinum. Two-dimensional echocardiography typically demonstrates an echo-free structure. On CT, a pericardial cyst manifests as a fluid attenuation mass with imperceptible or very thin walls that do not enhance. On MRI, a pericardial cyst has homogenous high T2 and low T1 signal without enhancement (Fig. 33-11). Occasionally, pericardial cysts may contain proteinaceous fluid or may be complicated by hemorrhage, thus leading to heterogeneous echotexture, high attenuation on CT, and high T1 and low T2 signal on MRI.

Pericardial Trauma

Blunt or penetrating trauma to the pericardium may result in pericardial rupture, hemopericardium, pneumopericardium, or hydropneumopericardium (Fig. 33-12).

Pericardial rupture is a rare consequence of trauma. It most often occurs along the left pleuropericardium

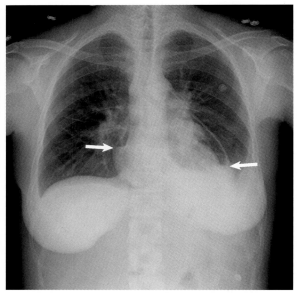

Figure 33-12 Upright chest radiograph in a 27-year-old woman after penetrating trauma demonstrates hemopneumopericardium. Note the bilateral intrapericardial air fluid levels *(arrows)*.

(50% of cases) and the diaphragmatic portion of the pericardium (27% of cases). Often, resultant lethal herniation of the heart occurs through these acquired pericardial sac defects (27% to 64% of cases of pericardial rupture). Herniation of abdominal contents, such as bowel, into the pericardial sac has been described.

Chest radiographs in the setting of pericardial rupture can demonstrate abnormal cardiac contour, prominent main pulmonary artery, displacement or rotation of the cardiac silhouette to the side of injury, pneumopericardium, hydropneumopericardium, and pneumomediastinum. Cardiac herniation is suggested by deviation of the normal cardiac axis, the "empty pericardial sac" sign (gas in the pericardial sac outlining the empty pericardium, vacated by herniation of the heart), and the "collar" sign (focal compression of the heart as it projects through the pericardial defect).

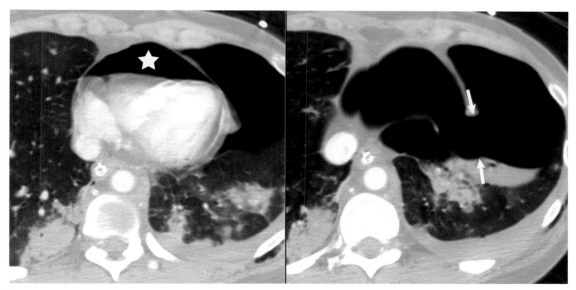

Figure 33-13 Axial computed tomography images of the chest after contrast enhancement in a 45-year-old man involved in a high-speed motor vehicle accident demonstrate pericardial rupture *(arrows)*, as well as pneumopericardium *(star)* and pneumothorax.

CT signs of pericardial rupture include discontinuity of the pericardium, interposition of the left lung between the aorta and the pulmonary artery, and pneumopericardium (see Fig. 33-12; Fig. 33-13).

Pericarditis

Pericarditis is an inflammatory condition of the pericardium. Common causes include infections (viral, bacterial, and fungal), myocardial infarction, lupus, uremia, paraneoplastic conditions, and idiopathic origin. On echocardiography, CT, and MRI, pericardial thickening is associated with pericardial effusion. On CT and MRI images with contrast, enhancement of the thickened pericardial layers can be seen (Fig. 33-14).

Calcified Pericardium

Earlier insult to the pericardium from surgery or infection can result in calcium formation. As with calcification in other parts of the body, this condition is best seen on conventional radiographs and CT.

Problem Solving: Pericardial Calcification Versus Myocardial Calcification

Myocardial necrosis from infarction leads to thinning, aneurysm formation, and calcification. On conventional radiographs, the key distinction between pericardial calcification and myocardial calcification is made by tracing the calcium in its entirety. Careful inspection of the calcified area usually reveals that the calcification (1) is thin and linear or curvilinear, (2) is found along the expected contour of the pericardium, and (3) crosses boundaries of the cardiac chambers or extends beyond the expected location of myocardium. This last observation is particularly important because it helps distinguish between pericardial calcification and myocardial calcification seen after infarction. Myocardial calcification from infarction is usually

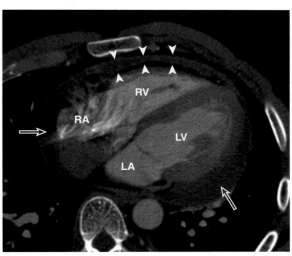

Figure 33-14 Axial image from a chest computed tomography with contrast in a 38-year-old man with chest pain demonstrates a moderate-size pericardial effusion *(arrows)* associated with enhancement of the visceral and parietal pericardial layers *(arrowheads)* consistent with pericarditis. The patient was treated with antiinflammatory medications, and the pericardial effusion resolved on subsequent echocardiograms. *LA,* Left atrium; *LV,* left ventricle; *RA,* right atrium; *RV,* right ventricle.

seen with aneurysm formation. True left ventricle (LV) aneurysms are more common at the apex. Chronic thrombus in the setting of remote infarct may also demonstrate calcification. Thick and irregular pericardial calcifications have classically been associated with earlier tuberculosis (Fig. 33-15).

Pericardial Constriction

Pericardial constriction results from fibrotic changes of the pericardium, with or without calcification, which limits heart motion and impairs diastolic filling. Although associated, the presence of pericardial calcification alone does not imply pericardial constriction

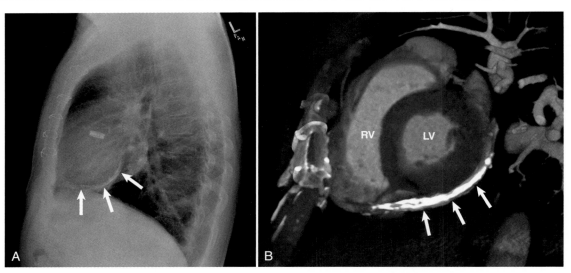

Figure 33-15 Lateral radiograph of the chest (**A**) and a corresponding volume rendered image from cardiac computed tomography (**B**) in a 67-year-old man demonstrate extensive pericardial calcifications involving the basal inferior pericardium and atrioventricular groove *(arrows)*. However, the patient did not have any symptoms of pericardial constriction with normal diastolic function on echocardiogram. Note changes from earlier open heart surgery with a single tilting disk prosthetic aortic valve (**A**). *LV,* Left ventricle; *RV,* right ventricle.

(see Fig. 33-15). The most common cause of pericardial constriction is previous cardiac surgery, followed by pericarditis and radiation therapy. Although thickened pericardium suggests constriction in the appropriate clinical setting, constriction can occur without pericardial thickening. The Doppler findings of pericardial constriction resemble those seen in cardiac tamponade.

Problem Solving: Echocardiographic Findings in Constrictive Disease

A brief discussion of some cardiac physiologic parameters is warranted to understand the echocardiographic findings in constrictive pericarditis. The following is what happens *normally*:

During inspiration, intrathoracic pressure falls. The purpose of this decrease is to increase blood flow to the lungs. The compliant walls of the SVC and IVC expand in response to negative intrathoracic pressure; thus, systemic venous return to the right heart is increased. Because the RV now has increased volume coming in, it expands circumferentially. Given that the pericardium is soft and compliant, most of this RV expansion occurs toward the pericardium, with minimal expansion toward the LV.

What happens if the pericardium is thickened, fibrosed, or calcified, as in constrictive disease? During inspiration, intrathoracic pressure again falls. However, because the pericardium is noncompliant, the RV cannot expand to accommodate this extra volume. As a result, during inspiration the ventricular septum bows toward the LV. As a result of this bowing, filling of the LV essentially depends on the amount of RV filling. This situation is known as ventricular interdependence. Exaggerated interdependence and abnormal ventricular septal motion explained by respiratory variation are hallmarks of constrictive disease.

A simple analogy is to consider a bag of water with two compartments, separated by a soft membrane. The bag is surrounded by compliant material, like a balloon. If the amount of fluid is increased in one compartment, the walls of that compartment will globally expand to accommodate the new fluid volume, without significantly affecting the other compartment. However, what if that balloon is encased within a rigid box? As the volume is increased in one chamber, the walls cannot expand beyond contact with the box. Any increase in volume within one chamber will cause the membrane to bulge toward the other chamber.

This situation is analogous to the septum bowing toward the LV during inspiration. Additionally, during expiration, the opposite happens, so with blood return to the left side, the septum bulges to the RV. Ventricular interdependence can be assessed during echocardiography when the patient is instructed to inspire and expire during the acquisition. MRI evaluation for *ventricular interdependence* uses echoplanar real-time cine MRI acquisition in a ventricular short-axis view during inspiration and expiration.

Adhesions between the parietal and visceral layers of the pericardium can result in constriction. Cine MRI with tagging is the only imaging modality that can demonstrate pericardial adhesions. Adequate interface between the pericardium and the mediastinal fat is needed to visualize the pericardium and detect changes in the tag lines during the cardiac cycle. For these reasons, tag lines orthogonal to the free wall of the RV and inferior wall are the preferred locations. During normal systolic ventricular shortening of the heart, unrestricted sliding motion occurs between the two pericardial layers and allows for normal cardiac motion. Tagged cine MRI images in physiologically normal patients demonstrate breaking of the tag lines at the level of the pericardium (dark line) during systole, except at the apex, where physiologic motion may be limited. In cases of constriction, adhesions between the two pericardial layers prevent the normal sliding motion between the

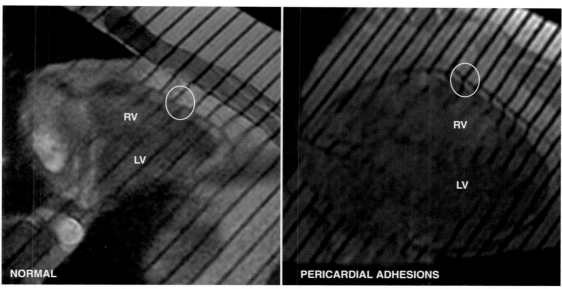

Figure 33-16 Tagged magnetic resonance imaging (MRI) images in a 35-year-old man demonstrate normal breaking of the tag lines at the level of the pericardium *(left)*. Tagged MRI images in a 63-year-old man with congestive heart failure demonstrate bending and stretching of the tag lines during systole consistent with pericardial adhesions *(right)*. *LV,* Left ventricle; *RV,* right ventricle.

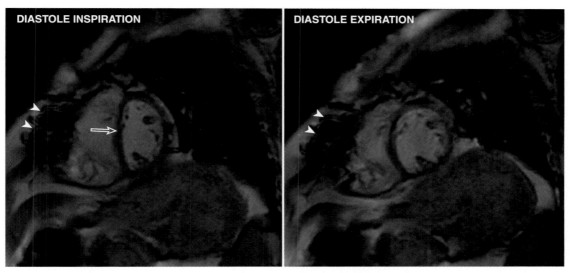

Figure 33-17 Short-axis balanced steady-state free precession cine images during deep inspiration *(left)* and expiration *(right)* in an 81-year-old man demonstrate diastolic flattening of the interventricular septum during inspiration consistent with interventricular interdependence. These findings, although not specific, suggest constrictive physiology. Note the deep position of the diaphragm during inspiration and the presence of sternal wires from earlier open heart surgery *(arrowheads)*.

layers and result in persistent continuity of the tag lines at the pericardium (dark line) and bending and stretching with cardiac motion, rather than breaking of the lines (Fig. 33-16). Other imaging findings on MRI suggestive of constriction are respirophasic septal flattening (Fig. 33-17) and septal bounce on cine-balanced steady-state free precession (SSFP) images. Secondary findings also include pericardial thickening (with or without calcification or enhancement), pleural effusions, and distention of the SVC, IVC, and hepatic veins.

A different entity is effusive constrictive pericarditis, in which pericardial inflammation and effusion result in constrictive physiology that persists despite drainage of the pericardial fluid. In both pericardial constriction and effusive constrictive pericarditis, the treatment of choice is pericardial stripping.

Problem Solving: Constrictive Pericarditis Versus Restrictive Cardiomyopathy

Restrictive cardiomyopathy can manifest with clinical signs and symptoms similar to those of constrictive disease. Both disorders are characterized by elevated venous pressure, low cardiac output, and a normal-sized LV chamber. Significant overlap also exists with imaging findings in these two disease categories. Differentiation of these two causes is important because treatment of constrictive disease is surgical removal of the pericardium, whereas treatment of restrictive disease

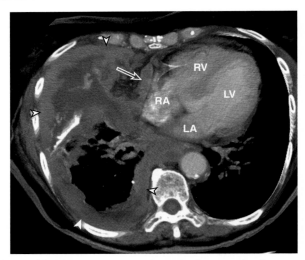

Figure 33-18 Axial contrast-enhanced volume rendered computed tomography image in a 59-year-old man with a history of asbestos exposure demonstrates thick nodular circumferential thickening of the right-side pleura extending into the major fissure consistent with pathologically proven malignant mesothelioma *(arrowheads)*. The nodular thickening of the right lateral pericardium *(arrow)* is consistent with metastatic disease. *LA,* Left atrium; *LV,* left ventricle; *RA,* right atrium; *RV,* right ventricle.

is medical. Constriction is favored when the following findings are seen: (1) pericardial calcification on conventional radiographs or CT; (2) pericardial thickening on CT or MRI; or (3) most important, ventricular interdependence (explained earlier) on echocardiography or cine MRI. Constriction may occur without thickening of the pericardium.

Pericardial Tumors

Primary pericardial tumors are rare and include lipomas, teratomas, fibromas, sarcomas, and mesotheliomas. Most pericardial tumors represent metastatic seeding (lymphatic seeding, vascular seeding, direct invasion) from primary breast and lung cancers, lymphomas, and melanomas. On CT and MRI, pericardial tumors may manifest as hemorrhagic effusions, pericardial thickening, or enhancing nodules or masses (Fig. 33-18).

■ PEARLS AND PITFALLS

- Reflections of the serous pericardium around the great vessels and the base of the heart are termed pericardial sinuses. The potential for fluid accumulation in these recesses is a pitfall that can be confused with lymphadenopathy.
- HU measurements should be made within pericardial effusions to check for accumulation of blood.
- Pericardial calcifications (1) are thin and linear or curvilinear, (2) are found along the expected contour of the pericardium, and (3) cross boundaries of the cardiac chambers.

- Failure of tag lines to break on cine-tagged MRI sequences suggests underlying adhesions resulting from fibrosis or inflammation of the pericardium.
- Ventricular interdependence is a key feature of constrictive pericarditis that helps distinguish this entity from restrictive cardiomyopathy.

■ ACKNOWLEDGMENTS

We would like to thank the following individuals for their contributions to this chapter: Jonathan Chung, MD; Brent Little, MD; and Avez Rizvi, MD.

Bibliography

Abbara S, Walker T. *Diagnostic Imaging: Cardiovascular.* Salt Lake City: Amirsys; 2008.

Abbas AE, Appleton CP, Liu PT, Sweeney JP. Congenital absence of the pericardium: case presentation and review of literature. *Int J Cardiol.* 2005;98:21-25.

Bogaert J, Francone M. Cardiovascular magnetic resonance in pericardial diseases. *J Cardiovasc Magn Reson.* 2009;11:14.

Borges AC, Gellert K, Dietel M, Baumann G, Witt C. Acute right-sided heart failure due to hemorrhage into a pericardial cyst. *Ann Thorac Surg.* 1997;63:845-847.

Clark DE, Wiles 3rd CS, Lim MK, Dunham CM, Rodriguez A. Traumatic rupture of the pericardium. *Surgery.* 1983;93:495-503.

Delille JP, Hernigou A, Sene V, et al. Maximal thickness of the normal human pericardium assessed by electron-beam computed tomography. *Eur Radiol.* 1999;9:1183-1189.

Glover LB, Barcia A, Reeves TJ. Congenital absence of the pericardium: a review of the literature with demonstration of a previously unreported fluoroscopic finding. *Am J Roentgenol Radium Ther Nucl Med.* 1969;106:542-549.

Groell R, Schaffler GJ, Rienmueller R. Pericardial sinuses and recesses: findings at electrocardiographically triggered electron-beam CT. *Radiology.* 1999;212:69-73.

Hill JK, Heitmiller 2nd RF, Askin FB, Kuhlman JE. Localized benign pleural mesothelioma arising in a radiation field. *Clin Imaging.* 1997;21:189-194.

Ivens E, Munt BI, Moss RR. Pericardial disease: what the general cardiologist needs to know. *Heart.* 2007;93:993-1000.

LeWinter M. Pericardial disease. In: Braunwald E, et al, ed. *Heart Disease: A Textbook of Cardiovascular Medicine.* 8th ed. Philadelphia: Saunders; 2008:1829-1853.

Ling LH, Oh JK, Tei C, et al. Pericardial thickness measured with transesophageal echocardiography: feasibility and potential clinical usefulness. *J Am Coll Cardiol.* 1997;29:1317-1323.

Miller S, Abbara S, Boxt L, eds. *Cardiac Imaging: The Requisites.* 3rd ed. St. Louis: Mosby; 2009:245-262.

Napolitano G, Pressacco J, Paquet E. Imaging features of constrictive pericarditis: beyond pericardial thickening. *Can Assoc Radiol J.* 2009;60:40-46.

Nassiri N, Yu A, Statkus N, Gosselin M. Imaging of cardiac herniation in traumatic pericardial rupture. *J Thorac Imaging.* 2009;24:69-72.

Netter FH. *Atlas of Human Anatomy.* 4th ed. Philadelphia: Saunders; 2006: 215.

Oh JK, Seward JB, Tajik AJ. *Echo Manual.* Baltimore: Lippincott Williams & Wilkins; 2006.

Otto C. *Textbook of Clinical Echocardiography.* 4th ed. Philadelphia: Saunders; 2009.

Rajiah P, Kanne JP, Kalahasti V, Schoenhagen P. Computed tomography of cardiac and pericardiac masses. *J Cardiovasc Comput Tomogr.* 2011;5:16-29.

Restrepo CS, Lemos DF, Lemos JA, et al. Imaging findings in cardiac tamponade with emphasis on CT. *Radiographics.* 2007;27:1595-1610.

Sherren PB, Galloway R, Healy M. Blunt traumatic pericardial rupture and cardiac herniation with a penetrating twist: two case reports. *Scand J Trauma Resusc Emerg Med.* 2009;17:64.

Sohn JH, Song JW, Seo JB, et al. Case report: pericardial rupture and cardiac herniation after blunt trauma. A case diagnosed using cardiac MRI. *Br J Radiol.* 2005;78:447-449.

Sparrow P, Merchant N, Provost Y, Doyle D, Nguyen E, Paul N. Cardiac MRI and CT features of inheritable and congenital conditions associated with sudden cardiac death. *Eur Radiol.* 2009;19:259-270.

Verhaert D, Gabriel RS, Johnston D, Lytle BW, Desai MY, Klein AL. The role of multimodality imaging in the management of pericardial disease. *Circ Cardiovasc Imaging.* 2010;3:333-343.

Yared K, Baggish AL, Picard MH, Hoffmann U, Hung J. Multimodality imaging of pericardial diseases. *JACC Cardiovasc Imaging.* 2010;3:650-660.

CHAPTER 34

Valves: Echocardiography

Niamh M. Kilcullen and Michael H. Picard

■ AORTIC VALVE

The normal aortic valve has three cusps: the right, left, and noncoronary cusps (Fig. 34-1, *A* and *B*). A bicuspid aortic valve occurs in 2% of the population, and these patients tend to present earlier with aortic stenosis or aortic regurgitation. In the case of a bicuspid valve, the right and left cusps are most commonly fused, followed by fusion of the right and noncoronary cusps (see Fig. 34-1, *C*). Unicuspid or quadricuspid aortic valves are less commonly seen in clinical practice (see Fig. 34-1, *D*). Lambl excrescences, which are thin filamentous strands commonly seen on the ventricular surface of the aortic valve cusps, are important to recognize. These features are regarded as normal and are thought to result from degenerative change (Fig. 34-2). These linear echodensities must be differentiated from abnormal masses such as vegetations and valve tumors.

Aortic Stenosis

The common cause of aortic stenosis is age-related degenerative disease; 3% of patients who are more than 75 years old have severe stenosis. In the parasternal long-axis view, leaflet thickening and calcification may be seen. As the disease progresses, reduced excursion of the aortic valve leaflets in systole is observed (Figs. 34-3 and 34-4, *A*). The examiner must assess the morphology of the aortic valve in systole because a bicuspid valve with raphe may appear tricuspid during diastole, when the valve is closed. Rheumatic aortic valve disease is no longer a common cause of aortic stenosis in the West, but it remains an important cause worldwide. Aortic sclerosis is common in older patients and is associated with jet velocities of up to 2.5 m/second. The normal aortic valve area is 3 to 4 cm² (Tables 34-1 and 34-2). As discussed in Chapter 1:

$$Flow = CSA \times Velocity$$

$$SV = CSA \times VTI$$

where CSA is the cross-sectional area, SV is the stroke volume, and VTI is the velocity time integral.

The continuity equation is based on the principle that the flow proximal and distal to a valve is equal, provided no intervening shunts are present. The continuity equation is routinely used to calculate aortic valve area in patients with aortic stenosis. To calculate the effective orifice area of the aortic valve, three measurements are required: (1) the left ventricular outflow tract (LVOT) diameter is measured in the parasternal long-axis view, in midsystole, from the septum to the anterior mitral leaflet, within 0.5 to 1.0 cm of the aortic valve; (2) in the apical, suprasternal, and right parasternal views, continuous wave Doppler across the aortic valve is obtained from which the peak velocity; and VTI may be calculated (Fig. 34-5, *A* and *B*); the outer edge of the "envelope" is traced to provide both the VTI and mean gradient; and (3) pulsed wave Doppler in the LVOT is obtained, from which the peak velocity and VTI are derived. Using the following continuity equation, the aortic valve area can be calculated:

$$AVA = \frac{LVOT\ area \times LVOT\ VTI}{Aortic\ valve\ VTI}$$

where AVA is the aortic valve area.

Aortic regurgitation often coexists with aortic stenosis (≤80% of patients) and should also be quantified. Left ventricular hypertrophy is present in almost all patients with severe aortic stenosis and reflects concentric remodeling of the left ventricle in response to the pressure load. The examiner must assess left ventricular systolic function and look for evidence of poststenotic dilatation in the ascending aorta. The continuity equation remains accurate in the presence of both aortic regurgitation and left ventricular impairment. Pulmonary hypertension may be present in patients with aortic stenosis and increases operative risk.

Low-dose dobutamine stress echocardiography is useful in patients with low-flow, low-gradient aortic stenosis. These patients typically have an aortic valve area smaller than 1 cm², a left ventricular ejection fraction lower than 40%, and a mean gradient of 30 to 40 mm Hg. Current recommendations suggest infusing a low dose (2.5 to 5.0 mcg/kg/minute) of dobutamine and increasing it up to 20 mcg/kg/minute. This approach enables differentiation of aortic leaflets that cannot open because of stenosis from those that do not open because of reduced stroke volume. The test should be stopped in the following situations: (1) symptoms of chest pain, shortness of breath, or dizziness occur; (2) heart rate is faster than 100 beats/minute or increases by

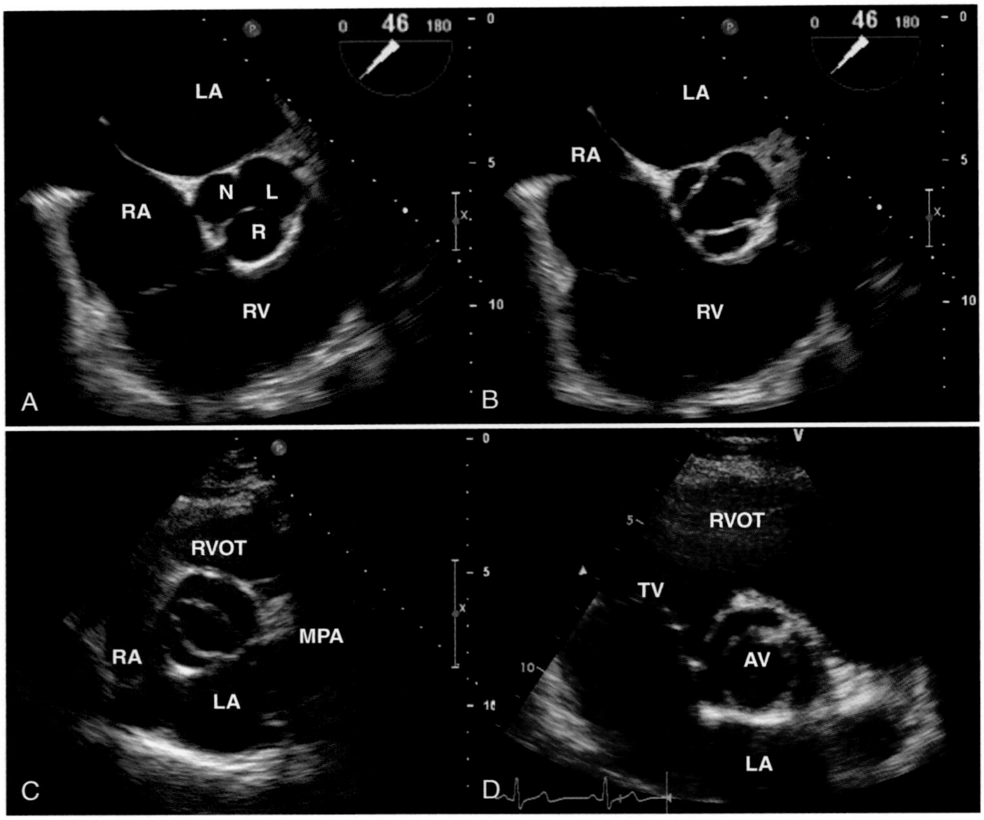

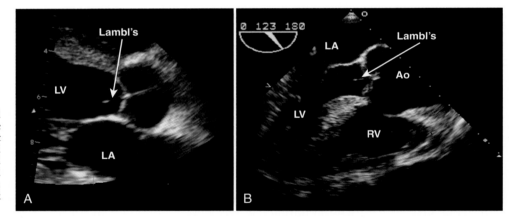

Figure 34-1 Transesophageal echocardiographic midesophageal short-axis view of the aortic valve (AV) that shows a normal valve closed in diastole (**A**) and open in systole (**B**). **C,** Transthoracic echocardiographic parasternal short-axis view at the level of the AV that shows a bicuspid AV. **D,** Transthoracic echocardiographic parasternal short-axis view at the level of the AV that shows a unicuspid AV. *L,* Left coronary cusp; *LA,* left atrium; *MPA,* main pulmonary artery; *N,* noncoronary cusp; *PV,* pulmonary valve; *R,* right coronary cusp; *RA,* right atrium; *RV,* right ventricle; *RVOT,* right ventricular outflow tract; *TV,* tricuspid valve.

Figure 34-2 Examples of Lambl excrescence on the ventricular side of the aortic valve. **A,** Transthoracic echocardiographic parasternal long-axis view. **B,** Transesophageal echocardiographic midesophageal long-axis view of the aortic valve. *Ao,* Aorta; *LA,* left atrium; *LV,* left ventricle; *RV,* right ventricle.

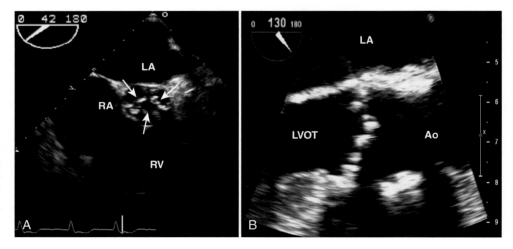

Figure 34-3 Transesophageal echocardiographic midesophageal short-axis (**A**) and long-axis (**B**) views of the aortic valve showing a heavily calcified and stenotic valve. The three cusps of the aortic valve are arrowed. *Ao,* Aorta; *LA,* left atrium; *LVOT,* left ventricular outflow tract; *RA,* right atrium; *RV,* right ventricle.

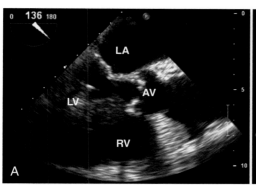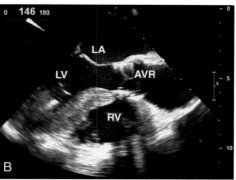

Figure 34-4 A, Transesophageal echocardiographic midesophageal long-axis view of the aortic valve (AV) that shows severe calcific aortic stenosis before transcatheter aortic valve implantation. **B,** Following deployment of a stent-mounted pericardial prosthesis under transesophageal echocardiographic guidance. *AVR,* Aortic valve replacement; *LA,* left atrium; *LV,* left ventricle; *RV,* right ventricle.

Table 34-1   Assessment of Aortic Stenosis

	Mild	Moderate	Severe
Jet velocity (m/sec)	2.6-3.0	3-4	>4
Mean gradient (mm Hg)	<20	20-40	>40
Aortic valve area (cm²)	>1.5	1.0-1.5	<1.0

more than 20 beats/minute from baseline; (3) hypotension develops; or (4) arrhythmias occur. Severe stenosis is confirmed if the jet velocity increases to more than 4 m/second, the mean gradient is more than 40 mm Hg, and the aortic valve area is less than 1 cm². The absence of contractile reserve, demonstrated by a failure to increase the stroke volume or ejection fraction to more than 20%, is a predictor of high mortality and overall poor prognosis.

LVOT obstructive lesions occur in 6% of patients with congenital heart disease. Most of these lesions are valvular. Subvalvular stenosis may result from the presence of a fibrous membrane and is often associated with other congenital anomalies (Fig. 34-6). It represents 10% to 14% of cases of congenital LVOT obstruction. Supravalvular stenosis is the least common form of LVOT obstruction and represents 8% to 14%. It is most commonly seen in children with Williams syndrome.

Aortic Regurgitation

Aortic regurgitation results from abnormalities of the aortic valve leaflets or the aorta. Trace aortic regurgitation is not regarded as physiologic and is observed in less than 1% of individuals less than 40 years old. Aortic regurgitation is associated with bicuspid valves, tricuspid valves with calcific degenerative change, rheumatic heart disease, myxomatous disease, and infective or noninfective endocarditis. Diseases affecting the aortic root and ascending aorta may also result in aortic regurgitation and include hypertension, aortic aneurysms, Marfan syndrome, aortic dissection, and inflammatory diseases. In chronic aortic regurgitation, the left ventricle is dilated as a result of chronic volume overload, whereas in acute aortic regurgitation, the left ventricle is usually normal in size. The most common causes of acute aortic regurgitation are endocarditis and aortic dissection.

Table 34-2   Tips and Tricks in Assessment of Aortic Stenosis

Problem	Solution
Underestimating peak velocity	Parallel orientation to beam required
	Peak velocity measured in several windows (apical, suprasternal, and right parasternal) to identify the highest
	Use of nonimaging continuous wave Doppler transducer in addition to standard imaging probe (higher signal-to-noise ratio)
	Averaging over several beats if irregular rhythm
Inaccurate aortic valve area	Careful measurement of left ventricular tract diameter required*
Mistaking mitral regurgitant jet for aortic velocity	Careful Doppler interrogation required with attention to timing of signal
If ascending aorta <30 mm	Pressure recovery taken into account†
Significant difference in serial measurements	Aortic jet velocity verified to be from same window
	Left ventricular tract size checked because this rarely changes in adult patients

*Small errors in the left ventricular tract diameter equate to significant errors in the calculated aortic valve area using the continuity equation because the radius of the left ventricular tract is squared.
†The conversion of potential energy to kinetic energy across a narrowed valve results in high velocity and a drop in pressure. Distal to the narrowed valve, flow decelerates. Some kinetic energy is reconverted into potential energy, with a resulting increase in pressure and a reduction in Doppler-derived gradient.

Assessment of the severity of aortic regurgitation tends to be more qualitative than quantitative in clinical practice, although several validated quantitative methods are available (Table 34-3). In the parasternal long-axis view, the degree of aortic regurgitation is assessed using color flow Doppler (Figs. 34-7 and 34-8, *A*). Color flow mapping is excellent for the detection of aortic regurgitation, with a sensitivity and specificity of 95% and almost 100%, respectively. The jet width in relation to the LVOT, rather than the length of the jet into the left ventricular cavity, allows assessment of severity. Severe aortic regurgitation is present when this jet width in the LVOT exceeds 65%. Eccentric jets, however, may be underestimated because the jet width may appear narrow and less significant. Furthermore, in patients with multiple jets, overestimating the severity of regurgitation is possible.

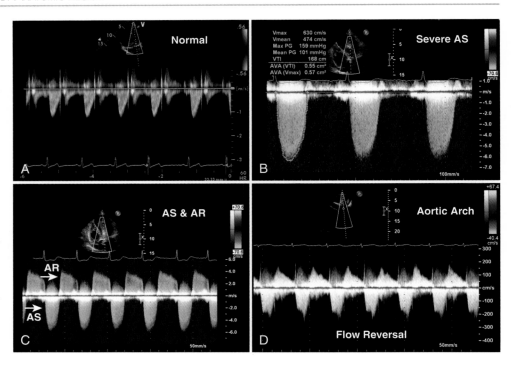

Figure 34-5 **A,** Example of normal continuous wave Doppler recording across the aortic valve in the apical five-chamber view. The peak velocity is 1.2 m/second. **B,** Example of continuous wave Doppler recording across the aortic valve in the apical five-chamber view in a patient with severe (critical) aortic stenosis (AS). The peak velocity is 6.3 m/second, with a peak gradient of 159 mm Hg. Note the different shape of the spectral trace in severe AS. **C,** Example of continuous wave Doppler recording across the aortic valve in the apical five-chamber view in a patient with both AS and aortic regurgitation (AR). **D,** Example of continuous wave Doppler recording showing holodiastolic flow reversal in the aortic arch in a patient with severe AR.

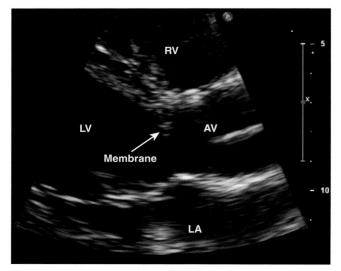

Figure 34-6 Transthoracic echocardiographic two-dimensional parasternal long-axis view showing a subaortic membrane. *AV,* Aortic valve; *LA,* left atrium; *LV,* left ventricle; *RV,* right ventricle.

The vena contracta is the narrowest portion of the jet at the level of the aortic valve and should be measured in the parasternal long-axis view. A vena contracta larger than 0.6 cm is associated with severe aortic regurgitation. Proximal isovelocity surface area (PISA) and effective regurgitant orifice area (EROA) may also be calculated, but these methods are more commonly used in the assessment of mitral regurgitation. When assessing aortic regurgitant jets, the examiner must be aware that parasternal views have a higher degree of axial resolution and are therefore preferable to apical views, which tend to make the jet appear larger as a result of beam spread.

Table 34-3   Assessment of Aortic Regurgitation

	Mild	Severe
Central jet width in left ventricular outflow tract (%)	<25	≥65
Vena contracta (cm)	<0.3	>0.6
Holodiastolic flow reversal in descending aorta	No	Yes
Pressure half-time (msec)	>500	<200

From apical views, a continuous wave Doppler recording across the aortic valve is obtained, and the signal density of the aortic regurgitation signal reflects the degree of regurgitation present (see Fig. 34-5, *C*). With increasing severity of aortic regurgitation, the aortic diastolic pressure falls rapidly. The pressure half-time is easily measured, and values lower than 200 msec reflect severe aortic regurgitation. The pressure half-time measurement is often the most useful marker of severity in acute aortic regurgitation because the left ventricular end-diastolic pressure rises quickly in the nondilated, less compliant left ventricle. Diastolic flow reversal in the descending aorta is easy to assess from suprasternal and subcostal views, by using pulsed wave Doppler, and can help confirm significant aortic regurgitation, if present. In severe aortic regurgitation, holodiastolic flow reversal may be seen in the descending aorta (see Fig. 34-8, *B*).

■ MITRAL VALVE

The mitral valve is a complex structure, consisting of anterior and posterior leaflets that are supported by a saddle-shaped annulus and subvalvular structures, namely, the chordae tendineae and the papillary muscles. By

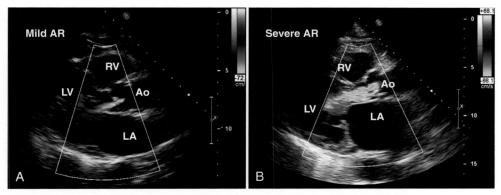

Figure 34-7 A, Transthoracic echocardiographic parasternal long-axis view showing a bicuspid aortic valve and mild central aortic regurgitation (AR). The jet width occupies less than 25% of the left ventricular outflow tract. **B,** Parasternal long-axis view showing severe AR. The jet width occupies greater than 65%, and the vena contracta is larger than 0.6 cm, indicating severe AR. *Ao,* Aorta; *LA,* left atrium; *LV,* left ventricle; *RV,* right ventricle.

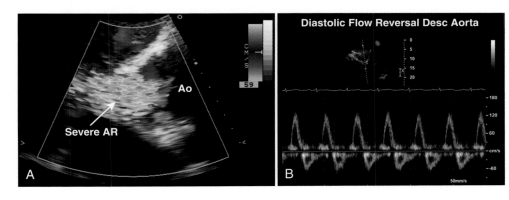

Figure 34-8 A, Transthoracic echocardiographic parasternal long-axis view of the aortic valve showing severe aortic regurgitation (AR). *Ao,* Aorta. **B,** Pulsed wave Doppler showing holodiastolic flow reversal in the descending (Desc) aorta that suggests severe AR.

convention, each leaflet is divided into three portions, with A1 and P1 laterally and A3 and P3 medially. The normal mitral valve area is 4 to 5 cm². The posteromedial papillary muscle is supplied by the right coronary artery, whereas the anterolateral papillary muscle has a dual blood supply from the left anterior descending and circumflex coronary arteries. Consequently, the posteromedial papillary muscle is most susceptible to ischemic injury.

Mitral Stenosis

The most common cause of mitral stenosis is rheumatic disease. Other rarer causes include connective tissue disease, drug-induced disease, infiltrative disease, and congenital mitral stenosis. Echocardiography is an excellent noninvasive tool for confirming the presence of mitral stenosis, determining the severity of stenosis, and assessing the suitability for percutaneous valvuloplasty. Patients with a mitral valve area larger than 1.5 cm² do not usually report symptoms. Exercise stress echocardiography is useful for patients with a valve area smaller than 1.5 cm² who do not report symptoms to objectively assess symptoms, functional capacity, and right ventricular systolic pressure.

In rheumatic mitral stenosis, the classic appearance comprises reduced mobility and doming of the leaflet tips, resulting in a "hockey-stick" appearance (Fig. 34-9, A). The leaflets may be thickened and calcified; however, commissural fusion is regarded as the hallmark of

rheumatic mitral stenosis. The chordae tendineae may also be thickened, calcified, and restricted. The examiner must look for evidence of other valve disease, specifically involving the aortic or tricuspid valves. The left atrium is usually significantly dilated, and evidence of spontaneous echo contrast reflecting sluggish blood flow may be present. Patients with mitral stenosis commonly have pulmonary hypertension, and therefore the right ventricular systolic pressure should be estimated from the tricuspid regurgitation continuous wave Doppler signal. Right atrial pressure is estimated from the assessment of inferior vena cava size and inspiratory collapse. The presence or absence of mitral regurgitation is also relevant when mitral valvuloplasty is considered because moderate or more mitral regurgitation is a contraindication to percutaneous intervention.

Assessment of Severity

Mitral valve area is calculated by direct planimetry using the parasternal short-axis view at the level of the mitral valve leaflet tips in mid-diastole (see Fig. 34-9, B). This measurement can be difficult if the valve is heavily calcified and may therefore not always be accurate. By using three-dimensional echocardiography, to the examiner can crop the image to obtain a true short-axis view, at the level of the mitral valve tips, increase the accuracy of the planimetered area (see Fig. 34-9, C). Alternatively, the mitral valve area can be derived from the pressure half-time, which is obtained by measuring the slope of the E wave. The mitral valve area is calculated as

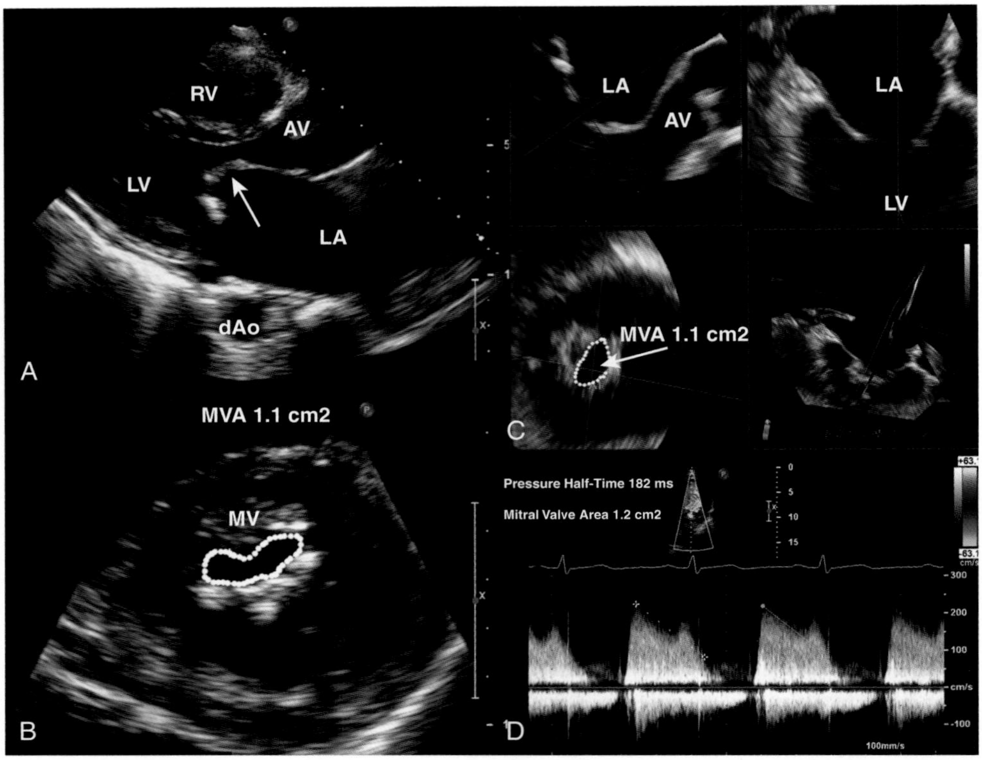

Figure 34-9 A, Transthoracic echocardiographic parasternal long-axis view in a patient with mitral stenosis, showing doming of the anterior mitral leaflet with the typical "hockey-stick" appearance *(arrow)*. **B,** Parasternal short-axis view at the level of the mitral valve (MV) in a patient with mitral stenosis. The mitral valve area (MVA) is calculated by direct planimetry of the valve. **C,** Transesophageal three-dimensional echocardiographic planimetry of the MV. **D,** Continuous wave Doppler showing measurement of the pressure half-time and derivation of the MVA. *AV,* Aortic valve; *dAo,* descending aorta; *LA,* left atrium; *LV,* left ventricle; *RV,* right ventricle.

Table 34-4 Assessment of Mitral Stenosis

	Mild	Moderate	Severe
Valve area (cm²)	>1.5	1.0-1.5	<1.0
Mean gradient (mm Hg)	<5	5-10	>10
Pressure half-time (msec)	100-150	150-220	>220
Right ventricular systolic pressure (mm Hg)	<30	30-50	>50

Table 34-5 Tips and Tricks in Assessment of Mitral Stenosis

Problem	Solution
Inaccurate valve area by planimetry	Use of pressure half-time Use of three-dimensional imaging (more accurate)
Inaccurate valve area by pressure half-time	Awareness of limitations of this method (assumption that atrial and ventricular compliance is normal)
Pressure half-time not always applicable (e.g., severe aortic regurgitation, ≤72 hours after valvuloplasty)	Awareness of limitations of this method Use of direct planimetry
Chordae tendineae not well seen in midesophageal view on transesophageal echocardiography	Assessment of chordae tendineae in transgastric views

220/pressure half-time and typically is automatically calculated by measurement software on the echocardiography machine or off-line work station (see Fig. 34-9, *D*).

$$MVA = \frac{220}{Pt\frac{1}{2}}$$

where MVA is the mitral valve area and $Pt\frac{1}{2}$ is the pressure half-time.

The peak and mean gradients are also obtained from the continuous wave Doppler mitral profile, but not from the pulse wave Doppler profile. The mean gradient is obtained by tracing the Doppler profile of the transmitral diastolic flow (see Fig. 34-9, *D*). The pressure gradient and pressure half-time measurements are accurate in the setting of normal atrial and ventricular compliance (Table 34-4). In patients with severe aortic regurgitation, the pressure half-time is shortened, and this may result in an overestimate of mitral valve area (Table 34-5).

Echocardiography is often used to assess suitability for percutaneous mitral valvuloplasty, and a scoring system has been devised for this purpose. Points are allocated (0 to 4) for valve thickening, valve calcification, leaflet mobility, and subvalvular thickening. A mitral valve score of less than 9 is associated with an optimal result following percutaneous mitral valvuloplasty (Fig. 34-10). A score of more than 11 is associated with a suboptimal result. Transesophageal echocardiography (TEE) is usually performed before mitral valvuloplasty, to ensure that the patient has no evidence of thrombus in the left atrium or left atrial appendage.

Mitral annular calcification is commonly seen in older patients and represents a form of degenerative mitral stenosis (Fig. 34-11, *A*). It is associated with hypertension and atherosclerotic disease and usually

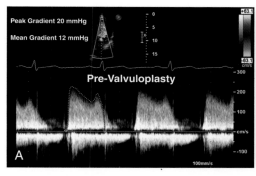
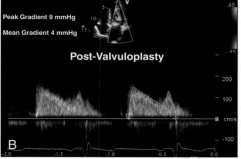

Figure 34-10 Continuous wave Doppler through the mitral valve obtained in the apical four-chamber view before (**A**) and after (**B**) mitral valvuloplasty. The peak and mean gradients are derived from the spectral trace obtained. Note the significantly lower gradients after valvuloplasty.

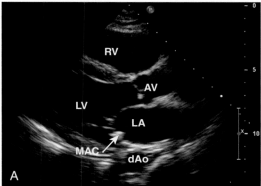
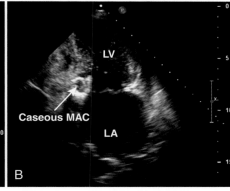

Figure 34-11 A, Transthoracic echocardiographic parasternal long-axis view showing posterior mitral annular calcification (MAC). **B,** Apical two-chamber view showing caseous MAC, a benign entity that should not be confused with a tumor. *AV,* Aortic valve; *dAo,* descending aorta; *LA,* left atrium; *LV,* left ventricle; *RV,* right ventricle.

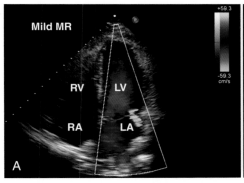
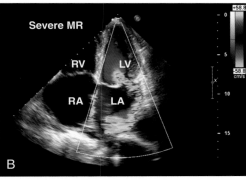

Figure 34-12 A, Transthoracic echocardiographic apical four-chamber view showing mild mitral regurgitation (MR) by color Doppler. **B,** Apical four-chamber view showing prolapse of the anterior mitral valve leaflet associated with severe eccentric mitral regurgitation by color Doppler. *LA,* Left atrium; *LV,* left ventricle; *RA,* right atrium; *RV,* right ventricle.

has no significant hemodynamic significance. Occasionally, extensive mitral annular calcification encroaches on the leaflets. This may result in restricted leaflet motion and reduced mitral orifice. Valve thickening and calcification involve the base of the leaflets, unlike in rheumatic mitral stenosis, where the tips are predominantly involved. Caseous mitral annular calcification is a rare variant occurring in less than 1% of patients with mitral annular calcification. It typically appears as a mass, involving the posterior mitral annulus, with an echolucent core representing central necrosis. Caseous calcification is benign and should not be misinterpreted as a tumor or abscess (see Fig. 34-11, *B*).

Mitral Regurgitation

Mitral regurgitation is common, and physiologic or trace mitral regurgitation is seen in up to 50% of physiologically normal individuals. Mitral regurgitation may result from valve leaflet abnormalities, including those caused by infection (rheumatic, endocarditis), myxomatous disease, drug treatment, or radiation therapy (Fig. 34-12). Functional mitral regurgitation can also arise from ventricular abnormalities such as left ventricular dilatation or papillary muscle ischemia.

Mitral valve prolapse is found in 2% of the population and is a common cause of mitral regurgitation (Fig. 34-13). Myxomatous valves appear thickened with redundant tissue, thus reflecting the increased mucopolysaccharides and leaflet disarray seen on histology. Mitral valve prolapse may also be associated with various connective tissue diseases such as Marfan syndrome, Ehlers-Danlos syndrome, and pseudoxanthoma elasticum. Mitral valve prolapse should be assessed only in the views that display the anterior and posterior portions of the mitral annulus, namely, the parasternal long-axis and apical long-axis views. In mitral valve prolapse, one or both leaflets are displaced at least 2 mm above the plane of the mitral annulus. For a diagnosis of classic mitral valve prolapse, mitral leaflet thickening (>5 mm)

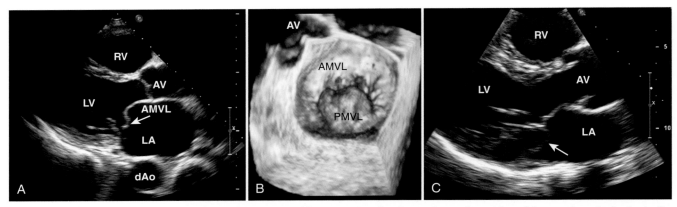

Figure 34-13 **A,** Transthoracic echocardiographic parasternal long-axis view showing prolapse of a portion of the anterior mitral valve leaflet (AMVL). **B,** Transesophageal echocardiographic midesophageal three-dimensional image of the mitral valve showing prolapse of P2, the middle scallop of the posterior mitral valve leaflet (PMVL). **C,** Transthoracic echocardiographic parasternal long-axis view showing prolapse of the PMVL *(arrow)*. *AV,* Aortic valve; *dAo,* descending aorta; *LA,* left atrium; *LV,* left ventricle; *RV,* right ventricle.

is also required. Mitral regurgitation associated with prolapse is often late systolic rather than holosystolic, and eccentrically directed jets are common. As stated previously, the assessment of eccentrically directed jets can be problematic, and the examiner should not rely on a single parameter or method when assessing severity of regurgitation. The severity of eccentrically directed jets of mitral regurgitation may be underestimated by up to 40%.

As a general rule, if the posterior mitral valve leaflet is prolapsed, the mitral regurgitant jet will be directed anteriorly and laterally. Similarly, if the anterior mitral valve leaflet is prolapsed, the mitral regurgitant jet will be directed posteriorly and medially (see Fig. 34-12, *B*). In clinical practice, a spectrum of mitral valve prolapse is seen, ranging from isolated P2 prolapse to severe myxomatous mitral valve disease (Barlow disease), in which most portions of the valve are involved. Disruption of a leaflet, or a portion of the anterior or posterior mitral valve leaflet, may result in a partial or complete flail. Not uncommonly, ruptured chordae tendineae are associated with a flail segment.

Mitral valve repair is currently the preferred treatment for mitral valve prolapse. Therefore, surgeons require detailed assessment of mitral valve anatomy before surgical intervention. Real-time three-dimensional imaging has proved extremely useful in the assessment of mitral valve disease because it can provide detailed views of the mitral valve from the left atrial perspective (see Fig. 34-13, *B*). In cases of prolapse, with three-dimensional imaging, surgeons have a unique opportunity to view mitral valve anatomy, identify the extent of the disease, and plan the operation ahead of time. In patients with myxomatous mitral valve disease, three-dimensional imaging is superior to two-dimensional imaging because it allows identification of mitral valve clefts, when present. This information is invaluable for surgeons and may in some cases alter the surgical strategy.

Functional mitral regurgitation is seen in patients with both ischemic and dilated cardiomyopathy. Apical and lateral papillary muscle displacement secondary to global or regional left ventricular enlargement

causes tethering and reduced closure of the mitral leaflets, resulting in varying degrees of mitral regurgitation. Patients not uncommonly have both mitral valve disease and left ventricular dysfunction, and a careful assessment of the mitral valve and its surrounding structures is therefore important. Left atrial size and volume provide helpful information regarding the chronicity of mitral regurgitation because the left atrium is typically not dilated in acute mitral regurgitation. In practice, differentiating between moderate and severe mitral regurgitation may be difficult, although several available quantitative methods are helpful in the assessment of mitral regurgitation (Table 34-6). However, these methods do make several assumptions, have limitations, and must be interpreted carefully, to avoid misdiagnosis.

Regurgitant Jet Area
Using color flow mapping, mitral regurgitation is seen in the left atrium in systole. The jet area gives an indication of severity; however, this qualitative assessment is not always accurate, for several reasons. The jet area may appear small if the left atrium is significantly dilated. A central jet may appear larger because of entrainment of red blood cells surrounding the jet. In contrast, eccentric jets that hug the left atrial wall may appear small and less significant (see Fig. 34-12).

Vena Contracta
The vena contracta is the narrowest portion of the jet at or just downstream from the mitral valve orifice.

Table 34-6   **Assessment of Mitral Regurgitation**

	Mild	Severe
Jet area	Small	Large
Vena contracta (cm)	<0.3	≥0.7
Effective regurgitant orifice area (cm²)	<0.2	≥0.4
Mitral E velocity (m/sec)	<1.2	>1.2
Systolic flow reversal in pulmonary vein	No	Yes

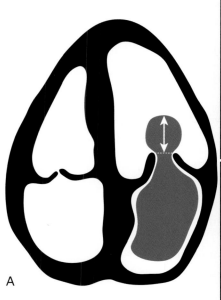

A

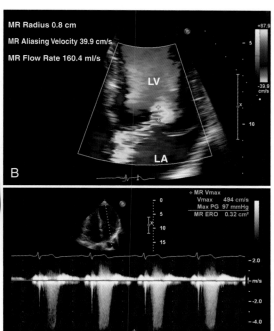

MR Radius 0.8 cm
MR Aliasing Velocity 39.9 cm/s
MR Flow Rate 160.4 ml/s

LV

LA

B

+ MR Vmax
Vmax   494 cm/s
Max PG   97 mmHg
MR ERO   0.32 cm²

C

Figure 34-14 Quantification of mitral regurgitation (MR). A, Schematic representation of proximal isovelocity surface area (PISA) measurement in the apical four-chamber view. **B,** Transthoracic echocardiographic apical four-chamber view zoomed on the mitral valve that shows PISA measurement. *LA,* Left atrium; *LV,* left ventricle. **C,** Continuous wave Doppler showing peak MR velocity and derivation of effective regurgitant orifice. A value of 0.3 cm² suggests moderate MR.

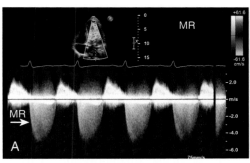

MR

MR

A

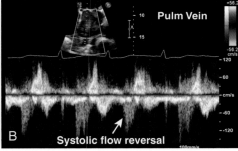

Pulm Vein

Systolic flow reversal

B

Figure 34-15 A, Continuous wave Doppler trace in a patient with severe mitral regurgitation (MR). Note the dense, triangular shape of the trace. **B,** Pulsed wave Doppler of a pulmonary vein (Pulm Vein) in the apical four-chamber view showing systolic flow reversal suggesting severe MR.

The CSA of the vena contracta reflects the EROA. The vena contracta diameter is measured in the parasternal long-axis view, ideally in magnified mode. A vena contracta diameter of less than 0.3 cm is associated with mild mitral regurgitation, and a value greater than 0.7 cm suggests severe mitral regurgitation. Inappropriate color gain settings, atrial fibrillation, and poor image quality may all affect the accuracy of the vena contracta measurement.

Flow Convergence or Proximal Isovelocity Surface Area

The flow convergence, or PISA, is used to estimate the regurgitant flow and regurgitant orifice area. This method is based on the continuity equation and is more accurate for central jets, in which the orifice area is circular. The Nyquist limit is reduced to increase the radius of the aliased velocity. This radius should be measured in midsystole (Fig. 34-14). The peak velocity of the mitral regurgitation signal is obtained from continuous wave Doppler imaging across the mitral valve in the apical four-chamber view (Fig. 34-15, *A*). The regurgitant flow

and EROA can then be calculated using the following equations:

$$\text{Regurgitant flow} = 2\pi r^2 \times Va$$

$$\text{EROA} \times \text{Pk Vreg} = 2\pi r^2 \times Va$$

$$\text{EROA} = \frac{(2\pi r^2 \times Va)}{\text{Pk Vreg}}$$

where Va is the aliasing velocity and Pk Vreg is the peak regurgitant velocity.

Pulmonary Vein Flow

In the apical four-chamber view, pulsed wave Doppler imaging is obtained from a pulmonary vein. As the left atrial pressure rises in severe mitral regurgitation, blood may be forced back into the pulmonary veins in systole. This finding is reflected by systolic flow reversal on the spectral trace and is specific, but not sensitive, for severe regurgitation (see Fig. 34-15, *B*). With an eccentrically directed jet, severe mitral regurgitation may be present

Table 34-7   Tips and Tricks in Assessment of Mitral Regurgitation

Problem	Solution
Entrainment of regurgitant jet	Awareness of this concept
Jet size affected by several parameters	Adjustment of pulse repetition frequency Setting of aliasing velocity 50-60 cm/sec Adjustment of color gain to eliminate color speckle
Inaccurate vena contracta	Use of zoom mode Use of narrow color flow sector width Adjustment of depth to maximize lateral and temporal resolution
Inaccurate PISA using color flow mapping	Adjustment of baseline toward direction of flow and/or lower Nyquist limit Awareness that PISA more accurate for central jets
Underestimation of severity in acute mitral regurgitation*	Maximizing of frame rate Vena contracta reliable in this setting
Severity of mitral regurgitation influenced by blood pressure	Recording of blood pressure at time of study
Possible underestimation of eccentric jets (out of plane)	Careful evaluation of mitral regurgitation Awareness of limitations of techniques Use of vena contracta Use of three-dimensional imaging (may be helpful)
Systolic flow reversal in pulmonary vein inaccurate in atrial fibrillation	Use of other parameters in assessment of severity of mitral regurgitation

PISA, Proximal isovelocity surface area.
*Insufficient temporal resolution in patient with tachycardia leading to small jet size despite significant mitral regurgitation.

without systolic flow reversal. This phenomenon reinforces the importance of not relying on a single parameter when assessing severity of valve disease (Table 34-7).

■ TRICUSPID VALVE

The tricuspid is larger than the mitral valve and consists of three leaflets. The free margins of the cusps are attached to the chordae tendineae, which are attached to three papillary muscles. In the right ventricle, the papillary muscles project from both the septum and lateral wall. The anterior leaflet is larger than the posterior and septal leaflets. The septal leaflet is more apically positioned than the other leaflets, and this morphology can help differentiate between the right and left ventricles in congenital heart disease. The normal tricuspid valve is 5 to 8 cm², and, therefore, the Doppler inflow velocity is lower than the transmitral velocity. In physiologically normal individuals, E and A waves are present in sinus rhythm, and the E/A ratio is 1.0.

Tricuspid Stenosis

Tricuspid stenosis is rare but may be seen in patients with rheumatic heart disease as thickened leaflets that dome in systole. Other rarer causes include carcinoid syndrome with coexistent tricuspid regurgitation. Mechanical obstruction from a tumor, vegetation, thrombus, or pacing wire may also rarely result in stenosis. Tricuspid stenosis is usually associated with a degree of tricuspid regurgitation. In cases of significant tricuspid stenosis, the right atrium and inferior vena cava are dilated (Table 34-8).

Tricuspid Regurgitation

Physiologic or trace central tricuspid regurgitation is seen in up to 70% of individuals and is regarded as

Table 34-8   Assessment of Tricuspid Stenosis

	Significant
Valve area (cm²)	<1.0
Mean gradient (mm Hg)	≥5
Tricuspid valve pressure half-time (msec)	≥190

normal. More severe tricuspid regurgitation may result from abnormalities of the valve, or more often it may be secondary to right ventricular dilatation and tricuspid annular dilatation. A common cause of tricuspid regurgitation is infection, specifically endocarditis, particularly in the setting of indwelling catheters or in intravenous drug users. Another common cause is secondary to right ventricular dilatation resulting from cardiomyopathy, chronic lung conditions, or pulmonary hypertension. A degree of tricuspid regurgitation is not uncommonly observed in patients with right ventricular pacing leads, although this regurgitation is usually mild. Less common causes of tricuspid regurgitation include tricuspid valve prolapse, carcinoid, and Ebstein anomaly (Figs. 34-16, *A*, 34-17, and 34-18).

Carcinoid tumors are rare (1 to 2 per 100,000) endocrine-secreting tumors associated with elevated serotonin and 5-hydroxytryptophan levels. Cardiac involvement may be seen in up to 50% of patients. Carcinoid is associated with thickening and retraction of tricuspid valve leaflets that result in relatively immobile or "frozen" leaflets and significant tricuspid regurgitation (see Fig. 34-17). Most patients also have pulmonary involvement with stenosis or regurgitation because the plaquelike fibrous deposits have a predilection for right-sided heart valves. The active metabolite is deactivated in the lungs, and, consequently, involvement of

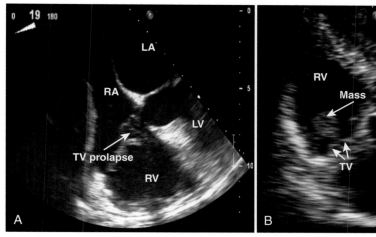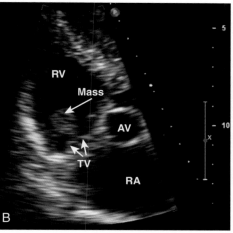

Figure 34-16 **A,** Transesophageal echocardiographic midesophageal view of the right ventricular inflow that shows prolapse of the tricuspid valve (TV). **B,** Transthoracic echocardiographic modified apical four-chamber view focused on the right side of the heart that shows a mass attached to the TV. This finding was confirmed as a papillary fibroelastoma following surgical resection. *AV,* Aortic valve; *LA,* left atrium; *LV,* left ventricle; *RA,* right atrium; *RV,* right ventricle.

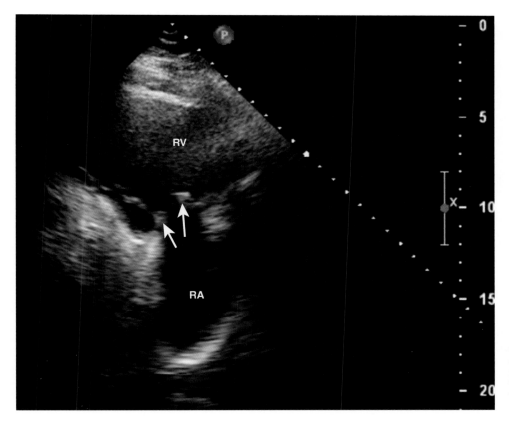

Figure 34-17 Transthoracic echocardiographic parasternal long-axis right ventricular inflow view showing thickened and retracted tricuspid valve leaflets *(arrows)* in a patient with carcinoid heart disease. *RA,* Right atrium; *RV,* right ventricle.

left-sided valves is rare. The two recognized exceptions are the presence of a left-to-right shunt and pulmonary metastases. Severe tricuspid regurgitation can be low-velocity, nonturbulent flow resulting from a large regurgitant orifice.

Ebstein anomaly is a congenital malformation with a prevalence of 1 in 50,000 to 200,000. It is more common in infants of mothers who take lithium. The anomaly primarily involves the tricuspid valve and right ventricle. The most important echocardiographic findings are (1) apical displacement of the septal tricuspid valve leaflet (≥8 mm/m² body surface area compared with the position of the mitral valve), (2) an decrease in right ventricular volume from atrialization

of a portion of the right ventricle, (3) paradoxical septal motion from right ventricular volume overload, and (4) the presence of tricuspid regurgitation (see Fig. 34-18). Ebstein anomaly may be associated with various other congenital defects such as atrial septal defects, ventricular septal defects, patent ductus arteriosus, coarctation of the aorta, and pulmonary stenosis or atresia.

Assessment of tricuspid regurgitation in practice is often more qualitative than quantitative, although the methods described previously for mitral regurgitation can all be used to assess the severity. The jet area is best evaluated in the apical four-chamber view; occasionally, however, eccentric jets may be better visualized in the

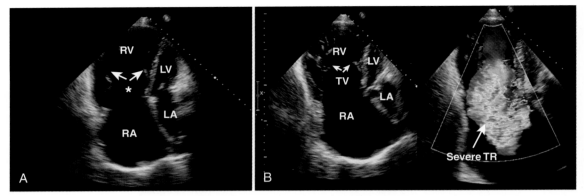

Figure 34-18 **A**, Transthoracic echocardiographic apical four-chamber view in a patient with Ebstein anomaly that shows apical displacement of the tricuspid leaflets *(arrows)* and atrialization *(asterisk)* of part of the right ventricle (RV). The right side of the heart is massively dilated in comparison with the left. **B**, Severe tricuspid regurgitation (TR) is seen by color Doppler imaging. *LA,* Left atrium; *LV,* left ventricle; *RA,* right atrium; *TV,* tricuspid valve.

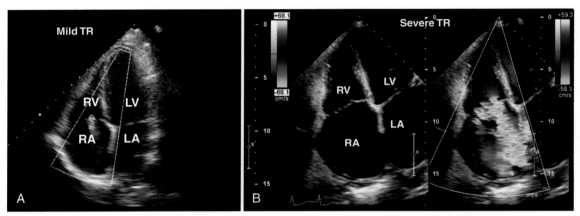

Figure 34-19 **A**, Transthoracic echocardiographic apical four-chamber view showing mild tricuspid regurgitation (TR) by color Doppler. **B**, Apical four-chamber view showing a dilated right atrium (RA) and severe TR by color Doppler. *LA,* Left atrium, *LV,* left ventricle; *RV,* right ventricle.

parasternal or subcostal views (Fig. 34-19). The shape and density of the continuous wave Doppler spectral trace also provide information regarding the severity of regurgitation. Mild tricuspid regurgitation is associated with a soft and parabolic profile, whereas severe tricuspid regurgitation often has a dense and triangular profile. In cases of severe tricuspid regurgitation, the vena contracta (narrowest diameter of the color jet as it passes through the valve) width is greater than 0.7 cm, and evidence indicates systolic flow reversal in the hepatic veins (provided the patient is not in atrial fibrillation, in which this sign is not reliable). The hepatic veins are well visualized in the subcostal view and allow good alignment for pulsed wave Doppler (Table 34-9). In severe tricuspid regurgitation, the elevated right atrial pressure causes blood to flow back into the hepatic veins (Fig. 34-20).

■ PULMONARY VALVE

The pulmonary valve consists of three leaflets: anterior, right, and left. It is best seen in the parasternal short-axis view at the level of the aortic valve. Trace or physiologic pulmonary regurgitation is commonly observed in physiologically normal individuals.

Table 34-9 **Tips and Tricks in Assessment of Tricuspid Regurgitation**

Problem	Solution
Underestimation of eccentric jets	Careful assessment for tricuspid regurgitant jet in different views
Possible inaccuracy of systolic flow reversal in atrial fibrillation	Assessment of jet area and vena contracta
Severe tricuspid regurgitation associated with low velocity from equalization of pressure between right atrium and ventricle	Awareness that right ventricular systolic pressure may be significantly underestimated

Pulmonary Stenosis

Pulmonary stenosis in most cases is congenital and is often associated with other, more complex congenital heart lesions such as tetralogy of Fallot (Fig. 34-21, *A*). Rarely, pulmonary stenosis may be caused by infiltrative disease, earlier surgical procedures or interventions, or compression by an adjacent tumor or mass. Carcinoid is the most common cause of acquired pulmonary valve disease. In the parasternal short-axis view

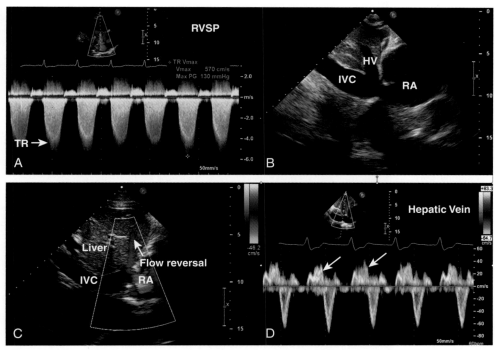

Figure 34-20 **A,** Continuous wave Doppler across the tricuspid valve. The peak velocity can be used to calculate the right ventricular systolic pressure (RVSP) by using the modified Bernoulli equation (pressure gradient = $4V^2$). Right atrial pressure is estimated from the assessment of inferior vena cava (IVC) size and the degree of inspiratory collapse. In this case, the RVSP was 150 mm Hg, indicating severe pulmonary hypertension. **B,** Subcostal view showing a dilated IVC and hepatic veins (HV). **C,** Subcostal view showing color Doppler of the HV. The blue flow indicates systolic flow reversal suggestive of severe tricuspid regurgitation (TR). **D,** Pulsed wave Doppler of the HV showing systolic flow reversal. The flow back into the HV is moving toward the ultrasound probe and so is displayed above the line on the Doppler trace *(arrows)*. *RA,* Right atrium.

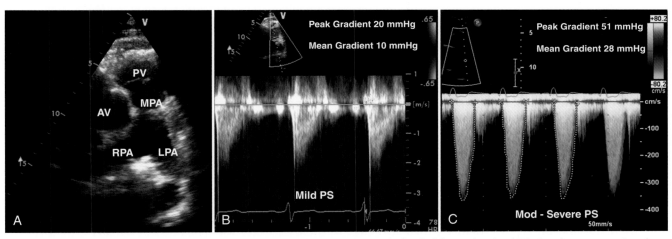

Figure 34-21 **A,** Transthoracic echocardiographic parasternal short-axis view, at the level of the aortic valve (AV), that shows a stenotic pulmonary valve (PV). *LPA,* Left pulmonary artery; *MPA,* main pulmonary artery; *RPA,* right pulmonary artery. Continuous wave Doppler in a patient with mild pulmonary stenosis (PS) **(B)** and moderate (Mod) to severe PS **(C).**

at the aortic valve level or in the subcostal short-axis view, continuous wave Doppler is used to obtain a peak and mean gradient (see Fig. 34-21, *B* and *C*). Pulsed wave Doppler may be used to determine the precise level of obstruction. As with aortic stenosis, Doppler derived peak gradients tend to be higher than peak-to-peak catheterization gradients in patients with pulmonary stenosis; however, unlike in aortic stenosis, the mean gradient is not commonly used in clinical practice (Table 34-10).

Table 34-10 Assessment of Pulmonary Stenosis

	Mild	Moderate	Severe
Peak velocity (m/sec)	<3	3-4	>4
Peak gradient (mm Hg)	<36	36-64	>64

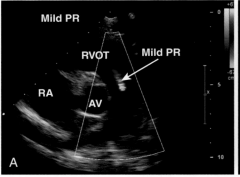
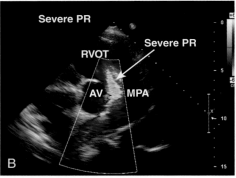

Figure 34-22 A, Transthoracic echocardiographic parasternal short-axis view, at the level of the aortic valve (AV), that shows mild pulmonary regurgitation (PR). **B,** Parasternal short-axis view of the pulmonary valve and main pulmonary artery (MPA) showing severe PR. *RA,* Right atrium; *RVOT,* right ventricular outflow tract.

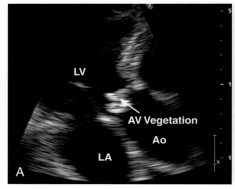
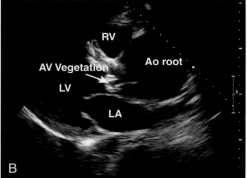

Figure 34-23 A, Transthoracic echocardiographic apical long-axis view showing a large vegetation on the aortic valve (AV). **B,** Parasternal long-axis view showing a vegetation on the AV and a markedly dilated aortic root (Ao root). *Ao,* Aorta; *LA,* left atrium; *LV,* left ventricle.

Pulmonary Regurgitation

As with tricuspid regurgitation, physiologic or trace pulmonary regurgitation is a normal finding, and jets are often eccentric (Fig. 34-22, *A*). The causes of pulmonary regurgitation are similar to those of tricuspid regurgitation and include infection (rheumatic disease, endocarditis), carcinoid, congenital defects, or conditions secondary to dilatation of the pulmonary artery (pulmonary hypertension). In clinical practice, the assessment of severity of pulmonary regurgitation is more qualitative than quantitative. Jet area is most commonly used to determine the severity of pulmonary regurgitation. The shape and density of the continuous wave Doppler spectral trace provide additional information regarding severity. Severe pulmonary regurgitation results in increased pulmonary artery flow, right ventricular volume overload, and progressive right ventricular dilatation (see Fig. 34-22, *B*).

■ ENDOCARDITIS

Echocardiography is an excellent imaging modality for the diagnosis and management of patients with endocarditis, for the following reasons:
- Identification of lesions at risk of endocarditis
- Detection of vegetations
- Assessment of complications and hemodynamics
- Serial evaluation
- Information regarding prognosis
    Vegetations are typically irregularly shaped echodensities that are independently mobile on echocardiography. TEE has a higher sensitivity (86% to 94%) and specificity

(88% to 100%) for the detection of vegetations; however, transthoracic echocardiography (TTE) is often adequate for the diagnosis of endocarditis (Figs. 34-23, 34-24, *A,* and 34-25). Vegetations as a rule are found on the ventricular side of the aortic valve and on the atrial side of the mitral valve. Tricuspid valve vegetations are often larger than left-sided lesions and are usually associated with intravenous drug abuse, indwelling catheters, or pacing leads. Large vegetations may also be seen in fungal endocarditis, which is more prevalent in immunocompromised patients. In the setting of endocarditis that does not respond to antimicrobial therapy, TEE may be indicated to look for evidence of an aortic root abscess (Fig. 34-26). In patients with aortic valve endocarditis, involvement of the conduction system, identified by a lengthening of the PR interval on the electrocardiogram, is particularly concerning for abscess formation, and these patients should be further evaluated with a TEE.
    Endocarditis is a serious infection, and complications occur in up to 40% of patients. Both TTE and TEE play an important role in assessing the risk and in detecting the following possible complications:
- Severe regurgitation (Figs. 34-27 and 34-28)
- Embolization (larger vegetations associated with a higher risk of embolization)
- Flail, aneurysmal, or perforated leaflet (see Fig. 34-27, *A*)
- Abscess formation (particularly associated with staphylococcal or enterococcal infection) (see Fig. 34-26)
- Fistula
- Dehiscence of prosthetic valve (both TTE and TEE usually required for adequate assessment of prosthetic valve)

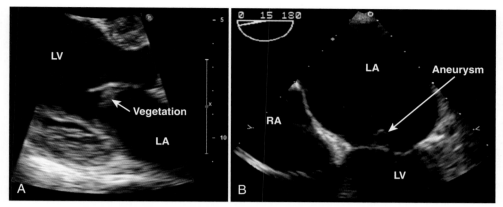

Figure 34-24 A, Transthoracic echocardiographic parasternal long-axis view, zoomed on the mitral valve, that shows a vegetation on the atrial side of the anterior mitral valve leaflet. **B,** Transesophageal echocardiographic midesophageal four-chamber view showing an aneurysm of the anterior mitral valve leaflet in a patient with endocarditis. Note the typical "wind sock" appearance of the aneurysm. *LA,* Left atrium, *LV,* left ventricle, *RA,* right atrium.

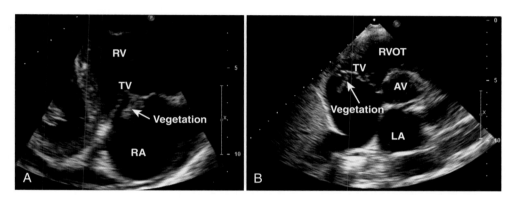

Figure 34-25 A, Transthoracic echocardiographic parasternal long-axis right ventricular inflow view showing a vegetation on the tricuspid valve (TV). **B,** Parasternal short-axis view at the level of the aortic valve (AV) that shows a vegetation on the TV. *LA,* Left atrium; *RA,* right atrium; *RV,* right ventricle; *RVOT,* right ventricular outflow tract.

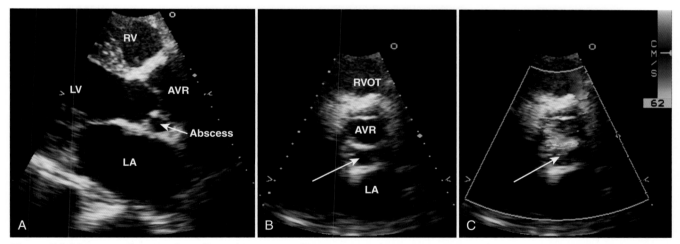

Figure 34-26 A, Transthoracic echocardiographic parasternal long-axis view showing an aortic root abscess in a patient with prosthetic aortic valve endocarditis. **B,** Parasternal short-axis view, at the level of the aortic valve, that shows the same echolucent space in the posterior aortic root with an abscess *(arrow).* **C,** Color flow Doppler showing flow within the echolucent space *(arrow). AVR,* Aortic valve replacement; *LA,* left atrium; *LV,* left ventricle; *RV,* right ventricle; *RVOT,* right ventricular outflow tract.

■ VALVE TUMORS

Papillary fibroelastomas are the second most common primary cardiac tumors in adults, and most of these tumors are attached to valves. Papillary fibroelastomas are typically small, homogenous tumors most commonly seen on the aortic valve (Fig. 34-29). They may be present on either surface of the aortic valve and often have a small stalk that makes them mobile. Tumors with a stalk are known to have a higher risk of embolization (Fig. 34-30). Papillary fibroelastomas attached to the mitral valve tend to be on the atrial side. Other less common locations for these tumors include the tricuspid and pulmonary valves, the right atrium and

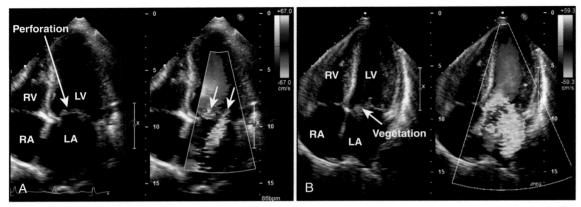

Figure 34-27 **A,** Transthoracic echocardiographic apical four-chamber view showing perforation of the anterior mitral valve leaflet associated with severe mitral regurgitation by color Doppler. The two separate jets of mitral regurgitation, central and through the perforation, are designated by *arrows* in the image on the *right*. **B,** Apical four-chamber view showing a vegetation on the anterior mitral valve leaflet associated with severe mitral regurgitation by color Doppler. *LA,* Left atrium; *LV,* left ventricle; *RA,* right atrium; *RV,* right ventricle.

Figure 34-28 **A,** Transesophageal echocardiographic midesophageal four-chamber view showing a calcified mass on the posterior mitral valve leaflet. The patient had a history of endocarditis, and the mass was thought to represent a healed vegetation. **B,** Color flow Doppler shows severe mitral regurgitation (MR). *LA,* Left atrium; *LV,* left ventricle; *RA,* right atrium; *RV,* right ventricle.

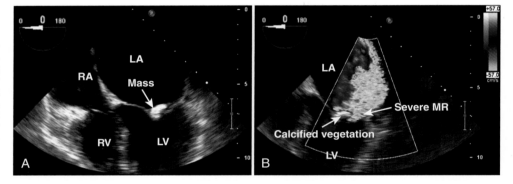

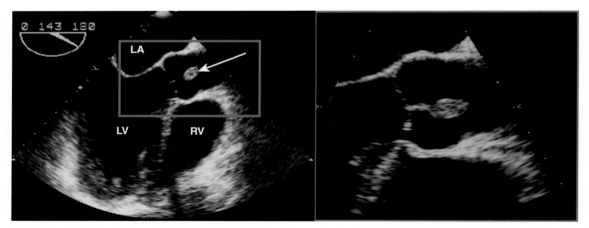

Figure 34-29 Transesophageal echocardiographic midesophageal long-axis view of the aortic valve that shows a papillary fibroelastoma attached to the aortic valve. *LA,* Left atrium; *LV,* left ventricle; *RV,* right ventricle.

ventricle, and, rarely, the interventricular septum or LVOT (see Fig. 34-16, *B*). Papillary fibroelastomas are often incidental findings, or they may be identified as a source of embolus in a patient presenting with a stroke. Asymptomatic patients with small (<1 cm) left-sided, nonmobile tumors are not usually referred for surgical treatment. Less common tumors are fibromyxosarcomas, which are highly malignant and are associated with a poor prognosis despite aggressive treatment (Fig. 34-31).

■ PROSTHETIC VALVES

Echocardiography is an excellent modality for the assessment of prosthetic valve function, although imaging can be challenging at times because of shadowing of the prosthesis and artifacts (Table 34-11). Normal opening and closing of the prosthetic valve must be ensured (see Fig. 34-4, *B*; Figs. 34-32 and 34-33). Abnormal rocking motion of the valve implies dehiscence. The velocity across a prosthetic valve is influenced by the position,

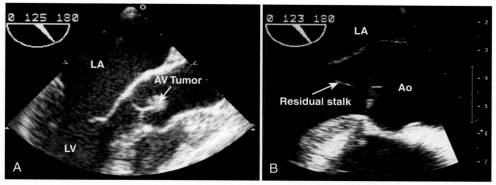

Figure 34-30 A, Transesophageal echocardiographic midesophageal long-axis view of the aortic valve (AV) that shows a papillary fibroelastoma attached to the AV. **B,** Midesophageal long-axis view of the AV in the same patient that shows a residual stalk following embolization of the tumor. Subsequent imaging with computed tomography showed the tumor occluding the ostium of the right coronary artery. *Ao,* Aorta; *LA,* left atrium; *LV,* left ventricle.

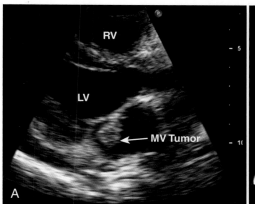 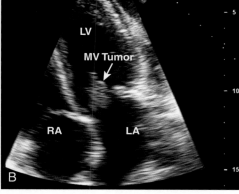

Figure 34-31 Mitral valve (MV) tumor seen in the transthoracic echocardiographic parasternal long-axis view (**A**) and transthoracic echocardiographic apical four-chamber view (**B**). This tumor was confirmed as a fibromyxosarcoma following surgical resection. *LA,* Left atrium; *LV,* left ventricle, *RA,* right atrium; *RV,* right ventricle.

Table 34-11   Tips and Tricks for Prosthetic Valves

Problem	Solution
Poor views on TTE from shadowing and/or artifacts	Modified views tried to reduce artifacts Use of TEE (especially for mitral valve prosthesis) Awareness of common artifacts with mechanical prosthetic valves
Misdiagnosis of aortic root abscess	Awareness aortic root may be thickened for ≤6 months postoperatively Comparison with intraoperative TEE
Underestimation of paravalvular regurgitation	Possible need for multiplanar TEE Use of three-dimensional TEE (can be helpful)
Difficulty in differentiating between pannus and thrombus	Attention to clinical history important (duration of symptoms, anticoagulation) Use of TEE imaging preferable Thrombus usually larger, with density similar to myocardium Thrombi associated with mitral prosthesis usually extending into left atrium or appendage Pannus more common in aortic prosthesis

TEE, Transesophageal echocardiography; *TTE,* transthoracic echocardiography.

type, and size of the valve. For all commercially available prosthetic valves, expected maximum velocities have been defined according to valve size. Therefore, the examiner must know the valve type and size when echocardiographic data are interpreted. As with native valves, continuous wave Doppler allows estimation of peak and mean gradients. Physiologic regurgitation is normal with prosthetic metallic valves, and characteristic patterns of washing jets are recognized for different valve types (Fig. 34-34, *B*). Pathologic regurgitation may be

central or paravalvular. As a general rule, central regurgitation is associated with bioprosthetic valves, whereas paravalvular regurgitation may be seen with both bioprosthetic and mechanical prosthetic valves (see Fig. 34-34; Fig. 34-35).

Complications of prosthetic valves may occur early or late and include infection, dehiscence, thrombosis, pannus formation, hemolysis from paravalvular leaks, and pseudoaneurysm formation. Endocarditis involving a prosthetic valve may result in significant regurgitation,

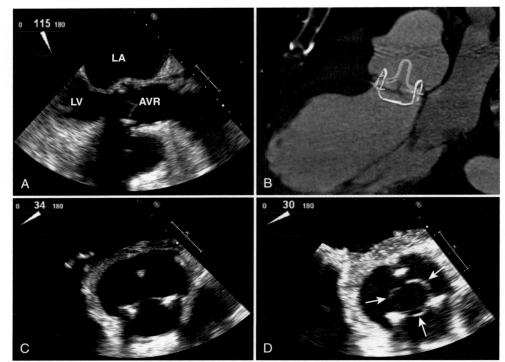

Figure 34-32 **A,** Transesophageal echocardiographic midesophageal long-axis view of the aortic valve showing a bioprosthetic aortic valve. *AVR,* Aortic valve replacement; *LA,* left atrium, *LV,* left ventricle. **B,** Computed tomography appearance of a bioprosthetic valve in the aortic position. Midesophageal short-axis view of a bioprosthetic aortic valve in diastole (**C**) and systole (**D**). The bioprosthetic leaflets are designated by *arrows.*

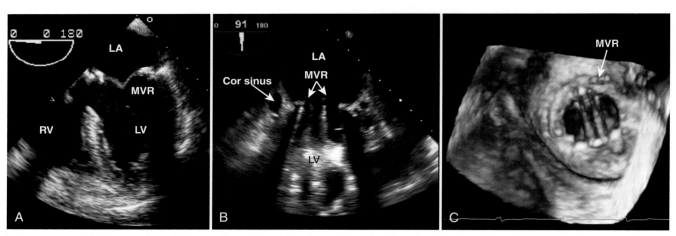

Figure 34-33 **A,** Transesophageal echocardiographic midesophageal four-chamber view showing a bioprosthetic mitral valve replacement (MVR). **B,** Midesophageal two-chamber view showing a mechanical prosthetic valve in the mitral position. Note the significant shadowing in the left ventricle (LV) as a result of the prosthesis. **C,** Midesophageal three-dimensional image of a bileaflet mechanical mitral valve prosthesis during diastole. *Cor,* Coronary; *LA,* left atrium; *RV,* right ventricle.

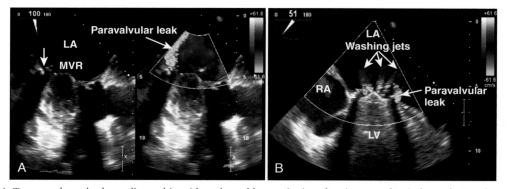

Figure 34-34 **A,** Transesophageal echocardiographic midesophageal long-axis view showing a mechanical prosthetic valve in the mitral position with evidence of a paravalvular leak by color Doppler. A small defect can be seen outside the sewing ring *(arrows).* **B,** Midesophageal four-chamber view showing a mechanical prosthetic valve in the mitral position. Color Doppler shows the normal washing jets; however, evidence of a paravalvular leak is also present. *LA,* Left atrium; *LV,* left ventricle; *MVR,* mitral valve replacement; *RA,* right atrium.

development of a shunt, or, in some cases, valve destruction. Echocardiography plays an important role in the diagnosis, management, and follow-up of patients with endocarditis. TTE and TEE are often helpful in cases of prosthetic valve endocarditis because anterior structures are often better visualized on TTE. Generally, TEE is superior for evaluation of mitral valve prosthesis and perivalvular abscesses in the posterior aortic root.

Current guidelines recommend TTE in the initial postoperative period to evaluate prosthetic valve function and to establish baseline gradients. Patients with prosthetic valves should also have a follow-up TTE study

3 years following surgical treatment to assess prosthetic valve function even if these patients are asymptomatic. Rising gradients usually indicate a degree of valve obstruction and require close examination of the prosthesis and surrounding structures (Fig. 34-36). The distinction between pannus ingrowth and thrombus can be extremely difficult. Clinical history and information regarding anticoagulation can be helpful in these cases. If prosthetic valve dysfunction is suspected, TEE should be considered to determine the mechanism and evaluate the degree of stenosis or regurgitation, if present. Pannus may be difficult to visualize but is more commonly seen in the aortic position, whereas thrombi tend to be larger and may extend into the surrounding chambers.

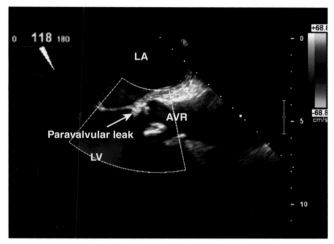

Figure 34-35 Transesophageal echocardiographic midesophageal long-axis view of the aortic valve that shows a prosthetic aortic valve with evidence of a trace posterior paravalvular leak by color Doppler. *AVR,* Aortic valve replacement; *LA,* left atrium; *LV,* left ventricle.

◼ RADIATION AND DRUG VALVULOPATHY

Radiation-induced valvulopathy may be seen in patients 10 to 15 years following radiation therapy. Because of their location, the aortic valve and anterior mitral valve leaflets are more likely to be affected. Valves may become thickened and fibrosed, resulting in regurgitation or stenosis.

In the 1990s, drugs such as fenfluramine and phentermine were implicated in causing significant valve disease in up to 33% of exposed patients. These drugs were subsequently removed from the market in 1997. Varying degrees of aortic and mitral regurgitation were observed in many of these patients, and a distinctive pattern of valve thickening was reported. Mild aortic regurgitation was the most common valve abnormality, and some studies reported regression of disease when the drug was discontinued.

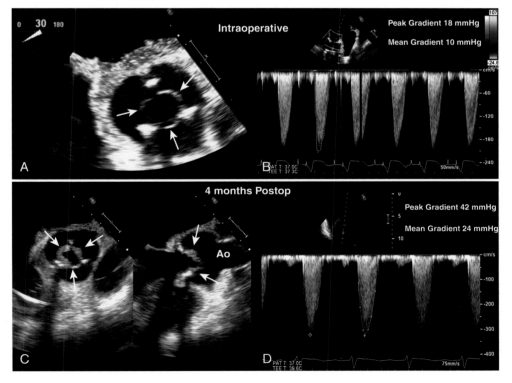

Figure 34-36 **A,** Transesophageal echocardiographic midesophageal short-axis view of the aortic valve that shows a normal bioprosthetic valve at the time of surgery. **B,** Continuous wave Doppler recording across the aortic bioprosthetic valve at the time of surgery that shows low gradients. **C,** Midesophageal short and long-axis views of the aortic bioprosthesis, 4 months postoperatively (Postop) that shows marked thickening of the leaflets *(arrows).* **D,** Continuous wave Doppler recording across the aortic bioprosthetic valve 4 months postoperatively that shows significantly higher trans–aortic valve gradients. The marked valve thickening was the result of endocarditis of the prosthetic valve, and the patient required further surgical intervention for definitive treatment. *Ao,* Aorta.

Bibliography

Allan LD, Desai G, Tynan MJ. Prenatal echocardiographic screening for Ebstein's anomaly for mothers on lithium therapy. *Lancet.* 1982;2:875-876.

Armstrong WF, Ryan R. *Feigenbaum's Echocardiography.* 7th ed. Philadelphia: Lippincott Williams & Wilkins; 2010.

Baumgartner H, Hung J, Bermejo J, et al. Echocardiographic assessment of valve stenosis: EAE/ASE recommendations for clinical practice. *J Am Soc Echocardiogr.* 2009;22:1-23.

Deluca G, Correale M, Ieva R, et al. The incidence and clinical course of caseous calcification of the mitral annulus: a prospective echocardiographic study. *J Am Soc Echocardiogr.* 2008;21:828-833.

Freed LA, Levy D, Levine RA, et al. Prevalence and clinical outcome of mitral valve prolapse. *N Engl J Med.* 1999;341:1-7.

Gussenhoven EJ, Stewart PA, Becker AE, et al. "Offsetting" of the septal tricuspid leaflet in normal hearts and in hearts with Ebstein's anomaly: anatomic and echographic correlation. *Am J Cardiol.* 1984;54:172-176.

Harpaz D, Auerbach I, Vered Z, et al. Caseous calcification of the mitral annulus: a neglected, unrecognized diagnosis. *J Am Soc Echocardiogr.* 2001;14:825-831.

Hoffman JIE, Kaplan S. The incidence of congenital heart disease. *J Am Coll Cardiol.* 2002;39:1890-1900.

Johri AM, Passeri JJ, Picard MH. Non-invasive imaging: three dimensional echocardiography: approaches and clinical utility. *Heart.* 2010;96:390-397.

Kitchiner D, Jackson M, Malaiya N, et al. Incidence and prognosis of obstruction of the left ventricular outflow tract in Liverpool (1960-91): a study of 313 patients. *Br Heart J.* 1994;71:588-595.

Levine RA, Stathogiannis E, Newell JB, et al. Reconsideration of echocardiographic standards for mitral valve prolapse: lack of association between leaflet displacement isolated to the apical four chamber view and independent echocardiographic evidence of abnormality. *J Am Coll Cardiol.* 1988;11:1010-1019.

Liu CW, Hwang B, Lee BC, et al. Aortic stenosis in children: 19-year experience. *Zhonghua Yi Xue Za Zhi(Taipei).* 1997;59:107.

Modlin IM, Sandor A. An analysis of 8305 cases of carcinoid tumors. *Cancer.* 1997;79:813-829.

Otto CM. *Textbook of Clinical Echocardiography.* 4th ed. Philadelphia: Saunders; 2009.

Pellikka PA, Tajik AJ, Khandheria BK, et al. Carcinoid heart disease: clinical and echocardiographic spectrum in 74 patients. *Circulation.* 1993;87:1188-1196.

Quiñones MA, Otto CM, Stoddard M, et al. Recommendations for quantification of Doppler echocardiography: a report. From the Doppler Quantification Task Force of the Nomenclature and Standards Committee of the American Society of Echocardiography. *J Am Soc Echocardiogr.* 2002;15:167-184.

Roberts WC. A unique heart disease associated with a unique cancer: carcinoid heart disease. *Am J Cardiol.* 1997;80:251-256.

Shiina A, Seward JB, Edwards WD, et al. Two-dimensional echocardiographic spectrum of Ebstein's anomaly: detailed anatomic assessment. *J Am Coll Cardiol.* 1984;3:356-370.

Sun JP, Asher CR, Yang XS, et al. Clinical and echocardiographic characteristics of papillary fibroelastomas: a retrospective and prospective study in 162 patients. *Circulation.* 2001;103:2687-2693.

Teramae CY, Connolly HM, Grogan M, et al. Diet drug-related cardiac valve disease: the Mayo Clinic Echocardiographic Laboratory experience. *Mayo Clin Proc.* 2000;75:456-461.

Wilkins GT, Weyman AE, Abascal VM, et al. Percutaneous balloon dilatation of the mitral valve: an analysis of echocardiographic variables related to outcome and the mechanism of dilatation. *Br Heart J.* 1988;60:299-308.

Wilson W, Taubert KA, Gewitz M, et al. Prevention of infective endocarditis: guidelines from the American Heart Association. A guideline from the American Heart Association Rheumatic Fever, Endocarditis, and Kawasaki Disease Committee, Council on Cardiovascular Disease in the Young, and the Council on Clinical Cardiology, Council on Cardiovascular Surgery and Anesthesia, and the Quality of Care and Outcomes Research Interdisciplinary Working Group. *Circulation.* 2007;116:1736-1754.

Zoghbi WA, Chambers JB, Dumesnil JG, et al. Recommendations for evaluation of prosthetic valves with echocardiography and Doppler ultrasound. *J Am Soc Echocardiogr.* 2009;22:975-1014.

Zoghbi WA, Enriquez-Sarano M, Foster E, et al. Recommendations for evaluation of the severity of native valvular regurgitation with two-dimensional and Doppler echocardiography. *J Am Soc Echocardiogr.* 2003;16:777-802.

CHAPTER **35**

Valves: Magnetic Resonance Imaging

Christopher M. Walker and Gautham P. Reddy

Echocardiography is the primary imaging method for the evaluation of patients suspected of having valvular dysfunction because this modality is relatively inexpensive, fast, and available in most hospitals. Its temporal resolution allows accurate depiction of valve morphology. However, echocardiography has limitations, including nondiagnostic or limited scans secondary to patient body habitus or emphysema, as well as interobserver variability of measurements of ejection fraction (EF) and valvular regurgitation.

Magnetic resonance imaging (MRI) is helpful to characterize valvular dysfunction further in certain patients. It is more accurate for quantifying ventricular mass and function, information that aids the cardiologist and surgeon in determining the appropriate timing of valvular surgery. Velocity encoded cine (VEC) phase contrast MRI allows highly accurate and reproducible quantification of regurgitant fraction in the setting of valvular insufficiency and pressure gradients across a valvular stenosis. In this chapter, the role of MRI in various conditions and diseases affecting the cardiac valves is explored (Box 35-1 and Table 35-1).

■ CLINICAL CONSIDERATIONS

Anatomy and Physiology

The four cardiac valves comprise two atrioventricular (mitral and tricuspid) and two semilunar (aortic and pulmonic) valves (Figs. 35-1 to 35-4). The aortic and mitral valves are adjacent and in fibrous continuity, whereas the pulmonic and tricuspid valves are separated by the muscular infundibulum of the right ventricle (Figs. 35-5 and 35-6).

Normal cardiac valves allow unidirectional unimpeded blood flow. If regurgitation or stenosis develops, the ventricle compensates with either dilatation or muscular hypertrophy. A cardinal rule of cardiology states that valvular regurgitation results in a dilated ventricle because of volume overload, whereas valvular stenosis results in a hypertrophied ventricle because of pressure overload. At first, these mechanisms compensate for the valvular abnormality, but over time, the ventricle eventually fails.

Clinical Pearl

Valvular regurgitation results in ventricular dilatation, and valvular stenosis results in ventricular hypertrophy.

■ SYSTEMATIC APPROACH TO VALVULAR ABNORMALITIES

Several questions are important to address in the imaging evaluation of the valves:
1. How does the valve look?
   Valve anatomy (unicuspid, bicuspid, tricuspid leaflets) (Fig. 35-7)
   Leaflet morphology (prolapsed, ruptured, fused, calcification, thickening, vegetation)
   Perivalvular abnormality (aneurysm, abscess)
   Valve cross-sectional area

BOX 35-1   Indications for Cardiac Valvular Magnetic Resonance Imaging

Assessment of severity of stenosis or regurgitation
Measurement of effects of volume overload on the heart and degree of myocardial hypertrophy
Assessment for complications of valvular endocarditis
Diagnosis and definition of valvular mass seen on echocardiography or computed tomography
Evaluation of postsurgical tetralogy of Fallot
Diagnosis of systolic anterior motion of the mitral valve and left ventricular outflow tract obstruction in hypertrophic cardiomyopathy

---

Table 35-1   Standard Cardiac Protocol for Valve Evaluation

Imaging View	Information Obtained
Longitudinal and perpendicular images through valve	Valve morphology and opening pattern
Outflow tract	Identification of stenosis or regurgitation
Cine four-chamber	Global cardiac wall motion
Phase contrast imaging perpendicular to valvular plane and proximal or distal to valve	Measurement of valvular gradient and construction of flow volume curves
Short axis	End-diastolic volume, end-systolic volume, and ejection fraction
Planimetry perpendicular to valve	Valve area
Late or delayed enhancement	Myocardial viability

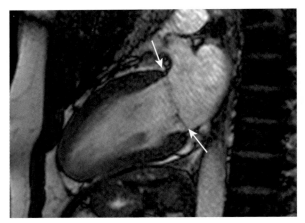

Figure 35-1 Normal mitral valve. Cine steady-state free precession vertical long-axis image shows a normal mitral valve *(arrows)*. Note the thin leaflets and lack of valve prolapse.

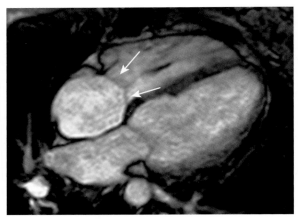

Figure 35-2 Normal tricuspid valve. Note the normal leaflet thickness *(arrows)*.

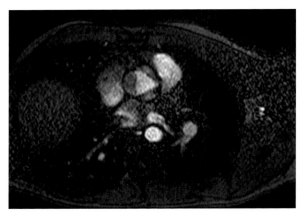

Figure 35-3 Normal aortic valve. Axial cine steady-state free precession image shows a normal three-leaflet aortic valve during systole. Note the lack of leaflet thickening and the normal valve opening.

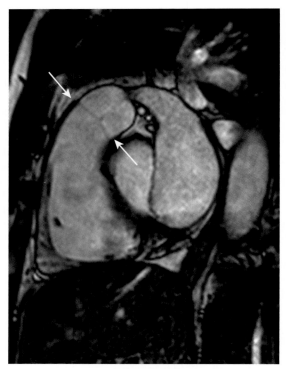

Figure 35-4 Normal pulmonary valve. Cine steady-state free precession right ventricular outflow tract image shows a normal pulmonary valve *(arrows)*.

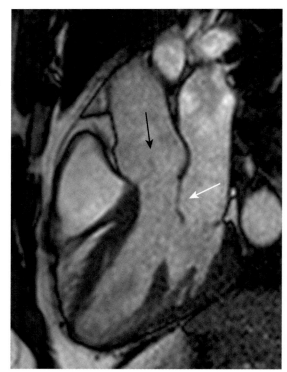

Figure 35-5 Aortic and mitral valve anatomy. Cine steady-state free precession left ventricular outflow tract image demonstrates close proximity of the mitral *(white arrow)* and aortic *(black arrow)* valves.

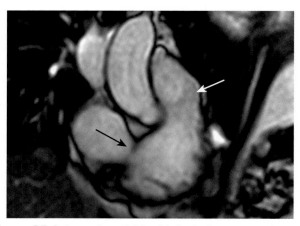

Figure 35-6 Separation of right-sided valvular structures by muscular infundibulum. Cine steady-state free precession right ventricular outflow tract image demonstrates separation of the tricuspid *(black arrow)* and pulmonary *(white arrow)* valves by a muscular infundibulum.

2. How does the valve function?
   Regurgitation or stenosis
   Opening and closing pattern
3. How does the valve affect cardiac function?
   EF and diastolic filling
   Wall motion
   Cardiac volumes
   Cardiac wall mass
4. Should additional points be addressed in the assessment of this particular valvular problem?
   Cardiac thrombus
   Coronary arterial disease
   Myocardial viability
   Associated conditions such as coarctation of the aorta with bicuspid aortic valve (Fig. 35-8)

■ REGURGITATION

Valvular regurgitation may have acute or chronic causes. Acute regurgitation is poorly tolerated, causes sudden and often severe symptoms, and is diagnosed primarily with echocardiography. It is rarely imaged with MRI. An example of a situation in which acute regurgitation is encountered is in the setting of mitral valve prolapse resulting from postinfarct papillary muscle rupture. This discussion focuses on chronic regurgitation.

Chronic mitral regurgitation is the most common valvular abnormality in industrialized countries. Its causes are myriad and include mitral valve prolapse, cardiomyopathies (ischemic, nonischemic, and hypertrophic obstructive [HCM]), rheumatic heart disease, and, rarely, left atrial myxoma. Mitral valve prolapse is the most common congenital cause of mitral regurgitation, characterized by myxomatous degeneration of the valvular apparatus without identifiable systemic connective tissue disease. It is defined by demonstration of leaflet bowing of greater than 2 mm beyond the valvular plane and by a maximal leaflet thickness greater than 5 mm (Figs. 35-9 to 35-11). Most patients with mitral regurgitation are asymptomatic until the development of atrial fibrillation, pulmonary hypertension, or ventricular failure.

Chronic aortic regurgitation is most often secondary to idiopathic degeneration and frequently occurs in conjunction with aortic stenosis. In patients less than 40 years old, Marfan syndrome with annuloaortic ectasia is the most frequent cause. Causes of aortic regurgitation are listed in Table 35-2. Symptoms secondary to aortic regurgitation include dyspnea, angina, and palpitations. Diagnosing aortic regurgitation before symptom onset is important because symptoms often herald the presence of irreversible left ventricular damage, a situation in which valvular replacement is no longer an effective treatment.

Pulmonary regurgitation and tricuspid regurgitation are most commonly associated with pulmonary arterial hypertension or congenital heart disease. Pulmonary regurgitation associated with repaired tetralogy of Fallot is a special situation and is described later. Patients are usually asymptomatic from these conditions unless regurgitation is severe. Severe pulmonic or tricuspid regurgitation manifests with symptoms of right ventricular failure, including ascites, fatigue, and lower extremity swelling.

Pathophysiology

Valvular regurgitation leads to a volume overload state in the heart. The body compensates with chamber dilatation that preserves the effective stroke volume and cardiac output initially. Over time, this adaptive response

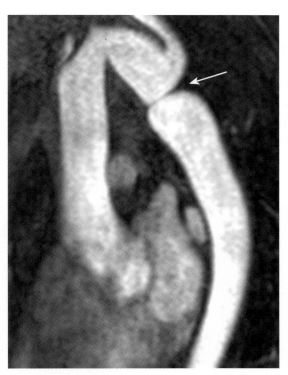

Figure 35-8 Coarctation of the aorta. Contrast-enhanced oblique sagittal magnetic resonance angiogram image through the aorta reveals narrowing *(arrow)* just distal to the takeoff of the left subclavian artery typical of coarctation. Velocity encoded cine phase contrast techniques can be used to measure the pressure gradient across the stenosis and collateral flow around the narrowing. Coarctation and pseudocoarctation are associated with a bicuspid aortic valve.

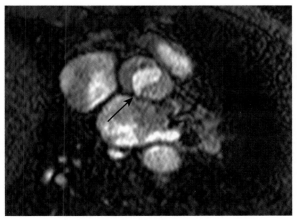

Figure 35-7 Axial turbo field echo image shows a bicuspid aortic valve *(arrow)*.

leads to irreversible ventricular damage or atrial dilation, resulting in symptoms.

Magnetic Resonance Imaging

Most patients have a diagnosis of valvular regurgitation before they present for cardiac MRI. Occasionally, regurgitation is identified during the imaging evaluation

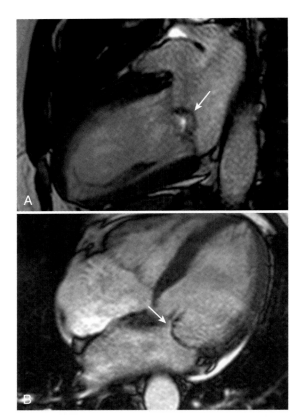

Figure 35-9 Myxomatous mitral valve prolapse. Cine steady-state free precession two-chamber (**A**) and four-chamber (**B**) views show prolapse of the posterior mitral valve leaflet *(arrows)* greater than 2 mm beyond the valvular plane. This patient had severe mitral regurgitation defined by a regurgitant fraction greater than 50%.

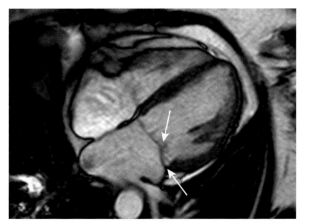

Figure 35-10 Mild mitral valve prolapse. Cine steady-state free precession four-chamber view shows mild mitral valve prolapse *(arrows)*.

for other indications, and the examiner must recognize the MRI appearance of a regurgitant valve. Currently, cine steady-state free precession (SSFP) is the primary technique used for the evaluation of cardiac valves. This sequence offers an excellent signal-to-noise ratio and high contrast between the blood pool and the myocardium. A disadvantage compared with cine fast gradient echo imaging is that a shorter echo time (TE) is used with SSFP. This disadvantage can be important because detection of a regurgitant flow jet depends on spin dephasing artifact secondary to turbulent flow. As the TE for the sequence decreases, turbulent flow from regurgitation has less dephasing artifact and creates less signal void. This issue is not necessarily significant in most patients undergoing valvular evaluation by MRI because they already carry a diagnosis of regurgitation.

Regurgitation shows a signal void directed away from the closed valve back into the chamber during diastole (Figs. 35-12 to 35-15). The size of the regurgitant jet is not an accurate quantifier of regurgitation because it

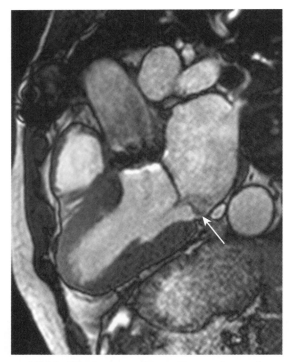

Figure 35-11 Mitral valve prolapse. Cine steady-state free precession left ventricular outflow tract image shows mitral valve prolapse defined by excursion of a mitral leaflet more than 2 mm beyond the valve orifice and myxomatous leaflet thickening *(arrow)*.

Table 35-2 Causes of Aortic Regurgitation

Leaflet Problems	Aortic or Annular Dilatation
Bicuspid aortic valve	Annuloaortic ectasia
Rheumatic valvular disease	Marfan syndrome
Myxomatous degeneration	Hypertension
Rheumatoid arthritis	Aortic aneurysm

varies with the TE value used in image acquisition and reflects turbulent blood flow and not the volume of regurgitation.

Clinical Pitfall

A TE value of less than 6 msec may not accurately depict a stenotic or regurgitant jet.

Quantification of Regurgitation in Patients With One Dysfunctional Valve

After identifying a regurgitant valve, the next step is quantification of the volume of regurgitation. This is accomplished with the use of either VEC MRI (the phase contrast technique) for direct quantification of retrograde diastolic flow or cine MRI to compare the stroke volumes of the two ventricles. In patients without regurgitation, the stroke volume of the right ventricle is equal to the stroke volume of the left ventricle. In patients with a single regurgitant valve, the difference in ventricular stroke volume is equal to the regurgitant volume. In any given patient, measurements using the two techniques can be compared, to serve as an internal control.

Quantification of Regurgitation in Patients With More Than One Dysfunctional Valve and Construction of a Flow Volume Curve

VEC MRI is the most widely used method to quantify regurgitation in patients with more than one regurgitant valve. The technique is similar for aortic and pulmonic regurgitation.

Velocity Encoded Cine Phase Contrast Technique

Information from the phase contrast sequence yields both magnitude and phase images. The velocity of flowing blood is encoded in each voxel, depicted in

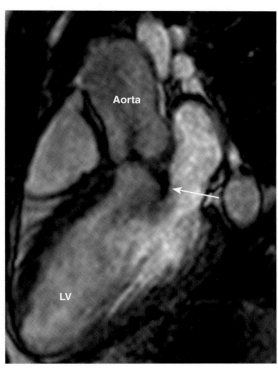

Figure 35-13 Aortic regurgitation. Cine steady-state free precession left ventricular outflow tract view during diastole shows a signal void *(arrow)* directed from the aortic valve into the left ventricle (LV), a finding indicative of aortic regurgitation.

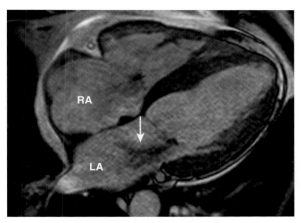

Figure 35-12 Mitral regurgitation. A signal void *(arrow)* emanates from the mitral valve into the left atrium (LA) during systole, a finding indicative of mitral regurgitation. *RA,* Right atrium.

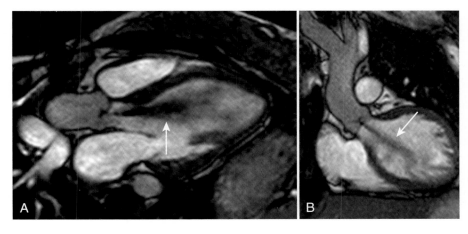

Figure 35-14 Aortic regurgitation. Cine steady-state free precession left ventricular outflow tract view (**A**) and oblique coronal view (**B**) obtained during diastole demonstrate a large signal void originating from the aortic valve directed into the left ventricle indicating aortic regurgitation *(arrows).*

grayscale on the phase images (Fig. 35-16). The magnitude images are a bright-blood gradient echo sequence used to define the anatomy and locate the vessel or outflow tract of interest. The vessel wall is a reference point for zero velocity, whereas flowing blood is depicted with varying degrees of white or black shading, depending on the velocity and direction of flow.

A region of interest (ROI) is drawn around the aorta or pulmonary artery perpendicular to flow and just superior to the valvular plane on each anatomic magnitude image. This ROI is then applied to the related phase image. Each voxel within the ROI has a specific encoded velocity (Venc) that is depicted by the corresponding grayscale value. The average velocity of the vessel of interest, measured just above the valvular plane, can be determined by measuring the cross-sectional area of the vessel; the product of vessel area and average mean velocity yields the flow volume for that particular frame of the cardiac cycle:

$$\text{Vessel area} \times \text{Average mean velocity} = \text{Flow volume}$$

This technique is applied over each frame of the cardiac cycle, and a flow volume curve is generated to represent flow over time during the cardiac cycle. Forward flow is depicted as flow above zero, whereas regurgitant flow is shown below the baseline (Fig. 35-17). Calculating the area outlined by the flow curve below the baseline yields the volume of regurgitation, and the area outlined by the curve above the baseline gives the volume of forward flow. Flow volume curves accurately determine the regurgitant fraction and have high interstudy reproducibility in patients with aortic or pulmonic regurgitation (Table 35-3).

Mitral regurgitation and tricuspid regurgitation are evaluated using slightly different methods because of the configuration of the valves and the multiple angles of the regurgitant flow. If only one valve is regurgitant, the difference between the right and left ventricular stroke volume calculated volumetrically with stacked short-axis images is equal to the volume of regurgitation. A useful

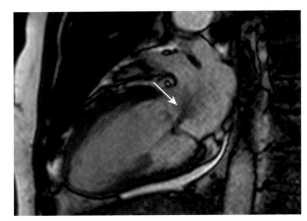

Figure 35-15 Ischemic mitral regurgitation. Cine steady-state free precession vertical long-axis view shows mitral regurgitation *(arrow)* and thinning of the left ventricular apex. In this patient with a history of multiple and recent myocardial infarctions, the regurgitation was deemed secondary to ischemia.

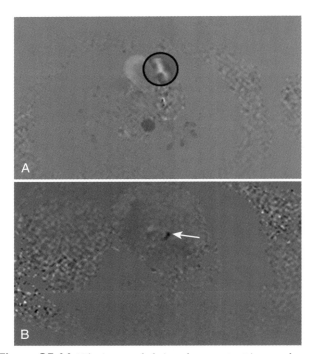

Figure 35-16 Velocity encoded cine phase contrast images show a bicuspid valve and aortic regurgitation. **A,** Phase contrast image during systole shows a bicuspid aortic valve *(black circle)* with forward flow depicted as white signal. **B,** Phase contrast image during diastole demonstrates regurgitant flow demonstrated by black signal *(arrow)*. The regurgitant fraction was 48%.

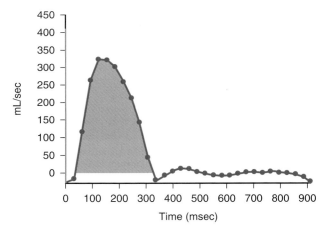

Figure 35-17 Normal aortic flow volume curve. Peak velocity obtained from phase images (not shown) was normal, measuring less than 2.0 m/second. The area above zero *(dark shaded area)* represents forward flow. During diastole, the forward flow stops.

Table 35-3 Grading Aortic Regurgitation

	Regurgitant Volume (mL)	Regurgitant Fraction (%)
Mild	<30	<30
Moderate	30-59	30-49
Severe	>60	>50

approach is to check this value internally with VEC phase contrast MRI as described later.

Two different methods using phase contrast MRI are available, and they are similar for the evaluation of mitral or tricuspid regurgitation; the aorta and left ventricle are assessed for mitral regurgitation, and the pulmonary artery and right ventricle are evaluated for tricuspid regurgitation. These methods hold in the absence of coexisting aortic or pulmonic regurgitation.

FIRST METHOD
1. An ROI is drawn around the proximal ascending aorta on the magnitude and phase VEC MRI images to determine forward flow.
2. Left ventricular stroke volume (end-diastolic volume minus end-systolic volume [EDV – ESV]) obtained from volumetric measurements is calculated.
3. Mitral regurgitant volume = Left ventricular stroke volume – Ascending aorta forward flow.
4. Mitral regurgitant fraction = Mitral regurgitant volume / Left ventricular stroke volume.

SECOND METHOD
1. An ROI is drawn around the mitral annulus to measure forward flow during diastole.
2. An ROI is drawn around the ascending aorta to determine forward flow during systole.
3. Mitral regurgitant volume = Forward flow mitral valve – Forward flow aorta.
4. Mitral regurgitant fraction = Mitral regurgitant volume/ Left ventricular stroke volume (Table 35-4).

Table 35-4 Grading Mitral Regurgitation

	Regurgitant Volume (mL)	Regurgitant Fraction (%)
Mild	<30	<30
Moderate	30-59	30-49
Severe	>60	>50

Clinical Pearl
A flow volume curve is derived from VEC phase contrast MRI and is useful for determining regurgitant fraction.

Cardiovascular Effects of Increased Volume

Ventricular mass and function are reliably documented using the cine SSFP technique. Contiguous short-axis images are acquired from the cardiac apex to the base of the heart in multiple phases of the cardiac cycle. When images are viewed as a cine loop, the examiner can assess global ventricular function and regional wall motion.

ESV and EDV are calculated using multislice short-axis images. ROIs are drawn around the ventricular cavity at end-systole and end-diastole and are multiplied by slice thickness and interslice gap to obtain ESV and EDV, respectively. ESV and EDV are used to calculate the EF (Fig. 35-18):

$$EF = (EDV - ESV) / EDV$$

Myocardial mass is measured with short-axis end-diastolic images obtained from the apex to the base of the heart. Myocardial volume is obtained by outlining the epicardial and endocardial surfaces from the base to the apex and multiplying this area by the slice thickness and interslice gap. Myocardial mass is the product of myocardial volume and the specific gravity of myocardium (1.05 g/mL):

$$Myocardial\ mass = Myocardial\ volume \times 1.05\ g\,/\,mL$$
$$(specific\ gravity\ of\ myocardium)$$

Boxes 35-2 and 35-3 provide a brief clinical overview of aortic and mitral regurgitation.

■ STENOSIS

Aortic stenosis, the most common valvular stenotic disease, affects 2% of the population that is more than 65 years old. When it occurs in older adults, aortic stenosis

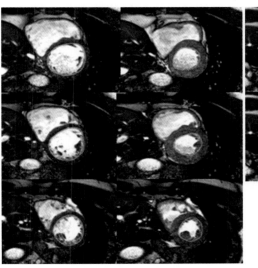
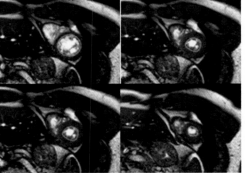

Figure 35-18 Calculation of left ventricular function. A region of interest *(green circle)* is drawn around the left ventricular cavity at end-diastole and end-systole for each anatomic level. The total volume at end-diastole and end-systole (all axial slices summed) is multiplied by the slice thickness to calculate end-diastolic volume (EDV) and end-systolic volume (ESV), respectively: Ejection fraction (EF) = (EDV – ESV) / EDV.

is most often secondary to calcific degeneration, whereas in younger individuals it is frequently related to congenital bicuspid aortic valve (Fig. 35-19). Less common causes of aortic stenosis are listed in Box 35-4. Symptoms secondary to aortic stenosis rarely occur unless the degree of stenosis is severe. Severe aortic stenosis is defined by a valvular systolic orifice area smaller than 1 cm^2, an aortic jet velocity greater than 4 m/second, and/ or a transvalvular gradient of more than 40 mm Hg. Critical stenosis is defined by an opening area of less than 0.7 cm^2. Severe stenosis is heralded by the onset of symptoms secondary to reduced cardiac output. Symptoms include angina, syncope, and dyspnea on exertion. When symptoms occur, valve replacement is usually indicated because survival without valve replacement is usually only 2 or 3 years after symptom onset (Table 35-5).

Mitral stenosis, which has a declining incidence in industrialized countries, is almost exclusively rheumatic in origin and is more commonly diagnosed in immigrant populations. Mitral stenosis dilates the left atrium and increases left atrial pressure; this increased pressure may cause atrial fibrillation. Patients can experience dyspnea and orthopnea secondary to pulmonary venous hypertension. Chronically elevated pulmonary pressures may eventually lead to right ventricular failure.

Grading of the severity of mitral stenosis is similar to that of aortic stenosis, with estimation of valve area and pressure gradient. The normal mitral valve is 4 to 6 cm^2 and has no significant valvular pressure gradient. Severe mitral stenosis is defined by a valvular area smaller than 1 cm^2 and a pressure gradient greater than 10 mm Hg (Table 35-6).

Pulmonic stenosis is a relatively uncommon congenital heart disease seen in isolation or in association with tetralogy of Fallot. Rare acquired causes include rheumatic fever and carcinoid syndrome. Mild or moderate pulmonic stenosis often causes no symptoms. Over time, chronic elevated pressure leads to right ventricular failure, and patients experience dyspnea, fatigue, and lower extremity edema.

Clinical Pearls

Severe aortic stenosis is defined by a valve area smaller than 1 cm^2, a peak aortic jet velocity greater than 4 m/second, or a transvalvular gradient of more than 40 mm Hg.

Aortic valve replacement is indicated if symptoms develop, when patients with moderate or severe stenosis undergo coronary artery bypass grafting, or occasionally in asymptomatic patients with severe or critical aortic stenosis.

BOX 35-2   What the Clinician Wants to Know: Aortic Regurgitation

1. Volume of regurgitation: regurgitant fraction quantified through phase contrast techniques and construction of a flow volume curve
2. Ejection fraction and ventricular volumes
3. Global ventricular function

BOX 35-3   What the Clinician Wants to Know: Mitral Regurgitation

1. Regurgitant fraction through phase contrast techniques
2. Cause of regurgitation: myxomatous valve and degree of valve prolapse, hypertrophic cardiomyopathy, tumor
3. Ventricular function, mass, and ejection fraction

BOX 35-4   Less Common Causes of Aortic Stenosis

Supravalvular stenosis (hourglass or diffuse narrowing)
Rheumatic valvular stenosis
Unicuspid valve
Subvalvular stenosis (thin membrane, thick fibromuscular ridge, diffuse tunnel-like obstruction)
Hypertrophic obstructive cardiomyopathy with asymmetric septal hypertrophy

---

Table 35-5   Grading Aortic Stenosis

	Maximal Jet Velocity (m/sec)	Valvular Area (cm^2)	Pressure Gradient (mm Hg)
Normal	<2.0	3.0-4.0	<5
Mild	2.0-3.0	1.6-2.9	5-24
Moderate	3.0-4.0	1.0-1.5	25-40
Severe	>4.0	<1.0	>40

Table 35-6   Grading Mitral Stenosis

	Valvular Area (cm^2)	Pressure Gradient (mm Hg)
Normal	4.0-6.0	0
Mild	1.6-3.9	<5
Moderate	1.0-1.5	5-10
Severe	<1.0	>10

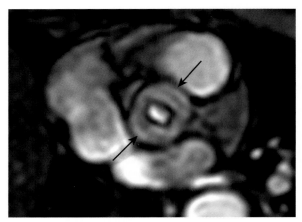

Figure 35-19 Bicuspid aortic valve. Cine steady-state free precession image demonstrates two leaflets *(arrows)* characteristic of a bicuspid aortic valve. This appearance has been likened to a fish mouth.

Severe mitral stenosis is defined by a transvalvular gradient greater than 10 mm Hg or a valve area of less than 1 cm^2.

Pathohysiology

The body counteracts valvular stenosis with myocardial hypertrophy, which reduces wall stress and compensates for reduced cardiac output. At first, this adaptation is beneficial. Over time, however, myocardial hypertrophy leads to congestive heart failure.

Identification

Poststenotic turbulent flow is represented by a signal void within the bright signal of moving blood. In aortic stenosis, the signal void is directed away from the valve into the ascending aorta (Figs. 35-20 to 35-22). Other valvular stenoses are similarly identified, with the signal void emanating from the valve into the receiving chamber or artery and away from the stenotic valve (Fig. 35-23).

Quantification

Quantification of valvular stenosis is important because surgical treatment is usually not performed until the stenosis is severe or the patient is symptomatic. Quantification can be accomplished in several ways using MRI.

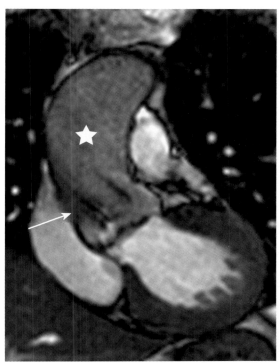

Figure 35-20 Severe aortic stenosis. Oblique coronal steady-state free precession image in systole shows a signal void *(arrow)* emanating from the aortic valve into the aorta, a finding indicating aortic stenosis. Note the ascending aortic enlargement *(star)*, which is commonly associated with valvular aortic stenosis.

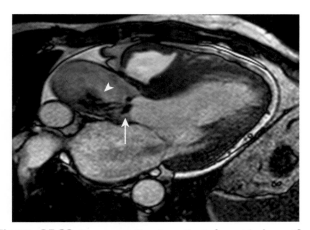

Figure 35-22 Severe aortic stenosis. Left ventricular outflow tract steady-state free precession image demonstrates a signal void *(arrowhead)* directed away from the aortic valve. The image also shows leaflet thickening *(arrow)*. Magnetic resonance imaging is used to assess the severity of aortic stenosis through phase contrast techniques with determination of the maximal jet velocity.

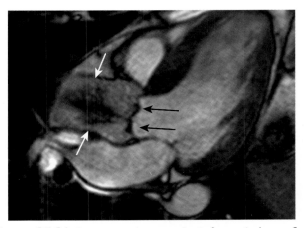

Figure 35-21 Severe aortic stenosis. Left ventricular outflow tract view demonstrates the typical findings of aortic valvular stenosis including leaflet thickening *(arrows)* and a signal void *(arrowheads)* emanating from the aortic valve into the ascending aorta. Severe aortic stenosis was diagnosed by velocity encoded cine phase contrast techniques with a transvalvular gradient of 63 mm Hg (not shown).

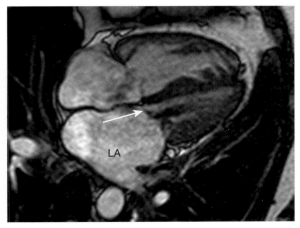

Figure 35-23 Mitral stenosis. The mitral valve leaflets are thickened *(arrow)*, the left atrium (LA) is dilated, and a signal void extends into the left ventricle, findings indicative of mitral stenosis. Mitral stenosis is usually secondary to rheumatic fever.

The most widely used method to calculate peak velocity across a stenosis is VEC phase contrast MRI (Fig. 35-24).

For aortic or pulmonic stenosis, an ROI is drawn around the aorta or pulmonary artery, just superior to the valvular plane and perpendicular to flow on both magnitude and corresponding phase images. After setting a Venc that is high enough to prevent aliasing, the phase contrast images are interrogated to determine the peak velocity. This peak velocity is used to determine the pressure gradient with use of the modified Bernoulli equation:

$$\Delta P = 4v^2$$

where ΔP is change in pressure across the valve and v = peak velocity in m/second.

For example, to calculate the pressure gradient for a peak velocity of 3 m/second:

$$\Delta P = 4v^2$$
$$\Delta P = 4\,(3)^2$$
$$\Delta P = 36 \text{ mm Hg}$$

Choosing too low a value for the Venc may result in aliasing and an artificially low peak velocity (Fig. 35-25).

Valve area can be directly measured by valve planimetry. Images are obtained perpendicular to the valve in a similar position to phase contrast measurements. Several valve areas are averaged at maximal opening to obtain the most accurate measurement (Fig. 35-26).

After quantifying valvular stenosis, the examiner must evaluate cardiac function, mass, and ventricular volumes as described in the earlier section on the cardiovascular effects of increased volume. These parameters are useful to the cardiologist and cardiac surgeon to determine the effectiveness of medical therapy and to guide timing of valvular replacement. MRI can also be used to demonstrate improvement in left ventricular function and reduction of left ventricular hypertrophy following valve replacement or other medical therapies (Box 35-5).

Clinical Pitfall
Too low a value for the Venc may cause aliasing and an artificially low peak velocity (see Fig. 35-25).

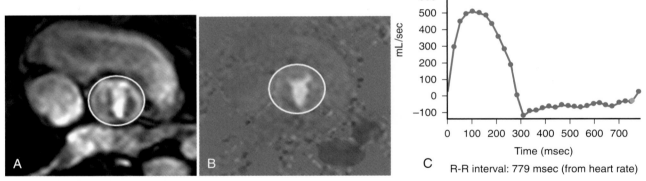

Figure 35-24 Velocity encoded cine phase contrast magnetic resonance imaging with flow volume curve. **A,** Axial magnitude image at end-systole shows a bicuspid aortic valve. The function of the magnitude image is to draw a region of interest (ROI) correctly around the aorta *(white circle).* The *white circle* is then applied to the corresponding phase image (**B**). **B,** The phase image encodes velocity, which is displayed as various shades of white and black. Peak velocity is interrogated within the ROI to calculate severity of aortic stenosis by using the modified Bernoulli equation. **C,** A flow volume curve is generated from the phase images obtained throughout the cardiac cycle. From the flow volume curve, the regurgitant flow and forward flow are obtained.

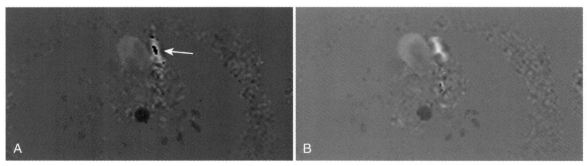

Figure 35-25 *Aliasing in pulmonic stenosis.* **A,** Velocity encoded cine phase contrast magnetic resonance imaging image obtained with an encoded velocity of 300 cm/second demonstrates aliasing identified by black signal within the surrounding white signal *(arrow)* in the proximal main pulmonary artery. **B,** An encoded velocity of 350 cm/second causes the internal black signal to disappear, thus indicating that 350 cm/second is the correct velocity setting.

■ SPECIAL SITUATIONS

Valve Assessment in Hypertrophic Obstructive Cardiomyopathy

HCM is an inherited condition responsible for one third of cases of sudden cardiac deaths in young athletes.

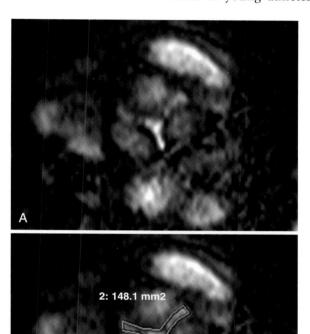

Figure 35-26 Moderate aortic valve stenosis diagnosed with planimetry. Axial turbo field echo image through the aortic valve during maximal opening shows a narrowed orifice (**A**) and a cross-sectional area of 1.48 cm² (**B**).

BOX 35-5   What the Clinician Wants to Know: Aortic Stenosis

1. Degree of stenosis: peak gradient measured by phase contrast techniques and maximal valve area by planimetry
2. Cardiac function: ejection fraction
3. Myocardial mass
4. Myocardial viability: to determine whether coronary artery bypass grafting is necessary at the same time of valve replacement

---

HCM often manifests with asymmetric septal hypertrophy, left ventricular outflow tract (LVOT) narrowing, and mitral regurgitation. LVOT narrowing is secondary to septal hypertrophy or systolic anterior motion (SAM) of the mitral valve leaflet. Patients with LVOT narrowing often present with exertional angina or syncope resulting from reduced cardiac output.

SAM is visualized on the cine four-chamber or LVOT (three-chamber) views and often causes a characteristic pattern of mitral regurgitation directed posteriorly into the left atrium. The cine LVOT view is helpful for the simultaneous demonstration of SAM, LVOT obstruction, and mitral regurgitation (Figs. 35-27 and 35-28). VEC phase contrast MRI techniques are able to quantify the volume of mitral regurgitation and the severity of aortic outflow tract stenosis.

Patients with symptomatic LVOT stenosis or a pressure gradient of more than 30 mm Hg may benefit from ethanol ablation, myotomy, or myomectomy of the hypertrophied septum. Posttreatment MRI readily demonstrates improvement in outflow tract stenosis and documents delayed hyperenhancement in the area treated by ethanol ablation.

Clinical Pearls

Phase contrast MRI can be used to quantify aortic outflow tract stenosis and mitral regurgitation in HCM.

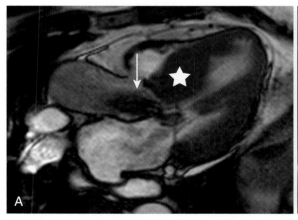
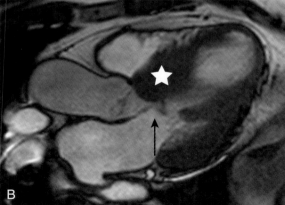

Figure 35-27 Hypertrophic cardiomyopathy (HCM) with subaortic stenosis and systolic anterior motion (SAM). **A,** Cine steady-state free precession left ventricular outflow tract (LVOT) image shows a hypertrophied interventricular septum *(star)* characteristic of HCM. Narrowing of the LVOT with a signal void *(arrow)* directed into the aorta indicates subaortic stenosis. **B,** Image obtained in early systole shows anterior motion of the mitral leaflet *(arrow)* also known as SAM. *Star,* Hypertrophied interventricular septum.

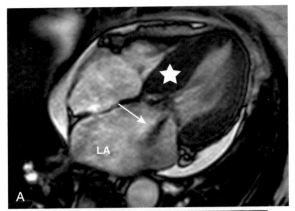

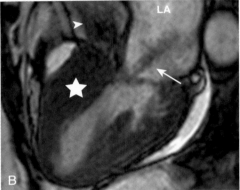

Figure 35-28 Hypertrophic cardiomyopathy with systolic anterior motion. Cine steady-state free precession four-chamber (**A**) and left ventricular outflow tract (**B**) views show a signal void directed retrograde into the left atrium originating from the mitral valve indicative of mitral regurgitation *(arrows)*. Note the hypertrophied septum *(stars)* and a flow void jet of aortic stenosis *(arrowhead)*. Incidentally noted is a small pericardial effusion. *LA,* Left atrium.

MRI accurately delineates infarcted myocardium in patients after alcohol ablation of the hypertrophied septum.

Valvular Evaluation After Surgical Repair of Tetralogy of Fallot

Pulmonary valve regurgitation is a common finding in patients after repair of tetralogy of Fallot. Most patients lead uneventful lives after repair of this defect until the third postoperative decade, when mortality and morbidity increase. During this time, patients who experience severe pulmonic regurgitation have increased rates of exercise intolerance, heart failure, arrhythmias, and sudden cardiac death. These symptoms are thought to be secondary to the effect of chronic right ventricular volume overload that leads to right ventricular dysfunction and arrhythmias (Fig. 35-29).

MRI plays a leading role in detecting and quantifying pulmonary valve regurgitation, and VEC phase contrast techniques can be used for direct measurement of the regurgitant fraction (Fig. 35-30). MRI plays a key role in depicting the morphologic and functional effects on the right ventricle, thereby guiding the surgeon in the appropriate timing of valve replacement. A pulmonic regurgitant fraction greater than 40% is considered severe in patients after repair procedures.

The goals of imaging in patients with tetralogy of Fallot include the following:

1. Quantification of pulmonic and tricuspid regurgitation
2. Demonstration of postsurgical anatomy with regard to the pulmonary arteries, right ventricular outflow tract, and systemic-to-pulmonary arterial collateral vessels
3. Quantification of right ventricular volume, mass, and EF (Fig. 35-31)
4. Evaluation for wall motion abnormalities
5. Assessment of myocardial viability with respect to areas separate from previous surgical scar

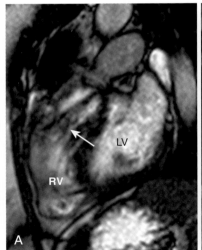

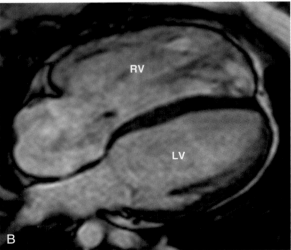

Figure 35-29 Pulmonary regurgitation in tetralogy of Fallot. Cine steady-state free precession right ventricular outflow tract view (**A**) and four-chamber view (**B**) show typical findings of pulmonary regurgitation in a patient who underwent repair of tetralogy of Fallot. A signal void *(arrow)* is directed into the dilated right ventricle (RV) from the pulmonary valve. *LV,* Left ventricle.

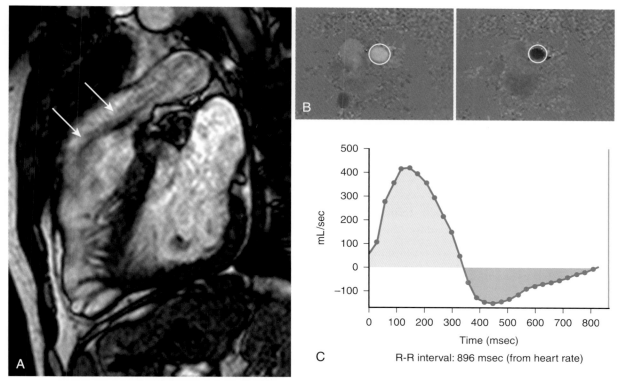

Figure 35-30 Severe pulmonary regurgitation in a patient post repair of tetralogy of Fallot. **A,** Cine steady-state free precession right ventricular outflow tract image demonstrates a signal void *(arrows)* directed into an enlarged right ventricle originating from the pulmonary valve, a finding indicating pulmonary regurgitation. **B,** Velocity encoded cine phase contrast images of pulmonary regurgitation *(white circles)*. The *left image* shows forward flow depicted as white pixels, and the *right image* shows regurgitant flow as black pixels. The software is then able to construct a flow volume curve from the multiple images obtained during the cardiac cycle. **C,** Flow volume curve of pulmonary regurgitation. The area above zero *(pale shading)* represents forward flow, whereas the area below zero *(dark shading)* represents regurgitant flow. The regurgitant fraction in this case measured 48%. Cardiac magnetic resonance imaging is an ideal method to measure pulmonary regurgitant fraction and its effects on right ventricular function in patients who have undergone repair of tetralogy of Fallot. A patient with a regurgitant fraction of greater than 35% can be considered for valvular replacement in the setting of right ventricular dysfunction or symptoms.

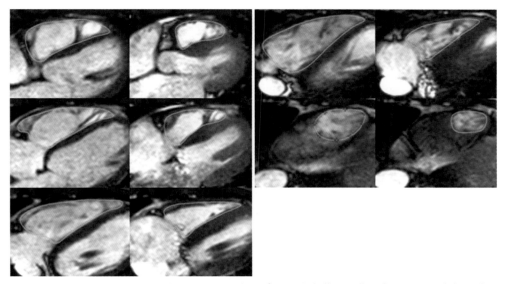

Figure 35-31 Calculation of right ventricular function. A region of interest *(yellow oval)* is drawn around the right ventricular cavity at end-diastole *(left images)* and end-systole *(right images)* for each anatomic level. The total volume at end-diastole and end-systole (all axial slices summed) is multiplied by the slice thickness to obtain end-diastolic volume (EDV) and end-systolic volume (ESV), respectively. Ejection fraction (EF) = (EDV – ESV) / EDV.

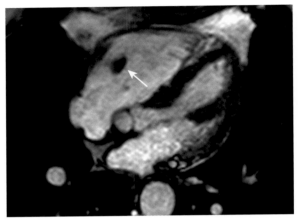

Figure 35-32 Tricuspid valve endocarditis. Cine steady-state free precession four-chamber image shows a mass *(arrow)* involving the tricuspid valve. No contrast enhancement occurred (not shown). This mass, which was thought to represent a vegetation from endocarditis in this intravenous drug user, resolved on follow-up imaging after antibiotics. The main differential diagnostic consideration was a thrombus, which also does not exhibit contrast enhancement.

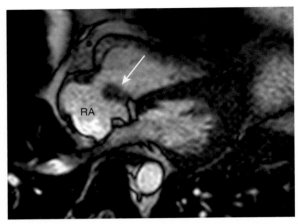

Figure 35-34 Tricuspid valve thrombus. Cine steady-state free precession four-chamber view shows a mass *(arrow)* involving the tricuspid valve. No enhancement occurred (not shown), and serial examinations showed resolution of the mass with anticoagulation. An additional diagnostic consideration for a nonenhancing mass includes vegetation related to infective endocarditis. *RA*, Right atrium.

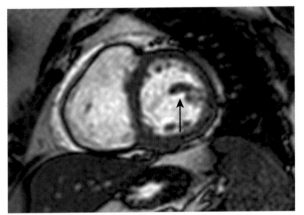

Figure 35-33 Mitral valve thrombus. Cine steady-state free precession short-axis image shows an isointense mass *(arrow)* involving the posterior mitral valve leaflet. No contrast enhancement occurred (not shown). This mass was clinically believed most likely to represent a thrombus, rather than a vegetation related to endocarditis.

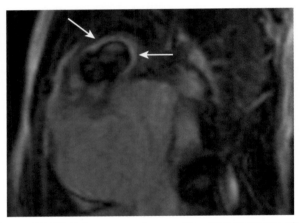

Figure 35-35 Pulmonary valve papillary fibroelastoma. Right ventricular outflow tract inversion recovery postgadolinium image shows a low-intensity mass attached to the pulmonary valve with peripheral delayed enhancement *(arrows)*. Unlike this case, most papillary fibroelastomas are less than 1 cm in size and occur on the left-sided valves. (Courtesy of Greg Kiscka, MD.)

Clinical Pearl

MRI can be used for the serial monitoring of regurgitant fraction and its effects on right ventricular function in postsurgical tetralogy of Fallot to determine the optimal timing of pulmonary valve replacement.

Appraisal of Valvular Masses and Endocarditis

Most valvular masses are not neoplasms but rather are vegetations related to endocarditis or thrombi. MRI of these lesions depicts an irregularly shaped mass with intermediate T2 signal intensity (Figs. 35-32 to 35-34). These diagnoses can be distinguished from valvular tumors with the use of gadolinium chelate contrast agent. Valvular thrombus and vegetations are characterized by lack of enhancement, whereas cardiac tumors demonstrate enhancement. Valvular vegetations and thrombus are often differentiated when clinical history is taken into account.

Complications of valvular endocarditis include regurgitation, pseudoaneurysm, fistula, and perivalvular or myocardial abscess. These complications can be readily and accurately diagnosed with MRI. A perivalvular abscess is best identified by a T2 bright fluid collection around the valve, with perilesion enhancement following administration of contrast agent.

Papillary fibroelastoma is rare, but it is the most common valvular tumor and the second most common primary cardiac neoplasm in adults. Although patients are generally asymptomatic, when symptoms are present, they are typically related to thromboembolism. Surgical treatment is curative. Tumors predominate on left-sided valves, usually the aortic

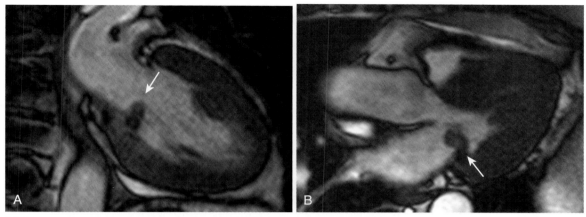

Figure 35-36 Degenerating calcified mitral valve myxoma. Two-chamber (**A**) and left ventricular outflow tract (**B**) cine steady-state free precession images show a mass *(arrows)* involving the posterior aspect of the mitral valve annulus. This mass displayed mild enhancement on postgadolinium images, as well as calcification on a computed tomography examination (not shown). It was presumed to be caseous necrosis of the mitral valve annulus; however, on pathologic examination, it was found to be a degenerating mitral valve myxoma. This is a rare location for a myxoma, which most commonly is attached to the left atrial side of the interatrial septum.

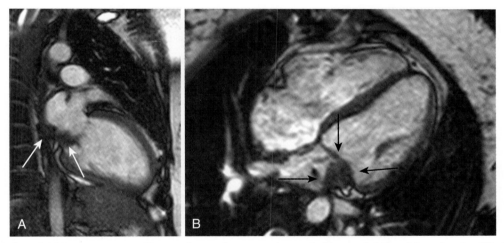

Figure 35-37 Left atrial leiomyosarcoma. Cine steady-state free precession vertical long-axis (**A**) and four-chamber (**B**) views show a mass *(arrows)* involving the posterior aspect of the left atrium and mitral valve annulus. It demonstrated contrast enhancement (not shown), thus distinguishing it from thrombus and vegetation. At surgical intervention, it was diagnosed as a leiomyosarcoma.

valve. Papillary fibroelastoma is typically less than 1 cm in size, has a low T2 signal on SSFP sequences, and enhances with contrast administration, an important distinguishing characteristic from thrombus and vegetations. This tumor tends to be connected to the valve by a thin stalk and is most frequently encountered on the aortic side of the aortic valve or on the atrial side of the mitral valve. The delayed gadolinium hyperenhancement technique has been used to identify these tumors (Fig. 35-35). Other primary and metastatic tumors may rarely involve the cardiac valves (Figs. 35-36 to 35-39).

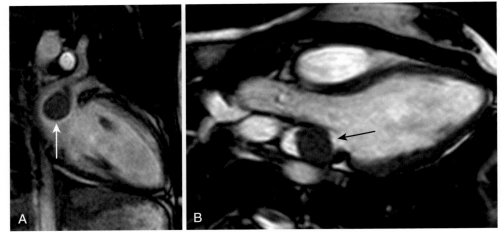

Figure 35-38 Pedunculated metastatic sarcoma. Cine steady-state free precession vertical long-axis (**A**) and left ventricular outflow tract (**B**) images show a pedunculated mass *(arrow)* abutting the mitral valve.

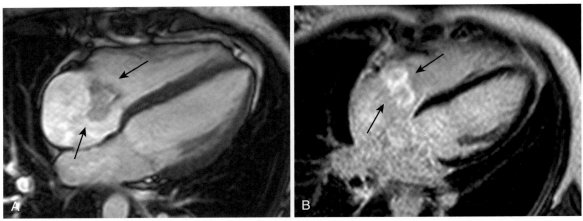

Figure 35-39 Tricuspid valve hemangioma. A, Cine steady-state free precession four-chamber view shows a mass *(arrows)* involving the tricuspid valve. **B,** Postcontrast inversion recovery image shows delayed enhancement *(arrows)*. Differential diagnostic considerations include papillary fibroelastoma and metastatic disease.

Bibliography

Geva T. Repaired tetralogy of Fallot: the roles of cardiovascular magnetic resonance in evaluating pathophysiology and for pulmonary valve replacement decision support. *J Cardiovasc Magn Reson.* 2011;13:9.

Glockner JF, Johnston DL, McGee KP. Evaluation of cardiac valvular disease with MR imaging: qualitative and quantitative techniques. *Radiographics.* 2003;23:e9.

Hansen MW, Merchant N. MRI of hypertrophic cardiomyopathy. Part I. MRI appearances. *AJR Am J Roentgenol.* 2007;189:1335-1343.

Masci PG, Dymarkowski S, Bogaert J. Valvular heart disease: what does cardiovascular MRI add? *Eur Radiol.* 2008;18:197-208.

Morris MF, Maleszewski JJ, Suri RM, et al. CT and MR imaging of the mitral valve: radiologic-pathologic correlation. *Radiographics.* 2010;30:1603-1620.

Vogel-Claussen J, Pannu H, Spevak PJ, et al. Cardiac valve assessment with MR imaging and 64-section multi-detector row CT. *Radiographics.* 2006;26:1769-1784.

CHAPTER 36

Valves: Computed Tomography

Daniel W. Entrikin

Shortly after the development of computed tomography (CT) in the early 1970s, great interest was expressed in applying this technology to imaging of the heart. In fact, less than a decade after Sir Godfrey Hounsfield developed the first CT scanner, he speculated about the future potential of his creation to be used as a tool for imaging the heart by synchronizing image acquisition with the diastolic phase of an electrocardiogram (ECG) tracing. In the late 1970s and early 1980s, some investigators were able to demonstrate the utility of both nongated and ECG-gated CT scans for evaluation of cardiac structure, myocardial perfusion, myocardial infarction, intracardiac masses, bypass graft patency, and pericardial diseases. However, the poor temporal and spatial resolution of early CT scanners was a major limiting factor that prevented routine use of CT in evaluation of cardiac disease. With the advent of electron beam CT (EBCT) in the 1980s, the potential clinical use of CT technology for assessment of cardiac disease was once again demonstrated for coronary calcium scoring, although the high cost of EBCT scanners and their limited utility for other imaging prevented their widespread use. Ultimately, in the early 1990s, a combination of slip-ring gantry technology and multidetector arrays led to the development of the first multidetector CT (MDCT) scanners capable of helical scanning at subsecond gantry rotation speeds.

When the first four-channel MDCT scanners were produced in 1998, a new era of cardiac imaging dawned, as many investigators employed ECG gating, rapid infusion of iodinated contrast material, and this new MDCT technology to perform the first cardiac computed tomography angiography (CTA) examinations. However, it was not until the development and widespread use of 64-channel MDCT scanners that clinical application of cardiac CTA became routine. Since that time, scanner manufacturers have diverged in their pursuit of the optimal cardiac CT scanner. Contemporary scanners offer a wide range of options that may include the following: large detector arrays that provide enough z-axis coverage to encompass the entire heart at one time; rapidly spinning gantries sometimes with multiple x-ray sources and detector arrays to improve temporal resolution; thinner detector elements and rapid focal spot modulation to improve spatial resolution in x-, y-, and z-axes; dual energy scanning capabilities that may reduce artifacts from calcium and offer promise of potential tissue characterization; and an ever increasing variety of iterative reconstruction algorithms to reduce image noise, improve image quality, and allow for substantial radiation dose reduction. Given the fast pace of advances in computer and CT technology, future applications of cardiac CTA seem limited only by imagination and ingenuity.

■ KEY CHALLENGES IN EFFECTIVE VALVE IMAGING WITH CARDIAC COMPUTED TOMOGRAPHY ANGIOGRAPHY

At present, direct assessment of blood flow or other hemodynamic information in a cardiac CTA examination is not possible. When compared with echocardiography and cardiac magnetic resonance imaging (MRI), the temporal resolution of cardiac CTA is substantially lower, particularly with a single source scanner. Cardiac CTA requires relatively low and regular heart rates and is therefore of limited value in patients with tachycardia or arrhythmias. Valve imaging with cardiac CTA also requires intravenous administration of iodinated contrast material, which carries some inherent risks to individuals with renal insufficiency, as well as a low risk of contrast reaction. Additionally, although significant progress has been made in reducing radiation exposure associated with cardiac CTA examinations by utilizing prospective triggering, high-pitch helical technique, advanced iterative reconstruction algorithms, limiting z-axis coverage, and customizing tube voltage (expressed in kilovolts [kV]) and tube current (expressed in milliamperes [mA]) settings for individual patients based on body mass index (BMI), retrospectively gated multiphase cardiac CTA examinations continue to result in relatively high radiation exposures to patients even with contemporary scanners. Because of these limitations, one could assume that cardiac CTA would have little value in the assessment of valvular function. However, cardiac CTA has several advantages that can be exploited to make it a useful alternative for valvular imaging when other first-line imaging modalities yield incomplete or conflicting results. In addition to being noninvasive, rapid, readily available, and easily tolerable, cardiac CTA has several fundamental strengths. These strengths include excellent spatial resolution (now as low as 0.3-mm isotropic voxel resolution), accurate depiction of calcification (which can be difficult to identify on cardiac MRI and can cause extensive artifacts on echocardiography), and the generation of true three-dimensional (3-D) or four-dimensional (4-D) data sets that allow thorough interactive assessment by the interpreting physician after the scan has been completed. As a result of these strengths, cardiac CTA offers an exceptional *anatomic* assessment of the structure and function of cardiac valves. In the setting of valvular dysfunction, this anatomic information derived from cardiac CTA can often accurately predict the hemodynamic effects of valvular lesions on blood flow. Therefore, optimizing scan protocols, injection protocols, and image postprocessing techniques is critically important, to ensure that accurate anatomic assessment of valves is achieved with each cardiac CTA examination.

Adjusting Scan and Injection Protocols to Ensure Optimal Image Acquisition

In general terms, optimization of cardiac CTA protocols for imaging heart valves is similar to optimization for evaluation of the coronary arteries. High temporal, spatial, and contrast resolution and low image noise are all of critical importance. However, heart valves are even more highly mobile and dynamic structures than are coronary arteries, and valves may be dysfunctional during systole, diastole, or both. Therefore, if a full functional assessment of a particular valve is desired, the heart must be imaged throughout the entire cardiac cycle (i.e., retrospective gating must be used while imaging through both systole and diastole). Additionally, when optimal visualization of the valve during systole is required, ECG-based tube current modulation is not recommended because the drop in tube current during systole results in increased image noise (so-called quantum mottle) and decreases diagnostic accuracy. Because of these requirements, cardiac CTA protocols to image the heart valves tend to result in higher radiation exposure to patients, given that the only means to reduce dose effectively are limited to BMI-based protocol modifications of kilovoltage and milliamperage. Newer scanners employing iterative reconstruction algorithms may further facilitate the acquisition of images at lower kilovoltage and milliamperage for any given BMI range. Because this technology is likely to continue to improve in the future, the use of cardiac CTA imaging for assessment of myocardial and valvular function should become more acceptable in terms of radiation exposure to patients.

Depending on the valve of interest, both bolus length and bolus timing must be adjusted to ensure optimal and uniform opacification of the blood pool surrounding the valve. Complete and uniform opacification of the blood pool with iodinated contrast material ensures the best delineation of delicate valvular structures, whereas poorly or heterogeneously opacified blood can blur discrimination of valvular structures from the adjacent blood pool. Because specifics of bolus length and timing vary extensively from one cardiac CTA laboratory to another, detailed instructions are not practical. However, the following suggestions may help to optimize visualization of the heart valves with cardiac CTA:

- For imaging the aortic valve, typical bolus length and image acquisition timing used for the coronary arteries are usually sufficient. However, if the patient has known severe aortic regurgitation (AR), elongation of the typical bolus and delay of image acquisition by 2 to 4 seconds will help to ensure optimal opacification of the blood pool around the aortic valve. In the setting of AR, mixing of blood that occurs at the level of the left ventricular outflow tract (LVOT) results in a delay to peak attenuation and thus necessitates this longer bolus and increased delay.

- For imaging the mitral valve, typical bolus length and image acquisition timing used for the coronary arteries are also usually sufficient. However, if the patient has known AR or mitral regurgitation (MR), elongation of the typical bolus and delay of image acquisition by 2 to 4 seconds may allow sufficient time for complete opacification of the blood pool within both the left ventricle and left atrium surrounding the mitral valve.

- For imaging the pulmonic valve, elongation of the typical bolus by 4 to 6 seconds without any change in image acquisition usually ensures optimal opacification of the blood pool surrounding the pulmonic valve while still allowing excellent evaluation of the coronary arteries.

- Because of the rapid inflow of unopacified blood from the inferior vena cava that which mixes violently with the opacified blood from the superior vena cava, to expect uniform opacification of blood in the region of the tricuspid valve is not reasonable. Therefore, consistent and accurate assessment of the tricuspid valve by cardiac CT is not always feasible.

Optimizing Image Postprocessing for Analysis

High temporal resolution is important for accurate valve imaging. Although the fundamental temporal resolution of a CT scanner cannot be significantly altered by the user (with the exception of selection of single segment versus multisegment reconstruction algorithms), the reconstruction window can be varied to allow for greater segmentation of valvular motion throughout the cardiac cycle. For most modern single source CT scanners, temporal resolution is roughly between 150 and 220 msec when a single segment reconstruction algorithm is used. For dual source CT (DSCT) scanners and single source CT scanners using a multisegment reconstruction algorithm, temporal resolution is lower than 100 msec. Although reconstructing 10 sets of images throughout the cardiac cycle (e.g., 10% increments from 5% to 95% of the R-R interval) has become routine, by reconstructing a greater number of phases throughout the cardiac cycle, a finer discrimination of valvular motion can be achieved. For example, assume a heart rate of 60 beats/minute during image acquisition. By reconstructing 10 phases, the relative temporal resolution in the image data set is 100 msec per phase (60 beats/minute = 1000 msec/beat; 1000 msec ÷ 10 phases = 100 msec/phase). If instead this same data set is taken and 25 phases are reconstructed, the relative temporal resolution is 40 msec/phase (1000 msec ÷ 25 phases = 40 msec/phase). Although the fundamental temporal resolution of the scan has not been altered, the way in which the reconstructed image data are presented has been changed, and a finer gradation of valvular motion can be analyzed. Several studies have demonstrated improved accuracy in assessment of both ventricular and valvular function by using a greater number of reconstructed phases.

Accurate assessment of valvular structure and function can also be augmented by the use of 4-D volume-rendered images. In particular, volume rendering techniques that are optimized to display the soft tissue structures of the heart but not display the contrast opacified blood in the chambers of the heart are extremely useful in assessment of valvular disease. This blood pool inversion (BPI) volume rendering technique can be performed on various different postprocessing systems and capitalizes on the ability of each system to designate a color (or color spectrum) and a percentage of opacity to a range of attenuation values by setting user-defined values called opacity transfer functions (OTFs). By defining OTFs to display low-attenuation soft tissue structures (40 to 150 Hounsfield units [HU]), and very-high-attenuation calcifications (often >700 HU), but not display the intermediate- to high-attenuation blood pool (often 300 to 600 HU), the user renders the blood pool completely transparent. Thick-slab 4-D BPI volumetric reconstructions can then be generated in an infinite number of potential imaging planes and perspectives to assess not only valvular anatomy and function but also other internal structures of the heart.

A thorough and systematic review of each valve requires a combined assessment that may involve the use of standard multiplanar reformation (MPR), minimal

intensity projection (MinIP), and BPI volume-rendered images. Each of these techniques has strengths and weaknesses in assessment of valvular anatomy and function, as demonstrated in Figure 36-1. For viewing each of the valves in the plane of the valve (i.e., in a plane perpendicular to the direction of blood flow), use of a thick-slab BPI volume-rendered technique offers a more comprehensive assessment of valvular structure and function than traditional techniques (also see Figs. 36-2 and 36-6). However, the BPI volume rendering technique does have significant limitations in some cases (discussed later) and generally offers no advantage over traditional MPR techniques for viewing valves in plane with blood flow (e.g., from a three-chamber perspective in assessment of the aortic or mitral valves), because the overlapping structures in a thick-slab BPI volume-rendered image may obscure subtle pathologic features. Under most circumstances, maximal intensity projection (MIP) images offer no advantages in assessment of cardiac valves because the thin valve cusps and leaflets are commonly obscured by the adjacent high-attenuation blood pool, particularly in thicker-slab MIPs.

■ PRACTICAL APPROACHES FOR IMAGING EACH OF THE HEART VALVES

Aortic Valve

By strict anatomic definition, the aortic root has three main components: the annulus, the cusps of the aortic valve, and the sinuses of Valsalva. Although commonly conceived as a planar structure, the anatomic annulus of

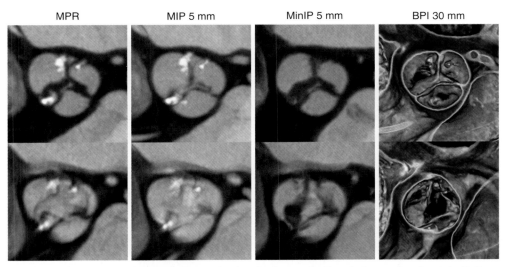

MPR   MIP 5 mm   MinIP 5 mm   BPI 30 mm

Figure 36-1 Comparison of postprocessing techniques. Aortic valve images in diastole *(top row)* and systole *(bottom row)* postprocessed with conventional multiplanar reformation (MPR), maximal intensity projection (MIP), and minimal intensity projection (MinIP) techniques, as well as volume rendered with a blood pool inversion (BPI) technique. Whereas MPR images are of minimal slice thickness (0.4 mm), MIP and MinIP reconstructions are thin slabs (5 mm thick). BPI images are a 30-mm-thick slab, representing 6 times more image data than MIP and MinIP images and 75 times more data than MPR images. Note how MPR images show clear delineation of calcium (white spots) and cusps in diastole, but with less delineation of cusps during systole. MIP images also demonstrate calcium well, but the cusps are incompletely visualized even during diastole. MinIP allows excellent delineation of cusps, particularly during systole, in which MinIP may facilitate planimetric measurements orifice area; however, MinIP overrepresents the degree of cusp thickening and does not allow visualization of calcium. BPI images demonstrate the extent of sclerosis and provide a four-dimensional overview of aortic root anatomy and valvular function. This excellent perspective on anatomy helps to identify the optimal plane for planimetry (which cannot be performed on volume-rendered images) on either MPR or MinIP images.

the aortic valve is a complex 3-D structure that is coronet shaped (i.e., crown shaped), in which each of the semilunar cusps attaches to the wall of the root (Fig. 36-2). The inferior border of the aortic root is at the basal attachments of the annulus of the valve. Because replacement of the valve or root necessitates complete removal of the native valve, the surgical annulus is typically considered to be at the inferior border of the aortic root just below the most inferior attachment of each cusp. The obtuse angle where the superior margins of the sinuses of Valsalva meet the ascending aorta constitutes the superior border of the aortic root and is called the sinotubular junction. The normal aortic valve comprises three semilunar cusps. The junctions between adjacent cusps are referred to as commissures, and the normal aortic valve has three commissures. A normally functioning aortic valve should have thin, pliable, noncalcified cusps that open well (>2 cm²) during systole and close completely during diastole.

Because cardiac CTA acquires complete 3-D or 4-D data sets, the aortic valve can be interrogated in various imaging planes to assess for anatomy and function. Routine imaging planes typically include those in plane with the valve, as well as one or two perpendicular to the plane of the valve, typically either three-chamber or LVOT planes. However, in the setting of valvular dysfunction, additional obliquities may be necessary to assess the severity of valvular dysfunction accurately (see the later discussion of AR and Fig. 36-6).

Aortic Stenosis

Although aortic stenosis (AS) has various causes, it is most commonly the result of degenerative aortic sclerosis: progressive thickening and calcification of the valve. The process of aortic sclerosis is very similar to that of atherosclerosis in that it involves inflammation, lipid deposition, and calcification within the valve cusps. Actually, this "calcification" of the cusps

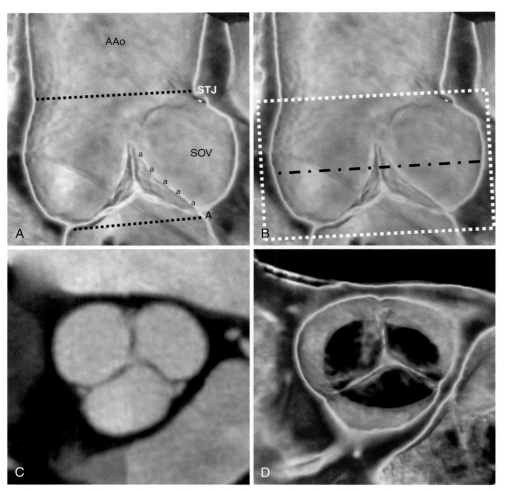

Figure 36-2 Normal anatomy of the aortic root. A, Longitudinal cross section through the aortic root demonstrating the surgical annulus (A) at the inferior margins of the true annulus (a), which is "coronet" shaped (i.e., crown shaped). The superior margin of the aortic root is at the junction between the sinuses of Valsalva (SOV) and the ascending aorta (AAo), the so-called sinotubular junction (STJ). **B,** The *black dotted line* indicates a thin two-dimensional imaging plane through the aortic valve that may be used to assess valvular anatomy and function with either two-dimensional echocardiography or multiplanar reformation images with cardiac computed tomography angiography, as is illustrated in **C.** The *white dotted box* in **B** indicates a volume of tissue that can be assessed with thick-slab blood pool inversion volume rendering, which allows assessment of the entire aortic root and adjacent anatomy in one imaging volume. **D,** Because normal aortic valve cusps are very thin, volumetric renderings often make them appear translucent (note how the dark ovoid left ventricular outflow tract can be seen deep to the valve cusps). By comparison, the thickened cusps of diseased valves are more easily volumetrically rendered, thus appearing more opaque (compare **D** with the valves in Fig. 36-3).

is metabolically active bone-forming tissue. Less commonly, rheumatic heart disease can cause AS, typically associated with scarring and fusion of the commissures, as well as significant retraction of the free edges of each cusp that results in concurrent regurgitation. Least commonly, congenital AS can be seen in children with bicuspid aortic valves (BAVs) or unicuspid aortic valves.

On gated noncontrast CT examinations used for calcium scoring of the coronary arteries, calcium scores of the aortic valve can also be assessed. Studies have shown a general trend that increasing aortic valve calcium scores (either by Agatston score, volume score, or mass score) correlate with increased severity of AS and have indicated reasonable accuracy in discriminating patients with severe stenosis from those with only mild or moderate stenosis. However, other studies have shown this relationship to be highly variable and have suggested that because of this variability, the clinical utility of this calcium scoring of the aortic valve is questionable, and additional correlative imaging will always be required to quantify the severity of stenosis more accurately.

Superior spatial resolution of cardiac CTA allows for excellent anatomic depiction of the aortic valve orifice during systole, even in the presence of significant calcification. Serial review of the aortic valve during systolic phases can be used to identify the reconstructed phase in which the aortic orifice is at its largest, and maximal aortic valve area (AVA) can then be measured during peak systole with planimetry (Fig. 36-3) to determine the presence and severity of AS (Table 36-1). However, planimetry, by its very nature, is a measurement of a two-dimensional area, when in reality the aortic valve orifice is a complex 3-D structure. Therefore, the examiner must thoroughly evaluate aortic valve anatomy to understand the optimal position for measurement of AVA. In the setting of only mild AS, the optimal level to perform planimetry is typically at the free edge of the aortic valve cusps in a plane that is orthogonal to the direction of blood flow. However, in the setting of severe or critical AS, the patient may have partial or complete fusion of cusps that may necessitate measurement at a lower level, or in a slightly oblique plane, to measure

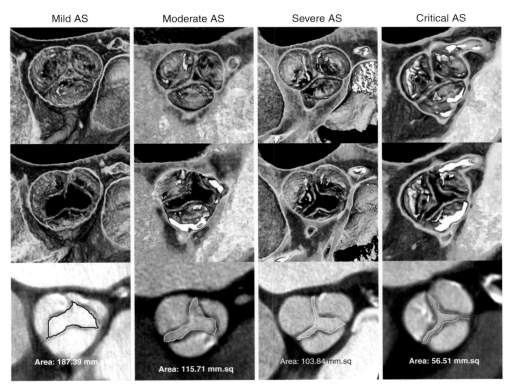

Figure 36-3 Aortic stenosis (AS) demonstrated by cardiac computed tomography angiography. These images demonstrate increasing severity of sclerosis (i.e., thickening and calcification of the cusps) and stenosis from *left* to *right*, with planimetric measurements of aortic valve area measuring 1.9, 1.2, 1.0, and 0.6 cm², respectively.

Table 36-1   *Grading Aortic Stenosis Severity*

	Mild	**Moderate**	**Severe**	**Critical**
Valve area	>1.5 cm²	1.0-1.5 cm²	<1.0 cm²	<0.7 cm²
Mean gradient	<25 mm Hg	25-40 mm Hg	>40 mm Hg	—
Jet velocity	<3.0 m/sec	3.0-4.0 m/sec	>4.0 m/sec	—

the true anatomic orifice area more accurately. In addition, even when the anatomic AVA is measured accurately with planimetry, the functional AVA (estimated by echocardiography) may be different because the functional AVA reflects blood flow through this complex 3-D orifice throughout systole and indicates not only the cross-sectional area but also the complex flow dynamics through this orifice.

PEARLS AND PITFALLS: ASSESSMENT OF LOW-GRADIENT AORTIC STENOSIS

Although many patients with so-called low-gradient AS have reduced resting left ventricular systolic function that results in low mean transvalvular gradients that tend to underestimate the severity of underlying aortic valve stenosis, a subset of individuals has normal resting left ventricular systolic function and low mean transvalvular gradient but calculated AVA (by use of the continuity equation) indicative of severe or critical AS. The conflicting low mean transvalvular gradient and small calculated AVA can be a diagnostic challenge. Studies with 3-D transesophageal echocardiography (TEE), cardiac MRI, and cardiac CTA have all demonstrated that the cause of this apparent discrepancy often is an *elliptic* cross-sectional geometry through the LVOT. For routine application of the continuity equation in echocardiography, the LVOT is assumed to be a tubular structure with a *circular* cross section.

On routine transthoracic echocardiography (TTE), the LVOT diameter is measured on the parasternal long-axis (three-chamber) view, and the cross-sectional area of the LVOT is then calculated using the formula for the area of a circle: πr^2. In fact, the diameter measured on the parasternal long-axis view is the *short* axis of the typically elliptic LVOT, such that use of this diameter to calculate a circular cross section usually results in significant underestimation of actual LVOT cross section (because the error of this smaller measurement is squared) and thereby causes significant underestimation of AVA by the continuity equation.

This concept is demonstrated in Figure 36-4, in which the LVOT area was further underestimated at echocardiography because the sonographer was not centered with respect to the LVOT; this error is common with TTE and is further worsened in the presence of any calcification of the aortic annulus and LVOT. In the example shown in Figure 36-4, the error resulted in an LVOT measurement that grossly underrepresented the true short-axis diameter of the LVOT ellipse and thereby resulted in a severe underestimation of actual LVOT cross-sectional area when this measurement was used to calculate the area of a circle (see Fig. 36-4, *D* to *F*). The cross section of the elliptic LVOT in this case was more than twice that of the assumed circular cross section used in the calculation of AVA, thus resulting in misclassification of someone with only mild to moderate AS as someone with near critical stenosis. Because of these types of errors, reporting specific LVOT measurements (long-axis and short-axis diameters, as well as cross-sectional area) during peak systole may be beneficial, given that these measurements can be combined with echocardiographic data to calculate

the functional AVA with the continuity equation more accurately (see Fig. 36-4).

Studies have demonstrated an excellent correlation between AVA measured by planimetry at cardiac CTA and similar planimetric measurements obtained during cardiac MRI and TEE. All these planimetric measurements of AVA tend to underestimate the severity of AS when compared with calculation of AVA derived from the continuity equation during TTE. However, this difference in many cases is likely related to the elliptic geometry of the LVOT, a finding suggesting that, in fact, the continuity equation tends to overestimate the severity of AS at echocardiography in some patients.

Aortic Regurgitation

AR has many potential causes, the most common of which include aortic sclerosis, congenital abnormalities of the aortic valve, rheumatic valve disease, Marfan syndrome, myxomatous degeneration, and infectious endocarditis. Regardless of the cause, the underlying problem is that during diastole, incompetence of the aortic valve results in retrograde flow of blood from the aorta into the left ventricle. Whether this condition is related to a region of malcoaptation between the valve cusps or is secondary to a perforation of the valve, the severity of regurgitation can be estimated by measurement of the regurgitant orifice area (ROA) by planimetry (Fig. 36-5 and Table 36-2). Studies of AR that used planimetric measurements of ROA in cardiac CTA examinations have demonstrated accurate discrimination between mild AR and moderate to severe AR by using a discriminatory cutoff value of a 0.25 cm², as well as accurate discrimination between mild to moderate AR and severe AR when they used a discriminatory planimetrically measured ROA cutoff of 0.75 cm². These values are significantly different from calculated effective ROA ranges proposed to represent various severities of AR measured by echocardiography (see Table 36-2). This difference has many potential causes, and a full discussion is beyond the scope of this text; however, the difference should be recognized when examiners report ROA values and comment on the potential severity of AR in cardiac CTA examinations. Additionally, a considerable gray area exists at the lower and upper limits of the moderate regurgitation range, such that planimetrically derived ROA values in these ranges may be more correctly reported with some degree of uncertainty as indicating mild to moderate AR and moderate to severe AR, respectively.

PEARLS AND PITFALLS: OPTIMIZING PLANIMETRY IN AORTIC REGURGITATION

Although some causes of AR result in relatively central and symmetric regions of malcoaptation (see Fig. 36-5), other processes such as prolapse in the setting of BAV disease often lead to very asymmetric regurgitant orifices that are not accurately measured in the typical plane of the aortic valve and instead require oblique imaging planes to measure the ROA properly with planimetry (Fig. 36-6). In these situations, using a combination of 4-D BPI volumetric reconstructions and MPRs in

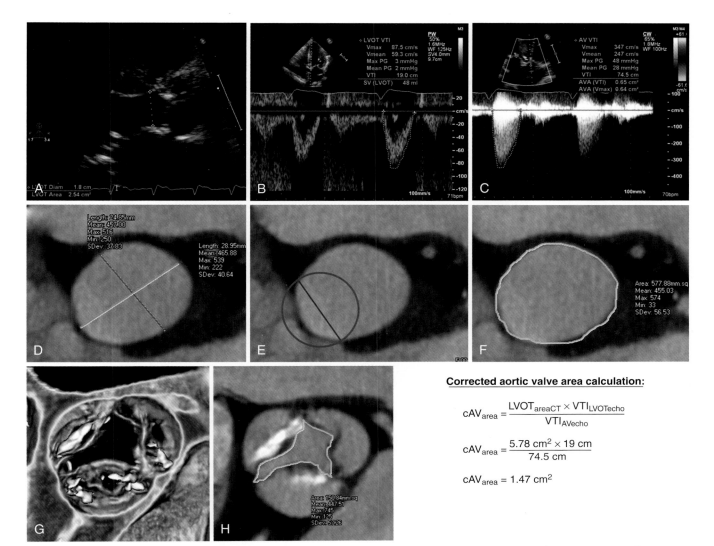

Corrected aortic valve area calculation:

$$cAV_{area} = \frac{LVOT_{areaCT} \times VTI_{LVOTecho}}{VTI_{AVecho}}$$

$$cAV_{area} = \frac{5.78 \text{ cm}^2 \times 19 \text{ cm}}{74.5 \text{ cm}}$$

$$cAV_{area} = 1.47 \text{ cm}^2$$

Figure 36-4 Use of left ventricular outflow tract (LVOT) planimetry to correct aortic valve area calculation by the continuity equation. **A to C,** Transthoracic echocardiography (TTE) data of patient with "low-gradient, critical aortic stenosis," with mean gradient of 28 mm Hg, LVOT diameter of 18 mm, and a calculated aortic valve area (AVA) of 0.65 cm² by the continuity equation. **D to F,** Images from cardiac computed tomography angiography (CTA) examination through the LVOT during peak systole demonstrate an elliptic LVOT measuring 25 × 29 mm. **E,** Demonstration of how a diameter of 18 mm may have been obtained slightly off-axis by the sonographer and how this results in significant underestimation of area as compared with the direct planimetric measurement of the LVOT (**F**). **G and H,** Blood pool inversion volume-rendered and multiplanar reformation images from the cardiac CTA examination demonstrate the aortic valve during peak systole with an estimated AVA of 1.51 cm². By taking the measured LVOT area from cardiac CTA and velocity time integral (VTI) data from TTE and using this in a "corrected" continuity equation, the calculated corrected aortic valve area (cAVarea) is 1.47 cm², suggesting mild to moderate (not critical) aortic stenosis; this calculation is also more consistent with the measured mean pressure gradient of 28 mm Hg.

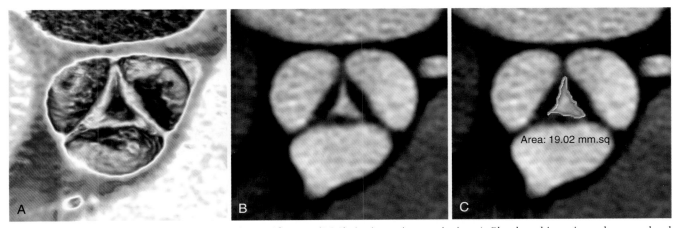

Figure 36-5 Use of planimetry to assess regurgitant orifice area (ROA) size in aortic regurgitation. **A,** Blood pool inversion volume-rendered image of a sclerotic aortic valve during diastole demonstrating marked thickening (but no calcification) and retraction of the free edge of the valve cusps that resulted in a central regurgitant orifice. **B,** Multiplanar reformation image oriented through the smallest portion of the regurgitant orifice. **C,** Planimetry used to measure the ROA as demonstrated by the *green outline* (ROA, 0.19 cm²).

various imaging planes can help to delineate the cause of valvular dysfunction and identify the most optimal imaging plane for performing planimetry to measure ROA. This multifaceted approach is useful not only with native valves, but also with dysfunctional bioprosthetic valves (Fig. 36-7, A to C), which can often be difficult to visualize clearly with echocardiography and cardiac MRI because of artifact from heavy calcification, support

Table 36-2   Grading Aortic Regurgitation Severity

	Mild	Moderate	Severe
CCTA-measured ROA	<0.25 cm^2	0.25-0.75 cm^2	>0.75 cm^2
TTE-calculated ROA	<0.1 cm^2	0.1-0.3 cm^2	>0.3 cm^2
Regurgitant fraction	<30%	30%-49%	≥50%

CCTA, Cardiac computed tomography angiography; *ROA,* regurgitant orifice area; *TTE,* transthoracic echocardiography.

structure (i.e., stented bioprostheses), or distorted tissue planes around the aortic root.

PEARLS AND PITFALLS: BIOPROSTHETIC AORTIC VALVES

Despite some of the advantages of cardiac CTA in the assessment of aortic valve structure and function, CTA does have a significant limitation when bioprosthetic valves are assessed for a cause of regurgitation. Although sclerosis of native aortic valves results in progressive thickening and calcification, degeneration of bioprosthetic valves is usually associated with severe calcification but minimal, if any, thickening of the cusps. Rather, the cusps of bioprosthetic valves progressively degenerate and are prone to development of small perforations (sometimes referred to as fenestrations), even in the absence of an underlying cause such as infective endocarditis. Because of the thin nature of bioprosthetic aortic valve cusps, and the limited spatial resolution of CT at this time, excluding the presence of significant valvular

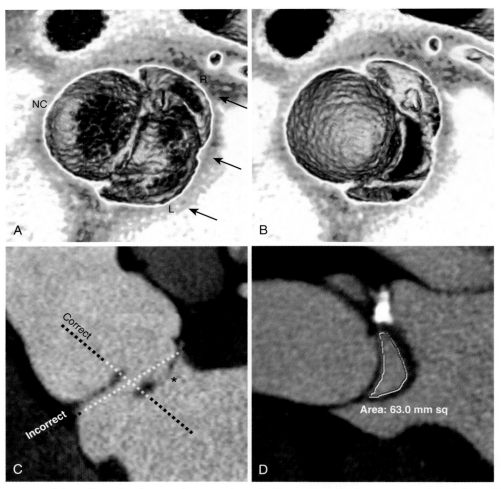

Figure 36-6 Importance of three-dimensional anatomic perspective to facilitate correct planimetry. **A,** Functionally bicuspid aortic valve with independent noncoronary (NC) cusp and fused left (L) and right (R) cusp moieties viewed from above (simulating an aortotomy perspective). From this perspective, no obvious region of malcoaptation is visualized. **B,** However, when viewed from a 65-degree oblique angle (as indicated by *arrows* in **A**) a large region of malcoaptation becomes apparent, related to prolapse of the fused cusp. **C,** Multiplanar reformation (MPR) in the left ventricular outflow tract plane demonstrates prolapse of the fused cusp (*asterisk*) and indicates both typical (incorrect) and very oblique (correct) imaging planes that could be used for planimetry to assess the regurgitant orifice area (ROA). **D,** Highly oblique MPR oriented to assess the ROA (as indicated by "correct" plane in **C**) demonstrates a large region of malcoaptation (ROA, 0.63 cm^2), a finding suggesting moderate to severe aortic regurgitation.

regurgitation related to one or more small perforations of the cusps is difficult when the assessment is based strictly on an anatomic evaluation of valvular structure and function by cardiac CTA. This situation is illustrated in Figure 36-7, *D* to *F,* which shows a 12-year-old aortic root allograft with severe regurgitation in which assessment by cardiac CTA appeared to demonstrate a relatively normally functioning bioprosthesis. Because of this limitation, if the patient has known or suspected AR, and no identifiable source on cardiac CTA, reporting should simply indicate a lack of an identifiable cause of AR (rather than stating that no evidence of regurgitation is noted). In such situations, correlation with complementary modalities such as echocardiography and cardiac MRI, which offer information regarding flow and hemodynamics, is recommended.

Congenital Aortic Valve Disease

Congenital abnormalities of the aortic valve involve variation in the number of cusps and commissures of the valve. As previously mentioned, the normal aortic valve has three cusps and three commissures. The most common congenital abnormality of the aortic valve is the BAV, which has several morphologic forms. Overall, BAV disease is the most common congenital heart lesion, with a prevalence of 0.5% to 2% in the population, and it is highly associated with other abnormalities such as aortic coarctation. Patients with BAV disease not only are prone to valvular dysfunction (with a higher incidence of stenosis or regurgitation) but also have an underlying connective tissue disease that increases their risk for aortic aneurysm and dissection. In the setting of aneurysmal dilatation of the thoracic aorta, recognition of BAV disease is important, given that surgical repair is indicated for a thoracic aortic diameter greater than 5 cm (as compared with 5.5 cm in the general population) because of the higher risk of aneurysm progression and rupture in these patients.

A few comments about terminology warrant discussion. The components of the aortic valve are properly

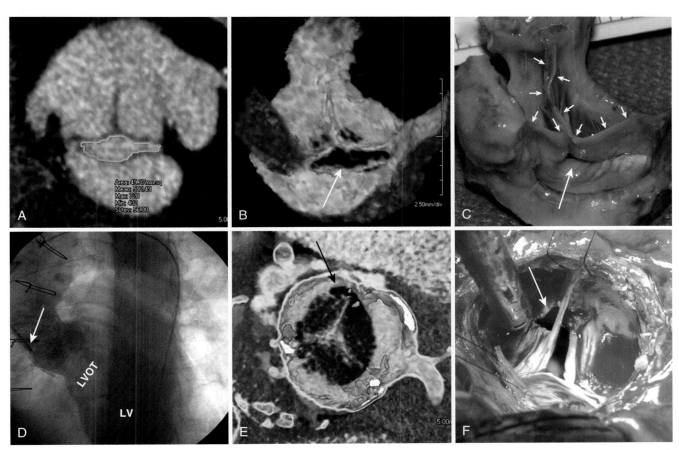

Figure 36-7 Bioprosthetic aortic valves. A to **C,** A 5-year-old aortic bioprosthesis. **A,** Highly oblique multiplanar reformation image through the aortic root during diastole demonstrating a large region of malcoaptation (regurgitant orifice area, 0.49 cm²) suggestive of moderate aortic regurgitation. **B,** Diastolic four-dimensional blood pool inversion (BPI) volume-rendered image of aortic root (note: other structures have been electronically dissected to show only the bioprosthesis) that demonstrates this region of malcoaptation caused by a prolapsing cusp *(white arrow).* **C,** Corresponding ex vivo photograph of bioprosthesis after surgical resection demonstrating two normal cusps (free edges indicated by *small white arrows*) and a prolapsing cusp with a regurgitant orifice *(large white arrow)* that would be larger with more severe prolapse in vivo under systemic arterial pressures. **D** to **F,** A 12-year-old aortic root allograft. **D,** Aortic root injection (catheter indicated by the *arrow*) demonstrating severe 4+ regurgitation of contrast material into the left ventricular outflow tract (LVOT) filling the left ventricle (LV). **E,** Diastolic phase BPI volume rendering of the aortic valve originally interpreted as normally functioning without obvious region of malcoaptation; in retrospect, a small fenestration *(arrow)* of the noncoronary cusp near the commissure was present and was later confirmed at surgery *(arrow* in the operative photograph, **F**). Multiple other small fenestrations of the valve were also visualized at surgery. Note how translucent the valve cusps are in **E,** thus making accurate assessment of small fenestrations exceedingly difficult on this and other bioprostheses when BPI volume rendering techniques are used.

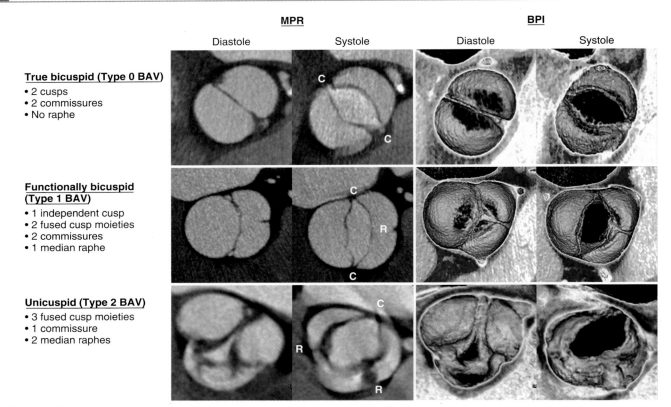

	MPR		BPI	
	Diastole	Systole	Diastole	Systole

True bicuspid (Type 0 BAV)
- 2 cusps
- 2 commissures
- No raphe

Functionally bicuspid (Type 1 BAV)
- 1 independent cusp
- 2 fused cusp moieties
- 2 commissures
- 1 median raphe

Unicuspid (Type 2 BAV)
- 3 fused cusp moieties
- 1 commissure
- 2 median raphes

Figure 36-8 Bicuspid aortic valves (BAV). Multiplanar reformation (MPR) and blood pool inversion (BPI) images demonstrating all forms of bicuspid aortic valves during both diastole and systole. Note the number of cusps, commissures (C), and raphes (R) in each form.

referred to as cusps, not leaflets. The term raphe is used to describe a malformed commissure that results in fusion between two typically underdeveloped cusp moieties. The most commonly used classification scheme for BAV is that of Sievers and Schmidtke, who described type 0, type 1, and type 2 BAVs, based on the presence of 0, 1, or 2 raphes, respectively (Fig. 36-8). According to this classification scheme, a type 0 BAV has two evenly sized cusps, two commissures, and no raphes; this type 0 BAV is sometimes referred to as a true BAV. A type 1 BAV has one normal or enlarged cusp and two (typically smaller) cusp moieties, two commissures, and one raphe; this type 1 BAV is commonly referred to as a functionally bicuspid aortic valve. A type 2 BAV has three cusp moieties all joined together by two raphes, thus resulting in one large functional cusp that has only one commissure. Notably, the type 2 BAV is sometimes referred to as a unicommissural unicuspid aortic valve (as opposed to a true unicuspid aortic valve, which consists of one broad membrane with a central orifice, with no commissures and no raphes).

Another extremely rare congenital variant of the aortic valve is the quadricuspid aortic valve, which has an unknown incidence estimated to be between 0.003% and 0.04%, based on necropsy and two-dimensional echocardiography studies. Reports of quadricuspid aortic valves in the literature indicate a high rate of regurgitation related to progressive degeneration, thickening, and retraction of the cusps that results in central regions of malcoaptation.

Mitral Valve

Discussion of the mitral valve is really a discussion of the mitral valve apparatus. This complex multifaceted anatomic structure consists of the mitral annulus, the mitral valve (anterior and posterior leaflets), and the subvalvular apparatus, which consists of both the chordae tendineae and the papillary muscles (Fig. 36-9). Dysfunction in any one of these components of the mitral valve apparatus can result in abnormal mitral valve function. For assessment of the mitral valve itself, most imagers and surgeons use the Carpentier classification system to assess for dysfunction in any one of the three segments (A1, A2, A3) of the anterior leaflet or three scallops (P1, P2, P3) of the posterior leaflet (see Fig. 36-9, C and D). Accordingly, accurate assessment of mitral valve disease and dysfunction requires a systematic approach to assess all portions of the mitral apparatus. With echocardiography, this assessment is typically achieved by the use of TEE; the echocardiographer rotates the probe through multiple degrees of rotation to sample all portions of the mitral apparatus systematically. Figure 36-10 demonstrates an analogous approach that can be used with cardiac CTA to evaluate each portion of the valve independently and thoroughly (i.e., A1-P1, A2-P2, and A3-P3). By using a combined approach that includes this systematic assessment of leaflet function, as well as an interactive assessment using a combination of 4-D BPI volume-rendered and MPR images to assess the

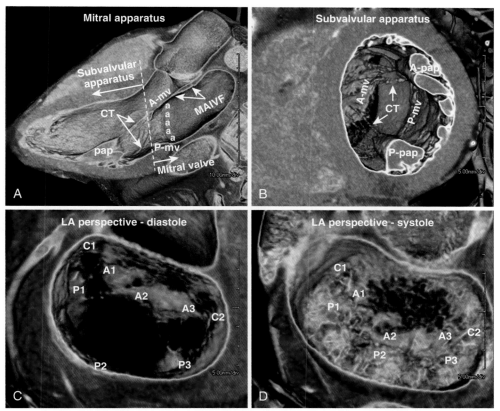

Figure 36-9 Mitral valve apparatus. A, Three-chamber thick-slab blood pool inversion (BPI) volume-rendered image providing an overview of the mitral valve apparatus. The *dotted yellow line* indicates the division between the subvalvular apparatus (chordae tendineae [CT] and papillary muscles [pap]) and the remainder of the mitral valve (anterior [A-mv] and posterior [P-mv] leaflets, as well as the annulus [a]). The mitral-aortic intervalvular fibrosa (MAIVF) is the fibrous continuity between the mitral and aortic valves. **B,** Thick-slab short-axis BPI image through the subvalvular apparatus to demonstrate the normally thin chordae tendineae (CT). **C** and **D,** Thick-slab short-axis BPI images through the mitral orifice at during diastole and systole, respectively, that demonstrate the two commissures (C1 and C2), as well as the three anterior leaflet segments (A1, A2, and A3) and three posterior leaflet scallops (P1, P2, and P3). Note how wide open the orifice is in this normal patient and compare with rheumatic (see Fig. 36-11, **D** to **G**) and parachute (see Fig. 36-12) mitral valves. *LA,* Left atrium.

annulus, commissures, chordae tendineae, and papillary muscles fully, the cardiac CTA reader can achieve a comprehensive overview of mitral valve structure and function.

Mitral Regurgitation

MR is a relatively common disorder. Although MR has numerous causes, one of the more common and the origin of some of the most severe cases of MR is myxomatous mitral valve disease (also known as Barlow syndrome or "floppy" mitral valve disease). In myxomatous mitral valve disease, the valve tissue has an abnormal accumulation of proteoglycans that results in thickening, elongation, and redundancy of the valve leaflets. This condition makes the leaflets prone to prolapse (in which the leaflet bows into the left atrium and the free edge breaks the plane of the annulus), and in severe end-stage disease, it can result in rupture of chordae tendineae and a frankly flail mitral valve leaflet (in which the free edge of the flail portion of the leaflet inverts and extends completely back into the left atrium during systole). Prolapse or flail mitral valve leaflets can involve one or more of the anterior segments or the posterior scallops of the valve and should be properly

preoperatively characterized to help facilitate optimal surgical planning and management.

Cardiac CTA can identify not only prolapse but also flail portions of the mitral valve leaflets preoperatively (Fig. 36-11, *A* to *C*). Although some cardiac CTA studies have demonstrated the utility of planimetric assessment of an ROA in cases of MR, because of the complex 3-D anatomy of the mitral apparatus, accurate assessment of the ROA is often challenging, particularly in the setting of a flail valve, in which the regurgitant orifice may have a complex 3-D shape not easily measured in a single plane. Despite this limitation, accurate assessment of severity of leaflet thickening, calcification, and any associated structural abnormalities (e.g., ruptured chordae tendineae) provides useful information that may be readily detected by cardiac CTA and may help guide surgical repair or replacement of the valve.

Mitral Stenosis

Mitral stenosis (MS) has various causes. In adult populations of Western societies, however, the most common cause is overwhelmingly rheumatic heart disease. Rheumatic MS has very characteristic imaging and pathologic findings; cardiac CTA is well suited to demonstrate these

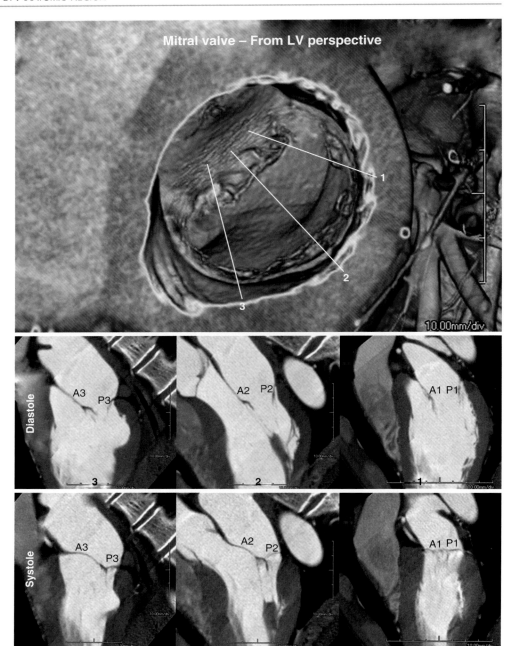

Figure 36-10 Systematic assessment of mitral valve segments and scallops. Each of the segment-scallop combinations of the anterior and posterior leaflets can be evaluated independently with cardiac computed tomography angiography by generating long-axis imaging planes through the mitral orifice as indicated by *lines 1 to 3* in the *upper image.*

findings and to quantitate the severity of MS (Table 36-3). Hallmark imaging findings of rheumatic MS include thickening and fusion of the chordae tendineae and mitral valve commissures. These features result in a significant reduction of the mitral valve orifice area, as well as a change in shape, from a wide open communication between the left atrium and ventricle to a constricted funnel-shaped orifice that is typically narrowest at the junction of the free edge of the valve leaflets with the chordae tendineae. This condition results in a very limited opening motion with a doming or "hockey stick" appearance of the anterior leaflet during diastole that is well demonstrated on cardiac CTA (see Fig. 36-11, *F*). Over time, this fusion of the chordae tendineae and

commissures worsens, and these structures may become heavily calcified. Figure 36-11, *D* to *G*, demonstrates a young patient with classic findings of rheumatic mitral valve disease, but only mild MS. Compare these cardiac CTA images with those of a normal mitral valve (see Figs. 36-9 and 36-10), and note the differences in the normally thin and unfused chordae tendineae and the normally well-separated commissures between A1 to P1 and A3 to P3, as well as the overall orifice size and shape. Optimal planimetry of the stenotic mitral orifice is achieved in early diastole when the valve is maximally opened, but at the position where the orifice is narrowest (typically at the junction of the chordae tendineae and the free edge of the leaflets, as demonstrated in Fig. 36-11, *F* to *G*).

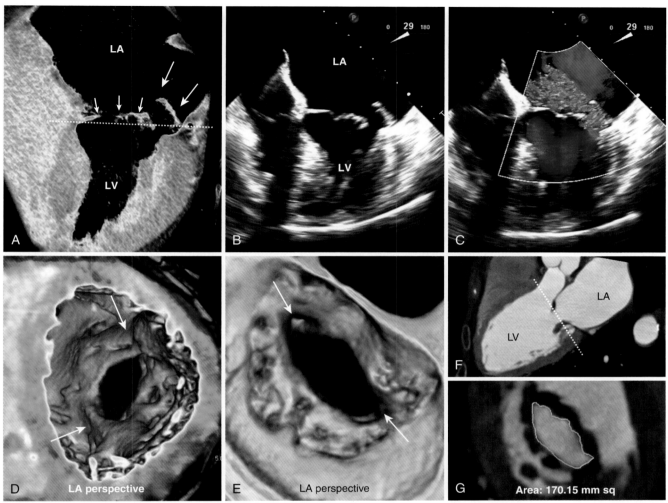

Figure 36-11 Evaluation of mitral regurgitation and stenosis with cardiac computed tomography angiography. **A** to **C,** Myxomatous insufficient mitral valve. **A,** Thin-slab blood pool inversion (BPI) volume rendering of a myxomatous mitral valve during systole that demonstrates mild prolapse of a thickened anterior leaflet *(small arrows)* that extends behind the plane of the mitral annulus (indicated by the *dotted white line*), as well as a flail P1 scallop *(large arrows)* of the posterior leaflet, which is a rare cause of mitral insufficiency and was an unexpected preoperative finding in this patient. **B** and **C,** Images from intraoperative transesophageal echocardiography obtained at 29 degrees of rotation without (**B**) and with (**C**) color Doppler also demonstrate the flail P1 scallop and associated mitral regurgitation. **D** to **G,** Rheumatic mitral valve. **D** and **E,** Thick-slab BPI images of a mitral valve from the left ventricular (**D**) and left atrial (**E**) perspectives, respectively, in a patient with a history of rheumatic fever. Note the marked thickening and fusion of the chordae tendineae *(arrows* in **D**; compare with Fig. 36-9, *B,* for normal reference). Also note the fusion of the commissures *(arrows* in **E**; compare with Fig. 36-9, *C,* for normal reference). **F,** Despite the impressive findings in **D** and **E,** planimetry performed in the diastolic phase, in which the valve was most open, but through the narrowest opening on that phase *(dotted white line),* demonstrated only mild stenosis (orifice area of 1.7 cm^2 in **G**). Also note the domed "hockey stick" appearance of the anterior leaflet in **F.** *LA,* Left atrium; *LV,* left ventricle.

Table 36-3 Grading Mitral Stenosis Severity

	Mild	Moderate	Severe
Valve area	>1.5 cm^2	1.0-1.5 cm^2	<1.0 cm^2
Mean gradient	<5 mm Hg	5-10 mm Hg	>10 mm Hg

Congenital Mitral Valve Disease: Using a Multifaceted Approach to Characterize the Valve

Many known congenital anomalies of the mitral valve are categorized based on their association with either MS or mitral insufficiency. Although a full discussion of these anomalies is beyond the scope of this text, one case example demonstrating two obstructive lesions

in a patient with Shone complex is used to illustrate the utility of cardiac CTA in assessment of congenital mitral valve disease. Figure 36-12 demonstrates cardiac CTA images from a patient with Shone complex who had both a parachute mitral valve and a midvalvular mitral ring. Patients with parachute mitral valve typically have the most severe form of congenital MS. In this particular patient, the anterior papillary muscle is hypoplastic and is not associated with any chordae tendineae; rather, all chordae tendineae from both the anterior and posterior mitral valve leaflets attach to the posterior papillary muscle, with a resulting stenotic tubular mitral orifice (see Fig. 36-12, *A* to *C*). This stenosis is further worsened by the presence of a midvalvular mitral ring (see Fig. 36-12, *D* to *F*) that is largest along the anterior mitral valve leaflet. These obstructing rings are different from the membranes seen with cor triatriatum sinister (which occur within the left atrial chamber) and can be either supravalvular (along the annulus) or midvalvular, as in this instance.

Correctly classification of these rings as supravalvular or midvalvular is critically important because surgical resection of a supravalvular ring is relatively easy and carries a low risk of injury to the valve, whereas resection of a midvalvular ring is more challenging and requires extra attention by the surgeon to reduce the risk of valvular injury and associated postoperative mitral insufficiency. By using a combined approach of BPI volume rendering and standard MPR techniques, both the parachute mitral valve and the midvalvular ring were correctly preoperatively characterized in the patient shown in Figure 36-12. This thorough combined approach can also aid in properly characterizing other obstructive and insufficient mitral valve variants.

Pulmonic Valve

Regardless of the imaging modality used, visualization and functional assessment of the pulmonic valve can be a challenge, for several reasons. With echocardiography, this difficulty is predominately related to the position of the valve within the thorax, a placement that makes obtaining optimal sonographic windows very challenging and in some cases impossible. With MRI, the limited spatial resolution and thin nature of the pulmonic valve cusps complicate accurate anatomic depiction of the valve; however, phase contrast MRI is very useful to assess pulmonic valve dysfunction. With multiphase cardiac CTA, the superior spatial resolution and 4-D data set obtained in many cases allow for excellent anatomic depiction of the valve; however, as with other valves, flow-related assessment of valvular function is not possible with cardiac CTA. Additionally, multiphase cardiac CTA is associated with significant radiation exposure to the patient, whereas echocardiography and cardiac MRI are not.

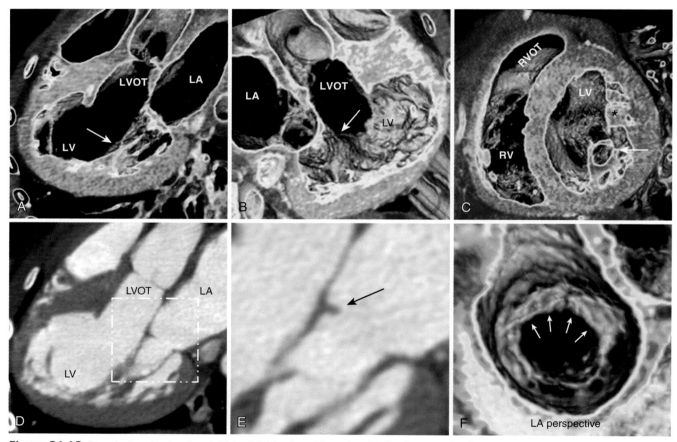

Figure 36-12 Parachute mitral valve. A, Thin-slab blood pool inversion (BPI) volume-rendered image in the three-chamber plane demonstrates convergence of all chordae tendineae toward one papillary muscle *(arrow)*. **B,** Thick-slab BPI in the three-chamber plane manipulated to view the mitral orifice from the left atrial perspective demonstrates a rounded orifice and convergence of the chordae tendineae on one papillary muscle *(arrow)*. **C,** Thick-slab short-axis BPI image again demonstrates convergence of the chordae tendineae on the posterior papillary muscle *(arrow)* and shows a hypoplastic anterior papillary muscle *(asterisk)* that is not associated with any chordae tendineae. **D,** Corresponding three-chamber plane when viewed with the multiplanar reformation technique. **E,** Magnified view of anterior leaflet of parachute mitral valve (as designated by *dotted white box* in **D**) that demonstrates a ridge of tissue on the anterior leaflet of the mitral valve *(arrow)* consistent with a midvalvular ring. **F,** Thick-slab short-axis BPI image from the left atrial perspective that demonstrates a circular orifice of the parachute mitral valve that is further narrowed by the midvalvular ring *(arrows)*. *LA,* Left atrium; *LV,* left ventricle; *LVOT,* left ventricular outflow tract; *RV,* right ventricle; *RVOT,* right ventricular outflow tract.

Congenital Pulmonic Valve Disease: Cardiac Computed Tomography Angiography Use in Preoperative Evaluation for Ross Procedure

Given the strengths of cardiac CTA in anatomic assessment of the pulmonic valve, one potential use is for evaluation of pulmonic valve morphology in patients under consideration for the Ross procedure: aortic root replacement with the patient's native pulmonic valve and subsequent replacement of the pulmonic valve with a bioprosthesis. Given the difficulties of both echocardiography and cardiac MRI for anatomic characterization of the pulmonic valve, cardiac CTA may play a specific role in the preoperative assessment of patients who are possible candidates for the Ross procedure. Figure 36-13 demonstrates a normal pulmonic valve with three cusps (see Fig. 36-13, B), as well as bicuspid and quadricuspid pulmonic valve variants (see Fig. 36-13, A and C, respectively).

Patients with bicuspid and quadricuspid pulmonic valve variants are not suitable candidates for the Ross procedure. Currently, most cardiothoracic surgeons perform arteriotomy of the pulmonic trunk for visual assessment of the pulmonic valve intraoperatively to determine suitability for the Ross procedure. Although this arteriotomy is simple to reverse and is generally well tolerated, preoperative characterization of the pulmonic valve with cardiac CTA can help avoid this unnecessary procedure in patients with congenital pulmonic valve variants and can thereby reduce potential operative complications and overall surgery time. As with the aortic valve, cardiac CTA may also allow preoperative identification of stenotic pulmonic valves, insufficient pulmonic valves, and pulmonic valves compromised by infectious endocarditis.

Tricuspid Valve

Accurate evaluation of tricuspid valve structure, function, and disease with cardiac CTA can be extremely challenging and is often limited by contrast bolus behavior. Specifically, whereas contrast-opacified blood enters the right atrium through the superior vena cava when intravenous injection is performed in a patient's upper extremity, a large volume of unopacified blood also enters the right atrium through the inferior vena cava. In this high-flow environment, the blood pool has a very heterogenous appearance within the right atrium and sometimes also within the right ventricle (i.e., on both sides of the tricuspid valve). Because of this heterogenous blood pool opacification, discriminating between unopacified blood and thin soft tissue structures such as the leaflets of the tricuspid valve may be

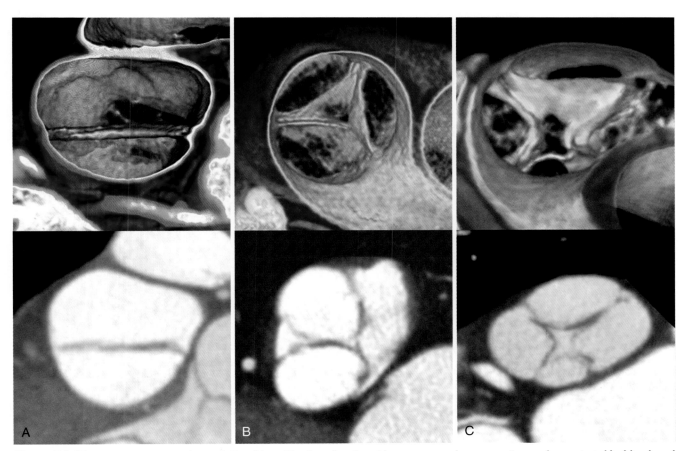

Figure 36-13 Pulmonic valve variants. A, True bicuspid pulmonic valve with two cusps and two commissures demonstrated by blood pool inversion volume rendering and multiplanar reformation. **B,** Normal tricuspid pulmonic valve. **C,** Quadricuspid pulmonic valve. Only the patient with the tricuspid pulmonic valve would be considered a potential candidate for a Ross procedure.

difficult; consequently, accurate assessment of the tricuspid valve is not always possible with cardiac CTA.

Most reports in the literature on the identification of tricuspid valve disease with cardiac CTA involve incidental identification of large vegetations on the tricuspid valve in patients with infectious endocarditis. Indeed, if a vegetation or tumor is large enough, it may be recognized as a mobile filling defect associated with the tricuspid valve leaflets on a cardiac CTA examination. Similarly, other lesions such as thrombi and papillary fibroelastomas (PFs) may also appear as mobile filling defects. Despite the general limitations of cardiac CTA in assessment of the tricuspid valve, the 3-D and 4-D data sets of cardiac CTA have demonstrated some utility in analysis of anatomic variants of the tricuspid valve.

Congenital Tricuspid Valve Disease: Ebstein Anomaly

Ebstein anomaly is a congenital variant of the tricuspid valve in which the leaflets are apically displaced, thus

resulting in a smaller than normal functional right ventricle and so-called atrialization of the remainder of the right ventricle. The degree of displacement of the tricuspid valve leaflets is highly variable, although the posterior leaflet is usually most severely apically displaced, the septal leaflet is usually slightly less displaced, and usually little or no displacement of the anterior leaflet occurs (Fig. 36-14). In addition, the posterior and septal leaflets are typically hypoplastic, whereas the anterior leaflet is often enlarged and sail-like in appearance and is sometimes tethered by multiple abnormal chordal attachments to the free wall of the right ventricle, with resulting in right ventricular outflow tract obstruction. When echocardiography and MRI are limited, cardiac CT can provide useful diagnostic information, by clearly defining the severity of apical displacement of the leaflets, the degree of leaflet hypoplasia, and the presence of anterior leaflet tethering (see Fig. 36-14). Additionally, cardiac CTA can allow volumetric assessment of the right ventricle. Overall, the prognosis is poor in Ebstein

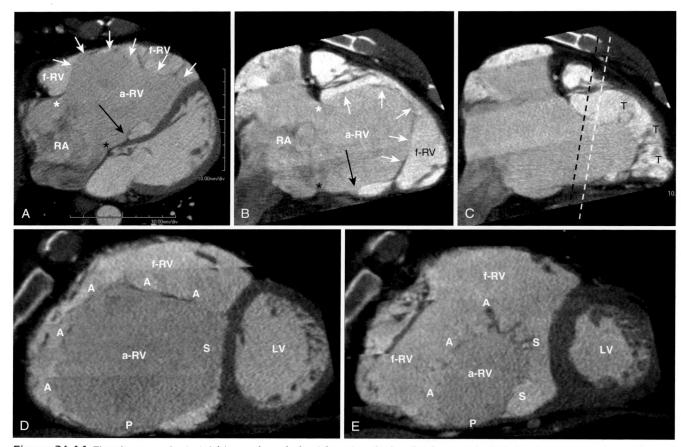

Figure 36-14 Ebstein anomaly. A, Axial image through the right atrium (RA) and right ventricle (RV) that demonstrates abnormal apical displacement of the attachment of the septal leaflet *(black arrow)* of the tricuspid valve compared with the normal location *(black asterisk)* in the tricuspid annulus. Note the severe apical displacement of the tricuspid valve (anterior leaflet indicated by *white arrows*) that results in a large atrialized portion of the right ventricle (a-RV) and small functional portion (f-RV). **B,** Diastolic vertical long-axis multiplanar reformation (MPR) through the right side of the heart that demonstrates a sail-like appearance of the anterior leaflet of the tricuspid valve *(white arrows),* as well as marked apical displacement of the attachment of the posterior leaflet *(black arrow)* compared with the normal location *(black asterisk),* with resulting atrialization of much of the RV. **C,** Systolic vertical long-axis MPR image through the right side of the heart demonstrates a tethering (T) of the anterior leaflet of the tricuspid valve. The *dotted black and white lines* represent the short-axis planes presented in **D** and **E,** respectively. **D,** Diastolic short-axis MPR image through the basal RV demonstrates the elongated anterior leaflet (A), but the septal and posterior leaflets (S and P) are not visualized because they failed to delaminate at this level. Note the large central atrialized portion of the RV. **E,** Systolic short-axis MPR image through the mid-RV demonstrates portions of both the anterior and septal leaflets (A and S), but still does not visualize the posterior leaflet (P). *LV,* Left ventricle.

anomaly if the volume of the functional right ventricle is less than one third the total (i.e., atrialized plus functional right ventricle) right ventricular volume.

Special Situations

Endocarditis: Evaluation of Valvular and Perivalvular Abnormalities

In the setting of suspected infectious endocarditis, many potential imaging findings can help to establish the diagnosis and indicate the extent of disease. Because multiphase cardiac CTA examinations are 4-D data sets, interactive use of different postprocessing techniques and infinite imaging planes allows thorough evaluation of both valvular and perivalvular anatomic complications of infectious endocarditis, such as vegetations, valvular perforations, perivalvular abscesses, and paravalvular leaks. This information can complement the anatomic and functional information obtained by other imaging modalities and in some cases may add incrementally to the understanding of the severity and extent of disease.

Imaging findings of infective endocarditis at cardiac CTA are completely analogous to those seen with other imaging modalities. Vegetations are typically irregularly shaped and highly variable in size, but most commonly they appear as hypermobile structures either associated with the free edge of valve cusps or leaflets or extending from the edges of a valvular perforation (Fig. 36-15, A and B). Occasionally, larger vegetations can have a more sessile appearance and may be less mobile (see Fig. 36-15, C to F). In the left side of the heart, vegetations are more common on the LVOT side of the aortic valve (see Fig. 36-15, B) and on the atrial side of the mitral valve. Vegetations are not exclusive to the valves and can also be seen on support apparatus (e.g., catheters and pacemaker leads), chamber walls, and chordae tendineae. Unfortunately, as with findings on echocardiography and cardiac MRI, no one single imaging characteristic on cardiac CTA can definitively identify

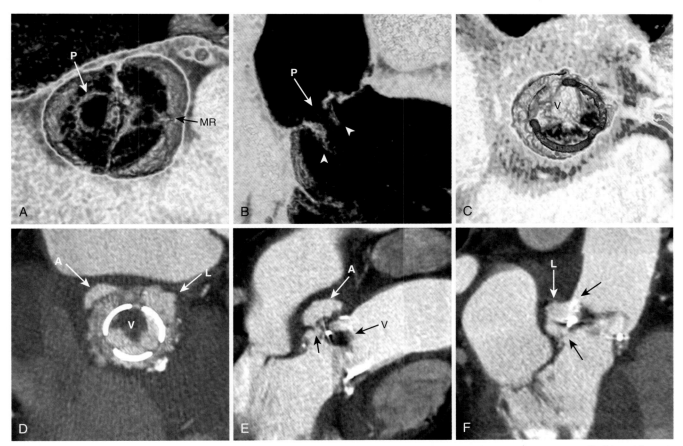

Figure 36-15 Endocarditis: perforations, vegetations, perivalvular abscesses, and paravalvular leaks. **A** and **B,** Functionally bicuspid aortic valve (BAV). **A,** Diastolic blood pool inversion (BPI) image of a type 1 BAV with a large perforation (P) in the noncoronary cusp opposite the fused left and right cusp moieties with the intervening median raphe (MR). **B,** Thin-slab BPI diastolic left ventricular outflow tract (LVOT) image through the same valve as in **A** that demonstrates wispy vegetations *(arrowheads)* extending into the LVOT beneath the perforation. **C** to **F,** Stented porcine aortic bioprosthesis. **C,** BPI volume-rendered image demonstrating a large, sessile vegetation (V) on the noncoronary cusp of the stented bioprosthesis. **D,** Multiplanar reformation (MPR) image in plane with the valve demonstrates two adjacent outpouchings representative of both a perivalvular abscess (A) and a paravalvular leak (L). Additional orthogonal MPR images oriented in directions of *arrows* through the abscess and leak are shown in **E** and **F,** respectively. **E,** MPR image oriented through an abscess (A) demonstrates a narrow neck *(small black arrow)* originating in the LVOT just beneath the large vegetation (V) of the noncoronary cusp of the valve; this abscess was pulsatile on multiphase images. **F,** By comparison, MPR image through the paravalvular leak demonstrates small communications both above and below the valve *(black arrows).*

a lesion as an infectious vegetation. Valvular perforations are defects in the body of valve cusps or leaflets that are commonly separate from their free edges and result in areas of regurgitation that are distinctly separate from the normal regions of valvular coaptation (see Fig. 36-15, A and B). As mentioned earlier, the edges of perforations commonly have associated vegetations extending from them (see Fig. 36-15, B), typically into the preceding heart chamber.

Perivalvular abnormalities in infective endocarditis include perivalvular abscesses and paravalvular leaks (sometimes referred to as valvular dehiscence). Surgeons use the term abscess to refer to infected blood-containing spaces adjacent to a valve. Because these abscesses are typically in direct communication with the adjacent cardiac chamber, these may more correctly be termed infected pseudoaneurysms; however, the term abscess is commonly used and clinically accepted. Abscesses can be highly variable in shape and size and can sometimes be elongated, forming fistulous tracts within the myocardium and adjacent tissues. Often, these abscesses have a narrow neck (see Fig. 36-15, E) and are dynamic structures that expand during systole and decompress during diastole. If an abscess fistulizes in a manner that develops communication with the blood pool on both sides of a valve, it becomes a paravalvular leak (see Fig. 36-15, F). As the name implies, paravalvular leaks allow bidirectional flow through the leak that bypasses the valve. These leaks may be slightly pulsatile (although less so than blind-ending abscesses), but they are best identified by recognition of the communication with the blood pool on both sides of the valve. Thorough evaluation of 4-D data sets with MPR images in various imaging planes facilitates discrimination between perivalvular abscesses and paravalvular leaks.

PEARLS AND PITFALLS: USING CARDIAC COMPUTED TOMOGRAPHY ANGIOGRAPHY TO COMPLIMENT OTHER IMAGING MODALITIES IN EVALUATION OF INFECTIOUS ENDOCARDITIS

The spectrum of imaging findings associated with infective endocarditis can be evaluated in several ways with cardiac CTA, including both typical MPR and 4-D BPI volume-rendered images. Figure 36-15 demonstrates use of cardiac CTA to evaluate all these complications of infective endocarditis in two different patients, one with a native type 1 BAV and one with a stented porcine bioprosthesis. In the example of the stented bioprosthesis, the perivalvular abscess and paravalvular leak were not recognized preoperatively by TTE, in part because both findings were in the far field of view and were obscured by artifact from the metallic stent of the valve, as well as by distortion of the surrounding tissue planes (which can adversely affect transmission and reflection of an ultrasound beam). These findings were confirmed during intraoperative TEE (because they were both then in the near field of view with the probe in the esophagus) and by direct surgical inspection. A companion case of a large paravalvular leak around the right cusp of the valve is not shown, but it was not identifiable on either preoperative TTE (because of large body habitus and suboptimal image quality) or intraoperative TEE (because it was in

the far field of view obscured by artifact from the stented bioprosthesis).

Preoperative recognition of the full extent of disease can be of critical importance to the surgeon attempting to treat patients with infectious endocarditis. Cardiac CTA shows great promise in this regard, although further studies are needed to define its role more clearly in preoperative evaluation of patients with infective endocarditis.

Valvular Masses: Papillary Fibroelastoma

In addition to vegetations from infective endocarditis, cardiac CTA can be useful in identification of valve-associated thrombi and tumors of the valves such as PFs. Although the appearance of vegetations is highly variable, and valve-associated thrombi appear as sessile lesions associated with valves that may reduce cusp or leaflet excursion, PFs have a characteristic appearance that can be easily recognized on cardiac CTA examinations.

PFs have been recognized in all age groups, but they are most commonly diagnosed in the sixth decade of life. These benign, slow-growing tumors are the second most common primary cardiac tumors (after myxomas), but they account for 75% of all valvular tumors. PFs arise from the endocardium and can occur anywhere in the heart, although they are located in the left side of the heart 95% of the time. Seventy-five percent of PFs arise from the cardiac valves, and the most common location of PFs is on the aortic valve. When PFs arise from the semilunar valves, they can project into either the ventricular or (more commonly) the arterial lumen. When PFs arise from the atrioventricular valves, they are most common on the atrial surface. PFs are typically solitary, but they can be multiple in rare cases. All PFs carry a risk of embolization, either from bland thrombus that was adherent to the surface of the PF or from embolization of the small, frondlike portions of the tumor nidus itself. This embolization can result in devastating complications, particularly for PFs located in the left side of the heart, including cerebrovascular infarct, myocardial ischemia (from either direct occlusion of a coronary artery ostium by an attached aortic valve lesion, or coronary artery embolization), and sudden death. Because of the risk of catastrophic consequences if left untreated, once they are recognized, most PFs are surgically resected.

Regardless of where they are located, PFs have a characteristic appearance on cardiac CTA. As demonstrated in Figure 36-16, PFs arise from a thin stalk that leads to the main tumor nidus that is typically approximately 10 mm in diameter (although PFs ≤70 mm in diameter have been described). PFs are hypermobile lesions that commonly appear to flutter on this thin stalk throughout the cardiac cycle. A comprehensive evaluation of cardiac CTA data sets using both 4-D BPI volume rendering and MPR images typically demonstrates these characteristic features and helps to discriminate PFs from other valvular lesions.

■ CONCLUSION

Valve imaging with cardiac CTA can offer useful correlative data in evaluation of patients with valvular heart

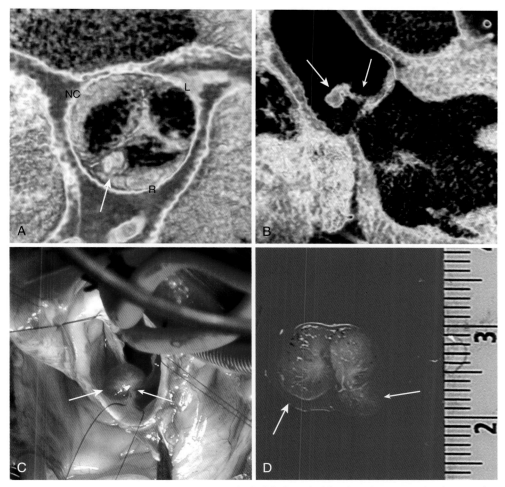

Figure 36-16 Papillary fibroelastoma of the aortic valve. A, Thick-slab diastolic blood pool inversion (BPI) image through the aortic root demonstrates a small lesion *(arrow)* associated with the right cusp (R) of the valve near the commissure with the noncoronary cusp (NC). *L*, Left. **B,** Thin-slab diastolic BPI image in the left ventricular outflow tract plane again demonstrates this nodular lesion *(large arrow)* which arises from a thin stalk *(small arrow)* from the arterial surface of the aortic valve. **C,** Intraoperative photograph demonstrates this lesion in vivo. **D,** Ex vivo photograph of the resected specimen. The nodular head and thin stalk are evident in both photographs *(large and small arrows,* respectively).

disease. CTA valve imaging is typically complementary to other imaging modalities, but it can sometimes offer incremental value. The benefits of valve imaging with cardiac CTA must be tempered by understanding its limitations and being conscious of the associated radiation exposure to the patient. As CT technology continues to evolve, improvements in spatial resolution, temporal resolution, and techniques to reduce radiation dose will undoubtedly improve both the clinical acceptability and the diagnostic utility of cardiac CTA in the assessment of valvular heart disease.

Bibliography

Abbara S, Pena AJ, Maurovich-Horvat P, et al. Feasibility and optimization of aortic valve planimetry with MDCT. *AJR Am J Roentgenol.* 2007;188:356-360.

Alkadhi H, Desbiolles L, Husmann L, et al. Aortic regurgitation: assessment with 64-section CT. *Radiology.* 2007;245:111-121.

Alkadhi H, Wildermuth S, Bettex DA, et al. Mitral regurgitation: quantification with 16-detector row CT: initial experience. *Radiology.* 2006;238:454-463.

Bonow RO, Carabello BA, Chatterjee K, et al. 2008 Focused update incorporated into the ACC/AHA 2006 guidelines for the management of patients with valvular heart disease: a report of the American College of Cardiology/American Heart Association Task Force on Practice Guidelines (Writing Committee to Revise the 1998 Guidelines for the Management of Patients With Valvular Heart Disease): endorsed by the Society of Cardiovascular Anesthesiologists, Society for Cardiovascular Angiography and Interventions, and Society of Thoracic Surgeons. *Circulation.* 2008;118:e523-e661.

Entrikin DW, Carr JJ. Blood pool inversion volume-rendering technique for visualization of the aortic valve. *J Cardiovasc Comput Tomogr.* 2008;2:336-371.

Gowda RM, Khan IA, Nair CK, et al. Cardiac papillary fibroelastoma: a comprehensive analysis of 725 cases. *Am Heart J.* 2003;146:404-410.

Halliburton SS, Abbara S. Practical tips and tricks in cardiovascular computed tomography: patient preparation for optimization of cardiovascular CT data acquisition. *J Cardiovasc Comput Tomogr.* 2007;1:62-65.

Lackner K, Thurn P. Computed tomography of the heart: ECG-gated and continuous scans. *Radiology.* 1981;140:413-420.

Morris MF, Maleszewski JJ, Suri RM, et al. CT and MR imaging of the mitral valve: radiologic-pathologic correlation. *Radiographics.* 2010;30:1603-1620.

Pouleur AC, le Polain de Waroux JB, Pasquet A, et al. Aortic valve area assessment: multidetector CT compared with cine MR imaging and transthoracic and transesophageal echocardiography. *Radiology.* 2007;244:745-754.

Sievers H, Schmidtke C. A classification system for the bicuspid aortic valve from 304 surgical specimens. *J Thorac Cardiovasc Surg.* 2007;133:1226-1233.

CHAPTER 37

Coronary Arteries: Anomalies, Normal Variants, Aneurysms, and Fistulas

Ronan Kileen and Jonathan D. Dodd

■ NORMAL ANATOMY

The sinuses of Valsalva are three adjacent dilatations or pouches of the aorta that have a cloverleaf configuration and lie above the level of the aortic valve but below the tubular portion of the ascending aorta. The sinotubular junction is where the sinuses of Valsalva meet the tubular segment of the ascending aorta. The right sinus of Valsalva is located anteriorly, and the left sinus of Valsalva is located more posteriorly and to the left. The right and left sinuses of Valsalva give rise to the right and left coronary arteries, respectively. There is also a noncoronary sinus called the *posterior sinus of Valsalva*, which in the normal configuration does not give rise to a vessel. The coronary arteries arise from the superior portions of the sinuses of Valsalva, just below the level of the sinotubular junction. The left main coronary artery (LMCA) normally arises more superiorly than the right coronary artery (RCA).

The proximal portion of the left coronary artery (LCA) is the LMCA. This segment is short (between 5 mm and 10 mm) and usually bifurcates into the left circumflex (LCx) and left anterior descending (LAD) arteries. The LMCA may trifurcate into LCx, LAD, and ramus intermedius in about 20% of people. The LAD usually descends in the anterior interventricular groove along the interventricular septum to the apex. The LAD gives rise to septal branches that course into the interventricular septum, supplying the superior two thirds of the septum. Diagonal branches arise from the LAD and descend toward the lateral margin of the left ventricular wall, supplying the anterior and sometimes anterolateral walls of the left ventricle. The septal branches may be difficult to see with cardiac computed tomography (CT), but the diagonal branches are consistently visualized. The diagonal branches are numbered sequentially (D1, D2, etc.).

The LCx branch descends in the left atrioventricular (AV) groove between the left atrium and left ventricle to supply obtuse marginal branches. There are a variable number of obtuse marginal branches, which supply the posterior and posterolateral walls of the left ventricle. The obtuse marginal branches are numbered sequentially (OM1, OM2, etc.).

The continuation of the LCx at this point can be variable. In left-dominant patients (10%) it travels all the way around the posterior wall of the heart, supplying both the posterior descending artery (PDA) and the posterior left ventricular branch, but more commonly it terminates as a small branch in the AV groove or continues as a small terminal posterior left ventricular branch.

The RCA originates from the right sinus of Valsalva at a slightly lower level than the LCA. The RCA then passes to the right, posterior to the pulmonary artery and under the right atrial appendage before descending in the anterior right AV groove between the right atrium and the right ventricle. In about 50% of patients the first branch from the RCA is the conus branch, which passes anteriorly and superiorly to supply the pulmonary outflow tract wall. The conus branch may also arise separately from the aorta or have a common origin from the aorta with the RCA. More rarely the conus branch may arise from the LCA. In 55% of patients the sinoatrial nodal artery is the next branch from the RCA. This vessel arises a few millimeters distal to the origin of the RCA and passes posteriorly toward the superior vena cava near the top of the interatrial septum. In 45% of patients the sinoatrial nodal artery arises from the proximal LCx. This is followed by two to three right ventricular wall branches. The acute marginal branch is the first large branch, which occasionally continues to the apex. In 70% of patients the RCA passes down the right AV groove to the crux of the heart, where it gives off the PDA and the posterior left ventricular branch. Approximately 20% of patients have a codominant supply, in which the PDA originates from the RCA but branches from the LCx also supply this territory. The PDA gives off inferior septal perforating branches which are not well visualized on cardiac CT.

■ ANOMALIES OF THE CORONARY ARTERIES

Congenital abnormalities of the coronary arteries are uncommon, with an incidence in the general population of approximately 1% to 2%. They are often found incidentally at angiography or autopsy, and many are of no clinical significance. However, a minority are an important cause of symptoms, including chest pain, palpitations, dyspnea, and sudden death. In patients with congenital heart disease there is an increased incidence of anomalies reported to be between 3% and 36%.

In the past, catheter angiography was used to diagnose and evaluate coronary anomalies, but complex anomalous courses may be difficult to interpret and the angiographer may be unable to find the location of the ostium of the anomalous vessel. Cardiac CT has proven highly accurate in the depiction of such anomalies and has become the noninvasive imaging gold standard.

Symptoms of Coronary Anomalies

Coronary anomalies have been associated with sudden death in young (<35 years) athletes, particularly those in whom the coronary artery arises from the wrong aortic sinus of Valsalva. Exercise-induced episodic myocardial ischemia is believed to be the cause of death in these patients. Most coronary anomalies are surgically correctable once identified, and thus sudden death in athletes may be preventable in many cases. Death typically occurs during or after 30 minutes of strenuous exercise. Antemorbid cardiovascular symptoms may be present in approximately one third of these patients. Episodes of syncope, dizziness, palpitations, and exertional chest pain have been reported in athletes who subsequently died suddenly, with symptoms in retrospect occurring up to 2 years before death. Symptoms of syncope and chest pain are more strongly associated with anomalous LMCA than anomalous RCA. Overall, up to one third of patients who die from an anomalous coronary artery have a history of exertional syncope or chest pain. Electrocardiograms (ECGs) may be normal or demonstrate premature ventricular contractions. Results of exercise stress tests performed before death in these athletes are frequently normal without ST-segment or T-wave changes, arrhythmias, or cardiac symptoms.

Pearl

Normal results for a maximal exercise stress test do not alter the likelihood of a coronary anomaly being present.

Several theories have been proposed to explain the mechanism of myocardial ischemia and sudden death in these patients. Pathologically, in patients with sudden cardiac death caused by anomalous coronary arteries, the origin of the anomalous vessel may have a fibrous ridge with an acute angle, and the orifice of the vessel is typically slitlike. Flaplike closure of the abnormal orifice and compression of the vessel between the aorta and pulmonary trunk may contribute to reduced myocardial perfusion, particularly during exercise. This may commence a cascade of distal myocardial ischemia, ventricular tachycardia, ventricular fibrillation, and subsequent cardiac arrest. Endothelial damage with resultant coronary spasm or thrombosis, or both, at the site of

anomalous vessels has also been suggested. Data from necropsies argue against the thrombosis theory because intraarterial thrombosis is rarely found in patients with sudden death and anomalous coronary arteries. By contrast, evidence of ischemic events is often identified at necropsy.

Pearl

The very proximal course of the anomalous vessel may be intramural within the myocardium. This is associated with a higher incidence of sudden death. Intramural courses allow for potential treatment with unroofing procedure of the anomalous vessel.

Pearl

Anomalous LCAs from the right sinus of Valsalva may have an intramyocardial course proximally (through the ventricular septum, resurfacing in the anterior interventricular groove). Such configurations are considered to be associated with a higher incidence of sudden death.

Congenital coronary anomalies are more commonly found as a cause of death in highly trained athletes than in nonathletes. The highest risk for death is in the first 30 years of life, and the risk increases if the aberrant coronary artery supplies a large area of myocardium. Because of the inherent lack of sensitivity of clinical examination, ECG, and exercise stress tests, these anomalies often become known only after death. In those patients who do have symptoms, the vast majority are exertional. In young trained athletes with exertional symptoms, the threshold for investigation of possible coronary anomalies should be low, given the catastrophic results that may occur if a malignant coronary anomaly is missed. Echocardiography has the ability to identify the location of the right and left coronary artery orifices in about 95% of young athletes. Failure to identify the proximal right and left coronary arteries at echocardiography in a young athlete with exertional symptoms should be followed by a second test to more clearly delineate the coronary artery origins, typically cardiac CT. Anomalous coronary arteries may also contribute to patient morbidity and mortality by increasing the incidence of complications during cardiac surgery and by increasing the technical difficulties encountered during angiography. There remains controversy over whether there is an association between coronary anomalies and increased risk for atherosclerotic disease.

Classification of Coronary Artery Anomalies

Coronary artery anomalies may be subdivided into three broad categories:
1. Anomalous aortic origin with benign course
2. Anomalous aortic origin with potentially "malignant" course
3. Anomalous origin from the pulmonary artery (serious)

High Takeoff of Coronary Arteries From Ascending Aorta

The coronary artery ostia may have abnormal takeoffs from the ascending aorta, which subsequently course in a normal direction. The most common is a "high-takeoff" coronary artery, which implies that the right or left coronary artery arises above the sinotubular junction (arises from the ascending aorta). This may be present in up to 6% of the population. This usually occurs a few millimeters above the sinotubular junction, but distances of up to 2.0 cm have been reported. Although this type of abnormality is not of major clinical significance, it may lead to difficulty in coronary artery cannulation during angiography.

Separate Ostia of the Left Circumflex and Left Coronary Arteries

The LCx and LCA may have separate ostia at the left sinus of Valsalva. This occurs in a small percentage of people (0.4%). Although this may lead to difficulties with cannulation at angiography, it also may provide collateral pathways in the event of proximal LCA disease. This anomaly has been reported to be associated with an increased incidence of aortic valve disease.

Absent Left Circumflex Artery

An absent LCx artery occurs in less than 0.005% of the population. In this anomaly a "superdominant" right coronary artery crosses the crux of the heart and ascends in the left AV groove in retrograde fashion to supply the posterolateral and lateral wall of the left ventricle.

Origin of the Left Circumflex Artery From the Right Sinus of Valsalva or Right Coronary Artery

Origin of the LCx from the right sinus of Valsalva or the proximal RCA is one of the most common of the coronary anomalies and constitutes between 30% and 60% of anomalies identified in angiographic studies. The prevalence of this anomaly is approximately 0.4%. The anomalous LCx more commonly arises from the right sinus of Valsalva (69%) than the proximal RCA (31%) and always courses posterior to the aorta. The LCx courses posterior to the aorta before supplying the left lateral wall of the heart. It may be an isolated anomaly with the LAD originating normally from the LCMA or may be associated with other branch anomalies such as the LAD originating from the anomalous LCx artery. At angiography contrast injection into the RCA may fail to opacify an anomalous LCx, and the catheter may need to be placed in the posterior aspect or the right sinus of Valsalva to visualize the vessel. Mismanagement may result if the angiographer assumes the LCx is occluded or congenitally absent. The cardiac surgeon should be informed of the presence of this anomaly to avoid injury during valve replacement surgery. This anomaly is benign.

Anomalous Origin of the Left Main Coronary Artery or Right Coronary Artery From the Posterior Sinus of Valsalva

Anomalous origin of the LMCA or RCA from the posterior sinus of Valsalva is extremely rare. This anomaly was identified in only 5 patients (RCA in 4 patients and LCA in 1 patient) in the study by Yamanaka and Hobbs of more than 126,000 patient angiograms. This anomaly is not associated with symptoms or complications and is considered benign.

■ ANOMALOUS AORTIC ORIGIN WITH POTENTIALLY "MALIGNANT" COURSE

Single Coronary Artery

A single coronary artery is a rare occurrence (<0.05%) in which all the coronary arteries arise from a single ostium (Fig. 37-1). This vessel may take the same proximal course as the normal right or left coronary artery before dividing into two branches that supply the same distributions as the right and left coronary arteries. This anomaly is associated with an increased risk for sudden death if a major coronary branch passes between the aorta and the right ventricular outflow tract. The Lipton classification scheme is used to further describe these anomalies. In group I anomalies there is a single coronary artery, which takes the course of the right or left coronary artery and supplies the entire myocardium. In group II anomalies the anomalous vessels arise from a normal proximal left or right coronary artery and take an interarterial or more commonly septal course before supplying their usual territory. In group III anomalies the LCx and LAD arise separately from the proximal RCA.

Origin of the Coronary Artery From the Opposite Coronary Sinus

In these anomalies the LCA arises from the right sinus of Valsalva or the RCA arises from the left sinus of Valsalva. The course that the vessel takes is described in relation to the ascending aorta and the right ventricular outflow tract or pulmonary trunk. The anomalous vessel can take four possible pathways:
1. Interarterial (between the pulmonary artery and the aorta)
2. Prepulmonic (anterior to the pulmonary artery)
3. Retroaortic (posterior to the aorta)
4. Septal (subpulmonic)

Pearl
The interarterial course carries a risk for sudden death, but prepulmonic, retroaortic, and septal courses are considered benign.

Anomalous Origin of Left Coronary Artery From Right Sinus of Valsalva

Origin of the left main trunk from the right sinus of Valsalva has an incidence of 0.02%, and origin of the LAD

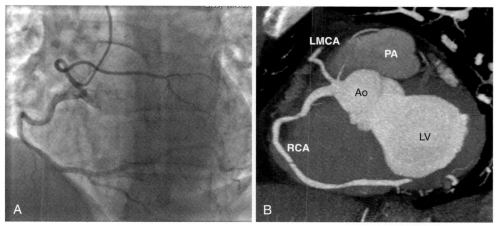

Figure 37-1 A 59-year-old man with chest pain. **A,** Invasive angiography suggested a single coronary origin from the right sinus of Valsalva. **B,** Cardiac computed tomography confirmed this to be the case, with the left main coronary artery passing anterior to the right ventricular outflow tract before bifurcating in the anterior interventricular groove into the left anterior coronary artery and the left circumflex coronary artery. *Ao,* Aorta; *LMCA,* left main coronary artery; *LV,* left ventricle; *PA,* pulmonary artery; *RCA,* right coronary artery.

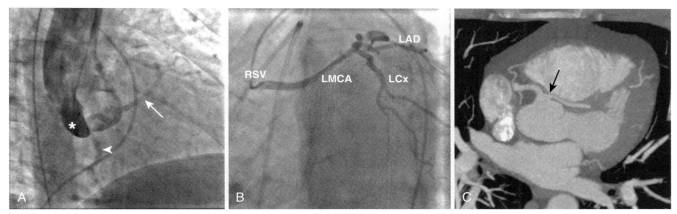

Figure 37-2 A 28-year-old man with palpitations during exercise. **A** and **B,** Invasive angiography suggested a common origin *(asterisk)* of the left main coronary artery *(arrow)* from the right sinus of Valsalva (note the right coronary artery *[arrowhead]*). **C,** Cardiac computed tomography confirmed that the left main coronary artery originated from the right sinus of Valsalva and passed between the great vessels *(arrow)*. *LAD,* Left anterior descending artery; *LCx,* left circumflex artery; *LMCA,* left main coronary artery; *RSV,* right sinus of Valsalva.

artery from the right sinus of Valsalva is more common, with an incidence of 0.03% in angiographic studies (Fig. 37-2). Passage of the left main trunk or LAD artery between the aorta and the pulmonary trunk may result in chest pain, syncope, myocardial ischemia, myocardial infarction, ventricular arrhythmias, and cardiac arrest as described earlier. In a right anterior oblique projection angiogram the anomalous left main trunk is seen as a "dot" on the anterior aspect of the ascending aorta as the vessel is seen end on (dot sign).

The septal course is the most common and has also been referred to as the *intramyocardial* or *tunneled* variant. In this anomaly the left main trunk crosses superior to the crista supraventricularis, then passes through the septum before typically becoming epicardial in the midseptum. Angiographically the vessels have the appearance of a "hammock" and are frequently confused with the interarterial variant. The septal course is considered benign.

In the prepulmonic variant the left main trunk courses anterior to the pulmonary trunk and then divides typically at the junction of the proximal and middle third of the septum. In the right anterior oblique projection at angiography the left main trunk with the LCx artery coursing posteriorly and inferiorly form the appearance of an "eye." Although this anomaly is considered benign, chest pain and myocardial infarction have been reported in association with it in the absence of atherosclerotic disease.

In the retroaortic subtype the left main trunk passes posterior to the aorta. This may be seen angiographically as a "dot" at the posterior aspect of the ascending aorta. This anomaly is considered benign. It may be difficult to elucidate the exact course of these anomalies with angiography using the indirect signs described, and cardiac CT is generally indicated in such cases.

Anomalous Origin of the Right Coronary Artery From the Left Sinus of Valsalva

Anomalous origin of the RCA from the left sinus of Valsalva is more common than an anomalous origin of the LCA from the right sinus of Valsalva and is seen in

0.1% of angiographic studies (Fig. 37-3). The ostium of the anomalous RCA usually lies anterior to the ostium of the left main trunk. Yamanaka and Hobbs reported 136 cases in their series of over 126,000 patients and reported that in all but 1 patient the RCA took an interarterial course. This anomaly is associated with chest pain, syncope, myocardial ischemia, myocardial infarction, ventricular arrhythmias, and cardiac arrest as described earlier. In one patient the RCA passed posterior to the aorta. Although considered by most to be malignant, it is less strongly associated with significant morbidity and mortality than the LMCA arising from the right sinus of Valsalva variant.

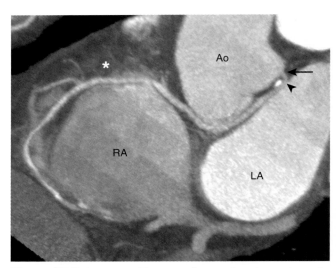

Figure 37-3 A 52-year-old man underwent invasive angiography for chest pain. The right coronary artery (RCA) was not found. Subsequent cardiac computed tomography demonstrated the RCA arising from the left sinus of Valsalva from a separate ostium *(arrow)* to the left main coronary artery. It followed a retroaortic course before resuming its normal configuration in the right atrioventricular groove *(asterisk)*. Note the sharp angulation *(arrowhead)* of the proximal segment characteristically seen in many coronary anomalies. Note also the nonobstructive calcified plaque in the proximal segment. *Ao,* Aorta; *LA,* left atrium; *RA,* right atrium.

Anomalous Coronary Origin From the Pulmonary Artery

Anomalous origin of the LCA from the pulmonary artery constitutes Bland-White-Garland syndrome. This entity is also referred to by the acronym *ALCAPA* (anomalous origin of the left coronary artery from the pulmonary artery). In this serious anomaly the LCA arises from the pulmonary artery instead of the aorta. As a result there is retrograde flow through the LMCA into the lower-pressure pulmonary artery system. The blood flow to the LCA is supplied by a dilated RCA via usually extensive enlarged and tortuous collaterals. The estimated prevalence of this condition is 1 in 300,000 live births. Few people with this anomaly reach adulthood, with 95% dying in infancy. The clinical symptoms and sequelae include angina, myocardial infarction, mitral regurgitation, arrhythmias, and cardiac arrest. Once this entity is identified, surgical correction is warranted because of the risk for sudden death. Treatment options include ligation of the LCA in conjunction with bypass grafting, construction of a conduit from the aorta to the LCA, and direct reimplantation of the LCA into the aorta. The choice of procedure is influenced by the age of the patient, with reimplantation preferred in infants rather than bypass grafting because of reports of vein graft failure with sudden death.

Anomalous origin of the RCA from the pulmonary artery (known as *ARCAPA*) is extremely rare, with origin of the LAD artery from the pulmonary artery even rarer (Fig. 37-4). In the first instance, flow passes from the LCA via collaterals retrograde through the RCA and then into the pulmonary artery. In the second instance, collaterals from the left main or right coronary artery supply the LAD with flow passing retrograde through the LAD into the pulmonary artery. Many patients with ectopic RCA or LAD from the pulmonary artery may remain asymptomatic, but angina, myocardial infarction, syncope, congestive cardiac failure, and sudden death have been reported.

If a coronary artery anomaly is identified with the right or left coronary artery arising from the wrong

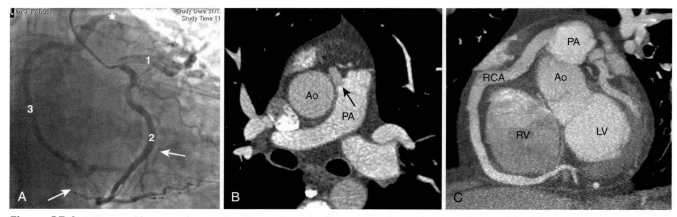

Figure 37-4 A 53-year-old man underwent invasive angiography for recurrent chest pain. Cannulation of the left main coronary artery demonstrated the entire coronary arterial tree. **A,** Note the right coronary artery *(3)* fills from collaterals *(arrows)* from the left coronary system before flushing into a large vessel *(asterisk)*. Note also the size of the left coronary vessels (left anterior descending artery *[1]*, left circumflex artery *[2]*), which are dilated, suggesting flow from a high-pressure to a low-pressure system. **B** and **C,** Cardiac computed tomography shows the right coronary artery (RCA) *(arrow)* arising from the main pulmonary artery (PA). *Ao,* Aorta; *LV,* left ventricle; *RV,* right ventricle.

coronary sinus, with an interarterial course, surgical treatment may be performed. Coronary artery bypass grafting may be performed to restore diminished distal coronary flow. Alternatively, surgical reimplantation of the vessel into the correct sinus can be performed. More recently, surgical unroofing (or marsupialization) of the anomalous orifice has been described when there is an aortic intramural course.

Myocardial Bridges

Myocardial bridging occurs when a normally epicardial coronary vessel has a segment with an intramyocardial course (Fig. 37-5). The reported prevalence of myocardial bridging varies widely between studies and on whether the study is based on autopsy (up to 85%), conventional angiography (up to 16%), or cardiac CT (up to 39%). This is considered a normal variant by many, and in the vast majority of patients no clinical consequences are evident. Because the vast majority of coronary blood flow occurs during diastole (85%), the systolic compression that occurs in myocardial bridging is not considered significant, although in rare instances ischemia, arrhythmias, acute coronary syndrome, coronary spasm, and sudden death have been associated with myocardial bridging. Tachycardia may elicit myocardial ischemia in the setting of a myocardial bridge because of alteration of flow dynamics by reducing the time for diastole and leading to increased reliance on systolic coronary flow for perfusion. Vessel luminal narrowing during dynamic contraction is typically between 30% and 50% but may be up to 100%. Clinical consequences occur almost exclusively with LAD myocardial bridging. Myocardial ischemia may result from myocardial bridging secondary to systolic compression, endothelial dysfunction and thrombus formation, and coronary vasospasm. It has been reported that dynamic compression is caused by the overlying myocardium compressing the vessel during systole. However, this does not explain the observation that dynamic compression can be seen in vessels without overlying muscle and two thirds of intramyocardial segments with overlying muscle do not demonstrate dynamic compression. More recently some authors have suggested that dynamic compression may relate to entrapment of the vessel within the interventricular gorge with squeezing of the vessel secondary to contraction of the two adjacent walls. It has been shown that the greater the total length of the myocardial bridge, the greater the chance of dynamic compression.

■ CORONARY ANEURYSMS

Coronary ectasia typically involves dilatation of the coronary artery but does not exceed 1.5 times the normal lumen diameter and usually involves more than 50% of the total length of the coronary artery (Fig. 37-6). Coronary artery aneurysms are defined as coronary artery segments that have a diameter that exceeds the diameter of normal adjacent coronary segments or the diameter of the patient's largest coronary vessel by 1.5 times and involve less than 50% of the total length of the vessel (Fig. 37-7). Cardiac CT is particularly suited to their evaluation, because the true size of the aneurysm may be underestimated on angiography, or the aneurysm may not even be seen when it is occluded or contains substantial thrombi or plaque (Fig. 37-8).

Vessel ectasia can be classified as follows: type I, indicating diffuse ectasia in two or three vessels; type II, indicating diffuse ectasia in one vessel and localized disease (i.e., aneurysm) in another; type III, indicating diffuse ectasia in only one vessel; and type IV, indicating coronary aneurysm in one vessel. Aneurysms can be classified as focal or diffuse. In the focal group they are termed *giant aneurysms* when they measure more than 20 mm to 150 mm in diameter in adults and more than 8 mm in diameter in children.

Numerous causes exist for the pathogenesis of coronary aneurysms. In adults the most common cause is atherosclerosis. In children the most important cause is Kawasaki disease. In this entity, spontaneous resolution occurs in 50%, and it is thought to be related to an autoimmune reactivity to a virus with subsequent vasculitis. Several inflammatory disorders may also affect the coronary arteries in children, including Takayasu arteritis, systemic lupus erythematosus, rheumatoid arthritis, Wegener granulomatosis, giant cell arteritis, Churg-Strauss syndrome, microscopic polyangiitis, antiphospholipid syndrome, Behçet syndrome, sarcoidosis, polyarteritis nodosa, CREST syndrome, ankylosing spondylitis, Reiter syndrome, and psoriatic arthritis.

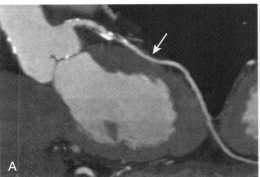
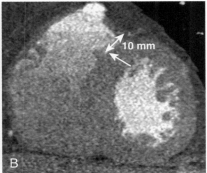

Figure 37-5 **A,** A 62-year-old man underwent cardiac computed tomography for chest pain. It revealed an obstructive stenosis in the proximal segment left anterior descending artery and a downstream shallow myocardial bridge *(arrow)*. **B,** Note that certain bridges may be very deep and may embed close to the right ventricular cavity *(arrows)*.

Connective tissue disorders may also affect younger patients' coronary arteries, specifically Ehlers-Danlos syndrome and Marfan syndrome, which are characterized by cystic medial necrosis. Other considerations include mycotic (*Staphylococcus aureus* or *Pseudomonas aeruginosa*, syphilis, Lyme disease); trauma/iatrogenic with coronary dissection; drugs (specifically cocaine), thought generally to be a result of direct endothelial damage from severe

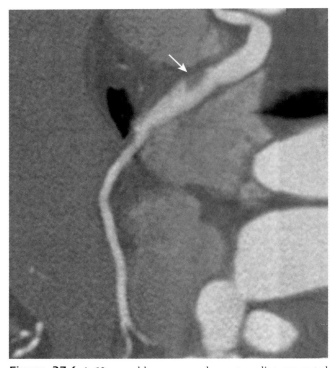

Figure 37-6 A 62-year-old woman underwent cardiac computed tomography for atypical chest pain. It revealed an ectatic, dilated right coronary artery involving most of the proximal segment and midsegment. Note the filling defect in the midsegment wall *(arrow)* consistent with mural thrombus. The patient was treated with anticoagulation and antiplatelet therapy.

episodic hypertension; vasoconstriction; and underlying atherosclerosis (Fig. 37-8).

Pearl

In the West, atherosclerosis, followed by congenital (17%) and infectious (10%) causes, is the most common cause of coronary aneurysms, whereas in Japan, Kawasaki disease is the predominant cause. Clinical presentation depends on the underlying cause. The atherosclerotic subtype tends to present in a way similar to other atherosclerotic coronary artery disease. Other factors that influence symptoms are the extent of atherosclerosis, the presence of poor distal vessel runoff, and the development of complications such as distal embolization with myocardial ischemia, rupture with associated fistula, cardiac tamponade or hemopericardium, thrombosis, dissection, and vessel compression. Patients with obstructive disease are treated as for any coronary stenosis. In those patients without obstructive disease, treatment is controversial. There are no randomized controlled trials of therapeutic agents in this setting. Medical therapy includes anticoagulant therapy and administration of antiplatelet drugs to minimize thromboembolic complications.

■ CORONARY ARTERY FISTULAS

A coronary artery fistula is an anomalous termination of a coronary vessel with an abnormal precapillary communication between one or more coronary arteries and a cardiac chamber, a pulmonary artery, a pulmonary vein, the coronary sinus, the superior vena cava, or even a bronchial artery or vein. If the connection is to a cardiac chamber, it is referred to as a *coronary-cameral fistula*. Fistulas may be congenital or acquired (most commonly iatrogenic), but most reported cases are of the congenital form. The estimated prevalence of coronary artery fistulas in the general population is 0.0002%, but at angiography the prevalence of coronary

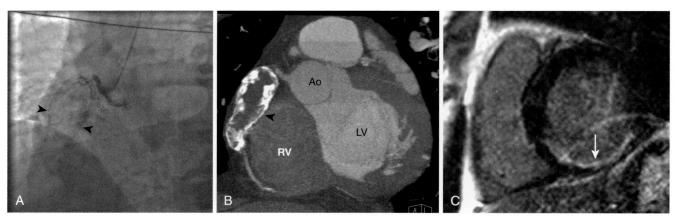

Figure 37-7 A 52-year-old man was admitted to the coronary care unit having been successfully resuscitated following a ventricular tachycardia arrest at home. He had a history of severe infection at age 4 years, characterized by pneumonia, severe mucositis, conjunctivitis, and skin desquamation of his palms and soles. **A,** Invasive coronary angiography demonstrated complete occlusion of the proximal segment right coronary artery (RCA) and a calcified linear opacity *(arrowheads)* suspicious for a giant calcified aneurysm distal to the occlusion. **B,** Coronary multidetector computed tomography confirmed the presence, location, and extent of a giant, calcified RCA aneurysm *(arrowhead)*. **C,** Cardiac delayed enhancement magnetic resonance imaging short-axis sequence following gadolinium demonstrated inferior wall hyperenhancement with wall thinning *(arrow)*, which is transmural in its epicenter, consistent with a chronic myocardial infarction in the RCA vascular territory. *RV,* Right ventricle.

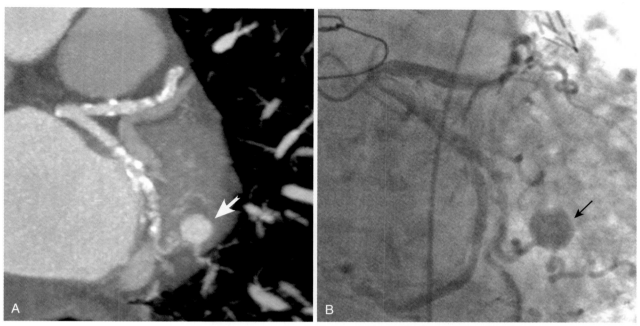

Figure 37-8 **A,** A 78-year-old woman had atypical chest pain and underwent cardiac computed tomography (CT). She had a history of three-vessel coronary artery bypass graft surgery 12 years previously. Cardiac CT revealed a focal aneurysm arising from the obtuse marginal branch. **B,** Invasive coronary angiography confirmed the aneurysm *(arrow)*, and she subsequently underwent surgical resection.

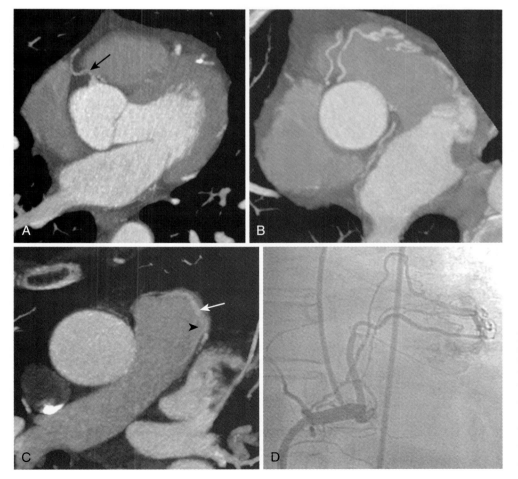

Figure 37-9 A 38-year-old man had atypical chest pain. Cardiac computed tomography (**A, B,** and **C**) revealed a small coronary fistula *(arrow)* from the right sinus of Valsalva, passing around the anterior wall of the RVOT in **B** before draining into the main pulmonary artery *(arrow* in **C**). Notice the blush of contrast in the main pulmonary artery from the fistula *(arrowhead* in **C**), also noted on the invasive angiogram (**D**).

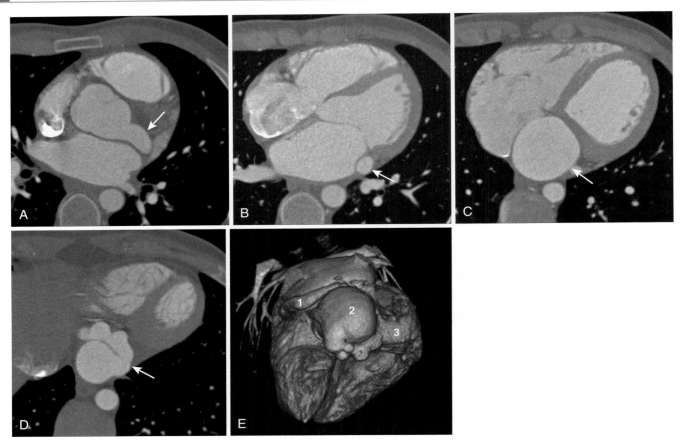

Figure 37-10 A 26-year-old man had palpitations and chest pain during exercise. **A,** Cardiac computed tomography revealed a dilated left circumflex coronary artery *(arrow)* leading into a giant aneurysmal fistula, which drained into the coronary sinus (**A, B, C,** and **D**). **E,** Volumetric three-dimensional reconstruction demonstrates the orientation in three dimensions and the feeding left circumflex artery *(1),* the giant aneurysmal fistula *(2),* and the draining coronary sinus *(3).*

artery fistulas is higher at 0.2%. There is no predilection for race or sex.

Both the RCA and the LCA have been reported in published series to be the most common site of origin of coronary artery fistulas, and it is likely that they give rise to coronary artery fistulas at approximately the same frequency. In less than 5% of reported cases both the RCA and LCA supply the fistula. The supplying artery is usually tortuous and dilated as a result of the increased blood flow into a low pressure system. At the distal end of the fistula there may be multiple draining vessels at the site of entry into the heart chamber or lower-pressure artery or vein, but most have a single communication. The right ventricle is the most common site of drainage (45%), followed by the right atrium and the pulmonary artery (Fig. 37-9). Rarer drainage sites include the coronary sinus (Fig. 37-10), the left atrium, the left ventricle, the superior vena cava, and a bronchial artery or vein. The diameter of coronary fistula varies throughout its length, ranging up to 4 cm, but is usually less than 1 cm.

Pearl

If a coronary-cameral fistula drains into a right cardiac chamber, it acts as a left-to-right shunt (90%). If a fistula drains into a left-sided heart chamber (10%), the hemodynamic changes that occur can mimic aortic regurgitation.

The most common presentation is a continuous heart murmur incidentally noted at auscultation. Symptoms typically occur late as a result of an enlarging coronary artery fistula with increasing shunt fraction and overload of the right heart with progressive right ventricular enlargement. Between 1 month old and 20 years old most patients are asymptomatic. Symptoms of a coronary artery fistula include exertional dyspnea, chest pain, fatigue, and cardiac failure. Cardiac failure is more common in neonates than infants and adults. Endocarditis, stroke, myocardial ischemia, and infarction have also been reported. The mechanism of myocardial ischemia is likely a steal phenomenon because of the low-resistance distal runoff within the fistula. Chronic left-to-right shunting may result in pulmonary hypertension, although this is rare. More commonly, aneurysmal dilatation of the distal vessel just before the fistulous connection is seen, and this may result in rupture. Aneurysm formation typically does not occur before the third decade and is most common in the seventh decade. Giant aneurysms have been reported, measuring over 20 cm in diameter. The fistula may thrombose, which may lead to myocardial infarction.

The draining component of a coronary artery fistula is within a low-pressure compartment and may be difficult to see at conventional angiography because of mixing of contrast within the distal compartment, unlike the proximal portion, which is reliably visualized at angiography. Echocardiography using microbubbles can also be used to delineate the extent of coronary artery fistulas. Cardiac CT has proven to be a valuable noninvasive test for depicting the full course of coronary fistulas. Use of three-dimensional volume-rendered images can provide the surgeon with an understanding of the complexity of the lesion and its relationship to adjacent cardiac and vascular structures, as well as extracardiac structures and the chest wall.

It is unclear if asymptomatic coronary artery fistulas should be treated, and some authors suggest surveillance with concomitant antiplatelet therapy and prophylaxis against endocarditis rather than definitive intervention. Elective closure in childhood has been recommended, given that patients with coronary artery fistulas may develop myocardial ischemia, congestive cardiac failure, endocarditis, or aneurysmal dilatation, although the incidence of cardiac complications is low with a small shunt.

Treatment options for symptomatic patients include surgical ligation or transcatheter embolization of the fistula. Both of these techniques have similar effectiveness, morbidity, and mortality. Surgical ligation is preferred for large coronary artery fistulas with high fistula flow or with aneurysm formation, or with large branches that may be embolized inadvertently. In patients with coronary artery fistula and additional complex heart disease, a surgical approach is also recommended. If transcatheter embolization is to be performed, it must be possible to cannulate the distal fistula without flow disturbance to the adjacent coronary branches. Long-term follow-up is indicated because of the possibility of recanalization of the fistula, continued dilatation of the coronary artery at the proximal aspect of the fistula, thrombus formation, and myocardial infarction.

Pearl

Unless flow within the fistula has completely ceased, antibiotic prophylaxis for bacterial endocarditis should be given before dental, urologic, or gastrointestinal procedures.

Bibliography

Angelini P, Velasco JA, Flamm S. Coronary anomalies: incidence, pathophysiology, and clinical relevance. *Circulation.* 2002;105:2449-2454.

Armsby LR, Keane JF, Sherwood MC, Forbess JM, Perry SB, Lock JE. Management of coronary artery fistulae: patient selection and results of transcatheter closure. *J Am Coll Cardiol.* 2002;39:1026-1032.

Basso C, Maron BJ, Corrado D, Thiene G. Clinical profile of congenital coronary artery anomalies with origin from the wrong aortic sinus leading to sudden death in young competitive athletes. *J Am Coll Cardiol.* 2000;35:1493-1501.

Dodd JD, Ferencik M, Liberthson RR, et al. Congenital anomalies of coronary artery origin in adults: 64-MDCT appearance. *AJR Am J Roentgenol.* 2007;188:W138-W146.

Kim PJ, Hur G, Kim SY, et al. Frequency of myocardial bridges and dynamic compression of epicardial coronary arteries: a comparison between computed tomography and invasive coronary angiography. *Circulation.* 2009;119:1408-1416.

Kim SY, Seo JB, Do KH, et al. Coronary artery anomalies: classification and ECG-gated multi-detector row CT findings with angiographic correlation. *Radiographics.* 2006;26:317-333;discussion 333–334.

Liberthson RR. Sudden death from cardiac causes in children and young adults. *N Engl J Med.* 1996;334:1039-1044.

Yamanaka O, Hobbs RE. Coronary artery anomalies in 126,595 patients undergoing coronary arteriography. *Cathet Cardiovasc Diagn.* 1990;21:28-40.

Zenooz NA, Habibi R, Mammen L, Finn JP, Gilkeson RC. Coronary artery fistulas: CT findings. *Radiographics.* 2009;29:781-789.

CHAPTER 38

Coronary Arteries: Coronary Atherosclerotic Disease

Stephan Achenbach

■ CORONARY ARTERY DISEASE

The definition of coronary artery disease is not uniform. Often any atherosclerotic plaque that is present in the coronary system, even if completely asymptomatic, will be labeled as coronary artery disease. Most physicians use the term if at least one flow-limiting stenosis is present, and the typical threshold assumed for a flow-limiting stenosis is a diameter reduction of 50%. Finally, some physicians argue that the term *coronary artery disease* should be reserved for individuals who have clinical symptoms because of the presence of coronary artery stenoses.

Similarly, there is no immediate relationship between the buildup of atherosclerotic plaque and narrowing of the coronary lumen, and not even a uniform understanding of the term *stenosis* (Fig. 38-1). When coronary atherosclerotic plaque develops, it is usually accompanied by a process called "remodeling," which expresses the fact that the overall vessel cross section typically dilates to compensate for the plaque volume. Rather large plaques can be present without substantial luminal narrowing. Thus the degree of stenosis when assessed by angiography ("luminal stenosis") will often be relatively mild, because the lumen is only slightly narrowed. However, if the lesion is visualized in cross section, for example by histologic examination or tomographic imaging (intravascular ultrasonography or corresponding reformats in cardiac computed tomography [CT]), the degree of stenosis that is obtained by comparing the area of the entire vessel cross section to the area of the remaining lumen can be substantial.

If, on the other hand, the process of remodeling fails to compensate for the growing plaque, the coronary artery lumen will be narrowed substantially, and angiographically detectable luminal stenosis is the consequence. Hence the degree of stenosis determined by investigating the coronary lumen will typically be less than stenosis determined by comparing vessel cross section to luminal cross section.

■ DETECTION OF CORONARY ARTERY DISEASE—ISCHEMIA VERSUS ANATOMY

It is important to note that clinically there are two different concepts for the detection of coronary artery stenoses in patients. On one hand, tests that determine ischemia or wall motion abnormalities during stress are often used (such as nuclear perfusion imaging, stress magnetic resonance imaging or stress echocardiography). It is important to note that the functional consequences of stenoses are not uniform and are difficult to predict. Even stenoses of more than 50% luminal reduction are not always associated with downstream ischemia, and the degree of stenosis is a relatively poor predictor of ischemia. Inducible ischemia has been demonstrated to be of prognostic significance, and clinical guidelines suggest ischemia testing as the first step in the workup of coronary artery disease. If no ischemia is present, there is relatively little to gain from revascularization, and hence further testing is generally not suggested.

Another method of diagnosing coronary artery disease is direct visualization of the coronary artery system and coronary stenoses, which is possible through invasive coronary angiography and coronary CT angiography (Fig. 38-2). Recently it has also become possible to use volumetric magnetic resonance imaging sequences for coronary imaging. Some applications exist in the context of coronary anomalies and Kawasaki disease, but coronary magnetic resonance imaging is not clinically used at the moment in patients with known or suspected coronary atherosclerotic disease.

■ CORONARY ARTERY IMAGING BY INVASIVE ANGIOGRAPHY AND COMPUTED TOMOGRAPHY

Invasive Coronary Angiography

In the vast majority of cases, invasive coronary angiography will be used to visualize the coronary arteries and detect coronary artery stenoses. It is an invasive procedure but relatively safe and with very few contraindications. A vascular access is required, which is typically between 4 French (Fr) and 6 Fr. The transfemoral access is used most frequently, but transradial procedures enjoy increasing popularity. Approximately 20 to 100 mL of iodinated contrast agent is required. Two main aspects speak for invasive coronary angiography as compared to CT angiography for the detection of coronary artery stenoses: the accuracy, for clinical purposes, can be considered to be close to 100%, and the method fails in almost no patients. If performed, a diagnostic

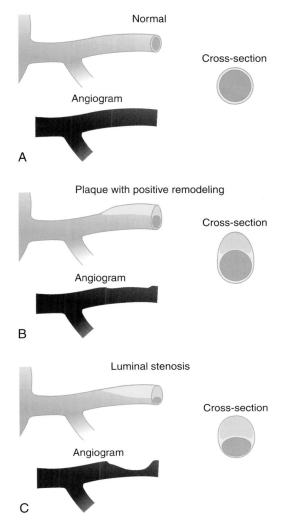

Normal

Cross-section

Angiogram

A

Plaque with positive remodeling

Cross-section

Angiogram

B

Luminal stenosis

Cross-section

Angiogram

C

Figure 38-1 Coronary atherosclerotic plaque and the process of "remodeling." A, Normal situation without plaque and without stenosis. **B,** Buildup of coronary atherosclerotic plaque with "positive remodeling." A large volume of atherosclerotic plaque develops in the coronary arterial wall (in the intimal layer of the vessel wall). As a compensatory mechanism, the overall vessel cross section increases so that the lumen is not substantially narrowed. "Stenosis degree" will therefore be substantially different, depending on whether it is assessed by angiography (which will show only mild luminal narrowing) or by imaging methods that generate cross-sectional views of the artery (such as intravascular ultrasonography or computed tomography). In the cross-sectional view, the degree of stenosis will be substantially more than in angiographic assessment based on lumen visualization alone. **C,** Coronary atherosclerotic plaque without compensation by remodeling. Vessel enlargement fails to compensate for the atherosclerotic plaque volume. Hence a substantial narrowing of the lumen occurs. Both in cross section and in angiographic luminal assessment, the vessel will appear significantly stenotic.

result is almost completely certain, except for extremely infrequent cases with access site problems or inability to engage the coronary arteries because of massive aortic enlargement or ectopic position of the coronary ostia. Potential disadvantages include the invasiveness, relatively high cost, and somewhat limited availability because not every hospital and practice has cardiac catheterization services.

Invasive coronary angiography will be the method of choice in all patients in whom it is questionable whether CT angiography will provide artifact-free images, either because of patient characteristics such as heart rate or obesity with poor breath-holding capability (see later discussion) or because of suspected very diffuse and severe coronary atherosclerosis. Further, invasive coronary angiography offers the possibility for immediate intervention. Hence it is the method of choice in patients with a high pretest likelihood of disease, whether based on clinical presentation or previous positive stress test results. In most cases, diagnostic coronary angiography can be immediately followed by revascularization.

Coronary Computed Tomography Angiography

Coronary CT angiography is a reasonable alternative to invasive coronary angiography if the clinical suspicion of stenoses is not very high (and hence the likelihood that revascularization will be required is low). Some further prerequisites should be fulfilled, including the availability of adequate hardware and software for coronary CT imaging. Importantly, the performing physician and staff should have sufficient expertise in data acquisition and interpretation, and patient characteristics should make a fully evaluable CT angiography examination highly probable (Table 38-1). The lack of any invasiveness, immediate ambulation, and lower cost are advantages of CT angiography as compared to invasive coronary angiography. The availability of coronary CT angiography as a noninvasive test has renewed interest in using direct anatomic visualization as a first-line diagnostic tool for coronary artery disease (as opposed to ischemia testing). However, the fact that not all stenoses produce ischemia (and hence not all stenoses require revascularization) has to be kept in mind. The threshold for noninvasive visualization of the coronary arteries should not be set too low.

■ SCENARIOS THAT REQUIRE DIAGNOSIS OF CORONARY ARTERY DISEASE

Clinically five major scenarios raise the question of the presence, extent, and distribution of coronary atherosclerosis and stenoses and may be reasons to visualize the coronary arteries:
1. Stable chest pain
2. Acute chest pain and acute coronary syndromes
3. Impaired left ventricular function
4. Risk stratification in asymptomatic individuals
5. Imaging of the coronary arteries in the context of coronary interventions (percutaneous coronary revascularization)

The majority of patients in whom imaging of the coronary arteries is considered are those with suspected coronary artery disease because of symptoms that occur during exercise (stable chest pain) or at rest (acute chest pain).

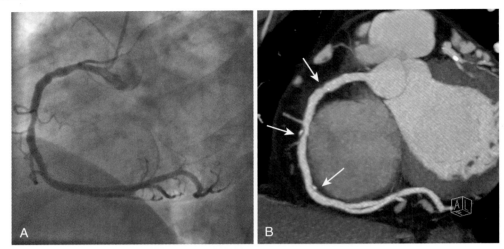

Figure 38-2 Coronary artery visualization by invasive angiography and coronary computed tomography (CT) angiography. A, Invasive coronary angiography is a projectional method that visualizes the coronary artery lumen with a spatial resolution of approximately 0.2 mm and a temporal resolution of approximately 8 msec. The vessel wall itself is not visible on invasive coronary angiography. **B,** CT coronary angiography is a cross-sectional imaging method with a spatial resolution of approximately 0.5 mm and a temporal resolution between 75 msec and 200 msec. Based on the cross-sectional images, two- or three-dimensional reconstructions can be rendered to show longer vessel segments. In two-dimensional reconstructions, atherosclerotic changes in the vessel wall can often be visualized *(arrows)*, whereas the normal vessel wall is typically not visible.

Table 38-1 Prerequisites for the Clinical Use of Coronary Computed Tomography Angiography

Institutional Characteristics

- Adequate hardware (usually at least 64-slice computed tomography)
- Adequate expertise in image acquisition
- Adequate expertise in image interpretation

Patient Characteristics

- Ability to follow breath-hold commands and perform a breath hold of approximately 10 sec
- Regular heart rate (sinus rhythm) with a frequency <65 beats/min, optimally <60 beats/min
- Lack of pronounced obesity
- Ability to establish a sufficiently large peripheral venous access (antecubital vein preferred)
- Absence of contraindications to radiation exposure and iodinated contrast media

Table 38-2 Pretest Likelihood of Coronary Artery Disease, Depending on Age, Sex, and Typicality of Symptoms

Age (yr)	Sex	Nonanginal Chest Pain (%)	Atypical Angina (%)	Typical Angina (%)
30-39	Male	4	34	76
	Female	2	12	26
40-49	Male	12	51	87
	Female	3	22	55
50-59	Male	20	65	93
	Female	7	31	73
60-69	Male	27	72	94
	Female	14	51	86

From Gibbons RJ, Balady FJ, Bricker JT, Chaitman BR, Fletcher GF, Froelicher VF, et al. ACC/AHA 2002 guideline update for exercise testing: summary article. A report of the American College of Cardiology/American Heart Association Task Force on Practice Guidelines (Committee to Update the 1997 Exercise Testing Guidelines). *J Am Coll Cardiol.* 2002;40:1531-1540.
"Typical angina" is assumed if chest pain meets all three of the following characteristics: (1) substernal chest discomfort with a characteristic and duration that is (2) provoked by exertion or emotional stress and (3) relieved by rest or nitroglycerin. "Atypical angina" meets two of these characteristics, and "nonanginal chest pain" is present if one criterion or no criteria are fulfilled.

■ PROBLEM SOLVING

Stable Chest Pain

Patients with stable chest pain typically report angina or shortness of breath when they exercise, but complaints vary substantially and can be rather nonspecific, especially in some patient groups such as diabetic patients. It is important to note that even in the presence of symptoms, the pretest likelihood of coronary stenoses being present varies substantially. Pretest likelihood is low in young persons and in women, and it is high in older persons and in men. Table 38-2 provides an estimate of pretest likelihood of coronary artery stenoses depending on age, sex, and typicality of symptoms.

The preferred clinical approach in patients with stable chest pain and suspected coronary artery disease is to perform a stress test to assess myocardial ischemia. The choice of stress testing (single photo emission CT [SPECT] myocardial perfusion imaging, magnetic resonance myocardial perfusion, stress echocardiography, or exercise electrocardiography [ECG]) will depend on local preference and patient characteristics. If stress test results are positive and indicate a relevant extent of ischemia, invasive coronary angiography is typically recommended to clarify the presence and extent of coronary artery stenoses. Medical management, percutaneous coronary intervention, and bypass surgery are treatment options when coronary artery stenoses are found.

Coronary CT angiography can be used to visualize the coronary arteries and detect coronary artery stenoses. However, its use has to be carefully considered. One important consideration is the pretest likelihood of disease.

Table 38-3 Appropriateness of Coronary Computed Tomography Angiography in Various Clinical Situations of Patients Presenting With Stable Disease

Clinical Situation	Appropriateness
Nonacute Symptoms Possibly Representing an Ischemic Equivalent—No Stress Test Done	
ECG interpretable **and** able to exercise	
▪ Low pretest likelihood (<10%)	Uncertain
▪ Intermediate pretest likelihood (10%-90%)	**Appropriate**
▪ High pretest likelihood (>90%)	Inappropriate
ECG uninterpretable **or** unable to exercise	
▪ Low pretest likelihood	**Appropriate**
▪ Intermediate pretest likelihood	**Appropriate**
▪ High pretest likelihood	Uncertain
Prior ECG Exercise Test	
Normal but continued symptoms	**Appropriate**
Abnormal	
▪ Low Duke treadmill score	Inappropriate
▪ Intermediate Duke treadmill score	**Appropriate**
▪ High Duke treadmill score	Inappropriate
Prior Stress Imaging Procedure	
Equivocal	**Appropriate**
▪ Mildly positive	Uncertain
▪ Moderately or severely positive	Inappropriate
▪ Discordant ECG exercise and stress imaging results	**Appropriate**
New or Worsening Symptoms With a Past Stress Imaging Study	
▪ Past study normal	**Appropriate**
▪ Past study abnormal	Uncertain
Patient With Previous Revascularization by CABG	
▪ Patient symptomatic, assessment of bypass patency required	**Appropriate**
▪ Patient asymptomatic, surgery <5 years ago	Inappropriate
▪ Patient asymptomatic, surgery ≥5 years ago	Uncertain
Patient With Previous Revascularization by PCI	
▪ Patient symptomatic, stent <3 mm	Inappropriate
▪ Patient symptomatic, stent ≥3 mm	Uncertain
▪ Asymptomatic, left main stent ≥3 mm	**Appropriate**
▪ Asymptomatic, other stents	Inappropriate

CABG, Coronary artery bypass graft; *CT,* computed tomography; *ECG,* electrocardiogram; *PCI,* percutaneous coronary intervention.

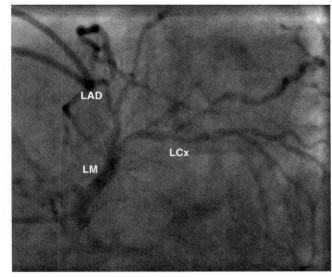

Figure 38-3 Severe and diffuse coronary artery disease with high-grade coronary artery stenoses in multiple coronary arteries as visualized by invasive coronary angiography in left anterior oblique caudal projection. *LAD,* Left anterior descending coronary artery; *LCx,* left circumflex coronary artery; *LM,* left main coronary artery.

When pretest likelihood for coronary artery disease is high, catheter-based invasive coronary angiography is the preferred test because it provides the option for immediate revascularization. On the other hand, when pretest likelihood is low, coronary CT angiography may be appropriate because it has a high negative predictive value and therefore allows the clinician to reliably rule out coronary artery stenoses. A second consideration of major importance is the question whether the patient is a suitable candidate for coronary CT angiography, will provide diagnostic image quality, and, especially if young, can be imaged with reasonably low radiation exposure. Table 38-3 lists situations in which coronary CT angiography is considered appropriate for the identification of stable coronary artery disease, according to expert consensus.

After clinical assessment the decision may be made that imaging of the coronary arteries is necessary. This can be the consequence of previous stress test results, which may be positive, equivocal, or negative with the suspicion of a false-negative result. It is also possible that the clinician might decide to forego stress testing and immediately ask for coronary visualization, for example, when stress testing cannot be performed to specific patient characteristics. As mentioned earlier, invasive coronary angiography and coronary CT angiography are the available options, and a decision must be made about which modality to use.

When to Use Invasive Angiography

Invasive coronary angiography will be the method of choice in all patients in whom CT is not expected to yield a fully diagnostic data set, either because of patient characteristics or because severe and diffuse disease is expected. (Fig. 38-3). More importantly, invasive angiography will be the method of choice if the clinical suspicion (pretest likelihood) of coronary artery disease is high. In this setting, noninvasive coronary angiography is not desirable. Invasive coronary angiography offers the possibility for immediate intervention, which CT angiography does not, and cardiac surgeons currently do not rely on CT angiography alone to plan bypass surgery.

When to Use Coronary CT Angiography

Coronary CT angiography (Fig. 38-4) is a reasonable alternative to invasive coronary angiography if the clinical suspicion of stenoses is not very high (and hence the likelihood that revascularization will be required is low). Importantly, patient characteristics must be considered, and CT angiography should be used only if fully diagnostic image quality can be expected (see Table 38-1). Many trials have demonstrated a high negative

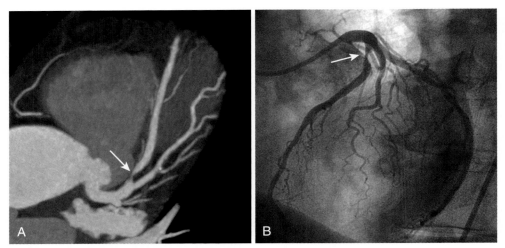

Figure 38-4 Coronary computed tomography (CT) angiography in a 53-year-old male patient with suspected coronary artery disease but low pretest likelihood because of relatively atypical symptoms. **A,** Coronary CT angiography shows a high-grade, eccentric stenosis of the proximal left anterior descending coronary artery *(arrow)*. **B,** Invasive coronary angiography confirms the high-grade stenosis of the proximal left anterior descending coronary artery *(arrow)*.

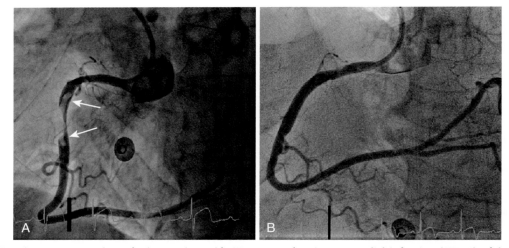

Figure 38-5 Invasive coronary angiography in a patient with ST-segment elevation myocardial infarction (STEMI) of the inferior wall. **A,** Invasive coronary angiography demonstrates a large thrombus in the right coronary artery with subtotal occlusion of the vessel *(arrows)*. **B,** After thrombus aspiration and stent placement, flow is restored and no luminal stenosis remains.

predictive value of coronary CT angiography in patients with suspected coronary artery disease. This means that a "negative" CT angiogram, which demonstrates absence of stenoses, very reliably rules out the presence of stenoses and thus no further testing is necessary. It is therefore possible to use coronary CT angiography in patients for whom clinical considerations suggest a relatively low likelihood that stenoses will actually be found (see Tables 38-2 and 38-3). Some experts consider the use of coronary CT angiography appropriate even as a first-line test, without prior stress testing, in selected patients.

Acute Chest Pain

Patients with acute chest pain have a very wide variability of coronary artery disease likelihood. They also have a very high variability of clinical risk. Coronary artery disease is almost certain in a patient who presents

with very typical anginal pain and who demonstrates ST-segment elevations in the resting ECG. Such patients require immediate (invasive) coronary angiography and intervention in order to re-open the presumably closed or sub-totally stenotic coronary artery (Fig. 38-5). Similarly, patients who have elevated serum markers of myocardial necrosis (troponin-positive patients) are typically at high risk and have high likelihood of coronary artery disease. Invasive coronary angiography is advised by guidelines and is clinically reasonable in these patients.

Coronary CT angiography is an alternative to invasive coronary angiography—or to a workup using stress testing—in selected individuals (Table 38-4). They should fulfill the criteria listed in Table 38-1 that permit a fully diagnostic CT coronary angiogram, and they should have a low-to-intermediate likelihood of coronary artery disease (Fig. 38-6). Several large clinical trials have demonstrated that CT angiography is a safe

Table 38-4 Use of Coronary Computed Tomography Angiography in Patients With Acute Symptoms and Suspicion of an Acute Coronary Syndrome (Urgent Presentation)

Symptoms	Appropriateness
Definite myocardial infarction	Inappropriate
Persistent ECG ST-segment elevation following acute MI	Uncertain
Normal ECG and normal cardiac biomarkers	
■ Low pretest likelihood	**Appropriate**
■ Intermediate pretest likelihood	**Appropriate**
■ High pretest likelihood	Uncertain
ECG uninterpretable	
■ Low pretest likelihood	**Appropriate**
■ Intermediate pretest likelihood	**Appropriate**
■ High pretest likelihood	Uncertain
Nondiagnostic ECG or equivocal biomarkers	
■ Low pretest likelihood	**Appropriate**
■ Intermediate pretest likelihood	**Appropriate**
■ High pretest likelihood	Uncertain
Acute chest pain of unknown cause (differential diagnosis includes pulmonary embolism, aortic dissection, and acute coronary syndrome)	Uncertain

CT, Computed tomography; *ECG,* electrocardiogram; *MI,* myocardial infarction.

method to rule out coronary artery stenoses in such patients and that they can be safely discharged (e.g., from the emergency department after a "negative" coronary CT angiogram).

There are considerations to use CT imaging to rule out several disease entities that could be responsible for chest pain, shortness of breath, or chest discomfort. The most prominent such diseases, next to coronary artery disease, are aortic dissection and pulmonary embolism. Combined protocols to rule out these three major diseases are sometimes termed *triple rule-out protocols.* They are not without controversy and not commonly recommended. Each of the three disease entities requires different scan ranges and contrast enhancement patterns, and optimization for one organ and disease will likely compromise the accuracy of investigating the others. Currently the use of triple rule-out protocols is not recommended, but this may change in the future.

Impaired Left Ventricular Function

Patients with heart failure may have coronary artery disease as the underlying reason. Impaired left ventricular function can be regional, in which case coronary artery disease is likely (but some differential diagnoses, such as scar after myocarditis, are possible). Alternatively, impaired left ventricular function can be global and diffuse, affecting all segments of the left ventricle equally, in which case dilated cardiomyopathy is a frequent reason, but diffuse, triple-vessel coronary artery disease may also be the underlying pathologic condition.

Invasive coronary angiography is part of the routine workup of patients with impaired left ventricular function. Some trials indicate that CT angiography has high accuracy—and especially high negative predictive value—for identifying patients with coronary artery stenoses as the underlying pathologic condition. Again, the use of coronary CT angiography instead of invasive coronary angiography can be considered if pretest likelihood for coronary artery stenoses is not high, if patient characteristics suggest good image quality, or if there are relative contraindications to the use of invasive coronary angiography.

Imaging for Risk Stratification

Deaths caused by coronary artery disease are usually secondary to arrhythmias, mainly ventricular fibrillation. Arrhythmia can occur spontaneously in patients with chronic coronary artery disease, typically as the consequence of electrically unstable myocardium in left ventricles that are dilated and display poor systolic function. Hence reduced left ventricular function is a strong predictor of sudden cardiac death.

Arrhythmia and death also occur as a direct consequence of "acute coronary syndromes," which comprise ST-segment elevation myocardial infarction (STEMI), non–ST-segment elevation myocardial infarction (NSTEMI), and unstable angina. The mortality risk of STEMI is greater than the risk of NSTEMI and unstable angina, but all three forms of acute coronary syndromes share a common pathomechanism. Either the sudden rupture of a coronary atherosclerotic plaque or, less frequently, erosion of its endothelial surface leads to thrombus formation and sudden total or near-total occlusion of the coronary artery. In many instances plaque rupture will occur at locations that do not display a "significant" stenosis (i.e., more than 50% luminal diameter reduction). This explains why patients often experience acute coronary syndromes without any previous symptoms, and patients may die suddenly. Acute coronary syndromes are difficult to predict. Risk stratification is usually based on the assessment of traditional cardiovascular risk factors. However, risk factors represent only a certain predisposition toward developing coronary atherosclerotic lesions, and they themselves are not the substrate of coronary events; their predictive accuracy for coronary events is limited. It is therefore an attractive approach to consider direct imaging of coronary atherosclerotic plaque for risk stratification purposes. Invasive coronary angiography is not well suited to visualizing coronary atherosclerotic plaque (Fig. 38-7); extensive plaque can be present without detectable luminal narrowing. CT offers the possibility of visualizing coronary atherosclerotic plaque in two different ways (Fig. 38-8). Without injection of contrast agent, and using very low-dose protocols, coronary artery calcification can be detected and quantified by ECG-gated CT. Coronary calcium is exclusively found in coronary atherosclerotic plaque, and the amount of calcium roughly correlates to the overall plaque extent. Numerous trials have conclusively shown that in asymptomatic individuals the

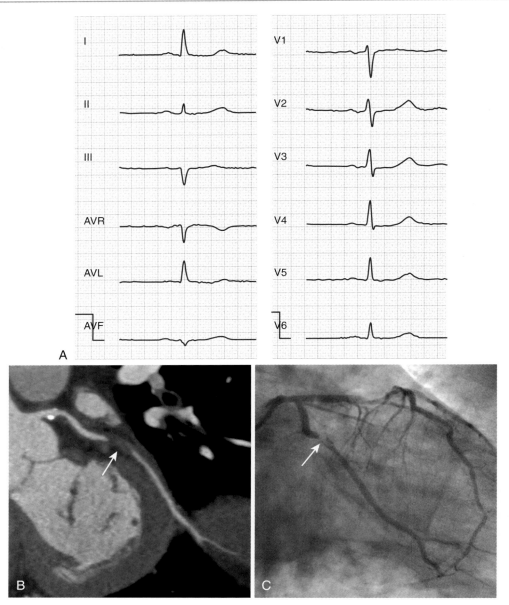

Figure 38-6 Coronary computed tomography (CT) angiography in a patient with acute chest pain, but somewhat atypical symptoms and lack of changes in the electrocardiogram (ECG). **A,** Twelve-lead ECG showing no changes typical for coronary ischemia or infarction. **B,** CT angiography shows a high-grade stenosis of the left circumflex coronary artery *(arrow)*. **C,** Invasive coronary angiography confirms a high-grade lesion with visible intracoronary thrombus in the left circumflex coronary artery *(arrow)*. It is important to note that especially the left circumflex coronary artery territory is often poorly reflected in the ECG. In acute coronary syndromes, even with a complete or near-complete occlusion of the left circumflex coronary artery or one of its side branches, ECG changes can be absent or very subtle.

presence and amount of calcium has strong predictive value concerning the occurrence of future hard cardiac events (death and myocardial infarction). The predictive value of coronary calcium is stronger than that of traditional risk factors (Table 38-5). According to official guidelines, the use of coronary calcium imaging can be considered by physicians who need additional information to achieve a decision about risk-modifying treatment (e.g., lipid-lowering therapy) in asymptomatic individuals at intermediate risk.

In addition to coronary calcification, coronary CT angiography (after injection of contrast agent and with higher-resolution acquisition protocols than those used for calcium detection) offers the possibility of visualizing noncalcified plaque components (see Fig. 38-8). To a limited extent, plaque can be quantified, typically by counting the number of coronary artery vessels or coronary artery segments that display detectable lesions. Several trials have shown that both the presence and extent of stenoses on coronary CT angiography (as a marker of especially pronounced plaque burden) and the presence and extent of nonobstructive plaque have strong prognostic value concerning mortality and hard cardiovascular events. Of importance, it has been demonstrated that prognosis is very good when detectable plaque is absent.

Good image quality is needed in coronary CT angiography to allow plaque detection. Some plaque characteristics, namely, pronounced positive remodeling, or

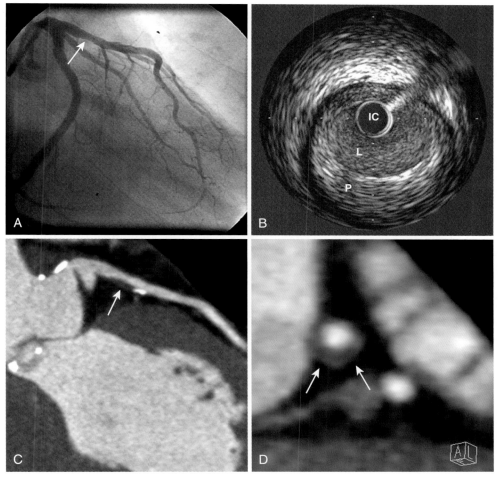

Figure 38-7 Visualization of nonobstructive coronary atherosclerotic plaque. A, Invasive coronary angiography of proximal left coronary artery in a 56-year-old man. No significant lumen narrowing is present. Invasive angiography merely demonstrates very mild luminal narrowing *(arrow)*. **B,** Intravascular ultrasound (IVUS) provides a cross-sectional image of the proximal left anterior descending coronary artery. It demonstrates substantial amounts of eccentric coronary atherosclerotic plaque that do not lead to luminal obstruction because of "positive remodeling" of the coronary artery. The vessel has expanded, allowing the plaque to grow in an outward direction, hence not leading to luminal obstruction. This explains why the substantial atherosclerotic burden is not detectable on the invasive coronary angiogram. Longitudinal two-dimensional display **(C)** and cross-sectional view of the left anterior descending coronary artery **(D)** obtained by 64-slice computed tomography angiography. On both reconstructions the atherosclerotic plaque *(arrows)* and the process of "positive remodeling" is clearly appreciated. *IC,* IVUS catheter; *L,* lumen; *P,* plaque.

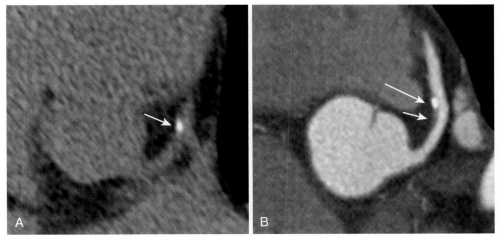

Figure 38-8 Coronary atherosclerosis in computed tomography (CT). A, Detection of coronary artery calcification *(arrow)* in nonenhanced CT scan. **B,** Same patient as in *A.* After injection of contrast agent and acquisition with a higher-resolution protocol, coronary CT angiography visualizes calcified *(large arrow)* and noncalcified plaque components *(small arrow).*

Table 38-5 Risk for Coronary Events (Adjusted for Risk Factors) Associated With Agatston Score in an Asymptomatic Population

Agatston Score	Hazard Ratio (Major Coronary Events)	No. of Individuals	
		With Events	Total
0	1	8	3409
1-100	3.89	25	1728
101-300	7.08	24	752
≥301	6.84	32	833

Modified from Detrano R, Guerci AD, Carr JJ, Bild DE, Burke G, Folsom AR, et al. Coronary calcium as a predictor of coronary events in four racial or ethnic groups. *N Engl J Med.* 2008;358:1336-1345.

Table 38-6 Characteristics of Coronary Atherosclerotic Plaques and the Rate of Acute Coronary Syndrome

Finding at Baseline	Total No. of Patients	ACS During Follow-Up	No ACS During Follow-Up
Plaques with positive remodeling **and** CT attenuation <30 HU	45	10 (22%)	35 (78%)
Plaques with positive remodeling **or** CT attenuation <30 HU	27	1 (4%)	26 (96%)
Plaques with **neither** positive remodeling **nor** CT attenuation <30 HU	822	4 (0.5%)	816 (99%)
No plaque	167	0 (0%)	167 (100%)

Modified from Motoyama S, Sarai M, Harigaya H, Anno H, Inoue K, Hara T, et al. Computed tomographic angiography characteristics of atherosclerotic plaques subsequently resulting in acute coronary syndrome. *J Am Coll Cardiol.* 2009;54(1):49-57.
ACS, Acute coronary syndrome; *CT,* computed tomography.

low CT densities (<30 Hounsfield units [HU]) measured within a coronary plaque have been shown to be very strongly associated with the risk for future cardiovascular events (Table 38-6 and Fig. 38-9).

It needs to be pointed out that the use of coronary CT angiography for risk stratification is not clinical routine or contained in official guidelines at the moment. Data concerning the predictive value of plaque seen in coronary CT angiography are strong, and evidence continues to accumulate. The strongest evidence is available in support of the fact that even in patients who are symptomatic, event rates are extremely low when coronary CT angiography demonstrates the absence of both coronary artery stenoses and coronary atherosclerotic plaque. Hence patients with entirely "normal" coronary CT angiography findings can be counseled as to their very low risk, and further diagnostic procedures, or specific medication, are not necessary.

Table 38-6 provides results of a prospective study by Motoyama et al in which 1059 patients were followed for a mean period of 27 months after a clinically indicated coronary CT angiogram. Coronary atherosclerotic plaques were identified and evaluated concerning the presence of positive remodeling and low CT attenuation (attenuation values <30 HU). It could be shown that the rate of acute coronary syndromes during follow-up was substantially higher in patients with plaques that demonstrated positive remodeling and low CT attenuation than in patients with other type of plaque or without plaque.

Imaging to Guide Coronary Interventions

A major application of coronary artery imaging is the support of coronary interventions. Coronary arteries are small, and diseased segments have luminal diameters

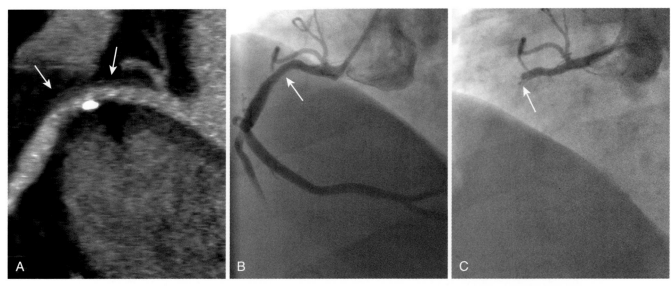

Figure 38-9 Example of a "high-risk" coronary atherosclerotic plaque in coronary computed tomography (CT) angiography. A, A coronary atherosclerotic plaque is visualized in the proximal right coronary artery *(arrows).* The plaque displays outward growth ("positive remodeling") and is of relatively low CT density but is not associated with a high-grade stenosis *(arrow)* **(B). C,** Three months later this atherosclerotic lesion results in a complete occlusion of the right coronary artery *(arrow),* with the consequence of inferior wall ST-segment elevation myocardial infarction (STEMI).

well below 0.5 mm. Percutaneous coronary revascularization requires real-time, high-resolution, and isotropic visualization of extremely fine details to permit adequate manipulation of guidewires, placement of balloons and stents, and immediate detection of even subtle complications such as small thrombi or dissections, which might otherwise rapidly turn into life-threatening complications. This is achieved by x-ray fluoroscopic imaging and repeated angiography during the procedure (Figs. 38-10 and 38-11). Some crude manipulations, such as placing a catheter into the coronary artery ostium or maneuvering a guidewire along a large and healthy coronary artery, have been described with alternative modes of imaging, for example, real-time magnetic resonance imaging. However, I have severe doubts that CT or magnetic resonance imaging will permit real-time guidance of coronary interventions in the foreseeable future because of their lack of temporal, spatial, and contrast resolution.

However, coronary CT angiography has a very valuable and specific application in the context of percutaneous coronary interventions. One area fraught with particular difficulty is the interventional reopening of chronically occluded coronary arteries ("chronic total occlusion"). The interventional success rate is approximately 75%, and it is difficult to predict success. CT imaging—in contrast to invasive angiography—visualizes the occluded segment (Fig. 38-12). The length of the occluded coronary artery segment, its tortuosity, and especially the extent of calcification seem to be predictors of the likelihood that interventional recanalization will succeed. Lack of severe calcification and the continuous visualization of a noncalcified vessel cross section throughout the entire occlusion are predictors of interventional success. Many experienced interventionalists appreciate visualization of occluded coronary segments before elective percutaneous recanalization and may order coronary CT angiography for this specific purpose (Figs. 38-12 and 38-13). If a coronary artery occlusion is found in a coronary CT angiogram performed for diagnostic purposes, it is helpful to comment on the length of the occluded segment, its course, and the extent of calcification.

■ PITFALLS AND PEARLS

Computed Tomographic Imaging

Artifacts Mimicking Stenoses
In coronary CT angiography, artifacts may occur that are caused by limited spatial resolution relative to the dimensions of the coronary arteries, by insufficient temporal resolution in order to freeze motion of the coronary

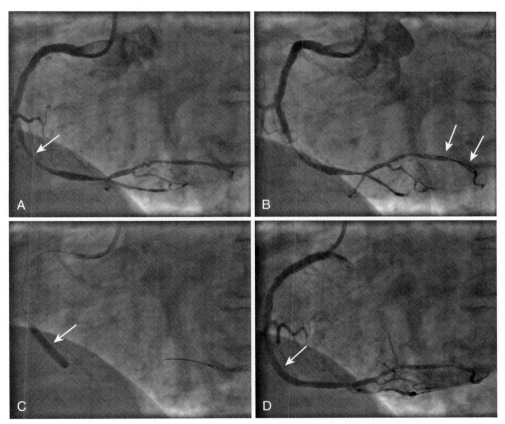

Figure 38-10 **Typical percutaneous coronary intervention, balloon angioplasty, and stent placement of a high-grade right coronary artery stenosis.** **A,** Invasive coronary angiography in left anterior oblique projection demonstrates a high-grade stenosis of the right coronary artery *(arrow).* **B,** A thin guidewire is passed down the narrowed coronary artery *(arrows* indicate the distal end of the guidewire in the distal right coronary artery). **C,** A coronary stent (diameter here, 3.5 mm) mounted on a balloon is advanced via the guidewire, inserted into the stenosis, and expanded by means of balloon inflation *(arrow).* **D,** After removal of the balloon the stent remains in place (not visible on the angiogram). The lesion has been treated successfully without residual luminal stenosis *(arrow).*

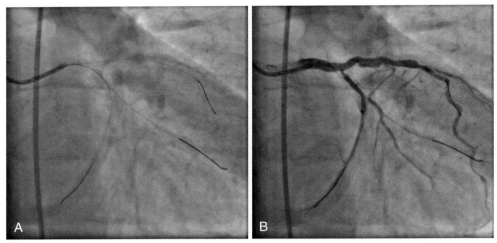

Figure 38-11 Complex percutaneous coronary interventions require extremely fine manipulation of the coronary guidewires over which balloons and stents are advanced into the lesion that is to be treated. It is very unlikely that the spatial resolution of cross-sectional imaging technologies such as computed tomography or magnetic resonance imaging will in the foreseeable future provide sufficient isotropic spatial resolution to serve as a real-time imaging modality for coronary interventions. In addition, cross-sectional imaging would need to overcome cardiac and respiratory motion. **A,** Placement of guidewires in the left anterior descending coronary artery, left circumflex coronary artery, and first obtuse marginal branch. Placing of such guidewires requires extremely fine manipulation under fluoroscopic control and with repeated contrast injections (**B**).

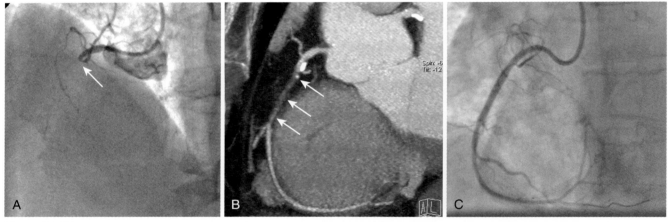

Figure 38-12 Computed tomography (CT) imaging has merit in the assessment of chronic total coronary artery occlusions. The length of the occluded segment, its tortuosity, and the extent of calcium can easily be determined based on CT angiography (but in most cases not from the invasive coronary angiogram) and have predictive value concerning the likelihood that interventional revascularization will be successful. **A,** Chronic total occlusion of a right coronary artery (invasive coronary angiogram in left anterior oblique projection). Invasive angiography visualizes the vessel only up to the occlusion site *(arrow)*. **B,** Coronary CT angiogram of the same patient. The occluded segment *(arrows)* is of intermediate length, not tortuous and lacks calcification, predictors that make successful recanalization rather likely. **C,** Invasive angiogram after successful interventional recanalization and stent placement.

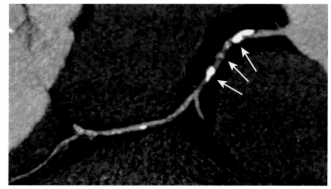

Figure 38-13 Severely calcified coronary artery occlusion *(arrows)* in coronary computed tomography angiography. The likelihood that interventional recanalization can be achieved is substantially lower than in the patient in Figure 38-12.

vessels, or by the fact that a typical coronary CT angiography data set is composed of multiple cardiac cycles. If artifacts occur, they are much more likely to cause false-positive impressions of high-grade coronary artery stenoses than to cause false-negative findings. It is important to recognize typical artifacts to avoid false-positive interpretations. The most frequent artifacts occur in the setting of pronounced coronary calcification, often in combination with residual motion Fig. 38-14), and as a consequence of "misalignment" at the border or image stacks acquired during two consecutive cardiac cycles (Fig. 38-15).

Overestimation of Stenosis Degree

Relative to invasive coronary angiography, coronary CT angiography tends to overestimate rather than

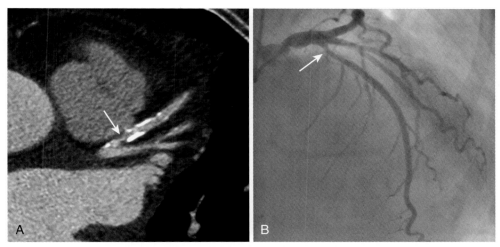

Figure 38-14 False-positive stenosis as a consequence of heavy calcification of a coronary arterial segment. Extensive coronary calcium, especially in combination with motion and potentially somewhat increased image noise, tends to lead to false-positive interpretations of stenosis degree. **A,** Severely calcified proximal segment of the left anterior descending coronary artery. Computed tomography angiography suggests the presence of a severe luminal stenosis *(arrow)*. Note relatively high image noise and some "unsharpness" caused by motion. **B,** Invasive coronary angiography confirms the presence of coronary atherosclerotic plaque with mild luminal narrowing, but no severe stenosis *(arrow)*.

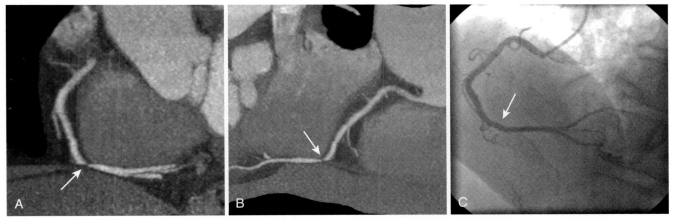

Figure 38-15 Misalignment is a potential reason for misinterpretation and false-positive coronary computed tomography (CT) angiography results. Misalignment can occur because a typical coronary CT angiography data set is made up of a stack of several hundred thin cross-sectional images that are acquired in a stepwise fashion in several consecutive cardiac cycles. If the heart does not return to exactly the same position from one cardiac cycle to the next, continuity is interrupted and misalignment artifacts can occur. **A,** Misalignment artifact in the distal right coronary artery *(arrow)*. It occurred because the vessel was offset by a few millimeters from one cardiac cycle to the next, potentially as a consequence of breathing, slightly changing heart rate, or inconsistent filling of the right ventricle. **B,** In a "curved multiplanar reconstruction" the artifact cannot be recognized as easily and creates the impression of a very high-grade stenosis. **C,** Invasive coronary angiography demonstrates that no stenosis *(arrow)* is present.

underestimate the degree of luminal stenosis. The effect is especially pronounced when cross-sectional images are used to evaluate coronary artery lesions (Fig. 38-16; see also Fig. 38-1), because the process of positive remodeling leads to the impression of a relevant luminal stenosis when the reference lumen proximal to the stenosis is not taken into account.

However, even in longitudinal views of coronary lesions, the impression of stenosis severity is often more severe in CT as compared to invasive angiography. This is probably a result of the limited spatial resolution that needs to be taken into account when reporting coronary CT angiography results (Fig. 38-17).

Coronary Artery Stents

Imaging of coronary artery stents by CT is challenging. The high-density–material stents can cause artifacts that may lead to false-positive interpretations of in-stent stenosis. The ability to evaluate stents by CT depends on many factors (Fig. 38-18). Next to image noise and heart rate, stent material and especially stent size have an influence on the likelihood of artifacts. Also, large stents (e.g., with a diameter of 3.5 mm or more) are less frequently affected by artifacts than stents with a smaller diameter. There is consensus that stents should not be evaluated by CT if their diameter is less than 3.0 mm, but even for larger stents most experts agree that artifacts

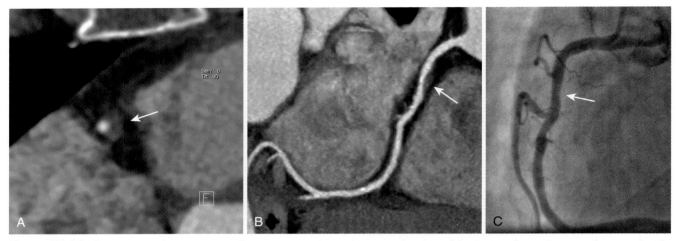

Figure 38-16 If cross-sectional images are used to assess stenosis severity, overestimation of the degree of stenosis can easily occur. **A,** Atherosclerotic lesion in the proximal right coronary artery *(arrow)*. Substantial amounts of noncalcified plaque are present and, with the small remaining residual lumen, the impression of a high-grade stenosis is created. **B,** A longitudinal view demonstrates that there is substantial positive remodeling (noncalcified plaque leading to vessel expansion) and that the degree of luminal stenosis is not as severe as it appears in the cross section *(arrow)*. **C,** Invasive coronary angiography. The degree of stenosis is very mild *(arrow)*.

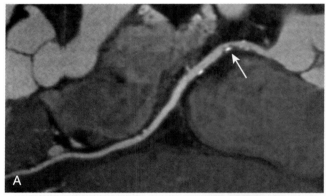

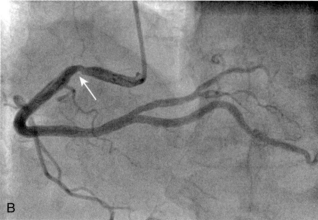

Figure 38-17 In coronary computed tomography (CT) angiography, the degree of stenosis frequently appears somewhat more severe than in the corresponding invasive coronary angiogram. **A,** CT angiography of a right coronary artery with a stenosis in the proximal segment *(arrow)*. **B,** Invasive coronary angiogram. The degree of stenosis appears less *(arrow)* than in CT angiography.

are too frequent to use CT clinically. A possible exception is a stent in the left main coronary artery, which is subjected to relatively little motion, so that the most recent expert consensus document on appropriate applications of coronary CT angiography rates CT assessment as "appropriate."

Invasive Coronary Angiography

Occluded Vessels

It is very infrequent that invasive coronary angiography is false-positive or false-negative as far as the presence of a significant coronary artery stenosis is concerned. A potential reason for a false-negative finding may be if, as a consequence of unsuitable projections, a stenotic vessel segment is superimposed by another artery and hence not visible. Also, albeit very infrequent, a completely occluded branch may be missed if the occlusion is at the very ostium and retrograde filling is so faint that it is missed and not detected (Fig. 38-19).

Coronary Artery Spasm

Invasive coronary angiography can be false-positive if focal coronary artery spasm occurs and is unnoticed. The visual impression can be the same as that of a stenosis because of atherosclerotic plaque (Fig. 38-20). Coronary spasms occur especially in young individuals and situations with high sympathetic drive. They can be resolved with intracoronary injection of nitroglycerin. Sometimes, repeated injections are necessary to resolve the luminal construction caused by spasm.

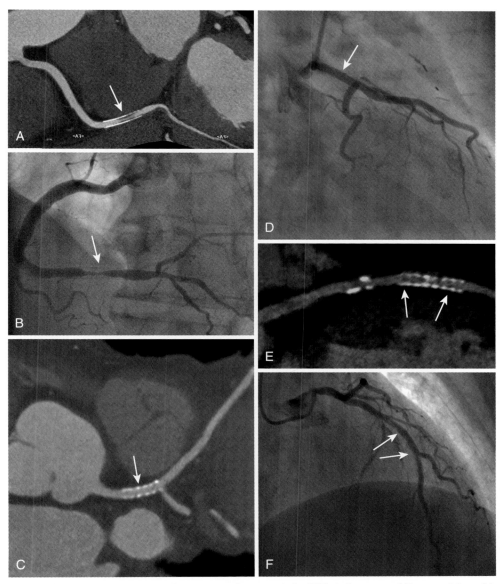

Figure 38-18 **Imaging of coronary artery stents by computed tomography (CT).** **A,** Large stent (diameter, 4.0 mm) in the right coronary artery. A diffuse in-stent stenosis is clearly detectable *(arrow)*. **B,** Invasive coronary angiography confirms the high grade in stent stenosis *(arrow)*. **C,** Good image quality of a stent with 3.0-mm diameter implanted in the left main coronary artery *(arrow)*. **D,** Corresponding invasive coronary angiogram. No in-stent stenosis. **E,** False-positive interpretation of in-stent stenosis in the mid left anterior descending coronary artery. Overall image quality is reduced as compared to the two previous examples, with some motion and increased image noise. Also, the stent is smaller (diameter, 2.75 mm). Artifacts lead to low CT attenuation inside the stent *(arrows)* and false-positive reading. **F,** Invasive angiography demonstrates that no significant in-stent stenosis is present *(arrows* indicate the location of the stent).

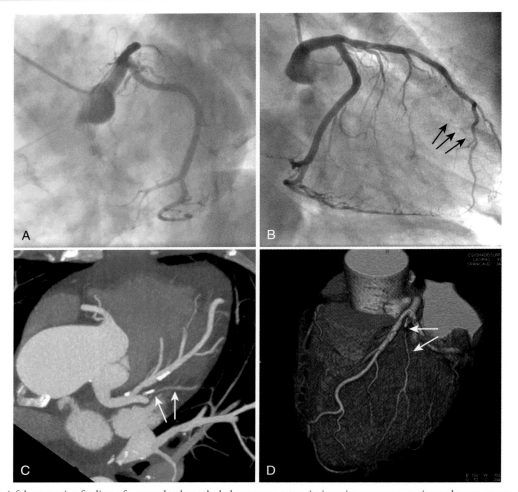

Figure 38-19 A false-negative finding of a completely occluded coronary artery in invasive coronary angiography can occur, albeit extremely infrequently. **A** and **B**, Invasive coronary angiography of the left coronary artery system in left anterior oblique caudal orientation ("spider view") and in RAO caudal projection shows no indication of an occluded, relatively large intermediate branch, except extremely faint filling of the distal vessel segments *(arrows)* in the RAO caudal projection. **C** and **D**, Coronary CT angiography in two-dimensional (**C**) and three-dimensional (**D**) reconstruction clearly demonstrates a relatively large intermediate branch *(arrows)* that is occluded directly at the ostium and was not detected in invasive angiography.

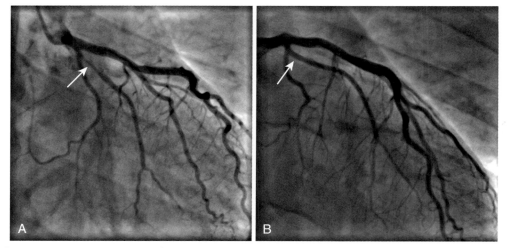

Figure 38-20 Coronary artery spasm. A, Invasive coronary angiogram in a young patient with atypical chest pain. A narrowing of the first obtuse marginal branch is seen *(arrow)*, and it is suggestive of an atherosclerotic coronary artery stenosis. **B,** After intracoronary application of nitrates, the luminal narrowing resolves completely *(arrow)*.

Bibliography

Abbara S, Arbab-Zadeh A, Callister TQ, Desai MY, Mamuya W, Thomson L, et al. SCCT guidelines for performance of coronary computed tomographic angiography: a report of the Society of Cardiovascular Computed Tomography Guidelines Committee. *J Cardiovasc Comput Tomogr.* 2009;3:190-204.

Chow BJ, Wells GA, Chen L, Yam Y, Galiwango P, Abraham A, et al. Prognostic value of 64-slice cardiac computed tomography severity of coronary artery disease, coronary atherosclerosis, and left ventricular ejection fraction. *J Am Coll Cardiol.* 2010;55:1017-1028.

Chung SH, Kim YJ, Hur J, Lee HJ, Choe KO, Kim TH, et al. Evaluation of coronary artery in-stent restenosis by 64-section computed tomography: factors affecting assessment and accurate diagnosis. *J Thorac Imaging.* 2010;25:57-63.

Detrano R, Guerci AD, Carr JJ, Bild DE, Burke G, Folsom AR, et al. Coronary calcium as a predictor of coronary events in four racial or ethnic groups. *N Engl J Med.* 2008;358:1336-1345.

Gibbons RJ, Abrams J, Chatterjee K, Daley J, Deedwania PC, Douglas JS, et al. ACC/AHA 2002 guideline update for the management of patients with chronic stable angina—summary article: a report of the American College of Cardiology/American Heart Association Task Force on practice guidelines (Committee on the Management of Patients With Chronic Stable Angina). *J Am Coll Cardiol.* 2003;41:159-168.

Goldstein JA, Chinnaiyan KM, Abidov A, Achenbach S, Berman DS, Hayes SW, et al. The CT-STAT (Coronary Computed Tomographic Angiography for Systematic Triage of Acute Chest Pain Patients to Treatment) Trial. *J Am Coll Cardiol.* 2011;58:1414-1422.

Hadamitzky M, Freissmuth B, Meyer T, Hein F, Kastrati A, Martinoff S, et al. Prognostic value of coronary computed tomographic angiography for prediction of cardiac events in patients with suspected coronary artery disease. *JACC Cardiovasc Imaging.* 2009;2:404-411.

Hoffmann U, Bamberg F, Chae CU, Nichols JH, Rogers IS, Seneviratne SK, et al. Coronary computed tomography angiography for early triage of patients with acute chest pain: the ROMICAT (Rule Out Myocardial Infarction using Computer Assisted Tomography) trial. *J Am Coll Cardiol.* 2009;53:1642-1650.

Hollander JE, Chang AM, Shofer FS, Collin MJ, Walsh KM, McCusker CM, et al. One-year outcomes following coronary computerized tomographic angiography for evaluation of emergency department patients with potential acute coronary syndrome. *Acad Emerg Med.* 2009;16:693-698.

Hulten EA, Carbonaro S, Petrillo SP, Mitchell JD, Villines TC. Prognostic value of cardiac computed tomography angiography: a systematic review and meta-analysis. *J Am Coll Cardiol.* 2011;57:1237-1247.

Meijboom WB, Meijs MF, Schuijf JD, Cramer MJ, Mollet NR, van Mieghem CA, et al. Diagnostic accuracy of 64-slice computed tomography coronary angiography: a prospective, multicenter, multivendor study. *J Am Coll Cardiol.* 2008;52:2135-2144.

Min JK, Dunning A, Lin FY, Achenbach S, Al-Mallah M, Berman DS, et al. Age- and gender-related differences in all-cause mortality risk based upon coronary computed tomographic angiography findings: results from the international multicenter CONFIRM registry of 23,854 patients without known coronary artery disease. *J Am Coll Cardiol.* 2011;58:849-860.

Motoyama S, Sarai M, Harigaya H, Anno H, Inoue K, Hara T, et al. Computed tomographic angiography characteristics of atherosclerotic plaques subsequently resulting in acute coronary syndrome. *J Am Coll Cardiol.* 2009;54:49-57.

Raff GL, Abidov A, Achenbach S, Berman DS, Boxt LM, Budoff MJ, et al. SCCT guidelines for the interpretation and reporting of coronary computed tomographic angiography. *J Cardiovasc Comput Tomogr.* 2009;3:122-136.

Rubinshtein R, Halon DA, Gaspar T, Jaffe R, Karkabi B, Flugelman MY, et al. Usefulness of 64-slice cardiac computed tomographic angiography for diagnosing acute coronary syndromes and predicting clinical outcome in emergency department patients with chest pain of uncertain origin. *Circulation.* 2007;115:1762-1768.

Taylor AJ, Cerqueira M, Hodgson JM, Mark D, Min J, O'Gara P, et al. ACCF/SCCT/ACR/AHA/ASE/ASNC/NASCI/SCAI/SCMR 2010 appropriate use criteria for cardiac computed tomography. *J Am Coll Cardiol.* 2010;56:1864-1894.

Wykrzykowska JJ, Arbab-Zadeh A, Godoy G, Miller JM, Lin S, Vavere A, et al. Assessment of in-stent restenosis using 64-MDCT: analysis of the CORE-64 Multicenter International Trial. *AJR Am J Roentgenol.* 2010;194:85-92.

CHAPTER 39

Coronary Artery Bypass Grafts

Darshan Raj Vummudi and Smita Patel

Coronary artery disease is the leading cause of death in the United States. Surgical revascularization for coronary artery disease (CAD) with coronary artery bypass graft (CABG) surgery is the recommended treatment for patients with significant left main disease, severe (≥70%) proximal left anterior descending (LAD) stenosis, significant two-vessel disease with involvement of the proximal LAD, and severe three-vessel CAD. The aim of CABG is to restore myocardial perfusion to the hypoperfused ischemic territories, which not only relieves angina and improves exercise tolerance but more importantly results in improved long-term survival.

Despite its obvious benefit, CABG over time may result in complications, particularly those of graft stenosis and occlusion, as well as progression of atherosclerotic disease in the native grafted and nongrafted coronary arteries. Saphenous venous grafts (SVGs) have a higher occlusion rate than internal mammary artery (IMA) grafts. The 1-year patency rates of IMA grafts and SVGs are not significantly different. However, 5 and 10 years after revascularization, patency rates for IMA grafts are superior at 88% and 83%, respectively, compared to 73% and 41% for SVGs. Invasive coronary angiography is considered the gold standard for evaluating CABGs and native coronary arteries. The risk for major complications is less than 1% for invasive coronary angiography. However, in postoperative CABG patients who have diffusely diseased coronary arteries, varying coronary and systemic atherosclerotic disease, and degenerated grafts, invasive coronary angiography is a complicated procedure that can result in life-threatening arrhythmias, damage to the vessel wall, and significant mortality in certain patient groups.

Given the high burden of CAD and greater than 470,000 CABGs performed annually in the United States, there is a need for an alternative accurate, reliable, relatively safe, and cheaper noninvasive option for evaluating patients after CABG. In the last decade rapidly evolving multidetector computed tomography (MDCT) technology, with significantly improved spatial and temporal resolution and near-isotropic imaging with submillimeter section thickness in a single breath hold, has resulted in easy, reliable, and accurate evaluation of bypass graft patency. Computed tomography (CT) has therefore emerged as a viable noninvasive imaging modality for evaluation of bypass grafts, especially with 64-detector and higher-generation electrocardiogram-gated MDCT scanners.

Bypass grafts are less challenging to evaluate on CT than native coronary arteries because they are less affected by cardiac motion, have a wider luminal diameter, and have less calcified plaque when compared to native coronary arteries. However, evaluation of the distal anastomotic site, distal runoff vessel, and heavily calcified, small-caliber nongrafted native coronary arteries can be a significant problem resulting in limited clinical utility of CT in some patients. Progressive advances in CT technology will probably overcome this problem and allow improved evaluation of these vessels.

A sensitivity of 85% to 100% and specificity of 89% to 100% for bypass graft occlusion and significant stenosis with 64-slice CT has been reported in a number of publications. A meta-analysis published by Hamon et al documented a pooled sensitivity of 98% and specificity of 97% for stenosis greater than 50% using 64-slice MDCT coronary angiography. Although the diagnostic accuracy for evaluation of bypass grafts is high with 64-slice CT, the diagnostic accuracy for detecting significant stenosis in native vessels following revascularization is lower than in native vessels of patients who have not undergone surgery. This is because the native coronary arteries in post-CABG patients are significantly calcified, are often of smaller caliber, and are prone to increased plaque burden. With 64-slice CT the sensitivity and specificity for significant stenosis in native and distal runoff vessels following CABG ranges from 77% to 97% and 76% to 100%, respectively. High diagnostic accuracy is reported by de Graaf et al for evaluation of graft stenosis and occlusion with a 320-detector scanner. Weustink et al report an even higher diagnostic accuracy (100%) for evaluation of not only the grafts but also native coronary arteries with dual-source CT, probably because of superior temporal resolution however, the patient population in this study was about 10 years younger and had revascularization surgery less than 10 years earlier.

For evaluation of bypass grafts with CT it is important to have an understanding of CABG surgical techniques and surgical conduits, specifically bypass graft anatomy and appearance of normal grafts, as well as graft complications. CT can also guide surgical approach if reoperation is being considered.

■ MULTIDETECTOR COMPUTED TOMOGRAPHY TECHNIQUE

A slow and steady heart rate ensures a diagnostic-quality CT scan. In patients with heart rates above 65 beats/minute, beta-blockers are administered orally or intravenously (e.g., metoprolol 100 mg orally or up to 25 mg intravenously) with the aim of achieving a heart rate of 65 beats/minute or less to minimize cardiac motion artifacts. As with invasive coronary angiography, 0.4 mg of sublingual nitroglycerin spray is often used just before scan acquisition, barring contraindications.

An 18-gauge angiocatheter in the right antecubital vein is preferred for contrast administration because significant streak artifact can result from contrast coursing through the left subclavian vein to the superior vena cava via the left brachiocephalic vein, which can limit evaluation of a left internal mammary artery (LIMA) graft or high SVG.

Scan delay can be determined by performing a timing bolus with 15 mL of nonionic high-concentration low- or iso-osmolar iodinated contrast medium at 5 to 7 mL/second followed by 20 mL saline flush at the same rate, with the region of interest in the aortic root at the left main coronary artery origin. Alternatively, automated bolus triggering can be applied, with scan acquisition beginning 5 to 10 seconds following achievement of a predefined threshold (usually 100 Hounsfield units [HU]) in the ascending or descending thoracic aorta.

An 80- to 100-mL volume of high-concentration, low- or iso-osmolar contrast agent is administered at 5- to 7-mL/second using a power injector to achieve adequate enhancement (>300 HU) of the coronary arterial lumen, followed by 50 mL of saline at the same flow rate. Higher flow rates are used in obese patients. Some centers calculate the amount of contrast to be used by the flow rate and contrast injection time.

Details of the prior surgical procedure are extremely useful in determining the z-axis coverage. Evaluation of the SVG should extend from the cephalad ascending aorta to the base of the heart, whereas imaging of the internal mammary graft begins at the lung apices to include the IMA origin from the subclavian artery and extends caudally to the cardiac apex. The scan is then acquired in a single breath hold from cranial-to-caudad direction during mid-to-end inspiration after initial hyperventilation to reduce heterogeneity of contrast in the right atrium, which occurs from inflow of unopacified blood from the inferior vena cava. Some centers use a caudal-to-cranial direction to minimize artifact from diaphragmatic motion.

Depending on the vendor and availability of the scanner, electrocardiogram gating is performed using prospective triggering or high-pitch (flash) acquisitions for patients with stable heart rates of less than 65 beats/minute to minimize radiation dose, and retrospective gating is reserved for patients with variable or higher than 65 beats/minute heart rates or if functional information is desired. Axial slices of the heart are acquired at 0.5- to 7-mm collimation and reconstructed at 0.5- to 1-mm collimation. For retrospectively gated scans, images are reconstructed at 60% to 80% R-R interval.

The raw data are transferred to an independent offline workstation with dedicated cardiac software for review.

The axial source images are evaluated first. All data are then visualized and analyzed using a number of reconstruction techniques: (1) multiplanar reformations, (2) maximum intensity projections, (3) curved multiplanar reconstructions, (4) linear lumen view, and (5) three-dimensional (3D) volume rendering (VR).

Each bypass graft is evaluated in turn for patency, stenosis, or occlusion with specific analysis of the (1) proximal anastomosis, (2) graft proper, (3) distal anastomosis, (4) distal runoff vessel, and (5) proximity of graft to the sternum or anterior chest wall. The native coronary arteries are also evaluated for stenosis.

Three dimensional VR images exquisitely depict the complex surgical anatomy of the bypass grafts, including the proximal and distal anastomosis and cardiac topography.

Coronary graft assessment broadly includes anatomy, patency, complications, and relationship to chest wall.

■ ANATOMY OF BYPASS GRAFT CONDUITS

Saphenous Venous Grafts

The first CABG in the early 1960s was performed with an SVG. SVGs are readily available, easy to harvest from the lower extremities, and less prone to vasospasm. However, they are prone to intimal hyperplasia when exposed to systemic blood pressure because of lack of nitric oxide and develop atherosclerosis over time that results in poor long-term patency rates. In a large angiographic follow-up study of 5065 patients after CABG, 88% of grafts were patent perioperatively, 81% at 1 year, 75% at 5 years, and only 50% at 15 years. However, with continuing improvements in surgical techniques along with the concomitant use of antiplatelet or anticoagulant therapy and lipid-lowering drugs, SVGs remain an important and frequently used conduit because of improved patency rates.

SVGs are attached proximally on the anterior wall of the ascending aorta and are grafted distally to the coronary artery beyond the significant stenosis or obstruction (Figs. 39-1 and 39-2). For revascularization of the right coronary artery (RCA), posterior descending artery (PDA), or distal LAD artery, SVG are anastomosed on the right side of the anterior ascending aorta proximally, either by being directly sutured to the aorta or by means of an aortovenous connector device that allows a quick, sutureless attachment without the need to clamp target vessels. The distal portion of the graft often lies on the diaphragmatic surface of the heart (see Fig. 39-1).

For revascularization of the anterior and lateral myocardium, the proximal anastomosis is made on the left side of the anterior ascending aorta and stabilized on the main pulmonary artery and the distal anastomosis to the mid-distal LAD, diagonal, ramus intermedius, left circumflex, or obtuse marginal arteries, beyond the significant stenosis or obstruction (see Fig. 39-2). SVGs can be used for sequential grafting to two or more vessels, when a side-to-side anastomosis is performed to

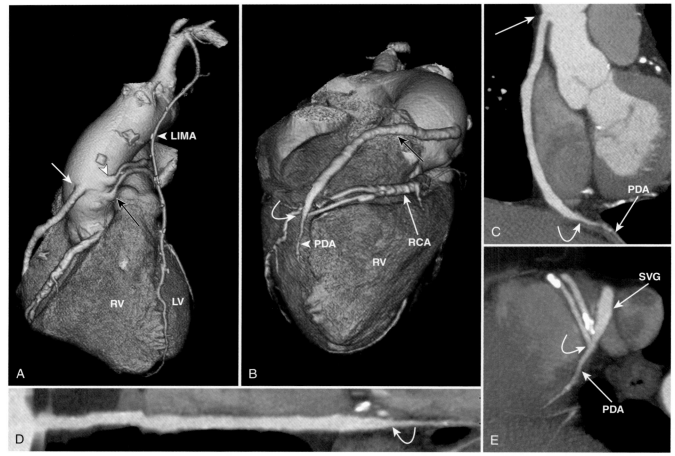

Figure 39-1 Seventy-two-year-old man, 12 years after coronary artery bypass graft, underwent computed tomography angiography to evaluate for bypass graft patency. Saphenous venous graft (SVG) to posterior descending coronary artery (PDA). **A,** Three-dimensional volume-rendered image demonstrates proximal anastomotic sites of the three SVGs sutured to the anterior aorta: SVG to PDA *(white arrow)*, SVG to obtuse marginal (OM) 1 *(black arrow)*, and SVG to OM2 *(arrowhead)*. Note the venous grafts (SVGs) are of larger caliber than the arterial graft (LIMA). **B,** Three-dimensional volume-rendered image demonstrates the SVG *(black arrow)* to the PDA. The *curved arrow* points to the distal anastomosis. Note the heavily calcified native right coronary artery (RCA) in the right atrioventricular groove. Curved multiplanar reformation (**C**), maximum intensity projection (**D**), and linear lumen view (**E**) demonstrate a mildly ectatic, widely patent SVG with proximal anastomosis to the anterior aorta *(white arrow)* and distal end-to-side anastomosis to the PDA *(curved arrow)*. Note small caliber of the distal runoff vessel (PDA). *LIMA,* Left internal mammary artery; *LV,* left ventricle; *RV,* right ventricle.

the proximal vessel and an end-to-side anastomosis to the distal vessel.

Venous grafts are larger than arterial grafts and are less prone to streak artifact from less use of surgical clips, hence are easily evaluated on CT when compared to arterial grafts. However, the distal anastomosis may sometimes be problematic to evaluate as a larger-caliber SVG anastomoses to a significantly smaller distal runoff vessel.

Arterial Grafts

Internal Mammary Grafts
IMA grafts have a significantly higher patency rate of greater than 90%, making them the graft of choice for revascularization of obstructed coronary arteries. The presence of endothelial prostacyclin and nitric oxides in arterial grafts leads to less vasospasm. Arterial grafts are better adapted to arterial pressures and have a lower incidence of intimal hyperplasia from the presence of nonfenestrated internal elastic lamina.

LEFT INTERNAL MAMMARY ARTERY
The left internal mammary artery (LIMA) is considered ideal for revascularization of the LAD and diagonal branches because of its location where it is used in situ, remaining connected at its origin at the left subclavian artery, and the mobilized distal portion is anastomosed to the LAD downstream to the critical occlusion. The LIMA can be used as a sequential graft with an end-to-side and end-to-end anastomosis to the LAD and diagonals, or both anastomoses on the LAD, one more distal than the other. The LIMA may also be used as a free graft. On CT the LIMA following its origin in the anterior inferior aspect of the proximal left subclavian artery is seen on the left side of the mediastinum, coursing down toward the anterior interventricular groove along the left heart border to anastomose to the LAD (Fig. 39-3). Multiple surgical clips are typically used to ligate collateral vessels throughout its course, which can result in streak artifacts from beam hardening and can limit evaluation

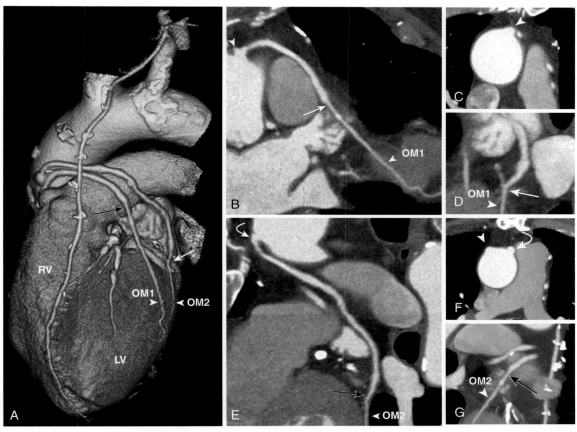

Figure 39-2 Seventy-two-year-old man, 12 years after coronary artery bypass grafts, underwent computed tomography angiography to evaluate for bypass graft patency. Saphenous venous grafts (SVG) to first obtuse marginal (OM) branch of the left circumflex (OM1) and OM2. **A,** Three-dimensional volume-rendered image demonstrates SVG to OM1 *(black arrow)* and SVG to OM2 *(white arrow)*. Both grafts are mildly ectatic. Curved multiplanar reformation (MPR; **B**) and maximum intensity projection (MIP; **C** and **D**) images demonstrate widely patent SVG to OM1. *Arrowhead* points to the proximal anastomosis at the left anterior aspect of the ascending thoracic aorta and *white arrow* to the end-to-side distal anastomosis to OM1. Curved MPR (**E**) and MIP images (**F** and **G**) demonstrate widely patent SVG to OM2. *Curved arrow* points to the proximal anastomosis at the left anterior aspect of the ascending thoracic aorta (just below the proximal anastomosis of SVG to OM1) and *black arrow* points to the end-to-side distal anastomosis to OM2. Note that the distal runoff vessel is of significantly smaller caliber than the SVG. *LV*, Left ventricle; *RV*, right ventricle.

of the LIMA. This is overcome to a certain degree with newer scan technology such as high-definition scanners and dual-energy scanners.

RIGHT INTERNAL MAMMARY ARTERY

The right internal mammary artery (RIMA), though less frequently used for the revascularization of the RCA or the left coronary arterial territory, can be used in many ways. It can be used as an in situ graft from its origin in the right subclavian artery to anastomose distally to the RCA or PDA, or it may course anterior to the ascending aorta and arch toward the left to anastomose to the LAD (Fig. 39-4). The RIMA can also be used as an in situ graft preserving its origin to the right subclavian artery to anastomose distally to the diagonal artery or obtuse marginal branches of the left circumflex artery by passing through the transverse sinus.

It is, however, more frequently used as a free or composite graft rather than an in situ graft, often sutured proximally onto the anterior ascending aorta and distally to the poststenotic coronary artery. It has also occasionally been used as a composite graft with a proximal anastomosis to a LIMA graft and distal anastomosis to the left circumflex arterial territory, resulting in total myocardial revascularization from a single inflow from the LIMA origin in the left subclavian artery. This technique results in improved 1-year patency rates when used for two-vessel disease versus treatment with a LIMA graft and an SVG.

Radial Artery

The radial artery is harvested from the nondominant arm and used in combination with other arterial grafts or as a third arterial graft for revascularization of the left ventricular myocardium instead of a venous graft. It is commonly used as an independent conduit in the form of a composite or free graft to perfuse the left ventricular territory, with the proximal anastomosis on the anterior ascending thoracic aorta, similar to the SVGs or RIMA. It can also be used as part of a Y configuration to perfuse the distal RCA or PDA. Despite falling out of favor because of increased vasospasm, the graft is again being used as a result of improved harvesting techniques that

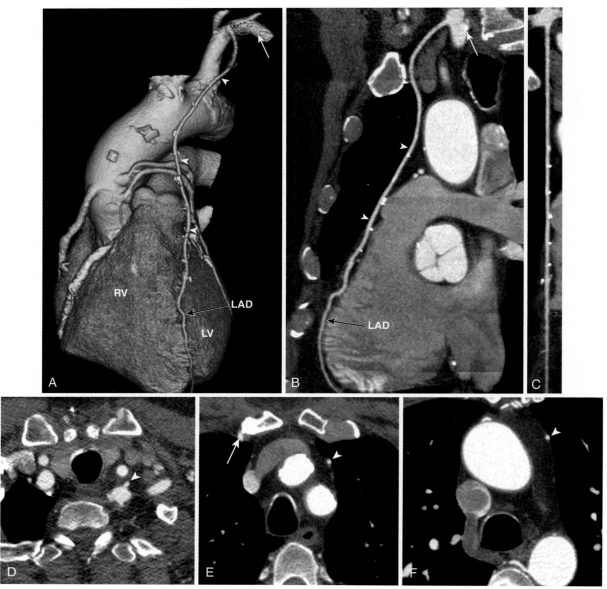

Figure 39-3 Seventy-two-year-old man, 12 years after coronary artery bypass graft, underwent computed tomography angiography to evaluate for bypass graft patency. Left internal mammary artery (LIMA) to left anterior descending (LAD) artery. Three-dimensional volume-rendered image (**A**) and curved multiplanar reformation (**B**) demonstrate the typical appearance of a patent LIMA graft *(arrowheads)* coming off the left subclavian artery *(white arrow)*, with end-to-side distal anastomosis to the mid-LAD *(black arrow)*. Note multiple surgical clips along the course of the LIMA, used to ligate collateral vessels. Axial computed tomography angiography demonstrates the LIMA origin *(arrowhead)* from the left subclavian artery (**D**), and well-opacified proximal LIMA *(arrowheads)* in the left paramediastinal region (**E** and **F**). The right internal mammary artery is located in its normal position *(arrow)*. *LV*, Left ventricle; *RV*, right ventricle.

avoid endothelial damage when used for two-vessel disease.

The radial artery has short-term patency rates similar to the LIMA but medium- and long-term patency rates similar to the SVG. The increased use of clips and staples needed during harvesting because of its muscular nature results in increased beam-hardening artifact on computed tomography angiography (CTA), which along with its small caliber, can result in limited evaluation.

Right Gastroepiploic Artery

The right gastroepiploic artery (RGEA) can be used as a second- or third-choice arterial conduit for total

myocardial revascularization or when no other viable grafts are available. For harvesting the RGEA the surgical incision extends from the median sternotomy caudally to the umbilicus, and the artery is harvested from the greater curvature of the stomach, which can lead to increased perioperative and long-term abdominal complications; hence it is rarely used as a conduit.

The RGEA is used as an in situ graft that is anastomosed on the distal PDA or left circumflex artery when it is directed in a retrograde fashion, or LAD in an antegrade fashion. On CTA the RGEA graft is the only vessel seen coursing anterior to the liver and through the diaphragm to the occluded target artery.

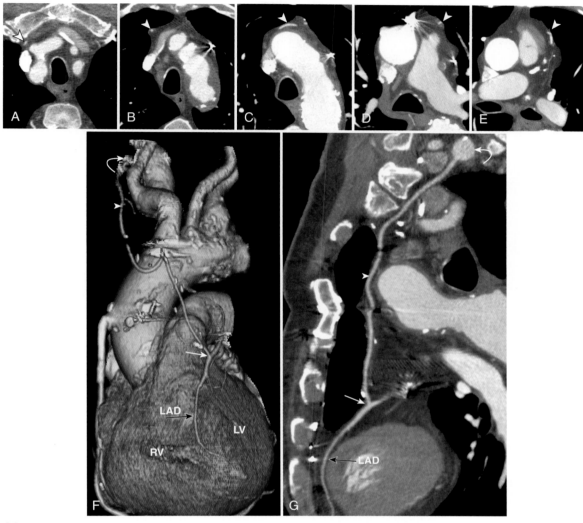

Figure 39-4 74-year-old man, 3 years after coronary artery bypass graft (CABG), with previously occluded left internal mammary artery to left anterior descending (LAD) artery, underwent redo CABG with right internal mammary artery (RIMA) to LAD. Axial images (**A** to **E**) demonstrate a patent RIMA *(arrowhead)* that, following its origin from the right subclavian artery *(curved arrow)*, courses from the right paramediastinal region, anterior to the distal ascending thoracic aorta, to the left paramediastinal region to reach the anterior interventricular groove. Three-dimensional volume-reduced image (**F**) and curved multiplanar reformation (**G**) demonstrate RIMA arising from the right subclavian artery with end-to-side anastomosis to the mid LAD *(black arrow)*. The distal anastomotic site is denoted by the *white arrow. LV,* Left ventricle; *RV,* right ventricle.

■ GRAFT COMPLICATIONS

Early Complications

Graft Thrombosis
Early occlusive complications within 1 month after surgery are invariably related to graft thrombosis from endothelial injury during harvesting/anastomosis. Storage procedures and mechanical trauma have also been linked to the triggering of coagulation cascade with resultant thrombosis. Within the first postoperative month, intimal hyperplasia on exposure to arterial pressures causes 25% of SVGs to stenose and 3% to 12% to occlude.

GRAFT MALPOSITION OR KINKING
An unduly long graft can result in early myocardial revascularization failure because of malpositioning or kinking of the graft. A short and stretched graft can result in graft failure in patients with severe chronic obstructive airway disease who have large-volume lungs. If an aortic connector used to attach the proximal anastomosis is not adequately supported, the conduit may kink. This kinking can often be observed on CTA.

Graft Vasospasm
The radial artery is most prone to vasospasm because of the presence of a prominent muscular wall. Intraoperative use of alpha-adrenergic blocking agents and postoperative administration of calcium channel blockers are supposedly effective in preventing graft vasospasm. On CTA, vasospasm could appear as a reduction in lumen diameter without evidence of intraluminal defects and is not always readily identified on CTA when compared with invasive coronary angiography.

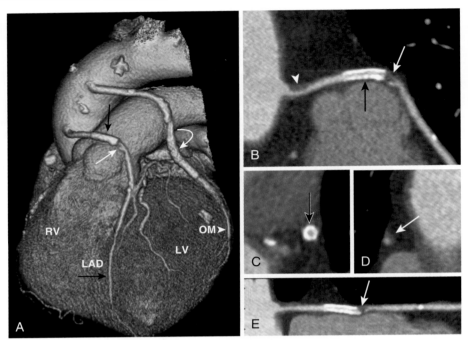

Figure 39-5 Seventy-four-year-old man had chest pain radiating to back. Patient had a third coronary artery bypass graft (CABG) 29 years ago and percutaneous stents placed 14 years later. Computed tomography angiography was performed to evaluate the aorta for aortic dissection. **A,** Three-dimensional volume-rendered (VR) image demonstrates saphenous venous graft (SVG) to the left anterior descending (LAD) artery and SVG to the obtuse marginal, with stents in both grafts (*black arrow* and *curved arrow*). Patency of grafts cannot be evaluated on the VR image. *White arrow* points to a significant stenosis that is not well seen on the VR image. **B,** Curved multiplanar reformation shows mild-to-moderate stenosis at the proximal anastomosis from noncalcified plaque (*arrowhead*) and severe stenosis (*white arrow*) in the SVG immediately distal to the patent stent (*black arrow*). **C,** Orthogonal cross-sectional view demonstrates the well-opacified patent stent (*black arrow*) in the SVG. Just distal to the stent there is a severe stenosis (*white arrow*) from noncalcified plaque shown on the orthogonal cross-sectional view (**D**) and the linear lumen view (**E**). Cardiac catheterization confirmed 80% stenosis of the SVG just distal to the graft. Patient underwent redo CABG with left internal mammary artery to LAD. *LV,* Left ventricle; *OM,* obtuse marginal; *RV,* right ventricle.

Long-Term Complications

Graft Patency

Recent studies have reported 15% to 20% of vein graft occlusions occur within the first year following revascularization. The graft occlusion rate thereafter is 1% to 2% between 1 and 6 years and 4% to 5% between 6 and 10 years. The patency rate after 10 years for SVGs is approximately 60%, and only 50% of these vein grafts remain free of stenosis. Antiplatelet therapy and lipid-lowering medications reduce the occlusion rate of SVGs.

Arterial grafts are relatively less involved by arteriosclerosis, and most occlusive complications occur at the distal anastomotic site. At 10 years 83% to 90% of LIMA grafts are patent. Arterial graft assessment can be precluded by surgical clips causing streak artifacts.

CTA is used to identify the presence or absence of atherosclerotic plaque; to characterize the plaque as calcified, partially calcified (previously referred to as mixed), or noncalcified; and to determine the degree of luminal diameter narrowing (Fig. 39-5). Plaque in SVGs is often eccentric in location. Qualitative and quantitative grading of stenosis can be performed for grafts, as well as native vessels. Percutaneous stenting is often performed to treat SVG stenosis. On CTA, stent patency and occlusion can be determined because caliber for SVGs is often bigger than for native vessels (see Fig. 39-5). In-stent stenosis may be difficult to see but is better visualized with the newer generation of scanners.

Complete occlusion of an SVG in an acute setting can manifest as an enlarged occluded SVG with nonopacified thrombus. Chronically thrombosed grafts are often of normal or smaller size (Fig. 39-6). A proximal SVG occlusion often appears as a contrast-filled outpouching, button, or nubbin at the proximal graft anastomosis on the anterior wall of the ascending thoracic aorta (Fig. 39-7) with nonvisualization of the remainder of the graft. Nonvisualization of SVGs or arterial grafts is indicative of complete occlusion.

Graft Aneurysm

Two types of CABG aneurysms have been reported in the literature: true aneurysms and pseudoaneurysms. True aneurysms are atherosclerotic in nature and appear 5 to 7 years after CABG (Fig. 39-8). Pseudoaneurysms usually occur within 6 months of surgery mainly at suture lines, from breakage/dehiscence of suture or infection, or from tension at the attachment site. Less commonly they could appear years later as a result of atherosclerosis. Aneurysms are incidentally detected on a chest x-ray examination as a mass. Up to 12% of pseudoaneurysms and 47% of true aneurysms are asymptomatic even when they are very large. Aneurysms should be evaluated for patency, size, and mass effect on adjacent structures. CTA is better at evaluating aneurysm size, because both the contrast-opacified lumen and associated thrombus can be well

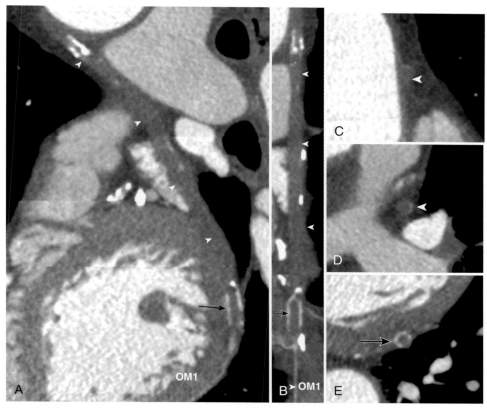

Figure 39-6 Seventy-year-old man with history of coronary artery bypass graft 10 years ago had atypical chest pain. Computed tomography angiography was performed to assess the bypass grafts. Curved reformat (**A**), linear lumen view (**B**), and orthogonal cross sectional views (**C** to **E**) of a completely thrombosed *(arrowheads)* saphenous venous graft to the obtuse marginal. Note the presence of a completely occluded stent *(black arrow)* in the distal graft just proximal to the distal anastomosis.

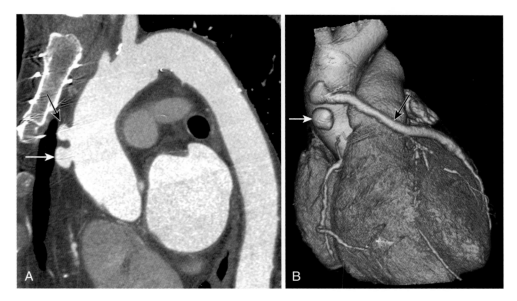

Figure 39-7 Seventy-five-year old man with chest pain 7 years after four-vessel coronary artery bypass graft. An oblique maximum intensity projection (**A**) and a three-dimensional volume-rendered image (**B**) shows a focal outpouching of contrast in the anterior wall of the ascending aorta from an occluded saphenous venous graft (SVG) resulting in the nubbin sign *(white arrow)*, and a patent mildly dilated SVG to the obtuse marginal *(black arrow)*. Three of the four grafts were completely occluded.

depicted on CT and the relationship to adjacent structures can be defined. At invasive coronary angiography only the contrast-opacified lumen is visualized, and the reported size of the aneurysm can be misleadingly small because the thrombosed portion of the aneurysm is not visualized. Although no consensus has been reached on the management of aneurysms, intervention to prevent complications may be considered based on patient presentation and aneurysm size. An aneurysm greater than 2 cm can be considered for potential surgery. Complications of graft aneurysms include embolization of thrombus, myocardial infarction, fistula formation to the right atrium or ventricle, and rupture of the aneurysm leading to hemopericardium, hemothorax, or even death.

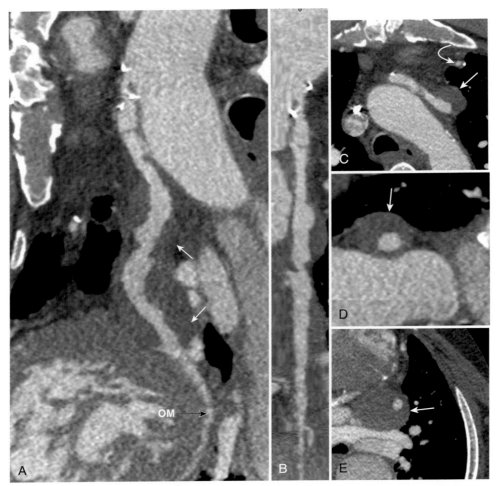

Figure 39-8 Fifty-four-year-old-man with four-vessel coronary artery bypass graft and known aortic dissection. Curved multiplanar reformation (MPR; **A**) and linear lumen view (**B**) demonstrate a diffusely aneurysmal *(arrows)* sequential saphenous venous grafts (SVG) to the obtuse marginal (OM) 1 and OM2. The limb to the OM2 was completely occluded. Oblique MPRs (**C** to **E**) demonstrate significant amount of thrombus in the partially thrombosed SVG aneurysm *(arrow)*, which is well depicted on computed tomography (CT), and the size of the aneurysm is also well assessed on CT. Cardiac catheterization depicted only the opacified portion of the lumen. The left internal mammary artery *(curved arrow)* was patent; however, the SVG to the right coronary artery was completely occluded.

■ REOPERATION

Reoperation is more complex than initial bypass grafting. Median sternotomy is a blind procedure that can lead to catastrophic bleeding in repeat operations because of injury to cardiac structures and extracardiac grafts. In a survey of 2046 catastrophic bleeding events in reoperations reported by 1116 surgeons, the most common cardiac structures injured were the right ventricle (39%), SVG (20%), aorta (15%), IMA (12%), and innominate vein (6%). The relative distribution of anatomic structures injured reflected their most common location in relation to the midline. A large proportion of reoperative patients with IMAs are graft dependent, and up to 5% injury and 50% reinfarction rates have been reported at the Cleveland Clinic.

Conventional coronary angiography provides luminal information but poor spatial information with relation to the sternum. MDCT with multiplanar reformats and 3D VR capability exquisitely depicts graft anatomy and its relationship to the sternum and chest wall (Fig. 39-9) and aids in planning reentry. MDCT angiography also affords the added advantage of identifying significantly calcified segments of the aorta that should be avoided during reentry. This leads to decreased embolic complications during cross clamping. Several modifications of the surgical approach in patients with a calcified aorta have been described, including off-pump CABG, "no-touch" off-pump total arterial revascularization, axillary artery cannulation, and mechanical or suture-based clampless proximal connectors.

In addition to commenting on graft patency, a description of the relationships of the graft to the sternum/midline should be provided. Multiplanar reformats with emphasis on sagittal maximum intensity projections, 3D VR, and sternal subtracted 3D VR, if possible, should be available to demonstrate graft course. In patients with renal dysfunction a gated noncontrast study is helpful to identify aortic calcification and right ventricular anatomy in relationship to the sternum.

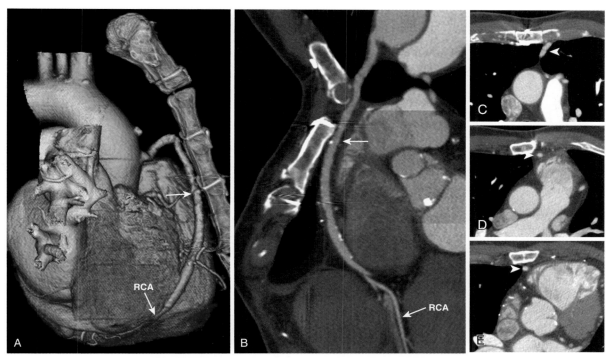

Figure 39-9 Sixty-nine-year-old man with history of severe aortic stenosis and history of prior coronary artery bypass graft. Computed tomography angiography was performed to evaluate aorta before surgery. Volume-rendered image (**A**), curved multiplanar reformation (**B**), and axial images (**C** to **E**) demonstrate a saphenous venous graft (SVG; denoted by *arrow* on CMPR and *arrowheads* on axial images) to the distal right coronary artery (RCA) with close approximation of the proximal/mid portion of the SVG to the sternum. Preoperative knowledge of the relationship of the graft to the sternum and chest wall is crucial when planning the surgical approach for aortic/cardiac surgery to avoid inadvertent resection or injury to the graft.

■ LIMITATIONS

Despite the high diagnostic accuracy for detection of graft stenosis or occlusion with 64-slice and higher-generation scanners, several limitations still exist.

In cases with rapid heart rate or arrhythmias, diagnosis can be difficult from cardiac motion artifacts. Metallic clips can result in significant streak artifact limiting evaluation. Evaluation of the native grafted and nongrafted vessels remains challenging because of significant calcified plaque in these vessels, limiting overall diagnostic accuracy. CT has limited ability to detect competitive or retrograde flow because of technical limitations and may erroneously misjudge an anastomotic site as having significant stenosis.

The other limiting factors common to both invasive coronary angiography and CTA are renal dysfunction and iodine allergy, which are both relative and not absolute contraindications to the use of iodinated contrast.

Radiation dose continues to be a cause for concern, particularly with retrospectively acquired scans. The radiation dose delivered by 64-MDCT varies from 2 to 15 mSv depending on the type of gating or triggering, body mass index and craniocaudal coverage, and type of scanner used. The increased z-axis coverage required to evaluate the entire course of the IMA or RGEA often results in higher doses. The use of prospective triggering, tube-current modulation, low kVp, iterative reconstruction methods, and high-pitch acquisitions where available have resulted in significant dose reduction, and graft assessment at 1 mSv is possible today in some patients.

■ CONCLUSION

Substantial improvements and refinement of MDCT technology have resulted in CT being used as an alternate imaging modality for assessment of bypass grafts, which is listed as an appropriate indication for use in the assessment of symptomatic patients. For accurate interpretation of CTA studies following revascularization, it is important to have knowledge of the CABG conduit anatomy and surgical procedure, and to recognize graft stenosis and occlusions, graft complications, and relationship of the graft to the sternum.

Bibliography

Bourassa MG, Fisher LD, Campeau L, Gillespie MJ, McConney M, Lespérance J. Long-term fate of bypass grafts: the Coronary Artery Surgery Study (CASS) and Montreal Heart Institute experiences. *Circulation*. 1985;72:V71-V78.

de Graaf FR, van Velzen JE, Witkowska AJ, Schuijf JD, van der Bijl N, Kroft LJ, et al. Diagnostic performance of 320-slice multidetector computed tomography coronary angiography in patients after coronary artery bypass grafting. *Eur Radiol*. 2011;21:2285-2296.

Dubois CL, Vandervoort PM. Aneurysms and pseudoaneurysms of coronary arteries and saphenous vein coronary artery grafts: a case report and literature review. *Acta Cardiol*. 2001;56:263-276.

Eagle, Guyton R, Davidoff, et al. ACC/AHA Guidelines for coronary artery bypass graft surgery: a report of the American College of Cardiology/American Heart Association Task Force on Practice Guidelines. *JACC*. 1999;110:1262-1347.

Eagle KA, Guyton RA, Davidoff R, Edwards FH, Ewy GA, Gardner TJ, et al. ACC/AHA 2004 guideline update for coronary artery bypass graft surgery: summary article: a report of the American College of Cardiology/American Heart Association Task Force on Practice Guidelines (Committee to Update the 1999 Guidelines for Coronary Artery Bypass Graft Surgery). *Circulation*. 2004;110:1168-1176.

Fitzgibbon GM, Kafka HP, Leach AJ, et al. Coronary bypass fraft fate and patient outcome: angiographic follow-up of 5065 frats related to survival and reoperation in 1388 patients during 25 years. *JACC*. 1996;26:616-626.

Follis FM, Pett Jr SB, Miller KB, Wong RS, Temes RT, Wernly JA. Catastrophic hemorrhage on sternal reentry: still a dreaded complication? *Ann Thorac Surg.* 1999;68:2215-2219.

Frazier AA, Qureshi F, Read KM, Gilkeson RC, Poston RS, White CS. Coronary artery bypass grafts: assessment with multidetector CT in the early and late postoperative settings. *Radiographics.* 2005;25:881-896.

Gilkeson RC, Markowitz AH, Ciancibello L. Multisection CT evaluation of the reoperative cardiac surgery patient. *Radiographics.* 2003;23:S3-S17.

Goetti R, Leschka S, Baumüller S, Plass A, Wieser M, Desbiolles L, et al. Low-dose high-pitch spiral acquisition 128-slice dual-source computed tomography for the evaluation of coronary artery bypass graft patency. *Invest Radiol.* 2010;45:324-330.

Hamon M, Lepage O, Malagutti P, Riddell JW, Morello R, Agostini D, et al. Diagnostic performance of 16- and 64-section spiral CT for coronary artery bypass graft assessment: meta-analysis. *Radiology.* 2008;247:679-686.

Hermann F, Martinoff S, Meyer T, Hadamitzky M, Jiang C, Hendrich E, et al. Reduction of radiation dose estimates in cardiac 64-slice CT angiography in patients after coronary artery bypass graft surgery. *Invest Radiol.* 2008;43:253-260.

Kamdar AR, Meadows TA, Roselli EE, Gorodeski EZ, Curtin RJ, Sabik JF, et al. Multidetector computed tomographic angiography in planning of reoperative cardiothoracic surgery. *Ann Thorac Surg.* 2008;85:1239-1245.

Khan NU, Yonan Y. Does preoperative computed tomography reduce the risks associated with re-do cardiac surgery? *Interact Cardiovasc Thorac Surg.* 2009;9:119-123.

Lee JH, Chun EJ, Choi SI, Vembar M, Lim C, Park KH, et al. Prospective versus retrospective ECG-gated 64-detector coronary CT angiography for evaluation of coronary artery bypass graft patency: comparison of image quality, radiation dose and diagnostic accuracy. *Int J Cardiovasc Imaging.* 2011;27:657-667.

Lu ML, Jen-Sho Chen J, Awan O, White CS. Evaluation of bypass grafts and stents. *Radiol Clin N Am.* 2010;48:757-770.

Malagutti P, Nieman K, Meijboom WB, van Mieghem CA, Pugliese F, Cademartiri F, et al. Use of 64-slice CT in symptomatic patients after coronary bypass surgery: evaluation of grafts and coronary arteries. *Eur Heart J.* 2007;28:1879-1885.

Marano R, Liguori C, Rinaldi P, Storto ML, Politi MA, Savino G, et al. Coronary artery bypass grafts and MDCT imaging: what to know and what to look for. *Eur Radiol.* 2007;17:3166-3178.

Nazeri I, Shahabi P, Tehrai M, Sharif-Kashani B, Nazeri A. Assessment of patients after coronary artery bypass grafting using 64-slice computed tomography. *Am J Cardiol.* 2009;103:667-673.

Onuma Y, Tanabe K, Chihara R, Yamamoto H, Miura Y, Kigawa I, et al. Evaluation of coronary artery bypass grafts and native coronary arteries using 64-slice multidetector computed tomography. *Am Heart J.* 2007;154:519-526.

Possati G, Gaudino M, Prati F, Alessandrini F, Trani C, Glieca F, et al. Long-term results of the radial artery used for myocardial revascularization. *Circulation.* 2003;108:1350-1354.

Weustink AC, Nieman K, Pugliese F, et al. Diagnostic accuracy of computed tomography angiography in patients after bypass grafting: comparison with invasive coronary angiography. *JACC Cardiovasc Imaging.* 2009;7:816-824.

Pulmonary Veins, Atria, and Atrial Appendage

Prabhakar Rajiah and Milind Y. Desai

The pulmonary veins and atria are affected by a variety of congenital and acquired abnormalities. Echocardiography is often the initial modality used in the evaluation of atria and atrial appendages. However, echocardiography is operator dependent, has limited field of view, and does not have tissue characterization capabilities. Computed tomography (CT) and magnetic resonance imaging (MRI) are increasingly used in the evaluation of atria and the atrial appendages. In addition, CT and MRI are the ideal noninvasive imaging modalities in the evaluation of pulmonary veins. Imaging plays an important role in the detection of abnormality and characterization of the lesion.

■ CROSS-SECTIONAL IMAGING TECHNIQUES

Pulmonary veins and the atria can be evaluated both by CT and MRI. Both CT and MRI have good spatial and temporal resolution, large field-of-view capabilities, and multiplanar reconstruction capabilities. CT is faster than MRI but requires the use of intravenous contrast media, which is potentially nephrotoxic in patients with predisposing conditions and is associated with a small but not insignificant risk for cancer because of ionizing radiation. MRI is not associated with radiation. MRI cannot be performed in patients with claustrophobia or those with contraindications such as metallic implants or pacemakers. Gadolinium-based contrast agents used in MRI are not nephrotoxic but can induce debilitating nephrogenic systemic fibrosis in patients with severe renal dysfunction. However, even in these patients angiography can be performed using the three-dimensional (3-D) whole heart steady-state free precession (SSFP) sequence.

Pulmonary veins and left atria are commonly imaged before and following radiofrequency ablation of the pulmonary venous ostia for atrial fibrillation. CT images are acquired at end expiration to enable mapping in the electrophysiology laboratory. Electrocardiogram (ECG) gating is preferred to avoid motion artifacts. In patients with low and stable heart rhythm, prospective ECG triggering can be performed to reduce the radiation dose. In patients with high heart rates and in large patients, retrospective ECG gating may be required. Non–ECG-gated helical scans are used in patients with atrial fibrillation and high heart rates. Non–ECG-gated technique has the least radiation dose of all the techniques available. Motion artifacts with this technique are trivial and do not compromise the ability to make a diagnosis. Pulmonary veins are typically imaged in the late systolic phase, when they have the largest caliber. Injection of 75 to 90 mL of nonionic iodinated contrast through an antecubital vein at the rate of 3.5 to 4.5 mL/second using a power injector is followed by 50 mL of normal saline to flush out the superior vena cava (SVC) to avoid obscuring the right superior pulmonary vein. Multiplanar reconstruction, volume rendering, shaded surface display, and endocardial (intraatrial) reconstructions are the postprocessing techniques used for evaluation of the left atrium and pulmonary veins.

MRI evaluation of the atria and pulmonary veins requires a combination of various sequences in different planes. Cine images are acquired through SSFP sequence. Characterization of a mass is performed using T1- and T2-weighted black-blood fast spin echo sequences. Early postcontrast images are acquired using T1-weighted spin echo sequence, and delayed postcontrast images are acquired using inversion recovery sequences, both following intravenous administration of 0.1 to 0.2 mmol/kg of gadolinium chelates. Evaluation of pulmonary veins can be done either using postcontrast MR angiography with T1-weighted spoiled gradient sequence or using a noncontrast whole heart 3-D SSFP sequence.

■ PULMONARY VEINS

Pulmonary Venous Anatomy and Drainage

In 80% to 85% of the normal population, four pulmonary veins are seen draining into the left atrium, namely, the right superior, right inferior, left superior, and left inferior pulmonary veins. The right middle vein drains into the right superior pulmonary vein (Fig. 40-1, *A*). Variations in pulmonary venous drainage are seen in 15% to 20% of the population. This includes variations in the number of ostia, the length of pulmonary veins, and branching patterns. In the conjoined pattern of drainage, the superior and inferior pulmonary veins of one side join before they drain into the left atrium, resulting in an ostium that is larger than normal (Fig. 40-1, *B*). This is more common on the left than the right. In accessory pattern of drainage, there are accessory ostia in addition to the normal four ostia. Although any of the pulmonary segmental branches can open directly into the left atrium, the right middle lobe and right lower lobe superior segmental branches are the most common accessory veins (Fig. 40-1, C). The accessory ostia are smaller than normal. Different patterns of drainage may be seen in the same individual. Occasionally a pulmonary vein drains into the pulmonary vein of the contralateral side (Fig. 40-1,D).

Anomalous pulmonary venous return is defined as drainage of pulmonary veins into a structure other than the left atrium. Anomalous drainage can either be partial or total. In partial anomalous pulmonary venous return (PAPVR), one to three of the pulmonary veins drain into the systemic venous circulation, either directly into the right atrium or into systemic veins, resulting in a partial left-to-right shunt. This is seen in 0.7% of the population and is usually asymptomatic. The left superior pulmonary vein is the most common vein to have anomalous drainage (47% of PAPVR cases), most commonly into the left brachiocephalic vein (Fig. 40-2, A), followed by right superior pulmonary vein draining into the SVC (Fig. 40-2, B). Anomalous drainage of the right inferior and the left inferior pulmonary veins is less common. The anomalous pulmonary vein may also drain into the coronary sinus, azygos vein, inferior vena cava (IVC), and very rarely into the right atrium. Sinus venosus defect is seen in 42% of patients with right upper lobe PAPVR. In the scimitar syndrome, there is anomalous pulmonary venous drainage of part of or the entire lung into the IVC,

coronary sinus, right atrium, azygos vein, portal vein, or hepatic vein. This is almost always seen on the right side and associated with hypoplasia of the right lung and right pulmonary artery. The anomalous pulmonary vein is seen in the shape of a scimitar, curving medially toward the diaphragm and the IVC in posteroanterior chest radiographs and coronal CT or MRI.

In total anomalous pulmonary venous return (TAPVR), all of the pulmonary veins drain directly into the right atrium or into a systemic venous channel that eventually drains into the right atrium. TAPVR is classified as supracardiac (typically a vertical vein draining into the brachiocephalic vein), cardiac (drainage directly into the right atrium or coronary sinus), or infradiaphragmatic (usually via the portal vein). Occasionally connections may exist at two or more levels. Obstruction to the pulmonary veins is seen most commonly in the infradiaphragmatic type, as the anomalous vein enters the portal vein, which has higher venous pressure than the right or left atrium and their tributaries.

Knowledge of variations in pulmonary venous drainage becomes crucial in patients being evaluated for radiofrequency ablation of pulmonary venous ostia for atrial fibrillation. Variations can be seen in the number of ostia, branching pattern, and length of branches. Because of the small size, accessory ostia may be easily missed during ablation procedures, resulting in recurrent atrial fibrillation caused by incomplete ablation of arrhythmogenic foci. Another variation to be recognized is the presence of an early or ostial branch that occurs

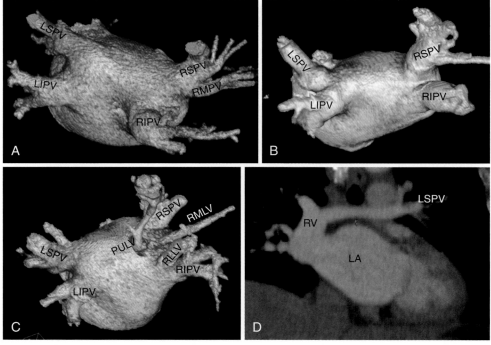

Figure 40-1 Variations in pulmonary venous drainage. A, Volume-rendered (VR) three-dimensional (3-D) computed tomographic (CT) image shows the most common pattern of pulmonary venous drainage, with separate ostia for the right superior pulmonary vein (RSPV), right inferior pulmonary vein (RIPV), left superior pulmonary vein (LSPV), and left inferior pulmonary vein (LIPV). The right middle vein (RMPV) opens into the right superior pulmonary vein. **B,** VR 3-D CT image of the left atrium shows a common ostium for the LSPV and the LIPV. There are separate ostia for the RSPV and the RIPV. **C,** VR 3-D CT image shows separate ostia for the LSPV and the LIPV. On the right, in addition to the RSPV and RIPV ostia, there are accessory ostia for the right middle pulmonary vein (RMPV), superior segment of the right lower lobe (RLLV), and posterior segment of the right upper lobe vein (PULV). **D,** Coronal reconstructed CT image shows the LSPV extending medially and crossing the midline to drain into a common venous trunk on the right (RV).

within 5 mm of the pulmonary venous ostia. This is most common in the right middle vein and has a high risk for the development of pulmonary stenosis following ablation. In the electrophysiology laboratory, 3-D reconstructions from CT or MRI angiographic images are typically integrated with electrophysiology data acquired from left atrium mapping catheters to establish a road map for catheter ablation procedures, including anatomic variations. Endocardial views also help in determining the presence of small accessory ostia.

Pulmonary venous stenosis is a well-recognized complication of ablation procedures for atrial fibrillation, seen in 1% to 3% of these procedures. Stenosis is caused by intimal thickening, thrombus, endocardial contraction, and elastic laminae proliferation. Symptoms are usually seen 2 to 5 months after the procedure, with the intensity related to the degree of obstruction. CT or MRI is used in the evaluation of pulmonary stenosis. With MRI, postcontrast MR angiography or noncontrast MR angiography using whole heart 3-D SSFP sequence can

be used. Based on the severity of the luminal narrowing, pulmonary venous stenosis can be graded as mild (<50% narrowing), moderate (50% to 69% narrowing), or severe (>70% narrowing) (Fig. 40-3, *A*). The veins are measured in short-axis images obtained using double axial reconstruction of two orthogonal images. Severe pulmonary vein stenosis is treated with balloon angioplasty with stent placement. CT is useful in the evaluation of patency of the stent (Fig. 40-3, *B*) and further development of complications.

■ ATRIA AND THE APPENDAGES

In normal individuals, the morphologic right and left atrium are located on the right and left sides, respectively. The right atrium receives the coronary sinus, the SVC, and the IVC, whereas the left atrium receives the pulmonary veins. The right atrium opens into the right ventricle through the tricuspid valve, and the left atrium opens into the left ventricle through the mitral valve.

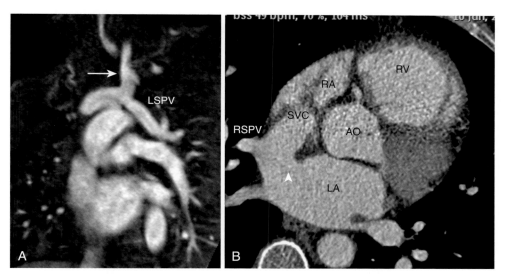

Figure 40-2 Partial anomalous pulmonary venous return. A, Coronal magnetic resonance angiographic image shows an anomalous left superior pulmonary vein (LSPV) draining into the left brachiocephalic vein *(arrow)*. **B,** Axial computed tomographic scan in a different patient shows partial anomalous drainage of the right superior pulmonary vein (RSPV) into the superior vena cava (SVC). There is an associated sinus venous defect *(arrowhead)*, with communication between the left atrium (LA) and the superior vena cava (SVC). *AO,* Aorta; *RA,* right atrium; *RV,* right ventricle.

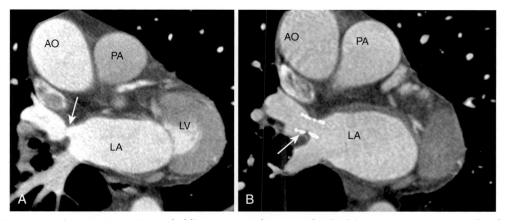

Figure-40-3 Pulmonary vein stenosis. A, Coronal oblique computed tomographic (CT) image in a patient 3 months after radiofrequency isolation of pulmonary venous ostia shows severe stenosis of the right superior pulmonary vein *(arrow)*. **B,** Coronal oblique CT image of the same patient following stent placement shows a patent stent with normal flow of contrast *(arrow)*. *AO,* Aorta; *LA,* left atrium; *LV,* left ventricle; *PA,* pulmonary artery.

The atria are smooth-walled chambers and are derived from outgrowth of pulmonary veins and sinus venosus. The morphologic atria can be distinguished based on the appearance of the atrial appendages.

Atrial appendages are trabeculated, muscular out-pouchings from the atrial chambers, which are remnants of the original embryonic atria. The right atrial append-age has a broad and triangular shape and has a wide junction with the right atrium. The left atrial append-age has a long, tubular, hook shape with crenellations and has a narrow junction with the left atrium. The atrial appendages are trabeculated, with muscle fibers oriented parallel to each other in the shape of a comb, called pectinate muscles, which are more pronounced in the right than the left. The atrial appendages are located within the confines of the pericardium and have only minimal useful function. The left atrial appendage is believed to act as a decompression chamber during left ventricular systole and when the left atrial pressure is elevated.

Accessory appendages or diverticula may be seen in the left atrium. An accessory appendage has ostium, body, and neck with an irregular contour because of pectinate muscle, more common in the left posterolat-eral wall. The accessory appendage may fibrillate inde-pendent of the rest of the heart and should be included in radiofrequency ablation. It can be a source of throm-boemboli. A diverticulum has a saclike appearance with broad-based ostium and smooth contour. Diverticulum is either a remnant of an accessory pulmonary vein or a varix at the distal end of a small accessory pulmo-nary vein. Diverticulum may cause mitral regurgitation, arrhythmias, thromboembolism, or pericarditis. In jux-taposition with atrial appendages, both atrial append-ages lie on one side of the great arteries. Diverticulum is associated with D-transposition of great arteries.

■ ATRIAL SIZE

Atrial measurements can be made in either CT or MRI. Atrial diameter and area are measured in the four-chamber images, usually in the end-systolic phase. Atrial volume can be measured using the area-length biplane or the prolate ellipsoid methods, both of which are less accurate than the modified Simpson method. Normal reference values have been established for atrial diameter,

area, and volume. The normal atrial diameter is less than 4.1 cm in males and 3.9 cm in females. The normal atrial area is 20 cm², and the normal volume is 59 mL in males and 53 mL in females. Volumes measured by CT have been noted to be higher than those measured by MRI. The atrial size varies with body surface area and less with age and sex. Based on area, 21 to 30 cm² is considered mild atrial enlargement, 31 to 40 cm² is considered moderate atrial enlargement, and greater than 40 cm² is considered severe atrial enlargement.

Left atrial enlargement is most commonly seen in mitral stenosis. Other causes include volume overload (mitral regurgitation, atrial septal defect with either shunt reversal or tricuspid atresia, ventricular septal defect, patent ductus arteriosus, aortopulmonary win-dow); pressure overload (noncompliant left ventricle [hypertrophic cardiomyopathy, hypertension, aortic stenosis], left ventricular dysfunction/failure, tumors); and miscellaneous (atrial fibrillation, idiopathic) (Fig. 40-4, A). Left atrial enlargement has been shown to be an indicator of the duration and severity of diastolic dysfunction and is a predictor of adverse cardiovascular outcomes such as atrial fibrillation, congestive cardiac failure, stroke, and cardiovascular death. It is a risk fac-tor for atrial fibrillation, stroke, and atrial fibrillation following therapy. Aneurysm of the left atrium is rare and can be congenital or result from rheumatic heart disease, tuberculosis, or syphilis. It most commonly involves the left atrial appendage. It is associated with pericardial defect and leads to mitral regurgitation, heart failure caused by pulmonary venous obstruction, respiratory distress, cardiac tamponade, thromboem-bolization, and arrhythmias. Small left atrium is seen in conditions with decreased pulmonary venous return such as hypoplastic left heart syndrome, TAPVR, and severe pulmonary venous stenosis.

Right atrial enlargement is seen because of either volume overload (tricuspid regurgitation, atrial sep-tal defect, atrioventricular canal defect, anomalous pulmonary venous return, pulmonary hypertension, sinus of Valsalva fistula) or pressure overload (right ventricular failure, tricuspid stenosis, tricuspid atre-sia, restrictive cardiomyopathy, myxoma) (Fig. 40-4, B). Cardiac failure, Ebstein anomaly, arrhythmogenic right ventricular dysplasia, and endocardial fibroelas-tosis are some of the causes of tricuspid regurgitation.

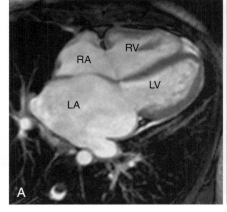
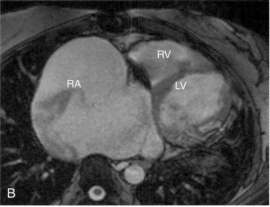

Figure 40-4 Atrial enlarge-ment. A, Four-chamber steady-state free precession (SSFP) magnetic resonance (MR) image in a patient with mitral stenosis shows severe enlargement of the left atrium (LA). **B,** Axial SSFP MR image in another patient with tricuspid valve replace-ment, severe tricuspid regurgita-tion, and pulmonary hypertension shows a giant right atrium (RA). *LV,* Left ventricle; *RV,* right ventricle.

Right atrial enlargement is usually accompanied by right ventricular enlargement, except in tricuspid atresia and Ebstein anomaly. Giant right atrium without underlying cardiac cause is rarely seen. It is usually asymptomatic but may be associated with arrhythmias or thromboembolism. Fontan operation is another cause of a giant right atrium.

Left atrial calcification may be seen in the endocardial and subendocardial layers as a sequel to chronic mitral disease, atrial fibrillation, or congestive cardiac failure. It may involve the left atrial appendage in mitral stenosis (type A), free wall and mitral valve in advanced mitral stenosis (type B), or the posterior wall in mitral regurgitation (type C).

■ CONGENITAL ABNORMALITIES

Congenital abnormalities of the atria include hypoplasia, dextrocardia, transposition of great arteries, cor triatriatum, and atrial septal defects.

In dextrocardia with situs solitus the cardiac apex is located on the right, the morphologic left atrium is located to the left of the morphologic right atrium, with preservation of the atrioventricular concordance (i.e., right atrium opens into right ventricle, left atrium opens into left ventricle). In dextrocardia with situs inversus the morphologic left atrium is located to the right of the morphologic right atrium, and there is atrioventricular concordance (Fig. 40-5). In situs ambiguus with left isomerism, bilateral morphologic left atrium is seen. In situs ambiguus with right isomerism, bilateral morphologic right atrium is seen. In D-transposition of great arteries there is atrioventricular concordance (right atrium opening into right ventricle, left atrium opening into left atrium), but there

is ventriculoarterial discordance (left ventricle opening into pulmonary artery, right ventricle opening into aorta), as a result of which a parallel circulation is seen. In L-transposition (congenitally corrected transposition), there is both ventriculoarterial and atrioventricular discordance (right atrium opening into left ventricle, left atrium opening into right ventricle).

Hypoplasia of the left atrium is seen in hypoplastic left heart syndrome, which is caused by diminished flow through the left heart structures during development. The left ventricle is small and nonfunctional, along with atresia of the aortic and mitral valves. The left atrium is either small or normal. The aortic arch is hypoplastic or has coarctation. Atrial septal defect is present, but the ventricular septum is usually intact. Hypoplasia of the right atrium is seen in hypoplastic right heart syndrome, in which there is pulmonary valve atresia, small right ventricle, small tricuspid valve, and small hypoplastic pulmonary artery. The right atrium is either small or normal in size.

Cor triatriatum sinister is a congenital anomaly in which a fibromuscular membrane divides the left atrium into a proximal posterosuperior chamber and a distal anteroinferior chamber (Fig. 40-6). The membrane has variable size and shape, and is either imperforate or fenestrated. The pulmonary veins typically open into the proximal chamber, and the distal chamber communicates with the mitral valve and the left atrial appendage. Very rarely, pulmonary veins may open in the distal chamber. In a subtotal cor triatriatum either the right or left pulmonary veins drain into the proximal chamber. Clinical symptoms depend on the size of the ostium and associated cardiac anomalies, such as anomalous pulmonary venous drainage. Cor triatriatum should be distinguished from a supravalvar membrane because in this condition the left atrial appendage is located proximal to the dividing membrane that is attached to the atrial surface of the mitral valve or superior to mitral annulus. Cor triatriatum dexter is a similar anomaly involving the right atrium.

Defect in the interatrial septum is the most common congenital disease presenting in adulthood. The most common type of atrial septal defect (80%) is the ostium secundum defect, which occurs in the midportion of the atrial septum at the location of fossa ovalis (Fig. 40-7, A). Ostium primum is the second most common type and is seen in the lower part of the interatrial septum (Fig. 40-7, B). This may be associated with atrioventricular canal defect, which also includes a high ventricular septal defect and cleft mitral and tricuspid valve. A sinus venosus defect is seen in the wall separating the left atrium and the SVC/IVC. This defect is located outside the interatrial septum and may be associated with PAPVR (Fig. 40-7, C and D). Coronary sinus defect (unroofed coronary sinus) is the least common type of atrial septal defect and is either a complete (Fig. 40-7, E and F) or partial communication between the coronary sinus and left atrium. It may be associated with a left-sided SVC. Septal defects are best assessed with MRI, which not only can assess the morphologic features of the defect but can also quantify the shunt, either by using the Qp-to-Qs ratio derived from phase contrast images performed through the main pulmonary artery and the ascending thoracic aorta or by directly measuring the flow through the defect.

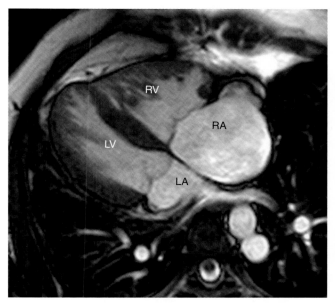

Figure 40-5 Dextrocardia. Axial steady-state free precession magnetic resonance image in a 18-year-old woman shows dextrocardia, with the cardiac apex located on the right hemithorax, with the right atrium (RA) located to the left of the left atrium (LA) and the right ventricle (RV) located to the left of the left ventricle (LV).

A patent foramen ovale (PFO) is seen in 25% to 30% of the population as a flaplike opening between the septum primum and septum secundum. This is not a septal defect because the septal tissue is intact. A right-to-left shunt may occur through a PFO during early systole, with inspiration, repetitive cough and straining, release phase of Valsalva maneuver, or with persistent Chiari network. PFO is not associated with higher risk for recurrent stroke or death in patients with previous cryptogenic stroke. On CT, PFO is seen as a channel-like appearance of the interatrial septum (Fig. 40-8, *A* and *B*) along with features of associated left-to-right shunt such

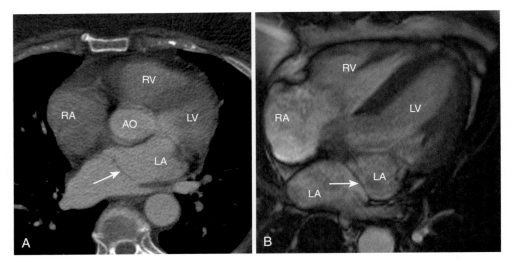

Figure 40-6 Cor triatriatum. A, Axial computed tomographic scan in a 68-year-old woman shows a vertical membrane *(arrow)* extending across the left atrium (LA), consistent with a cor triatriatum. **B,** Axial steady-state free precession magnetic resonance image in a 37-year-old woman shows a membrane *(arrow)* in the left atrium, consistent with cor triatriatum. *AO,* Aorta; *LV,* left ventricle; *RA,* right atrium; *RV,* right ventricle.

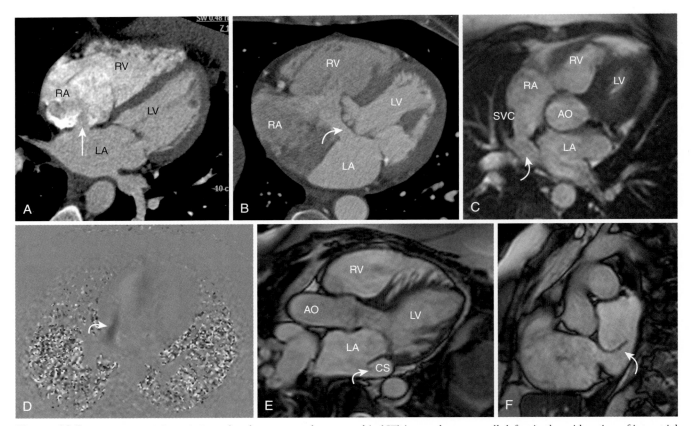

Figure 40-7 Arial septal defect. A, Four-chamber computed tomographic (CT) image shows a small defect in the midportion of interatrial septum *(arrow)*, consistent with an ostium secundum defect. **B,** Four-chamber CT image shows a defect in the lower part of the interatrial septum *(arrow)*, consistent with an ostium primum defect. **C,** Four-chamber steady-state free precession (SSFP) magnetic resonance (MR) image in a 32-year-old woman shows a defect between the superior vena cava (SVC) and the left atrium (LA; *arrow*) consistent with a superior sinus venosus defect. **D,** Four-chamber phase contrast MR image of the same patient shows low-velocity (velocity encoding, 50 cm/sec) flow across the defect *(arrow).* **E,** Axial SSFP MR image in a 51-year-old woman shows complete unroofing *(arrow)* of the coronary sinus (CS), with direct communication between the coronary sinus and the left atrium. **F,** Sagittal SSFP MR image in the same patient shows communication *(arrow)* between coronary sinus and the left atrium. *AO,* Aorta; *LV,* left ventricle; *RA,* right atrium; *RV,* right ventricle.

as contrast jet extending from the left to the right atrium (Fig. 40-8, *C*). Presence of left-to-right shunt with a short flap valve or atrial septal aneurysm is an indicator of bidirectional shunt. On MRI a flap or channel-like appearance of the interatrial septum is indicative of PFO. A shunt is less commonly seen in MRI because of its small size. Interatrial septal aneurysm is mobile interatrial septal tissue in the region of the fossa ovalis, which has a combined excursion of greater than 1.5 cm into the atria (Fig. 40-9). It is seen in 37% of patients with PFO on MRI. Atrial septal aneurysm is associated with migraine. However, there is no conclusive evidence for increased risk for subsequent stroke. CT and MRI show bulging of the interatrial septum into the atria, measuring greater than 1.5 cm, more commonly into the right atrium.

■ PROBLEM SOLVING: DISTINGUISHING ATRIAL MASSES

The questions that need to be answered in the evaluation of atrial masses are the following:

1. Is there is a mass?
2. Is it a normal variant or a real mass?
3. Is it nonneoplastic or neoplastic?
4. If neoplastic, is it benign or malignant?
5. Can you narrow the differential diagnosis?

Atrial masses should be distinguished from normal variants. Masses can be nonneoplastic or neoplastic, which can be benign or malignant. Normal variants that can mimic masses include the crista terminalis, Chiari network, and the Coumadin ridge. The crista terminalis is a muscular ridge seen in the posterolateral aspect of the

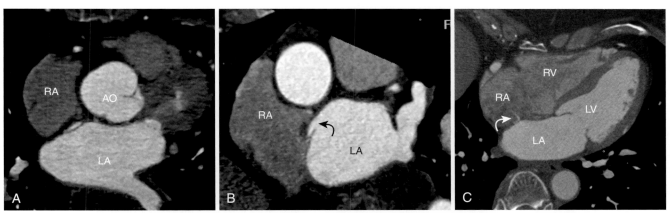

Figure 40-8 Patent foramen ovale. Four-chamber (**A**) and coronal reconstruction (**B**) computed tomographic (CT) images in a 64-year-old woman show a flaplike appearance in the region of fossa ovalis *(arrow)*, consistent with a patent foramen ovale (PFO). **C,** Four-chamber CT image in another patient shows a small PFO with a small jet of contrast *(arrow)* extending from the left atrium (LA) to the right atrium (RA). *AO,* Aorta; *LV,* left ventricle; *RV,* right ventricle.

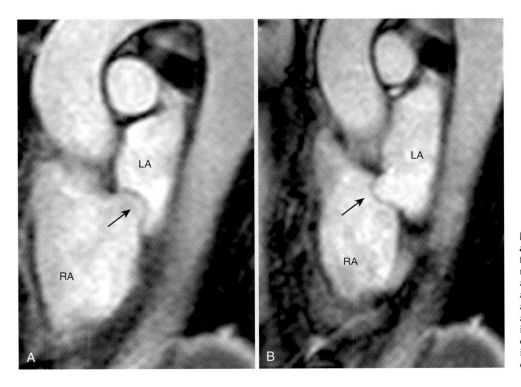

Figure 40-9 Interatrial septal aneurysm. Sagittal steady-state free precession (SSFP) magnetic resonance (MR) image of the interatrial septum shows bulging of the atrial septum *(arrow)* into the left atrium (LA) during diastole (**A**) and into the right atrium (RA) during systole (**B**). The combined total excursion of the interatrial septum in systole and diastole is 15 mm, consistent with a septal aneurysm.

right atrium (Fig. 40-10, *A*), extending from the SVC to the IVC orifice. It has a broad nodular appearance, with signal intensity similar to that of the myocardium. A prominent eustachian valve may be seen at the junction of the IVC with the right atrium (Fig. 40-10, *B*). The Chiari network is a remnant of the eustachian valve, is more mobile and fenestrated than the eustachian valve, and extends from the inferior aspect of the crista terminalis to the base of the interatrial septum. It has signal intensity similar to the myocardium. The Coumadin ridge ("Q-tip sign") is an embryologic remnant of the left atrium. It is seen in MRI as a ridge of smooth muscle with a bulbous tip that separates the left atrial appendage from the left superior pulmonary vein. In the normal atrial septum, fat is seen but is less than 10 mm in thickness and is more prominent in the anteromedial part anterior to the fossa ovalis than the posterior portion. There is no fat in the fossa ovalis, and this should not be interpreted as a septal defect.

Nonneoplastic atrial masses include lipomatous hypertrophy and thrombus. In lipomatous hypertrophy the interatrial septum is thickened with excessive fat deposition, measuring greater than 2 cm. It is seen in older and obese patients. On CT and MRI the septum has a dumbbell shape with signal characteristics of fat and characteristic sparing of the fossa ovalis (Fig. 40-11).

Thrombus is a common mass in the atrium, more commonly seen in the left than the right atrium. In the left atrium it is commonly seen with atrial fibrillation, mitral valvular disease, left atrial dilation, and left ventricular dysfunction. It is most commonly seen in the extreme posterior wall of the left atrium (MacCallum patch) (Fig. 40-12, *A*) and the left atrial appendage (Fig. 40-12, *B*). Left atrial thrombus is a common cause of stroke. Right atrial thrombus is commonly seen in association with indwelling catheters, particularly at the junction of the SVC and the right atrium (Fig. 40-12, *C* and *D*). Right atrial appendage thrombus is less common. On CT, thrombus is seen as a low-attenuation filling defect. A similar appearance can be seen as a result of slow flow caused by incomplete mixing of contrast and blood. However, the attenuation of thrombus (<50 Hounsfield units [HU]) is lower than that of slow flow (>70 HU).

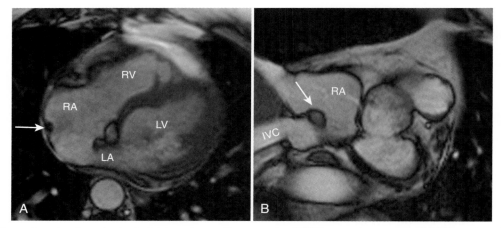

Figure 40-10 Normal anatomic variants. A, Axial steady-state free precession (SSFP) magnetic resonance (MR) image in a 54-year-old woman shows a broad-based small nodular structure with signal intensity similar to the myocardium in the right atrial wall, consistent with the crista terminalis *(arrow)*. **B,** Sagittal SSFP MR image in a 35-year-old woman shows an intermediate signal intensity structure *(arrow)* at the junction of the inferior vena cava (IVC) and the right atrium (RA), which is consistent with a prominent eustachian ridge or valve. *LA,* Left atrium; *LV,* left ventricle; *RV,* right ventricle.

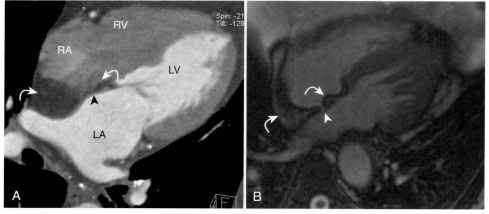

Figure 40-11 Lipomatous hypertrophy of the interatrial septum. A, Four-chamber computed tomographic image shows dumbbell-shaped fatty infiltration and thickening of the interatrial septum *(arrows)* with characteristic sparing of the fossa ovalis *(arrowhead)*. **B,** Four-chamber steady-state free precession magnetic resonance image in another patient shows the dumbbell-shaped fatty infiltration *(arrows)* and septal thickening with sparing of the fossa ovalis *(arrowhead)*. *LA,* Left atrium; *LV,* left ventricle; *RA,* right atrium; *RV,* right ventricle.

In addition, the low attenuation of thrombus is seen both in early and delayed phases, whereas slow flow is seen only in the early phase. Although there is no significant difference between the ratio of left atrial appendage attenuation to that of ascending aorta between thrombus and stasis in early phase (a ratio <0.75 has high sensitivity of prediction of either thrombosis or stasis), the ratio is lower for thrombus (0.29 ± 12) than slow flow (0.85 ± 12) in the delayed phase. Calcification may be seen in chronic thrombus. On MRI the thrombus has intermediate signal intensity on SSFP images. There is no contrast enhancement, either in the early or delayed phases, which distinguishes a thrombus from a neoplasm, which shows at least some enhancement. The low signal intensity in a thrombus persists even at high inversion times (e.g., 600 msec), unlike the normal myocardium or a solid tumor, both of which will have increasing signal intensity with higher inversion times. However, chronic thrombus may be vascularized, in which case it shows heterogeneous intermediate signal intensity and patchy areas of enhancement. Thrombus may occasionally be pedunculated, when it might be confused for a myxoma. In the left atrium, thrombus originates from the posterior wall of the left atrial appendage, is typically small, and never prolapses into the valve, whereas a myxoma originates from the fossa ovalis, is larger and polypoidal/villous, and typically prolapses into the mitral valve.

Neoplastic masses can be benign or malignant. Location, size, margin, and invasion are features that enable distinguishing benign from malignant lesions.

Benign lesions are more common in the left side; are small; have smooth, well-defined margins; and may have a pedicle. Calcification is unusual, and there is no invasion or pericardial effusion or metastasis.

Benign atrial masses include myxoma, lipoma, hemangioma, fibroelastoma, paraganglioma, rhabdomyoma, and fibroma. Myxoma is the most common benign cardiac neoplasm. Seventy-five percent of myxomas are seen in the left atrium (Fig. 40-13, A and B), and 20% are seen in the right atrium (Fig. 40-13, C and D). It is more common in the 30- to 60-year age group without any particular sex predilection. On CT myxoma is seen as a well-defined, lobulated, smooth mass that is mobile and attached by a narrow pedicle to the fossa ovalis. Calcification and hemorrhage may be seen. On MRI myxoma has a heterogeneous, intermediate signal intensity on T1-weighted and high signal intensity on T2-weighted images. A mobile myxoma may obstruct the mitral valve (see Fig. 40-13, B), and this is associated with a higher risk for embolism. Occasionally myxoma may have a broad base or frondlike appearance.

Lipoma can be seen in any age group and does not have sex predilection. It has well-defined margins and is composed of mature fat. On CT lipoma has homogenous fat attenuation (Fig. 40-14). On MRI it shows signal characteristics of fat in all the sequences, high in T1-weighted images, intermediate to high in T2-weighted images, and loses signal with fat saturation. There is no contrast enhancement. Obstruction and compressive effects are uncommon, except in very large lipomas.

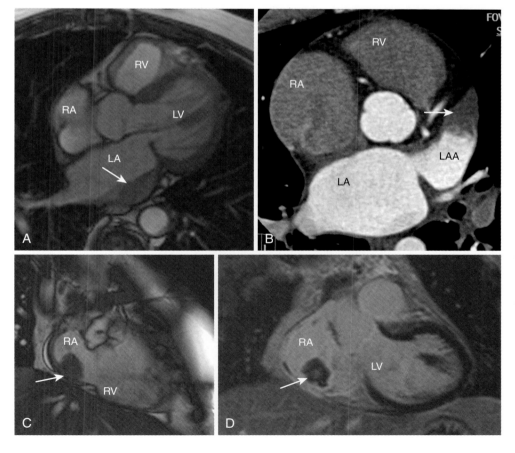

Figure 40-12 Thrombus. A Four-chamber steady-state free precession (SSFP) magnetic resonance (MR) image shows a layered thrombus *(arrow)* in the posterior wall of the left atrium (LA). **B,** Four-chamber computed tomographic image in a 38-year-old woman shows a hypodense thrombus within the left atrial appendage (LAA; *arrow*). **C,** Coronal SSFP MR image in a 53-year-old woman shows an isointense thrombus *(arrow)* attached to the free wall of the right atrium (RA). **D,** Delayed enhancement inversion recovery image in the same patient following gadolinium administration shows no enhancement of the hypointense thrombus *(arrow)*. LV, Left ventricle; RV, right ventricle.

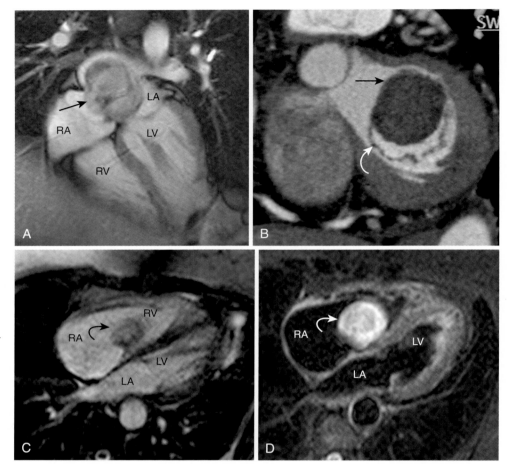

Figure 40-13 Myxoma. **A,** Four-chamber steady-state free precession (SSFP) magnetic resonance (MR) image in a 37-year-old woman shows a large, lobulated intermediate signal intensity mass *(arrow)* attached to the interatrial septum by a stalk. **B,** Short-axis computed tomographic (CT) image in a 65-year-old woman shows a myxoma *(straight arrow)* originating from the mitral valve *(curved arrow)* and protruding through the valve apparatus. **C,** Four-chamber SSFP MR image in a 42-year-old man showing a pedunculated mass *(arrow)* attached to the right side of the interatrial septum, prolapsing into the tricuspid valve. **D,** Four-chamber short tau inversion recovery MR image in the same patient as **C** shows the pedunculated mass having high T2-weighted signal *(arrow)*. This is a case of right atrial myxoma. *LA,* Left atrium; *LV,* left ventricle; *RA,* right atrium; *RV,* right ventricle.

Hemangioma is a vascular tumor composed of dilated vascular channels. It can be seen at any age and is more common in females. On CT it is seen as a well-marginated mass with heterogeneous attenuation, with areas of fat signal. On MRI it has heterogeneous intermediate to high signal on T1-weighted images because of slow flow and high signal intensity on T2-weighted images. Contrast enhancement depends on the flow, with low or no enhancement in low-flow lesions, but heterogeneously intense enhancement in high-flow lesions.

Paraganglioma is a benign tumor originating from the chromaffin cells of the parasympathetic ganglia. It is seen in young adults, in their 30s and 40s, and is more common in females. It is more commonly seen in the roof of the left atrium and in the interatrial septum. On CT a well-defined, smooth mass with heterogeneous attenuation is seen. On MRI flow voids may be seen in T1-weighted spin echo images because of the high vascularity of the lesion (Fig. 40-15, *A*). High signal intensity is seen in T2-weighted images (Fig. 40-15, *B*). Intense contrast enhancement is seen in both CT and MRI.

Fibroelastoma is a benign tumor that is seen in middle and older age, with no sex predilection. It is composed of papillary fronds of connective tissue. It is typically seen on the cardiac valves and occasionally arises from endocardial surface. Twenty-five percent of fibroelastomas originate from the mitral valve and may protrude into the left atrium. Fibroelastomas are

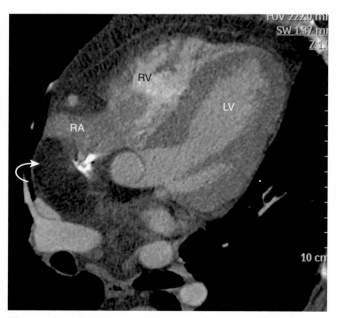

Figure 40-14 Lipoma. Axial computed tomographic image of a 68-year-old man shows a well-defined fatty mass *(arrow)* with mean attenuation of −110 Hounsfield units in the right atrium (RA). There is no soft tissue component in the mass, and this is consistent with a lipoma. *LV,* Left ventricle.

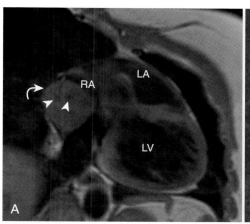

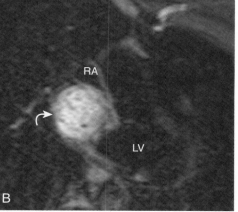

Figure 40-15 Paraganglioma. **A,** Coronal oblique T2-weighted black-blood image in a 37-year-old woman shows a well-defined mass with intermediate signal intensity *(arrow)* and small flow voids *(arrowheads)* in the right interatrial groove compressing the right atrium (RA). **B,** Coronal oblique short tau inversion recovery image in the same patient shows intense high signal within the mass. Biopsy results showed that this was a paraganglioma. *RA,* Right atrium; *LV,* left ventricle.

usually small (1 to 2 cm), homogeneous, and pedunculated. Thrombus may be seen on the surface of the neoplasm.

Malignant lesions are more common in the right atrium; they are usually large and may even fill the chamber; they tend to be lobulated with ill-defined margins and broad based; calcification is frequently seen; and invasion of myocardium, pericardium, or extracardiac structures may be present. Pericardial effusion and metastasis may be seen. Direct extension of tumors may occur into the left atrium from lung cancer or the right atrium from hepatocellular or renal carcinoma through the IVC (Fig. 40-16). Metastasis is the most common malignant tumor to involve the atria. Melanoma, sarcoma, and cancers of the lung, breast, esophagus, and kidney spread to the heart. Spread can be direct from adjacent structures, hematogenous, transvenous, or lymphatic. On CT and MRI metastasis is seen either as nodules or focal masses. Pericardial effusion, thickening, and invasion of adjacent structures are seen. Lymphomatous involvement of the heart is more often secondary than primary and is often of highly aggressive non-Hodgkin B-cell type. It is more common in the right atrium, pericardium, subepicardial fat, and atrioventricular groove. It can be a large focal mass, diffusely infiltrative, or multiple nodules. Pericardial effusion may be the only finding. Heterogeneous contrast enhancement and mediastinal adenopathy may be seen.

Sarcoma is the most common primary malignancy to involve the atria. Angiosarcoma, rhabdomyosarcoma, undifferentiated sarcoma, leiomyosarcoma, osteosarcoma, liposarcoma, and malignant fibrous histiocytoma are the sarcomas that affect the heart. Angiosarcoma is the most common sarcoma of the heart. It is most commonly seen in the right atrium. It is more common between 20 and 50 years and in women. On CT and MRI it is seen as a focal, irregular, nodular, and broad-based mass in the right atrium (Fig. 40-17). Heterogeneous enhancement may be seen because of hemorrhage and necrosis. Pericardial infiltration and invasion of surrounding structures is seen. Undifferentiated sarcoma is a sarcoma with no specific pathology. It is more common in the fourth and fifth decade. It is more common in the left atrium.

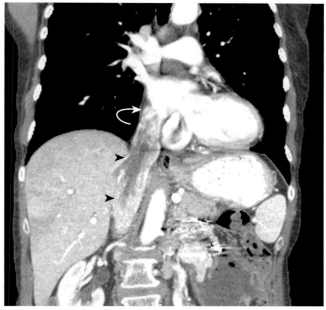

Figure 40-16 Direct extension of tumor. Coronal CT image in a 52-year-old-man shows extension of left renal cancer through the renal vein into the inferior vena cava *(arrowheads)* and the right atrium *(arrow).*

On CT and MRI it is seen as a focal, discrete mass or irregular infiltration. Spindle cell sarcoma is a type of undifferentiated sarcoma (Fig. 40-18). Rhabdomyosarcoma is seen in any age group and has no sex predilection. It is the commonest primary malignant tumor of childhood. Leiomyosarcoma is most common in the left atrium. Osteosarcoma is a rare tumor, also common in the left atrium. It has a broad base with irregular margins and has heterogeneous attenuation with areas of calcification (Fig. 40-19). Heterogeneous contrast enhancement is seen. Invasion of adjacent structures and distal metastasis may be present. Liposarcoma presents as heterogeneous mass with areas of fat and soft tissue attenuation that may show infiltration of heart and adjacent structures. Mild contrast enhancement may be observed. Malignant fibrous histiocytoma is composed of malignant mesenchymal and fibroblastic cells. It is more common in the posterior wall of the left atrium and may extend to the

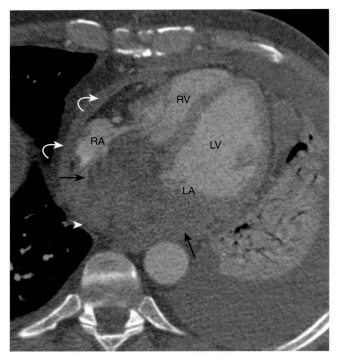

Figure 40-17 Angiosarcoma. Axial computed tomographic scan in a 46-year-old woman shows an irregular mass in the right atrium *(black arrows)*, extending to the left atrium. The mass is also seen extending outside the heart *(arrowhead)*, with associated pericardial infiltration and pericardial effusion *(curved arrow)*. There is left pleural effusion and underlying atelectasis.

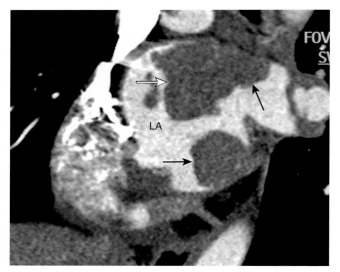

Figure 40-18 Spindle cell sarcoma. Coronal reconstructed computed tomographic image of a 43-year-old woman shows multiple heterogeneous, irregular masses *(arrows)* in the left atrium (LA), with infiltration of the wall, indicating a malignant lesion. Biopsy results showed spindle cell sarcoma.

pulmonary veins. Imaging findings are nonspecific. Fibrosarcoma and myxosarcoma are less common.

Extrinsic compression of the atria can be seen as a result of lesions in the mediastinum, such as hiatal hernia (Fig. 40-20), aneurysm, and solid and cystic tumors.

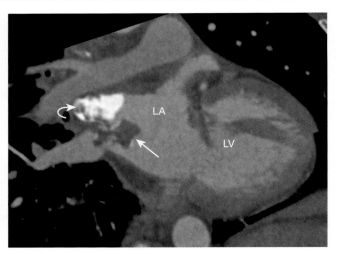

Figure 40-19 Osteosarcoma Coronal oblique reconstructed computed tomographic image shows a heterogeneous mass in the left atrium (LA), containing areas of soft tissue *(straight arrow)* and calcification *(curved arrow)*, with extension into the right superior pulmonary vein. Biopsy results showed that this was an osteosarcoma. *LV*, Left ventricle.

■ MISCELLANEOUS CONDITIONS

Amyloidosis is an infiltrative disorder with deposition of beta pleated sheet fibrillar proteins. Cardiac amyloidosis is characterized by diffuse myocardial thickening with restrictive cardiomyopathy. There is also thickening of the atrial walls and interatrial septum (Fig. 40-21, A). There is diffuse enhancement of the myocardium, which involves only the subendocardial layer in the early stages but progresses to involve the entire myocardial thickness (transmural) in advanced stages. There is also enhancement of the atria and interatrial septum (Fig. 40-21, B). Extensive scarring of the atria is also seen in chronic atrial fibrillation. Areas of scarring are seen in patients who undergo radiofrequency ablation of pulmonary venous ostia.

Fistulas may be seen opening into the atria. Coronary artery, aorta, and pulmonary artery may open into the right (Fig. 40-22) or left atrium. Rarely fistula may be seen between mediastinal arteries or the internal mammary arteries and the left atrium. Mediastinal malformation rarely drains into the left atrium.

■ ABNORMALITIES OF THE ATRIAL APPENDAGE

The atrial appendage is the most common location of thrombus formation in the left atrium (90% of all left atrial thrombi), usually secondary to stasis resulting from atrial fibrillation. Thrombus in the left atrial appendage accounts for 25% of all strokes, and the resulting strokes are usually more lethal and disabling than those with other causes. Thrombus is less common in the right atrial appendage than in the left atrial appendage. Aneurysm has been reported in the left atrial appendage, caused by congenital dysplasia of the pectinate muscles and the left atrial muscle bundles related to them. This may be associated with cerebral thromboembolism and arrhythmia. The tumors described earlier can involve the atrial appendages.

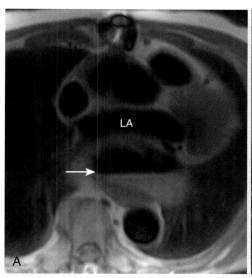

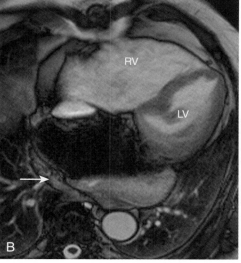

Figure 40-20 Extrinsic compression. Axial steady-state free precession (**A**) and T2-weighted black-blood magnetic resonance images (**B**) in a 47-year-old man with suspected left atrial mass in echocardiography show a large gas-filled hiatal hernia (*arrow*) in the posterior mediastinum, which is causing extrinsic compression of the atria, particularly the left atrium (LA). *LV,* Left ventricle; *RA,* right atrium; *RV,* right ventricle.

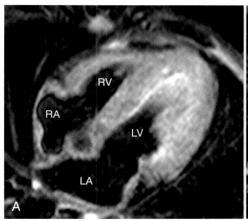

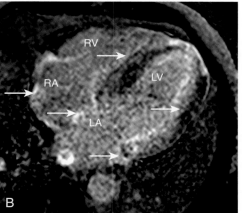

Figure 40-21 Amyloidosis. A, Four-chamber short tau inversion recovery magnetic resonance (MR) image shows moderate thickening of the atrial walls, interatrial septum, and myocardium, indicating an infiltrative process. **B,** Four-chamber delayed enhancement inversion recovery MR image of the same patient shows subendocardial enhancement of the atrial walls, interatrial septum, and the ventricles (*arrows*), consistent with cardiac amyloidosis. *LA,* Left atrium; *LV,* left ventricle; *RA,* right atrium; *RV,* right ventricle.

■ SURGERIES AND INTERVENTIONS

Atrial anatomy and function are altered following surgical and interventional procedures.

Atrial switch procedure was performed in patients with D-transposition of great arteries. Baffles were used to divert the systemic venous return into the right atrium, and the pulmonary venous return was diverted into the left atrium. Serial circulation is thus established, because in these patients the left ventricle opens into the pulmonary artery and the right ventricle into the aorta. There are two types of atrial switch techniques, the Mustard procedure in which a pericardial patch is used (Fig. 40-23, *A*) and the Senning procedure, in which native atrial tissue is used for baffle (Fig. 40-23, *B*). Atrial septal defects can be closed percutaneously or surgically with occluder devices that have a central waist to close the defect and two disks for fixation. CT can be used before the procedure to determine if the patient is suitable and following the procedure to detect complications such as perforation, device erosion, or device migration.

As discussed earlier, atrial fibrillation can be treated with radiofrequency ablation of the pulmonary venous ostia. CT or MRI is used for determining the pulmonary

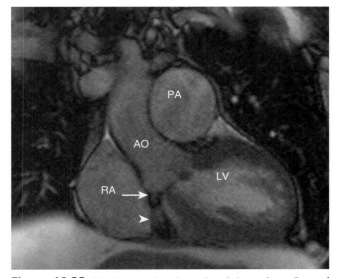

Figure 40-22 Fistula opening into the right atrium. Coronal steady-state free precession magnetic resonance image in a 47-year-old man with recent history of aortic valve replacement shows a communication between the aortic root and the right atrium (*arrow*) with a dark jet extending into the right atrium (*arrowhead*), consistent with a fistulous communication.

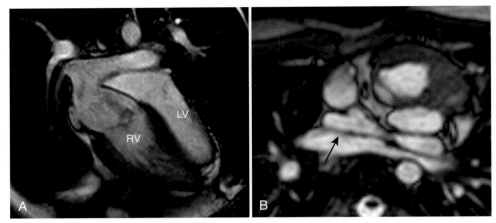

Figure 40-23 Atrial switch procedures. A, Four-chamber steady-state free precession (SSFP) magnetic resonance image in a patient who underwent the Mustard procedure for D-transposition of great arteries shows the pulmonary vein baffled to the right atrium, which opens into the right ventricle (RV), which gives origin to the aorta (not shown here). The right ventricle is hypertrophied because it is supplying the high-resistance systemic circulation. The systemic flow to the right atrium has been diverted through a baffle into the left atrium, which then opens into the left ventricle (LV), which gives origin to the pulmonary artery. As a result of these baffles the blood flow becomes a serial circuit. **B,** Four-chamber SSFP image in another patient who underwent the Senning procedure for D-transposition of great arteries shows the atrial baffle (*arrow*), which diverts blood from the pulmonary veins to the right heart and blood from the superior vena cava and the inferior vena cava to the left heart.

venous anatomy and variations, left atrial size, left atrial thrombus, and position of the esophagus in relation to the left atrium. CT or MRI is also used following the procedure to evaluate complications such as pulmonary venous stenosis, left atrial thromboembolism, or esophageal fistulas. MRI is increasingly used to evaluate the adequacy of ablation using delayed enhancement technique, in which a circumferential scar about the pulmonary venous ostia indicates good ablation.

The left atrial appendage may be excised or excluded by sutures or staples to reduce the incidence of thromboemboli, which is a risk factor for stroke. Following left atrial appendage closure, stump measurement of more than 10 mm or persistent flow into the appendage indicates failure of the closure procedure. Partial anomalous pulmonary veins can be reimplanted into the left atrial appendage when a significant shunt is present. In the classic Fontan procedure the right atrium is anastomosed to the pulmonary artery. This is performed in patients with single ventricle physiology, particularly in patients with tricuspid atresia.

■ CONCLUSION

CT and MRI are very useful imaging tools in the evaluation of a variety of congenital and acquired abnormalities involving the pulmonary veins, atria, and appendages. Imaging is often required for evaluation of form and structure before cardiovascular surgeries or interventions and following these procedures for the assessment of complications.

Bibliography

Al-Saady NM, Obel OA, Camm AJ. Left atrial appendage: structure, function, and role in thromboembolism. *Heart.* 1999;82:547-554.

Choi SII, Seo JB, Choi SH, Lee SH, Do KH, Ko SM, et-al. Variation of the size of pulmonary venous ostia during the cardiac cycle: optimal reconstruction window at ECG gated multidetector row CT. *Eur Radiol.* 205;15:1441–1445.

Ho ML, Bhalla S, Bierhals A, Gutierrez F. MDCT of partial anomalous pulmonary venous return in adults. *J Thorac Imaging.* 2009;24:89-95.

Hoey ET, Gopalan D, Ganesh V, Agarwal SK, Screaton NJ. Atrial septal defects: magnetic resonance imaging and computed tomographic appearances. *J Med Imaging Radiat Oncol.* 2009;53:261-270.

Johnson DW, Ganjoo AK, Stone CD, Srivyas RC, Howard M. The left atrial appendage; our most lethal human attachment; surgical implications. *Eur J Cardiothorac Surg.* 2000;17:718-722.

Kim YJ, Hur J, Shim CY, Lee HJ, Ha JW, Choe KO, et al. Patent foramen ovale: diagnosis with multidetector CT—comparison with transesophageal echocardiography. *Radiology.* 2009;250:61-67.

Ko SF, Liang CD, Yip HK, Huang CC, Ng SG, Huang CF, et al. Amplatzer septal occluder closure of the atrial septal defect: evaluation of transthoracic echocardiography, cardiac CT, transesophageal echocardiography. *AJR Am J Roentgenol.* 2009;193:1522-1529.

Kroft LJ, de Roos A. MRI diagnosis of giant right atrial aneurysm. *AJR Am J Roentgenol.* 2007;189:W94-W95.

Lacomis JM, Wigginton W, Fuhrman C, Shwartzman D, Armfield DR, Pealer KM. Multi-detector row CT of the left atrium and pulmonary veins before radio-frequency catheter ablation for atrial fibrillation. *Radiographics.* 2003;23:S35-S50.

Mas JL, Arquizan C, Lamy C, et al. Patent foramen ovale and atrial septal aneurysm study group: Recurrent cerebrovascular events associated with patent foramen ovale, atrial septal aneurysm, or both. *N Engl J Med.* 2001;345:1740-1746.

Messe SR, Silverman ID, Kizer J, Homma S, Zahn C, Gronseth G, et al. Practice parameter: recurrent stroke with patent foramen ovale and atrial septal aneurysm: report of the Quality Standards Subcommittee of the American Academy of Neurology. *Neurology.* 2004;62:1042-1050.

Mulder BJ, van der Wall EE. Size and function of the atria. *Int J Cardiovasc Imaging.* 2008;24:713-716.

O'Donnell DH, Abbara S, Chaithirraphan V, Yared K, Killeen RP, Cury RC, et al. Cardiac tumors: optimal cardiac MR sequences and spectrum of imaging appearances. *AJR Am J Roentgenol.* 2009;193:377-387.

Patel A, Au E, Donegan K, Kim RJ, Lin FY, Stein KM, et al. Multi-detector row computed tomography for identification of left atrial appendage filling defects in patients undergoing pulmonary vein isolation for treatment of atrial fibrillation: comparison with transesophageal echocardiography. *Heart Rhythm.* 2008;5:253-260.

Rajiah P, Kanne JP. Computed tomography of septal defects. *J Cardiovasc Comput Tomogr.* 2010;4:231-245.

Rajiah P, Kanne JP, Kalahasti V, Schoenhagen P. Computed tomography of cardiac and pericardiac masses. *J Cardiovasc Comput Tomogr.* 2011;5:16-29.

Sparrow PJ, Kurian JB, Jones TR, Sivanathan MU. MR imaging of cardiac tumors. *Radiographics.* 2005:1255-1276.

Victor S, Nayak VM. Aneurysm of the left atrial appendage. *Tex Heart Inst J.* 2001;28(2):111-118.

CHAPTER 41

Septal Defects and Other Cardiovascular Shunts

Carlos Andres Rojas

The typical challenges a radiologist confront when evaluating a patient with a shunt are to decide the location, type, and size of the defect, as well as rim size and associated anomalies, and to detect signs of right ventricular flow and pressure overload. These questions can be answered for the most part with echocardiography. The use of magnetic resonance imaging (MRI) and computed tomography (CT) is growing in these patients because of the excellent anatomic depiction with these techniques and the reliable quantification of the shunt with MRI.

Physiologic and morphologic separation between the systemic (arterial) and pulmonary (venous) circulation is essential for the normal function of the cardiovascular system. Abnormal communication between these two systems results in shunting of blood from the high-pressure system (arterial) to the low-pressure system (venous), thereby creating a left-to-right shunt. The direction and magnitude of shunting are determined by the size of the defect and the relative compliance of the ventricles. Small defects are associated with a small shunt volume and no hemodynamic sequelae. Conversely, large defects may be associated with a large shunt volume that causes right ventricular volume overload and heart failure. Communications between the venous and arterial systems can happen at the level of the heart, in the setting of atrial septal defects (ASDs) and ventricular septal defects (VSDs) (Fig. 41-1), or at the level of the great vessels, as in the setting of a patent ductus arteriosus (PDA). Certain vascular malformations (abnormal pulmonary venous return, pulmonary arteriovenous malformations, and vein of Galen aneurysm) or vascular tumors (infantile hemangioendothelioma) can also result in similar physiologic features, although these lesions are beyond the scope of this chapter.

Shunts can be congenital (PDA, ASDs, patent foramen ovale [PFO], VSDs) or acquired (traumatic, infectious, or infarct-related VSDs). Their long-term effects relate to their size and amount of blood shunted per cardiac cycle. In cases of significant shunting (ratio of pulmonary flow [Qp] to systemic flow [Qs]) >1.5), overload of the right-side or venous system can result in increased right-sided pressures and ultimately in right-sided heart failure.

Intracardiac shunts can result from deficient morphogenesis of the cardiac septa (congenital ASDs and VSDs) or injury to the cardiac septa (myocardial infarction, trauma, or iatrogenic causes), or they can be secondary to persistence of fetal communications.

Shunting between the pulmonary and systemic circulation is necessary during fetal life to provide oxygen-rich blood from the venous system (which brings oxygen-rich maternal blood to the fetus through the umbilical veins) into the arterial system, thus bypassing the high-pressure prenatal pulmonary circulation. Persistence of fetal circulation (foramen ovale and ductus arteriosus) beyond the first months of life can result in pathologic left-to-right shunting.

Small shunts may go undetected for many years and may manifest as incidental findings on physical examination or imaging studies. Patients with larger defects can present with fatigue or dyspnea on exertion. On chest radiography, the finding of enlargement of the right-side chamber and pulmonary arteries with prominent peripheral pulmonary branches and distended veins is consistent with shunt vascularity suggestive of intracardiac shunts. Transthoracic echocardiography (TTE) is the initial diagnostic examination in the evaluation of intracardiac shunts given its widespread availability and high sensitivity. Transesophageal echocardiography (TEE) is reserved for guidance during placement of closure devices, given its invasiveness. MRI is a great tool for evaluating morphology and potentially associated anomalies and for quantification of shunts. CT imaging is an excellent tool in the morphologic analysis of cardiac shunts and their associated anomalies in patients in whom echocardiography is limited or MRI is contraindicated.

■ DEFINITION OF THE INTERATRIAL SEPTUM

The definition of the interatrial septum is controversial and varies in the literature from the classic definition of a partition separating the upper chambers of the heart (atria) to the more accurate revised definition of a structure that divides the right and left atria that can be removed without exiting from the cardiac chambers. The cardiac imager, and particularly the interventional cardiologist and cardiac surgeon, must understand this concept because percutaneous or surgical treatments of pathologic conditions performed outside the "true" interatrial septum result in extension outside the cardiac chambers. From this perspective, the true atrial septum

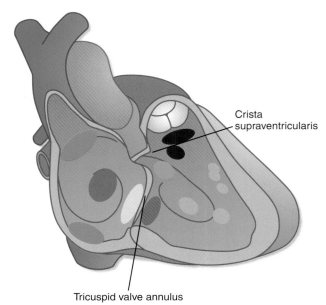

Crista
supraventricularis

Tricuspid valve annulus

Figure 41-1 Schematic diagram depicting the various types of atrial septal defect (ASD) and ventricular septal defect (VSD): ostium primum ASD *(yellow)*, ostium secundum ASD *(red)*, sinus venosus ASD *(blue)*, membranous VSD *(green)*, supracristal VSD *(black)*, muscular VSD *(orange)*, and inlet VSD *(purple)*.

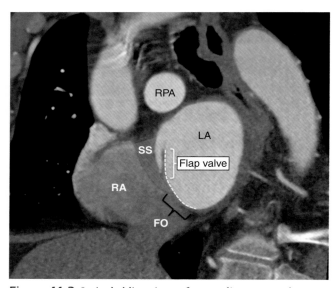

Figure 41-2 Sagittal oblique image from cardiac computed tomography in a 66-year-old man with lipomatous hypertrophy of the interatrial septum. The excess accumulation of fat in the septum secundum (SS; *orange*) helps delineate the anatomy of the interatrial septum. Fossa ovalis (FO), septum primum *(dashed line)*, and flap valve *(dotted line)*. *LA*, Left atrium; *RA*, right atrium; *RPA*, right pulmonary artery.

is exclusively made up of the flap valve of the fossa ovale (septum primum) and part of its bulbous anteroinferior base. The superior, posterior, and anterior rim of the fossa ovale, commonly referred to as the septum secundum, is the infolded wall between the superior vena cava (SVC) and the right pulmonary veins and is not considered part of the true interatrial septum as is commonly described (Fig. 41-2).

DEVELOPMENT OF THE INTERATRIAL SEPTUM

During early fetal life, a common atrium divides into right and left atria by the development of two overlapping structures, the septum primum and septum secundum, as depicted in Figure 41-3.

PATENT FORAMEN OVALE

The foramen ovale is a normal communication between the right and left atrium during fetal development. A PFO results from failure of fusion between the septum primum (which forms a flaplike valve over the fossa ovale) and the septum secundum. PFOs are common, occurring in up to one third of the population. This condition is not considered a true ASD, but rather a potential communication between the two atria, given the lack of structural deficiency of the atrial septum. Atrial shunting through a PFO has been associated with cryptogenic stroke, arterial hypoxemia, migraine headaches, and decompression illness. A PFO, which is probe patent, can exist with or without detectable shunting. Shunting through a PFO can be bidirectional (Fig. 41-4). Under normal physiologic conditions, the slightly higher pressures in the left atrium translate into a left-to-right shunt. During coughing, Valsalva maneuver, or pathologic conditions with increased right-sided pressures, a right-to-left shunt can result.

Treatment of PFO is controversial. Some groups prefer a conservative approach with anticoagulation, whereas others use closure devices.

ATRIAL SEPTAL DEFECTS

The different types of ASDs can be characterized by imaging techniques such as echocardiography, conventional angiography, cardiac CT, and MRI. Information regarding the morphology of these defects, their associations, and physiologic significance is needed to determine the most appropriate treatment. To understand the morphology of the different types of ASDs, the examiner must review the embryology. As with many other developmental defects, ASDs comprise a spectrum of disease with widely ranging morphologic and physiologic presentations. Before surgical correction of ASDs, morphologic assessment is needed to determine the presence of single versus multiple defects, shape, size, rim size, and associated anomalies.

Types of Defects and Imaging Appearances

ASDs are morphologic abnormalities that result in shunting at the level of the cardiac atria. The four types of ASDs can be classified as defects resulting from abnormal development of the atrial septum (ostium primum and ostium secundum [OS]) and as defects resulting in interatrial communication with normally developed atrial septum (sinus venosus and coronary sinus subtypes).

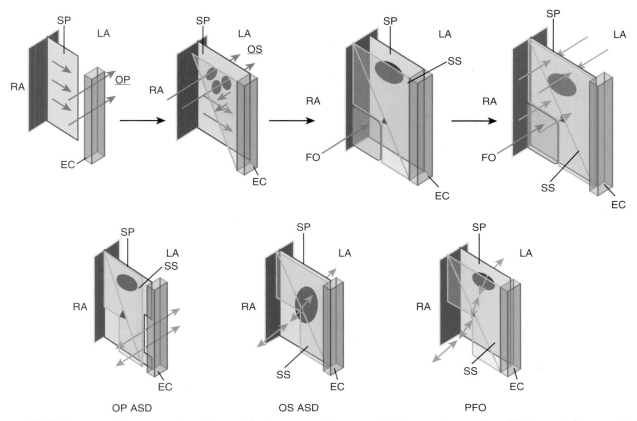

OP ASD

OS ASD

PFO

Figure 41-3 Diagrammatic representation of normal development and common developmental anomalies of the interatrial septum. Beginning at the fifth week of gestation, the septum primum (SP) begins to develop growing toward the endocardial cushions (EC). The gap between the EC and SP is known as the ostium primum (OP) *(green arrows)*. Postnatal persistence of this gap is known as an OP atrial septal defect (ASD). Before the SP fuses with the EC, fenestrations develop in the cephalic portion of the SP that create a window called ostium secundum (OS). Meanwhile, the septum secundum (SS) begins to form as an infolding of the ventrocranial atrial wall, to the right of the SP. While the SS continues its caudal descent overlapping the OS, the OS fenestrations coalesce to form a larger fenestration. The lack of overlap of the SS over the OS results in an OS ASD. The SS stops its growth, thus leaving a small gap known as fossa ovale (FO). Eventually, in most of the population within the first 2 years of life, the SS fuses *(blue arrows)* with the SP to create a physiologic and morphologic separation between the two atria. The lack of fusion between the SS and SP results in a patent foramen ovale (PFO). *LA,* Left atrium; *RA,* right atrium.

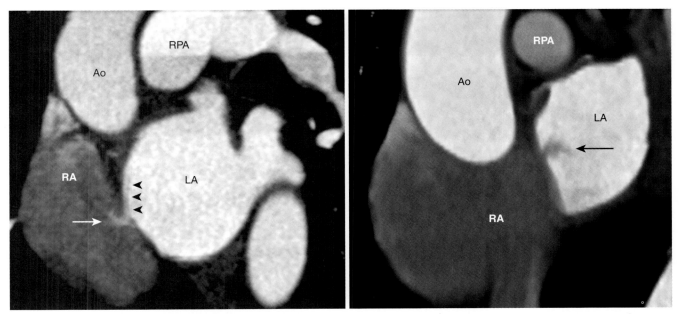

Figure 41-4 *Left,* Sagittal oblique image from cardiac computed tomography (CT) in a 45-year-old man with atypical chest pain incidentally demonstrates a high-density jet of contrast material extending from the left atrium (LA) to the right atrium (RA) consistent with a patent foramen ovale (PFO). *Right,* Sagittal oblique image from cardiac CT in a 53-year-old man with chest pain incidentally demonstrates a low-density jet extending from the RA into the LA consistent with a PFO. *Ao,* Aorta; *RPA,* right pulmonary artery.

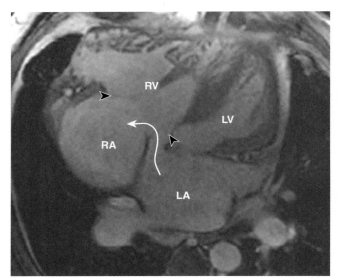

Figure 41-5 Four-chamber balanced steady-state free precession image from a 29-year-old man with a known ostium primum atrial septal defect *(curved arrow)*. Note the location of the defect, immediately posterior to the insertion site of the tricuspid valve leaflets *(arrowheads)*. Also note the secondary right ventricular enlargement. *LA,* Left atrium; *LV,* left ventricle; *RA,* right atrium; *RV,* right ventricle.

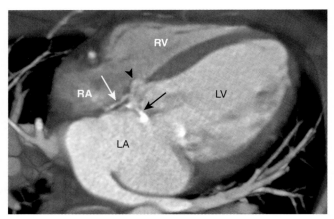

Figure 41-6 Four-chamber view from cardiac computed tomography in a 39-year-old man with a history of endocardial cushion defect after surgical repair. Note the patch repair of the ostium primum atrial septal defect *(white arrow)*, postsurgical calcifications along the anterior leaflet of the mitral valve *(black arrow)*, and a small membranous septal aneurysm *(arrowhead)*. *LA,* Left atrium; *LV,* left ventricle; *RA,* right atrium; *RV,* right ventricle.

Ostium primum ASDs correspond to 2% to 3% of all ASDs. These defects are considered the mildest form of atrioventricular septal defects (AVSDs) or endocardial cushion defects (ECDs). During normal embryology, the endocardial cushions contribute to the development of the medial portions of the mitral and tricuspid valves, the portion of the atrial septum adjacent to the atrioventricular valves and the inlet portion of the ventricular septum. When the defect results from failure of fusion between the free edge of the septum primum and the atrioventricular cushions, it is termed ostium primum ASD (Fig. 41-5). If the defect associates with abnormal development of the atrioventricular valves or ventricular septum, it is known as an AVSD or ECD (Fig. 41-6). Because ostium primum ASDs occur secondary to the lack of fusion between the septum primum and the endocardial cushions, they are seen as interatrial communications located immediately posterior to the mitral valve annulus.

On electrocardiogram (ECG)–gated multidetector CT (MDCT) images after contrast with saline chaser, ostium primum ASDs can be seen as an abnormal communication between the right and left atria located immediately posterior to the mitral valve annulus. Depending on the size of the defect, relative equalization of contrast density in the right and left chambers can be seen. Associated enlargement of the right-sided chambers is usually present.

OS-type ASDs are the most common, accounting for 80% to 90% of ASDs. These defects are centered in the fossa ovalis of the interatrial septum. They result from excessive apoptosis of the cephalic portion of the septum primum (a large OS) or incomplete development of the septum secundum (Fig. 41-7).

OS ASDs can be seen as defects of variable size in the region of the fossa ovalis. Differentiating a small OS

ASD from a PFO can sometimes be difficult. Important imaging findings that can help in the diagnosis are the horizontally oriented flow in OS ASDs compared with the cephalad or caudal direction of flow in patients with PFO. The tunnel appearance of the PFO can also help in the diagnosis, whereas OS ASDs are seen as a hole in the interatrial septum.

Sinus venosus ASDs are defects located between the venous inflow of either the SVC or the inferior vena cava (IVC) and the left atrium. The superior sinus venosus ASD accounts for 2% to 3% of all interatrial communications. It is located at the superior cavoatrial junction and is frequently associated with anomalous drainage of the right-sided pulmonary veins into the SVC (Fig. 41-8). Contrast-enhanced MDCT images can demonstrate concentrated contrast material accumulating in the posterior wall of the left atrium resulting from the abnormal communication between the SVC-right atrial junction and the left atrium consistent with the "fallen contrast sign."

An inferior sinus venosus ASD is located at the junction of the IVC and right atrium and may involve unroofing of the coronary sinus. This subtype may be associated with anomalous drainage of a right inferior pulmonary vein to the intrapericardial segment of the IVC or right atrium (Fig. 41-9).

Unroofed coronary sinus ASDs are uncommon. They occur when septation is lacking between the back wall of the left atrium and the coronary sinus because of abnormal cell death during embryologic development; the result is abnormal drainage of venous blood into the left atrium. The unroofed portion of the coronary sinus connects to the inferior aspect of the left atrium before draining into the right atrium. Patients often have a persistent left SVC resulting from failure in degeneration of the left anterior cardinal vein. ECG-gated coronary MDCT images typically reveal low attenuation of the coronary sinus upstream from the defect and equalization with the enhanced left atrium at the level of the defect secondary to free communication between these

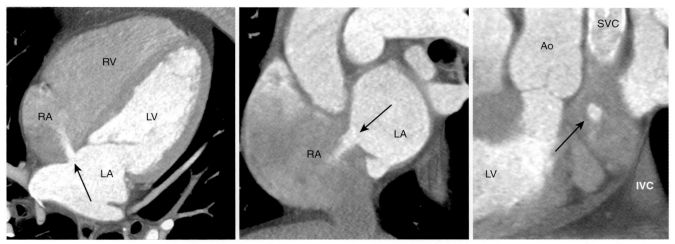

Figure 41-7 *From right to left,* Four-chamber, coronal oblique, and sagittal oblique views from cardiac computed tomography demonstrate a high attenuation jet of contrast material extending from the left atrium (LA) to the right atrium (RA) consistent with a secundum type atrial septal defect. Associated mild enlargement of the right-side chambers is visible. The secundum defect measured 9 × 7 mm with a sufficient anterosuperior rim measuring 9 mm amenable for endovascular closure. No associated anomalies were identified. *Ao,* Aorta; *IVC,* inferior vena cava; *LV,* left ventricle; *RV,* right ventricle; *SVC,* superior vena cava.

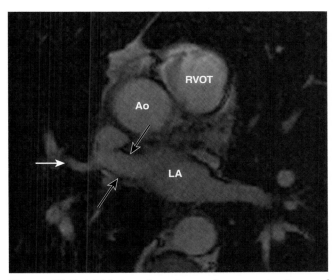

Figure 41-8 Axial balanced steady-state free precession image of the heart demonstrates a communication between the superior aspect of the left atrium (LA) and the superior vena cava–right atrial junction consistent with a superior sinus venosus defect *(outlined arrows).* Also note the presence of an abnormally draining pulmonary vein into the defect *(white arrow)* consistent with partial anomalous pulmonary venous return. *Ao,* Aorta; *LVOT,* left ventricular outflow tract.

two structures, as well as shunting of high attenuation blood downstream into the right atrium.

Imaging Techniques

Echocardiography is the primary modality for the diagnosis, morphologic assessment, and follow-up of patients with ASDs, although the role of MRI and CT continues to evolve.

Currently, CT serves as an additional tool to assess morphology and associated anomalies when echocardiography is limited. Imaging of ASDs by CT requires

appropriate intracardiac opacification. In general, contrast material is administered using a biphasic protocol consisting of an initial contrast bolus at a rate of 4 to 7 mL/second, followed by 40 to 50 mL of saline solution to flush out the contrast material from the right side of the heart. This method provides ideal opacification of the left side of the heart for the detection of left-to-right shunts. Using this same technique, right-to-left shunts can be seen as low attenuation jets entering the opacified left atrium.

Images can be acquired in a prospectively triggered or retrospectively gated fashion. Retrospectively gated acquisition uses helical scanning and thus exposes the patient to radiation during the entire cardiac cycle. Conversely, prospectively triggered acquisition obtains information during a specific point in time and significantly reduces radiation exposure. Given that intracardiac shunting in patients with ASDs commonly occurs in late diastole (70% R-R interval), prospective triggering is preferred whenever feasible (in patients with a regular, slow heart rate).

MRI is a versatile tool to assess morphologic and physiologic data of ASDs. With the use of T1-weighted or T2-weighted double inversion recovery images, balanced steady-state free precession (SSFP) imaging, and gadolinium-enhanced angiograms in the pulmonary venous and systemic arterial phases, MRI can assess for the presence of shunts or abnormalities in the pulmonary venous return. The examiner must be aware of the intrinsic limitations of MRI related to spatial resolution, such as decreased visualization of the septum primum at the fossa ovalis, which could simulate an ASD. Velocity encoded, phase sensitive contrast imaging is used to assess differences in flow volumes between the pulmonary and systemic circulations (Qp/Qs ratio). Furthermore, phase contrast imaging perpendicular to the shunt jet can also assess the volume and peak gradient across the defect. Balanced steady-state free precession (SSFP) images in the short-axis plane covering the

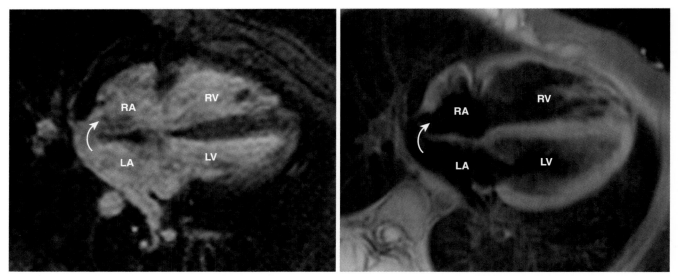

Figure 41-9 Contrast-enhanced magnetic resonance imaging and triple inversion recovery T2-weighted images in the four-chamber plane demonstrate an abnormal communication between the inferior left atrium (LA) and the inferior vena cava–right atrial junction *(curved arrow)*, consistent with an inferior sinus venosus atrial septal defect. Note minimal enlargement of the right ventricle (RV). *LV,* Left ventricle; *RA,* right atrium.

ventricles are used to determine biventricular volumes and function using the Simpson method. This method of volume quantification and stroke volume analysis allows detection of increased flow or shunting in one of the systems when the defect is located at the atrial level. On the contrary, defects at the ventricular level cannot be quantified this way because of the maintained stroke volumes in both ventricles. Furthermore, flow quantification using the Simpson method assumes the absence of valvular regurgitation, and this is another limitation.

Treatment

Management of ASDs depends on multiple factors, including the patient's symptoms and degree of shunting. Shunts with a Qp/Qs ratio greater than 1.5 are known to have an increased risk of right-sided volume and pressure overload that can result in heart failure and arrhythmias, and therefore these defects are usually closed. Symptoms of patients with shunts vary from dyspnea on exertion, arrhythmias, and heart failure to paradoxical embolism resulting in stroke, or rarely myocardial infarction.

Surgical treatment with an atrial approach and patch repair is performed for primum ASDs and unroofed coronary sinus ASDs. The type of surgical repair used for sinus venosus ASDs depends on the presence or absence of associated partial anomalous pulmonary venous return. Surgical correction of secundum ASDs is preferred in patients with associated anomalies, insufficient rim size, and large or multiple defects.

Endovascular closure of secundum ASDs can be performed with self-centered closure devices (Amplatzer Septal Occluder (AGA, Plymouth, Minn.) or the NMT CardioSEAL STARFlex Septal Occluder (NMT Medical, Boston, Mass.)). These devices are preferred over non–self-centered or pin devices, which are used for off-label closure of PFO. Self-centered devices can be recognized

on imaging by the presence of a waist between the two disks that stabilizes their position within the interatrial septum.

Not all secundum defects are amenable to endovascular closure, given their location, number of defects, defect size, and rim size. Defects larger than 36 mm are not considered amenable for endovascular repair. Moreover, a rim size greater than 3 to 4 mm in all directions (anterosuperior and aortic valve, anteroinferior and tricuspid valve, posterosuperior and SVC, and posteroinferior and IVC) is needed for successful deployment and seating of the closure device.

■ DEVELOPMENT OF THE INTERVENTRICULAR SEPTUM

The interventricular septum is formed from three separate septa: muscular, outlet, and inlet septa, as depicted in Figure 41-10.

■ VENTRICULAR SEPTAL DEFECTS

Types of Defects and Imaging Appearances

VSDs are the most common congenital abnormalities found in children. The various classifications and names for each one of the types of VSDs can make this subject a bit confusing. The four main types of VSDs are perimembranous, muscular, subarterial, and inflow.

Perimembranous VSDs are the most common type of VSDs, accounting for 75% to 80% of cases. They are also known as infracristal, subaortic, membranous, or paramembranous VSDs. They occur in the upper part of ventricular septum immediately under the crista supraventricularis and anterior to the septal leaflet of the tricuspid valve. Membranous VSDs close spontaneously in a large percentage of the population, either completely

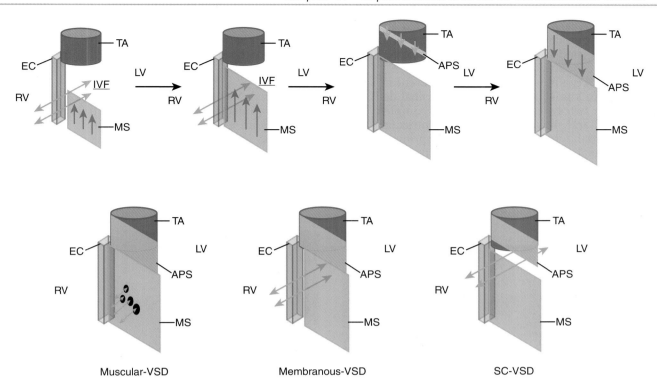

Muscular-VSD   Membranous-VSD   SC-VSD

Figure 41-10 Diagrammatic representation of normal development and common developmental anomalies of the interventricular septum. The interventricular septum is formed from three separate septa: muscular, outlet, and inlet septa. Early in embryologic development, the muscular septum (MS) grows upward from the floor of the ventricles toward the already fused endocardial cushions (EC). The gap between the edge of the muscular interventricular septum and endocardial cushion tissue is called the interventricular foramen (IVF). Defects in the fusion of the MS and EC result in membranous ventricular septal defect (VSD). Meanwhile, two spiral ridges of tissue appear on the sides of the truncus arteriosus (TA), known as the conotruncal ridges (truncoconal swellings). The conotruncal ridges grow toward each other and fuse, making a spiral-shaped septum termed the aortopulmonary septum (APS). The APS divides the TA into the pulmonary trunk and the aorta. The conotruncal ridges also grow downward into the ventricles and meet with the already fused EC and the ventricular MS. Incomplete fusion of the APS with the EC-MS septum results in supracristal VSD (SC-VSD). By the seventh to eighth week of gestation, the membranous septum is formed when the APS, EC, and MS completely fuse, thus closing off the interventricular septum. *LV,* Left ventricle; *RV,* right ventricle.

or partially, because of apposition of the septal leaflet of the tricuspid valve or by prolapse of an aortic cusp into the defect. Apposition of the septal leaflet of the tricuspid valve can produce an aneurysm of the ventricular septum with or without residual shunt (Fig. 41-11). On ECG-gated MDCT images after contrast with saline chaser, membranous defects are seen as defects in the region of the membranous septum that are bounded by both membranous and muscular septum. High attenuation contrast can be seen crossing through the defect and entering the infracristal right ventricle (Fig. 41-12).

Muscular VSDs account for 20% of VSDs. They can be single or multiple, small or large. Two thirds of these defects are located in the apical third. They are most common in children, and 75% of muscular VSDs close at age 2 years. They are seen as defects in the muscular septum; therefore, each defect is bounded by muscular tissue. On ECG-gated MDCT images after contrast with saline chaser, high attenuation contrast is noted crossing through the muscular defects into the washed-out right ventricle. Associated dilation of the right ventricle can be seen in patients with large defects. Small defects usually do not produce dilation of the right ventricle (Fig. 41-13).

Subarterial VSDs account for 5% of the VSDs. They are also known as outlet VSDs, subpulmonary, infundibular, doubly committed, or conoseptal VSDs. They are most

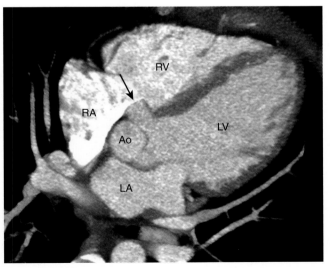

Figure 41-11 Five-chamber view from cardiac computed tomography demonstrates the presence of an interventricular septal aneurysm *(arrow),* without a residual ventricular septal defect. *Ao,* Aorta; *LA,* left atrium; *LV,* left ventricle; *RA,* right atrium; *RV,* right ventricle.

common in Asians. These defects are located above the crista supraventricularis (Fig. 41-14). Subarterial VDSs can be associated with prolapse of unsupported aortic valve and secondary aortic insufficiency.

Inflow VSDs almost exclusively are present in ECDs. They are also known as atrioventricular canal defects or AVSDs. The two types of ECDs are the complete ECD (ASD, VSD, and single common atrioventricular valve) and the partial or incomplete ECD (only primum ASD).

The normal tricuspid valve septal leaflet attachment is more apically located than the opposite mitral valve. Hence, a small segment of right atrium is opposite the left ventricle at this portion of the membranous septum. A defect in this particular portion of the membranous

septum results in a communication of the left ventricle with the right atrium, usually resulting in shunting of blood from the left ventricle into the right atrium during the entire cardiac cycle. This defect is called a Gerbode defect.

Acquired VSDs may be secondary to myocardial infarction, infective endocarditis, and trauma. VSD formation is an uncommon complication of myocardial infarction, with a reported incidence of 1% to 2%. A transmural myocardial infarction in the vascular distribution supplying the septum (left anterior descending coronary artery or PDA) can cause significant weakness of the wall that can ultimately result in myocardial

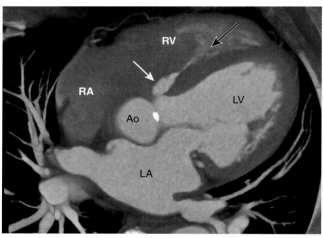

Figure 41-12 Five-chamber view of cardiac computed tomography in a 67-year-old man with a history of membranous ventricular septal defect (VSD). Note a ventricular septal aneurysm *(white arrow)* with a high attenuation jet entering the right ventricular apical region *(outlined arrow)* consistent with a partially closed membranous VSD. *Ao,* Aorta; *LA,* left atrium; *LV,* left ventricle; *RA,* right atrium; *RV,* right ventricle.

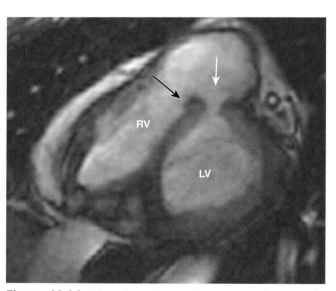

Figure 41-14 Balanced steady-state free precession image in the short-axis plane demonstrates the presence of a supracristal ventricular septal defect *(white arrow)*. Note the small muscular ridge below the defect consistent with the crista supraventricularis *(black arrow)*. *LV,* Left ventricle; *RV,* right ventricle.

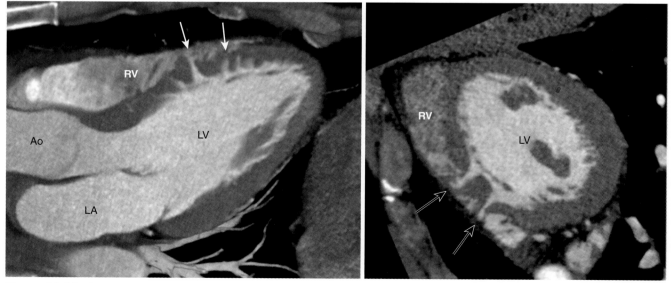

Figure 41-13 Three-chamber *(left)* and short-axis *(right)* images demonstrate multiple small muscular ventricular septal defects *(arrows)*. No right chamber enlargement is noted. *Ao,* Aorta; *LA,* left atrium; *LV,* left ventricle; *RV,* right ventricle.

rupture and the creation of a VSD. These defects are typically small and occur during the first week after a myocardial infarction. The vascular territory most commonly involved is the left anterior descending coronary artery (60%), with infarcts involving the posterior and inferior wall corresponding the other 40% of cases. Posterior inferior wall myocardial infarctions can be accompanied by injury or rupture of the posteromedial papillary muscle because of its single blood supply. Traumatic VSDs can happen in penetrating and nonpenetrating chest trauma. The mechanism of injury in nonpenetrating trauma is not well understood, but investigators have postulated that acute compression of the heart during late diastole (closed valves) could result in tearing of the myocardium (Fig. 41-15).

Treatment of VSDs depends on the patient's symptoms, the size and morphology of the defect, the presence of right ventricular dilation or pulmonary hypertension, and the presence of associated anomalies. Endovascular closure of selected membranous and muscular VSDs can be performed, thus avoiding the morbidity and mortality of open heart surgery.

■ PATENT DUCTUS ARTERIOSUS

PDA is a relatively common congenital malformation, accounting for approximately 10% of cases of congenital heart disease. The incidence of PDA is higher than average in pregnancies complicated by persistent perinatal hypoxemia or maternal rubella infection, as well as in infants born at high altitude or prematurely.

The ductus arteriosus is a normal in utero communication between the aorta and the pulmonary artery, necessary to provide oxygen-rich blood from the pulmonary artery to the systemic circulation, thereby bypassing the lungs. Embryologically, the ductus arteriosus has its

origin from the left sixth arch. The ductus arteriosus normally closes during the first few weeks of extrauterine life secondary to hormonal stimulation. Persistence of the ductus can be necessary in cases of congenital heart disease when left-to-right communication is needed, such as in transposition of the great vessels and single ventricle.

Patients with a small PDA tend to be asymptomatic and have a normal chest radiograph. Patients with a large PDA can present with fatigue, palpitations, and dyspnea on exertion. On chest radiography, these patients have shunt vascularity with proximal pulmonary arterial dilatation and a prominent ascending aorta. On a long-term basis, pulmonary vascular obstruction may develop with secondary increase in right-sided pressures and reversal of the shunt. In a small percentage of patients, the ductus arteriosus may become aneurysmal and calcified, which predisposes to rupture (Fig. 41-16).

On radiographs or CT images, the physiologically closed ductus arteriosus can be seen as a focal calcification between the aortic arch and the main or left pulmonary artery known as the ligamentum arteriosum.

On imaging studies, a PDA is seen as a vascular communication between the distal aortic arch or descending aorta junction region and the main or left pulmonary artery. On echocardiography, a continuous color flow jet can be seen entering the pulmonary artery. Similar findings can be seen on MRI SSFP images. CT images with intravenous contrast are needed to determine patency of the ductus (Fig. 41-17).

Treatment of PDA consists of either surgical or endovascular closure. In patients with ductal aneurysm formation or calcification, resection using cardiopulmonary bypass may be required. Closure is contraindicated in patients with severe pulmonary vascular obstructive disease.

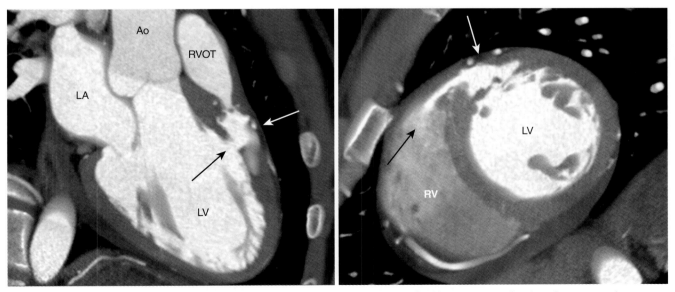

Figure 41-15 Three-chamber *(left)* and short-axis *(right)* views in a 21-year-old man after blunt trauma to the chest demonstrate the presence of a contained rupture of the anterior wall of the left ventricle (LV; *white arrow*) extending posteriorly to involve the interventricular septum. High attenuation contrast is noted entering the washed-out right ventricle (RV) consistent with a traumatic ventricular septal defect *(black arrow)*. *Ao,* Aorta; *LA,* left atrium; *RVOT,* right ventricular outflow tract.

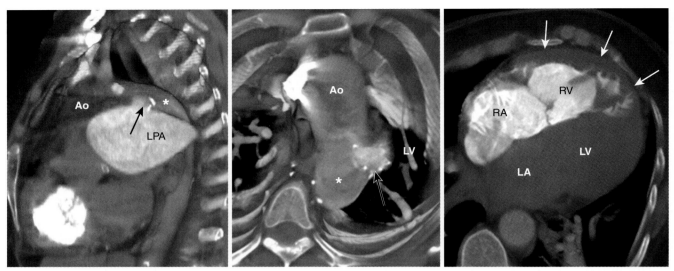

Figure 41-16 Sagittal and axial computed tomography images with contrast in a 49-year-old man with a history of long-standing patent ductus arteriosus (PDA). Note the presence of a large, partially calcified PDA *(black arrow)* associated with right ventricular hypertrophy *(white arrows)* and right-to-left shunting evidenced by the high attenuation contrast in the aorta (Ao) distal to the PDA *(asterisk)*. *LA,* Left atrium; *LPA,* left pulmonary artery; *LV,* left ventricle; *RA,* right atrium; *RV,* right ventricle.

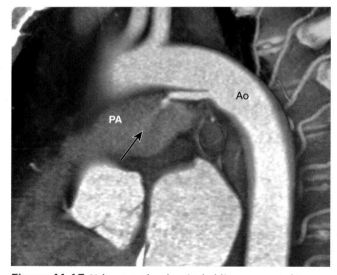

Figure 41-17 Volume rendered sagittal oblique computed tomography angiography image in a 65-year-old woman demonstrates a high attenuation jet directed from the aorta (Ao) to the main pulmonary artery (PA; *arrow*) consistent with a left-to-right shunt from a patent ductus arteriosus.

Bibliography

Anderson RH, Brown NA. The anatomy of the heart revisited. *Anat Rec.* 1996;246:1-7.

Anderson RH, Brown NA, Webb S. Development and structure of the atrial septum. *Heart.* 2002;88:104-110.

Anderson RH, Cook AC. The structure and components of the atrial chambers. *Europace.* 2007;9(suppl 6):vi3-vi9.

Anderson RH, Ho SY, Becker AE. Anatomy of the human atrioventricular junctions revisited. *Anat Rec.* 2000;260:81-91.

Anderson RH, Lenox CC, Zuberbuhler JR. Mechanisms of closure of perimembranous ventricular septal defect. *Am J Cardiol.* 1983;52:341-345.

Anderson RH, Webb S, Brown NA. Clinical anatomy of the atrial septum with reference to its developmental components. *Clin Anat.* 1999;12:362-374.

Attenhofer Jost CH, Connolly HM, Danielson GK, et al. Sinus venosus atrial septal defect: long-term postoperative outcome for 115 patients. *Circulation.* 2005;112:1953-1958.

Bright EF, Beck CS. Nonpenetrating wounds of the heart. *Am Heart J.* 1935:293-321.

Church W. Congenital malformations of the heart: abnormal septum in the left auricle. *Trans Pathol Soc Lond.* 1868:188-190.

Davia JE, Cheitlin MD, Bedynek JL. Sinus venosus atrial septal defect: analysis of fifty cases. *Am Heart J.* 1973;85:177-185.

Fisher DC, Fisher EA, Budd JH, Rosen SE, Goldman ME. The incidence of patent foramen ovale in 1,000 consecutive patients: a contrast transesophageal echocardiography study. *Chest.* 1995;107:1504-1509.

Gatzoulis MA. *Cases in Adult Congenital Heart Disease.* New York: Churchill Livingstone; 2010.

Hagen PT, Scholz DG, Edwards WD. Incidence and size of patent foramen ovale during the first 10 decades of life: an autopsy study of 965 normal hearts. *Mayo Clin Proc.* 1984;59:17-20.

Handke M, Harloff A, Olschewski M, Hetzel A, Geibel A. Patent foramen ovale and cryptogenic stroke in older patients. *N Engl J Med.* 2007;357:2262-2268.

Hara H, Virmani R, Ladich E, et al. Patent foramen ovale: current pathology, pathophysiology, and clinical status. *J Am Coll Cardiol.* 2005;46:1768-1776.

Hidalgo A, Ho ML, Bhalla S, Woodard PK, Billadello JJ, Gutierrez FR. Inferior type sinus venosus atrial septal defect: MR findings. *J Thorac Imaging.* 2008;23:266-268.

Hoey ET, Gopalan D, Ganesh V, Agrawal SK, Screaton NJ. Atrial septal defects: magnetic resonance and computed tomography appearances. *J Med Imaging Radiat Oncol.* 2009;53:261-270.

Hoffman JI, Kaplan S. The incidence of congenital heart disease. *J Am Coll Cardiol.* 2002;39:1890-1900.

Hundley WG, Li HF, Lange RA, et al. Assessment of left-to-right intracardiac shunting by velocity-encoded, phase-difference magnetic resonance imaging: a comparison with oximetric and indicator dilution techniques. *Circulation.* 1995;91:2955-2960.

Johri AM, Passeri JJ, Picard MH. Three dimensional echocardiography: approaches and clinical utility. *Heart.* 2010;96:390-397.

Johri AM, Witzke C, Solis J, et al. Real-time three-dimensional transesophageal echocardiography in patients with secundum atrial septal defects: outcomes following transcatheter closure. *J Am Soc Echocardiogr.* 2011;24:431-437.

Kim YJ, Hur J, Shim CY, et al. Patent foramen ovale: diagnosis with multidetector CT—comparison with transesophageal echocardiography. *Radiology.* 2009; 250:61-67.

Lechat P, Mas JL, Lascault G, et al. Prevalence of patent foramen ovale in patients with stroke. *N Engl J Med.* 1988;318:1148-1152.

Luotolahti M, Saraste M, Hartiala J. Saline contrast and colour Doppler transoesophageal echocardiography in detecting a patent foramen ovale and right-to-left shunts in stroke patients. *Clin Physiol.* 1995;15:265-273.

Mohrs OK, Petersen SE, Erkapic D, et al. Dynamic contrast-enhanced MRI before and after transcatheter occlusion of patent foramen ovale. *AJR Am J Roentgenol.* 2007;188:844-849.

Mohrs OK, Petersen SE, Erkapic D, et al. Diagnosis of patent foramen ovale using contrast-enhanced dynamic MRI: a pilot study. *AJR Am J Roentgenol.* 2005;184:234-240.

Oliver JM, Gallego P, Gonzalez A, Dominguez FJ, Aroca A, Mesa JM. Sinus venosus syndrome: atrial septal defect or anomalous venous connection? A multiplane transesophageal approach. *Heart.* 2002;88:634-638.

Ootaki Y, Yamaguchi M, Yoshimura N, Oka S, Yoshida M, Hasegawa T. Unroofed coronary sinus syndrome: diagnosis, classification, and surgical treatment. *J Thorac Cardiovasc Surg.* 2003;126:1655-1656.

Revel MP, Faivre JB, Letourneau T, et al. Patent foramen ovale: detection with nongated multidetector CT. *Radiology.* 2008;249:338-345.

Rojas CA, El-Sherief A, Medina HM, et al. Embryology and developmental defects of the interatrial septum. *AJR Am J Roentgenol.* 2010;195:1100-1104.

Rojas CA, Jaimes CE, El-Sherief AH, et al. Cardiac CT of non-shunt pathology of the interatrial septum. *J Cardiovasc Comput Tomogr.* 2011;5:93-100.

Rootman DB, Latter D, Admed N. Case report of ventricular septal defect secondary to blunt chest trauma. *Can J Surg.* 2007;50:227-228.

Rostad H, Sorland S. Atrial septal defect of secundum type in patients under 40 years of age: a review of 481 operated cases. Symptoms, signs, treatment and early results. *Scand J Thorac Cardiovasc Surg.* 1979;13:123-127.

Saremi F, Channual S, Raney A, et al. Imaging of patent foramen ovale with 64-section multidetector CT. *Radiology.* 2008;249:483-492.

Schwinger ME, Gindea AJ, Freedberg RS, Kronzon I. The anatomy of the interatrial septum: a transesophageal echocardiographic study. *Am Heart J.* 1990;119:1401-1405.

Sojak V, Sagat M, Balazova E, Siman J. Outcomes after surgical repair of sinus venosus atrial septal defect in children. *Bratisl Lek Listy.* 2008;109:215-219.

Stoddard MF, Keedy DL, Dawkins PR. The cough test is superior to the Valsalva maneuver in the delineation of right-to-left shunting through a patent foramen ovale during contrast transesophageal echocardiography. *Am Heart J.* 1993;125:185-189.

Strunk BL, Cheitlin MD, Stulbarg MS, Schiller NB. Right-to-left interatrial shunting through a patent foramen ovale despite normal intracardiac pressures. *Am J Cardiol.* 1987;60:413-415.

Sun JP, Stewart WJ, Hanna J, Thomas JD. Diagnosis of patent foramen ovale by contrast versus color Doppler by transesophageal echocardiography: relation to atrial size. *Am Heart J.* 1996;131:239-244.

Van Praagh S, Carrera ME, Sanders SP, Mayer JE, Van Praagh R. Sinus venosus defects: unroofing of the right pulmonary veins—anatomic and echocardiographic findings and surgical treatment. *Am Heart J.* 1994;128:365-379.

Wang ZJ, Reddy GP, Gotway MB, Yeh BM, Higgins CB. Cardiovascular shunts: MR imaging evaluation. *Radiographics.* 2003;23:S181-S194.

Warden HE, Gustafson RA, Tarnay TJ, Neal WA. An alternative method for repair of partial anomalous pulmonary venous connection to the superior vena cava. *Ann Thorac Surg.* 1984;38:601-605.

Warnes CA, Williams RG, Bashore TM, et al. ACC/AHA 2008 guidelines for the management of adults with congenital heart disease: a report of the American College of Cardiology/American Heart Association Task Force on Practice Guidelines (Writing Committee to Develop Guidelines on the Management of Adults With Congenital Heart Disease). Developed in Collaboration With the American Society of Echocardiography, Heart Rhythm Society, International Society for Adult Congenital Heart Disease, Society for Cardiovascular Angiography and Interventions, and Society of Thoracic Surgeons. *J Am Coll Cardiol.* 2008;52:e1-121.

Webb G, Gatzoulis MA. Atrial septal defects in the adult: recent progress and overview. *Circulation.* 2006;114:1645-1653.

Wessels A, Markman MW, Vermeulen JL, Anderson RH, Moorman AF, Lamers WH. The development of the atrioventricular junction in the human heart. *Circ Res.* 1996;78:110-117.

Williamson EE, Kirsch J, Araoz PA, et al. ECG-gated cardiac CT angiography using 64-MDCT for detection of patent foramen ovale. *AJR Am J Roentgenol.* 2008;190:929-933.

CHAPTER 42

Pulmonary Arteries

Brett W. Carter and Gerald F. Abbott

■ NORMAL ANATOMY

The main pulmonary artery arises from the right ventricle at the level of the pulmonic valve and travels approximately 5 cm before bifurcating into the left and right pulmonary arteries. The right pulmonary artery passes anterior to the right main bronchus and divides into the truncus anterior, which extends into the right upper lobe of the lung, and the interlobar branch, which divides into segmental arteries extending into the right middle and right lower lobes. A branch of the interlobar artery supplies the posterior segment of the right upper lobe in approximately 90% of patients. The left pulmonary artery is typically a shorter vessel and passes cephalad to the left main bronchus; it continues as an interlobar artery and extends into the left upper and lower lobes of the lung through segmental branches. A separate branch supplying the left upper lobe may arise from the left pulmonary artery before continuing as the interlobar artery.

Comparisons of pulmonary arterial size in physiologically normal patients and in those with pulmonary arterial hypertension (PAH) resulted in suggested measurements for the upper limits of normal vessel diameters. These values are 28.6 mm for the main pulmonary artery, 28 mm for the left pulmonary artery, and 24.3 mm for the right pulmonary artery. Distal to the origin of the upper lobe bronchi, the ratio of the sizes of the pulmonary artery and adjacent bronchus is approximately 1.3:1 to 1.4:1. This ratio approaches 1:1 in the periphery. Pulmonary arterial branching is dichotomous, with approximately 17 separate divisions from the bifurcation of the main pulmonary artery. Three main types of pulmonary arteries have been described: elastic, muscular, and transitional. Elastic arteries measure greater than 0.5 mm and are composed of internal and external elastic laminae around central circular muscle and connective tissue. These vessels receive the blood ejected from the right ventricle. Muscular arteries measure less than 0.5 mm and are composed of fewer internal and external elastic laminae around more substantial central circular muscle and connective tissue. These vessels course with the peripheral airways to the level of the terminal bronchioles. Transitional arteries are characterized by composition between the elastic and muscular types. Pulmonary arterioles typically measure less than 0.15 mm, but arterioles as small as 300 μm may be seen in the periphery on high-resolution computed tomography (HRCT).

■ ACUTE PULMONARY EMBOLISM

Pathogenesis

Acute pulmonary embolism (PE), one of the most common causes of cardiovascular morbidity and mortality, ranks behind only myocardial infarction and stroke in prevalence. Approximately 300,000 patients die of PE each year. Because patients with PE may be asymptomatic, the diagnosis often goes undetected and may be made only at autopsy. The most common presenting clinical symptoms include dyspnea, pleuritic chest pain, tachypnea, and tachycardia. Only one half of the patients with PE present with one component of the classic triad of chest pain, dyspnea, and hemoptysis.

PEs are typically the result of dislodged thrombus that originally formed within the deep veins of the calf. Approximately 79% of patients with PE have evidence of thrombus formation, and PE occurs in approximately 50% of patients with deep venous thrombosis (DVT).

Common clinical manifestations of DVT include leg pain, warmth, and swelling. Acute medical illness may be the most common clinical situation in which PE is encountered. Surgical procedures for hip fracture, knee and hip replacement, and cancer, as well as trauma and spinal cord injury, are associated with a high risk of PE. Other risk factors include prolonged immobilization, advanced age, cerebrovascular accident, pregnancy, and genetic or acquired thrombophilia. PE involving the lower lobes of the lung has a higher incidence.

The D-dimer test measures the levels of a specific derivative of cross-linked fibrin and is commonly used to evaluate the probability of DVT and PE. However, this test is nonspecific, and elevated levels may be encountered in trauma, inflammatory states, infection, malignancy, and pregnancy, as well as during the postoperative period. The clinical probability of PE can be assessed with one of several clinical prediction scores, the most commonly used of which are the Canadian (Wells) prediction score and the Revised Geneva score. Imaging studies are not indicated in patients with low to moderate pretest probability because the pretest probability of DVT and PE is low. However, further evaluation with imaging is recommended if the pretest probability is high.

The strongest prognostic implications for short-term mortality are derived from the hemodynamic status of the patient at the time of presentation. The mortality rate in normotensive patients without evidence of right ventricular dysfunction at the time of presentation is approximately 2%. The short-term mortality rate of massive PE, characterized by arterial hypotension or shock, ranges from 15% to 30% and increases to 65% in patients presenting with cardiac arrest.

Imaging Evaluation

Chest Radiography

The chest radiograph is often the first imaging examination performed in the evaluation of a patient with suspected PE. Although no specific abnormalities may be detected on the chest radiograph in a patient with PE, other potential causes of symptoms simulating PE may be detected. These include abnormalities such as pneumonia, pulmonary edema, and pneumothorax.

Many classic signs of PE on chest radiography have been described, but they are infrequently encountered. These include the Westermark sign, which is characterized by lucency within all or a portion of a lung and represents oligemia secondary to vasoconstriction distal to the site of PE (Fig. 42-1). Pulmonary infarction, which is encountered approximately 10% to 15% of the time, may appear as a peripheral consolidation adjacent to the pleura that is also known as the Hampton hump (Fig. 42-2). Additional imaging manifestations of infarction include atelectasis, pleural effusion, and diaphragmatic elevation. Focal enlargement and abrupt tapering of the central pulmonary artery comprise the Fleischner sign. However, these imaging findings are nonspecific for the diagnosis of PE, and additional imaging is usually required.

Ventilation-Perfusion Scintigraphy

Ventilation-perfusion (V/Q) scintigraphy is most valuable in the absence of cardiopulmonary disease and in the setting of a normal chest radiograph. The examination involves the intravenous injection of technetium-99m–macroaggregated human albumin (MAA) and the inhalation of either xenon-133 or aerosolized technetium-99m diethylenetriamine pentaacetate. PE is suggested by the appearance of a V/Q mismatch. However, other abnormalities such as lung cancer, vasculitis, fat emboli, and PAH may result in similar imaging characteristics.

The Prospective Investigation of Pulmonary Embolism II (PIOPED II) interpretation scheme is used in the evaluation of the V/Q scan. The diagnostic categories include normal, very low probability, low probability, intermediate probability, and high probability. This technique has a sensitivity of 98%, but a specificity of 10%, for the diagnosis of PE. A normal perfusion scan result virtually excludes the possibility of PE, whereas a high-probability scan is considered diagnostic of PE. However, most patients undergoing V/Q scanning have results that lie between these two categories and usually require an additional imaging test for definitive diagnosis.

Pulmonary Angiography

Once considered the gold standard for diagnosing PE, pulmonary angiography has largely been replaced by contrast-enhanced multidetector computed tomography (MDCT) at most institutions. The procedure involves percutaneously accessing the femoral vein and extending a catheter through the right atrium and ventricle into the pulmonary arteries. After the injection of intravenous contrast material, fluoroscopic images are obtained. The most common imaging manifestation of PE is a filling defect. Other findings include abrupt vessel cutoff and regions of oligemia with pruning of vascular branches.

Computed Tomography

TECHNIQUE

MDCT has emerged as the gold standard for the detection of PE in many institutions and has supplanted pulmonary angiography and V/Q scintigraphy. Contrast-enhanced

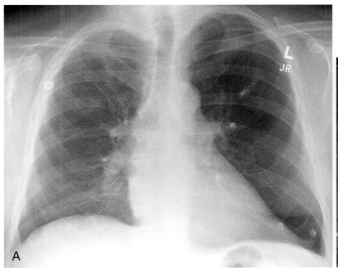
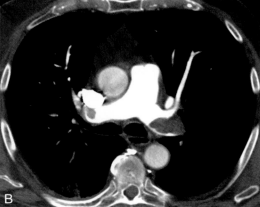

Figure 42-1 *Acute pulmonary embolism with the Westermark sign.* **A,** Anteroposterior chest radiograph demonstrates lucency within the left lung, consistent with diminished vascularity. **B,** Axial computed tomography image shows a large pulmonary embolism (PE) within the left pulmonary artery. A smaller PE is also present within the right pulmonary artery.

MDCT has the highest sensitivity and specificity for the detection of PE in the main, lobar, and segmental pulmonary arteries, with sensitivities ranging from 55% to 100% and specificities ranging from 83% to 100%. Other primary advantages of MDCT include its widespread availability, fast scan times, noninvasiveness and the ability to visualize the subsegmental pulmonary arteries. Additionally, CT can be used to evaluate the remainder of the thorax for possible alternative diagnoses resulting in symptoms mimicking PE such as pneumonia, congestive heart failure, and pneumothorax, as well as to evaluate the lungs and mediastinum for nodules and masses.

Careful selection of scan protocol and timing of contrast material administration are the most important factors in obtaining high-quality CT images through the thorax. Modern MDCT scanners are able to image the entire thorax in a single breath hold, thus resulting in shorter acquisition times. Shorter acquisition times lead to maximal spatial and temporal resolution and decreased artifacts secondary to respiratory and cardiac motion. The shortest rotation time and the highest pitch are recommended to maximize resolution. Dual source MDCT scanners, in which two tubes and detector configurations are present, have been shown in studies to optimize temporal resolution and offer higher pitches than those available on standard MDCT scanners. The amount and rate of iodinated contrast material injected are greater than those administered for routine CT scanning of the thorax, although the details vary among institutions. Optimal timing of the scan acquisition following contrast injection, the most important factor in obtaining adequate opacification of the pulmonary arterial system, may be achieved through either bolus tracking technology or the use of a test injection. Following image acquisition, multiplanar reformations may be constructed with modern MDCT scanners to optimize visualization of the pulmonary arterial system.

FINDINGS

Central hypodense filling defects within opacified pulmonary arterial branches are the most common imaging manifestations of PE. Sharp interfaces between the filling defects and the contrast material and acute angles between the filling defects and the vessel wall are usually present. Serpiginous filling defects within pulmonary arteries may result in a tram-track appearance, and occluded branches may dilate. Emboli bridging the main pulmonary arteries, known as saddle emboli, may be seen. Less specific findings include complete arterial occlusion and abrupt cutoff of vessels, which may be seen in either acute or chronic PE.

The most common imaging manifestations within the lung parenchyma are segmental and subsegmental atelectasis, which may obscure visualization of the adjacent lung parenchyma and the presence of PE within pulmonary arterial branches. Pulmonary infarction, reported to occur in 10% to 15% of cases, manifests as wedge-shaped opacities of solid, ground glass, or mixed density abutting the pleural surface in the lung periphery. Although insensitive, this finding is the most specific sign of acute PE. Pleural effusions, which may

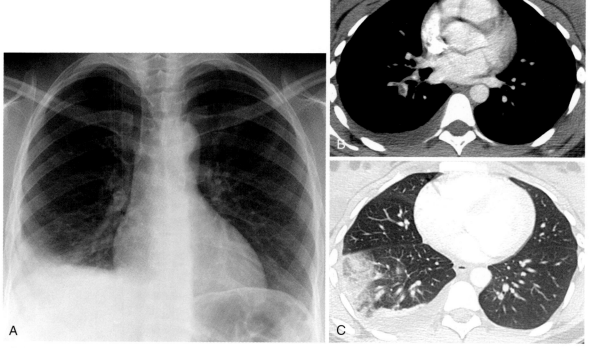

Figure 42-2 Acute pulmonary embolism with the Hampton hump. A, Anteroposterior chest radiograph shows consolidation within the right costophrenic sulcus. **B** and **C,** Axial computed tomography images demonstrate a pulmonary embolism within a right lower lobe pulmonary arterial branch and a small right pleural effusion. Mixed solid and ground glass consolidation abutting the pleura in the peripheral right lung base is consistent with infarction.

be transudative or hemorrhagic, have been reported to occur in approximately 30% of cases.

The term massive PE is used to characterize the association of right ventricular dysfunction and systemic hypotension with acute PE. These patients have been shown to benefit from additional systemic thrombolysis. Right ventricular dysfunction is manifested on contrast-enhanced MDCT as cardiac strain, the most specific feature of which is dilation of the right-sided cardiac chambers as compared with the left-sided cardiac chambers (Fig. 42-3). This measurement is made at the point of maximal diameter, typically near the base of the heart at the level of the atrioventricular valves. Straightening of the anterior interventricular septum, bowing of the interatrial septum toward the left atrium, and right atrial dilation may also be seen. A less specific sign of right-sided cardiac strain is enlargement of the pulmonary arteries, most commonly the main pulmonary artery, to more than 3.5 cm. Dilation between 3.0 and 3.5 cm also suggests right-sided cardiac strain if the pulmonary artery is larger than the ascending aorta at the same level. Additional findings may include reflux of contrast into the inferior vena cava and diminished pulmonary vascularity.

Magnetic Resonance Imaging

Magnetic resonance imaging (MRI) provides an alternative way to evaluate for the presence of PE, but it is less commonly used than MDCT because of longer scan times and increased cost. Additionally, sensitivity for the detection of PE has been demonstrated only within the main, lobar, and segmental pulmonary arteries. Studies comparing the use of contrast-enhanced MDCT and multitechnique MRI have been performed. One of these studies, employing real-time MRI, MRI perfusion imaging, and contrast-enhanced magnetic resonance angiography (MRA) separately and in combination, demonstrated sensitivities and specificities ranging from 77% to 100% and 91% to 100%, respectively.

The Prospective Investigation of Pulmonary Embolism III (PIOPED III) trial evaluated the efficacy of using gadolinium-enhanced MRA to diagnose acute PE. Adequate studies were defined as those demonstrating adequate opacification of the pulmonary arteries to the subsegmental level. However, only 25% of the examinations performed were deemed adequate for diagnostic

purposes averaged across all participating institutions. Technically inadequate examinations correctly identified PE in 57% of cases. Technically adequate examinations demonstrated a sensitivity and specificity of 78% and 99%, respectively. The combination of technically adequate contrast-enhanced MRA and magnetic resonance venography (MRV) had a sensitivity of 92%, higher than that of MRA alone, and a specificity of 96%, slightly lower than that of MRA alone. However, 52% of patients who had MRA and MRV had inadequate examinations. The investigators of PIOPED III concluded that MRA should be used for the evaluation of PE only if patients have contraindications to other tests, such as contrast allergy in the case of contrast-enhanced MDCT, and in those institutions that routinely perform the test and perform it adequately.

■ CHRONIC PULMONARY EMBOLISM

Approximately 90% of PEs resolve fully without sequelae. In the remainder of cases, however, PEs may organize, retract, and recanalize. One of the most common imaging manifestations of chronic PE on contrast-enhanced MDCT is complete occlusion of a pulmonary arterial branch, which is usually smaller than the adjacent branches. In contrast to acute PE, the filling defects of chronic PE are eccentrically located within the pulmonary arteries and demonstrate obtuse angles with respect to the vessel wall (Fig. 42-4). Thrombus may become incorporated into the vessel wall, and intraluminal webs and flaps may be visualized. Recanalized pulmonary arterial branches demonstrate contrast opacification of a smaller lumen when compared with the adjacent vessels, and the vessel walls may be thickened. Similar findings may be seen on MRI, although the limited spatial resolution of MRI may impair identification of residual disease if thrombus is incorporated into the wall of the vessel. Manifestations of chronic PE on MDCT, apart from those involving the pulmonary arteries, include the formation of prominent collateral vessels, usually of bronchial origin, and mosaic perfusion within the lung parenchyma (see Fig. 42-4). Although most pulmonary infarctions resolve completely over the course of several weeks, patchy opacities representing scar may persist at the site of infarction.

Chronic PE may result in the development of PAH, which may manifest clinically as dyspnea and fatigue.

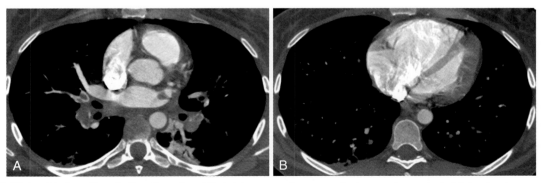

Figure 42-3 Right-sided cardiac dysfunction. A and **B,** Axial computed tomography images demonstrate bilateral pulmonary emboli. The right ventricle is enlarged. The straightening and bowing of the interventricular septum toward the left ventricle indicate cardiac strain.

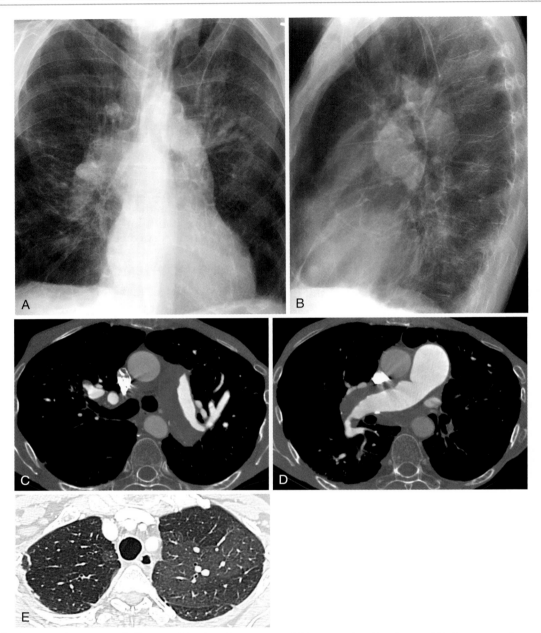

Figure 42-4 Chronic pulmonary embolism resulting in pulmonary arterial hypertension (PAH). **A** and **B,** Posteroanterior and lateral chest radiographs demonstrate enlargement of the main, left, and right pulmonary arteries, consistent with PAH. **C** and **D,** Axial computed tomography images demonstrate low-attenuation thrombus within the peripheral aspects of the pulmonary arteries bilaterally. Foci of calcification are present within the thrombus. The pulmonary arteries are enlarged. **E,** Axial computed tomography image shows mosaic attenuation of the lung parenchyma, which can be seen in chronic PAH.

PAH may be suggested by enlargement of the main, left, and right pulmonary arteries on chest radiography. Additionally, MDCT may demonstrate dilation of the main pulmonary artery to more than 3 cm (see Fig. 42-4).

■ PULMONARY ARTERIAL HYPERTENSION

Pathogenesis

PAH is an abnormality characterized by elevated pulmonary vascular resistance and pulmonary artery pressure. It is defined as mean pulmonary artery pressure greater than 25 mm Hg at rest or greater than 30 mm Hg during exercise. Mean pulmonary capillary wedge pressure and left ventricular end-diastolic pressure are typically less than 15 mm Hg. The World Health Organization has classified PAH into five separate groups on the basis of mechanism. PAH has been designated as group 1 in the classification scheme and comprises idiopathic PAH (IPAH); PAH in the setting of collagen vascular disease, portal hypertension, congenital left-to-right cardiac shunts, and infection with the human immunodeficiency virus (HIV); and persistent PAH of the newborn. Group 2 includes pulmonary hypertension (PH) with left heart disease. Group 3 comprises PH secondary to lung diseases such as chronic obstructive pulmonary disease (COPD) and interstitial lung disease. Group 4 includes PH due to pulmonary emboli or other blood clotting disorders. Group 5 comprises PH secondary to blood disorders such as polycythemia vera, systemic diseases such as sarcoidosis and vasculitides, and metabolic disorders.

Another common scheme used to categorize the causes of PAH is to partition them into precapillary and postcapillary etiologic groups. In IPAH, the cause of PAH is unknown. The most common clinical presentation is dyspnea on exertion. Other presenting symptoms include fatigue, syncope, and chest pain. Women are affected more often than are men. Sporadic and familial forms of IPAH have been described. The familial form of IPAH is responsible for approximately 10% of cases and is inherited in an autosomal dominant fashion. Plexogenic pulmonary arteriopathy is the term given to describe the pathologic abnormalities involving the pulmonary arteries in IPAH, and it consists of medial hypertrophy, intimal proliferation and fibrosis, and necrotizing arteritis.

Most cases of PAH, however, are secondary to a known cause. Common precapillary causes of PAH include chronic thromboembolic disease, congenital heart diseases resulting in left-to-right shunts such as patent ductus arteriosus and atrial and ventricular septal defects, hepatic disease, infection with HIV, and drugs and toxins. Abnormalities of the lung parenchyma such as emphysema and interstitial lung disease are additional precapillary causes of PAH. Common postcapillary causes of PAH include left-sided cardiac failure, mitral stenosis, fibrosing mediastinitis, and pulmonary veno-occlusive disease. The diagnosis and assessment of the severity of PAH are most reliably made with right-sided heart catheterization, in which right-sided pressures may be directly measured. However, several noninvasive modalities are often used to screen for PAH. They can provide estimates of pulmonary arterial pressures at rest and at exercise, and they can demonstrate secondary imaging findings suggestive of the diagnosis. Echocardiographic findings that are consistent with right ventricular pressure overload include enlargement of the right ventricle and atrium, right ventricular hypertrophy, and global right ventricular dysfunction. Systolic flattening and increased thickness of the interventricular septum, as well as an abnormally increased ratio of the interventricular septum to the posterior wall of the left ventricle greater than 1, may be present.

The radiologic manifestations of IPAH are often indistinguishable from those of secondary PAH. The most common finding on chest radiography is enlargement of the main pulmonary artery, which appears convex. The left and right pulmonary arteries may also be enlarged, as well as the right atrium and right ventricle. Evaluation of the pulmonary arteries and right-sided cardiac chambers is more accurately performed with MDCT, and dilation of the main pulmonary artery to more than 3 cm suggests PAH (Fig. 42-5). Pruning of the peripheral pulmonary arteries is usually present. Electrocardiogram-gated CT angiography has demonstrated substantially decreased distensibility of the pulmonary arterial wall, defined as the change in cross-sectional area between systole and diastole, in PAH. In chronic PAH, atherosclerotic calcifications may develop within the peripheral

aspect of the central pulmonary arteries (Fig. 42-6). Such calcifications are most commonly seen in patients with PAH secondary to Eisenmenger syndrome, in which a long-standing left-to-right shunt is reversed.

Mosaic attenuation of the lung parenchyma, representing differential perfusion, may be present, with diminished vascularity in the regions of decreased attenuation. HRCT may demonstrate centrilobular ground glass nodules, representing hemorrhagic foci or cholesterol granulomas. Additionally, interlobular septal thickening, pleural effusions, and airspace opacities may be seen in postcapillary causes of PAH. MDCT has been used in attempts to predict which patients with PAH may benefit from treatment with epoprostenol or prostacyclin. These drugs may be used as an alternative to heart-lung transplantation, based on pretreatment and posttreatment imaging findings. In one such study, pretreatment findings such as centrilobular ground glass nodules, interlobular septal thickening, pleural effusions, pericardial effusions, and lymphadenopathy were substantially more common in patients whose disease worsened with therapy and ultimately resulted in death.

Both precapillary and postcapillary causes of PAH may result in pulmonary venous hypertension, the most common radiographic finding of which is cephalization of the pulmonary vasculature. This phenomenon is characterized by increased caliber of the upper lobe pulmonary vessels in which the arterial diameter is larger than the adjacent bronchus. The lower lobe pulmonary vessels are usually more prominent, and the arterial diameter is typically equal to the adjacent bronchus in physiologically normal subjects.

Phase contrast MRI provides a noninvasive method of evaluating the morphology of the pulmonary arterial system and characterizing blood flow direction and velocities. Studies have demonstrated the potential use of parameters when interrogating the pulmonary trunk such as pulmonary regurgitant fraction, pulmonary artery dimensions, and pulmonary artery strain. Studies have also shown that increased resistance to flow and decreased average flow velocity may be useful parameters in evaluating the severity of PAH noninvasively.

■ PULMONARY ARTERY DISSECTION

Pulmonary artery dissection is a very rare, potentially fatal entity usually encountered in the setting of chronic PAH. Less common causes include pulmonary arterial inflammation, atherosclerosis, trauma, endocarditis of the right side of the heart, and amyloidosis. The most common clinical presentation is exertional dyspnea, followed by retrosternal chest pain and central cyanosis. The diagnosis is usually made at autopsy because the dissection may propagate into the pericardium and result in acute cardiac tamponade.

Because of its noninvasiveness and widespread availability, echocardiography may be the first examination performed, and it typically demonstrates the origin and extension of the intimal flap. Contrast-enhanced MDCT may also be used as the initial examination, given that it may demonstrate intimal flaps not detected on echocardiography, show the extent of dissection, and allow the

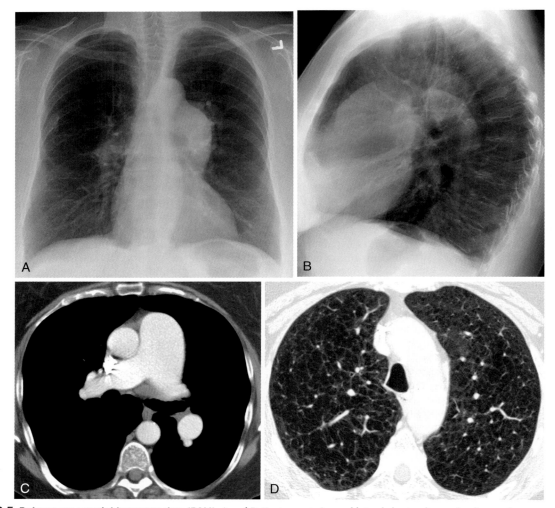

Figure 42-5 Pulmonary arterial hypertension (PAH). A and B, Posteroanterior and lateral chest radiographs show enlargement of the main pulmonary artery. C and D, Axial computed tomography images demonstrate enlargement of the main pulmonary artery. Emphysema is present within the lungs, consistent with a postcapillary origin of PAH.

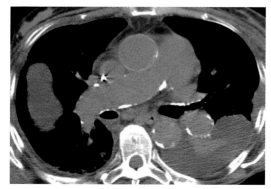

Figure 42-6 Chronic pulmonary arterial hypertension (PAH). Axial computed tomography image demonstrates enlargement of the main and right pulmonary arteries. Calcifications are present within the peripheral aspects of the right pulmonary artery, consistent with chronic PAH.

examiner to evaluate other causes of acute chest pain, such as PE. CT can also be used to evaluate for the presence of thrombus and hemopericardium. Multiplanar reconstruction and three-dimensional rendering provide more detailed anatomic information. Dissection usually occurs

at a site of aneurysm or dilation, a finding suggesting that the tissue at the site of origination is unable to support the tension of the pulmonary arterial wall. In contrast to aortic dissection, in pulmonary artery dissection the false lumen tends to rupture, rather than to develop a reentry site.

■ CONGENITAL ANOMALIES

Anomalies of the Pulmonary Arteries

Pulmonic Stenosis
Pulmonic stenosis is most commonly congenital and accounts for approximately 10% of patients with congenital heart disease. Valvular pulmonic stenosis is the most common type, comprising 90% of cases, followed by subvalvular and supravalvular types. The anomaly is characterized by thickening and fusion of the leaflets at the commissures that restricts opening of the leaflets during systole. Patients may be asymptomatic for many years, although symptoms of chronic right ventricular failure may manifest early in severe cases.

The most characteristic radiographic finding of congenital pulmonic valvular stenosis is enlargement of

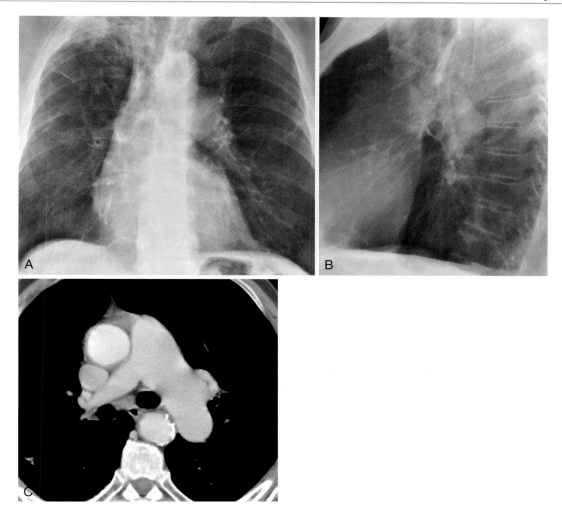

Figure 42-7 Congenital pulmonic valvular stenosis. A and **B,** Posteroanterior and lateral chest radiographs demonstrate enlargement of the main and left pulmonary arteries. **C,** Axial computed tomography image confirms enlargement of the main and left pulmonary arteries, consistent with congenital pulmonic valvular stenosis.

the main and left pulmonary arteries, representing post-stenotic dilatation (Fig. 42-7). The right pulmonary artery may be normal in size, thus resulting in an asymmetric appearance of the pulmonary hila that distinguishes this entity from PAH, in which all three vessels are typically enlarged. The right ventricle may also be enlarged. However, no radiographic abnormality may be detected in some patients. MDCT may demonstrate leaflet thickening and enlargement of the main and typically only the left pulmonary artery, although sometimes only right pulmonary arterial enlargement may be present. Pulmonary arterial wall calcification in the vicinity of the site where the systolic stenotic jet hits the wall may be present. Occasionally, valvular calcifications or a calcified pericardial ring surrounding the pulmonary artery at the level of the valve may result in severe stenosis and poststenotic dilatation of the main and left pulmonary arteries. Doppler echocardiography can demonstrate the degree of valve restriction during systole and the maximal flow velocity within the pulmonary artery. MRI is useful for evaluating the severity of the stenosis by characterizing the direction and size, by quantifying the flow velocities of the abnormal flow jet associated with pulmonic steno-

sis, and by calculating the gradient across the valve. Additional morphologic abnormalities, such as valve bulging, leaflet thickening, reduced valve movement, and right ventricular hypertrophy and thickening, may be observed.

Idiopathic Dilation of the Pulmonary Trunk

Idiopathic dilation of the pulmonary trunk is a rare developmental anomaly that is characterized by abnormal enlargement of the main pulmonary artery that may be present in isolation or associated with enlargement of the left and right pulmonary arteries. The diagnosis is made by excluding other causes of pulmonary arterial enlargement, primarily congenital pulmonic valvular stenosis and PAH. The diagnosis of PAH is excluded by the demonstration of normal right ventricular and pulmonary arterial pressures.

Chest radiography demonstrates an abnormal convexity along the left aspect of the mediastinum in the expected position of the main pulmonary artery. Contrast-enhanced CT or MRI in conjunction with echocardiography is effective in demonstrating enlargement of the main pulmonary artery, with or without involvement of the left and right pulmonary arteries.

Proximal Interruption of the Pulmonary Artery

Proximal interruption of the left or right pulmonary artery is an uncommon congenital anomaly in which the vessel terminates at the level of the hilum. Collateral systemic vessels consisting primarily of the bronchial arteries, but also branches of the internal thoracic, intercostal, internal mammary, and subclavian arteries, deliver blood to the lung. Interruption of the right pulmonary artery is more common than is interruption of the left and is usually an isolated finding, whereas interruption of the left pulmonary artery is commonly associated with a right aortic arch and other congenital anomalies.

Chest radiography typically demonstrates varying degrees of pulmonary hypoplasia and shift of the heart and mediastinum toward the affected side. Reticular opacities may be present, representing bronchial collateral vessels supplying the abnormal lung. Rib notching may be noted on the affected side when branches of the intercostal arteries serve as collateral vessels. CT can illustrate the abnormal pulmonary artery as it blindly ends at the level of the hilum and can characterize the network of collateral vessels supplying the lung. However, various parenchymal abnormalities have been described with proximal interruption of the pulmonary artery, the most common of which include pleural thickening, subpleural parenchymal bands, reticular opacities, and mosaic attenuation. Other abnormalities include bronchial wall thickening, bronchiectasis, and honeycombing.

Anomalous Origin of the Left Pulmonary Artery

In this rare developmental anomaly, the left pulmonary artery arises from the extrapericardial segment of the right pulmonary artery and extends between the trachea anteriorly and the esophagus posteriorly on its path to the left lung. The proximal portion of the anomalous vessel may compress the right main bronchus and impede respiration to all or portions of the right lung, thus resulting in a pulmonary sling. This anomaly is potentially fatal when it is associated with long-segment tracheal stenosis secondary to complete tracheal rings. Tracheal reconstruction is required in this group of patients.

The most characteristic radiographic finding is the identification of a rounded opacity between the trachea and the esophagus on the lateral radiograph (Fig. 42-8). Barium esophagram may demonstrate indentation of the anterior wall of the esophagus by the anomalous vessel. CT is diagnostic of the anomaly by demonstrating the abnormal origin and course of the vessel, and it facilitates evaluation of the airway for complete tracheal rings through three-dimensional reconstructive techniques such as virtual bronchoscopy. MRI can also be used to delineate the vascular anatomy and generate volumetric reconstructions of the airway.

Abnormalities of the Pulmonary Arteries and Veins

Hypogenetic Lung Syndrome

Hypogenetic lung syndrome, also known as scimitar syndrome and congenital venolobar syndrome, is a rare anomaly that predominantly affects the right lung. The primary components of the syndrome include hypoplasia of the right lung, hypoplasia of the right pulmonary artery, anomalous systemic arterial supply to the right lower lobe (usually from the subdiaphragmatic aorta or one of its branches), and anomalous pulmonary venous drainage of all or a portion of the right lung into the inferior vena cava. However, not all these components may be seen when the syndrome is present, and great variations may be encountered. The hypoplastic right lung commonly demonstrates abnormal segmentation, and other developmental abnormalities of the bronchi, diaphragm, spine, and genitourinary tract are frequently encountered. Three types of hypogenetic lung syndrome have been described. In the infantile form, a connection exists between the anomalous artery supplying the right lower lobe and the subdiaphragmatic aorta. The adult form is characterized by a shunt between the right pulmonary veins and the inferior vena cava. The third form is distinguished by additional cardiac and extracardiac abnormalities.

Approximately 40% of patients with hypogenetic lung syndrome are asymptomatic. When patients are symptomatic, fatigue, dyspnea, and recurrent pulmonary infection are the most common clinical presentations. Although the syndrome is much more common on the right, cases of hypogenetic lung syndrome on the left side have been reported. In these cases, the anomalous vein drains into the coronary sinus. The characteristic finding on chest radiography is a vertically oriented opacity within the right middle and lower lung zones paralleling the right cardiac border and extending toward the right diaphragmatic surface (Fig. 42-9). This opacity represents the anomalous draining vein and often resembles a scimitar (Turkish sword). Contrast-enhanced MDCT better demonstrates the anomalous vein, which may drain the entire right lung and is closely related to the right major interlobar fissure. Other common components of the syndrome, including pulmonary parenchymal and arterial hypoplasia, and anomalous arterial supply of a portion of the right lung, usually of the right lower lobe, are typically seen.

Arteriovenous Malformations

Pulmonary arteriovenous malformations (AVMs) are anomalies characterized by the lack of an intervening capillary network between pulmonary artery and vein. Approximately 80% of cases are congenital, and 70% of these cases are associated with hereditary hemorrhagic telangiectasia (HHT), also known as Osler-Weber-Rendu syndrome. This syndrome includes additional malformations of the skin, nasal, oral, and conjunctival mucosa, and abdominal viscera. Acquired lesions may be secondary to thoracic trauma, surgery, infection, or malignant disease. Pulmonary AVMs are usually diagnosed in adult life and enlarge slowly over time. Small malformations may be asymptomatic. However, as malformations increase in size, hypoxemia, cyanosis, and the risk of paradoxic emboli increase. Cerebrovascular accidents secondary to paradoxic embolus are potentially fatal. Rupture of pulmonary AVMs may result in

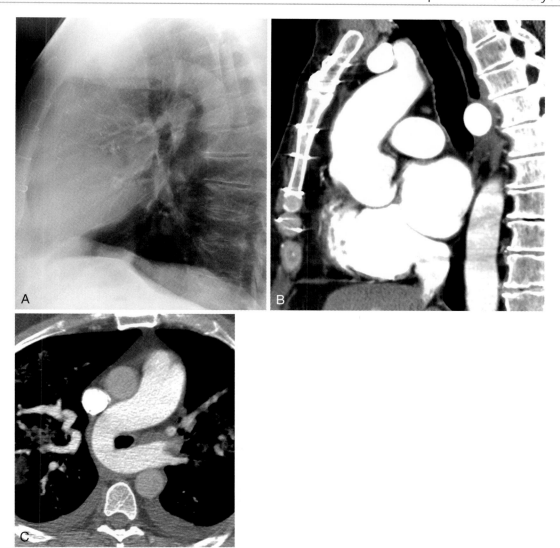

Figure 42-8 Pulmonary sling. A, Lateral chest radiograph demonstrates an opacity between the trachea anteriorly and the esophagus posteriorly. **B** and **C,** Axial and sagittal computed tomography images demonstrate the left pulmonary artery arising from the right pulmonary artery and insinuating itself between the trachea and esophagus as it travels toward the left hemithorax.

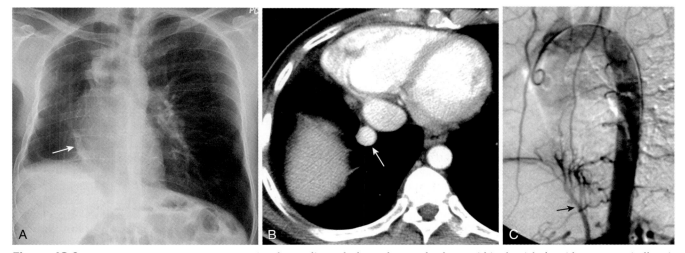

Figure 42-9 Scimitar syndrome. A, Anteroposterior chest radiograph shows decreased volume within the right hemithorax. A vertically oriented opacity *(arrow)* paralleling the right cardiac border extends toward the right hemidiaphragm. **B,** Axial computed tomography shows the anomalous draining vein *(arrow)* proximal to its insertion into the inferior vena cava. **C,** Aortic angiogram demonstrates an anomalous arterial branch *(arrow)* extending into the right lower lung zone.

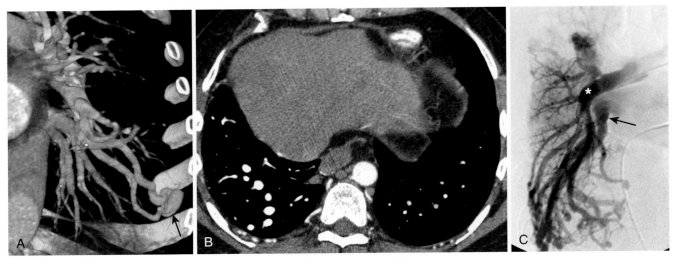

Figure 42-10 Arteriovenous malformations. A, Reconstructed image from contrast-enhanced computed tomography (CT) demonstrates a simple arteriovenous malformation (AVM, *arrow*) with a single feeding artery, nidus, and single draining vein. B, Axial CT image shows asymmetric prominence of the veins within the right lower lobe, suggestive of AVM. C, Pulmonary angiogram demonstrates a complex AVM with feeding arteries (*asterisk*) and draining veins.

pulmonary hemorrhage and hemothorax. Approximately two thirds of AVMs are located within the lower lobes of the lung, often in a subpleural location. These anomalies are multiple 35% of the time and bilateral in approximately 10% of patients.

AVMs may be characterized as simple or complex, depending on the number of feeding arteries (Fig. 42-10). A simple AVM is characterized by a single feeding artery and a single draining vein, whereas a complex AVM is characterized by more than one feeding artery. Simple AVMs are much more common than are complex AVMs.

The chest radiograph may be normal in patients with small pulmonary AVMs. The most commonly detected abnormality on chest radiography is a sharply defined nodular opacity, usually located within the lung periphery. Pulmonary angiography was once considered the gold standard for detection and characterization of pulmonary AVMs. However, noncontrast MDCT with maximum intensity projection (MIP) reconstruction has demonstrated greater sensitivity in detection, although a significant radiation dose is associated with this modality, especially for younger patients. The most common imaging manifestation of a simple AVM on MDCT is a well-circumscribed, round or elliptical nodule usually located within the subpleural lung. Complex AVMs appear as lobulated masses secondary to the presence of multiple feeding arteries, which may become tangled and tortuous. Feeding arteries become much more apparent in larger AVMs, such as those greater than 1 to 2 cm. Although the administration of intravenous contrast material is usually not necessary for diagnosis, pulmonary AVMs demonstrate rapid contrast opacification and washout in phase within the main pulmonary artery and right ventricle when contrast material is infused.

Breath-hold enhanced three-dimensional MRA has been shown to be accurate in diagnosing pulmonary AVMs greater than 5 mm in diameter and AVMs in which the feeding artery measures at least 3 mm in diameter.

Small series employing MRA have demonstrated excellent sensitivity and specificity in these situations.

Twenty-five percent of patients with pulmonary AVMs experience progression of symptom severity, and up to 50% of patients eventually die of complications. The primary indication for treatment of pulmonary AVMs is the prevention of neurologic complications. Thirty to 40% of patients with malformations and a feeding artery at least 3 mm in diameter experience transient ischemic attack, stroke, and brain abscess. Therefore, most of these AVMs are treated. AVMs with a feeding artery less than 3 mm in diameter may be monitored and treated only if expansion is observed. Other indications for treatment include exercise intolerance and prevention of hemoptysis and hemothorax. Pulmonary angiography is often performed before treatment and at the time of embolization, which may be performed with coils or detachable balloons. Surgical excision may be performed if attempts at embolization have failed or in the event of rupture. The use of nonferromagnetic embolization coils permits follow-up with MRI.

■ PULMONARY ARTERY ANEURYSMS AND PSEUDOANEURYSMS

Aneurysms

Aneurysms of the pulmonary artery are characterized by focal dilation of the vessel that involves all three layers and may be congenital or acquired. Common congenital causes include abnormalities of the vessel wall, valvular and postvalvular stenosis, and congenital anomalies resulting in left-to-right shunts. Depending on their size and location within the thorax, pulmonary artery aneurysms may result in compression of the left main bronchus, left main coronary artery, and left pulmonary vein. Thrombus formation may be present. Potentially life-threatening complications include

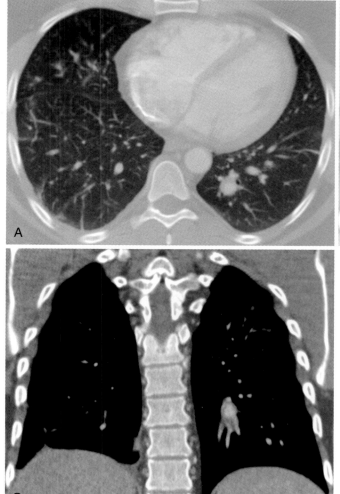

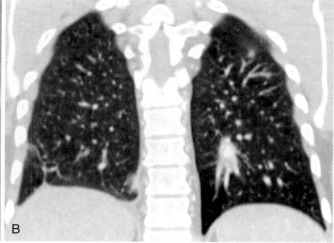

Figure 42-11 *Pulmonary artery aneurysm in Behçet disease.*
A, Axial computed tomography (CT) shows a nodular opacity within the left lower lobe. **B** and **C,** Coronal CT images with contrast demonstrate an enhancing nodular opacity in the left lower lobe that is in phase with the adjacent pulmonary arterial branches.

thromboembolic phenomena such as cerebrovascular accident and aneurysm rupture. Up to 50% of reported cases are associated with congenital heart disease, typically disorders resulting in left-to-right shunts such as patent ductus arteriosus and atrial and ventricular septal defects. Aneurysms in these patients are the result of volume and pressure overload. The aneurysms associated with Eisenmenger complex, which is characterized by flow reversal in long-standing left-to-right shunts, have the highest risk of rupture. Other associated congenital anomalies include tetralogy of Fallot, valvular pulmonic stenosis, pulmonary valvular regurgitation, bicuspid pulmonic valve, and transposition of the great vessels.

Vasculitides such as Behçet disease and Hughes-Stovin syndrome may result in pulmonary artery aneurysms (Fig. 42-11). Behçet disease is a multisystemic type of vasculitis that typically manifests as oral and genital ulcers and uveitis and usually affects both arteries and veins. The aorta, inferior vena cava, and pulmonary arteries are affected in approximately one fourth of cases. Sixty-five percent of arterial lesions manifest as aneurysms, and 35% manifest as occlusion. Aneurysms may be single or multiple and unilateral or bilateral.

Some studies have demonstrated a greater proportion of multiple and bilateral aneurysms in Behçet disease. Hughes-Stovin syndrome is characterized by multiple pulmonary artery aneurysms with a propensity to rupture and venous thrombosis. Significant overlap of the predominant features of these two syndromes is reported, including increased incidence in young men, abnormalities of both arteries and veins, and similar pathologic abnormalities identified within pulmonary artery aneurysms.

Intrinsic abnormalities of the vessel wall, such as those seen in conditions such as Marfan syndrome, Ehlers-Danlos syndrome, and cystic medial necrosis, result in weakening of the pulmonary arteries and can lead to aneurysm formation. Other causes include PAH, pulmonary thromboemboli, and trauma.

Pseudoaneurysms

Pseudoaneurysms of the pulmonary arteries are not contained by all three layers of the vessel wall and are therefore at an increased risk of rupture. The most common clinical presentation of pulmonary artery pseudoaneurysms is hemoptysis, which may be massive. One

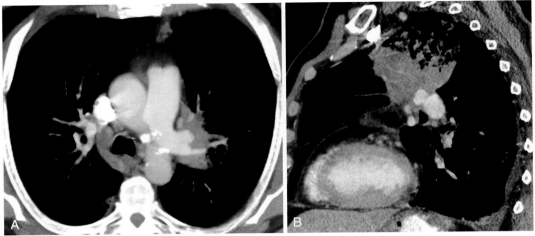

Figure 42-12 Mycotic pulmonary artery pseudoaneurysm. A, Axial computed tomography (CT) image with contrast demonstrates focal outpouching of the anterior aspect of the proximal left pulmonary artery. **B,** Sagittal CT image with contrast again shows this focal outpouching, as well as consolidation within the left upper lobe. These findings are consistent with mycotic pseudoaneurysm

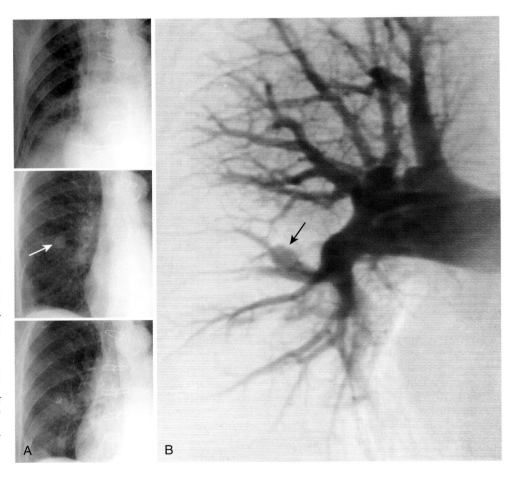

Figure 42-13 Iatrogenic pulmonary artery pseudoaneurysm. A, The initial anteroposterior chest radiograph *(top)* demonstrates a pulmonary artery catheter terminating within the right pulmonary artery at the level of the right hilum. A subsequent chest radiograph *(middle)* shows removal of the catheter. Interval development of a nodular opacity *(arrow)* within the right lower lobe has occurred, consistent with pseudoaneurysm. The final chest radiograph *(bottom)* demonstrates multiple embolization coils following treatment of the pseudoaneurysm. **B,** Pulmonary angiogram demonstrates focal outpouching *(arrow)* from a right lower lobe pulmonary arterial branch, consistent with pseudoaneurysm.

of the most common causes is infection with bacterial, mycobacterial, and fungal organisms. Mycotic pseudoaneurysms from bacterial infection are most commonly seen in intravenous drug users, usually with concomitant endocarditis and septic emboli (Fig. 42-12). Pseudoaneurysms in the setting of tuberculosis, also known as Rasmussen aneurysms, usually involve the upper lobes of the lung at the site of reactivation.

Lung cancer and metastases from other primary malignant diseases may invade the pulmonary arteries and result in pseudoaneurysm formation. Primary malignant diseases of the pulmonary arteries, the most common of which is angiosarcoma, may expand and dilate the pulmonary arteries. Malpositioned Swan-Ganz catheters are among the most common iatrogenic causes of pulmonary artery pseudoaneurysms (Fig. 42-13). One study reported a 0.2% incidence of rupture and hemorrhage following Swan-Ganz catheter placement. Pseudoaneurysms are most commonly encountered when the distal end of the catheter has been advanced into the peripheral pulmonary arterial system, resulting in erosion and weakening of the vessel wall. Complications such as thrombus formation or rupture may be seen. Other iatrogenic causes of pseudoaneurysm include thoracic surgery and biopsy, chest tube insertion, and conventional angiography.

Imaging Evaluation of Aneurysms and Pseudoaneurysms

The initial radiographic examination usually performed in the patient presenting with hemoptysis is the chest radiograph. However, visualization of aneurysms and pseudoaneurysms on chest radiography is variable and depends on the size and location of the abnormality. Therefore, the chest radiograph may appear normal. In the early stages, these entities may appear as patchy, poorly circumscribed opacities. Over time, these opacities become more circumscribed and may appear as discrete nodular opacities. Hilar enlargement or perihilar nodules may be identified. Aneurysms and pseudoaneurysms should be suspected in patients presenting with hemoptysis and in whom the chest radiograph demonstrates stable or enlarging nodular opacities.

Contrast-enhanced MDCT is the noninvasive imaging modality of choice in the identification and characterization of pulmonary artery aneurysms and pseudoaneurysms because their number, size, and location may be accurately determined. One of the primary advantages of MDCT is the short scan time, which is important in making a timely diagnosis, especially given that the mortality rate for rupture is 100%. Inflammation of the pulmonary arteries may manifest as thickening of the vessel wall on MDCT and MRI and 18-fluorodeoxyglucose (18-FDG) uptake on 18-FDG positron emission tomography with CT (PET/CT).

MRI may demonstrate abnormal thickening and enhancement of the pulmonary arterial wall in patients with vasculitis and connective tissue disorders resulting in aneurysms and pseudoaneurysms. In patients with aneurysms and pseudoaneurysms secondary to congenital abnormalities of the pulmonic valve, MRI may assess direction and velocity of blood flow.

■ NEOPLASMS OF THE PULMONARY ARTERY

Neoplastic involvement of the pulmonary arteries may result from primary malignant disease of the vessel, tumor emboli, or direct extension into the vessels by tumors of the lung, hila, or mediastinum.

Primary Malignant Disease

Pulmonary artery sarcomas are rare tumors of the cardiovascular system, but they are the most common primary malignant tumor of the pulmonary arteries. These tumors most commonly arise from the main or proximal left or right pulmonary arteries. Most cases are diagnosed at autopsy or at the time of surgery. The most common clinical symptoms include dyspnea, cough, chest pain, and hemoptysis. The prognosis is poor, with a mean survival time of 12 months following initial presentation.

Findings on chest radiography depend largely on tumor size and the extent of spread. If the sarcoma is entirely intraluminal and does not result in pulmonary artery dilation, the chest radiograph may be normal. If the tumor remains intraluminal but expands the pulmonary artery, the appearance may be that of a hilar mass. Distal oligemia may be present. If the mass extends outside the pulmonary artery, it may mimic lung cancer or metastatic disease.

Conventional angiography may demonstrate polypoid filling defects within the pulmonary arteries. However, distinguishing tumor from thrombus may be difficult. Movement of the filling defects during the cardiac cycle suggests malignancy. Additionally, bronchial arteriography may demonstrate tumor neovascularity.

Contrast-enhanced MDCT may demonstrate filling defects within the pulmonary arteries, although tumor may be indistinguishable from acute or chronic PEs in this setting. The pulmonary artery may be enlarged, a finding that may also be present in setting of acute PEs. A mosaic pattern of lung attenuation reported in the setting of pulmonary artery sarcoma may result from extension of tumor into small pulmonary arteries or occlusion of small peripheral vessels by tumor emboli or thrombi that formed on the surface of the tumor. This finding is nonspecific, however, and can be seen in patients with primary PAH, pulmonary capillary hemangiomatosis, pulmonary veno-occlusive disease, polyarteritis nodosa, and scleroderma. Extraluminal extension of tumor may also be visualized.

Intravascular ultrasound and transesophageal echocardiography can be used to characterize the morphology of the mass and evaluate for involvement of the pulmonic valve. Gadolinium-enhanced MRI may be useful for distinguishing tumor from thrombus because tumor is more likely to demonstrate enhancement than is thrombus (Fig. 42-14). However, enhancement may be seen in the setting of acute thrombus. Reports of increased 18-FDG uptake within intravascular pulmonary artery sarcomas on 18-FDG PET/CT have suggested that the modality may be able to distinguish this entity from bland PEs. Nonetheless, 18-FDG uptake within PEs has been described, as has uptake within segments of the pulmonary arterial wall affected by vasculitis and connective disease.

Tumor Emboli

Pulmonary intravascular tumor emboli are often difficult to diagnose clinically and radiographically, and the diagnosis is commonly made at autopsy. An autopsy study showed that approximately 2.4% of solid neoplasms demonstrated microscopic tumor emboli in the pulmonary arteries in the absence of other metastatic disease. Other studies have demonstrated the presence of pulmonary tumor emboli in up to 26% of patients.

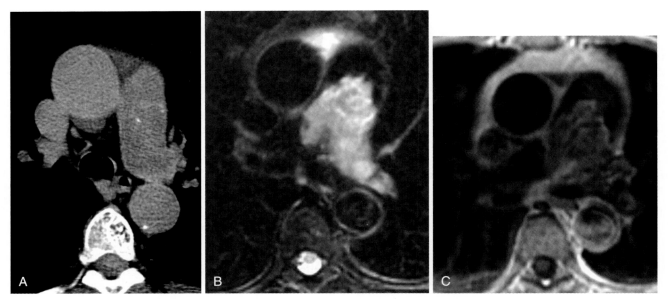

Figure 42-14 Pulmonary artery sarcoma. A, Axial computed tomography image without contrast demonstrates low attenuation and scattered foci of calcification in the main pulmonary artery with extension into the proximal left pulmonary artery. These findings can be seen with malignant disease or chronic pulmonary embolism. **B,** T2-weighted fat saturation, fast spin echo oblique axial image. A heterogeneously T2 hyperintense mass is centered within the main pulmonary artery and extends into the proximal left and right pulmonary arteries. **C,** T1-weighted postgadolinium axial image shows heterogeneous enhancement of the mass, consistent with malignant disease.

The radiographic diagnosis of pulmonary intravascular tumor emboli is difficult to make because most chest radiographs are normal. Cardiomegaly and enlargement of the central pulmonary arteries have been described. These features may be secondary to occlusion of the main, lobar, or segmental pulmonary arteries and resultant PAH. The perfusion portion of V/Q scintigraphy may demonstrate multiple subsegmental perfusion defects, whereas the ventilation portion is usually normal. Pulmonary angiography may demonstrate delayed filling of the segmental pulmonary arteries, pruning and tortuosity of small vessels, and occasional subsegmental filling defects. Contrast-enhanced CT has demonstrated single and multifocal regions of pulmonary artery dilation and beading in patients with intravascular tumor emboli (Fig. 42-15). Small wedge-shaped opacities within the peripheral lungs have been described, representing pulmonary infarction.

Direct Extension

Invasion of the pulmonary artery by lung cancer is very rare and is most likely to occur in patients with malignant tumors arising near the pulmonary hila. Although small cell carcinoma and squamous cell carcinoma are more likely to occur within the central lung near the hila, the pathologic types previously reported include small cell, squamous cell, adenosquamous cell, and large cell neuroendocrine carcinoma. Primary malignant diseases and lymphadenopathy of the mediastinum may rarely invade the pulmonary artery.

The chest radiograph may demonstrate a nodule or mass within the central lung or hila. However, chest radiography is unlikely to reveal invasion of the pulmonary artery. Contrast-enhanced MDCT has been used to define the relationship between the tumor and the adjacent lung, hila, and mediastinum, including the pulmonary artery (see Fig. 42-15). In one reported case, MDCT demonstrated a large central lung mass invading the left pulmonary artery and filling defects within the main pulmonary artery. In other cases, MDCT demonstrated the primary lung cancer, but no evidence of pulmonary artery invasion, although such involvement was identified at the time of surgical resection. In one of these reported cases, pulmonary angiography demonstrated diminished vascularity in two lobes of the lung on the same side as the tumor. In another case, V/Q scintigraphy demonstrated diminished perfusion of the portion of the lung supplied by the invaded pulmonary arterial segment.

Multiple signs of pulmonary artery invasion were described in a study comparing the CT and MRI findings of lung cancer invading the pulmonary arteries with surgical and pathologic findings. These findings included thickening of the pulmonary artery wall (present in 73.7% of CT and 84.6% of MRI images), luminal narrowing (present in 55.3% of CT and 69.2% of MRI images), and stranding within the perivascular fat (present in 100% of both CT and MRI images). In this study, CT and MRI findings were found to correlate well with surgical and pathologic findings, with kappa values of 0.61 for CT and 0.84 for MRI.

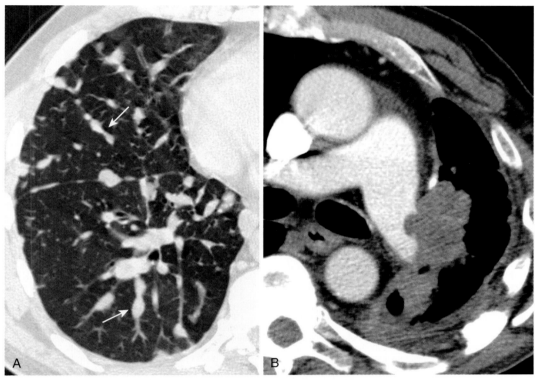

Figure 42-15 Tumor emboli and direct invasion of the pulmonary artery. A, Axial computed tomography (CT) image through the lower thorax demonstrates irregular beading and dilation of pulmonary arterial branches *(arrow)* in the lower lobes of the lung in this patient with a history of metastatic disease. These findings are consistent with tumor emboli. **B,** Axial CT image with contrast demonstrates a small cell carcinoma of the left lung invading the left pulmonary artery. The fat plane between the left pulmonary artery and the mediastinum has been obliterated and the posterior wall of the vessel is thickened.

Bibliography

Badesch DB, Raskob GE, Elliott CG, et al. Pulmonary arterial hypertension: baseline characteristics from the REVEAL Registry. *Chest.* 2010;137:376-387.

Berden WE, Baker DH, Wung JT. Complete cartilage-ring tracheal stenosis associated with anomalous left pulmonary artery; the ring-sling complex. *Radiology.* 1984;152:57-64.

Blackmon SH, Rice DC, Correa AM, et al. Management of primary pulmonary artery sarcomas. *Ann Thorac Surg.* 2009;87:977-984.

Bossone E, Bodini BD, Mazza A, et al. Pulmonary arterial hypertension: the key role of echocardiography. *Chest.* 2005;127:1836-1843.

Castañer E, Gallardo X, Rimola J, et al. Congenital and acquired pulmonary artery anomalies in the adult: radiologic overview. *Radiographics.* 2006;26:349-371.

Chalazonitis AN, Lachanis SB, Mitseas P, et al. Hughes-Stovin syndrome: a case report and review of the literature. *Cases J.* 2009;2:98.

Chan CK, Hutcheon MA, Hyland RH, et al. Pulmonary tumor embolism: a critical review of clinical, imaging, and hemodynamic features. *J Thorac Imaging.* 1987;2:4-14.

Cho YK, Lee W, Choi SI, et al. Cardiovascular Behçet disease: the variable findings of rare complications with CT angiography and conventional angiography and its interventional management. *J Comput Assist Tomogr.* 2008;32:679-689.

Chong S, Kim TS, Kim BT, et al. Pulmonary artery sarcoma mimicking pulmonary thromboembolism: integrated FDG PET/CT. *AJR Am J Roentgenol.* 2007;188:1691-1693.

Coche EE, Muller NL, Kim KI, et al. Acute pulmonary embolism: ancillary findings at spiral CT. *Radiology.* 1998;207:753-758.

Coche EE, Verschuren F, Hainaut P, et al. Pulmonary embolism findings on chest radiographs and multislice spiral CT. *Eur Radiol.* 2004;14:1241-1248.

Collomb D, Paramelle PJ, Calaque O, et al. Severity assessment of acute pulmonary embolism: evaluation using helical CT. *Eur Radiol.* 2003;13:1508.

Contractor S, Maldjian PD, Sharma VK, et al. Role of helical CT in detecting right ventricular dysfunction secondary to acute pulmonary embolism. *J Comput Assist Tomogr.* 2002;26:587.

Cox JE, Chiles C, Aquino S, et al. Pulmonary artery sarcomas: a review of clinical and radiologic features. *J Comput Assist Tomogr.* 1997;21:750-755.

Dennie CJ, Veinot JP, McCormack DG, et al. Intimal sarcoma of the pulmonary arteries seen as a mosaic pattern of lung attenuation on high-resolution CT. *AJR Am J Roentgenol.* 2002;178:1208-1210.

Dikensoy O, Kervancioglu R, Bayram NG, et al. Horseshoe lung associated with scimitar syndrome and pleural lipoma. *J Thorac Imaging.* 2006;21:73-75.

Dupont MV, Drăgean CA, Coche EE. Right ventricle function assessment by MDCT. *AJR Am J Roentgenol.* 2011;196:77-86.

Elliott CG, Goldhaber SZ, Visani L, et al. Chest radiographs in acute pulmonary embolism: results from the International Cooperative Pulmonary Embolism Registry. *Chest.* 2000;118:33-38.

Elliott FM, Reid L. Some new facts about the pulmonary artery and its branching pattern. *Clin Radiol.* 1965;16:193-198.

Erkan F, Gul A, Tasali E. Pulmonary manifestations of Behçet's disease. *Thorax.* 2001;56:572-578.

Farber HW, Loscalzo J. Pulmonary arterial hypertension. *N Engl J Med.* 2004;351:1655-1665.

Ferretti GR, Thony F, Link RM, et al. False aneurysm of the pulmonary artery induced by a Swan-Ganz catheter: clinical presentation and radiologic management. *AJR Am J Roentgenol.* 1996;167:941-945.

Frazier AA, Galvin JR, Franks TJ, et al. From the archives of the AFIP: pulmonary vasculature: hypertension and infarction. *Radiographics.* 2000;20:491-524.

Groves AM, Win T, Charman SC, et al. Semi-quantitative assessment of tricuspid regurgitation on contrast-enhanced multidetector CT. *Clin Radiol.* 2004;59:715.

Haimovici JB, Trotman-Dickenson B, Halpern EF, et al. Relationship between pulmonary artery diameter at computed tomography and pulmonary artery pressures at right-sided heart catheterization: Massachusetts General Hospital Lung Transplantation Program. *Acad Radiol.* 1997;4:327-334.

Han D, Lee KS, Franquet T, et al. Thrombotic and nonthrombotic pulmonary arterial embolism: spectrum of imaging findings. *Radiographics.* 2003;23:1521-1539.

Jefferson KE. The normal pulmonary angiogram and some changes seen in chronic nonspecific lung disease. I. The pulmonary vessels seen in the normal pulmonary angiogram. *Proc R Soc Med.* 1965;58:677.

Jiménez D, Aujesky D, Yusen RD. Risk stratification of normotensive patients with acute symptomatic pulmonary embolism. *Br J Haematol.* 2010;151:415-424.

Khalil A, Farres MT, Mangiapan G, et al. Pulmonary arteriovenous malformations. *Chest.* 2000;117:1399-1403.

Khattar RS, Fox DJ, Alty JE, Arora A. Pulmonary artery dissection: an emerging cardiovascular complication in surviving patients with chronic pulmonary hypertension. *Heart.* 2005;91:142-145.

Kieffer SA, Amplantz K, Anderson RC, et al. Proximal interruption of a pulmonary artery. *AJR Am J Roentgenol.* 1965;95:592-597.

King MA, Bergin CJ, Yeung DW, et al. Chronic pulmonary thromboembolism: detection of regional hypoperfusion with CT. *Radiology.* 1994;191:359-363.

King MA, Ysrael M, Bergin CJ. Chronic thromboembolic pulmonary hypertension: CT findings. *AJR Am J Roentgenol.* 1998;170:955-960.

Kluge A, Luboldt W, Bachmann G. Acute pulmonary embolism to the subsegmental level: diagnostic accuracy of three MRI techniques compared with 16-MDCT. *AJR Am J Roentgenol.* 2006;187:W7-W14.

Kuriyama K, Gamsu G, Stern RG, et al. CT-determined pulmonary artery diameters in predicting pulmonary hypertension. *Invest Radiol.* 1984;19:16-22.

Kuzo RS, Goodman LR. CT evaluation of pulmonary embolism: technique and interpretation. *AJR Am J Roentgenol.* 1997;169:959-965.

Mastora I, Remy-Jardin M, Masson P, et al. Severity of acute pulmonary embolism: evaluation of a new spiral CT angiographic score in correlation with echocardiographic data. *Eur Radiol.* 2003;13:29.

Mattoo A, Fedullo PF, Kapelanski D, et al. Pulmonary artery sarcoma: a case report of surgical cure and 5-year follow-up. *Chest.* 2002;122:745-747.

Miao J, Zhou H, Zhu P, et al. CT and MRI findings of cancerous invasion of the main pulmonary artery in lung cancer: the correlation with pathologic features and the value in making surgical plan. *Zhongguo Fei Ai Za Zhi.* 2003;6:3-7:[in Chinese].

Murata K, Itoh H, Todo G, et al. Centrilobular lesions of the lung: demonstration by high-resolution CT and pathologic correlation. *Radiology.* 1986;161:641-645.

Naidich DP, Rumancik WM, Ettenger NA, et al. Congenital anomalies of the lungs in adults: MR diagnosis. *AJR Am J Roentgenol.* 1988;151:13-19.

Neimatallah MA, Hassan W, Moursi M, et al. CT findings of pulmonary artery dissection. *Br J Radiol.* 2007;80:e61-e63.

Nguyen ET, Silva CI, Seely JM, et al. Pulmonary artery aneurysms and pseudoaneurysms in adults: findings at CT and radiography. *AJR Am J Roentgenol.* 2007;188:W126-W134.

Nikolaou K, Schoenberg SO, Attenberger U, et al. Pulmonary arterial hypertension: diagnosis with fast perfusion MR imaging and high-spatial-resolution MR angiography—preliminary experience. *Radiology.* 2005;236:694-703.

Okamoto Y, Tsuchiya K, Nakajima M, et al. Primary lung cancer with growth into the lumen of the pulmonary artery. *Ann Thorac Cardiovasc Surg.* 2009;15:186-188.

Park HS, Im JG, Jung GW, et al. Anomalous left pulmonary artery with complete cartilaginous ring. *J Comput Assist Tomogr.* 1997;21:478-480.

Piazza G, Goldhaber SZ. Chronic thromboembolic pulmonary hypertension. *N Engl J Med.* 2011;364:351-360.

Pineda LA, Hathwar VS, Grant BJ. Clinical suspicion of fatal pulmonary embolism. *Chest.* 2001;120:791-795.

Pollak JS, Saluja S, Thabet A, et al. Clinical and anatomic outcomes after embolotherapy of pulmonary arteriovenous malformations. *J Vasc Interv Radiol.* 2006;17:35-44.

Remy-Jardin M, Duhamel A, Deken V, et al. Systemic collateral supply in patients with chronic thromboembolic pulmonary hypertension: assessment with multi-detector row helical CT angiography. *Radiology.* 2005;235:274-281.

Remy-Jardin M, Louvegny S, Remy J, et al. Acute central thromboembolic disease: posttherapeutic follow-up with spiral CT angiography. *Radiology.* 1997;203:173.

Remy-Jardin M, Remy J, Artaud D, et al. Peripheral pulmonary arteries: optimization of the spiral CT acquisition protocol. *Radiology.* 1997;204:157-163.

Remy-Jardin M, Remy J, Artaud D, et al. Spiral CT of pulmonary embolism: technical considerations and interpretive pitfalls. *J Thorac Imaging.* 1997;12:103-117.

Resten A, Maître S, Humbert M, et al. Pulmonary arterial hypertension: thin-section CT predictors of epoprostenol therapy failure. *Radiology.* 2002;222:782-788.

Revel MP, Faivre JP, Remy-Jardin M, et al. Pulmonary hypertension: ECG-gated 64-section angiographic evaluation of new functional parameters as diagnostic criteria. *Radiology.* 2009;250:558-566.

Romero CS, Hernandez BL, Soler MJ, et al. Biochemical and cytologic characteristics of pleural effusions secondary to pulmonary embolism. *Chest.* 2002;121:465-469.

Ryu DS, Spirn PW, Trotman-Dickenson BEA. HRCT findings of proximal interruption of the right pulmonary artery. *J Thorac Imaging.* 2004;19:171-175.

Sanz J, Kuschnir P, Rius T, et al. Pulmonary arterial hypertension: noninvasive detection with phase-contrast MR imaging. *Radiology.* 2007;243:70-79.

Sbano H, Mitchell AW, Ind PW, et al. Peripheral pulmonary artery pseudoaneurysms and massive hemoptysis. *AJR Am J Roentgenol.* 2005;184:1253-1259.

Schneider G, Uder M, Koehler M, et al. MR angiography for detection of pulmonary arteriovenous malformations in patients with hereditary hemorrhagic telangiectasia. *AJR Am J Roentgenol.* 2008;190:892-901.

Schoepf UJ, Costello P. CT angiography for diagnosis of pulmonary embolism: state of the art. *Radiology.* 2004;230:329.

Schoepf UJ, Costello P. Multidetector-row CT imaging of pulmonary embolism. *Semin Roentgenol.* 2003;38:106.

Senbaklavaci O, Kaneko Y, Bartunek A, et al. Rupture and dissection in pulmonary artery aneurysms: incidence, cause, and treatment—review and case report. *J Thorac Cardiovasc Surg.* 2001;12:1006-1008.

Shepard JA, Moore EH, Templeton PA, et al. Pulmonary intravascular tumor emboli: dilated and beaded peripheral pulmonary arteries at CT. *Radiology.* 1993;187:797-801.

Sherrick AD, Swensen SJ, Hartman TE. Mosaic pattern of lung attenuation on CT scans: frequency among patients with pulmonary artery hypertension of different causes. *AJR Am J Roentgenol.* 1997;169:79-82.

Stein PD, Chenevert TL, Fowler SE, et al. Gadolinium-enhanced magnetic resonance angiography for pulmonary embolism: a multicenter prospective study (PIOPED III). *Ann Intern Med.* 2010;152:434-443.

Stone DN, Bein ME, Garris JB. Anomalous left pulmonary artery: two new adult cases. *AJR Am J Roentgenol.* 1980;135:1259-1263.

Tacelli N, Remy-Jardin M, Flohr T, et al. Dual-source chest CT angiography with high temporal resolution and high pitch modes: evaluation of image quality in 140 patients. *Eur Radiol.* 2010;20:1188-1196.

Tapson VF. Acute pulmonary embolism. *N Engl J Med.* 2008;358:1037-1052.

Tsai KL, Gupta E, Haramati LB. Pulmonary atelectasis: a frequent alternative diagnosis in patients undergoing CT-PA for suspected pulmonary embolism. *Emerg Radiol.* 2004;10:282-286.

Tunaci M, Ozkorkmaz B, Tunaci A, et al. CT findings of pulmonary artery aneurysms during treatment for Behçet's disease. *AJR Am J Roentgenol.* 1999;172:729-733.

van Gent MW, Post MC, Luermans JG, et al. Screening for pulmonary arteriovenous malformations using transthoracic contrast echocardiography: a prospective study. *Eur Respir J.* 2009;33:85-91.

Wittram C, Scott JA. 18F-FDG PET of pulmonary embolism. *AJR Am J Roentgenol.* 2007;189:171-176.

Yamaguchi T, Suzuki K, Asamura H, et al. Lung carcinoma with polypoid growth in the main pulmonary artery: report of two cases. *Jpn J Clin Oncol.* 2000;30:358-361.

Yi CA, Lee KS, Choe YH, et al. Computed tomography in pulmonary artery sarcoma: distinguishing features from pulmonary embolic disease. *J Comput Assist Tomogr.* 2004;28:34-39.

CHAPTER 43

Carotid and Vertebral Arteries

Jason M. Johnson, Anna Meader, David T. Hunt, and Javier M. Romero

Noninvasive imaging of the carotid and vertebral arteries is achieved with duplex ultrasonography, computed tomography angiography (CTA), and magnetic resonance angiography (MRA). This chapter focuses on pearls and pitfalls of these modalities in the evaluation of steno-occlusive disease of the carotid and vertebral arteries.

■ ULTRASONOGRAPHY

Justification

Carotid artery duplex ultrasonography is a noninvasive, affordable screening test that is devoid of radiation for patients at high risk for severe carotid disease, and hence at high risk for acute stroke. Duplex ultrasonography of the internal carotid arteries (ICAs) is indicated in several clinical settings, including patients who have experienced transient ischemic attacks, patients with ischemic stroke, and asymptomatic patients who possess cervical carotid bruits, and as a preoperative evaluation before coronary artery bypass graft surgery or aortic valve replacement.

Although carotid screening is not recommended for all coronary artery bypass graft surgery or aortic valve replacement candidates, patients over the age of 60 years or those presenting with a minimum of two cardiovascular risk factors, such as elevated cholesterol levels or hypertension, should undergo carotid evaluation to reduce the risk for perioperative stroke. Noninvasive carotid imaging is also important for those patients who have experienced transient ischemic attacks because of the significantly increased risk for stroke in the months following a transient ischemic attack. Approximately 20% to 30% of embolic strokes originate from the carotid arteries, and it is recommended that patients suffering from acute stroke also undergo carotid artery duplex ultrasonography to serve as a baseline for future evaluations. Although a carotid bruit in itself is neither a specific nor sensitive indication of carotid disease, it has been documented that up to one third of patients with bruits do have severe ICA stenosis. Therefore noninvasive duplex ultrasonography to assess the degree of carotid stenosis is important to determine those patients who will benefit the most from carotid artery revascularization.

Standard Evaluation

A standard carotid duplex ultrasonography consists of a bilateral examination of the common carotid arteries (CCAs), ICAs, external carotid arteries (ECAs), and the vertebral arteries (VAs).

Transverse grayscale images are typically obtained at the carotid artery bulb and carotid artery bifurcation, and in the case of any significant lesions, both grayscale images and color Doppler images are obtained in the transverse plane. Images in the longitudinal plane are obtained throughout the course of the CCA and ICA, ECA, and VA. Grayscale imaging is conducted separately from the spectral Doppler evaluation. Spectral Doppler waveforms are obtained with a defined technique; the waveforms should be obtained by placing the cursor in the longitudinal view of the artery with the cursor placed in the center of the stream of flow, the "flow jet." The recommended Doppler angle is between 40 and 60 degrees. Nine standardized sites are imaged: the proximal, middle, and distal CCA; the proximal, middle, and distal ICA; the proximal ECA; and the proximal and middle VA. According to the American College of Radiology and American Institute of Ultrasound in Medicine, blood-flow velocity measurements should be recorded at a minimum of one site in the CCA, ECA, and VA, and two sites in the ICA. If significant stenoses are detected, spectra should be sampled within and distal to each stenosis, with the highest velocity determined and recorded.

Normal Waveform Characteristics

Each vessel has a characteristic normal waveform pattern based on the vascular bed distal to the artery. The ICA demonstrates a low-resistance waveform with continuous forward flow throughout diastole; in contrast, the ECA displays a high-resistance waveform with a sharp systolic upstroke and decreased diastolic flow. Waveforms in the CCA are hybrids of the ICA and ECA waveforms, generally displaying a sharp systolic upstroke and continuous flow throughout the diastole. The VA in a healthy patient demonstrates a low-resistance waveform with continuous forward flow in the diastole. Changes in the waveforms of the VA are further discussed later.

Grayscale and color flow imaging and spectral Doppler evaluation provide the necessary tools to determine the severity of carotid stenosis. Multiple studies have defined significant carotid stenosis as greater than 70%. We use the guidelines listed in Table 43-1 at our laboratory to determine the degree of carotid artery stenosis.

Postoperative Evaluation

For those patients who have undergone carotid endarterectomy or stenting, subsequent follow-up should also be performed to assess for restenosis, occlusion, and development of intimal hyperplasia. Intimal hyperplasia is probably the most frequent complication after surgery and results secondary to operative trauma, usually peaking at 3 months post surgery. It generally does not progress after the first year and is characterized by scar tissue or redundant granulation. Intimal hyperplasia with smooth muscle cell and matrix accumulation is the prominent feature in all these situations. Primary carotid atheromatous disease is associated with intense cell proliferation and cell death without evidence of inflammation.

The evaluation of the revascularized carotid artery should be focused on the expected areas of surgical incision and clamping. For instance, the evaluation of the postendarterectomy carotid artery should be concentrated on the near wall, which is usually the area of carotid artery incision, and special attention should be paid to the distal portion of the ICA, where a clamp is usually placed and intraoperative inspection is often limited.

Principal Indications for Sequential Carotid Artery Studies

Although CTA and MRA are the tests of choice in the workup of acute ischemic events, radiation and cost limit these techniques for sequential follow-up of carotid artery lesions. Ultrasonography may be ideal for long-term follow-up of patients at high risk for atheromatous disease of the carotid arteries and postsurgical complications.

Sequential carotid artery imaging is suggested for the following:
- To assess for progression of carotid artery stenosis caused by atheromatous disease
- To monitor the revascularized carotid artery for evidence of intimal hyperplasia or recurrent atheromatous disease
- To evaluate dissected carotid arteries for evidence of progression or resolution of occlusive process

Carotid Artery Duplex Ultrasonography Pitfalls

Problems occurring with carotid artery duplex ultrasonography may be divided into three general groups: technical pitfalls, limitations of the technology, and interpretation pitfalls.

Technical Pitfalls
Technical pitfalls include equipment difficulties such as choosing the correct probe according to patient body habitus and selecting appropriate imaging parameters (pulse repetition frequency [PRF], color gain, filters, speckle-reduction software) for the highest diagnostic image quality.

APPROPRIATE TRANSDUCER
As the Doppler beam propagates through tissues, its intensity decreases with increasing penetration in a process referred to as attenuation. Although attenuation is quite high for muscle and skin, in fluid-filled structures such as the carotid arteries, attenuation is very low. Higher frequencies in duplex ultrasonography typically offer improved image resolution. A 7- to 9-MHz probe is the most commonly used and is appropriate for most patients; however, in a patient with a large body habitus or in a patient with deep vessels, a 5-MHz probe will allow for greater penetration. In a patient with very superficial vessels, a higher frequency transducer such as a 10- or 12-MHz probe may be more appropriate.

ANGLE OF INSONATION
The angle of insonation must be considered when performing and interpreting carotid ultrasonography. If the

Table 43-1 Guidelines for Determining Degree of Vessel Stenosis in Carotid Duplex Ultrasonography

Degree of Stenosis	Peak Systolic Velocity (cm/sec)	Approximate Degree of Stenosis (%)	Luminal Diameter (mm)	Other Indirect Signs
Normal limits	<150	<50	>3	
Mild	150-200	50-60	2.5-3	
Moderate	200-300	60-70	2-2.5	
Severe	300-400	70-80	1-2	Reversal flow ipsilateral ACA (TCD)
Critical	>400	80-90	0.7-1	Reversal flow ophthalmic artery (TCD)
	Falling off	>90	<0.7	MRA shows absent distal ICA signal (slow flow versus occlusion); consider CTA

Modified from the Neurovascular Laboratory, Massachusetts General Hospital, Boston, Mass.
ACA, Anterior cerebral artery A1 segment; *CTA,* computed tomography angiography; *ICA,* internal carotid artery; *MRA,* magnetic resonance angiography; *TCD,* transcranial Doppler ultrasonography.

correct angle is used, the sampling cursor will be parallel to the vessel wall. The recommended Doppler angle is between 40 and 60 degrees; an angle that is too low or too high results in inaccurate insonated peak systolic velocities. Tortuous vessels can be especially difficult to insonate; keeping the angle between 40 and 60 degrees may at times be impossible. In cases in which the vessel "dives deeply," using an angle of zero degrees may be the most appropriate. Because of the inherent difficulty in placing the Doppler probe, velocities are often overestimated secondary to vessel tortuosity. When interpreting the degree of stenosis in a tortuous vessel, it is important to note that although peak systolic velocities may be consistent with stenosis, velocities may also be simply overestimated because of the limitations of the Doppler angle. As always, the best angle to use is one in which the cursor is parallel to the vessel wall and located in the middle of the flow jet.

LUMINAL ECHO (REVERBERATION ARTIFACT)
The reverberation artifact results from the differences in impedances of two different objects. In the context of the carotid artery, these two materials are the near wall of the carotid artery and a small carotid plaque or a calcified nodule within the soft tissue of the neck. When the transducer scans to the left or right of the high-impedance object, in this case the plaque or calcified nodule, the normal image of the top surface of this object is displayed over the image of the object below, in this case the carotid artery wall. If the impedance differences are of the proper magnitude when the transducer is above the object, the ultrasound pulse will reflect back and forth several times between the top and bottom surfaces. This gives rise to a series of echoes, equally spaced in dimension, received by the transducer. This appears on the grayscale images as a series of lines within the carotid lumen that may be mistaken for a dissection with an intraluminal flap.

The correction for this artifact is usually dynamic and is easily discovered; when changes in the angle of insonation are performed and the luminal echo disappears or changes in location, this is consistent with reverberation artifact.

MIRROR IMAGE ARTIFACT
The mirror image artifact is usually present when the ultrasonic beam of insonation intersects within the oblique surface and the echoes from this oblique surface do not return to the transducer. The time elapsed for these echoes from the oblique structure is longer than for those that are perpendicular; however, they may be interpreted as deeper given the time difference. The resulting artifact is an image that displays a mirror image at an artifactual depth compared to the true surface. The simplest correction for this artifact is again dynamic imaging; mirror image artifact is easily discovered when changes to the angle of insonation are performed.

EXCESSIVE COLOR GAIN
Excessive color gain results in overestimation of the residual lumen given that the increased color gain surpasses and covers the boundaries of the stenosis and

vessel (Fig. 43-1). This prevents accurate assessment of plaque composition and thickness. Appropriate color gain is especially important in the imaging of a carotid dissection involving the intima, when excessive color gain artifact may overshadow an intimal flap. Narrowing of the vessel lumen diameter should be evaluated based on the peak systolic velocities and not solely on color flow or grayscale imaging.

APPROPRIATE PULSE REPETITION FREQUENCY
In the case of a carotid pseudo-occlusion (hairline lumen), it is especially important that an appropriate PRF is used in the insonation of the vessel. In a typical hairline lumen, pseudonormalization will be observed, and in such a "slow-flow" situation, a PRF between 10 and 40 is typically most appropriate. A PRF below 10 will result in excess color artifact (Fig. 43-2); this could potentially resemble color flow within the vessel, which could be misconstrued as normal carotid flow. A PRF above 40 will likely diminish all low-level flow, and images could be misinterpreted as true arterial occlusion.

Limitations of the Technology
Limitations of the technology include physical limitations such as the inability to insonate the CCA origin or the ICA at the skull base, as well as flow limitations, as seen during the imaging of ICA tandem lesions.

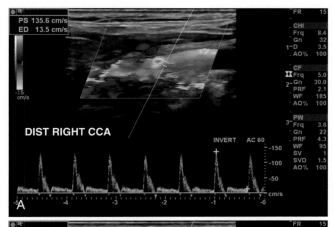

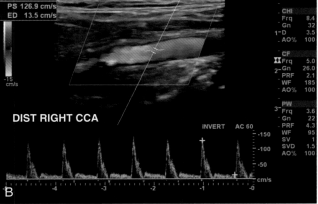

Figure 43-1 A, Normal vessel insonated with excessive color gain. Note that the color flow exceeds the boundaries of the vessel wall. **B,** After correction. *CCA,* Common carotid artery.

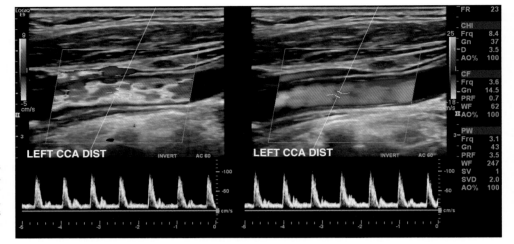

Figure 43-2 Comparison images of a healthy vessel. *Left,* Image is insonated with a low pulse repetition frequency (PRF), resulting in excess color artifact. *Right,* Image is insonated with an appropriate PRF. *CCA,* Common carotid artery.

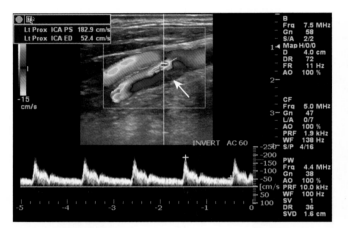

Figure 43-3 A large hypoechoic plaque *(arrow)* in the internal carotid artery correctly insonated using color flow Doppler.

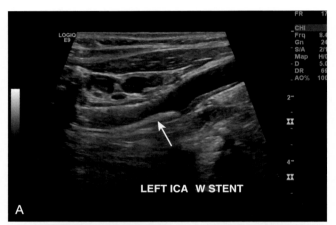

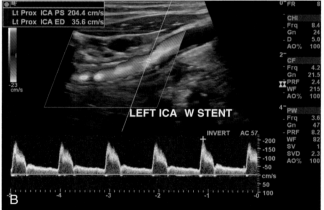

Figure 43-4 Imaging of internal carotid artery stent *(arrow in A).* The stent is seen as linear echogenic focus along the inner surface of the internal carotid artery. Color Doppler evaluation (**B**) shows flow through the stent, suggesting patent stent.

B-MODE (GRAYSCALE) ULTRASONOGRAPHY

B-mode alone is not a reliable measure of the degree of stenosis in the carotid arteries. Although B-mode is useful in determining plaque location, composition, and length, dense hypoechoic plaque is not well identified on B-mode alone (Figs. 43-3 and 43-4); the use of color flow is necessary to demonstrate hemodynamic significance. Peak systolic velocities should be used to determine the degree of stenosis.

HEAVILY CALCIFIED PLAQUE

Heavily calcified plaque impedes Doppler measurements of the underlying vessel. This limitation is of great importance when a calcified plaque extends greater than 1 cm down the course of the vessel; such lesions cannot be thoroughly imaged using duplex ultrasonography, and distal Doppler measurements are not reliable to infer the degree of proximal stenosis. MRA and dual energy CTA with calcium removal are useful to evaluate these segments.

TANDEM LESIONS

Tandem lesions in the carotid arteries are defined as two separate stenoses occurring at least 3 cm apart, resulting in a severe stenosis of the vessel. The second lesion, located downstream from the insonated lesion, causes dampening of the peak systolic velocity between the two lesions. This phenomenon is secondary to increased pulse pressure between the two lesions, which eliminates the pressure gradient necessary to increase velocities immediately distal to the initial lesion. In this situation,

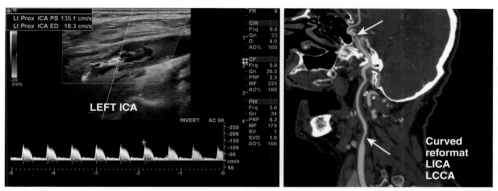

Figure 43-5 The internal carotid artery (ICA) of a patient with tandem lesions imaged using duplex ultrasonography, juxtaposed with the patient's computed tomography angiogram (CTA). Note that the duplex ultrasonography image does not display elevated velocities despite heavy calcification and hypoechoic plaque. The CTA demonstrates stenotic lesions (arrows) at the origin and distal cervical right ICA.

although B-mode imaging is consistent with a severe stenosis, velocities and spectral configuration of flow of the poststenotic segment (between the two lesions) remain within normal or slightly abnormal limits (Fig. 43-5). It is the stenosis with the greatest narrowing that determines the hemodynamic compromise. When tandem lesions are suspected because of the discrepancy between the B-mode images and Doppler flow, CTA or contrast-enhanced MRA or conventional angiography of the neck should be used for a definitive diagnosis.

ANATOMIC LIMITATIONS

Carotid duplex ultrasonography is limited in its ability to evaluate the entire ICA. The distal ICA, defined as the ICA at the skull base, cannot be imaged with duplex ultrasonography because of anatomic limitation. The presence or absence of stenosis in this vessel segment must be determined by MRA or CTA. However, changes in the proximal ICA waveforms can provide clues about the presence of stenosis distal to the area of insonation in this specific scenario. High-resistance waveforms demonstrating sharp systolic upstrokes are suggestive of a more distal stenosis of the ICA, likely in the intracranial portion, when not visualized in the area of sampling (Fig. 43-6).

Alternatively, delayed systolic upstrokes and low peak systolic velocities noted throughout the course of the ICA are suggestive of more proximal stenosis at the ICA origin, in the bulb, or in the more proximal CCA. Similarly, the CCA origin cannot be insonated secondary to anatomic limitations; however, changes in the CCA waveform are useful in determining the presence of more proximal stenosis. Again, delayed systolic upstrokes and low peak systolic velocities are suggestive of a more proximal stenosis, either of the aorta or at the CCA origin, whereas highly resistant waveforms with sharp systolic upstrokes are suggestive of severe distal stenosis within the ICA. Tandem lesions could also be considered an anatomic limitation for ultrasound coverage.

Interpretation Pitfalls

INTERNAL CAROTID ARTERY VERSUS EXTERNAL CAROTID ARTERY

During interpretation it is essential that the ICA and ECA are correctly identified. The worst-case scenario is

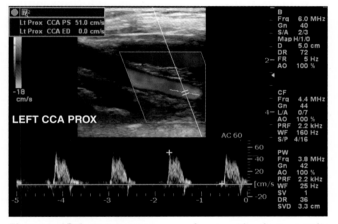

Figure 43-6 High-resistance waveforms with sharp systolic upstrokes insonated in the common carotid artery (CCA) secondary to ipsilateral internal carotid artery occlusion.

that the two vessels are confused, and a patient with severe stenosis is recommended for carotid revascularization, only to find out that the diseased vessel is an ECA. There are four anatomic and waveform patterns that help distinguish the ECA from the ICA. It is important that during the course of carotid duplex ultrasonography the sonographer uses a temporal tap to prove that the vessel being insonated is an ECA; an ECA will respond to a temporal tap, whereas the ICA will not. In addition, the ECA may have visible branches and will most likely be located medial to the ICA. Lastly, as previously discussed, the ECA will demonstrate high-resistance waveforms, whereas the ICA demonstrates low-resistant waveforms.

PSEUDO-OCCLUSION VERSUS COMPLETE OCCLUSION OF THE INTERNAL CAROTID ARTERY

Vessel occlusion is indicated by lack of Doppler shift within the vessel lumen; however, very slow flow may not be detected during routine examination. Routine duplex ultrasonography may be insensitive to such low velocities. Carotid duplex ultrasonography displays a sensitivity of 80% to 90% for detecting hairline lumina when correct parameters are followed (Fig. 43-7); technique should be optimized by placing the Doppler signal in the ghost vessel while increasing color gain to the maximum level and decreasing filters and PRF. When there is clinical suspicion for ICA or CCA occlusion with duplex ultrasonography, CTA may be required for a definitive diagnosis, although conventional catheter angiography remains the standard for accurately determining between true occlusion and pseudo-occlusion/residual hairline lumen.

VELOCITIES FALLING OFF

In general, as the vessel lumen diameter decreases and the degree of stenosis increases, peak systolic velocities within or just distal to the lesion will correspondingly increase because of elevation of the pressure gradient. Vessels demonstrating a critical stenosis of more than 99% may display a sudden decrease in velocity, which is referred to as "velocities falling off," or pseudonormalization. Pseudonormalization results in a decrease in peak systolic velocities into a range associated with less-severe stenosis or absence of stenosis. If velocities alone are considered in a description of vessel health, pseudonormalization is problematic in that it may lead to an inaccurate description of vessel stenosis; in extreme cases there is the risk for a severely stenotic vessel being overlooked. To ensure that a diseased vessel does not go unnoticed, other factors must be considered as indications of pseudonormalization, such as turbulent flow, a pinpoint residual lumen on color flow images in either the longitudinal or transverse plane, dampening of the distal vessel waveform, and spectral broadening found in the presence of "normal" velocities. Transcranial Doppler ultrasonography may also be used when pseudonormalization is suspected. Indirect signs of collateral circulation may be found; for example, retrograde flow in an ophthalmic artery is consistent with a severe stenosis or occlusion of the ipsilateral CCA or ICA.

HEMODYNAMIC CHANGES SECONDARY TO A CONTRALATERAL OCCLUSION OR HIGH-DEGREE STENOSIS

Often when an ICA is occluded or demonstrates a severe stenosis, elevated peak systolic velocities are noted in the contralateral vessel. These elevated velocities reflect hemodynamic changes in the healthy vessel secondary to the contralateral occlusion and are not representative of stenosis (Fig. 43-8). Collateral flow should be suspected when elevated velocities are noted but no lesion is noted on B-mode and color Doppler ultrasonography. This increase of velocity is a reflection of compensatory collateral flow in the contralateral vessel to supply the cerebral hemisphere with the diseased vessel via the circle of Willis.

INTERNALIZED EXTERNAL CAROTID ARTERY

When an ICA is occluded or demonstrates very slow flow consistent with a hairline lumen, flow in the ipsilateral ECA may also demonstrate hemodynamic changes. It is not uncommon for the waveforms in the ECA to demonstrate increased diastolic flow and lower resistance; this is referred to as internalization of the ECA. This phenomenon is also secondary to compensatory collateral flow through an internal maxillary artery–ophthalmic artery–distal ICA anastomosis. This abnormality is usually identified with chronic critical stenosis or complete occlusion of the ICA. Based on this change of blood flow direction, transcranial Doppler ultrasonography is able to detect retrograde flow within the ophthalmic artery. These indirect findings can prove extremely helpful in the evaluation of suspected severe ICA disease.

CAROTID OR VERTEBRAL ARTERY DISSECTION

The incidence of spontaneous carotid artery dissection is approximately 2.6 to 2.9 per 100,000. Spontaneous carotid artery dissection carries significant risk for embolic strokes, secondary to the thrombogenic

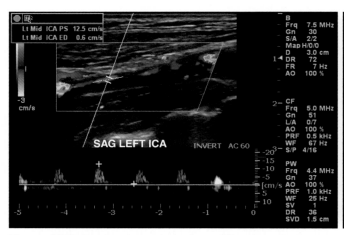

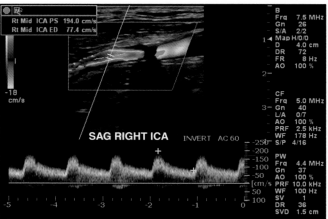

Figure 43-7 Despite a hypoechoic plaque filling the entire lumen on B-mode, Doppler insonation of the left internal carotid artery (ICA) displays minimal color flow and tardus parvus waveforms with velocities falling off, consistent with a hairline lumen.

Figure 43-8 Increased velocities are noted in the right internal carotid artery (ICA), likely representing collateral flow secondary to the hairline lumen noted in the left internal carotid artery.

nature of the injured vessel where a tear within the endothelium results in the release of thrombogenic factors by the damaged intima to promote thrombus formation. However, spontaneous ICA dissection usually occurs at the level of the skull base, which is distal to and likely out of the anatomic scope of duplex ultrasonography. For these cases an evaluation of the entire course of the ICA with CTA or MRA is recommended. A diagnosis of spontaneous dissection is usually supported with axial fat-saturated T1-weighted images of the neck demonstrating the intramural clot as a hyperintense intravascular lesion.

Traumatic carotid artery dissection is one of the most feared complications of craniocervical trauma. This category of dissection may likely be evaluated by duplex ultrasonography, given that the trauma is usually at the level of the exposed cervical segment. Ultrasonography is also the elected modality when direct arterial punctures are suspected after intended venous approach for central line placement. B-mode allows for imaging of the endothelial flap, likely representing the dissection (Fig. 43-9), whereas hemodynamic significance may be determined via pulsed wave Doppler. While imaging a carotid dissection in the longitudinal plane, the false lumen created by the entry of blood into the vessel wall should be insonated; unless occluded by thrombus, flow in the lumen will demonstrate high-resistance flow (Fig. 43-10). Dissection should be considered if a smooth tapering stenosis is noted in the ICA of a patient who demonstrates no other atheromatous disease. Occasionally the ICA may appear normal; however, an increase in the resistance of the waveform should alert one to the possibility of dissection.

CAROTID BODY TUMOR

Carotid body tumors are a specific type of paragangliomas with an incidence of approximately 0.012%. They originate from epithelial cells derived from the neural crest of the carotid bifurcation. These lesions, despite a slow growth rate, frequently become symptomatic through local carotid compression and mass effect. Although these are benign lesions, carotid body tumors

may progressively enlarge and can involve the arterial wall and neighboring cranial nerves. (Fig. 43-11).

The normal carotid body is a small mass of neurovascular tissue located bilaterally in the medial valley of the carotid artery bifurcation. The fetal carotid body develops within the arterial wall between the medial and adventitial layers. The carotid body is a minute conglomerate of cells 1.5 mm in diameter located on the posterior aspect of the carotid bifurcation. The blood supply is mostly via a small vessel from the carotid bifurcation and branches of the ECA.

Afferent branches of the glossopharyngeal nerve, vagus nerve, and the cervical sympathetic ganglia innervate the carotid body. As a carotid body tumor enlarges, it may lead to cranial nerve palsies, including paralysis of the hypoglossal, glossopharyngeal, recurrent laryngeal, spinal accessory nerve, or the sympathetic chain. Carotid body tumors may therefore be associated with pain, hoarseness, dysphagia, Horner syndrome, or shoulder drop.

Bilateral carotid body tumors are uncommon but occur more frequently in familial cases. The prevalence of local recurrence and local invasion is estimated at about 10% for carotid body tumors. Surgical removal of carotid body tumors is regarded as the only curative option.

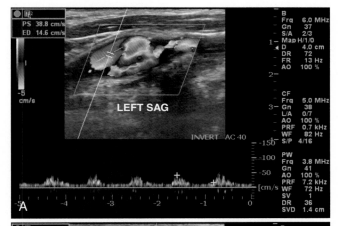

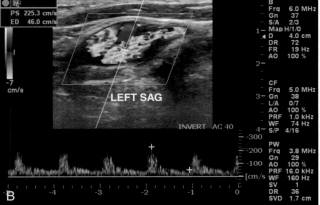

Figure 43-10 A, High-resistance waveforms with low peak systolic velocities noted in the false lumen created by an internal carotid artery dissection. **B,** Elevated velocities and turbulent blood flow in the true lumen.

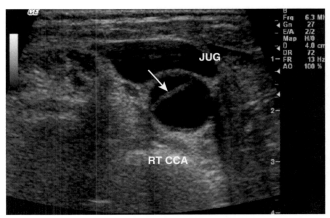

Figure 43-9 An intimal flap *(arrow)* noted in a transverse view of the common carotid artery (CCA).

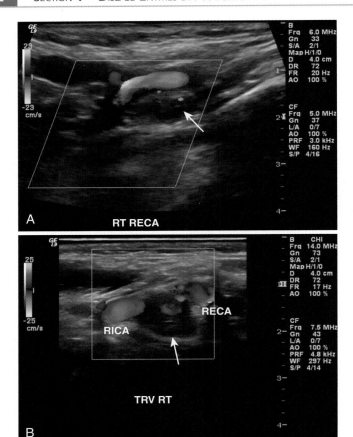

Figure 43-11 Longitudinal (**A**) and transverse (**B**) insonations of a carotid body tumor (*arrow*).

CHANGES OF THE VERTEBRAL ARTERY WAVEFORMS

Changes in the waveforms of the VA are especially important to note, because they can be not only indicative of stenosis of the VA but also suggestive of subclavian artery stenosis. The VA origin is the most commonly stenosed segment of the extracranial vessel; the segment of the VA distal to the stenosis demonstrates delayed systolic upstrokes. If the occlusion of the VA is at the origin, usually no flow will be seen within the cervical segment and multiple collateral cervical vessels are visualized. Stenosis in the cervical section is much less common; if severely elevated velocities are noted, one should consider VA dissection or severe atheromatous disease as a possibility. The intracranial segment of the VA is also a common location for atheromatous disease; insonation of the cervical segment in this case will reveal high-resistance waveforms with sharp systolic upstrokes. A challenging diagnosis of exclusion for high-resistance waveforms within the VA is hypoplastic VAs. These vessels are congenitally small, measuring less than 3 mm in diameter, and also have decreased peak systolic and diastolic velocities.

Bilateral elevation of velocities within the VAs may be present; technical thoroughness requires insonation of each of the VAs at multiple levels to confirm that the elevation is diffuse and not solely focal. Diffusely elevated velocities within the VAs is often a sign of severe stenosis

of the ICAs bilaterally (anterior circulation) and likely represents collateral flow supply via hyperperfusion of the VAs and the vertebrobasilar system.

The ipsilateral subclavian artery should be insonated when retrograde flow is noted in a VA, or when a systolic notch is noted in the VA waveforms, because these changes are suggestive of subclavian stenosis. There are four types of subclavian steal phenomena (Fig. 43-12), each with its own subtle characteristic changes in the ipsilateral VA. The characteristic waveforms are defined by the ratio of flow velocity at the midsystolic notch to flow velocity at end diastole, with a higher ratio suggesting a more advanced steal phenomenon. A mild notch between systolic peaks characterizes the most mild form of the subclavian steal phenomenon, type I. As the degree of steal increases, the severity of the systolic notch increases; a type II steal demonstrates a more pronounced systolic notch, and a type III steal is characterized by a systolic notch extending to or slightly below baseline, although forward flow resumes before diastole. In the most severe subclavian steal phenomenon, type IV, flow in the ipsilateral VA is completely retrograde.

Changes in the waveforms of the subclavian artery may also be suggestive of subclavian stenosis. A healthy subclavian artery demonstrates triphasic flow, with end-systolic flow in the retrograde direction before returning to the forward direction in diastole. In a subclavian artery demonstrating a greater than 50% stenosis, waveforms in the subclavian artery will generally be monophasic, occurring only above the baseline. In addition, in a subclavian artery with a segment of greater than 50% stenosis, multiple insonations along the course of the vessel will reveal that the area of stenosis displays velocities at least double of those velocities in the healthy proximal vessel segment.

INTIMA-MEDIA THICKNESS

Patients with increased thickness of the intima-media layer of the carotid artery present not only a higher incidence of myocardial infarction but also a higher incidence of stroke. With a carotid intima-media thickness increase of 0.1 mm, the future risk for myocardial infarction increases by 10% to 15%, and the stroke risk increases by 13% to 18%. B-mode imaging may be used to determine both the carotid intimal and medial thickness (Fig. 43-13). The advantages of using carotid duplex ultrasonography are that it is both a reproducible and an economical method and has the benefit of being an easily accessible measure of intima-media thickness.

INTIMAL HYPERPLASIA

Intimal hyperplasia, as previously discussed, is a result of vessel trauma following carotid endarterectomy. Because of the risk for intimal hyperplasia, it is recommended that carotid endarterectomy patients receive sequential followup with duplex ultrasonography following carotid revascularization. Increased thickness of the vessel wall results in increased peak systolic velocities in the affected vessel; follow-up examinations should be compared to assess the severity of intimal hyperplasia or restenosis.

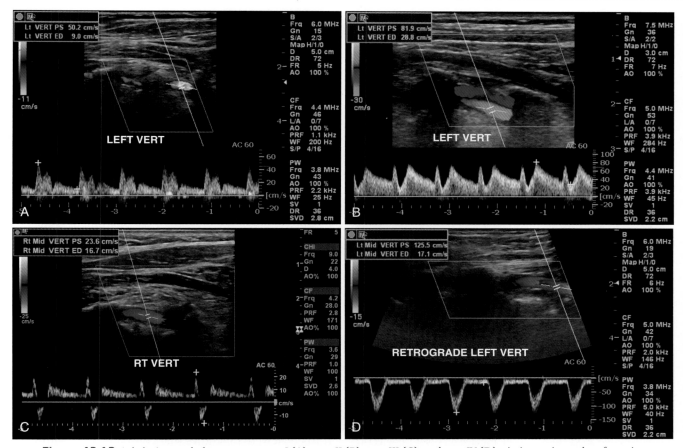

Figure 43-12 Subclavian steal phenomena—type I (**A**), type II (**B**), type III (**C**), and type IV (**D**)—in increasing order of severity.

CAROTID ARTERY PSEUDOANEURYSM

Although aneurysms or pseudoaneurysms of the carotid arteries are rare, carotid duplex ultrasonography is often requested following a failed venous access or a direct penetrating injury to rule out aneurysm or pseudoaneurysm. The diagnostic suspicion increases when a pulsatile mass or enlarging mass is noted after a cervical procedure. Aneurysms are present in approximately one third of carotid artery dissections. Because the walls of aneurysms that form as a result of a subadventitial dissection contain vessel wall structures, the term *dissecting aneurysm* is more appropriate than *pseudoaneurysm*. Dissecting aneurysms are most often treated surgically.

■ COMPUTED TOMOGRAPHY ANGIOGRAPHY

CTA is a widely available imaging modality; its major strengths are high-resolution imaging, minimal to no invasiveness, and quick acquisition times. This technique has major advantages over other modalities in the detection of arteriovenous malformations, aneurysms, stenosis, and occlusions in the arteries of the neck and head in patients with symptoms related to stroke given its high vascular resolution. The development of multidetector CT has made CTA a viable imaging modality for assessment of the intracranial and extracranial vasculature in the emergency department.

Technique

The technical details pertain to that practiced at our institution. Initially a standard noncontrast CT is performed with a 64-detector CT scanner using 120 kVp, 170 mA, 2-second scan time, and 5-mm slice thickness. The extent of the scan ranges from the skull base to the vertex. Contiguous axial slices parallel to the inferior orbitomeatal line are obtained. This is followed by CTA using a helical scan technique. Images are acquired after a single bolus injection of 90 to 120 mL of nonionic contrast material into an antecubital vein at 3 to 4 mL/second and a scan delay of approximately 20 to 25 seconds from the start of the contrast material injection to the start of image acquisition. The scan extends from the upper chest to the centrum semiovale or vertex with a scan field of view of 25.0 cm. Other technical parameters are as follows: 140 kVp; 170 mA; table speed 3.75 mm/second; detector thickness of 0.625 mm and 1 second gantry rotation time. Source images are reconstructed to 1.25-mm slice thickness at 0.625-mm intervals.

Safety

CTA is a noninvasive to minimally invasive procedure. The administration of intravenous nonionic iodinated contrast material in patients with stroke has demonstrated no immediate adverse reactions in a large series

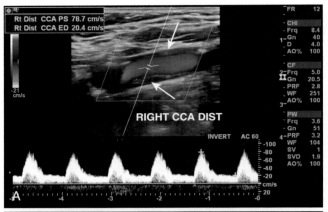

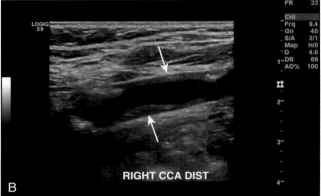

Figure 43-13 Intima-media thickening *(arrows)* of the distal right common carotid artery (CCA) is demonstrated on Color Doppler **(A)** and grayscale ultrasonography **(B)**.

of patients. Historically, contrast material–associated concerns were related to the administration of ionic contrast material. The clinical and experimental administration of nonionic contrast material has been demonstrated not to worsen the symptoms of stroke or to enlarge brain infarction volumes.

Recent publications have evaluated the utility of decreasing the volume of the contrast material and kilovolts peak required to achieve diagnostic-quality images to reduce the risks for nephrotoxicity and radiation-induced skin changes. Bahner et al demonstrated improved signal-to-noise ratio of the intracranial vessels at 80 kVp compared to 120 kVp despite an increased image noise at 80 kVp. Multiphasic injection method with decreased contrast material volume for uniform prolonged vascular enhancement at CTA has also been experimented with to reduce nephrotoxicity without deteriorating vessel enhancement.

Assessment of Major Vessel Occlusion

CTA demonstrates excellent sensitivity and specificity in the assessment of large vessel occlusion compared with other noninvasive techniques such as MRA and transcranial Doppler ultrasonography. Compared to the gold standard of conventional angiogram for the detection of large vessel occlusion, Lev et al demonstrated a sensitivity and specificity of 98.4% and 98.1%, respectively, for CTA (Figs. 43-14 and 43-15). A meta-analysis on diagnostic accuracy of CTA for the assessment of carotid stenosis reviewed 28 studies that compared CTA with DSA and found similar results. CTA was found to be highly accurate for diagnosing the degree of carotid occlusion, with an overall sensitivity of 97% and specificity of 99%.

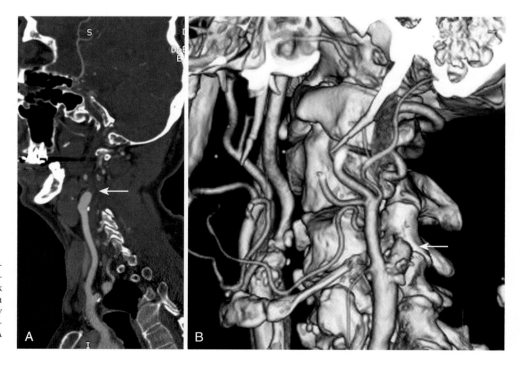

Figure 43-14 A, Curved reformation from computed tomography angiography (CTA) of the neck demonstrates a proximal occlusion of the left internal carotid artery (ICA; *arrow*). **B,** Volume rendering of the CTA shows the left ICA occlusion *(arrow)*.

For severe stenoses (70–99% range), CTA was found to be reliable, with sensitivity of 85% and specificity of 93%. Measurement of residual lumen diameter by CTA compares favorably to digital subtraction angiography (DSA), MRA, and ultrasonography.

Novel postprocessing algorithms have improved the visualization of stented carotid arteries, which has traditionally been a weakness of CTA (Fig. 43-16). In addition, CTA is significantly more sensitive and specific in the detection of basilar artery patency in patients with clinical symptoms of basilar artery ischemia compared to Doppler ultrasonography. CTA not only demonstrates the exact site of occlusion or stenosis but also provides information on the length of basilar artery occlusion and collateral pathways (Figs. 43-17 and 43-18).

Transcranial Doppler ultrasonography has also been compared to CTA in the evaluation of middle cerebral artery stenosis; a small review demonstrates that abnormal transcranial Doppler results are highly suggestive of MCA stenosis. However, normal transcranial Doppler findings do not exclude MCA stenosis, especially in patients with distal M1 or M2 segment disease (Fig. 43-19). A systematic review of the literature demonstrates a high degree of accuracy of CTA in the detection of ICA occlusion and distinction with hairline residual lumen. For detection of an ICA occlusion the sensitivity and specificity is 97% (95% confidence interval [CI], 93% to 99%) and 99% (95% CI, 98% to 100%), respectively.

Limitations

CTA is limited in demonstrating distal branch occlusion, compared to conventional angiogram. Smaller, M3 branch occlusions are difficult to visualize; however, these abnormalities are still more readily detected than with other noninvasive modalities.

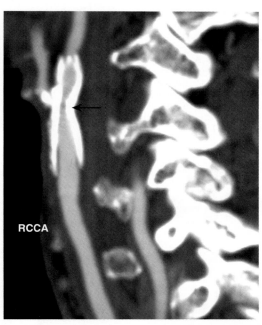

Figure 43-16 Curved reformat from computed tomography angiography of the neck demonstrates a stent extending from the distal right common carotid artery (RCCA) to the proximal right internal carotid artery. There is a midstent failure with moderate narrowing *(arrow)* of the lumen.

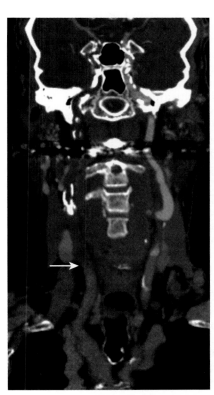

Figure 43-15 Computed tomography angiography of the neck demonstrates a proximal occlusion of the right common carotid artery *(arrow)*.

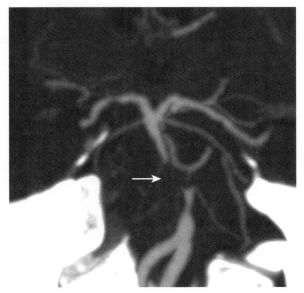

Figure 43-17 Maximum intensity projection reformat of computed tomography angiography of the posterior fossa demonstrates a mid basilar artery occlusion *(arrow)*.

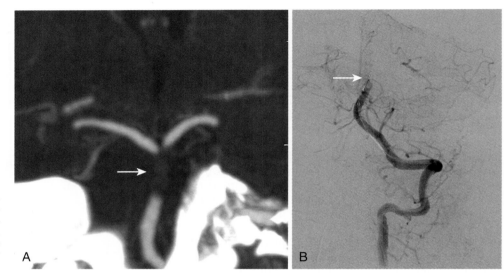

Figure 43-18 A, Computed tomography angiography demonstrates occlusion *(arrow)* of mid basilar artery. **B,** Conventional catheter angiogram in the same patient confirms the site of basiliar artery occlusion *(arrow)*.

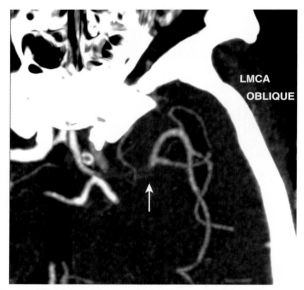

Figure 43-19 Computed tomography angiography shows a proximal *(arrow)* occlusion of the left middle cerebral artery (LMCA).

■ MAGNETIC RESONANCE ANGIOGRAPHY

MRA is a safe, convenient, and noninvasive screening tool for carotid artery stenosis. Duplex ultrasonography, CTA, and MRA all show similar accuracy in the diagnosis of symptomatic carotid artery stenosis; however, contrast-enhanced MRA (CE-MRA) appears to be the most accurate noninvasive modality and is regarded by some as the noninvasive gold standard for assessing ICA narrowing. However, in some centers, because MRA is not as accessible as ultrasonography or CTA, it is not the imaging method of choice. Although no single technique is currently accurate enough to replace DSA, two noninvasive techniques in combination, with a third one performed if the first two disagree, appear to improve accuracy over a single technique. In patients for

whom duplex ultrasonography and CE-MRA are discordant, CTA is an appropriate troubleshooter.

Technique

Unenhanced MRA is frequently used to evaluate the carotid vasculature and is usually performed as a time of flight (TOF) or phase contrast flow-sensitive imaging, which can be either a two-dimensional (2-D) or 3-D volumetric acquisition (Fig. 43-20). Although these methods have the benefit of no contrast material administration, there are issues with the diagnostic quality of this technique, particularly in the setting of pulsation artifact (e.g., from the aorta), diminutive vessels, or slow flow. These sequences are also vulnerable to signal-intensity dropout artifacts in the stenotic vascular segments, which can cause issues with distinguishing near from total occlusion. In general, unenhanced TOF MRA has the same diagnostic accuracy as that of CTA when compared to DSA but has a tendency to overestimate the degree of stenosis.

The addition of intravenous gadolinium for CE-MRA helps to overcome the limitations seen with unenhanced MRA; however, it also adds to the cost and complexity of imaging. CE-MRA is increasingly used for evaluation of the carotid and vertebral arteries because of high sensitivity and specificity compared with DSA. CE-MRA is an attractive imaging option when used as a complementary modality to duplex ultrasonography, by enhancing the already high sensitivity/specificity and cost-effectiveness of duplex ultrasonography. CE-MRA is superior to 2-D TOF MRA in visualizing long-segment carotid artery morphologic and anatomic characteristics. For screening and identification of patients with greater than 70% ICA stenosis, however, CE-MRA does not offer significant advantages over 2-D TOF MRA (Fig. 43-21).

Contrast-enhanced and unenhanced MRA acquisitions can be viewed as a series of images or reconstructed in a variety of maximum intensity projection formats. Lesion detection is typically maximized using

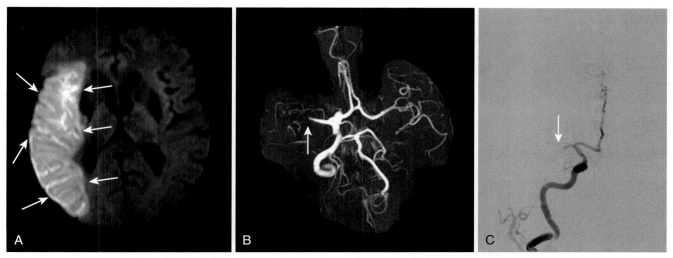

Figure 43-20 A, Magnetic resonance imaging of the brain. Diffusion-weighted image demonstrates a large area *(arrows)* of restricted diffusion in the right middle cerebral artery territory, likely representing an acute infarction. **B,** Magnetic resonance angiography of the same patient performed with three-dimensional time of flight of the circle of Willis shows a proximal occlusion *(arrow)* of the proximal right middle cerebral artery. **C,** Conventional catheter angiogram confirms the site of the occlusion *(arrow)*.

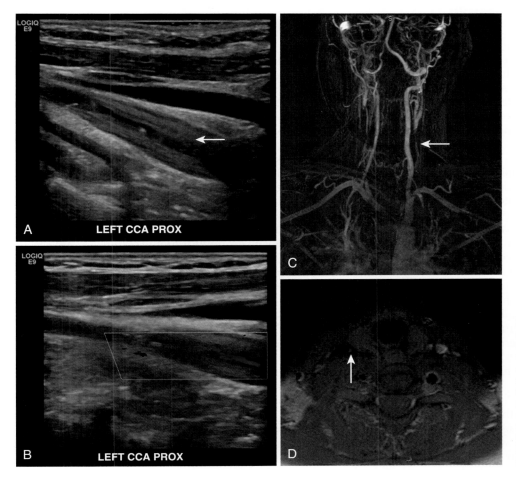

Figure 43-21 A and **B,** Carotid ultrasonography demonstrates thickening *(arrow)* of the carotid wall, likely the intima-media layer of the proximal common carotid artery (CCA), probably representing a large vessel arteritis. **C** and **D,** Magnetic resonance angiography of the neck demonstrates multiple areas of decreased flow or no flow *(arrows)* in the carotid arteries bilaterally, likely representing a diffuse large vessel vasculitis.

a combined review of "raw" data and maximum intensity projection reformations. Several different methods have been used for measuring the degree of stenosis: North American Symptomatic Carotid Endarterectomy Trial (NASCET), European Carotid Surgery Trial, and minimal residual lumen size. When comparing these methods for CE-MRA and DSA, the NASCET criteria performed most consistently between the examinations and therefore is the standard method of assessing CE-MRA images.

Safety

The major safety issues related to MRA include contra-indications to gadolinium-based contrast materials and general magnetic resonance imaging (MRI) contraindications, including metallic foreign bodies, claustrophobia, and patient issues related to remaining motionless during the imaging procedure. Contraindications to gadolinium-based contrast materials include a history of anaphylactic reaction upon prior administration and renal failure. The concern for patients with poor renal function is a reaction called nephrogenic systemic fibrosis, which is exclusively seen in patients with glomerular filtration rate of less than 15 mL/minute/1.73 m^2. At our institution, patients in acute or chronic renal insufficiency with glomerular filtration rate of less than 30 mL/minute/1.73 m^2 must receive clearance from the nephrology department before receiving gadolinium-based contrast materials. In these cases the diagnostic information must be considered essential and not available from non–contrast-enhanced MRI.

Limitations and Interpretation Pitfalls

MRA has limitations, most notably flow-related signal dropout in regions of turbulence or vortex flow. Although CE-MRA may improve flow-related enhancement, turbulence (see Fig. 43-21, *C*) and susceptibility effects from metallic stents, subclavian steal (and other high-flow shunts), motion, and metal continue to be limiting factors in the assessment of carotid artery stenosis.

Stents

MRI in the presence of metallic stents is problematic despite improvement in stent design, stent materials, and MRI parameters. To differentiate between artifact and stenosis, knowledge of the degree of signal intensity reduction and artificial lumen narrowing within vascular stents is essential. Stent geometry, the relative orientation to the magnetic field, and alloy composition influence signal intensity alteration within the stent lumen. Thus far, nitinol- and tantalum-based stents have shown the least artifacts in both in vitro and in vivo experiments. Platinum-based, commercially available balloon-expandable stents allow assessment of luminal patency on CE-MRA using standard sequences. Stent-induced artifacts resulting in luminal narrowing do not reach a degree that would be considered hemodynamically significant.

Subclavian Steal

Several studies have shown the utility of MRA for the effective and noninvasive diagnosis of subclavian steal syndrome. Subclavian steal syndrome is a condition secondary to an occlusion in the proximal subclavian artery that leads to upper extremity blood supply being derived by reversal of flow within the ipsilateral VA. Several MRA techniques are able to demonstrate reversal of flow in a VA. These include 2-D TOF MRI with a selective presaturation pulse applied first above and then below the volume of interest. Phase contrast MRI can also be used to detect reversal of flow, but there are

issues related to susceptibility or aliasing effects with this technique. 3-D CE-MRA is now commonly used to evaluate the proximal aortic arch vessels and the VAs. However, although this technique can be used to evaluate the anatomic characteristics of the VAs and to assess for stenosis and occlusion, it cannot reliably be used to directly determine flow direction. The exact anatomic relationships of the vascular structures can be well demonstrated on CE-MRA with the associated flow reversal visible on flow-sensitive (unenhanced) MRA.

Metal

Local magnetic field inhomogeneity caused by metal can degrade the image quality of MRA. Care is necessary in evaluating MRA because the recorded signal is based on flow characteristics and not necessarily "true" anatomy. Dephasing artifacts related to local magnetic field inhomogeneity can cause signal intensity that can mimic either focal flow or occlusion. If the reconstructed MR angiograms show arterial stenosis, the source images must be viewed. The source images may show less stenosis than the maximum intensity projection. When a discrepancy is identified between the source images and the maximum intensity projection reconstructions, attention to the patient history and comparison examinations is recommended to evaluate for artifact-causing material such as vascular clips, bullet fragments, or shunt tube joints.

Overestimation of Stenosis

MRA has limitations, most notably flow-related signal dropout in the regions of turbulence or vortex flow. These are more prominently seen with 2-D TOF MRA, which has more vulnerability to signal-intensity dropout (or flow-void) artifacts resulting from intravoxel dephasing related to turbulent flow associated with the stenotic segments of vasculature. Vascular areas of signal-intensity dropout are found in approximately 15% of all 2-D TOF MRA studies. The presence of these signal-intensity dropouts is highly correlated with severe (>70%) ICA stenosis. The limitations lay in the inability for further evaluation and differentiation (i.e., between severe, critical, and hairline) stenoses.

■ CONCLUSION

Noninvasive carotid artery assessment has significantly improved in the recent years. The combined use of duplex ultrasonography with either MRA or CTA has almost completely replaced DSA in the evaluation of carotid artery disease. With careful multimodality evaluation and avoidance of the imaging pitfalls described earlier, appropriate patient triage and treatment recommendations can be performed in a cost-efficient and noninvasive manner.

Bibliography

Aaslid R, Lindegaard K, Sorteberg W, Nornes H. Cerebral autoregulation dynamics in humans. *Stroke*. 1989;20:45-52.
Aaslid R, Markwalder T-M, Nornes H. Noninvasive transcranial Doppler ultrasound recording of flow velocity in basal cerebral arteries: <http://dxdoiorg/103171/jns19825760769>; 1982.

Ackermann H, Diener H, Seboldt H, Huth C. Ultrasonographic follow-up of subclavian stenosis and occlusion: natural history and surgical treatment. *Stroke*. 1988;19:431-435.

AIUM practice guideline for the performance of an ultrasound examination of the extracranial cerebrovascular system. *J Ultrasound Med*. 2012;31: 145-154.

Babiarz LS, Romero JM, Murphy EK, Brobeck B, Schaefer PW, González RG, et al. Contrast-enhanced MR angiography is not more accurate than unenhanced 2D time-of-flight MR angiography for determining > or = 70% internal carotid artery stenosis. *AJNR Am J Neuroradiol*. 2009;30:761-768.

Bae K, Tran H, Heiken JP. Multiphasic injection method for uniform prolonged vascular enhancement at CT angiography: pharmacokinetic analysis and experimental porcine model. *Radiology*. 2000;216:872-880.

Bahner ML, Bengel A, Brix G, Zuna I, Kauczor H-U, Delorme S. Improved vascular opacification in cerebral computed tomography angiography with 80 kVp. *Invest Radiol*. 2005;40:229-234.

Barnett H, Taylor D, Eliasziw M, Fox AJ, Ferguson GG, Haynes RB, et al. Benefit of carotid endarterectomy in patients with symptomatic moderate or severe stenosis. North American Symptomatic Carotid Endarterectomy Trial Collaborators. *N Engl J Med*. 1998;339:1415-1425.

Beneficial effect of carotid endarterectomy in symptomatic patients with high-grade carotid stenosis. North American Symptomatic Carotid Endarterectomy Trial Collaborators. *N Engl J Med*. 1991;325:445-453.

Bishop CC, Powell S, Rutt D, Browse NL. Transcranial Doppler measurement of middle cerebral artery blood flow velocity: a validation study. *Stroke*. 1986;17:913-915.

Borisch I, Horn M, Butz B, Zorger N, Draganski B, Hoelscher T, et al. Preoperative evaluation of carotid artery stenosis: comparison of contrast-enhanced MR angiography and duplex sonography with digital subtraction angiography. *AJNR Am J Neuroradiol*. 2003;24:1117-1122.

Brandt T, Knauth M, Wildermuth S, Winter R, von Kummer R, Sartor K, et al. CT angiography and Doppler sonography for emergency assessment in acute basilar artery ischemia. *Stroke*. 1999;30:606-612.

Carr JC, Shaibani A, Russell E, Finn JP. Contrast-enhanced magnetic resonance angiography of the carotid circulation. *Top Magn Reson Imaging*. 2001;12:349-357.

Carriero A, Salute L, Tartaro A, Iezzi A, Dragani M, Tamburri L, et al. The role of magnetic resonance angiography in the diagnosis of subclavian steal. *Cardiovasc Intervent Radiol*. 1995;18:87-91.

Cirillo F, Leonardo G, Renzulli A, Crescenzi B, Irace C, Gnasso A, et al. *Int J Angiol*. 2002;11:210-215.

Doerfler A, Engelhorn T, von Kummer R, Weber J, Knauth M, Heiland S, et al. Are iodinated contrast agents detrimental in acute cerebral ischemia? An experimental study in rats. *Radiology*. 1998;208:211-217.

Drutman J, Gyorke A, Davis WL, Turski PA. Evaluation of subclavian steal with two-dimensional phase-contrast and two-dimensional time-of-flight MR angiography. *AJNR Am J Neuroradiol*. 1994;15:1642-1645.

Flynn PD, Delany DJ, Gray HH. Magnetic resonance angiography in subclavian steal syndrome. *Br Heart J*. 1993;70(2):193-194.

Fusco MR, Harrigan MR. Cerebrovascular dissections—a review part I: spontaneous dissections. *Neurosurgery*. 2011;68:242-257:discussion 257.

Hagspiel KD, Leung DA, Nandalur KR, Angle JF, Dulai HS, Spinosa DJ, et al. Contrast-enhanced MR angiography at 1.5 T after implantation of platinum stents: in vitro and in vivo comparison with conventional stent designs. *AJR Am J Roentgenol*. 2005;184:288-294.

Işık AC, İmamoğlu M, Erem C, Sari A. Paragangliomas of the head and neck. *Med Princ Pract*. 2007;16:209-214.

Klemm T, Duda S, Machann J, Seekamp-Rahn K, Schnieder L, Claussen CD, et al. MR imaging in the presence of vascular stents: a systematic assessment of artifacts for various stent orientations, sequence types, and field strengths. *J Magn Reson Imaging*. 2000;12:606-615.

Kliewer MA, Hertzberg BS, Kim DH, Bowie JD, Courneya DL, Carroll BA. Vertebral artery Doppler waveform changes indicating subclavian steal physiology. *AJR Am J Roentgenol*. 2000;174:815-819.

Kluytmans M, van der Grond J, van Everdingen KJ, Klijn CJ, Kappelle LJ, Viergever MA. Cerebral hemodynamics in relation to patterns of collateral flow. *Stroke*. 1999;30:1432-1439.

Koelemay MJW, Nederkoorn PJ, Reitsma JB, Majoie CB. Systematic review of computed tomographic angiography for assessment of carotid artery disease. *Stroke*. 2004;35:2306-2312.

Kuta A, Smoker W, Cole T. MR angiography artifact due to metal joint of ventriculoperitoneal shunt mimicking severe carotid stenosis. *J Magn Reson Imaging*. 1995;5:125-126.

Leclerc X, Gauvrit JY, Nicol L, Pruvo JP. Contrast-enhanced MR angiography of the craniocervical vessels: a review. *Neuroradiology*. 1999;41:867-874.

Lee VH, Brown RD, Mandrekar JN, Mokri B. Incidence and outcome of cervical artery dissection: a population-based study. *Neurology*. 2006;67: 1809-1812.

Lenhart M, Völk M, Manke C, Nitz WR, Strotzer M, Feuerbach S, et al. Stent appearance at contrast-enhanced MR angiography: in vitro examination with 14 stents. *Radiology*. 2000;217:173-178.

Lev MH, Farkas J, Rodriguez VR, Schwamm LH, Hunter GJ, Putman CM, et al. CT angiography in the rapid triage of patients with hyperacute stroke to intraarterial thrombolysis: accuracy in the detection of large vessel thrombus. *J Comput Assist Tomogr*. 2001;25:520-528.

Lorenz MW, Markus HS, Bots ML, Rosvall M, Sitzer M. Prediction of clinical cardiovascular events with carotid intima-media thickness: a systematic review and meta-analysis. *Circulation*. 2007;115:459-467.

Maeda H, Etani H, Handa N, Tagaya M, Oku N, Kim BH, et al. A validation study on the reproducibility of transcranial Doppler velocimetry. *Ultrasound Med Biol*. 1990;16:9-14.

Magarelli N, Scarabino T, Simeone AL, Florio F, Carriero A, Salvolini U, et al. Carotid stenosis: a comparison between MR and spiral CT angiography. *Neuroradiology*. 1998;40:367-373.

Maldonado TS. What are current preprocedure imaging requirements for carotid artery stenting and carotid endarterectomy: have magnetic resonance angiography and computed tomographic angiography made a difference? *Semin Vasc Surg*. 2007;20:205-215.

Meairs S, Hennerici M. Long-term follow-up of aneurysms developed during extracranial internal carotid artery dissection. *Neurology*. 2000;54:2190.

Meyer JM, Buecker A, Schuermann K, Ruebben A, Guenther RW. MR evaluation of stent patency: in vitro test of 22 metallic stents and the possibility of determining their patency by MR angiography. *Invest Radiol*. 2000;35:739-746.

Mustert BR, Williams DM, Prince MR. In vitro model of arterial stenosis: correlation of MR signal dephasing and trans-stenotic pressure gradients. *Magn Reson Imaging*. 1998;16:301-310.

Nederkoorn PJ, van der Graaf Y, Eikelboom BC, van der Lugt A, Bartels LW, Mali WPTM. Time-of-flight MR angiography of carotid artery stenosis: does a flow void represent severe stenosis? *AJNR Am J Neuroradiol*. 2002;23:1779-1784.

Patel S, Collie D, Wardlaw J. Outcome, observer reliability, and patient preferences if CTA, MRA, or Doppler ultrasound were used, individually or together, instead of digital subtraction angiography before carotid endarterectomy. *J Neurol Neurosurg Psychiatry*. 2002;73:21-28.

Pellitteri P. Paragangliomas of the head and neck. *Oral Oncol*. 2004;40:563-575.

Reinhard M, Müller T, Roth M, Guschlbauer B, Timmer J, Hetzel A. Bilateral severe carotid artery stenosis or occlusion—cerebral autoregulation dynamics and collateral flow patterns. *Acta Neurochir (Wien)*. 2003;145:1053-1060.

Remonda L, Senn P, Barth A, Arnold M, Lövblad K-O, Schroth G. Contrast-enhanced 3D MR angiography of the carotid artery: comparison with conventional digital subtraction angiography. *AJNR Am J Neuroradiol*. 2002;23:213-219.

Reynolds PS, Greenberg JP, Lien L-M, Meads DC, Myers LG, Tegeler CH. Ophthalmic artery flow direction on color flow duplex imaging is highly specific for severe carotid stenosis. *J Neuroimaging*. 2002;12:5-8.

Ringelstein EB, Sievers C, Ecker S, Schneider PA, Otis SM. Noninvasive assessment of CO_2-induced cerebral vasomotor response in normal individuals and patients with internal carotid artery occlusions. *Stroke*. 1988;19:963-969.

Romero JM, Ackerman RH, Dault NA, Lev MH. Noninvasive evaluation of carotid artery stenosis: indications, strategies, and accuracy. *Neuroimaging Clin N Am*. 2005;15:351-365.

Romero JM, Lev MH, Chan ST, Connelly MM, Curiel RC, Jackson AE, et al. US of neurovascular occlusive disease: interpretive pearls and pitfalls. *Radiographics*. 2002;22:1165-1176.

Rosenthal D, Ellison Jr RG, Clark MD, Lamis PA, Nilsen BR. Carotid artery aneurysm diagnosed by duplex scanning. *J Clin Ultrasound*. 1986;14:732-734.

Rouleau PA, Huston J, Gilbertson J, Brown RD, Meyer FB, Bower TC. Carotid artery tandem lesions: frequency of angiographic detection and consequences for endarterectomy. *AJNR Am J Neuroradiol*. 1999;20:621-625.

Rydberg J, Charles J, Aspelin P. Frequency of late allergy-like adverse reactions following injection of intravascular non-ionic contrast media:a retrospective study comparing a non-ionic monomeric contrast medium with a non-ionic dimeric contrast medium. *Acta Radiol*. 1998;39:219-222.

Schürmann K, Vorwerk D, Bücker A, Neuerburg J, Grosskortenhaus S, Haage P, et al. Magnetic resonance angiography of nonferromagnetic iliac artery stents and stent-grafts: a comparative study in sheep. *Cardiovasc Intervent Radiol*. 1999;22:394-402.

Sevilla García MA, Llorente Pendás JL, Rodrigo Tapia JP, García Rostán G, Suárez Fente V, Coca Pelaz A, et al. Head and neck paragangliomas: revision of 89 cases in 73 patients. *Acta Otorrinolaringologica*. 2007;58:94-100:[English ed].

Shrier D, Tanaka H, Numaguchi Y, Konno S, Patel U, Shibata D. CT angiography in the evaluation of acute stroke. *AJNR Am J Neuroradiol*. 1997;18:1011-1020.

Sturzenegger M, Mattle H, Rivoir A, Baumgartner RW. Ultrasound findings in carotid artery dissection: analysis of 43 patients. *Neurology*. 1995;45:691-698.

Suwanwela NC, Phanthumchinda K, Suwanwela N. Transcranial Doppler sonography and CT angiography in patients with atherothrombotic middle cerebral artery stroke. *AJNR Am J Neuroradiol*. 2002;23:1352-1355.

Thanvi B. Carotid and vertebral artery dissection syndromes. *Postgrad Med J*. 2005;81:383-388.

Thiele BL, Young JV, Chikos PM, Hirsch JH, Strandness DE. Correlation of arteriographic findings and symptoms in cerebrovascular disease. *Neurology*. 1980;30:1041-1046.

Timaran CH, Rosero EB, Valentine RJ, Modrall JG, Smith S, Clagett GP. Accuracy and utility of three-dimensional contrast-enhanced magnetic resonance angiography in planning carotid stenting. *J Vasc Surg*. 2007;46:257-264.

Turjman F, Tournut P, Baldy-Porcher C, Laharotte JC, Duquesnel J, Froment JC. Demonstration of subclavian steal by MR angiography. *J Comput Assist Tomogr*. 1992;16:756-759.

U-King-Im JM, Hollingworth W, Trivedi RA, Cross JJ, Higgins NJ, Graves MJ, et al. Contrast-enhanced MR angiography vs intra-arterial digital subtraction angiography for carotid imaging: activity-based cost analysis. *Eur Radiol*. 2004;14:730-735.

U-King-Im JM, Trivedi RA, Cross JJ, Higgins NJ, Hollingworth W, Graves M, et al. Measuring carotid stenosis on contrast-enhanced magnetic resonance angiography: diagnostic performance and reproducibility of 3 different methods. *Stroke.* 2004;35:2083-2088.

U-King-Im JM, Trivedi RA, Graves MJ, Higgins NJ, Cross JJ, Tom BD, et al. Contrast-enhanced MR angiography for carotid disease: diagnostic and potential clinical impact. *Neurology.* 2004;62:1282-1290.

Van Grimberge F, Dymarkowski S, Budts W, Bogaert J. Role of magnetic resonance in the diagnosis of subclavian steal syndrome. *J Magn Reson Imaging.* 2000;12:339-342.

Wang SH, Chiu KM, Cheng PW. Bilateral carotid body paragangliomas. *CMAJ.* 2011;183:E606.

Wieneke JA, Smith A. Paraganglioma: carotid body tumor. *Head Neck Pathol.* 2009;3:303-306.

Wu C, Zhang J, Ladner CJ, Babb JS, Lamparello PJ, Krinsky GA. Subclavian steal syndrome: diagnosis with perfusion metrics from contrast-enhanced MR angiographic bolus-timing examination—initial experience. *Radiology.* 2005;235:927-933.

Yang CW, Carr JC, Futterer SF, Morasch MD, Yang BP, Shors SM, et al. Contrast-enhanced MR angiography of the carotid and vertebrobasilar circulations. *AJNR Am J Neuroradiol.* 2005;26:2095-2101.

Young B, Moore WS, Robertson JT, Toole JF, Ernst CB, Cohen SN, et al. An analysis of perioperative surgical mortality and morbidity in the asymptomatic carotid atherosclerosis study. ACAS Investigators. Asymptomatic Carotid Atherosclerosis Study. *Stroke.* 1996;27:2216-2124.

Zubilewicz T, Wronski J, Bourriez A, Terlecki P, Guinault AM, Muscatelli-Groux B, et al. Injury in vascular surgery—the intimal hyperplastic response. *Med Sci Monit.* 2001;7:316-324.

CHAPTER 44

Thoracic Aorta and Its Branches

Jonathan H. Chung, Martin L. Gunn, Sanjeeva P. Kalva, and Suhny Abbara

The aorta, the largest artery in the body, pumps up to 200 million L of blood in an average lifetime. Thoracic aortic diseases range from chronic to acute and have a wide variation in symptoms. Consequently, pathologic features of the aorta may be detected incidentally (as in an aneurysm incidentally detected on imaging) or as a result of severe chest pain (as in acute aortic dissection). The increase in the reported prevalence of aortic disease in developed countries is most likely the result of improved clinical awareness and increased life expectancy.

Noninvasive imaging is central to the diagnosis and management of disorders of the thoracic aorta. Initial examination of the aorta should include the entire aortoiliac system. Aortic diseases such as aneurysm or dissection frequently often extend along large portions of the aorta or may be multifocal.

■ RADIOGRAPHY

Chest radiographs have a limited role in the assessment of the thoracic aorta, given its low inherent contrast. The main utility of radiography in aortic diseases is in the emergency setting in which an anteroposterior (AP) chest radiograph acts as a screening tool to exclude actionable traumatic aortic injury. The negative predictive value of a normal chest radiograph is 98% in the setting of blunt trauma. Imaging abnormalities are based on the assumption that aortic injuries result in mediastinal hematomas. Common findings include superior mediastinal widening, right paratracheal stripe thickening, abnormal aortic morphology, obliteration of the aorto-pulmonary window, rightward deviation of mediastinal structures or thickening of the left paraspinal interface (given that the descending aorta is a left-sided structure), left hemothorax, and inferior displacement of the left mainstem bronchus (Fig. 44-1). Intimal injuries, however, cannot be detected without the use of intravenous contrast.

Severe calcification of the aorta, its branches, and aortic valve leaflets is readily detected on radiography, although mild calcification may be subtle or undetectable. Aortic valve calcification is better demonstrated on lateral radiographs and when present, it is highly suggestive of significant aortic stenosis (Fig. 44-2). The aortic valve is located above an imaginary line drawn along the long axis of the heart on the lateral view. One often sees associated dilation of the ascending aorta from a poststenotic jet phenomenon, which manifests as broad convexity just superior to the right heart border. Aortic dilation and congenital anomalies may also be detected using posteroanterior and lateral chest radiographs; however, detailed imaging assessment of the thoracic aorta requires further evaluation with cross-sectional imaging. Rarely, displacement of the calcified intimal surface can be detected on radiography, and this finding is essentially diagnostic of aortic dissection (Fig. 44-3).

■ COMPUTED TOMOGRAPHY IMAGING PROTOCOL

In the 1990s, single detector spiral computed tomography (CT) was introduced into clinical practice. This technique allowed for excellent visualization of vessels in multiple planes. However, CT was still limited by long breath holds, motion artifacts from slow gantry rotation time, and limited z-plane coverage. Later in the 1990s, multidetector row CT (MDCT) was introduced to wide acclaim. MDCT resulted in improved z-axis resolution, rapid gantry rotation, increased coverage in the z-axis, and increased table speed. Modern 64- to 320-row MDCT can evaluate the entire aorta and its branches in a single short acquisition. Unlike with catheter angiography, the walls of vessels are also well assessed with MDCT. Catheter angiography is essentially a study of the vessel lumen (luminography). Given the nearly isotropic acquisition of current MDCT, two-dimensional and three-dimensional reconstructions can be made retrospectively in any orientation.

Noncontrast Computed Tomography

Inclusion of a noncontrast CT scan is mandatory in aortic imaging because intramural hematomas (IMHs) are more evident without intravascular contrast (Fig. 44-4). In addition, calcified atherosclerotic plaque is more easily detected. A noncontrast phase may also be helpful in patients with calcified lymph nodes or metallic surgical material or felt pledgets or rings, which can simulate vascular disease during the arterial phase. Finally, in the rare case of a vascular mass, noncontrast acquisition is necessary to assess the degree of

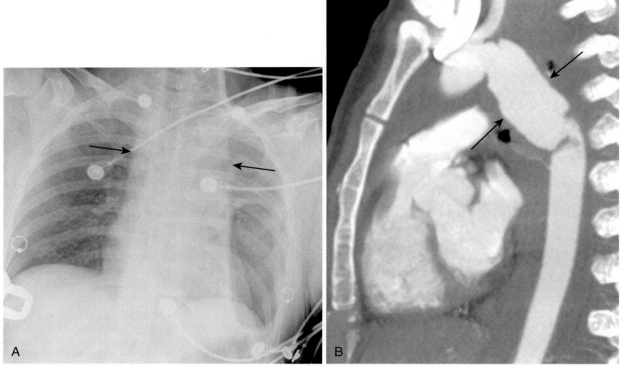

Figure 44-1 **A,** Anteroposterior chest radiograph shows widening of the superior mediastinum *(arrows)* with silhouetting of the aortic contour in this patient with a history of a recent high-speed motor vehicle collision. **B,** Sagittal maximum intensity projection reformation from contrast-enhanced computed tomography angiography of the thorax shows a pseudoaneurysm of the aortic isthmus *(arrows)* diagnostic of acute aortic injury. The patient was taken for immediate aortic repair.

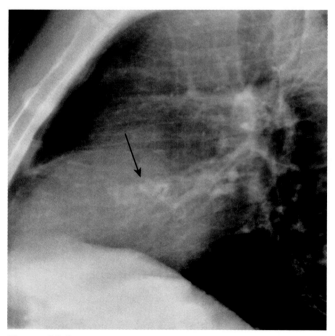

Figure 44-2 Aortic stenosis. Lateral chest radiograph shows coarse calcification *(arrow)* in the expected location of the aortic valve in this patient with history of aortic stenosis. If aortic valve calcification is evident on radiography, it usually indicates significant aortic valvular stenosis, which can be corroborated with more detailed imaging.

enhancement within the lesion confidently. Internal enhancement is more suggestive of neoplasm, whereas thrombus or iatrogenic material typically does not demonstrate significant enhancement. The radiation dose can be reduced during this phase by increasing collimation, decreasing peak kilovoltage, or increasing the noise index.

Computed Tomography Angiography

Thoracic aortic CT angiography (CTA) is usually performed with a pitch of 1 to 1.5, a collimation of 0.5 to 1.0 mm, and reconstruction thickness of 1.0 to 1.5 mm with spacing of 0.75 to 1 mm. The tube potential is usually between 120 and 140 kVp. Lower tube potential (80 to 100 kVp) may be used in pediatric patients or in those with a lower body mass index. Automated tube current modulation should be used when available; tube current is automatically decreased while scanning areas with lower attenuation (the midchest, where much of the anatomy consists of air-filled lungs) and is increased for areas with higher attenuation (upper chest and shoulders, upper abdomen). A desired noise index is set, defined as the standard deviation of Hounsfield units in the center of an image using soft tissue kernel reconstruction.

A threshold-based bolus tracking strategy is typically used with a region of interest in the ascending aorta. Intravenous contrast material is injected at rates of 3 to 5 mL/second. The overall contrast volume can be

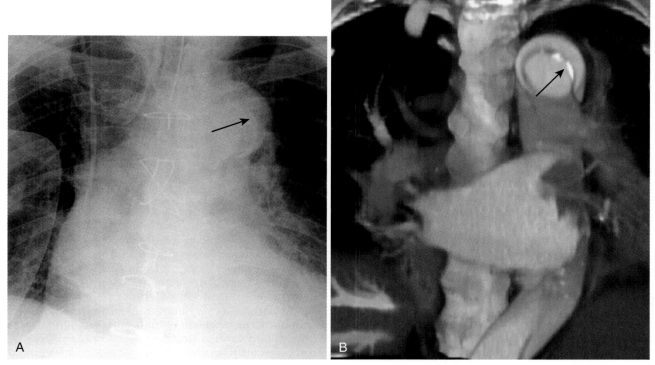

Figure 44-3 Aortic dissection. A, Anteroposterior chest radiograph after sternotomy and coronary artery bypass grafting shows internal displacement of intimal calcification *(arrow)* in the aorta that was new compared with preoperative films. **B,** Coronal volume rendered image from contrast-enhanced chest computed tomography angiography shows aortic dissection internally displacing intimal calcification *(arrow)* medially. The dissection was repaired on an emergency basis.

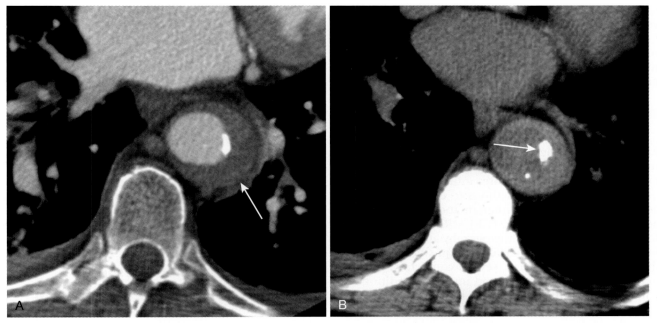

Figure 44-4 Intramural hematoma. A, Contrast-enhanced computed tomography (CT) of the chest shows asymmetric, nearly circumferential soft tissue density *(arrow)* around the aorta suggestive of an intramural hematoma. **B,** Noncontrast chest CT more clearly demonstrates the inherent hyperdensity of the intramural hematoma; inward displacement of intimal calcification *(arrow)* is visible. Treatment of intramural hematomas is similar to that of aortic dissections.

calculated as injection rate (in milliliters per second) multiplied by [scan duration in seconds + 5 to 10 seconds]. The contrast material must be injected for an additional 5 to 10 seconds to compensate for the time it takes for gantry movement from the position of the bolus tracking in the ascending aorta and the start position of the CTA scan in the neck. Alternatively, a fixed amount of contrast—based on an injection period of 20 to 35 seconds—can be used and usually results in similar image quality. Reconstructing a small field of view in x-y dimension is advantageous for optimizing spatial resolution of the aorta and its branches. However, a full field of view is mandatory to detect potentially significant incidental findings or secondary findings within the end organs. Initial evaluation of the thoracic aorta should include the abdominal aorta and iliac arteries because aortic disease may be multifocal or may extend throughout the thoracic and abdominal aorta, unless the status of the abdominal and pelvic vessels is known.

Delayed Scan

A delayed scan 2 minutes after injection is useful to assess for late filling of a false lumen in dissections, slow endoleaks in endovascular aneurysm repair, or contrast extravasation from aortic rupture.

Postprocessing

Multiplanar maximum intensity projections (MIPs) in the sagittal plane, sagittal oblique plane (candy cane view), coronal plane, aortic short axis, and aortic root long axis are routinely acquired. Three-dimensional volume rendered images are often acquired and can be helpful to identify major disease or for surgical planning. However, axial reconstruction and interactive multiplanar reformations are usually clinically more useful.

■ MAGNETIC RESONANCE IMAGING PROTOCOL

As opposed to imaging of the thoracic aorta with CT, magnetic resonance angiography (MRA) of the thoracic aorta most often requires multiple magnetic resonance imaging (MRI) methods to evaluate the aorta adequately. The most utilitarian tool in MRI of the aorta is contrast-enhanced (CE) MRA. Images similar to conventional invasive angiography are reconstructed from a single three-dimensional acquisition or from a dynamic MRA acquisition (several consecutive breath-held acquisitions). Black-blood imaging (traditionally with spin echo imaging, which has been supplanted with more advanced techniques) is used primarily to evaluate the walls of the aorta, given the high contrast between signal in the fixed mediastinal structures and flowing blood. Gradient echo sequences allow for qualitative functional and morphologic evaluation of the aortic valve. In addition, quantitative data on vascular flow can also be acquired using velocity encoded cine MRI.

Contrast-Enhanced Magnetic Resonance Angiography

With the advent of rapid gradient systems, three-dimensional CE MRA is the most often used means to evaluate the aorta. Time of flight (TOF) imaging may also be used as a concomitant sequence; however, given its limitations in areas of slow or turbulent flow, TOF imaging is rarely used in isolation unless the patient has a contraindication to gadolinium contrast administration. CE MRA relies on the T1 shortening effect of gadolinium contrast and is less prone to imaging artifact. The exact protocol for CE MRA differs among institutions and MRI scanners. As a general rule, however, contrast material is injected through an antecubital vein with a power injector at a rate of approximately 2 mL/second (0.2 mmol/kg of body weight). The injection rate should be adjusted to avoid unnecessary injection of contrast material beyond the scan time. Bolus timing is mandatory, given the short intravascular phase of maximal contrast enhancement. Imaging before the peak plateau of contrast enhancement may result in ringing artifact, whereas delayed imaging leads to venous contamination, which complicates differentiation of arterial and venous structures. Real-time imaging or a test bolus technique can be employed to determine the optimal time point to scan the patient after injection of the contrast material. A T1-weighted gradient echo sequence is acquired using short repetition time (TR; 3 to 5 msec) and echo time (TE; 1 to 2 msec) with a large flip angle (45 degrees). Images are acquired using a single breath hold lasting from 20 to 30 seconds. Supplemental oxygen as well as hyperventilation can aid patients in achieving this breath hold, which can be challenging in patients with cardiorespiratory disease. Electrocardiogram (ECG) gating is not necessary to perform this sequence.

A precontrast mask image before the CE acquisition is often helpful for background suppression. The precontrast sequence method is similar to that of the CE sequence. The precontrast mask images are then subtracted from the CE images before MIP images are postprocessed from the source data. Most often, the MIP images are reconstructed as projection images that resemble conventional angiographic images. Given the nearly isovolumetric acquisition of the CE MRA sequence, reformation can be created in any plane that is advantageous in vascular imaging, considering the high variation in the course and size of the vasculature in different patients.

Noncontrast Magnetic Resonance Angiography

Although noncontrast MRA has been available for many years, it was initially inferior to CE MRA and therefore was not frequently used. However, the more recently recognized risk of nephrogenic systemic fibrosis and nephrogenic fibrosing dermopathy with administration of gadolinium compounds in renally impaired patients led to renewed focus on noncontrast MRA techniques. Most of the noncontrast MRA use bright-blood imaging techniques that show bright signal in an voxel through which fluid flows.

Gradient Echo Imaging

Also known as bright-blood imaging, gradient recalled echo imaging results in high signal in flowing blood. Combined with retrospective or prospective gating, cine sequences at specific points in the anatomy can be acquired that provide both dynamic and functional data, albeit at the expense of less detail within the walls of the vessels. High signal in flowing blood is achieved with a very short TR (4 msec) and a low flip angle (20 to 30 degrees). TE is also short (1 to 2 msec). Signal in vessels is reduced with slow flow; nonlaminar turbulent flow results in spin dephasing and concomitant low signal that often suggest the presence of an underlying structural abnormality. Filling defects within the aorta, as well as aortic valvular dysfunction, are readily identifiable using this method.

Black-Blood Imaging

Black-blood imaging of the thoracic aorta is essential in the assessment of the aortic wall. The high contrast between flowing blood and the aorta is valuable in the evaluation of acute aortic syndrome, vasculitis, and atherosclerosis. Traditionally, black-blood imaging was obtained with a spin echo technique, using a pair of slice-selective radiofrequency pulses at 90 and 180 degrees. Protons in flowing blood resulted in a signal void in vessels not in the plane of acquisition. More advanced techniques, such as fast spin echo and breath-hold inversion recovery, have largely supplanted simple spin echo imaging in thoracic aortic evaluation, given their superior resolution and decreased susceptibility to motion artifact.

■ NORMAL ANATOMY

The thoracic aorta extends from the aortic annulus to the diaphragm. The thoracic aorta can be divided into three major parts: the ascending aorta, the aortic arch, and the descending thoracic aorta (Fig. 44-5). The aortic root and the tubular ascending aorta comprise the ascending aorta. The aortic root lies between the aortic annulus and the sinotubular junction. The sinuses of Valsalva are found in the aortic root. The tubular ascending aorta consists of the portion of the aorta between the sinotubular junction and the brachiocephalic artery. The first 3 cm of the proximal ascending aorta is within the confines of the pericardium. The ascending aorta is devoid of branches except for the coronary arteries. The aortic arch is between the brachiocephalic trunk and the origin of the left subclavian artery. The isthmus is a small segment of the aorta extending from the left subclavian artery to the ligamentum arteriosum. Three branches most commonly arise from the aortic arch: the brachiocephalic artery (innominate artery), the left common carotid artery, and the left subclavian artery. The descending thoracic aorta extends from the isthmus to the diaphragm. In contradistinction to the

ascending aorta, the descending aorta has multiple branches including the bronchial, intercostal, spinal, superior phrenic arteries and various small mediastinal branches.

Anatomic Variants (Asymptomatic)

In approximately 7% of people, the left vertebral artery arises directly from the aortic arch. This finding is of limited clinical significance in most instances, although knowledge of this normal variant anatomy may be helpful before neuroangiography procedures. The bovine arch is another normal variant in which the left common carotid artery arises directly from the brachiocephalic artery and occurs in up to one fourth of the population (see Fig. 44-5). The bovine arch is, in fact, a misnomer for this aortic variant. Cows have a single brachiocephalic trunk that splits into the subclavian arteries and a bicarotid trunk. A common arch variant is the ductus diverticulum, which is a focal convexity along the inner aspect of the aortic isthmus that represents a remnant of the ductus arteriosus. Uncommonly, the aorta may extend above the level of the clavicles into the lower aspect of the neck (Fig. 44-6). Known as a cervical aortic arch, this anomaly is usually an isolated finding. However, cervical aortic arches may occur in patients with cardiac defects (most commonly ventricular septal defects or conotruncal abnormalities). In addition, cervical aortic arches may

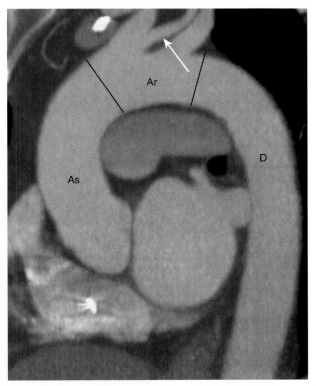

Figure 44-5 Normal aorta and bovine arch. Oblique sagittal view of the aorta during contrast-enhanced computed tomography angiography shows a normal aortic contour. The thoracic aorta can be divided into the ascending aorta (As), the aortic arch (Ar), and the descending aorta (D). The left common carotid artery *(arrow)* arises from the innominate artery, diagnostic of a bovine arch.

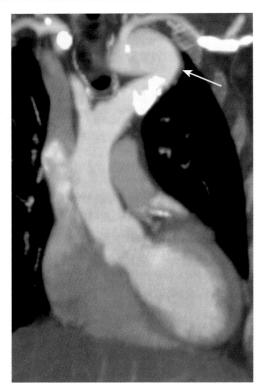

Figure 44-6 Cervical arch. The atherosclerotic aortic arch *(arrow)* is redundant and extends more superiorly than expected into the lower aspect of the cervical neck on contrast-enhanced chest computed tomography.

result in a vascular ring when the cervical arch and the descending thoracic aorta are contralateral (most often the case), thus leading to chronic tracheoesophageal compression and asthma-like symptoms.

In approximately 0.5% of people, the right subclavian artery may arise anomalously from the proximal aspect of the descending thoracic aorta and almost always passes into the right hemithorax behind the esophagus (Fig. 44-7). This anomaly does not typically result in a vascular ring and is therefore often asymptomatic or minimally symptomatic. However, dysphagia may result from compression of posterior aspect of the esophagus (dysphagia lusoria).

Pseudocoarctation is a normal variant of the aortic arch and proximal descending artery that occurs when the third to seventh embryonic dorsal segments fail to fuse appropriately; the resultant high proximal arch leads to kinking of the redundant aorta where it is tethered to the pulmonary artery by the ligamentum arteriosum (Fig. 44-8).

Anatomic Variants (Symptomatic)

The right aortic arch, the most common asymptomatic arch anomaly, is thought to result from persistence of the entire right dorsal arch and involution of a segment of the left arch. Chest radiography shows abnormal leftward deviation of the trachea. In normal circumstances, the trachea is pushed slightly toward the right by a left-sided aortic arch. Cross-sectional imaging (CT or MRI)

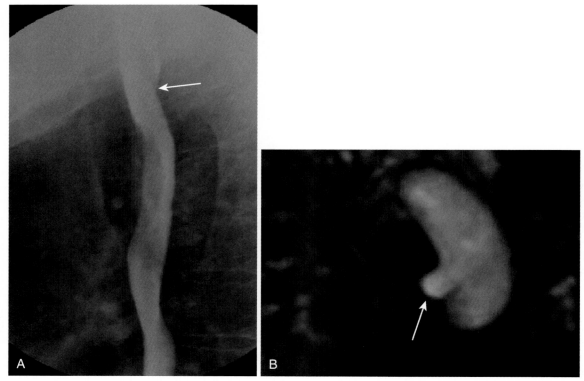

Figure 44-7 Aberrant right subclavian artery. A, Lateral view from an esophagogram shows extrinsic indentation *(arrow)* along the posterior aspect of the esophagus. **B,** Axial image from contrast-enhanced magnetic resonance angiography shows an aberrant right subclavian artery *(arrow)* arising from the left-sided aortic arch.

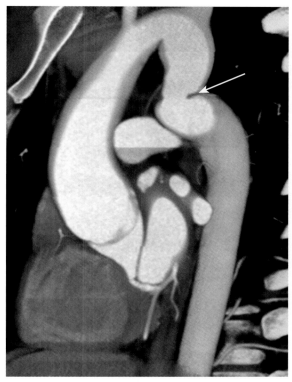

Figure 44-8 Pseudocoarctation. Candy cane volume rendered image of the thoracic aorta from contrast-enhanced, electrocardiogram-triggered computed tomography angiography shows redundancy of the aortic arch resulting in a kinked appearance at the level of the ligamentum arteriosum *(arrow)*. No collateral arteries are apparent, a finding implying that no hemodynamically significant stenosis is present at the level of the pseudocoarctation.

is usually diagnostic. The two main types are right aortic arch with aberrant left subclavian artery and right aortic arch with mirror image branching. In cases of right aortic arch with an aberrant left subclavian artery, the aberrant left subclavian almost always passes behind the esophagus and is often seen on lateral chest radiograph or esophagogram (Fig. 44-9). A ring usually results from the left-sided ligamentum arteriosum. Patients commonly present with tracheal symptoms resembling asthma. In mirror image branching, the normal branching pattern of the aorta is completely reversed, and no vascular ring is present. However, this anomaly is highly associated with congenital heart disease (most commonly tetralogy of Fallot).

A double aortic arch results from persistence of both fourth aortic arches during development. This anomaly is the most common symptomatic vascular ring; patients usually present in the early months of life with inspiratory stridor that is worse with feeding. On radiography, the trachea is abnormally at midline or deviated away from the dominant arch. Cross-sectional imaging is again most often diagnostic (Fig. 44-10). More commonly, the right aortic arch is larger and more superiorly located than the left aortic arch. The carotid and subclavian arteries arise from the ipsilateral aortic arch and result in the four artery sign: symmetric branching of the carotid and subclavian arteries in the superior thorax. In a minority of cases, a portion of the double aortic arch may be atretic, although the ring remains intact because of a persistent fibrous band of tissue in the atretic portion of the aorta.

Interrupted aorta results from regression of both fourth arches during development such that the ascending aorta

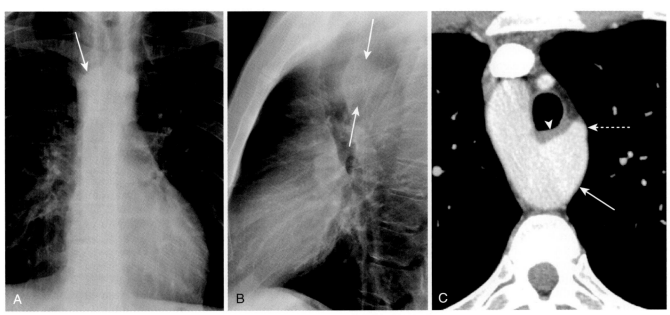

Figure 44-9 Right aortic arch with aberrant left subclavian artery. A, Posteroanterior chest radiography (windowed to delineate the mediastinal structures more clearly) shows rounded soft tissue density *(arrow)* to the right of the aortic arch with leftward deviation of the trachea, suggestive of a right aortic arch. **B,** Lateral chest radiography shows soft tissue density *(arrows)* posterior to the trachea that causes focal anterior displacement of the superior aspect of the trachea. **C,** Axial image from contrast-enhanced computed tomography angiography shows a large outpouching *(solid arrow)* along the posterior aspect of the right aortic arch passing behind the esophagus *(arrowhead),* diagnostic of a diverticulum of Kommerell. The left subclavian artery *(dashed arrow)* arises directly from the diverticulum of Kommerell.

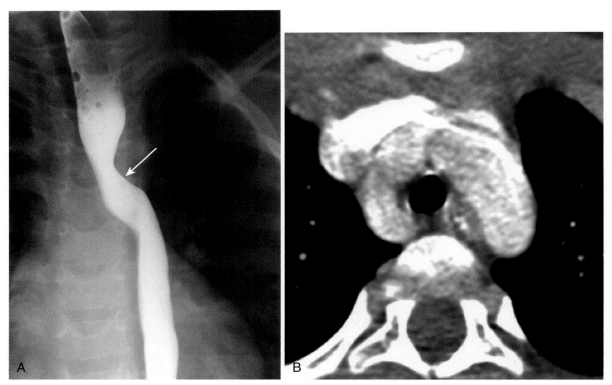

Figure 44-10 Double aortic arch. A, Frontal view from an esophagogram shows extrinsic compression on the esophagus *(arrow)* most consistent with a vascular anomaly. **B,** Contrast-enhanced computed tomography shows a double aortic arch. The resultant vascular ring often leads to respiratory symptoms and is usually diagnosed early in life, as in this case.

and descending aorta are no longer in continuity. The descending aorta is perfused by the patent ductus arteriosum or collateral arteries (Fig. 44-11). A strong association exists between interrupted aortic arch and congenital heart defects (most commonly ventricular septal defects). Other anomalies may also occur (truncus arteriosus, transposition of the great arteries, and aortopulmonary window).

Aortic coarctation represents narrowing of the aorta that is usually focal, although it can also be segmental. The narrowing results from a fibrous ridge, which arises from abnormal hyperplasia of the tunica media. Aortic coarctations are relatively common malformations and affect men two to five times more often than women. Coarctations are most often juxtaductal in location, just distal to the origin of the left subclavian artery. A strong association exists with bicuspid aortic valve (30% to 40%) and patent ductus arteriosus. Aortic coarctation is also moderately associated with Turner syndrome, ventricular septal defects, and intracranial berry aneurysms. This diagnosis can be suggested on radiographs. Poststenotic dilation distal to the coarctation along with the focal area of narrowing of the aorta manifests as contour irregularity along the left superior mediastinum on a frontal chest radiograph, which often demonstrates a reversed-3 configuration. In long-standing coarctations, dilation of the intercostal arteries may lead to inferior rib notching. Increased afterload may progress to left ventricular hypertrophy.

Aortic coarctation is well demonstrated on CT or MRI, given their ability to image in any plane. Typically, the narrowing is best measured in aortic short-axis views, which can be derived from an oblique sagittal view (candy cane view) orthogonal to the long axis of the segment in question to gauge the severity of narrowing relative to normal aortic diameter. In addition, enlarged collateral arteries are easily identified using cross-sectional imaging (Fig. 44-12). Gated CT and MRI delineate the aortic valve to advantage. The aortic valve should be assessed both in diastole and systole because bicuspid aortic valves may appear falsely tricuspid during end-diastole. Gradient echo (bright-blood) MRI across the coarctation provides qualitative functional data. Using velocity encoded phase contrast MRI, the pressure gradient across the stenotic portion of the aorta can be calculated, as can the degree of aortic valvular disease in cases of bicuspid aortic valves. Velocity encoded phase contrast MRI can also be used to gauge the collateral flow through the intercostal arteries by measuring flow volumes in a plane just distal to the coarctation and in another plane at the level of the diaphragmatic crura. In the setting of intercostal collateral flow, the flow volume in the distal aorta is greater (by the amount of collateral flow contribution) compared with the flow in the proximal descending aorta. Circle of Willis CTA or MRA is helpful in excluding occult berry aneurysms, which may become symptomatic longer after successful aortic coarctation repair.

Rarely, aortic narrowing may be acquired. Takayasu aortitis is a well-known cause of acquired aortic stenosis, and it often involves the midthoracic or abdominal aorta. Takayasu aortitis tends to affect younger women

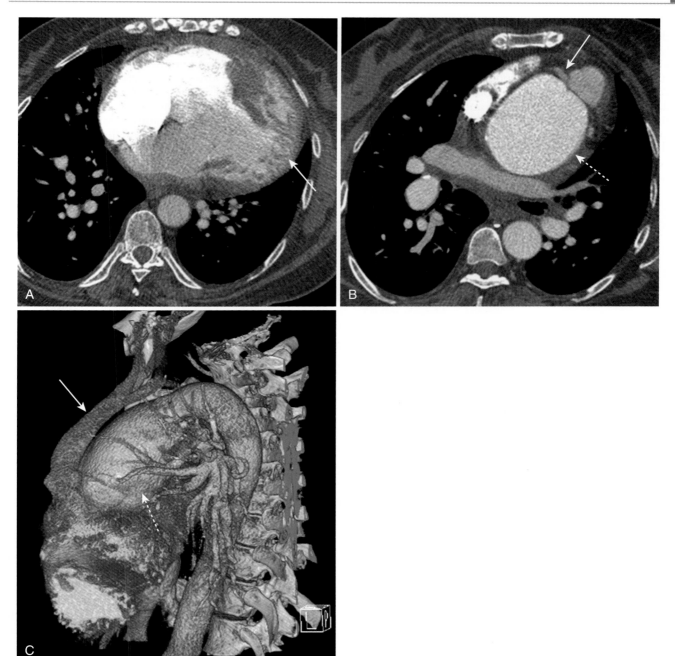

Figure 44-11 *Aortic interruption with transposition of the great arteries after surgical correction.* A, Contrast-enhanced chest computed tomography shows atrioventricular discordance; the heavily trabeculated right ventricle *(arrow)* has inflow from the left atrium. **B,** More superiorly, the aorta (the right coronary artery is visualized *[solid arrow]*) is abnormally positioned anterior and to the left of the enlarged pulmonary artery *(dashed arrow)*. **C,** Sagittal three-dimensional reformation shows the small ascending aorta *(solid arrow)* and an aortic arch (note branches superiorly) that does not connect to the descending aorta. The enlarged pulmonary artery *(dashed arrow)* supplies blood to the descending thoracic aorta through a large patent ductus arteriosus.

(mean age, <30 years). Asians are more often affected. Imaging findings consistent with Takayasu aortitis include smooth thickening of the walls of the aorta and its branches (Fig. 44-13), patchy and symmetric stenosis of the aorta and arch branches, aneurysmal dilation of the aorta and its branches, and aortic regurgitation secondary to aortic root dilation. Occasionally, pulmonary artery involvement may be present (Fig. 44-14). Because of the frequent presentation with ostial stenoses or occlusions of the aortic arch vessel, the disease has also been referred to as the pulseless disease or aortic arch syndrome.

Problem Solving: Differentiating Pseudocoarctation from Aortic Coarctation
Differentiation of aortic coarctation and pseudocoarctation can be challenging on cursory inspection. Both conditions most commonly occur in the postductal portion

of the aorta, distal to the left subclavian artery. Both may demonstrate a reversed-3 configuration on chest radiography. Both can lead to apparent narrowing of the aorta. However, whereas aortic coarctations represent inherent narrowing of the aorta, pseudocoarctations result from congenital elongation of the aortic arch that produces a kinked appearance where the aorta is tethered to the ligamentum arteriosum. Therefore, in the candy cane view (oblique sagittal plane), pseudocoarctations do not demonstrate significant luminal narrowing relative to

the normal adjacent aorta, and no poststenotic dilation results. Therefore, no development of collateral arteries or left ventricular hypertrophy occurs. Furthermore, the elongated and tortuous aortic arch is apparent, often extending into the lower neck; augmentation of the normal flow across the aortic arch may result in an aortic aneurysm. Finally, bicuspid aortic valves are substantially more often present in true aortic coarctation than in pseudocoarctation, although isolated cases of bicuspid aortic valve in association with pseudocoarctation have been reported.

Problem Solving: Differentiating Right Aortic Arch With Mirror Image Branching From Double Aortic Arch With Atretic Distal Left Segment

An incomplete double aortic arch with an atretic distal left segment is a rare vascular anomaly that results in a vascular ring. Patients may present with airway manifestations similar to asthma (stridor or wheezing) or with dysphagia. Two subsets of an incomplete double aortic arch with distal left atretic segment are recognized: one in which atresia occurs distal to the left ligamentum arteriosum and the other in which atresia occurs between the left subclavian artery and the left ligamentum arteriosum. However, differentiation of these two entities on cross-sectional imaging is nearly impossible. As long as both the ligamentum arteriosum and the fibrous atretic left segment are transected during surgery, differentiation is academic.

Differentiation of this anomaly from a right aortic arch with mirror image branching is also challenging but has clinical ramifications. Whereas the double aortic arch with atretic distal left segment results in a ring and can be treated surgically, a right aortic arch with mirror image branching does not typically result in a vascular ring. The right aortic arch with mirror image branching is highly associated with serious congenital heart defects, as aforementioned, of which tetralogy of Fallot is most common. Further evaluation with ECG-gated cardiac CTA, MRI, or echocardiography is mandatory.

Double aortic arch with atretic distal left segment is associated with three findings on cross-sectional imaging that aid in differentiation from right aortic arch with mirror image branching: symmetric branching of

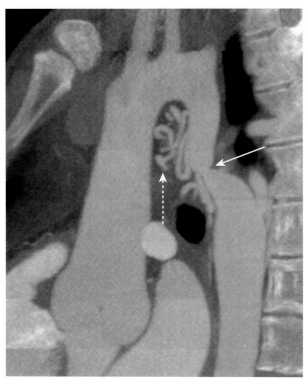

Figure 44-12 Aortic coarctation. Sagittal oblique volume rendered image from electrocardiogram-gated computed tomography angiography of the aorta shows focal narrowing *(solid arrow)* of the aorta along the proximal aspect of the descending thoracic aorta essentially diagnostic of aortic coarctation. An enlarged bronchial arterial *(dashed arrow)* and intercostal collateral arteries are also present.

Figure 44-13 *Takayasu aortitis.* **A,** Axial image from contrast-enhanced chest computed tomography angiography shows circumferential soft tissue thickening *(arrow)* around the aorta with associated mild narrowing of the aorta. **B,** More inferiorly, the aorta demonstrates normal caliber and no abnormal periaortic soft tissue thickening.

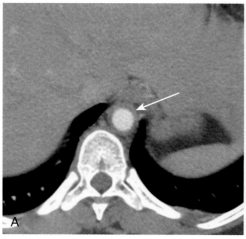

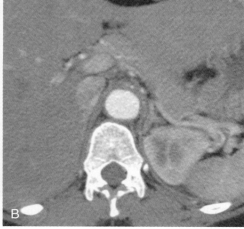

the carotid and subclavian arteries, posterior position of the atretic left arch (from posterior tethering by the atretic fibrous cord) relative to the innominate artery in right aortic arch with mirror image branching, and aortic diverticulum along the left aspect of the descending thoracic aorta (Fig. 44-15). Of these findings, symmetric branching of the carotid and subclavian arteries and aortic diverticulum of the descending thoracic aorta appear to be the most reliable means to differentiate these two entities.

■ ACUTE AORTIC SYNDROME

Acute aortic syndrome (penetrating atherosclerotic ulcer [PAU], IMH, aortic dissection, rupturing aneurysms, and traumatic aortic injury) comprises emergency conditions that usually require immediate intervention. Early identification of these entities is imperative, given the lifesaving ramifications. MDCT

is the current diagnostic modality of choice because of its wide availability and rapid acquisition. MRI is also often diagnostic; however, it is often not feasible in patients who may require cardiorespiratory support. ECG-gated MDCT scans are superior to nongated scans. In most cases, the majority of the thoracic aorta can be adequately evaluated without ECG gating; however, the ascending aorta is difficult to image without motion artifact even with the current high temporal resolution of MDCT. At present, accurate evaluation of the aortic root requires ECG gating or triggering.

Intramural Hematoma

IMH represents hemorrhage located in the aortic media without a visible intimal tear. The treatment and prognosis of IMH are similar to those of aortic dissection because IMH may progress to aortic dissection and rupture. IMHs most often develop secondary to spontaneous rupture of

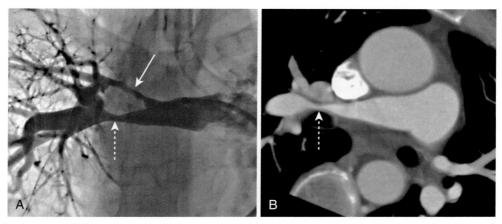

Figure 44-14 Takayasu arteritis involving the pulmonary artery. A, Pulmonary angiogram shows severe narrowing of the right ascending pulmonary artery *(solid arrow)* and the descending pulmonary artery *(dashed arrow)*. **B,** Oblique axial volume rendered image from contrast-enhanced computed tomography angiography shows severe narrowing of the right descending pulmonary artery *(dashed arrow)* with surrounding soft tissue rim in this patient with Takayasu arteritis.

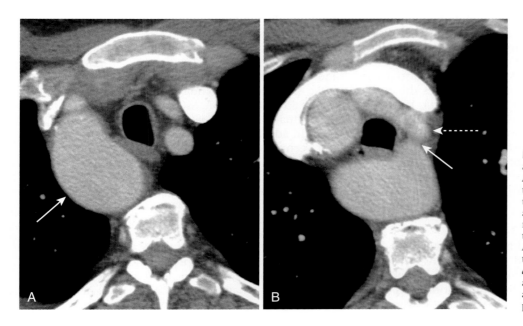

Figure 44-15 Double aortic arch with atretic left segment. **A** and **B,** Axial images from contrast-enhanced chest computed tomography show the right aortic arch *(solid arrow* in **A)**, which is more superior to and larger than the left aortic arch *(dashed arrow)*. Although the posterior aspect of the left aortic arch is atretic *(solid arrow* in **B)**, this anomaly results in a vascular ring that puts the patient at risk for tracheoesophageal compression.

vasa vasorum of the medial aortic layer; however, PAU, blunt trauma, and iatrogenic conditions may also cause IMHs. Hypertension is the most often cited predisposing risk factor.

Unenhanced CT is essential in identifying IMHs. Usually, CT shows circumferential or crescent-shaped hyperdense thickening of the aortic wall that represents hematoma within the media of the aorta (see Fig. 44-4). Intimal calcification from atherosclerosis may be internally displaced, but this rarely allows for diagnosis on radiography. On CE studies, IMHs are often much more subtle; instead of being hyperdense, IMHs are hypodense relative to the CE aortic lumen. No significant enhancement of the hematoma should be present. On MRI, IMHs typically manifest as regions of T1 hyperintensity in the aortic wall that mirror their appearance on noncontrast CT. Similarly, postgadolinium MRI sequences typically show low intensity in the IMH relative to the CE aortic lumen. Although differentiating IMHs from the thrombosed false lumen of aortic dissection may be challenging, several findings may be helpful: IMHs do not enhance, they have no intimal tears, and they maintain a constant relationship with the aortic wall, as opposed to the longitudinal spiral geometry of a false lumen of a dissection. IMHs with involvement of the ascending aorta, concomitant pericardial or pleural effusion, and an aortic diameter greater than 5 cm are at risk of progression to true aortic dissection.

Problem Solving: Differentiating Intramural Hematoma From Vasculitic Aortitis

Based purely on imaging, the differentiation of IMH from vasculitis of the aorta may be challenging. Both lead to thickening of the aortic wall, may mildly narrow the lumen of the aorta (although severe narrowing or occlusion of the aorta would be highly atypical of IMH and most suggestive of a long-standing aortitis), and progress to local aneurysm formation. First and foremost, one must recall that vasculitis is relatively rare compared with IMHs and therefore should be seriously considered only after IMHs has been deemed unlikely. Takayasu arteritis, the most common cause of aortic vasculitis, tends to occur in younger Asian women. Conversely, IMHs tends to occur in older patients in their seventh decade of life. Giant cell arteritis may also occur in older patients, but more often it involves the extracranial carotid system, rather than the aorta. IMHs do not enhance unless they are associated with a PAU. The walls of the aorta may enhance with vasculitic conditions and sometimes demonstrate a double ring configuration (avid enhancement of the outer aspect of aortic wall thickening with a relatively hypodense central ring outlining the opacified aortic lumen).

Aortic Dissection

Aortic dissections are caused by intimal tears extending into the aortic media. Blood flows into this abnormal space and leads to two aortic lumina, the false and true lumen, which are separated by a thin intimal flap. The false lumen may be thrombosed. Acute aortic dissection is a potentially fatal condition but is relatively uncommon (incidence, 2.9 per 100,000 persons per year). Persons at risk for aortic dissections include patients with a thoracic aortic aneurysm, hypertension, Marfan syndrome, bicuspid aortic valve, and earlier cardiovascular surgery. Aortic dissections most commonly occur in the ascending aorta (approximately 65% of cases). Approximately 20% of aortic dissections occur in the descending thoracic aorta, 10% in the aortic arch, and 5% in the abdominal aorta. The caliber of the dissected aorta varies from normal to dilated.

Classification systems for aortic dissections carry prognostic information. Involvement of the ascending aorta implies a worse prognosis, and it usually requires surgical management. The DeBakey and Stanford classifications are most commonly used. In type I DeBakey dissections, the intimal flap involves the ascending and descending thoracic aorta. In type II DeBakey dissections, the intimal flap involves the ascending aorta only, proximal to the left subclavian artery origin. In type III DeBakey dissections, the intimal flap is isolated to the descending thoracic aorta. In Stanford type A dissections, the intimal flap involves the ascending thoracic aorta with variable involvement of the descending aorta. In Stanford type B dissections, the intimal flap is isolated to the descending aorta. Dissections involving the ascending aorta (Stanford A; DeBakey I and II) are surgical emergencies because these dissections are at risk of catastrophic rupture. This rupture, in turn, can lead to hemopericardium, pericardial tamponade, or even death. Ascending aortic dissections may also lead to aortic valve tear, aortic insufficiency, coronary artery dissection, stroke, and myocardial infarction. Surgery in type B dissection is usually not mandatory. Cases with obstruction of aortic branches and end-organ ischemia, continued expansion or extension of the dissection, or frank aortic rupture in addition to an acute dissection in a patient with Marfan syndrome warrant surgical intervention. Watchful waiting is not a viable option in the setting of acute ascending aortic dissections. Mortality rates for untreated Stanford A dissections are 1% to 2% per hour during the first day and approximately 80% during the first 2 weeks.

The high sensitivity of MDCT for the detection of aortic dissections, the wide availability of this technique, and its ability to detect alternative reasons for chest pain make it an excellent choice in the evaluation of suspected aortic dissection. MDCT also shows the extent of the intimal flap, which is essential in preoperative planning. In addition, MDCT often helps identify the entry and reentry sites, relationships between the true and false lumina, patency of aortic branches, aortic valve function, and coronary artery extension. MRI is also highly accurate in the detection of aortic dissections, with nearly perfect sensitivity. However, widespread use of MRI in this setting has not occurred because of long and cumbersome acquisition, which may not be feasible in the emergency setting. Moreover, many medical devices used in gravely ill patients are ferromagnetic, which is a major contraindication to MRI.

Radiography has a limited (if any) role in the robust evaluation of patients with suspected aortic dissection.

Given the relatively low contrast ratio from overlap of multiple anatomic structures, dissections of the aorta can neither be reliably excluded nor identified radiographically. In fact, up to one fourth of patients with aortic dissection actually have normal chest radiographs. Catheter aortography performs well in the diagnosis of aortic dissection (sensitivity, 77% to 90%; and specificity, 90% to 100%) and was the original modality of choice for vascular imaging before the advent of cross-sectional imaging. However, the risks associated with invasive catheter-based imaging and high-flow contrast injection make this modality less attractive. Transesophageal echocardiogram (TEE) is an alternative modality that is useful in unstable patients who cannot be transferred readily onto the gurney of a CT or MRI scanner. TEE is accurate, with a sensitivity of 90% to 100% and a specificity of 77% to 100%. However, TEE relies on operator skill, is prone to ultrasound artifacts, and is limited by inconsistent visualization of the distal ascending aorta and proximal arch because of acoustic window and other restrictions.

The main cross-sectional finding in aortic dissection is the intimal flap, which is a thin linear filling defect that separates the true and false lumina (Fig. 44-16). In patients with atherosclerosis, intimal plaque acts as inherent contrast showing the internally displaced intimal layer. Differentiation of the false and true lumina is important in treatment planning. Most of the time, the true lumen can be delineated by its continuity with the undissected aspect of the aorta. Furthermore, true lumen spirals across the level of the aortic arch (posteriorly located in the ascending aorta and anteriorly located in descending aorta).

The false lumen is usually larger than the true lumen and often demonstrates delayed enhancement relative to the true lumen or even thrombosis. Moreover, the cobweb sign (thin strands of low density regions representing residual media) is specific for the false lumen (see Fig. 44-16). Finally, the beak sign (the section of hematoma that cleaves a space for the propagation of the false lumen) is another helpful sign that helps

identify the false lumen (see Fig. 44-16). Intimointimal intussusception is a rare subtype of aortic dissection; circumferential dissection of the aorta results in invagination of the intimal layer into the more distal aorta, similar to a windsock. Neurologic impairment may be more common in this entity and should be excluded.

Traumatic Aortic Transection

Traumatic aortic transection (traumatic aortic laceration or traumatic aortic injury) results in disruption of all three layers of the aortic wall and is most often caused by violent deceleration (typically from a high-speed motor vehicle accident or a fall from height). Most afflicted individuals die at the scene of injury. Survival is thought to be highest for tears at the aortic isthmus, given that this is the most common manifestation of aortic transection on imaging. Aortic injury may also occur at the level of the aortic root and the diaphragm; however, these patients likely do not survive long enough to be imaged by cross-sectional imaging. Shearing forces, rapid deceleration, aortic hydrostatic forces, or osseous pinching (or a combination thereof) likely play a role in aortic transection injury. Currently, MDCT is the modality of choice in the setting of suspected acute aortic injury because of its wide availability and rapid acquisition. In most level I trauma centers, the AP chest radiograph is used as a screen for acute aortic transection. Imaging findings of acute aortic injury on radiography are based on the assumption that aortic injuries result in mediastinal hematomas. Common findings again include superior mediastinal widening, right paratracheal stripe thickening, abnormal aortic morphology, obliteration of the aortopulmonary window, rightward deviation of mediastinal structures or thickening of the left paraspinal interface (given that the descending aorta is a left-sided structure), left hemothorax, and inferior displacement of the left mainstem bronchus (see Fig. 44-1).

CE MDCT imaging findings of traumatic aortic injury include abrupt change in aortic contour at the isthmus,

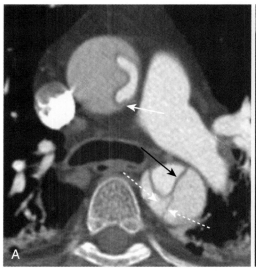 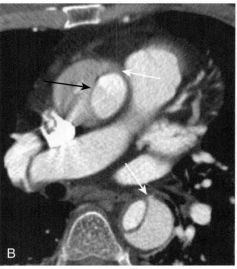

Figure 44-16 Type A aortic dissection. A and B, Axial images from contrast-enhanced computed tomography angiography show the dissection flap in high detail (*black arrows*). Thin linear opacities (*dashed arrows* in A) in the false lumen of the descending aortic dissection (cobweb sign) are specific for the false lumen. In addition, the beak sign (*white arrows* in A and B) is another finding that helps to identify the false lumen.

intramural ridge or flap, focal pseudoaneurysm, mediastinal hematoma, and contrast extravasation (see Fig. 44-1). IMH may also result from blunt trauma and is best appreciated on noncontrast chest CT. At times, a residual ductus diverticulum can mimic the appearance of a traumatic pseudoaneurysm. A normal CE MDCT study is highly reassuring, considering its nearly 100% negative predictive value in the evaluation of traumatic aortic injury.

Problem Solving: Differentiating Traumatic Aortic Injury From Ductus Diverticulum

Traumatic aortic transection and aortic diverticula both occur at the level of the aortic isthmus. In the setting of violent blunt trauma, differentiating between these two entities may be difficult. However, the ductus diverticulum has smooth margins with obtuse angles relative to the adjacent aorta (Fig. 44-17). Aortic transection from blunt trauma has irregular margins with acute angles relative to the adjacent aorta. Although aortic transection may be present in the absence of mediastinal hematoma, it often results in adjacent mediastinal hematoma that manifests as amorphous hyperdense fluid within the mediastinum. In such cases, the fat plane between the involved portion of the aorta and the mediastinal hematoma is usually lost. When the fat plane between the aorta and hyperdense fluid is intact, the mediastinal hematoma is likely the result of bleeding from mediastinal veins or

from musculoskeletal injuries (sternal or spinal fractures), which are often evident on CT.

Penetrating Atherosclerotic Ulcers

PAUs are ulcerated atheromas that disrupt the aortic intima. PAU develops when an atheromatous plaque ruptures, thus leading to disturbance of the elastic lamina that may extend into the media. Hypertension and age are the most important risk factors. The descending aspect of the aorta is the most often affected. Extensive atherosclerosis is often present throughout the aorta. PAUs can be multifocal. On cross-sectional imaging, a discrete contrast-filled outpouching beyond the normal confines of the aorta is often noted (Fig. 44-18). A PAU may extend into the medial layer of the aorta, and this extension can result in an IMH, aortic dissection, saccular pseudoaneurysm, or mediastinal hematoma. Surgery or endovascular repair is considered in patients with pain, cardiovascular instability, or signs of acute or subacute aortic expansion. Asymptomatic patients are usually followed with optimization of medical management.

Problem Solving: Differentiating Penetrating Atherosclerotic Ulcer From Ulcerated Atherosclerotic Plaque

PAUs may be difficult to differentiate from ulcerated atherosclerotic plaque. Careful attention should be paid to the extension of the ulceration relative to the margins of the aortic wall. PAU, by definition, must extend beyond the intimal layer of the aorta. An irregular aortic

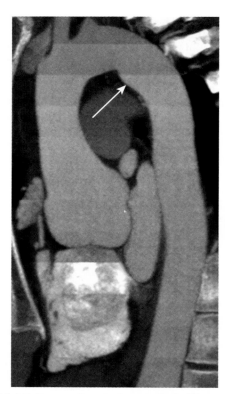

Figure 44-17 Ductus diverticulum. Sagittal oblique image from electrocardiogram-triggered computed tomography angiography of the aorta shows smooth dilation *(arrow)* of the aortic isthmus with smooth margins that form obtuse angles with the normal aorta most consistent with a normal ductus diverticulum. Mild ectasia of the ascending aorta is present.

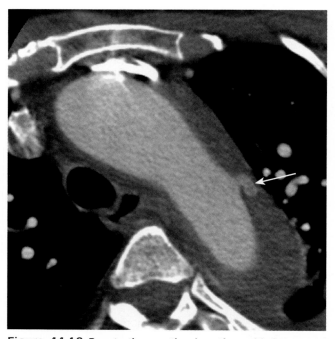

Figure 44-18 Penetrating aortic ulceration with intramural hematoma. Contrast-enhanced chest computed tomography shows a small outpouching *(arrow)* along the lateral wall of the aortic arch that extends beyond the expected confines of the aortic lumen, essentially diagnostic of a penetrating aortic ulceration. Soft tissue thickening along the aortic arch represents intramural hematoma.

contour is highly suggestive of PAU, rather than a simple ulcerated atherosclerotic plaque. In addition, in acute PAUs, patients often present with tearing chest pain not dissimilar to that in aortic dissection. Furthermore, PAUs often result in subintimal hematomas, which cause local thickening of the aortic wall; noncontrast images demonstrate relative hyperdensity in this region. In some cases, this subintimal hematoma enhances after administration of intravenous contrast, given its communication with the aortic lumen.

Thoracic Aortic Aneurysm

In a true aortic aneurysm, greater than 50% of the aorta is dilated. The intima, media, and adventitia in true aneurysms remain intact, as opposed to false aneurysms (pseudoaneurysms). Rupture of an aortic aneurysm is a surgical emergency, given the rapid resultant hemodynamic compromise. As life expectancy has increased, so have the incidence and prevalence of aortic aneurysms. The incidence of aortic aneurysms is approximately 10.9 cases per 100,000 persons per year; between 3% and 4% of patients more than 65 years of age are affected. Men are more often affected than are women. Hypertension is present in 60% of patients, and atherosclerosis is present in approximately 75%. Thoracic aortic aneurysms are less common than are abdominal aortic aneurysms, although it is not uncommon for both to occur concomitantly (up to 25% of patients with thoracic aneurysm also have an abdominal aortic aneurysm).

Patients are usually asymptomatic. However, when large, aneurysms of the ascending aorta or the aortic arch may lead to hoarseness from mass effect on the left vagus or left recurrent laryngeal nerve, diaphragmatic dysfunction from phrenic nerve compression, asthma-like symptoms from tracheobronchial distortion, dysphasia from mass effect on the esophagus, and facial swelling from superior vena cava compression. Rarely, patients may present with hematemesis or hemoptysis in the setting of fistula formation to the esophagus or airway, respectively.

The aortic root and ascending aorta (aortic valve to the brachiocephalic artery) are affected in 60% (Fig. 44-19), the aortic arch in 10%, the descending thoracic aorta (distal to left subclavian artery) in 40%, and the thoracoabdominal aorta in 10% of patients with thoracic aortic aneurysms. The purpose of imaging is not only to identify the presence of thoracic aortic aneurysms, but also to determine their extent, location, and size. Size is most accurately reported in the double oblique aortic short axis (orthogonal to the aortic segment long axis). MDCT and MRI can also accurately detect the presence of complications such as rupture, infection, and fistulas. However, in the acute setting, MDCT is likely more appropriate and is usually more widely available than is MRI. Furthermore, MDCT or MRI can detect aneurysmal involvement of branches of the aorta, a finding that is helpful to surgeons before surgical intervention.

Thoracic aortic aneurysms can be classified based on their extent or morphology. The Crawford classification contains four subtypes. Type I aneurysms extend from the left subclavian artery to the renal artery. Type II aneurysms extend from the left subclavian artery to the aortic bifurcation and have the worst postsurgical outcome. Type III aneurysms extend from the mid-thorax to the aortic bifurcation. Type IV aneurysms extend from the diaphragm to the aortic bifurcation. Thoracic aneurysms can also be subdivided morphologically into fusiform aneurysms (smooth dilation of the entire circumference of the involved portion of the aorta), saccular aneurysms (focal outpouching of the aorta), and pseudoaneurysms (contained rupture of the aortic wall with disruption of at least the intima and media and contained by adventitia or periadventitial tissue).

Size is the only risk factor predicting aortic rupture in true thoracic aortic aneurysms. Aortic aneurysms larger than 4 cm are at risk of rupture. An incremental increase in the risk of aortic rupture is associated with increased aneurysmal size. Aneurysms between 4 and 5.9 cm carry a 16% risk of rupture, and aneurysms larger than 6 cm carry a 31% risk of rupture. On average, thoracic aneurysms grow 1 to 10 mm per year. In general, larger aortic aneurysms have the fastest growth rates. Aneurysms larger than 5 cm grow on average 7.9 mm per year compared with 1.7 mm per year for smaller aneurysms. Larger aneurysms have higher wall tension, given fixed vascular pressure resulting from Laplace law. Therefore, larger aneurysms are at higher risk for rapid growth and rupture. Thoracic descending midaortic aneurysms tend to have the fastest growth rate, whereas ascending aneurysms tend to have the slowest growth

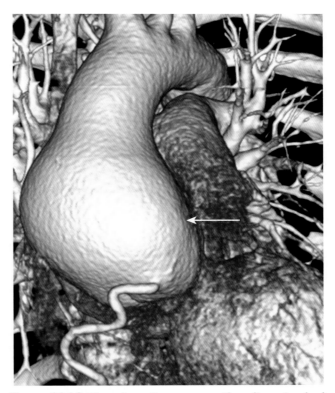

Figure 44-19 *Thoracic aortic aneurysm.* Three dimensional volume rendered reformation from contrast-enhanced computed tomography angiography shows marked dilation of the ascending aorta *(arrow).*

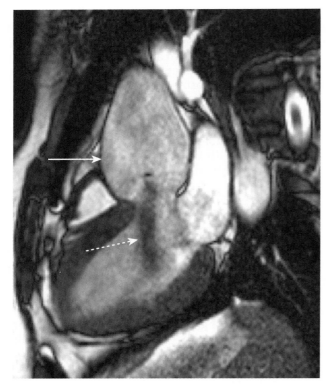

Figure 44-20 Annuloaortic ectasia. Oblique sagittal cine magnetic resonance gradient echo image of the ascending aorta shows dilation of the ascending aorta *(solid arrow)* that extends from the annulus beyond the effaced sinotubular junction. Also visible is an associated regurgitation jet *(dashed arrow)* from aortic insufficiency.

Table 44-1   Normal Values for the Thoracic Aorta

Aorta	Normal Values
Left ventricular outflow tract	20.3 ±3.4 mm (2 SD)
Sinus of Valsalva	34.2 ± 4.1 mm (2 SD) 36.9 ± 3.8 mm (2 SD) (end-diastolic, gated)
Aortic root	25-37 mm (95% CI) (end-diastolic) 26.3 ± 2.8 mm (coronal) 23.5 ± 2.7 mm (sagittal)
Sinotubular junction	29.7 ± 3.4 mm (2 SD)
Ascending aorta	32.7 ± 3.8 mm (2 SD) 33.6 ± 4.1 mm (2 SD) (male/intraluminal/end-systolic) 31.1 ± 3.9 mm(2 SD) (female/intraluminal/end-systolic) 21-35 mm (95% CI) (end-diastolic)

Data from Lu et al, Ocak et al, Lin et al, Tops et al, and Mao et al.
CI, Confidence interval; *SD*, standard deviation.

rate despite larger initial diameters. The risk of dissection is related to the size of the aneurysm, which is also likely related to increased wall tension with increased aortic diameter. The risk of dissection per year is 2% for aneurysms less than 5 cm, 3% for aneurysms 5 to 5.9 cm, and more than 7% for aneurysms more than 6 cm in diameter, with a 5-year survival rate of only 54% without surgery.

Aortic aneurysms in Marfan syndrome and Ehlers-Danlos syndrome may efface the sinotubular junction (annuloaortic ectasia), thus resulting in a classic tulip bulb configuration (Fig. 44-20). Aortic root aneurysms may also occur in patients with bicuspid aortic valves or familial thoracic aortic aneurysm syndrome (FTAAS). Tubular ascending aortic aneurysms are usually idiopathic but may also occur in patients with bicuspid aortic valve, FTAAS, temporal arteritis, and syphilis. Bicuspid aortic valves are an independent predictor of ascending aortic aneurysm formation even in the absence of aortic stenosis. Dilation of the aortic root or the ascending aorta is present in half the patients with normally functioning bicuspid aortic valves. As in most diseases, a hereditary component is present. Up to 20% of patients with thoracic aneurysms have a positive family history.

Ascending aneurysms greater than 5 to 6 cm and descending aneurysms greater than 6 to 7 cm are typically repaired surgically. Alternatively, an aortic size index (ratio of aortic diameter over body surface area

in square meters) greater than 2.75 cm/m^2 can also be used as a cutoff value for surgical intervention. Greater than 1 cm growth in a year for aneurysms smaller than 5 cm is also an indication that surgical repair may be necessary. Risk factors for rapid aneurysmal growth include female sex, advanced age, low forced expiratory volume in 1 second (<1.5 L/min), smoking, and the presence of a bicuspid aortic valve. Concomitant aortic valve replacement is often performed in the setting of aortic root or ascending aortic aneurysms in patients with aortic regurgitation.

Problem Solving: Estimation of True Aortic Size Across Different Modalities and Normal Aortic Size

Published normal measurements of the aorta are listed in Table 44-1. Previously quoted normal aortic diameters were based on various imaging modalities prone to motion artifact or inaccuracy. In addition, measurements based on anatomic axis from cross-sectional imaging are inaccurate, given the oblique plane through the aortic lumen. This is particularly true of the ascending aorta and aortic arch, which are naturally curved structures and may be of variable tortuosity. In most patients, the ascending aorta at the level of the pulmonary artery is the only portion of the aorta that can be accurately measured on true body axial images. Therefore, the "normal" aortic size is somewhat uncertain. Both ECG-gated MDCT and MRI are free of motion artifact and allow for true short-axis (double oblique) measurement throughout the aorta.

Sinus of Valsalva Aneurysm

Sinus of Valsalva aneurysms are rare congenital anomalies that are thought to arise from incomplete fusion of the distal bulbar septum, which connects to the anulus fibrosus of the aortic valve. The right coronary

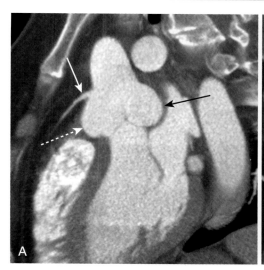
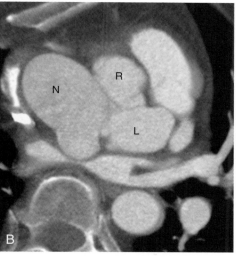

Figure 44-21 Sinus of Valsalva aneurysms. A, Oblique sagittal reformation from electrocardiogram-gated computed tomography angiography shows aneurysmal dilation of the right *(dashed arrow)* and noncoronary *(black arrow)* sinuses of Valsalva. Also visible is high origin of the right coronary artery *(white arrow).* **B,** Short-axis image through the aortic valve shows dilated right (R), noncoronary (N), and left (L) sinus of Valsalva aneurysms.

sinus of Valsalva is most common. Noncoronary sinus involvement is less common, and left coronary sinus involvement is rare. Right sinus of Valsalva aneurysms usually rupture into right-sided cardiac chambers and lead to left-to-right shunting. Rupture into the pericardial sac is rare and may occur in left sinus of Valsalva aneurysms, and it can lead to acute cardiac tamponade and death. Obstruction of the right ventricular outflow tract may occur in patients with large aneurysms. Ventricular septal defect, aortic insufficiency, aortic coarctation, and bicuspid aortic valve are unusual, but have all been described in the setting of sinus of Valsalva aneurysms. On CT or MRI, asymmetric dilatation of one or more of the sinuses of Valsalva is visible (Fig. 44-21). Progression in size is often more influential in proper timing of surgical intervention than is a single time point measurement in asymptomatic patients.

Problem Solving: Differentiating Ascending Aortic Aneurysms in the Setting of Marfan Syndrome Versus Loeys-Dietz Syndrome

Loeys-Dietz syndrome (LDS) is an autosomal dominant connective tissue disease caused by defects in the genes encoding the type I or II transforming growth factor-β (TGF-β) receptor. Phenotypically, these patients resemble patients with Marfan syndrome, Shprintzen-Goldberg syndrome, and vascular Ehlers-Danlos syndrome. Two types of LDS are recognized. Type 1 disease is characterized by hypertelorism, bifid uvula, cleft palate, musculoskeletal abnormalities, and craniosynostosis. Patients with type 2 disease also have a bifid uvula, but the other craniofacial abnormalities in type 1 disease are typically absent. In both subtypes, however, patients are predisposed to general arterial tortuosity, ascending aortic aneurysms, and aortic dissection. Patients with Marfan syndrome also develop ascending aortic aneurysms, as previous described. In addition, in both syndromes, pulmonary arterial dilation may occur. However, patients with LDS also tend to develop aneurysms in other arteries that are also prone to rupture. This finding is in contradistinction to Marfan syndrome.

Furthermore, aneurysms in LDS dissect and rupture at a younger age and at a smaller size than in Marfan syndrome. Whereas 5 cm is the cutoff at which patients with Marfan syndrome are considered for elective ascending aortic aneurysm repair, more aggressive treatment is the norm in LDS.

Bibliography

Abbara S, Kalva S, Cury R, Isselbacher E. Thoracic aortic disease: spectrum of multidetector computed tomography imaging findings. *J Cardiovasc Comput Tomogr.* 2007;1:40-54.

Adams J, Trent R. Aortic complications of Marfan's syndrome. *Lancet.* 1998;352:1722-1723.

Armerding M, Rubin G, Beaulieu C, et al. Aortic aneurysmal disease: assessment of stent-graft treatment-CT versus conventional angiography. *Radiology.* 2000;215:138-146.

Attenhofer Jost C, Schaff H, Connolly H, et al. Spectrum of reoperations after repair of aortic coarctation: importance of an individualized approach because of coexistent cardiovascular disease. *Mayo Clin Proc.* 2002;77: 646-653.

Batra P, Bigoni B, Manning J, et al. Pitfalls in the diagnosis of thoracic aortic dissection at CT angiography. *Radiographics.* 2000;20:309-320.

Berko N, Jain V, Godelman A, Stein E, Ghosh S, Haramati L. Variants and anomalies of thoracic vasculature on computed tomographic angiography in adults. *J Comput Assist Tomogr.* 2009;33:523-528.

Bonow R, Carabello B, Chatterjee K, et al. ACC/AHA 2006 guidelines for the management of patients with valvular heart disease: a report of the American College of Cardiology/American Heart Association Task Force on Practice Guidelines (writing Committee to Revise the 1998 guidelines for the management of patients with valvular heart disease) developed in collaboration with the Society of Cardiovascular Anesthesiologists endorsed by the Society for Cardiovascular Angiography and Interventions and the Society of Thoracic Surgeons. *J Am Coll Cardiol.* 2006;48:e1-e148.

Bonser R, Pagano D, Lewis M, et al. Clinical and patho-anatomical factors affecting expansion of thoracic aortic aneurysms. *Heart.* 2000;84:277-283.

Brickner M, Hillis L, Lange R. Congenital heart disease in adults: first of two parts. *N Engl J Med.* 2000;342:256-263.

Burkhart H, Gomez G, Jacobson L, Pless J, Broadie T. Fatal blunt aortic injuries: a review of 242 autopsy cases. *J Trauma.* 2001;50:113-115.

Cigarroa J, Isselbacher E, DeSanctis R, Eagle K. Diagnostic imaging in the evaluation of suspected aortic dissection: old standards and new directions. *N Engl J Med.* 1993;328:35-43.

Clouse W, Hallett JJ, Schaff H, Gayari M, Ilstrup D, Melton L. Improved prognosis of thoracic aortic aneurysms: a population-based study. *JAMA.* 1998;280:1926-1929.

Coady M, Davies R, Roberts M, et al. Familial patterns of thoracic aortic aneurysms. *Arch Surg.* 1999;134:361-367.

Coady M, Rizzo J, Goldstein L, Elefteriades J. Natural history, pathogenesis, and etiology of thoracic aortic aneurysms and dissections. *Cardiol Clin.* 1999;17:615-635, vii.

Coady M, Rizzo J, Hammond G, Kopf G, Elefteriades J. Surgical intervention criteria for thoracic aortic aneurysms: a study of growth rates and complications. *Ann Thorac Surg.* 1999;67:1922-1926: discussion 1953-1928.

Dapunt O, Galla J, Sadeghi A, et al. The natural history of thoracic aortic aneurysms. *J Thorac Cardiovasc Surg.* 1994;107:1323-1332. discussion 1332-1323.

Davies R, Gallo A, Coady M, et al. Novel measurement of relative aortic size predicts rupture of thoracic aortic aneurysms. *Ann Thorac Surg.* 2006;81:169-177.

Davies R, Goldstein L, Coady M, et al. Yearly rupture or dissection rates for thoracic aortic aneurysms: simple prediction based on size. *Ann Thorac Surg.* 2002;73:17-27. discussion 27-18.

Dyer DS, Moore EE, Ilke DN, et al. Thoracic aortic injury: how predictive is mechanism and is chest computed tomography a reliable screening tool? A prospective study of 1,561 patients. *J Trauma.* 2000;48:673-682: discussion 682-683.

Fan Z, Zhang Z, Ma X, Guo X. Acute aortic dissection with intimal intussusception: MRI appearances. *AJR Am J Roentgenol.* 2006;186:841-843.

Fawzy M, Awad M, Hassan W, Al Kadhi Y, Shoukri M, Fadley F. Long-term outcome (up to 15 years) of balloon angioplasty of discrete native coarctation of the aorta in adolescents and adults. *J Am Coll Cardiol.* 2004;43:1062-1067.

Feczko J, Lynch L, Pless J, Clark M, McClain J, Hawley D. An autopsy case review of 142 nonpenetrating (blunt) injuries of the aorta. *J Trauma.* 1992;33:846-849.

Gomes AS, Bettmann MA, Boxt LM, et al. Acute chest pain--suspected aortic dissection. American College of Radiology. ACR Appropriateness Criteria. *Radiology.* 2000;215 (suppl):1-5.

Gott V, Pyeritz R, Magovern GJ, Cameron D, McKusick V. Surgical treatment of aneurysms of the ascending aorta in the Marfan syndrome: results of composite-graft repair in 50 patients. *N Engl J Med.* 1986;314:1070-1074.

Greenberg R, Secor J, Painter T. Computed tomography assessment of thoracic aortic pathology. *Semin Vasc Surg.* 2004;17:166-172.

Hagan P, Nienaber C, Isselbacher E, et al. The International Registry of Acute Aortic Dissection (IRAD): new insights into an old disease. *JAMA.* 2000;283:897-903.

Hayashi H, Matsuoka Y, Sakamoto I, et al. Penetrating atherosclerotic ulcer of the aorta: imaging features and disease concept. *Radiographics.* 2000;20:995-1005.

Heinemann M, Laas J, Karck M, Borst H. Thoracic aortic aneurysms after acute type A aortic dissection: necessity for follow-up. *Ann Thorac Surg.* 1990;49:580-584.

Hellenbrand W, Allen H, Golinko R, Hagler D, Lutin W, Kan J. Balloon angioplasty for aortic recoarctation: results of Valvuloplasty and Angioplasty of Congenital Anomalies Registry. *Am J Cardiol.* 1990;65:793-797.

Isselbacher E. Thoracic and abdominal aortic aneurysms. *Circulation.* 2005;111:816-828.

Johnson PT, Chen JK, Loeys BL, Dietz HC, Fishman EK. Loeys-Dietz syndrome: MDCT angiography findings. *AJR Am J Roentgenol.* 2007;189:W29-W35.

Johnston K, Rutherford R, Tilson M, Shah D, Hollier L, Stanley J. Suggested standards for reporting on arterial aneurysms: Subcommittee on Reporting Standards for Arterial Aneurysms, Ad Hoc Committee on Reporting Standards, Society for Vascular Surgery and North American Chapter, International Society for Cardiovascular Surgery. *J Vasc Surg.* 1991;13:452-458.

Kaatee R, Van Leeuwen M, De Lange E, et al. Spiral CT angiography of the renal arteries: should a scan delay based on a test bolus injection or a fixed scan delay be used to obtain maximum enhancement of the vessels? *J Comput Assist Tomogr.* 1998;22:541-547.

Kaji S, Nishigami K, Akasaka T, et al. Prediction of progression or regression of type A aortic intramural hematoma by computed tomography. *Circulation.* 1999;100(suppl II):II281-II286.

Kazerooni E, Bree R, Williams D. Penetrating atherosclerotic ulcers of the descending thoracic aorta: evaluation with CT and distinction from aortic dissection. *Radiology.* 1992;183:759-765.

Layton K, Kallmes D, Cloft H, Lindell E, Cox V. Bovine aortic arch variant in humans: clarification of a common misnomer. *AJNR Am J Neuroradiol.* 2006;27:1541-1542.

Lee C, Goo J, Ye H, et al. Radiation dose modulation techniques in the multidetector CT era: from basics to practice. *Radiographics.* 2008;28:1451-1459.

LePage M, Quint L, Sonnad S, Deeb G, Williams D. Aortic dissection: CT features that distinguish true lumen from false lumen. *AJR Am J Roentgenol.* 2001;177:207-211.

Lin F, Devereux R, Roman M, et al. Assessment of the thoracic aorta by multidetector computed tomography: age- and sex-specific reference values in adults without evident cardiovascular disease. *J Cardiovasc Comput Tomogr.* 2008;2:298-308.

Lobato A, Puech-Leão P. Predictive factors for rupture of thoracoabdominal aortic aneurysm. *J Vasc Surg.* 1998;27:446-453.

Lu T, Huber C, Rizzo E, Dehmeshki J, von Segesser L, Qanadli S. Ascending aorta measurements as assessed by ECG-gated multi-detector computed tomography: a pilot study to establish normative values for transcatheter therapies. *Eur Radiol.* 2009;19:664-669.

Maksimowicz-McKinnon K, Hoffman GS. Takayasu arteritis: what is the long-term prognosis? *Rheum Dis Clin North Am.* 2007;3:777-786, vi.

Mao S, Ahmadi N, Shah B, et al. Normal thoracic aorta diameter on cardiac computed tomography in healthy asymptomatic adults: impact of age and gender. *Acad Radiol.* 2008;15:827-834.

Meier J, Seward J, Miller FJ, Oh J, Enriquez-Sarano M. Aneurysms in the left ventricular outflow tract: clinical presentation, causes, and echocardiographic features. *J Am Soc Echocardiogr.* 1998;11:729-745.

Mészáros I, Mórocz J, Szlávi J, et al. Epidemiology and clinicopathology of aortic dissection. *Chest.* 2000;117:1271-1278.

Moore A, Eagle K, Bruckman D, et al. Choice of computed tomography, transesophageal echocardiography, magnetic resonance imaging, and aortography in acute aortic dissection: International Registry of Acute Aortic Dissection (IRAD). *Am J Cardiol.* 2002;89:1235-1238.

Morgan-Hughes G, Marshall A, Roobottom C. Refined computed tomography of the thoracic aorta: the impact of electrocardiographic assistance. *Clin Radiol.* 2003;58:581-588.

Nelsen K, Spizarny D, Kastan D. Intimointimal intussusception in aortic dissection: CT diagnosis. *AJR Am J Roentgenol.* 1994;162:813-814.

Nienaber C, von Kodolitsch Y, Nicolas V, et al. The diagnosis of thoracic aortic dissection by noninvasive imaging procedures. *N Engl J Med.* 1993;328:1-9.

Nienaber C, von Kodolitsch Y, Petersen B, et al. Intramural hemorrhage of the thoracic aorta: diagnostic and therapeutic implications. *Circulation.* 1995;92:1465-1472.

Nihoyannopoulos P, Karas S, Sapsford R, Hallidie-Smith K, Foale R. Accuracy of two-dimensional echocardiography in the diagnosis of aortic arch obstruction. *J Am Coll Cardiol.* 1987;10:1072-1077.

Nistri S, Sorbo M, Marin M, Palisi M, Scognamiglio R, Thiene G. Aortic root dilatation in young men with normally functioning bicuspid aortic valves. *Heart.* 1999;82:19-22.

Nuenninghoff D, Hunder G, Christianson T, McClelland R, Matteson E. Incidence and predictors of large-artery complication (aortic aneurysm, aortic dissection, and/or large-artery stenosis) in patients with giant cell arteritis: a population-based study over 50 years. *Arthritis Rheum.* 2003;48:3522-3531.

Ocak I, Lacomis J, Deible C, Pealer K, Parag Y, Knollmann F. The aortic root: comparison of measurements from ECG-gated CT angiography with transthoracic echocardiography. *J Thorac Imaging.* 2009;24:223-226.

Pagni S, Denatale R, Boltax R. Takayasu's arteritis: the middle aortic syndrome. *Am Surg.* 1996;62:409-412.

Parikh S, Hurwitz R, Hubbard J, Brown J, King H, Girod D. Preoperative and postoperative "aneurysm" associated with coarctation of the aorta. *J Am Coll Cardiol.* 1991;17:1367-1372.

Quint L, Francis I, Williams D, et al. Evaluation of thoracic aortic disease with the use of helical CT and multiplanar reconstructions: comparison with surgical findings. *Radiology.* 1996;201:37-41.

Quint L, Williams D, Francis I, et al. Ulcerlike lesions of the aorta: imaging features and natural history. *Radiology.* 2001;218:719-723.

Rojas C, Restrepo C. Mediastinal hematomas: aortic injury and beyond. *J Comput Assist Tomogr.* 2009;33:218-224.

Roos J, Willmann J, Weishaupt D, Lachat M, Marincek B, Hilfiker P. Thoracic aorta: motion artifact reduction with retrospective and prospective electrocardiography-assisted multi-detector row CT. *Radiology.* 2002;222:271-277.

Rubin G. MDCT imaging of the aorta and peripheral vessels. *Eur J Radiol.* 2003;45(suppl 1):S42-S49.

Safir J, Kerr A, Morehouse H, Frost A, Berman H. Magnetic resonance imaging of dissection in pseudocoarctation of the aorta. *Cardiovasc Intervent Radiol.* 1993;16:180-182.

Sebastià C, Quiroga S, Boyé R, Perez-Lafuente M, Castellà E, Alvarez-Castells A. Aortic stenosis: spectrum of diseases depicted at multisection CT. *Radiographics.* 2003;23:S79-S91.

Stanson A, Kazmier F, Hollier L, et al. Penetrating atherosclerotic ulcers of the thoracic aorta: natural history and clinicopathologic correlations. *Ann Vasc Surg.* 1986;1:15-23.

Steenburg S, Ravenel J, Ikonomidis J, Schönholz C, Reeves S. Acute traumatic aortic injury: imaging evaluation and management. *Radiology.* 2008;248:748-762.

Svensson L, Crawford E, Hess K, Coselli J, Safi H. Experience with 1509 patients undergoing thoracoabdominal aortic operations. *J Vasc Surg.* 1993;17:357-368:discussion 368-370.

Takach T, Reul G, Duncan J, et al. Sinus of Valsalva aneurysm or fistula: management and outcome. *Ann Thorac Surg.* 1999;68:1573-1577.

Therrien J, Thorne S, Wright A, Kilner P, Somerville J. Repaired coarctation: a "cost-effective" approach to identify complications in adults. *J Am Coll Cardiol.* 2000;35:997-1002.

Tops L, Wood D, Delgado V, et al. Noninvasive evaluation of the aortic root with multislice computed tomography implications for transcatheter aortic valve replacement. *JACC Cardiovasc Imaging.* 2008;1:321-330.

Van Hoe L, Baert A, Gryspeerdt S, et al. Supra- and juxtarenal aneurysms of the abdominal aorta: preoperative assessment with thin-section spiral CT. *Radiology.* 1996;198:443-448.

von Kodolitsch Y, Aydin M, Koschyk D, et al. Predictors of aneurysmal formation after surgical correction of aortic coarctation. *J Am Coll Cardiol.* 2002;39:617-624.

von Kodolitsch Y, Csösz S, Koschyk D, et al. Intramural hematoma of the aorta: predictors of progression to dissection and rupture. *Circulation.* 2003;107:1158-1163.

Williams M, Farrow R. Atypical patterns in the CT diagnosis of aortic dissection. *Clin Radiol.* 1994;49:686-689.

CHAPTER 45

Bronchial Arteries

Khashayar Farsad, Mathew P. Cherian, and Sanjeeva P. Kalva

The bronchial arteries represent approximately 1% of the blood supply to the lungs and do not participate in gas exchange. They provide systemic blood supply to the airways, esophagus, posterior mediastinum, portions of the visceral pleura, and mediastinal lymph nodes, as well as to the pulmonary arteries themselves through their vasa vasorum. When normal, the bronchial arteries are not typically well visualized on thoracic aortography. In patients with various cardiopulmonary disorders, including chronic lung infections, lung tumors, inflammatory lung disease, pulmonary vasculitis, congenital heart disease, and chronic pulmonary vascular obstruction, the bronchial arteries can become enlarged as a major source of collateral circulation. In these settings, the risk of hemoptysis from a bronchial artery source exists. Imaging of the bronchial arteries is therefore an important step in the management of these patients. Although evaluation of the bronchial arteries has relied on thoracic aortography and selective bronchial artery angiography, computed tomography (CT) imaging of the bronchial arteries has become more technically feasible and can yield valuable information in the diagnostic workup of a patient with hemoptysis.

■ KEY ISSUES FOR PROBLEM SOLVING IN BRONCHIAL ARTERY IMAGING

- Anatomy of the bronchial arteries
- Technique for CT imaging in hemoptysis: how to optimize visualization of the bronchial arteries
- CT findings in bronchial artery imaging
- CT evaluation of nonbronchial systemic collateral vessels
- CT evaluation of bronchial-to-systemic artery communications
- Bronchial artery embolization: technique and considerations

■ ANATOMY

The bronchial arteries are variable in number and origin (Box 45-1). Certain typical features may be seen, however. The bronchial arteries arise from the descending thoracic aorta in approximately 70% of individuals, usually at the T5 to T6 thoracic vertebral body level. This configuration is considered the orthotopic origin of the bronchial arteries. Based on cadaveric studies, the most common orthotopic pattern is of a right intercostobronchial trunk and two separate left bronchial arteries. The right intercostobronchial trunk has branches supplying the bronchi and the chest wall, and it typically originates from the posteromedial wall of the aorta. The left bronchial arteries typically arise along the anterior wall of the aorta, although an origin from the right posteromedial aorta or even the right intercostobronchial trunk has been observed. Occasionally, a right and left bronchial artery will arise from a common trunk along the anterior thoracic aorta (Fig. 45-1). Less common or aberrant sites of origin of the bronchial arteries include the thoracic aortic arch (typically from the concavity, but also from the convexity), the subclavian artery and its branches, the internal thoracic artery, the brachiocephalic trunk, and the abdominal aorta (see Fig. 45-1). Important anastomoses of the bronchial arteries include contributions to the anterior spinal artery, branches to the esophagus, anastomoses to the coronary arteries, and anastomoses to the pulmonary arteries, particularly in the setting of chronic lung disease. Of these anastomoses, contributions to the anterior spinal artery are the most feared aspect of bronchial artery intervention because inadvertent embolization results in potential paralysis. Evaluation of the bronchial arteries has traditionally required catheter angiography. The improved quality of high-resolution multidetector row CT (MDCT) has enabled visualization of the origin and course of the bronchial arteries before intervention and can be a helpful aid in the evaluation of hemoptysis.

Pearls and Pitfalls

- Bronchial artery anatomy is variable; 70% of bronchial arteries arise from the descending aorta at the T5 to T6 vertebral body level.
- Aberrant origins of the bronchial arteries are commonly seen from the concavity of the thoracic aortic arch, but they can also be found from the convexity of the arch, the subclavian artery and its branches, the internal thoracic artery, and the abdominal aorta.
- A potential communication of the bronchial arteries with the anterior spinal artery should always be scrutinized before intervention.

BOX 45-1   Bronchial Artery Origins

Orthotopic Bronchial Artery Origin

Right intercostobronchial trunk; two left bronchial arteries

Right intercostobronchial trunk; one left bronchial artery

Right intercostobronchial trunk and one additional right bronchial artery; two left bronchial arteries

Right intercostobronchial trunk and one additional right bronchial artery; one left bronchial artery

Common trunk supplying a right and left bronchial artery

Aberrant Bronchial Artery Origin

Aortic arch (mostly from concavity)

Subclavian artery (ipsilateral or contralateral)

Descending aorta; abdominal aorta

Brachiocephalic trunk

Internal thoracic artery

Thyrocervical trunk

■ COMPUTED TOMOGRAPHY TECHNIQUE FOR IMAGING THE BRONCHIAL ARTERIES

If CT is being performed for a case of hemoptysis, the examiner must obtain high-resolution images with thin-slice collimation and considerable overlap. MDCT angiographic protocols are preferable, particularly because evaluation of lung parenchyma, with its intrinsic high contrast, is less dependent on the phase of vessel opacification. Slice thickness of 1.25 mm with 0.625-mm overlapping increments allows for high-resolution reformations, to visualize the origin and course of the bronchial arteries most clearly. Imaging parameters with most 16- and 64-row MDCT scanners include 80- to 140 kilovolt peak (kVp) range, 90 to 140 mA, a 10-mm beam width, and a beam pitch of 1.2 to 1.5. A contrast injection rate of at least 3.5 mL/second with a power injector through an 18-gauge cannula is suggested. Typically, 80 to 120 mL high-density nonionic contrast agent (300 to 350 mg/dL) is used with either bolus tracking or an 18-second delay to begin scanning at peak arterial enhancement. These parameters usually provide adequate opacification of both systemic and pulmonary arterial vasculature in the regions of interest.

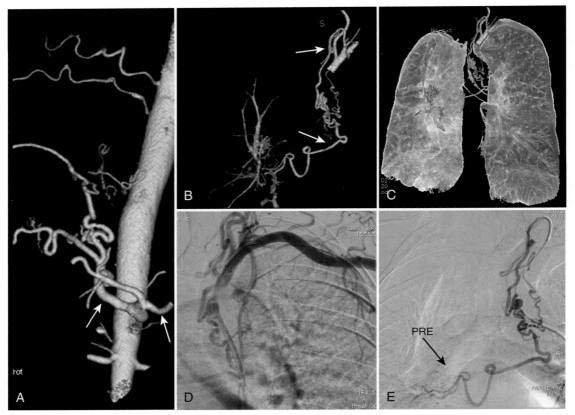

Figure 45-1 Bronchial artery variation. A, Three-dimensional reformatted computed tomography (CT) angiogram demonstrates the descending thoracic aorta with enlarged, tortuous bronchial arteries *(arrows)*. Left and right bronchial arteries arise from a common trunk originating from the anterior aspect of the aorta. **B,** In addition, a right bronchial artery arises from the left subclavian artery and thyrocervical trunk *(arrows)*. Evaluation of **B** and **C** shows an aberrant origin of a bronchial artery as it travels into the right hilum and courses with the bronchi. **D** and **E,** Corresponding angiograms in the same patient demonstrate the aberrant origin of this right bronchial artery. Preprocedural CT scanning is very helpful in identifying these anatomic variants before intervention.

The scan should ideally span the base of the neck to the level of the renal arteries, to capture potential aberrant origins of the bronchial arteries, as well as major sources of potential nonbronchial systemic collateral vessels. With 16- or 64-detector row scanners, the entire scan may be performed in a single breath hold. Sagittal and coronal reformations are routinely performed using the raw data in the axial thin-section images, with additional two-dimensional and three-dimensional reformations and volume rendered images as necessary on a case by case basis. Imaging the origin and course of the bronchial arteries in this way provides information valuable to the interventionalist in planning potential embolization, and it may also assist a surgeon for planning potential vessel ligation.

Pearls and Pitfalls

- Thin-collimation MDCT technique provides the best current resolution for identifying the origin and course of the bronchial arteries.
- Sagittal, coronal, two-dimensional, and three-dimensional reformation techniques may all be used to improve visualization of the origin and course of the bronchial arteries.
- Scan should extend from the base of the neck to the level of the renal artery origins, to identify any aberrant origins of the bronchial arteries and common sources of potential nonbronchial systemic collateral vessels.

■ COMPUTED TOMOGRAPHY EVALUATION OF BRONCHIAL ARTERIES

Bronchial arteries 3 mm or greater in diameter are considered dilated and may be the source of bleeding in a patient with hemoptysis, particularly if parenchymal findings lateralize to the same side as the dilated bronchial artery. CT can provide very useful information regarding parenchymal findings and areas of hemorrhage to help in preprocedural planning for bronchial artery embolization. Some of these findings include bronchiectasis, ground glass opacities indicating hemorrhage, malignant disease, chronic lung infection, and cavitary changes. The airways should be evaluated for air-fluid levels as a potential sign of hemorrhage. Occasionally, extravasated contrast material may collect in the airways, a finding that may be seen both on CT and angiography. Finally, a pulmonary arterial source of hemoptysis may be identified in patients with central cavitation, known tuberculosis (i.e., Rasmussen aneurysm), known pulmonary vasculitis such as Behçet disease, a history of pulmonary artery catheterization, or identification of a pulmonary arteriovenous malformation. If extensive hemorrhage obscures the parenchyma, a follow-up CT scan a few weeks after cessation of hemoptysis may be performed, to evaluate for a potentially obscured underlying parenchymal lesion more accurately.

Dilated and tortuous bronchial arteries, which often represent the source of hemoptysis, can readily be seen on CT (Fig. 45-2). In addition, the ability to visualize a bronchial artery clearly from its origin to its respective lung hilum has independently been described as a CT imaging finding identifying the likely bronchial artery causing hemoptysis at angiography (Figs. 45-3 and 45-4). Aneurysms of the bronchial arteries, either in an intrapulmonary location or in the mediastinum, can also be identified by CT (Figs. 45-5 and 45-6). When in an intrapulmonary location, bronchial artery aneurysms indicate a potential source of hemoptysis. Furthermore, CT imaging can identify the rare pseudosequestration,

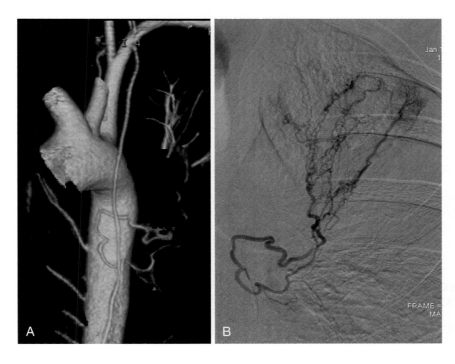

Figure 45-2 Three-dimensional computed tomography (CT) (**A**) and corresponding angiography (**B**) in another patient with hemoptysis. An early bifurcating left bronchial artery is seen on both CT and angiography.

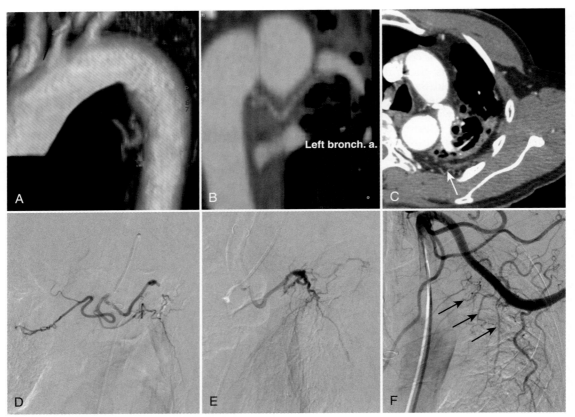

Figure 45-3 A to F, *Nonbronchial systemic collateral vessels.* A and B, Computed tomography reformatted imaging using volumetric and curved reformation techniques demonstrates a common trunk of the right and left bronchial arteries arising from the anterior aorta. The left bronchial artery in **B** is clearly visualized from its origin to the hilum, and this was the bleeding source at angiography (**D** and **E**). In cases with disease extending to pleural surfaces such as this, prominent vessels in the extrapleural fat (**C**, *arrow*) suggest nonbronchial systemic collateral vessels, seen clearly at angiography from branches of the left subclavian artery (**F**, *arrows*). Changes of chronic lung disease as seen in **C** also help to lateralize the search for the bleeding source. Comparison of Figure 45-1 with Figure 45-2 demonstrates differences between a bronchial artery with an aberrant origin and a dilated nonbronchial systemic collateral vessel.

a pure vascular pulmonary sequestration, as a source of hemoptysis. In this entity, a systemic branch of the descending thoracic aorta typically supplies an otherwise normal portion of the lung base (no associated bronchial or parenchymal sequestration) and drains through a pulmonary vein.

Pearls and Pitfalls

- MDCT can accurately identify the origin and course of the bronchial arteries, particularly the arteries involved in hemoptysis, in most cases.
- Aberrant origins of the bronchial arteries can be seen on CT.
- Associated pulmonary parenchymal findings can help direct the search for abnormal bronchial arteries.
- A pulmonary arterial source of hemoptysis may be identified in selected cases.

■ COMPUTED TOMOGRAPHY EVALUATION OF NONBRONCHIAL SYSTEMIC COLLATERAL VESSELS

When pulmonary parenchymal disease extends to or involves the pleura, nonbronchial systemic collateral vessels are recruited across pleural adhesions to supply the areas of abnormality. CT can evaluate for recruitment of these nonbronchial systemic collateral vessels to the bronchial circulation, typically from the intercostal arteries, branches of the subclavian or axillary artery, the internal thoracic artery, or the inferior phrenic arteries (Box 45-2). Dilated, tortuous arteries in the extrapleural space should be followed for collateralization, especially when they are associated with adjacent pleural abnormalities (see Fig. 45-3). Parenchymal findings on CT may help direct the search for associated nonbronchial systemic collateral vessels. For example, lower lobe findings should prompt a search for inferior phrenic artery collateral vessels, posterior lung findings should prompt a search for intercostal artery collateral vessels, and anterior lung findings should prompt a search for internal thoracic artery collateral vessels. Nonbronchial systemic collateral vessels are differentiated from a bronchial artery with an aberrant origin by recognizing that the bronchial artery with an aberrant origin will still enter the hilum and course along the major bronchi, as opposed to systemic collateral vessels, which penetrate the pleura or pulmonary ligament and do not travel along the bronchi.

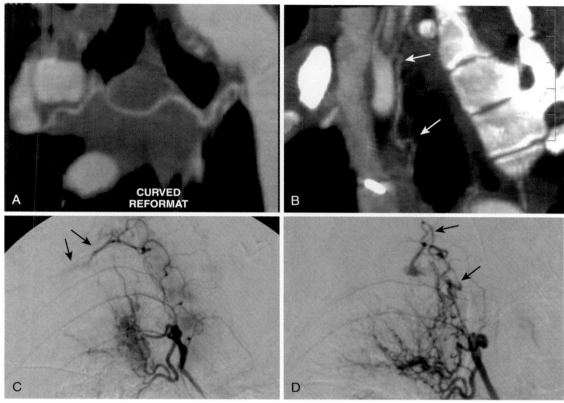

Figure 45-4 Bronchial artery anastomoses. **A,** Curved reformatted computed tomography image in a patient with chronic lung disease from cystic fibrosis demonstrates an enlarged, tortuous right bronchial artery clearly visualized from its origin into the right hilum. **B,** Tracing this intercostobronchial trunk more peripherally demonstrates communication with a branch of the right subclavian artery *(arrows).* **C** and **D,** Findings at angiography confirm anastomoses with the right subclavian artery (**C,** *arrows*) through multiple small vessels (**D,** *arrows*). Care must be taken to embolize distal to these anastomoses at intervention to prevent nontarget embolization to the right upper extremity.

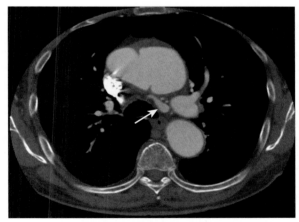

Figure 45-5 Bronchial artery aneurysm. Axial computed tomography scan demonstrates an aneurysm of an enlarged and tortuous bronchial artery extending from the mediastinum toward the left hilum *(arrow)*. Mediastinal bronchial artery aneurysms are more likely to be identified as mass lesions on imaging. Hemoptysis may not be present.

Pearls and Pitfalls

- Dilated and tortuous arteries in the extrapleural fat should be evaluated to see whether they represent nonbronchial systemic collateral vessels.

- CT findings may help direct the source of nonbronchial systemic collateral vessels based on the proximity of the abnormality to potential collateral arteries.
- Aberrant origins of the bronchial arteries are differentiated from nonbronchial systemic collateral vessels by their course along the major bronchi.

■ COMPUTED TOMOGRAPHY EVALUATION OF BRONCHIAL-TO-SYSTEMIC ARTERY COMMUNICATIONS

Bronchial-to-systemic artery communications in critical vascular beds exist and should be recognized. Among the most important of these communications are contributions to anterior medullary spinal branches, which reinforce the anterior spinal artery along the thoracic aorta. The artery of Adamkiewicz is the dominant of these communications to the anterior spinal artery from the thoracic aorta. Although it typically arises more inferiorly, between the T9 and T12 vertebral bodies, the artery of Adamkiewicz may arise at midthoracic vertebral body levels, close to the orthotopic origin of the bronchial arteries. Communication of the bronchial arteries to the anterior spinal artery and the classic hairpin loop configuration of the communicating branch described on

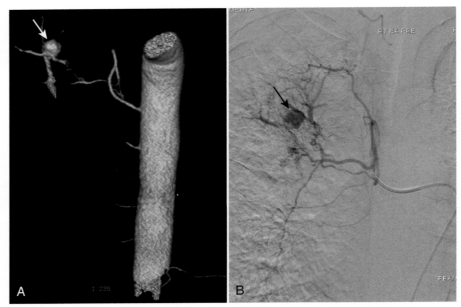

Figure 45-6 Bronchial artery aneurysm. Computed tomography imaging (**A**) and corresponding angiography (**B**) in a patient with hemoptysis clearly demonstrate an aneurysm *(arrows)* along an intrapulmonary segment of the right bronchial artery.

BOX 45-2 Typical Origins of Nonbronchial Systemic Collateral Arteries

Brachiocephalic trunk
Subclavian artery
Thyrocervical or costocervical trunk
Axillary artery
Internal thoracic artery
Inferior phrenic artery
Intercostal arteries
Abdominal aorta branches

---

angiography are not always well evaluated on CT imaging, and further intervention requires close scrutiny of potential spinal branches before embolization.

Another important bronchial-to-systemic artery communication involves anastomoses to branches communicating with the coronary arteries. These communications generally occur in the retrocardiac region and can involve branches of both coronary arteries. Coronary-to-bronchial artery communication may be stimulated in the setting of decreased pulmonary perfusion, in which the coronary circulation contributes to the pulmonary circulation through bronchial artery collateral vessels, or in the setting of coronary atherosclerosis, in which the bronchial artery circulation contributes to coronary perfusion. Anastomoses between the coronary arteries and the bronchial arteries can often be seen on CT angiographic imaging, and they constitute an important consideration for further intervention.

Pearls and Pitfalls

- Important bronchial-to-systemic artery anastomoses include those to the anterior spinal artery and those to the coronary arteries.

- Spinal artery communications are often difficult to see on CT, and close angiographic evaluation is required before embolization.
- Bronchial-to-coronary artery anastomoses typically occur with arteries coursing in the retrocardiac region.

■ BRONCHIAL ARTERY EMBOLIZATION

Massive hemoptysis, variably defined as hemoptysis of approximately 200 to 600 mL in 24 hours, often has a bronchial artery source. Bronchial artery embolization is a useful procedure to arrest bleeding. With adequate chest CT, the origins of the bronchial arteries can be ascertained before the procedure, and the appropriate catheter shapes for effective catheterization can be selected. If CT findings are bilateral, or if the source of bleeding is unclear, a preprocedural bronchoscopic evaluation may help determine the likely site of bleeding and assist the interventionalist with targeting the appropriate source. Findings at angiography to suggest the involved bronchial artery include enlargement to 3 mm or more, tortuosity and irregularity, hypervascularity and neovascularity of the lung parenchyma, bronchial-to-pulmonary artery or vein shunting, and bronchial artery aneurysm. Although active extravasation akin to that seen in gastrointestinal or solid organ bleeding is a rare finding, parenchymal staining, which is essentially a form of extravasation, can be seen. On occasion, contrast material can accumulate in the airways, as described earlier, and this feature is also consistent with extravasation. Nonbronchial systemic collateral vessels contributing to hemoptysis share the same findings at angiography.

When findings consistent with a bronchial artery source for hemoptysis are seen at angiography, embolization is typically undertaken. Coaxial catheter technique with a 3-French microcatheter is used to cannulate the bronchial artery securely and to avoid important bronchial-to-systemic collateral vessels and reflux into the aorta. Diagnostic imaging should be performed at the proposed site of treatment to evaluate these findings. As mentioned earlier, care is taken to look for a vessel with a hairpin loop configuration coursing along the midline, to identify a possible spinal artery branch. Once catheter positioning is optimized, embolization is undertaken using particulate embolic materials such as polyvinyl alcohol particles, spheric embolic agents, or a Gelfoam slurry. Liquid embolic agents, such as n-butyl cyanoacrylate glue, are less favored by interventionalists because of the potential difficulty of controlling their administration. Metallic coils are avoided, to facilitate retreatment in these patients, in whom recurrent bleeding often occurs. Occasionally, coils may be used to close a large bronchopulmonary vascular shunt before particulate embolization; however, larger particulate embolic materials can also be used for the same purpose.

In general, bronchial artery embolization is effective, with a 90% technical success rate and 70% to 95% initial control of hemoptysis. Treatment failures usually result from unsuccessful catheterization, failure to identify the correct bleeding artery, and failure to recognize additional contributing vessels to bleeding. A pulmonary arterial source of hemoptysis should also be considered in the appropriate setting. The late recurrence rate is relatively high, at 20% to 30%; again, this is why particulate agents are preferred over coils. Causes of recurrence include incomplete initial embolization, recanalization of embolized vessels, progression of disease, unidentified additional sources of bleeding, and recruitment of new collateral vessels. A postembolization syndrome of fever, chest wall pain, or dysphagia can occur. The complication rate is approximately 2% to 5%, including spinal cord infarction, nontarget embolization, esophageal necrosis from embolization of collateral branches to the esophagus, and pulmonary infarction in the setting of pulmonary artery obstructive disease.

Pearls and Pitfalls

- Findings at angiography implicating a bronchial arterial source for hemoptysis are enlargement to 3 mm or more, tortuosity and irregularity, hypervascularity and neovascularity, bronchial to pulmonary artery or vein shunting, and bronchial artery aneurysm. Active extravasation is rarely seen.
- Bronchial-to-systemic collateral vessels with the anterior spinal artery and the coronary arteries are important considerations when intervention is planned.
- Embolization with particles is favored over coils to facilitate repeat intervention if necessary.
- A possible pulmonary arterial source of hemoptysis may be considered in the appropriate clinical setting if no evident abnormality is seen in the bronchial arteries.

Bibliography

Bruzzi JF, Remy-Jardin M, Delhaye D, et al. Multi-detector row CT of hemoptysis. *Radiographics.* 2006;26:3-22.

Cauldwell EW, Siekert RG. The bronchial arteries; an anatomic study of 150 human cadavers. *Surg Gynecol Obstet.* 1948;86:395-412.

Chung MP, Yi CA, Lee HY, et al. Imaging of pulmonary vasculitis. *Radiology.* 2010;255:322-341.

Kalva SP. Bronchial artery embolization. *Tech Vasc Interv Radiol.* 2009;12:130-138.

Kalva SP, Wicky S. Mediastinal bronchial artery aneurysms: endovascular therapy in two patients. *Catheter Cardiovasc Interv.* 2006;68:858-861.

Khalil A, Fartoukh M, Tassart M, et al. Role of MDCT in identification of the bleeding site and the vessels causing hemoptysis. *AJR Am J Roentgenol.* 2007;188:W117-W125.

Remy-Jardin M, Bouaziz N, Dumont P, et al. Bronchial and nonbronchial systemic arteries at multi-detector row CT angiography: comparison with conventional angiography. *Radiology.* 2004;233:741-749.

Valji K. *Vascular and Interventional Radiology.* Philadelphia: Saunders; 1999.

Wilson SR, Winger DI, Katz DS. CT visualization of mediastinal bronchial artery aneurysm. *AJR Am J Roentgenol.* 2006;187:W544-W545.

Yildiz AE, Ariyurek OM, Akpinar E, et al. Multidetector CT of bronchial and nonbronchial systemic arteries. *Diagn Interv Radiol.* 2011;17:10-17.

Yoon YC, Lee KS, Jeong YJ, et al. Hemoptysis: bronchial and nonbronchial systemic arteries at 16-detector row CT. *Radiology.* 2005;234:292-298.

CHAPTER 46

Abdominal Aorta and Branches

Khashayar Farsad

The abdominal aorta and its primary branches are involved in many diseases and conditions that affect large and medium-sized arteries. Traditional evaluation of the abdominal aorta relied on catheter aortography; however, with the advent of multislice computed tomography (CT), rapid and robust CT angiography (CTA) imaging of the abdominal aorta and its branches has increasingly rivaled catheter angiography as a primary diagnostic imaging modality, particularly in hemodynamically stable patients. Knowledge of the radiologic appearance of the abdominal aorta and branches is helpful in differentiating various pathologic states.

■ KEY ISSUES FOR PROBLEM SOLVING IN IMAGING OF THE ABDOMINAL AORTA AND ITS BRANCHES

- Features of occlusive disease
- Differentiating aneurysmal disease
- Imaging the postoperative aorta
- Differentiating causes of the acute aortic syndrome
- Features of iatrogenic and traumatic disease
- Findings in inflammatory vascular disease
- Imaging the visceral arteries

■ OCCLUSIVE DISEASE

Aortoiliac Atherosclerosis

Mural calcification of the abdominal aorta and primary branches is a common finding on CT scanning. In fact, the prevalence of calcific changes in the abdominal aorta has been reported to be more than 90% in certain ethnic groups by age, including non-Hispanic whites and Chinese populations. Common causes of mural calcification include hypercholesterolemia, diabetes, smoking history, hypertension, and renal disease. Atherosclerotic aortoiliac stenotic or occlusive disease has been reported to occur in slightly more than half of all patients who are evaluated for peripheral arterial disease.

Although identifying changes of atherosclerosis is typically not a diagnostic imaging dilemma, certain features are helpful in assessing the significance of the affected arterial segments. For example, chronic aortoiliac occlusive disease is characterized by numerous collateral pathways for reconstitution of the pelvic vessels and the lower extremity runoff. Dominant collateral pathways are typically through arteries running along the body wall, such as the internal mammary arteries, epigastric arteries, and lumbar arteries, or by arteries supplying viscera, such as branches of the inferior mesenteric artery. These structures are best seen by angiography, but the astute imager also recognizes many of these pathways on CT or magnetic resonance imaging (MRI) as abnormally dilated collateral vessels (Fig. 46-1). Without the real-time benefit of flow dynamics seen on catheter angiography, the presence of these collateral vessels is a good cross-sectional clue to severe focal stenosis or occlusion. Focal stenosis or occlusion can be missed in the axial dimension if the lesion is very short and good collateral runoff opacifies the vessel distal to the diseased segment. Evaluation of reformatted images in the coronal and sagittal planes should therefore be performed because a focal hemodynamically significant lesion, which was otherwise subtle on axial CTA, may be better demonstrated. Common sites of such lesions in the peripheral circulation include the superficial femoral artery at the adductor hiatus, where short focal lesions are often associated with dilated collateral vessels through the profunda femoris or genicular branches to supply the runoff. Viewing well-opacified distal runoff vessels in this setting as indicative of no significant disease would be a mistake.

Coral Reef Aorta

One particularly significant form of aortic occlusive disease is known as the "coral reef" aorta, so named because of the bulky, frondlike calcifications seen primarily to involve the visceral segment of the abdominal aorta (Fig. 46-2). This condition may result in hemodynamically significant stenoses of the visceral and mesenteric arteries, as well as compromised flow to the lower extremities. Recognizing this finding is important because it may be a cause of significant distal embolic disease. In addition, given that the coral reef aorta increases the risk of embolic disease during endovascular procedures, awareness of this finding is important for the interventionalist.

Rare Entities

Nonatherosclerotic forms of aortic stenosis are rare. These include the coarctation or middle aortic syndromes,

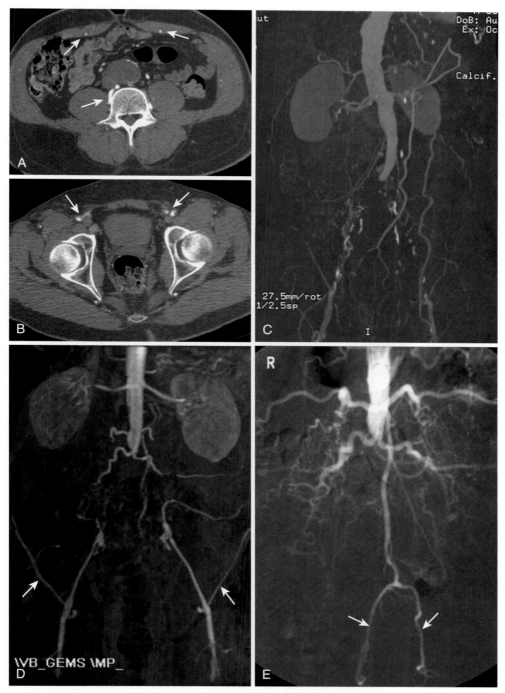

Figure 46-1 Aortoiliac occlusive disease. Computed tomography angiography (**A** to **C**), magnetic resonance angiography (**D**), and angiographic (**E**) images of aortoiliac occlusive disease demonstrate a dilated body wall and visceral collateral vessels that provide the runoff to the lower extremities. Prominent collateral pathways include the inferior epigastric artery (*oblique paired arrows* in **A**), deep circumflex iliac artery (*paired arrows* in **D**), and visceral collateral arteries through the inferior mesenteric artery (*paired arrows* in **E**) to branches of the internal iliac followed by the external iliac arteries. Paired arrows (**A** and **B**) highlight inferior epigastric artery collateral vessels to the common femoral arteries, and the arrow in **A** adjacent to the vertebral body demonstrates a prominent lumbar artery collateral vessel. Especially with chronic occlusions, these collateral arteries should be readily seen on cross-sectional imaging and three-dimensional reformations.

such as Takayasu arteritis, neurofibromatosis, mucopolysaccharidoses, and the hypoplastic aortic syndrome. Differentiating features of these conditions include the relative lack of atherosclerotic change, although concurrent atherosclerosis may still be present, and the younger age of the affected individuals. Some conditions, such as the hypoplastic aortic syndrome, have a predilection for young to middle-aged female patients (Fig. 46-3). Other rare causes of nonatherosclerotic aortic stenosis include retroperitoneal fibrosis and radiation aortitis. Retroperitoneal fibrosis can be recognized by stranding and cicatrization in the surrounding retroperitoneal fat,

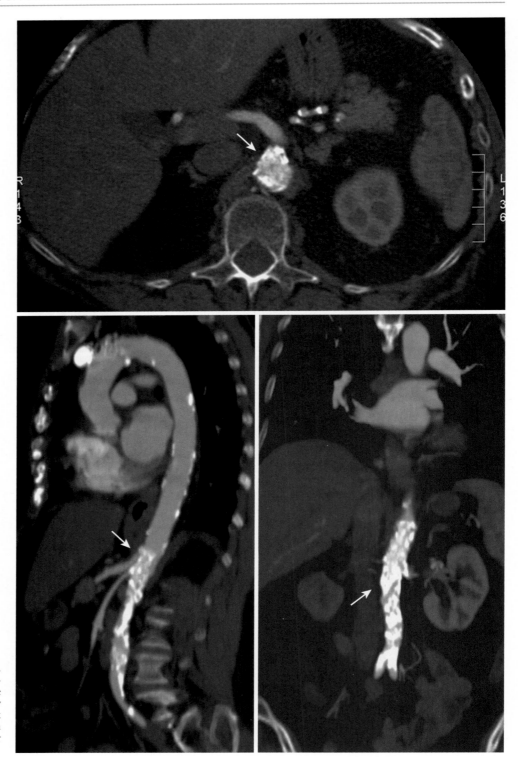

Figure 46-2 Coral reef aorta. Computed tomography angiography showing dense, proliferative calcification of the aorta, especially involving the visceral segment *(arrows)*. Endovascular intervention in this condition carries a higher risk of embolic complications.

classically associated with medial displacement of the ureters and possible hydronephrosis. Radiation aortitis can usually be suggested from the patient's history. Aortic angiosarcoma can manifest with peripheral or visceral ischemia and a polypoid intraluminal mass on imaging. This mass may appear as polypoid thrombus and plaque and can be difficult to distinguish by CT. Clues to the diagnosis include an atypical polypoid appearance and

lack of extensive atherosclerotic change or aneurysm. MRI with contrast is optimal for soft tissue characterization and enhancement.

Pearls and Pitfalls

■ Aortoiliac stenotic and occlusive disease is common in patients with peripheral arterial disease.

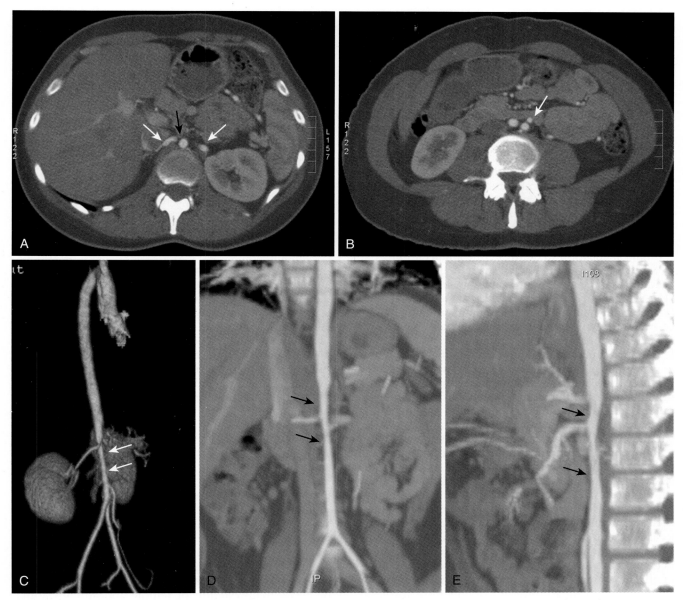

Figure 46-3 Hypoplastic aortic syndrome. A to C, Computed tomography angiography shows smooth narrowing of the infrarenal abdominal aorta in a patient with middle aortic syndrome (**A**, *black arrow,* and **C**, *arrows*). Note the relative diameter of the aorta (**A**, *black arrow,* and **C**, *arrows*) compared with the renal arteries (**A**, *white arrows*). The markedly hypertrophied inferior mesenteric artery (**B**, *arrow*) is compensating for the decreased flow through the superior mesenteric artery, which originates from the hypoplastic segment (not shown). **D** and **E**, Coronal and sagittal reformatted CT images in a different patient with neurofibromatosis demonstrate similar findings *(arrows).*

- Atherosclerosis is the most common cause, but other rare entities should be entertained in certain demographic groups such as younger individuals.
- The coral reef aorta poses an increased risk of thromboembolic disease during intervention.

■ ANEURYSMAL DISEASE

Degenerative Abdominal Aortic Aneurysm

Degenerative aneurysmal disease of the abdominal aorta is thought to affect approximately 8% of the population, men much more commonly than women. The infrarenal abdominal aorta is primarily involved. The definition of aneurysm is generally accepted as a vessel that is more than 1.5 times its normal diameter. Therefore, for a typical 2-cm abdominal aorta, an aneurysm is defined as an aorta with a maximal cross-sectional diameter of more than 3 cm. Because the normal abdominal aorta tapers as it approaches the iliac bifurcation, an infrarenal abdominal aorta that does not meet size criteria for aneurysm but does not appropriately taper may herald early aneurysmal change. Although abdominal aortic aneurysm was originally thought to represent a sequela of atherosclerosis, it may represent a focal manifestation of a generalized vascular disease. Atherosclerotic changes are often concurrently present. CTA is the modality of choice for evaluation and follow-up of abdominal aortic aneurysms. CT clearly demonstrates aneurysm size and other potentially significant associated findings such as mural thrombus, calcifications, focal ulceration, or dissection (Fig. 46-4). In addition, CT allows for evaluation of associated structures, such as the retroperitoneum for signs of hemorrhage or inflammation, the kidneys, and the ureters. Retroperitoneal stranding and high-density fluid in a patient presenting with acute back pain should suggest a ruptured or leaking abdominal aortic aneurysm (Fig. 46-5). Contrast-enhanced CT may also demonstrate extravasation of contrast material or a focal outpouching from the aneurysm. Ultrasound is also useful as an imaging modality with its ability to demonstrate cross-sectional size and mural thrombus (Fig. 46-6). Radiographs are less reliable for primary evaluation because they mainly rely on intimal calcification to delineate the aneurysm sac.

Multiplanar CT has become very helpful in preprocedural planning for endovascular aneurysm repair (EVAR), and several proprietary software products exist for accurately sizing graft components. A crucial aspect of evaluating aneurysm size is understanding that the aneurysmal process affects both aortic diameter and length. Tortuosity is therefore a frequent finding with aneurysmal dilation. As a result, care must be taken to measure the diameter of the aneurysm in its true orthogonal plane, rather than in the cross-sectional image seen on a representative CT slice. Obliquities in the plane of view can lead to gross overestimation and measurement variability. For this reason, using the current multiplanar features in electronic imaging is important for assessing true aneurysm diameter (Fig. 46-7). Most interventionalists and surgeons believe that the risk of aneurysm rupture at 5 cm equals or exceeds the risk of procedural complications, and they therefore recommend treatment for aneurysms that reach that size threshold. For treatment planning, particularly for EVAR, certain measurements, such as diameter and length of the infrarenal neck, angulation of the neck, and diameter and length of the iliac arteries, are of paramount importance for assessing the compatibility of the aneurysm for endovascular repair and for sizing of the appropriate components (Fig. 46-8). As technology and device engineering improve, these measurements will also change, and each manufacturer will have its own measurement profile for the device's instructions for use. Because of this variability, even though reporting the relevant measurements is appropriate, the diagnostic radiologist should avoid commenting on suitability for endovascular repair in the radiology report.

Mycotic Abdominal Aortic Aneurysm

Other rare causes of abdominal aortic aneurysm formation include mycotic aneurysm, pseudoaneurysm, inflammatory aneurysm, and connective tissue disease related aneurysm. A mycotic aneurysm can arise either from infectious destruction of the aortic wall leading to mural weakening and aneurysmal degeneration or from secondary infection of a preexisting aneurysm. Mycotic

aneurysms are typically irregular, lobulated, and saccular in morphology, and they can have perivascular inflammatory changes. These morphologic findings in a rapidly expanding aneurysm should raise the suspicion of an infectious origin. Common organisms include *Salmonella* and *Staphylococcus* species, and risk factors include vascular intervention, intravenous drug use, and immunosuppression including from diabetes or steroid use. If a mycotic aneurysm is suspected by clinical findings and cross-sectional morphology, a useful problem-solving modality would be an indium-111–tagged leukocyte scan to look for uptake in the aneurysm wall (Figs. 46-9 and 46-10). This technique is also useful for identifying suspected surgical graft infection.

Inflammatory Abdominal Aortic Aneurysm

Inflammatory aortic aneurysms are associated with an elevated erythrocyte sedimentation rate, and they demonstrate a thickened mural rind surrounding the aneurysm. Occasionally, the rind enhances on contrast-enhanced CT and MRI during delayed phase imaging. This mural thickening can resolve after treatment (Fig. 46-11). Recognizing and reporting features of an inflammatory aneurysm are important because these patients often have associated adhesions to the bowel and ureters that may make surgery more complicated. A very rare cause of inflammatory aneurysm caused by immunoglobulin G4–mediated disease has also been described (Fig. 46-12).

Abdominal Aortic Pseudoaneurysm

Pseudoaneurysms of the abdominal aorta are typically sequelae of iatrogenic or blunt abdominal trauma. What differentiates a pseudoaneurysm from a true aneurysm is lack of all three components of the vascular wall. Pseudoaneurysms are typically contained only by adventitia, and as such they carry a significant risk of rupture. Pseudoaneurysm of the abdominal aorta may be a late manifestation of remote abdominal trauma. Iatrogenic causes include aortic surgery and spinal surgery. Finding an aneurysm adjacent to an anastomotic margin or area of spinal instrumentation therefore can be a clue to pseudoaneurysm (Fig. 46-13).

Ultrasound, if performed, may show typical to and fro flow on Doppler imaging characteristic of pseudoaneurysms elsewhere in the body. This finding is likely less specific for an abdominal aortic pseudoaneurysm, however, because any saccular aneurysm may demonstrate this finding. If a high-velocity neck is also identified, diagnostic confidence increases.

Connective Tissue Disorders

Patients with congenital connective tissue disorders such as Marfan syndrome or Ehlers-Danlos syndrome are at risk of dissection and aneurysm formation of the entire aorta, including the abdominal aorta. Abdominal aortic findings in this setting are often extensions of thoracic aortic dissections and aneurysms; therefore, any such

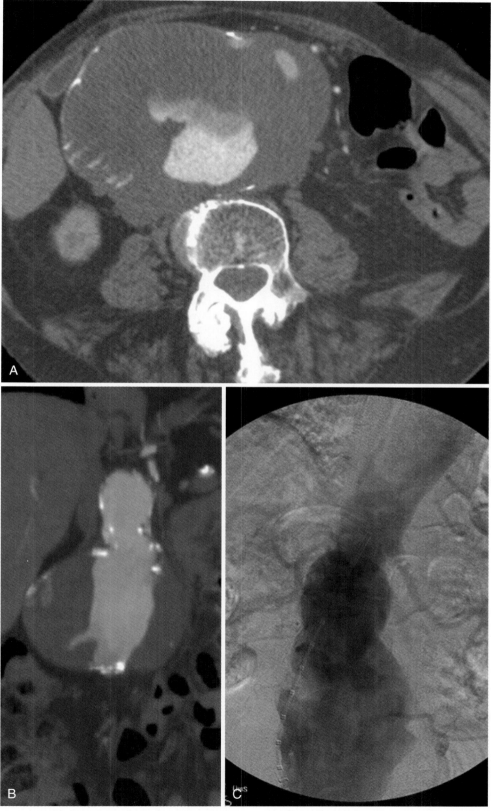

Figure 46-4 *Abdominal aortic aneurysm.* A and **B,** Computed tomography demonstrating a 12-cm aneurysm of the infrarenal abdominal aorta with extensive mural thrombus. **C,** The extent of the aneurysm is underestimated on angiography because of opacification of only the central lumen.

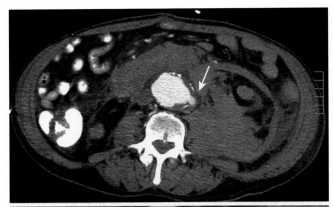

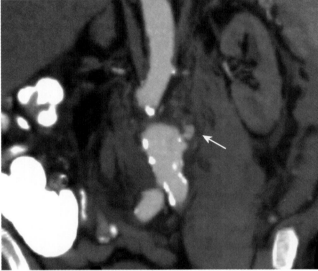

Figure 46-5 Ruptured abdominal aortic aneurysm. Computed tomography angiography of a patient presenting with hypotension and severe back pain. Extensive hematoma surrounds the abdominal aortic aneurysm extending anteriorly and posterolaterally in the perirenal space. The psoas margin has been obliterated. Note the focal "nipple" along the left posterolateral margin of the aneurysm *(arrows)* that represents a focal pseudoaneurysm at the likely rupture site.

finding on an abdominal CT should be further evaluated with dedicated imaging of the thoracic aorta (Fig. 46-14). Finding dissection and aneurysm in the aorta of a young patient who was not otherwise involved in trauma should raise the suspicion of an underlying connective tissue disorder if the diagnosis has not been considered.

Pearls and Pitfalls

- Ultrasound and CTA are useful imaging modalities for abdominal aortic aneurysm disease; however, CTA is usually required for preprocedural planning.
- Mycotic aneurysms should be suspected in lesions with saccular morphology, rapid expansion, and periaortic inflammatory changes. Nuclear scintigraphy with indium-labeled leukocytes can be a helpful problem-solving tool.
- Aneurysms near suture margins should raise the suspicion of pseudoaneurysm.

- Dissection and aneurysm formation in a young individual may represent underlying collagen vascular disease. The examiner should look for patency of the true and false lumina and the branches arising from both.

■ POSTOPERATIVE AORTA

Open and endovascular procedures of the abdominal aorta and branches have proliferated, and as a result, radiologists must be aware of the various imaging findings in the postoperative aorta. Knowing the radiologic appearance of bypass grafts, endovascular grafts, and combination procedures is helpful for understanding the expected imaging findings and therefore for rendering a helpful interpretation.

Aortobifemoral Bypass Graft

The traditional open operation for abdominal aortic aneurysms consists of aneurysm resection and repair with a tube graft or an aortobifemoral bypass graft. The sac is wrapped around the graft to provide a biologic barrier. The components of these grafts are not typically radiopaque and are therefore relatively easy to miss. Clues include subtle caliber differences at anastomotic margins and a double barrel appearance of the proximal iliac limbs as they course through the wrapped aneurysm sac (Fig. 46-15).

Stent Graft Endovascular Aneurysm Repair

Endovascular stent grafts are easy to identify on CT because of the metallic stent struts. Various manufacturers for stent grafts exist, each with their own designs and configurations. Examiners should familiarize themselves with the CT cross-sectional appearance of these different products. In EVAR, because the aneurysm sac is excluded and not resected, the aneurysm sac is still visible. In fact, sizing the sac is a principal component of follow-up imaging to evaluate adequate exclusion of the aneurysm and the presence of ongoing pressurization of the aneurysm sac.

Key elements to evaluate on post-EVAR imaging are aneurysm sac size, possible endoleak, and possible stent graft migration or distortion (Fig. 46-16). Although CTA is the primary diagnostic imaging modality for follow-up imaging after EVAR, the combination of ultrasound and radiography may also be performed if concern for an endoleak is minimal. Although duplex ultrasound has been shown to detect endoleaks, sensitivity is low, and evaluation for endoleak in the presence of an enlarging sac requires an additional study. The aneurysm sac size may stay stable or preferably decrease over time, but it should never increase after EVAR. If the sac size increases, it heralds the presence of an endoleak and persistent flow or pressurization within the aneurysm sac.

Five types of endoleak are recognized. Endoleak types 1 and 3 involve leakage at the junctions of the graft and native vessels or at the junction between graft components and are assessed carefully at the time of stent graft

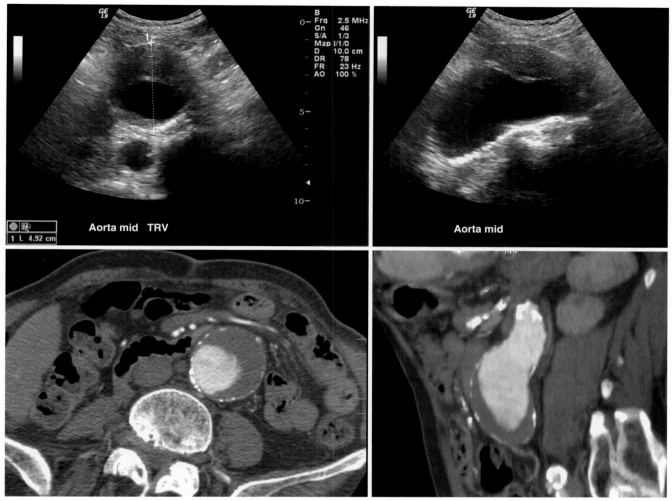

Figure 46-6 Ultrasound of abdominal aortic aneurysm. *Top panels* demonstrate transverse and longitudinal images of an abdominal aortic aneurysm. Note the hypoechoic patent central lumen, with the moderately echogenic mural thrombus. Correlative computed tomography from the same patient is shown in the *bottom panels.*

placement. When found, these endoleaks are corrected immediately. Endoleak type 4 is considered periprocedural secondary to systemic anticoagulation. Endoleak type 2 represents delayed opacification of the aneurysm sac from retrograde filling by branch vessels. Endoleak type 5 is controversial and is considered to represent ongoing pressurization of the aneurysm sac without a definite source of inflow. Of the endoleak types, endoleak type 2 is best evaluated on follow-up CT imaging with both arterial and delayed imaging. If contrast material is seen accumulating within the aneurysm sac, the examiner should look carefully for a feeding vessel. If the contrast material is accumulating posteriorly, it is often from a lumbar artery, and if the contrast material is accumulating anteriorly, it is often from a patent inferior mesenteric artery (Fig. 46-17).

Although the reported incidence of a type 2 endoleak is relatively high, most of these endoleaks either spontaneously resolve or do not cause persistent aneurysm dilation. A type 2 endoleak in the presence of an enlarging aneurysm sac, however, should be brought to the attention of the interventionalist or surgeon because

these endoleaks often require embolization or additional treatment. If the aneurysm sac is noted to be expanding, but no opacification of the sac is seen on either arterial or delayed phase imaging, then the possibility of a type 5 endoleak may be entertained. Validity of a type 5 endoleak is debated by some who believe that this entity usually has an underlying cause that has not been fully assessed. For example, magnetic resonance angiography (MRA) has been shown to demonstrate type 2 endoleaks when CTA has failed to show a source of aneurysm sac expansion, and it has been shown to be much more sensitive at detecting various endoleaks compared with CTA. MRA may therefore be a useful problem-solving tool if the patient's renal function does not prohibit administration of gadolinium. The distinction between endoleak types 2 and 5 is important because a type 2 endoleak may lend itself to a percutaneous procedure, whereas a true type 5 endoleak may require surgical revision.

In certain patients who either have an extremely narrow aortic bifurcation or an unsuitable iliac artery system on one side to accommodate a bifurcated stent

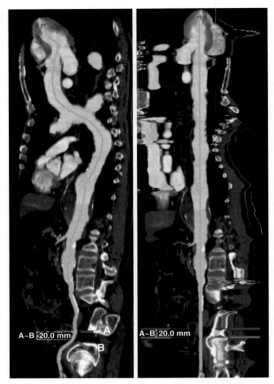

Figure 46-7 True aneurysm diameter on computed tomography. Example of postprocessing using proprietary software to assess the true diameter of the aorta from a centerline extrapolation. Looking at the sagittal reformatted image in the *left panel*, obliquities of measurement on axial imaging would lead to false measurements. More accurate measurements can be made after postprocessing to assess the true centerline of the aorta, as seen in the *right panel.*

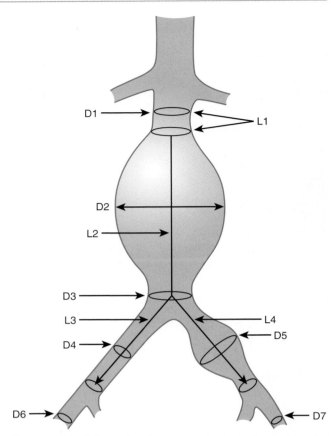

Figure 46-8 Schematic of common important diameter (D) and length (L) measurements for evaluating an abdominal aortic aneurysm for endovascular repair. Different manufacturers may have specific sites of measurement that may vary somewhat from this general scheme.

graft, different endovascular solutions exist. One solution employs an aorto-uni-iliac stent graft used in conjunction with a femoral-femoral bypass graft. In these cases, the contralateral iliac limb is excluded from the circulation by the stent graft proximally and with coils or plugs distally. This solution may also be employed if a limb of a bifurcated graft becomes thrombosed and is not amenable to percutaneous thrombolysis (Fig. 46-18).

Occasionally, the access vessels (i.e., the common femoral and external iliac arteries) are too narrow to accommodate the large delivery systems for the stent grafts. With most current stent graft delivery systems, a minimum diameter of 6 to 7 mm is needed for the access arteries. In patients with narrow access arteries, a synthetic graft conduit is surgically anastomosed to the common iliac artery or aorta where the diameters are larger, and the stent graft delivery system is then introduced through the conduit. This appears on CT as a tubular structure spanning laterally from the body wall to the aortoiliac system. When the conduit is not in use, it is tied off peripherally, and thus it often appears on CT as a tubular structure with thrombus (Fig. 46-19). The radiologist must know why the conduit is in place, to avoid rendering a confusing interpretation on post-EVAR CT scanning.

The typical landing zone of the stent graft proximally is in the infrarenal aorta, and most systems in use today require a 10- to 15-mm neck to achieve a proper proximal seal for the stent graft. If this neck is shorter or if the aneurysm arises immediately below the renal arteries, the term juxtarenal aneurysm is used. These aneurysms have traditionally required open repair; however, some endovascular options have been devised that are important to recognize on postoperative imaging. One solution to the juxtarenal aneurysm is a fenestrated stent graft that can accommodate perfusion to the renal and mesenteric arteries and allow for a suprarenal seal zone for the stent graft without compromising blood flow to the renal or mesenteric arteries. Another option is to deploy a stent graft over flexible stents placed into the renal and mesenteric arteries that extend above the proximal stent graft body. Termed "chimneys" or "snorkels," these stents maintain perfusion to the renal and mesenteric arteries while providing additional seal length for the stent graft (Fig. 46-20).

Another option for juxtarenal or thoracoabdominal aneurysms takes advantage of both open and endovascular techniques involving a combination of visceral artery debranching with bypass grafts followed by stent graft repair. Although the debranching procedure is still a major operation, it is thought to be less intensive than an open thoracoabdominal

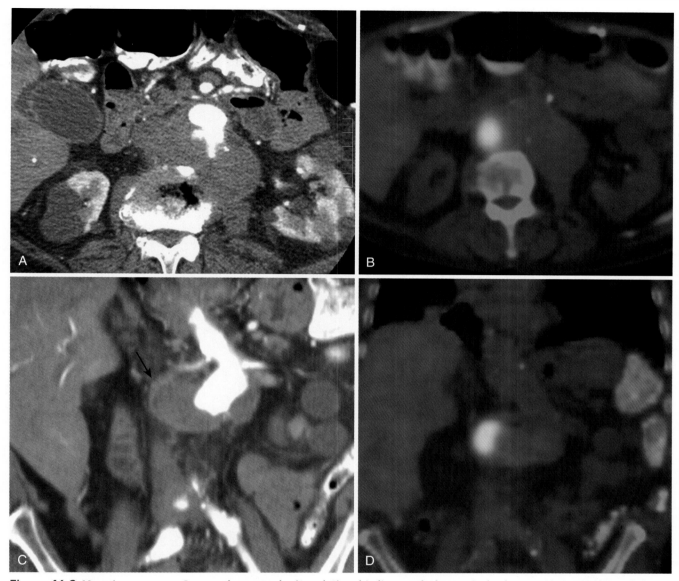

Figure 46-9 Mycotic aneurysm. Computed tomography (**A** and **C**) and indium-111 leukocyte single photon emission CT (SPECT) (**B** and **D**) imaging of a mycotic aneurysm. The aneurysm has lobulated saccular morphology, with surrounding inflammatory changes. Note the rind of enhancement along the right aspect of the aneurysm sac *(arrow)* that correlates with the area of radiotracer uptake by SPECT.

operation in selected patients. The postoperative appearance of these cases includes a combination of a stent graft with multiple visceral artery bypass grafts (Fig. 46-21).

Pearls and Pitfalls

- The postoperative abdominal aorta can have many appearances with various endovascular and open bypass graft options. Familiarity with these procedures is essential for postprocedure imaging evaluation.
- Evaluation of the aorta after stent grafting is currently best performed by CTA, to assess for sac size measurement, endoleak, and graft migration and morphology. Ultrasound and radiography may be used in combination to evaluate sac size and graft migration if concern for endoleak is minimal.

- Type 2 endoleaks are relatively common, and most are supplied by lumbar arteries or the inferior mesenteric artery. Arterial and delayed phase CT imaging is helpful for evaluating sac opacification. MRI may be a useful problem-solving tool for slow endoleaks not seen by CT.

■ ACUTE AORTIC SYNDROME

Acute aortic syndrome comprises three entities that can give the same clinical picture of an acute tearing chest or abdominal pain radiating to the back. This syndrome includes aortic dissection, penetrating aortic ulcer (PAU), and intramural hematoma (IMH). Many of the symptomatic cases of acute aortic syndrome occur in the thoracic aorta; however, involvement of the abdominal aorta is also seen. The three

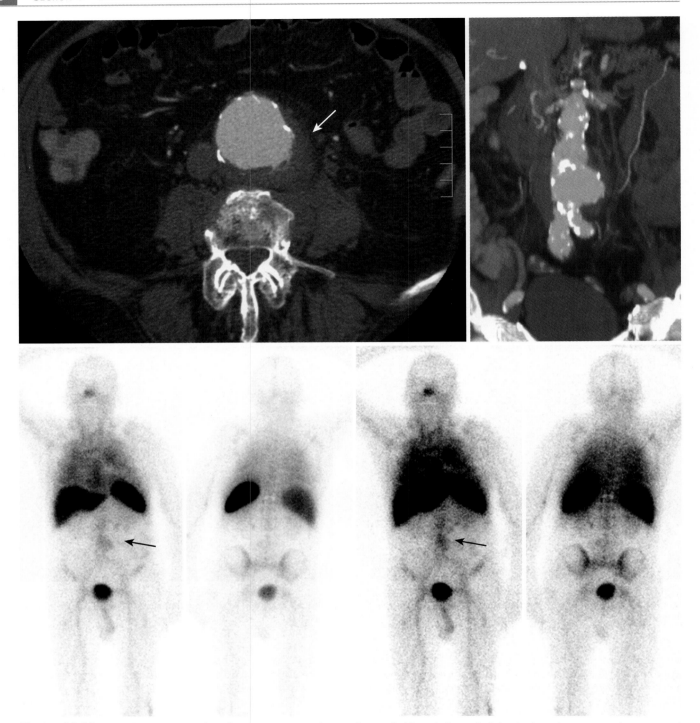

Figure 46-10 Mycotic aneurysm. Saccular aneurysm superimposed on a fusiform infrarenal abdominal aortic aneurysm by computed tomography angiography, with focal radiotracer uptake in this region on indium-111 leukocyte planar scintigraphy *(arrows)*. *Escherichia coli* was cultured from the aneurysm at repair.

entities comprising the acute aortic syndrome may represent a continuum of disease. The causes of acute aortic syndrome are not able to be distinguished on a clinical basis, and therefore imaging studies are an integral part of the diagnosis. The best evaluation for a patient with suspected acute aortic syndrome includes dedicated three-phase CTA with a noncontrast study to

assess for IMH, an arterial phase to assess the involved segments and communication with intramural components, and a venous delayed phase to assess for a possible rupture with extravasation and accumulation of contrast. At the least, a noncontrast study followed by an arterial phase study is helpful for differentiating these entities.

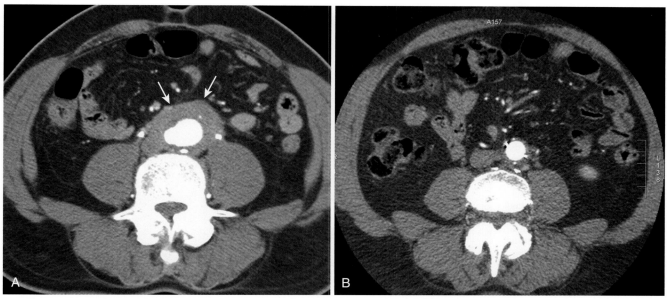

Figure 46-11 Inflammatory aneurysm. A, Computed tomography image of an inflammatory aneurysm. Note the marked thickened rind surrounding the aneurysm *(arrows)*. B, Nearly complete resolution of this thickened rind is evident after treatment and stent grafting.

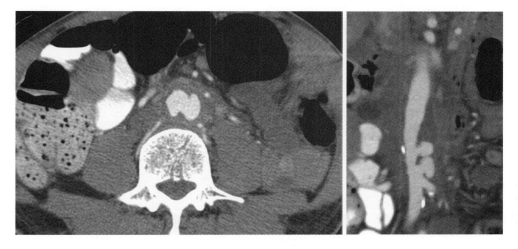

Figure 46-12 immunoglobulin G4 (IgG4) aneurysm. Rare autoimmune-mediated inflammatory aneurysm from IgG4. Note the lobulated aneurysms in the infrarenal abdominal aorta.

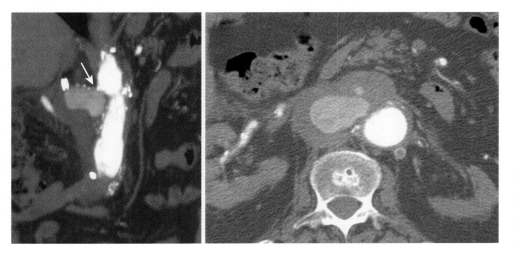

Figure 46-13 Abdominal aortic pseudoaneurysm. Focal saccular outpouching of contrast at the suture margin of a previous renal artery bypass graft *(arrow)* represents a postoperative pseudoaneurysm.

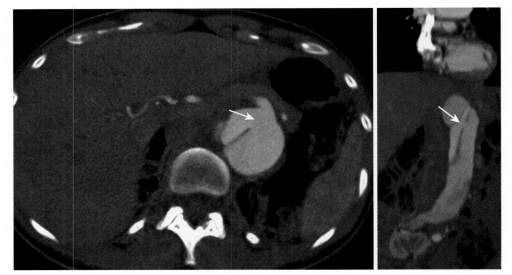

Figure 46-14 Connective tissue disease. Computed tomography angiography in a patient with Marfan syndrome demonstrating thoracoabdominal aortic dissection with secondary aneurysmal degeneration. Note the prominent fenestration allowing opacification of both true and false lumina through the extent of the dissection *(arrows)*.

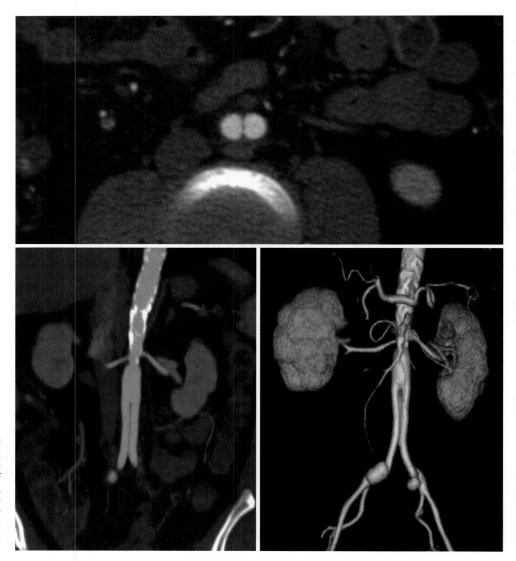

Figure 46-15 Aortobifemoral bypass graft. The synthetic grafts are not radiodense; therefore, the appearance may be confusing if one does not have the history. A "double barrel" appearance of the high-bifurcating iliac limbs as they course through the resected and oversewn aneurysm sac is a clue to this postoperative appearance.

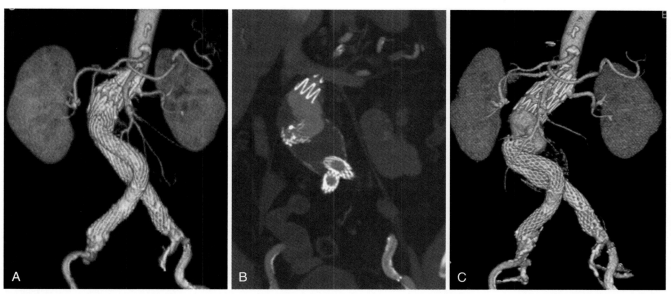

Figure 46-16 *Stent graft migration.* A, Three-dimensional shaded surface rendering of a stent graft repair of an abdominal aortic aneurysm. **B,** Follow-up computed tomography (CT) several years later demonstrates separation of the cuff component from the body and limb components, with an enlarging aneurysm sac. **C,** Shaded surface rendering of this CT clearly shows migration of the body and limb components compared with the original CT scan.

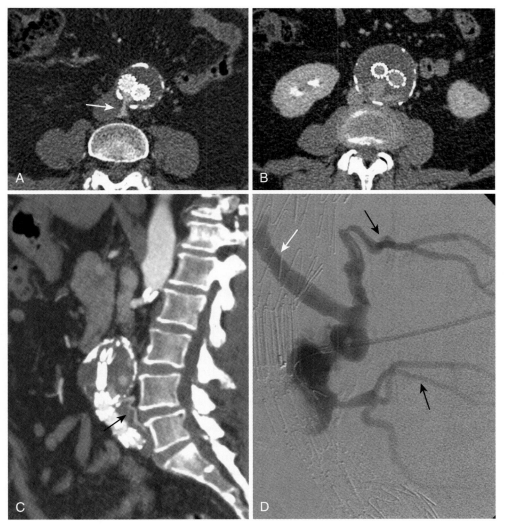

Figure 46-17 Type 2 endoleak. A and **C,** Computed tomography (CT) angiogram after endovascular repair of an abdominal aortic aneurysm demonstrating clear backfilling of the aneurysm sac through the median sacral artery *(arrows).* **B,** Delayed images demonstrate increasing contrast opacification of the aneurysm sac, thus confirming the endoleak. **C** and **D,** Comparison of the sagittal reformatted images from the CT with the subsequent angiogram obtained by direct percutaneous puncture of the aneurysm sac clearly correlates the findings. Additional sources of type 2 endoleak from paired lumbar arteries *(black arrows* in **D)** posteriorly and the inferior mesenteric artery *(white arrow* in **D)** anteriorly are better appreciated on the angiogram.

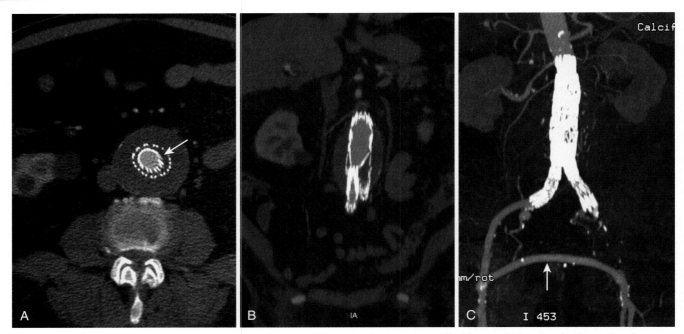

Figure 46-18 Aorto-uni-iliac graft with femoral-femoral bypass graft. Patient presented with acute limb ischemia after earlier placement of an endovascular stent graft. Satisfactory thrombectomy could not be performed through the left iliac limb; therefore, conversion to an aorto-uni-iliac graft was performed on the right side, with femoral-femoral bypass grafting (*arrow* in **C**) to preserve flow to the left lower extremity. Note the contrast-opacified new aorto-uni-iliac graft inside the earlier stent graft body on the axial image (*arrow* in **A**).

Aortic Dissection

Aortic dissection can be seen in the setting of trauma or spontaneously in the setting of hypertension or underlying connective tissue disease. Most abdominal aortic dissections are continuations of thoracic aortic dissections. The hallmark of aortic dissection is visualization of the intimal flap, which appears on CT as a linear low-density structure traversing the vessel. This feature is best appreciated on the arterial phase of CTA (Fig. 46-22). Often, fenestrations in the intimal flap allow for blood flow in both the false and true lumina. The dissection flap may continue into the visceral vessels and past the iliac bifurcation. Vessels can be supplied by both the false and true lumina. In most instances of thoracic aortic dissection extending into the abdominal aorta, the true lumen is the smaller lumen along the smaller curvature of the aortic arch. The true lumen often supplies the superior mesenteric artery and right renal artery, and the false lumen may supply the left renal artery through a fenestration. Variations to the flow distribution exist, and the radiologist should determine whether a visceral vessel has thrombosed or is severely stenotic as a result of the dissection.

A noncontrast study can help to identify IMH associated with the dissection. Delayed images can help to determine whether differential phases of renal enhancement are present, and these images may be a useful way of deciphering whether flow to one of the renal arteries is limited as a result of dissection. The target organs should be evaluated for evidence of infarction. The natural history of dissection is subsequent aneurysmal dilation of the false lumen with the potential for thrombosis and rupture.

Penetrating Aortic Ulcer

PAU is a condition that can cause the acute aortic syndrome, and its symptoms can be similar to those of acute aortic dissection. A PAU typically represents ulceration of an atherosclerotic plaque through the intima into the media and is often associated with an IMH. Some authorities believe that this entity can be the source of dissection, and, indeed, PAUs often dissect caudad or cephalad to a certain degree along the media. The distinguishing feature of PAU is ulceration into the media (Fig. 46-23). This feature should help differentiate PAU from an ulcerated or polypoid plaque that maintains the integrity of the intima. Often, coronal or sagittal CT reformations can help evaluate the depth of ulceration.

Intramural Hematoma

IMH represents a hematoma either without intraluminal communication or from a communication that is too small to capture on imaging. Some authorities believe that IMH represents spontaneous rupture of the vasa vasorum. IMH can be associated with aortic dissection, as well as with PAU. Most cases of isolated IMH are seen in the ascending thoracic aorta. A noncontrast CT scan can identify a crescent-shaped high-density IMH; however, the contrast phase is equally important to evaluate the lumen and exclude an intraluminal communication or thrombosed dissection, as well as to differentiate the hematoma from mural thrombus associated with an abdominal aortic aneurysm (Fig. 46-24). MRI can also demonstrate the hematoma either against the signal void background of the

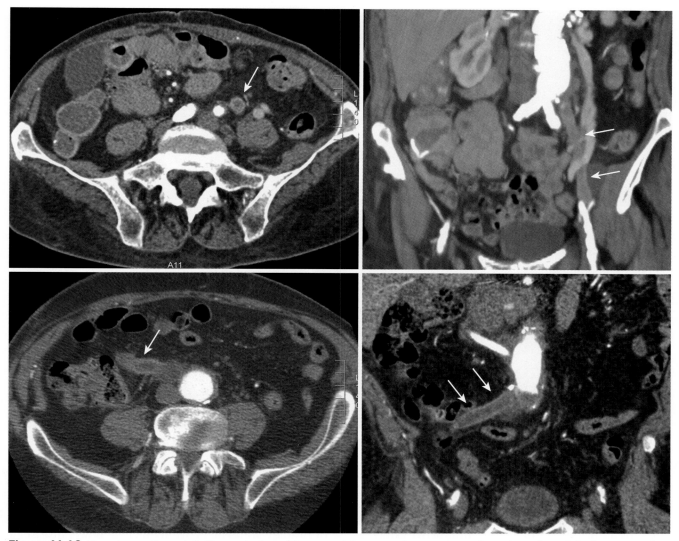

Figure 46-19 *Vascular graft conduit.* Demonstration of the computed tomography appearance of vascular graft conduits that are occasionally used to deploy endovascular devices with large delivery systems unsuitable for transfemoral approach if the patient has unfavorable anatomy. Once the conduit is tied off, it stays internally and thromboses, thus giving the appearance of a thrombosed vessel *(arrows)*.

lumen when no gadolinium is used or against intraluminal contrast when gadolinium is used. In addition, the radiologist can predict the age of the hematoma by the methemoglobin level contribution to T1- and T2-weighted imaging.

Pearls and Pitfalls

- The three entities comprising the acute aortic syndrome may represent a similar pathologic process in various stages.
- Two- or three-phase CT imaging is best for evaluating the presence of hematoma and defining the anatomy.
- In the setting of dissection, patency of branch vessels with end-organ evaluation should be performed to look for thrombosis and infarcts.
- The presence of intimal calcification may be a useful landmark to distinguish PAU from polypoid plaque.

■ IMAGING OF AORTIC TRAUMA AND IATROGENIC INJURY

Aortic Rupture

Abdominal aortic trauma can manifest as rupture, dissection, or IMH. Often, clues to know to look carefully for abdominal aortic trauma include the appropriate clinical setting (i.e., seatbelt injury, high-velocity impact, penetrating trauma) and associated imaging findings such as retroperitoneal stranding, associated midline visceral injuries, and spine injuries. Rupture is the greatest emergency, and it manifests as retroperitoneal stranding and fluid, particularly within the perirenal space, with or without active contrast extravasation. Again, three-phase CT imaging is the preferred means of evaluation, particularly if the patient is hemodynamically stable enough to undergo scanning. The noncontrast phase evaluates for IMH, as well as retroperitoneal

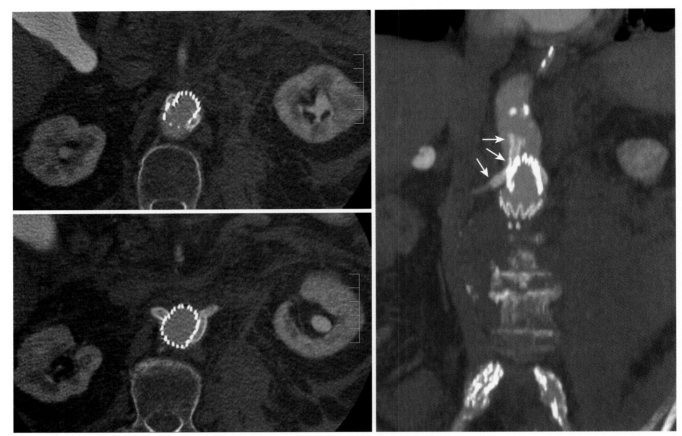

Figure 46-20 Renal artery "chimneys" or "snorkels." Juxtarenal abdominal aortic aneurysms pose a unique challenge for endovascular repair. One newer technique employed for certain selected cases involves coverage of the renal segment of the aorta with a stent graft while maintaining flow to the renal arteries by stents coursing along the outer aspect of the stent graft. The appearance is akin to a chimney or snorkel *(arrows)* and allows for blood flow to the renal arteries from above the sealed zone of the aneurysm.

and intraabdominal hematoma. The arterial phase evaluates the aortic lumen and may identify active extravasation, and delayed phase imaging identifies an expanding hematoma and persistent contrast leak.

Aortic Fistula

Various forms of aortic fistula include aortocaval fistula, aortoenteric fistula, and aortoureteric fistula. The most common causes of fistula formation are iatrogenic, although these entities may also happen in the setting of aneurysmal disease or trauma. Common iatrogenic sources include surgery or procedures involving the aorta, retroperitoneum, or spine. Aortocaval fistula can manifest clinically as high-output heart failure, and CT imaging may demonstrate loss of a normal fat plane between the aorta and inferior vena cava (IVC), with arterial phase opacification of the IVC (Fig. 46-25). For this reason, intravenous contrast material use in the arterial phase is imperative, and noncontrast or delayed phase imaging is less helpful. Duplex ultrasound may also demonstrate turbulent arterialized flow in the IVC and may potentially identify the point of communication.

Aortoenteric fistula often occurs after aortic graft placement (secondary aortoenteric fistula) and manifests

clinically as massive gastrointestinal bleeding. Causes of primary aortoenteric fistula include bowel disease or inflammation, aortic aneurysm or inflammation, and rarer causes. The most common location of the fistula is along the third or fourth portion of the duodenum, where it is in close proximity to the infrarenal abdominal aorta. Aortoenteric fistula is a difficult diagnosis to make by imaging, and it requires very high clinical suspicion. Clues to the diagnosis include air within the aneurysm sac or postoperative graft, with a closely apposed adjacent bowel loop (Fig. 46-26).

Aortoureteric fistula is very rare and usually results from erosion caused by either a ureteral stent or an aneurysm pulsating on the ureter. The clinical presentation can be massive or intermittent hematuria. Imaging by ureterography or aortography may identify the communication, and CT imaging may identify early opacification of the ureter. Preexcretory renal phase imaging is required; otherwise, contrast material in the ureters obscures any possibility of identifying the fistula.

Pearls and Pitfalls

- Stranding and fluid in the retroperitoneum, particularly in the perirenal space, should raise the suspicion

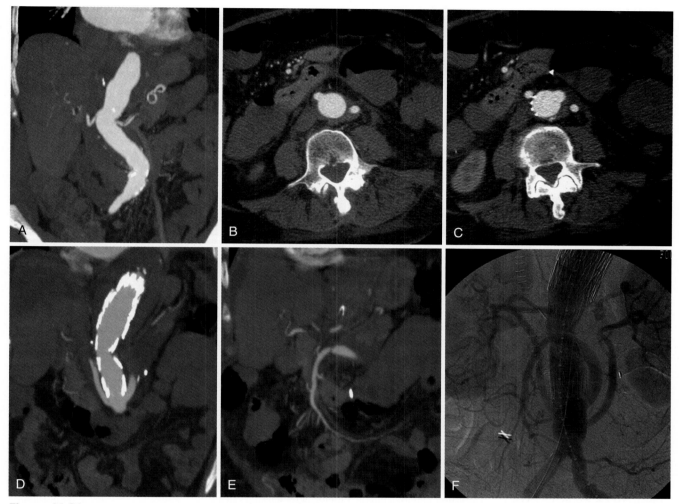

Figure 46-21 A to F, Hybrid thoracoabdominal aneurysm repair with visceral debranching and stent graft. **A,** Computed tomography (CT) coronal reformatted image of a thoracoabdominal aortic aneurysm. The patient first underwent a visceral debranching procedure in which the mesenteric and renal arteries were bypassed to a lower segment of the abdominal aorta, followed by a second procedure in which the thoracoabdominal aneurysm was excluded with a stent graft. Final angiography (**F**) correlates well with postprocedure CT angiography (**B** to **E**), demonstrating patency of the bypassed visceral arteries.

of aortic injury in the setting of trauma. Three-phase scanning can assess for hematoma and active extravasation.

■ Aortic fistulas may be traumatic or iatrogenic and are often difficult to diagnose. Air within an aneurysm sac or graft remote from surgery suggests aortoenteric fistula.

■ INFLAMMATORY DISEASE AND ARTERITIS

Takayasu Arteritis and Giant Cell Arteritis

Takayasu arteritis, also termed pulseless disease, is a condition that more typically involves the thoracic aorta and arch vessels. Involvement of the abdominal aorta can be seen as an extension of the descending thoracic aorta, and involvement of the infrarenal aorta and branches may also be seen. Takayasu arteritis is a

cause of abdominal aortic coarctation, and it can also result in infrarenal aortic occlusion, as just described. Tortuous aneurysmal dilation of the aorta and visceral branches may be a component of this process. Aortography may demonstrate typical features such as areas of smooth, tapered narrowing and occlusions. CT can demonstrate concentric mural thickening in the involved segments. MRI improves characterization by demonstrating a thickened edematous wall during the acute phase or a thickened enhancing wall during the chronic phase (Fig. 46-27).

Giant cell arteritis has many features resembling those of Takayasu arteritis. In addition to mural thickening and inflammation, the association of giant cell arteritis with aneurysm formation, including abdominal aortic aneurysm, and dissection, is high. Typically, age of onset is older, and patients have involvement of upper extremity and carotid artery branches, such as the temporal and ophthalmic arteries. Angiography and MRI have been most often used for imaging

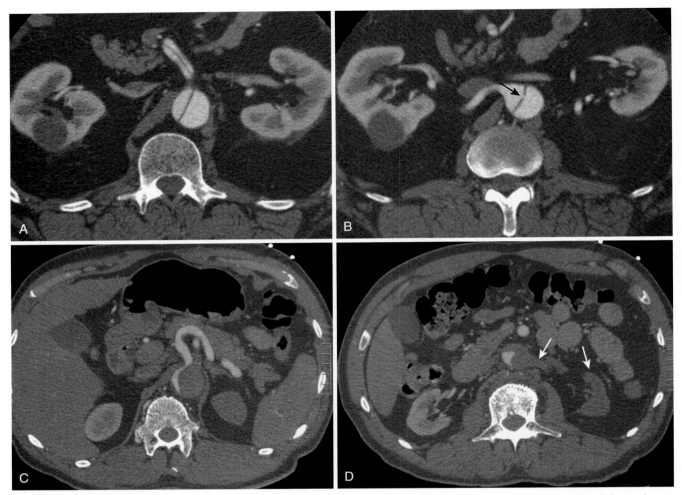

Figure 46-22 Aortic dissection. A, Dissection flap on computed tomography imaging extends longitudinally down the abdominal aorta and includes the origin and proximal aspect of the superior mesenteric artery coming off anteriorly. **B,** Patency of the false lumen is maintained by fenestrations in the dissection flap, seen as focal discontinuity in the dissection flap *(arrow)*. **C** and **D,** When this situation is not adequate to maintain patency of the false lumen, the false lumen and branches arising from it may undergo thrombosis. Note the lack of opacification of the left renal artery and the resultant lack of contrast perfusing the left kidney (**D,** *arrows*).

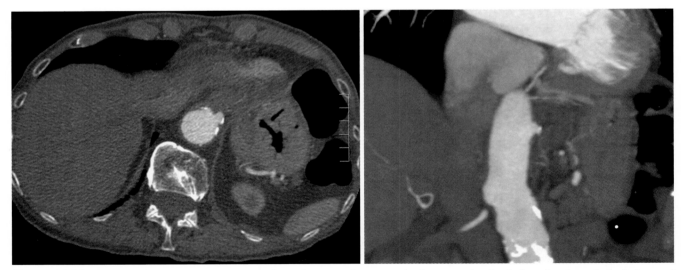

Figure 46-23 Penetrating aortic ulcer. Contrast-enhanced computed tomography demonstrating focal ulceration through the intima and into the media in the left anterolateral aspect of the abdominal aorta. Calcification can be used as a marker for the location of the intima for differentiating an ulcer from polypoid, irregular mural thrombus.

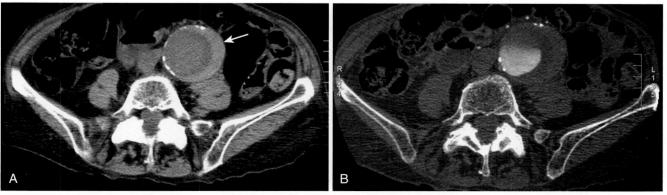

Figure 46-24 Intramural hematoma (IMH). Noncontrast (**A**) and contrast-enhanced (**B**) computed tomography scan of the abdomen demonstrating an IMH. The crescent-shaped hematoma appears dense relative to luminal blood on the noncontrast study (**A**, *arrow*), and this characteristic can help distinguish IMH from active extravasation after administration of contrast material.

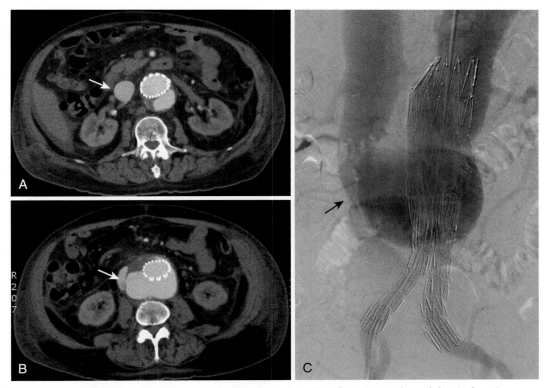

Figure 46-25 Aortocaval fistula. A and **B,** Computed tomography angiography of a patient with an abdominal aortic aneurysm persistently filling despite attempted endovascular repair using a stent graft. Aneurysm filling was through a descending thoracic aortic dissection (not shown). *Arrow* in **A** demonstrates arterial opacification of the inferior vena cava (IVC) from an aortocaval fistula. A direct communication between the aneurysm sac and the IVC is demonstrated more inferiorly (**B**, *arrow*). **C,** Angiography in the same patient demonstrates rapid shunting of contrast through the aneurysm sac into the IVC *(arrow),* a finding consistent with an aortocaval fistula.

evaluation, and they yield clear demonstration of stenoses, beading, aneurysm formation, and perivascular inflammatory changes. A hypoechoic halo, likely representing perivascular inflammation, that surrounds the temporal arteries of patients with giant cell arteritis has been described on ultrasound with subsequent resolution after corticosteroid treatment. Other systemic inflammatory or autoimmune conditions, such as relapsing polychondritis, rheumatoid arthritis, and reactive arthritis, can also be associated with large and medium vessel vasculitis.

Retroperitoneal Fibrosis

Retroperitoneal fibrosis is an uncommon inflammatory condition that results in fibrotic changes and cicatrization of the retroperitoneal fat. Many causes have been proposed, but most cases are idiopathic. Commonly involved structures include the abdominal aorta and ureters. Distortion from fibrosis can be severe enough to cause ureteric obstruction, hydronephrosis, and renal failure. This distortion results in the classic radiographic appearance of medial displacement of the

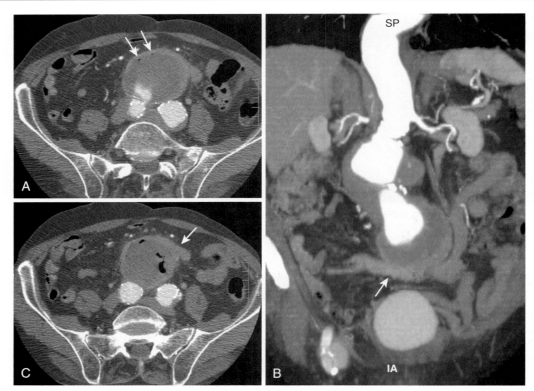

Figure 46-26 Aortoenteric fistula. Computed tomography images of an infrarenal abdominal aortic aneurysm demonstrate foci of gas (*arrows* in **A**) within the aneurysm sac. Note the presence of a small bowel loop draped across the aneurysm *(arrows* in **B** and **C**). An aortoenteric fistula was found at operation. *IA,* Inferoanterior; *SP,* superoposterior.

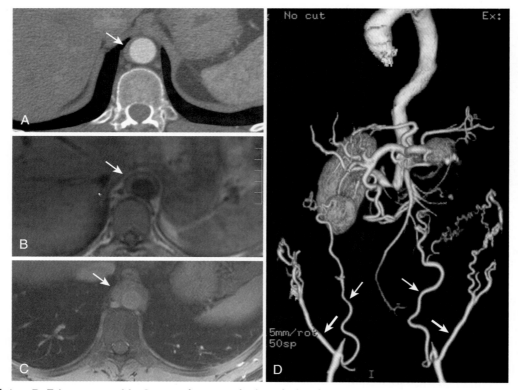

Figure 46-27 A to D, Takayasu arteritis. Computed tomography (**A** and **D**) and T1-weighted (**B**) and T2-weighted (**C**) magnetic resonance images of Takayasu arteritis. The axial images demonstrate an inflammatory rind surrounding the thoracoabdominal aorta *(arrows)*, isointense to liver on T1, and hyperintense on T2. Takayasu arteritis can progress to aortoiliac occlusion, as seen on the three-dimensional reformatted image (**D**). Note the supply of the lower extremity runoff by way of body wall collateral vessels including the inferior epigastric arteries (*white arrows* in **D**) and deep circumflex iliac arteries (**D**, *thick arrows*).

bilateral ureters on excretory pyelography. The nonmalignant and malignant causes of retroperitoneal fibrosis are difficult to distinguish from each other by imaging. Nonmalignant causes include inflammatory aortitis, granulomatous infections, severe atherosclerotic periaortitis, radiation, surgery, autoimmune disease, histiocytoses, and drug-induced conditions.

One rare form of histiocytosis known to cause retroperitoneal fibrosis is Erdheim-Chester disease (Fig. 46-28). Erdheim-Chester disease is also associated with sclerosis in the metadiaphyses of the long bones, interstitial lung disease, and central diabetes insipidus. Rare benign causes of retroperitoneal fat stranding that mimic retroperitoneal fibrosis also include retroperitoneal amyloidosis (see Fig. 46-28).

Malignant causes of retroperitoneal fibrosis include lymphoma, adenocarcinoma (e.g., from lung, breast, prostate, and gastrointestinal primary tumors), and sarcoma. In addition, certain malignant diseases can have a periaortic distribution with no associated fibrosis. The radiologist must always consider malignant disease in the differential diagnosis of periaortic soft tissue thickening (Fig. 46-29).

Ultrasound imaging of retroperitoneal fibrosis demonstrates a hypoechoic or anechoic periaortic halo, similar to that described earlier for the temporal artery in giant cell arteritis. CT and MRI demonstrate periaortic thickening and retroperitoneal stranding. A key feature is noting that the vessels are engulfed, rather than displaced, by the process. In addition, relatively little mass effect on other adjacent structures, such as the psoas muscle, is noted. Enhancement may indicate active disease, whereas relative nonenhancement represents a more quiescent, fibrotic stage of the disease. Nuclear scintigraphy with gallium has also been demonstrated to indicate active disease with significant uptake of radiotracer in the affected region. MRI demonstrating inhomogeneous enhancement of the surrounding tissues and plaque may indicate underlying malignant disease. In nonmalignant retroperitoneal fibrosis, the changes in the retroperitoneum can often dramatically improve with steroid or immunosuppressive therapies.

Pearls and Pitfalls

- Takayasu arteritis may manifest as aortic coarctation and aortic and visceral artery aneurysm or stenosis. An inflammatory soft tissue rind around the vessel wall is often seen. MRI may help to differentiate active from chronic disease.
- Retroperitoneal fibrosis has multiple causes, and it is a contractile process that can often result in ureteral obstruction and hydronephrosis. Malignant disease should always be considered, especially if the process appears expansile.

■ VISCERAL ARTERIES

Mesenteric Artery Occlusive Disease

Mesenteric artery occlusive disease is typically atherosclerotic or embolic. Atherosclerotic occlusion results from ostial stenosis with superimposed thrombosis. Embolic disease is typically from a cardiac source. In the mesenteric vessels, if underlying stenosis is already present, collateral pathways have typically developed, and the presentation of superimposed thrombosis is more chronic. Classic clinical findings include postprandial abdominal pain, fear of food, and weight loss.

The general rule of thumb is that chronic disease is not likely to be clinically significant unless two of the three mesenteric vessels are involved. In embolic disease, the presentation is typically acute because of the lack of developed collateral vessels. A typical site of embolic disease in the superior mesenteric artery is distal to the origin of the middle colic artery (Fig. 46-30). In this setting, the radiologist must look at the supplied

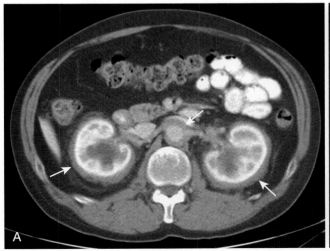
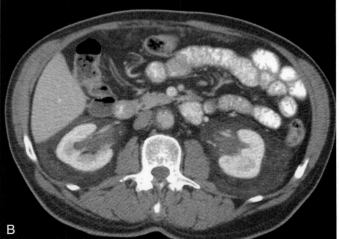

Figure 46-28 Retroperitoneal fibrosis. A, Contrast-enhanced axial computed tomography scan of the abdomen demonstrates soft tissue density *(arrows)* in the retroperitoneum surrounding the abdominal aorta and perinephric structures in a patient with Erdheim-Chester disease, a rare form of histiocytosis associated with retroperitoneal fibrosis. **B,** A similar pattern is seen in a different patient. Biopsy of the retroperitoneum in this individual yielded amyloidosis, a rare condition with imaging findings mimicking retroperitoneal fibrosis.

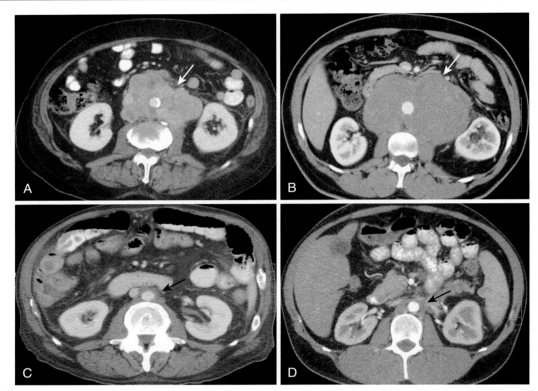

Figure 46-29 Malignant periaortic thickening. Axial computed tomography images of malignant diseases with periaortic soft tissue thickening *(arrows):* lymphoma (**A**), testicular seminoma (**B**), metastatic colonic adenocarcinoma (**C**), and Kaposi sarcoma (**D**). Malignant disease should always be a consideration in the differential diagnosis of periaortic soft tissue thickening.

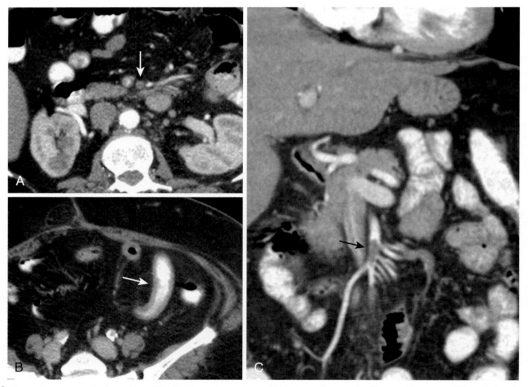

Figure 46-30 Superior mesenteric artery (SMA) thrombus. Acute SMA thrombus typically manifests as a filling defect in the SMA, often just distal to the origin of the middle colic artery. **A** to **C,** Computed tomography images demonstrate a focal filling defect seen in the SMA (**A** and **C,** *arrows*), with evidence of small bowel wall thickening in the left lower quadrant (**B,** *arrow*).

bowel and carefully evaluate for signs of bowel ischemia, including bowel wall thickening, lack of bowel wall enhancement, pneumatosis, and fluid or stranding in the mesentery. Exploratory laparotomy may be necessary when these findings are noted in the appropriate clinical setting.

One form of mesenteric artery stenosis in patients complaining of chronic abdominal pain involves impingement of the celiac artery origin by the median arcuate ligament traversing the diaphragmatic crura.

This condition typically causes mass effect on the superior aspect of the celiac axis that becomes more exaggerated during expiration as the diaphragmatic excursion increases impingement on the celiac axis. A poststenotic dilated segment can also be seen (Figs. 46-31 and 46-32). That this finding can be seen in asymptomatic individuals calls into question the true origin of the patients' pain. Some investigators have considered whether mechanical impingement on the celiac neural plexus, rather than mesenteric ischemia, is truly the cause of

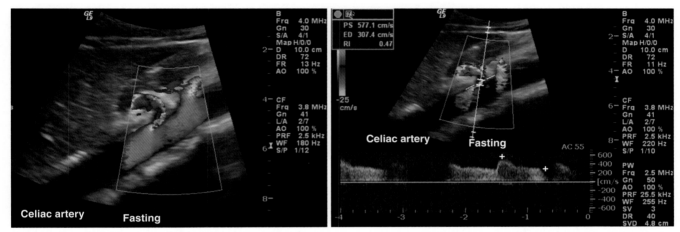

Figure 46-31 Median arcuate ligament syndrome. Ultrasound can demonstrate the visceral segment of the abdominal aorta, and, as in this case, demonstrate elevated velocities at the origin of the celiac axis in a patient with median arcuate ligament syndrome.

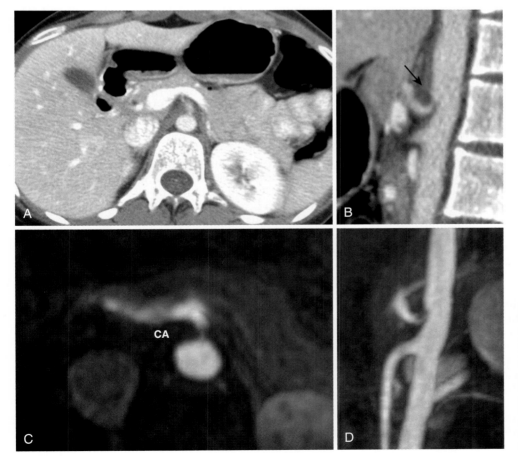

Figure 46-32 Median arcuate ligament syndrome. Contrast-enhanced computed tomography (**A** and **B**) and magnetic resonance imaging (**C** and **D**) show the anatomic relationships, in the same patient as in Figure 46-31, of severe proximal celiac artery (CA) stenosis with the median arcuate ligament passing just ventral to the abdominal aorta above the celiac axis (**B,** *arrow*). Note the lack of other atherosclerotic changes.

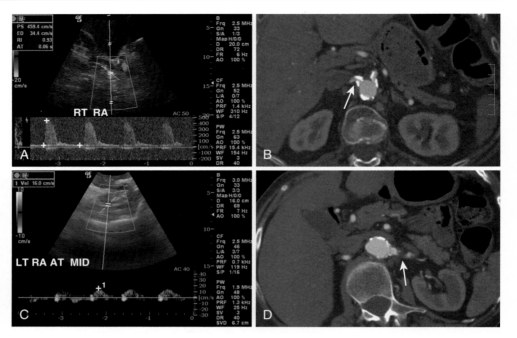

Figure 46-33 Renal artery stenosis. A, Ultrasound examination of the right (RT) renal artery (RA) demonstrates markedly elevated velocities and spectral broadening. **B,** Correlative computed tomography (CT) in the same patient demonstrates a severe, calcified, ostial stenosis in the right renal artery *(arrow).* **C,** Ultrasound examination of the left (LT) renal artery in a different patient demonstrates a very slow velocity with a parvus et tardus waveform in the midarterial (MID) segment. **D,** Correlative CT image demonstrates severe stenosis in the proximal left renal artery *(arrow).*

pain in this setting. When these morphologic findings are noted in a patient with appropriate clinical symptoms, CT or angiography in inspiration and expiration can help to confirm the findings. Definitive treatment usually involves dividing the median arcuate ligament, although percutaneous treatment with angioplasty and stenting may also have a role in selected patients.

Renal Artery Stenosis

In the renal arteries, atherosclerotic occlusive disease, accounting for 90% of stenotic disease, is typically ostial and may result in renal insufficiency and hypertension. Duplex ultrasound has become a commonly used screening modality for renal artery stenosis. Although duplex ultrasound is limited by operator proficiency and a range of relatively nonspecific published metrics, relatively reliable signs of renal artery stenosis include elevated velocities (typically >200 cm/second), a parvus et tardus waveform with spectral broadening distal to the stenotic segment, and a ratio of renal artery to aorta peak systolic velocity greater than 3.5.

Because of a relative lack of specificity, if ultrasound identifies certain criteria of renal artery stenosis, the patient is typically referred for a more definitive anatomic evaluation such as CTA, MRA, or catheter angiography (Fig. 46-33). CTA and MRA may show ostial stenosis and poststenotic dilation. In addition, careful examination for stenotic accessory renal arteries should be made because these also trigger the renin-angiotensin axis to increase blood pressure and can be the source of false-negative ultrasound examinations. Severe stenosis on MRA is often overestimated and appears as a loss of signal that may be misinterpreted as an occlusion. Moreover, gadolinium-based MRI contrast agents have been associated with nephrogenic systemic fibrosis in patients with compromised renal function, thus limiting the utility of this technique

for renal artery evaluation in many patients. Noncontrast MRI protocols are evolving for effective anatomic evaluation of the renal arteries. Catheter angiography remains the gold standard and has the added benefit of directly measuring pressure gradients across a stenosis to ascertain hemodynamic significance. Physiologically significant and reversible renal artery stenosis can also be demonstrated with a nuclear captopril nephrogram.

Fibromuscular Dysplasia

Fibromuscular dysplasia (FMD) of the renal arteries is a cause of poorly controlled hypertension in young to middle-aged female patients. FMD accounts for 10% of cases of renal artery stenosis. Various histologic subtypes of FMD are recognized, the most common of which is medial fibroplasia. Characteristic features include involvement of the middle and distal thirds of the renal artery, in contradistinction to atherosclerotic disease, which involves the ostium and proximal thirds of the artery, and a beaded pattern of stenoses and ectasia (Fig. 46-34). Although cross-sectional imaging may suggest the diagnosis based on morphology, hemodynamically significant flow dynamics across the artery cannot be reliably assessed, and catheter angiography with pressure gradient measurement remains the gold standard. The radiologist should still look for ancillary findings such as dissections, emboli, and renal infarcts on CT. Sequelae of embolic disease to the renal arteries are typically seen as segmental renal infarcts with wedge-shaped areas of peripheral hypoperfusion or atrophy. If FMD is found by imaging in the renal arteries, the carotid arteries may also be involved and thus may require further diagnostic workup.

Rare Causes

Segmental arterial mediolysis (SAM) is a poorly understood noninflammatory process typically affecting visceral

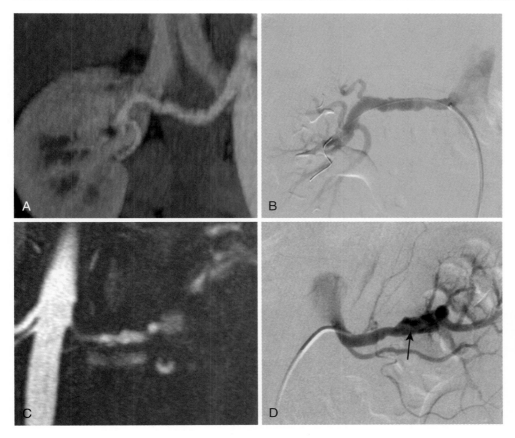

Figure 46-34 Fibromuscular dysplasia (FMD). Reformatted computed tomography (**A**) and corresponding right renal angiogram (**B**) in a patient with fibromuscular dysplasia. Note the beaded appearance affecting the midportion of the renal artery, classic for the more common medial fibroplasia subtype of FMD. High-pressure gradients were recorded across this segment on angiography. **C,** Contrast-enhanced magnetic resonance imaging demonstrates irregularity and beading in the middle and distal portions of the left renal artery. **D,** Corresponding angiogram in the same patient confirms these findings and demonstrates dissection of the middle to distal portion of the artery *(arrow)*. Dissections are more common in the intimal and perimedial subtypes of FMD.

arteries. Histologically, destruction of mural muscular elements is noted, and the clinical presentation can be acute, resulting from dissection, occlusion, or rupture. Distinguishing SAM affecting the renal arteries from other causes of spontaneous dissection, including intimal or perimedial subtypes of FMD or Ehlers-Danlos syndrome, may be difficult. Multiple affected visceral branches may be clues to the diagnosis (Figs. 46-35 and 46-36). Similar findings may be seen in patients with collagen vascular disease (Fig. 46-37). Another rare cause of renovascular hypertension is involvement of the renal arteries with neurofibromatosis. Caused by intimal proliferation of smooth muscle cells and fibrous tissue, neurofibromatosis typically causes proximal renal artery stenosis in affected individuals (Fig. 46-38). Additional rare causes of renovascular hypertension include Takayasu arteritis, Williams syndrome, Marfan syndrome, congenital rubella, Kawasaki disease, and Crohn disease.

Visceral Artery Aneurysms

Aneurysms of the visceral arteries are relatively rare. These aneurysms can be either fusiform, when they are associated with underlying vessel degeneration (e.g., in FMD or SAM), or saccular, when they are seen at vessel bifurcations or as part of medium vessel vasculitis (e.g., periarteritis nodosa). Reformatted images on CT, including maximum intensity projection reformations, are helpful for characterizing the aneurysm and its relationships with parent and branch vessels, particularly when

involving a tortuous artery such as the splenic artery (Fig. 46-39). Many interventionalists and surgeons use 2.5 cm as a guideline for intervention or surgery in the splenic or renal beds.

Pseudoaneurysms

Pseudoaneurysms of the visceral arteries are often iatrogenic, such as from percutaneous biopsy or intervention, and they can be a significant source of bleeding. Although angiography remains the gold standard once the clinical suspicion of pseudoaneurysm is high, findings on ultrasound and CT are also present that are helpful for making the diagnosis. Characteristic findings on ultrasound include a cystic-appearing vascular lesion with to and fro flow, possibly demonstrating a yin-yang sign on color Doppler imaging. For CT, typically, a three-phase study is warranted. Patients with suspected bleeding often undergo noncontrast CT scanning because of the inherently high density of blood clots. If high-density clot surrounds an abdominal organ or is present in the ureter, for example, the noncontrast scan should be followed by an arterial phase and 2-minute delayed phase scan to look for an arterial source of bleeding (Fig. 46-40). At angiography, multiple obliquities are often necessary to identify the parent vessel unambiguously, and failure to obtain sufficient oblique images during the diagnostic portion of the study may lead to inappropriate embolization of overlying branches without treating the feeding artery to the pseudoaneurysm.

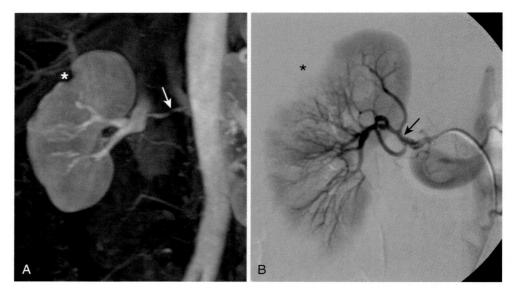

Figure 46-35 Segmental arterial mediolysis. A, Renal magnetic resonance imaging (MRI) demonstrates a spiral narrowing in the right renal artery consistent with dissection *(arrow)*. A focal cortical defect in the upper pole of the right kidney is also seen *(asterisk)*, consistent with secondary infarction. **B,** Renal angiogram in the same patient with the dissection seen as a linear filling defect in the right renal artery *(arrow)*. Note also the lack of parenchymal blush in the right upper pole of the kidney *(asterisk)* that represents the infarct seen on MRI.

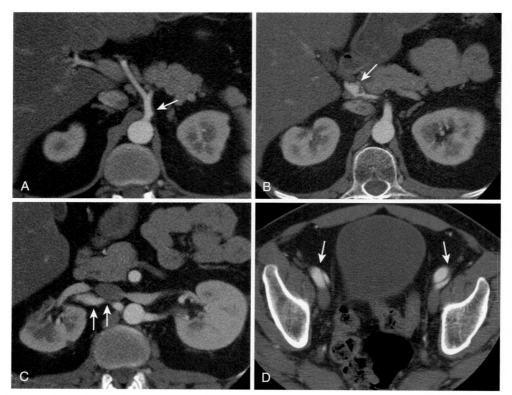

Figure 46-36 Segmental arterial mediolysis. Computed tomography images of a patient with multisegmental arterial irregularities *(arrows)* seen in the celiac axis (**A**), hepatic artery with aneurysm (**B**), right renal artery with dissection and aneurysm formation (**C**), and dissections in the bilateral common iliac arteries (**D**). This broad distribution of arterial irregularity suggests segmental arterial mediolysis.

Arteriovenous Malformation

Arteriovenous malformations (AVMs) of visceral branches are rare and most often sporadic. When multiple AVMs are identified, the radiologist should consider a congenital syndrome such as hereditary hemorrhagic telangiectasia. The AVM is identified by dilated tortuous vessels and early venous opacification. In the kidney, causes of AVMs include congenital lesions and acquired lesions from earlier iatrogenic or blunt trauma (Fig. 46-41). Hypoenhancement in a segment of the kidney adjacent to an AVM, presumed to represent hypoperfusion from steal phenomena across the AVM, has been described, but it should not exclude evaluation for an associated relatively hypodense renal mass. On ultrasound, a renal AVM can often resemble a cyst in the hilum, and the examiner must always use color Doppler techniques to exclude a vascular lesion. Treatment of AVMs can

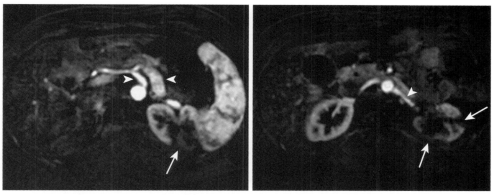

Figure 46-37 Ehlers-Danlos syndrome. Contrast-enhanced magnetic resonance imaging of the abdomen demonstrating fusiform aneurysmal ectasia in the celiac axis, splenic artery aneurysm, and irregularities in the midleft renal artery *(arrowheads)*. This condition has resulted in distal embolization with wedge-shaped areas of nonperfusion and infarct in the spleen and left kidney *(arrows)*. These findings can also be seen in segmental arterial mediolysis.

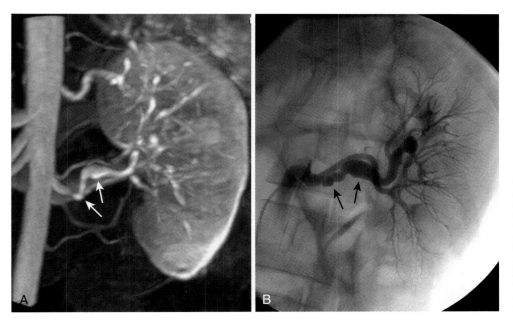

Figure 46-38 Neurofibromatosis of the renal artery. Magnetic resonance imaging (**A**) and angiography (**B**) in the same patient with neurofibromatosis and hypertension. Note the irregularity and beaded appearance involving the proximal renal artery, with aneurysm formation along the midaspect of the artery *(arrows)*. These findings are similar to those seen in fibromuscular dysplasia.

be either open surgery or percutaneous intervention using various embolic agents.

Visceral Artery Stents

Vascular stents can be either bare metal or covered, typically with Dacron (polyethylene) or polytetrafluoroethylene (PTFE). Stents can be recognized by their meshwork or lattice appearance on CT. Usually, the segment of artery with the stent appears very regular in caliber, and extremely wide windows are required to view the lattice appearance of the stent (Fig. 46-42). If contrast is used, patency of the stent and the presence of in-stent stenosis with low-density neointimal thickening can be seen and should be reported. Evaluation for stent migration or fracture should be made. However, many stents, especially in the renal or mesenteric arteries, are placed such that 1 to 2 mm of the stent prolapses into the aorta. This finding should not be misinterpreted as misplacement or stent migration. Stents cause significant

signal void on MRI, and MRA is therefore not useful for assessing stent patency. Stents can also be evaluated by ultrasound. However, the examiner should wait at least 24 hours after stent placement before ultrasound evaluation, especially in patients with covered stents, because small amounts of introduced air between the stent and the vessel wall during deployment may limit the ability to insonate across the stent and may give the false appearance of occlusion resulting from the lack of Doppler signal.

Pearls and Pitfalls

- Atherosclerotic visceral and renal artery stenosis is often ostial. Other causes of stenosis and aneurysms such as FMD or SAM can affect variable segments of the arteries.
- Ultrasound findings include elevated velocities at the site of stenosis and a parvus et tardus waveform distal to the site of stenosis.

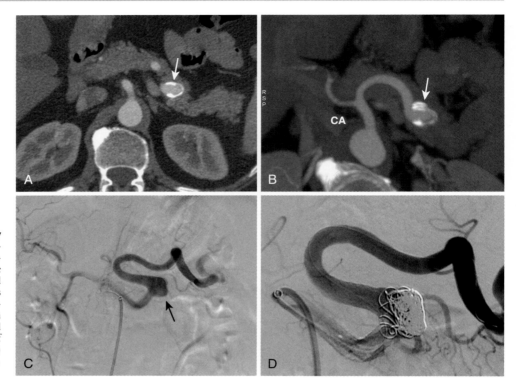

Figure 46-39 Splenic artery aneurysm. A, Computed tomography image demonstrates a partially calcified aneurysm of the splenic artery *(arrow)*. **B,** A curved multiplanar reformatted image is helpful to illustrate the relationship of the aneurysm *(arrow)* with the tortuous splenic artery. **C** and **D,** Angiographic appearance of this aneurysm before (**C,** *arrow*) and after coil embolization. *CA,* Celiac artery.

- Visceral artery stents are placed prolapsing into the aorta by 1 to 2 mm to maintain radial strength at the ostium.
- Three-phase CT is helpful for evaluating iatrogenic visceral pseudoaneurysm.

■ CONCLUSION

CTA has become a valuable diagnostic tool for imaging of the abdominal aorta and branches, and it has largely supplanted diagnostic angiography in many instances. Specific features helpful for problem-solving strategies in vascular imaging include obtaining precontrast images in addition to early arterial phase and 2-minute venous delayed phase imaging, rather than the standard portal venous phase imaging of most conventional diagnostic abdominal CT scans. Ultrasound is a useful screening modality in many cases, and it may be the definitive study in certain cases. Typically, however, a confirmatory study with CTA or MRA is helpful. Finally, maintaining a differential diagnosis and looking for root causes of the findings are always important because the radiologist may be the first to render the appropriate diagnosis in many cases.

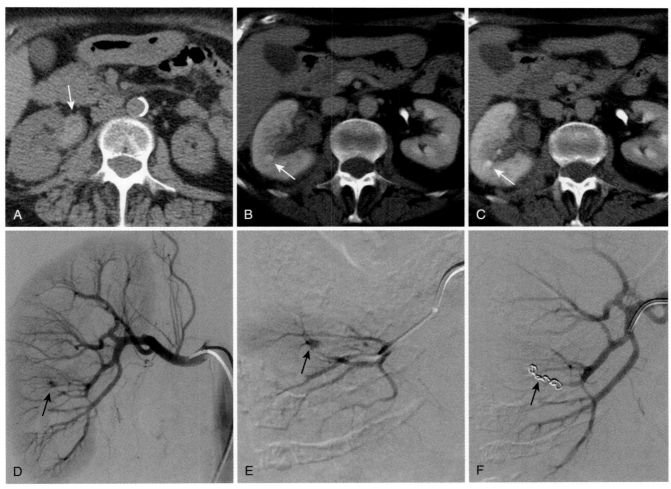

Figure 46-40 Renal artery pseudoaneurysm. Computed tomography images in precontrast (**A**), portal venous (**B**), and 2-minute delayed (**C**) phases in a patient with hematuria after percutaneous renal biopsy. The noncontrast image is useful because it demonstrates the hyperdense hematoma in the renal collecting system (**A,** *arrow*). The contrast-enhanced and delayed studies show a small pool of contrast material (**B** and **C,** *arrows*) consistent with a pseudoaneurysm. **D** to **F,** Angiography in the same patient that demonstrates the pseudoaneurysm and subsequent coil embolization of the feeding artery *(arrows)*.

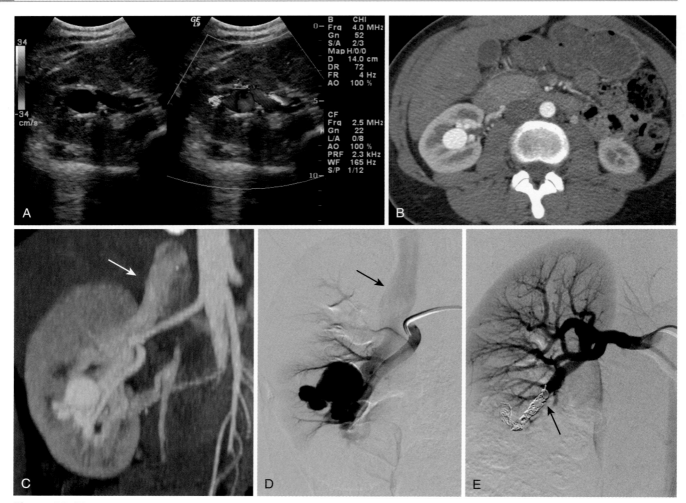

Figure 46-41 Renal arteriovenous malformation. A, Ultrasound demonstrates a rounded anechoic structure in the right kidney, potentially easily confused with a cyst until color Doppler is used, thus demonstrating a vascular lesion. **B,** Contrast-enhanced axial computed tomography (CT) image shows a rounded focus of contrast with dilated adjacent vessels. **C** and **D,** Coronal reformatted image from the CT scan clearly (**C**) demonstrates early opacification of the renal vein *(arrow)* and correlates well with the angiogram of the same patient (**D,** *arrow*). **E,** Coil embolization *(arrow)* of the arteriovenous malformation was successful. The lower pole of the kidney was supplied by an accessory renal artery (not shown).

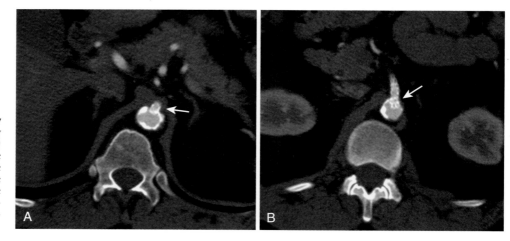

Figure 46-42 Visceral artery stents. Computed tomography images demonstrate stents *(arrows)* within the celiac axis (**A**) and the superior mesenteric artery (**B**). Wide windows demonstrate the lattice pattern of the stent. Slight prolapse into the aorta is expected and purposeful at the time of stent placement to achieve optimal patency.

Bibliography

Akino H, Gobara M, Suzuki Y, et al. Report of a case of a renal arteriovenous malformation presenting an unusual computed tomographic finding. *Hinyokika Kiyo*. 1987;33:757-761.

Allison MA, Budoff MJ, Nasir K, et al. Ethnic-specific risks for atherosclerotic calcification of the thoracic and abdominal aorta (from the Multi-Ethnic Study of Atherosclerosis). *Am J Cardiol*. 2009;104:812-817.

Brandenburg VM, Frank RD, Riehl J. Color-coded duplex sonography study of arteriovenous fistulae and pseudoaneurysms complicating percutaneous renal allograft biopsy. *Clin Nephrol*. 2002;58:398-404.

Daniels SR, Loggie JM, McEnery PT, et al. Clinical spectrum of intrinsic renovascular hypertension in children. *Pediatrics*. 1987;80:698-704.

Dieter RS, Dieter RA, Dieter RA. *Peripheral Arterial Disease*. New York: McGraw-Hill Medical; 2009.

Duncan AA. Median arcuate ligament syndrome. *Curr Treat Options Cardiovasc Med*. 2008;10:112-116.

Glynn Jr TP, Kreipke DL, Irons JM. Amyloidosis: diffuse involvement of the retroperitoneum. *Radiology*. 1989;170:726.

Hiramoto JS, Chang CK, Reilly LM, et al. Outcome of renal stenting for renal artery coverage during endovascular aortic aneurysm repair. *J Vasc Surg*. 2009;49:1100-1106.

Johnsen SH, Joakimsen O, Singh K, et al. Relation of common carotid artery lumen diameter to general arterial dilating diathesis and abdominal aortic aneurysms: the Tromso Study. *Am J Epidemiol*. 2009;169:330-338.

Kalva SP, Mueller PR. Vascular imaging in the elderly. *Radiol Clin North Am*. 2008;46:663-683:v.

Kasashima S, Zen Y. IgG4-related inflammatory abdominal aortic aneurysm. *Curr Opin Rheumatol*. 2011;23:18-23.

Kranokpiraksa P, Kaufman JA. Follow-up of endovascular aneurysm repair: plain radiography, ultrasound, CT/CT angiography, MR imaging/MR angiography, or what? *J Vasc Interv Radiol*. 2008;19:S27-S36.

Macedo TA, Stanson AW, Oderich GS, et al. Infected aortic aneurysms: imaging findings. *Radiology*. 2004;231:250-257.

Malav IC, Kothari SS. Renal artery stenosis due to neurofibromatosis. *Ann Pediatr Cardiol*. 2009;2:167-169.

Nordon I, Brar R, Taylor J, et al. Evidence from cross-sectional imaging indicates abdominal but not thoracic aortic aneurysms are local manifestations of a systemic dilating diathesis. *J Vasc Surg*. 2009;50:171-176. e1.

Nordon IM, Hinchliffe RJ, Loftus IM, et al. Pathophysiology and epidemiology of abdominal aortic aneurysms. *Nat Rev Cardiol*. 2011;8:92-102.

Ohrlander T, Sonesson B, Ivancev K, et al. The chimney graft: a technique for preserving or rescuing aortic branch vessels in stent-graft sealing zones. *J Endovasc Ther*. 2008;15:427-432.

Ozkan U, Oguzkurt L, Tercan F. Atherosclerotic risk factors and segmental distribution in symptomatic peripheral artery disease. *J Vasc Interv Radiol*. 2009;20:437-441.

Ozkan U, Oguzkurt L, Tercan F, et al. The prevalence and clinical predictors of incidental atherosclerotic renal artery stenosis. *Eur J Radiol*. 2009;69:550-554.

Parker MV, O'Donnell SD, Chang AS, et al. What imaging studies are necessary for abdominal aortic endograft sizing? A prospective blinded study using conventional computed tomography, aortography, and three-dimensional computed tomography. *J Vasc Surg*. 2005;41:199-205.

Pitton MB, Schmiedt W, Neufang A, et al. Classification and treatment of endoleaks after endovascular treatment of abdominal aortic aneurysms. *Rofo*. 2005;177:24-34.

Safian RD, Textor SC. Renal-artery stenosis. *N Engl J Med*. 2001;344:431-442.

Schmidt WA, Kraft HE, Vorpahl K, et al. Color duplex ultrasonography in the diagnosis of temporal arteritis. *N Engl J Med*. 1997;337:1336-1342.

Schurch W, Messerli FH, Genest J, et al. Arterial hypertension and neurofibromatosis: renal artery stenosis and coarctation of abdominal aorta. *Can Med Assoc J*. 1975;113:879-885.

Soulen MC, Cohen DL, Itkin M, et al. Segmental arterial mediolysis: angioplasty of bilateral renal artery stenoses with 2-year imaging follow-up. *J Vasc Interv Radiol*. 2004;15:763-767.

Sprouse 2nd LR, Meier 3rd GH, Parent FN, et al. Is three-dimensional computed tomography reconstruction justified before endovascular aortic aneurysm repair? *J Vasc Surg*. 2004;40:443-447.

Taylor DB, Blaser SI, Burrows PE, et al. Arteriopathy and coarctation of the abdominal aorta in children with mucopolysaccharidosis: imaging findings. *AJR Am J Roentgenol*. 1991;157:819-823.

Thalheimer A, Fein M, Geissinger E, et al. Intimal angiosarcoma of the aorta: report of a case and review of the literature. *J Vasc Surg*. 2004;40:548-553.

Vaglio A, Salvarani C, Buzio C. Retroperitoneal fibrosis. *Lancet*. 2006;367:241-251.

Valji K. *Vascular and Interventional Radiology*. Philadelphia: Saunders; 1999.

van Bommel EF. Retroperitoneal fibrosis. *Neth J Med*. 2002;60:231-242.

Wicky S, Fan CM, Geller SC, et al. MR angiography of endoleak with inconclusive concomitant CT angiography. *AJR Am J Roentgenol*. 2003;181:736-738.

Zeller T, Bonvini RF, Sixt S. Color-coded duplex ultrasound for diagnosis of renal artery stenosis and as follow-up examination after revascularization. *Catheter Cardiovasc Interv*. 2008;71:995-999.

CHAPTER 47

Upper Extremity Arteries

Sanjeeva P. Kalva, Sandeep Hedgire, and Arthur C. Waltman

Upper extremity arteries are affected by a myriad of vascular disorders. Atherosclerosis is the most common arterial disease, but other conditions, such as vasculitis, chronic repetitive traumatic injuries, and trauma, constitute a significant portion of the arterial diseases. This chapter summarizes the salient features of these disorders.

■ ATHEROSCLEROSIS

Atherosclerosis is less commonly encountered in the upper extremities than in the lower extremities. The risk factors for atherosclerosis include diabetes, hypercholesterolemia, smoking, and hypertension. Subclinical disease is common, but symptomatic disease is rare given the small muscle mass and lower demand for oxygen in the upper extremities. Asymptomatic disease is often discovered when asymmetrical arm blood pressures are found during clinical examination. Symptoms include arm pain with exertion, rest pain, and digit ulceration. Coldness, nail and skin atrophy, and hair loss can be indicative of long-term ischemic change. Patients with proximal subclavian artery stenosis may have symptoms of subclavian steal syndrome—dizziness, vertigo, and syncope during arm exertion (Fig. 47-1). Similarly, ischemic symptoms may occur following creation of an arteriovenous fistula or graft in the upper extremity that steals the blood and brings out subclinical atherosclerotic disease caused by decreased flow to the distal arterial bed (Fig. 47-2).

A clinical diagnosis of upper extremity arterial stenosis may be suspected when a blood pressure difference of greater than 10 mm Hg between the arms is identified during physical examination. Noninvasive vascular laboratory tests such as segmental limb pressures, pulse volume recordings, and wrist-brachial index measurement should be performed. On measurement of segmental limb pressures, a difference of greater than 10 mm Hg between the arms suggests proximal disease affecting the brachiocephalic or subclavian or axillary arteries, whereas a difference of greater than 10 to 20 mm Hg between the successive arm levels suggests intervening occlusive disease. On pulse volume recordings, mild disease is characterized by loss of dicrotic notch and an outward bowing of the downstroke. Decreased amplitude of the waveform suggests severe disease. The normal wrist-brachial index is 1.0 and a value of less

than 0.85 is indicative of arterial disease. Noninvasive tests after exercise are helpful to detect subclinical disease. Similarly, vasospastic disorders can be tested after exposing the hands to the appropriate stimuli (cold water in cases of Raynaud syndrome).

Imaging evaluation of upper extremity atherosclerosis can be performed with duplex ultrasonography, computed tomography angiography (CTA), and magnetic resonance angiography (MRA). Catheter angiography is reserved for evaluation of small vessel disease in the hand and for interventions. An occlusion is suspected on duplex ultrasonography with appropriate technical settings (low pulse repetition frequency and appropriate wall filters) when there is no color flow on color Doppler and absence of flow on spectral Doppler. A stenosis of 50% or more luminal narrowing is suspected when the peak systolic velocity at the site of narrowing is more than two times that of the proximal normal segment. A ratio of the peak systolic velocity in the stenotic segment to the peak systolic velocity in the proximal normal segment that is more than 4:1 suggests greater than 75% luminal narrowing. The waveforms distal to the stenosis show decreased peak systolic velocity, increased acceleration time (tardus parvus pattern), and monophasic flow pattern. The proximal subclavian artery is often difficult to evaluate with duplex ultrasonography. However, the presence of a hemodynamically significant stenosis can be suspected when a tardus parvus monophasic waveform is seen in the distal subclavian artery or the axillary artery. A reversal of flow in the vertebral artery may be seen if the stenosis is proximal to the origin of the vertebral artery. This is often referred to as subclavian steal syndrome. In patients with a coronary bypass graft using the internal mammary artery, coronary-subclavian steal may occur, wherein there is reversal of flow through the internal mammary artery on duplex ultrasonography with exertion of the upper extremity.

CTA with multidetector computed tomography is highly accurate in localization and estimation of percentage of stenosis or occlusion of peripheral arterial disease affecting the upper extremity (see Fig. 47-1). Caution should be exercised when performing these studies. The contrast material should be injected through the asymptomatic arm to prevent streak artifacts from the contrast material–filled subclavian veins. Plaques are identified as mural-adherent calcified or noncalcified linear structures protruding into the lumen. Ulceration of the plaque may be seen as a central or paracentral acutely

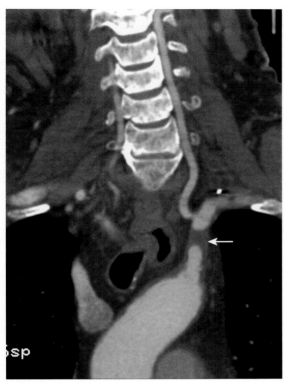

Figure 47-1 Reformatted computed tomography angiogram shows short segment occlusion *(arrow)* of the left subclavian artery. The distal subclavian artery fills through retrograde flow from the left vertebral artery.

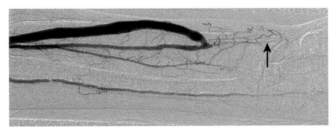

Figure 47-2 Steal following creation of an arteriovenous fistula. Digital subtraction angiography of the forearm arteries reveals decreased flow to the distal radial artery *(arrow)* as significant amount of flow is shunted through the arteriovenous fistula.

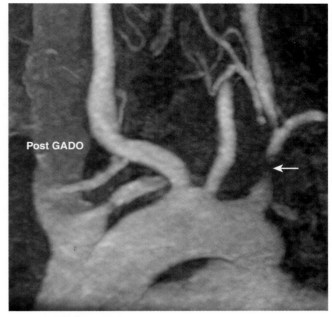

Figure 47-3 Maximum intensity projection from a contrast-enhanced magnetic resonance angiography shows short segment occlusion *(arrow)* of the left subclavian artery.

angulated depression within the plaque surface. Occlusions may be seen as filling defects within the arteries. Collateral vessels may be identified in the presence of occlusion or hemodynamically significant stenosis. As with other locations in the body, atherosclerosis tends to affect the vessel origins and bifurcation points.

MRA with gadolinium is one of the best methods of assessing the extent of atherosclerotic disease in the upper extremities (Fig. 47-3). Noncontrast methods are not adequate for the assessment of proximal subclavian artery disease; however, the reversal of flow in the vertebral arteries may be seen with two-dimensional time of flight sequences. Arterial disease affecting the arm and forearm may be assessed with various noncontrast methods; however, the arteries of the hand require high-resolution imaging that is often inadequate on noncontrast MRA. Time-resolved techniques allow detection

of collateral flow pattern and help assess the hemodynamic significance of a stenosis.

Catheter angiography is reserved for assessment of small vessels in the hand. Digital arterial occlusive disease secondary to atherosclerosis is common but rarely symptomatic, unless the disease is severe or the proximal arterial flow is diverted (such as after creation of an arteriovenous fistula or graft in patients with renal failure), when it leads to gangrene or ulceration of the fingers. Catheter angiography may demonstrate luminal narrowing, irregularity of the luminal surface in the presence of ulcerated plaques, collateral flow, and arterial occlusions (Fig. 47-4). Catheter angiography of the carotid arteries demonstrates the reversal of flow in the vertebral artery in the presence of proximal subclavian artery stenosis (Fig. 47-5). Similarly, coronary angiography may demonstrate reversal of flow through the internal mammary artery bypass graft in patients with coronary-subclavian steal syndrome. Catheter angiography is part of endovascular and open interventional procedures on the blood vessels. It is useful for assessing the patency of stents and bypass grafts (see Fig. 47-4).

Pearls and Pitfalls

1. Upper extremity atherosclerosis is often subclinical, rarely causes symptoms, and is incidentally discovered on physical examination when a difference in blood pressure between the arms prompts further investigation.

2. Proximal subclavian artery disease leads to subclavian steal syndrome; patients have dizziness, vertigo, and syncope, especially after upper extremity exertion. Duplex ultrasonography, MRA, and catheter angiography are helpful in diagnosing this condition.

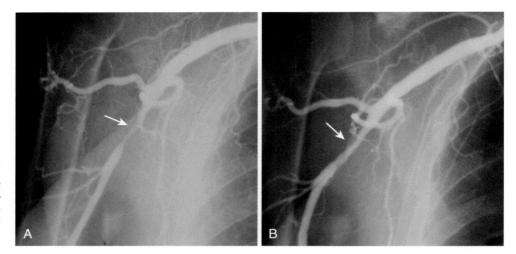

Figure 47-4 Atherosclerotic disease of the upper extremity. A, Catheter angiography shows luminal narrowing *(arrow)* of right axillary artery. **B,** Following balloon angioplasty.

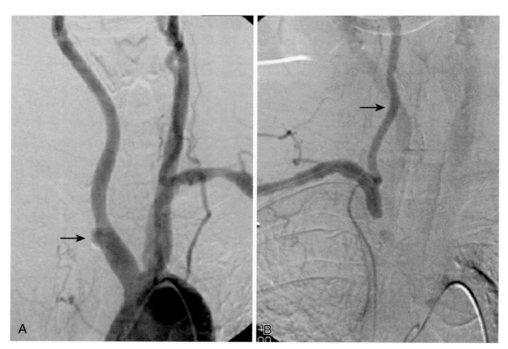

Figure 47-5 Subclavian steal syndrome. A, Arch aortography shows occlusion *(arrow)* of the right subclavian artery. **B,** During the late phase of the injection there is reversal of flow in the right vertebral artery *(arrow)*, filling the right subclavian distal to the occluded segment.

3. Digital artery atherosclerosis is best evaluated with catheter angiography.
4. Steal phenomenon from hemodialysis fistula or graft is best assessed through angiography. A catheter is positioned above the level of the arteriovenous anastomosis, and contrast material is injected before and after compression of the venous outflow. A significant improvement of distal flow with venous outflow occlusion and immediate improvement in clinical symptoms suggest steal phenomenon.

■ NONATHEROSCLEROTIC, NONINFLAMMATORY ARTERIAL OCCLUSIVE DISEASE

Dissection

Dissection affecting the upper extremity arteries is usually secondary to extension of an aortic dissection. It usually affects the brachiocephalic and subclavian arteries, and rarely does this extend to the axillary artery. Isolated dissections without the involvement of the aorta should raise the possibility of collagen vascular disorders such as Marfan and Ehlers-Danlos syndromes. Dissections involving the brachial and forearm arteries are rare and are usually secondary to trauma or vascular interventions (Fig. 47-6). Dissection flap is rarely visible on ultrasonography but can be well recognized on CTA and MRA. The true lumen is recognized by its small size and early filling with contrast material.

Fibromuscular Dysplasia

Fibromuscular dysplasia affects the medium and small arteries. Commonly observed in young and middle-aged females, it affects the renal arteries, extracranial cerebral arteries, iliofemoral arteries, and splanchnic arteries. Upper extremity arteries are rarely affected.

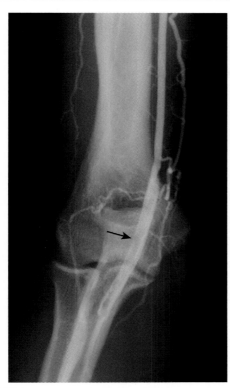

Figure 47-6 Conventional angiography shows a traumatic dissection *(arrow)* of the brachial artery following attempted arterial access.

Among the upper extremity arteries, the subclavian artery is the most commonly affected artery, followed by the brachial, axillary, and forearm arteries. Patients are usually asymptomatic, and the disease is discovered incidentally on imaging. Rarely patients may present with distal embolism. Duplex ultrasonography, CTA, and MRA may show the beaded appearance of the artery (Fig. 47-7). Ultrasonography is useful to assess the presence of hemodynamically significant stenosis. Catheter angiography confirms the diagnosis (see Fig. 47-7). Both upper extremities should be assessed to rule out the presence of bilateral disease (see Fig. 47-7). In addition, evaluation of the renal and carotid arteries must be performed to detect the presence of subclinical disease in these territories, because fibromuscular dysplasia tends to involve multiple territories in one third of the patients. Hemodynamically significant, symptomatic lesions respond well to angioplasty.

Raynaud Syndrome

In this condition an abnormal vasoconstriction of the digital arteries to cold temperature or emotional stress results in color changes in the skin of the digits. With exposure to cold temperature the digits become cold, with sharply demarcated pallor (paleness) or cyanosis (blue discoloration), or both. With rewarming the skin becomes red because of reperfusion. The symptoms usually involve a single finger and spread to other fingers symmetrically in both hands. Patients may complain of numbness, ache, or a sensation of pins and needles. Diagnosis is usually clinical, but noninvasive vascular

tests and color Doppler ultrasonography may demonstrate changes in the digital flow. Such changes include decreased amplitude on pulse volume recordings in the digits in response to exposure to cold temperature (Fig. 47-8) and decreased amplitude with monophasic flow and absent diastolic flow on Doppler ultrasonography. Catheter angiography may also demonstrate vascular spasm of the digital arteries with exposure to cold that reverses on rewarming. The secondary form of Raynaud syndrome refers to the presence of underlying diseases such as atherosclerosis or connective tissue disorders that disrupt the normal complex regulation of regional blood flow to the digits and skin.

Frostbite

Frostbite is a severe localized cold-induced injury resulting from freezing of tissue on exposure to cold weather. On exposure to subfreezing temperatures, ice crystals form extracellularly and sometimes intracellularly, leading to cellular disruption and inflammation. Depending on the severity, frostbite is classified into first degree (superficial involvement with pallor and anesthesia of the skin), second degree (blisters with edema and erythema), third degree (hemorrhagic blisters with black skin eschar), and fourth degree (complete tissue necrosis involving muscles and bone). There is associated vascular thrombosis of the affected tissue. Vascular occlusion may be seen on MRA. However, catheter angiography is highly sensitive in identifying the extent of vascular occlusion in the hands (Fig.47-9, *A*) and for institution and follow-up of thrombolytic therapy (Fig.47-9, *B*).

Pearls and Pitfalls

1. The presence of noncontiguous dissections in the distal arteries suggests iatrogenic trauma from repeated arterial access.
2. The thumb is seldom involved in primary Raynaud syndrome. Secondary Raynaud phenomenon results from a large variety of conditions.
3. Fibromuscular dysplasia often involves both upper extremities and is often associated with other arterial involvement.
4. Arterial injuries in frostbite are best evaluated with catheter angiography.
5. Arterial injuries following arterial access to the brachial artery are secondary to the small size and anatomic variations (high bifurcation) of the brachial artery.

■ ANEURYSMS

Aneurysms of the upper extremity are uncommon. True aneurysms from atherosclerosis or arterial degeneration affect the proximal subclavian and axillary arteries. Distal aneurysms are usually secondary to trauma and iatrogenic injuries. Patients may be asymptomatic or may present with symptoms resulting from extrinsic compression of adjacent structures or distal thromboembolism. CTA and MRA are accurate in localizing the aneurysms and demonstrating the characteristic

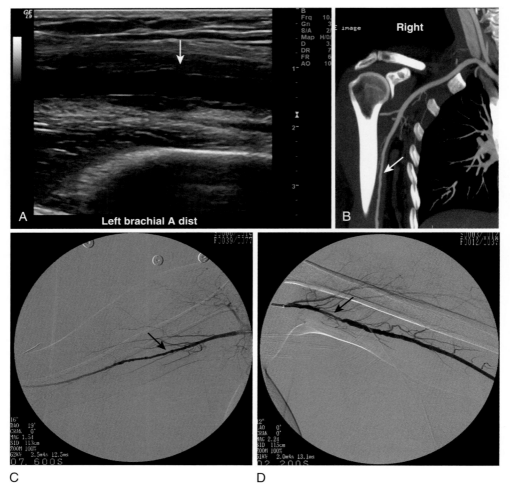

Figure 47-7 Fibromuscular dysplasia affecting upper extremity arteries. Ultrasonography (**A**) shows irregular appearance *(arrow)* of the brachial artery intima. Reformatted computed tomography angiography (**B**) shows a characteristic beaded appearance *(arrow)*, which is confirmed on catheter angiography (**C** and **D**; *arrows*). Note bilaterally symmetrical appearance of the disease.

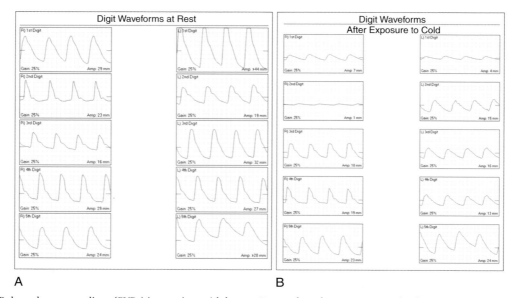

Figure 47-8 Pulse volume recordings (PVRs) in a patient with known Raynaud syndrome. **A,** At rest the digits show normal PVRs. **B,** Following exposure to cold, there is dampening of PVRs in the first and second digits consistent with Raynaud syndrome.

features: vessel dilatation, mural thrombus, calcification, extrinsic compression over the adjacent structures, and distal emboli (Fig. 47-10). Abnormal dilatation (>2 cm) of the proximal segment of an aberrant right subclavian artery is referred to as Kommerell diverticulum (Figs. 47-11 and 47-12). Patients may have dysphagia or distal thromboembolism. These diverticula are usually treated surgically. Pseudoaneurysms from trauma may be treated surgically or with stent grafts.

■ EMBOLISM

Upper extremity arterial embolism results in acute ischemic symptoms, digital gangrene, or ulceration. The sources of emboli are usually the heart (left atrial fibrillation, left ventricular thrombus from aneurysm, or myocardial infarction); aorta (mural thrombus from aortic aneurysm); proximal arterial diseases such as thoracic outlet syndrome, fibromuscular dysplasia, and atherosclerosis; arterial trauma; or following thrombectomy of an arteriovenous fistula or graft. Emboli tend to lodge at the vessel bifurcation points.

Ultrasonography, CTA, and MRA are useful to assess the location and extent of the emboli and the source of the emboli. Digital arterial emboli are best evaluated with catheter angiography. Emboli are seen as intravascular filling defects on CTA, MRA, and catheter angiography (Fig. 47-13). Similarly, extensive thrombosis of the vessels is seen as lack of expected enhancement of the arteries with injection of contrast material. Unless the disease has been chronic with repetitive emboli, collateral vessels are rarely identified. Extensive thrombosis of the upper extremity arteries is usually treated with surgical thrombectomy, given the poor quality of life associated with delayed reperfusion. However, thrombolysis may be attempted in selected cases, and results are promising.

■ VASCULITIS

Various types of vasculitis affect the upper extremity arteries. A detailed description of vasculitis is given in Chapter 25. Large vessel involvement is seen with Takayasu arteritis, giant cell arteritis, and Behçet syndrome. Buerger disease affects the medium and small arteries. Small vessel arteritis is seen with systemic lupus erythematosus, scleroderma, rheumatoid arthritis, polyarteritis nodosa,

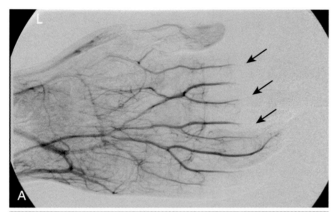

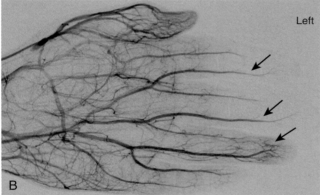

Figure 47-9 Frostbite. Occluded digital arteries *(arrows)* in a patient with frostbite (**A**) with subsequent improvement (**B**) following thrombolytic therapy.

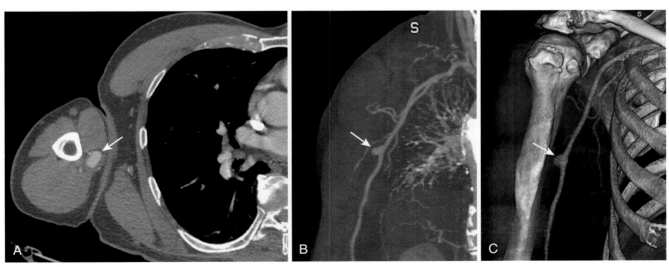

Figure 47-10 Degenerative aneurysm of the brachial artery *(arrow)* seen on axial contrast-enhanced computed tomography (CT; **A**), maximum intensity projection (**B**), and on volume-rendered three-dimensional CT angiogram (**C**).

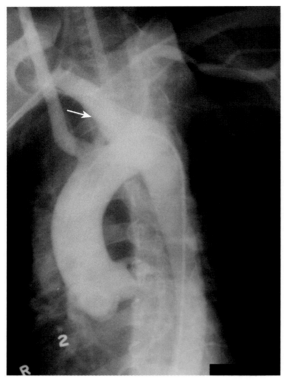

Figure 47-11 Aortic arch angiography shows an aberrant origin of the right subclavian artery with abnormal dilatation *(arrow)* of the proximal segment (Kommerell diverticulum).

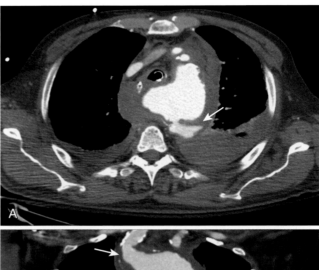

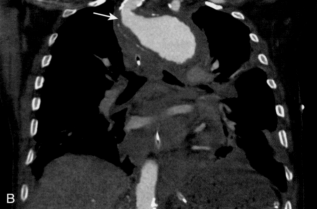

Figure 47-12 Axial (**A**) and coronal contrast-enhanced chest computed tomography (CT; **B**) shows a ruptured Kommerell diverticulum. Soft tissue around the subclavian artery *(arrow* in **B**) and active extravasation of the contrast material *(arrow* in **A**) are important signs on CT that signify a ruptured diverticulum.

and other connective tissue disorders. Radiation arteritis involves the arteries included in the radiation therapy portal.

Takayasu Arteritis

Takayasu arteritis involves the branches of the aorta: brachiocephalic, carotid, subclavian, and renal arteries. The affected vessel shows mural thickening with diffuse long-segment narrowing or occlusion of the vessel. Multiple vessels may be involved with asymmetrical distribution. Aneurysmal dilatation is also seen in some patients. The active phase is characterized by enhancement of the affected vessel wall and increased metabolic activity on 2-fluoro-2-deoxyglucose positron emission tomography (FDG-PET). Serologic markers of inflammation such as erythrocyte sedimentation rate and C-reactive protein level may be elevated. Computed tomography and magnetic resonance imaging (MRI) are excellent in depicting the vessel wall thickening (Fig. 47-14) and enhancement and extent of luminal narrowing or occlusion (Fig. 47-15). Catheter angiography is reserved for planning therapy and should be avoided when active inflammation is suspected.

Giant Cell Arteritis

Giant cell arteritis affects older adults (in the sixth and seventh decades) and involves the large and medium vessels. Patients have headaches, visual changes, symptoms of polymyalgia rheumatica, jaw claudication, fever,

or anemia. The superficial temporal artery (a branch of the external carotid artery) is commonly affected. In the upper extremity the subclavian and axillary arteries are often affected. The disease appears to be symmetrical, involving both upper extremities (Fig. 47-16). Patients may be asymptomatic or may have ischemic symptoms in the upper extremities. CTA and MRA show focal or short segment vessel narrowing, mural thickening, and vessel wall edema and enhancement (see Fig. 47-16). Ultrasonography shows hypoechoic vessel wall thickening (the halo sign), luminal narrowing, and occlusion. Catheter angiography shows luminal abnormalities in the form of stenosis and occlusions (see Fig. 47-16). Collateral vessels bypassing the stenosis or occlusion may be seen.

Buerger Disease

Also known as thromboangiitis obliterans, Buerger disease affects medium and small vessels. It is a segmental inflammatory disease in which highly cellular and inflammatory thrombus occludes vessel lumen, sparing the vessel wall. Young male smokers are commonly affected, and the use of tobacco or cannabis is essential for diagnosis. Patients present with distal extremity ischemia,

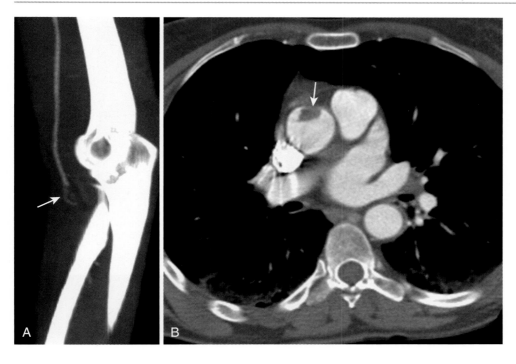

Figure 47-13 Brachial artery embolism is seen as a filling defect (*arrow* in **A**) on this reformatted computed tomography image. Aortic thrombosis (*arrow* in **B**) was the underlying cause in this case.

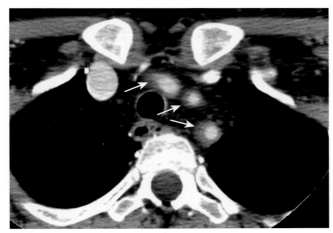

Figure 47-14 Contrast-enhanced chest computed tomography shows mural thickening involving the brachiocephalic, left common carotid, and left subclavian arteries (*arrows*) in a patient with Takayasu arteritis.

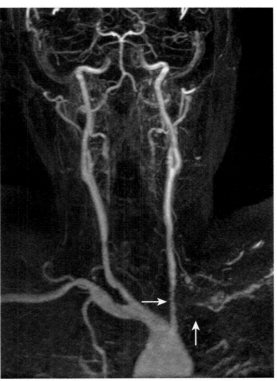

Figure 47-15 Coronal magnetic resonance angiography shows occlusion of left subclavian artery (*vertical arrow*) along with luminal narrowing of left common carotid artery (*horizontal arrow*) in a patient with Takayasu arteritis.

digital ulcers, or gangrene. Clinically Allen test results may be positive. Ultrasonography, CTA, and MRA may demonstrate segmental occlusion of the radial and ulnar arteries. Associated lower extremity disease is commonly seen. Catheter angiography is diagnostic. It demonstrates segmental vascular occlusion with corkscrew collaterals within the vessel wall (Fig. 47-17).

Radiation Arteritis

Radiation arteritis affects the arteries within the radiotherapy portal. This is frequently encountered after radiation therapy to the breast and axilla and commonly involves the axillary and brachial arteries. Catheter angiography demonstrates artery occlusion or irregular luminal narrowing, or both (Fig. 47-18).

Small Vessel Arteritis

Small vessel arteritis involving the hand is seen with inflammatory vasculitis. Catheter angiography shows normal-appearing large vessels with segmental narrowing and occlusions of the distal forearm and hand

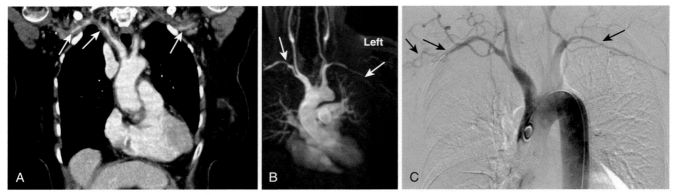

Figure 47-16 Giant cell arteritis. Coronal computed tomography angiography (**A**) shows mural thickening *(arrow)* involving the brachioce-phalic, left common carotid, and subclavian arteries. Magnetic resonance angiography (**B**) shows luminal narrowing *(arrows)* involving bilateral subclavian arteries. Digital subtraction angiography (**C**) of the aortic arch confirms the occlusion in the right subclavian artery with multiple collaterals *(arrows)* along with involvement of the left subclavian artery in the form of luminal narrowing *(arrow)*.

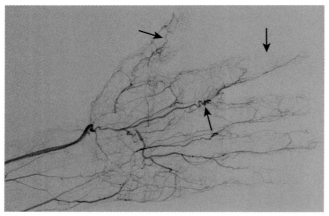

Figure 47-17 Catheter angiography of the hand shows multiple corkscrew collaterals *(oblique arrows)* with digital artery occlusion *(vertical arrow)* in a patient with Buerger disease.

arteries, vessel wall irregularity, and lack of collaterals. Absence of intravascular filling defects distinguishes this from distal embolic disease.

■ TRAUMA

Acute Trauma

Arterial injuries following trauma to the upper extremities occur with penetrating injuries, gunshot wounds, fracture dislocations, and stretch injuries. Arterial injuries may be suspected in the presence of an enlarging hematoma, active hemorrhage, extremity ischemia, bruit, and loss of pulse. Such injuries include vasospasm, active extravasation (Fig. 47-19) from rupture or transection of a vessel (Fig. 47-20), intimal tear or dissection, pseudoaneurysm (Fig. 47-21), arteriovenous fistula, and thrombosis. Hemodynamic stability and access to the area of injury determine the optimal imaging modality. In a stable patient duplex ultrasonography and CTA may be performed to assess the arterial injuries. When noninvasive modalities are inconclusive about the arterial injury (especially intimal tears) and the clinical suspicion is high, catheter angiography is

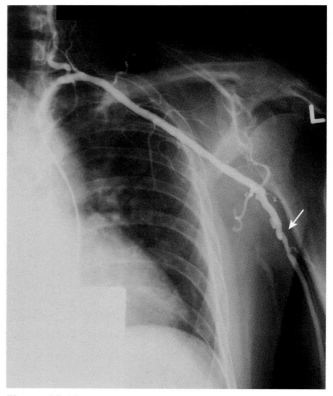

Figure 47-18 Radiation arteritis. Note irregular luminal narrowing and dilatations of the left brachial artery *(arrow)* in this patient with history of radiation to the axilla.

recommended. It can be combined with appropriate endovascular interventions. Stretch injuries result from stretching of the upper extremity when one tries to hold onto something while falling down a hill or tree or with fracture dislocation. The arterial wall is stretched, leading to intimal and medial tears that result in thrombosis and distal embolization. Thoracic trauma may result in injuries to the great vessels—the brachiocephalic artery and the subclavian artery. The imaging findings include regional hematoma, abnormal arterial contour, pseudoaneurysm, thrombosis (Fig. 47-22), and dissection. Iatrogenic injuries from arterial catheterization (axillary

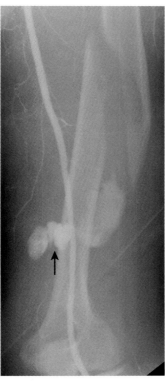

Figure 47-19 Active contrast material extravasation *(arrow)* during catheter angiography of the left upper extremity in a patient with humeral fracture.

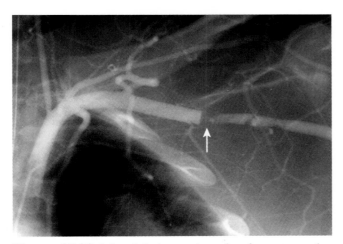

Figure 47-20 Left subclavian angiography shows transection *(arrow)* of the distal subclavian artery secondary to trauma.

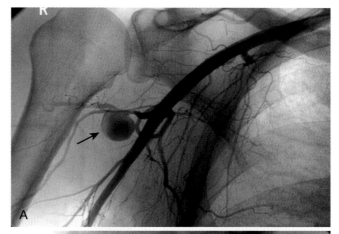

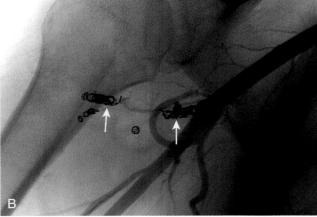

Figure 47-21 Traumatic pseudoaneurysm *(arrow)* of right circumflex humeral artery seen on this subclavian angiogram **(A)**. This was successfully treated by coil embolization *(arrows)* **(B)**.

or brachial or radial arteries) may result in dissection, thrombosis, pseudoaneurysm, and arteriovenous fistula. Inadvertent arterial injury may occur with other surgical procedures such as venous access, chest tube placement, and bone interventions.

Chronic Repetitive Trauma

Thoracic Outlet Syndrome

The thoracic outlet extends from the cervical spine and mediastinum to the lower border of the pectoralis minor and includes three spaces: the interscalene triangle, the costoclavicular space, and the retropectoral space. Symptoms result from dynamic compression of the brachial plexus and subclavian artery and vein in these spaces because of either the hypertrophy of normal structures or abnormal bony structures (cervical rib, callus from fracture of the clavicle or first rib, bony exostosis from the first rib or clavicle) or muscular or ligamentous structures (fibrous bands, variations in the insertion of scalene muscles, supernumerary muscles, posttraumatic or postoperative fibrous scarring). The most common location for arterial compression is the interscalene triangle, followed by the costoclavicular space. Chronic repetitive compression of the artery caused by arm motion results in arterial stenosis, poststenotic dilatation, thrombus formation, and distal embolization. Arterial symptoms occur in 5% to 10% of patients with thoracic outlet syndrome. Patients often have neurologic symptoms because of coexistent neural compression. When the arterial compression is isolated, patients present late with distal embolic symptoms. Arterial compression can be suspected clinically when the radial pulse becomes feeble or no more palpable with hyperabduction and external rotation of the arm.

The role of imaging is to assess the arterial compression, to detect the underlying structural abnormality, and to evaluate the arterial changes. Plain radiograph

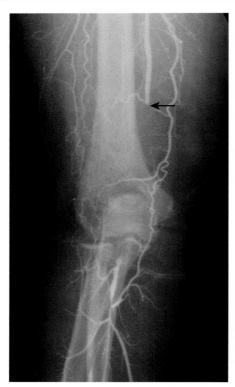

Figure 47-22 Upper extremity trauma. Left brachial angiogram shows abrupt cutoff *(arrow)* of the brachial artery consistent with thrombosis.

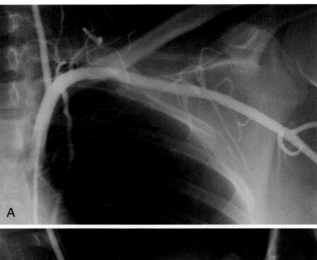

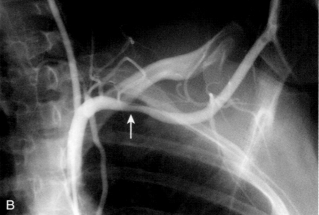

Figure 47-23 Left subclavian angiogram shows normal-appearing artery at neutral position (**A**). Note compression of the artery between the clavicle and the first rib when the arm is abducted and externally rotated (**B**), consistent with thoracic outlet syndrome.

of the neck may show presence of cervical rib or other bony abnormalities as described earlier. MRI is highly useful for assessing muscular and ligamentous abnormalities. Color Doppler ultrasonography and noninvasive vascular test results may demonstrate changes in the distal vascular bed from dynamic compression of the vascular bed. Changes in pulse volume recording (decreased amplitude and loss of dicrotic notch) and a change in the flow pattern (monophasic, tardus parvus pattern from triphasic flow) within the axillary and brachial arteries on color Doppler ultrasonography following provocative positioning of the arm raise the suspicion of arterial compression. CTA and MRA are useful to detect arterial wall changes: stenosis, poststenotic dilatation, aneurysm, thrombus within the dilated segment, and distal embolization. Arterial compression on CTA and MRA may be elicited with hyperabduction and external rotation of the arm. It is important to assess the opposite arm in positive cases because the disease tends to be bilateral. Catheter angiography is highly useful for assessing the dynamic compression of the artery (Fig. 47-23) and detecting arterial stenosis, aneurysm, and thromboembolism (Fig. 47-24). Treatment is usually surgical with resection of underlying bony or soft tissue abnormality, resection of the aneurysm, and creation of an arterial bypass.

Quadrilateral Space Syndrome
Axillary nerve and posterior circumflex humeral artery compression within the quadrilateral space (bounded by the long head of the triceps, the teres minor and teres major muscles, and the cortex of the humerus) in the upper arm results in the quadrilateral space syndrome. Fibrous bands and large paralabral cysts within this space compress the nerve and result in teres minor atrophy and clinical symptoms. The clinical manifestations include poorly localized shoulder pain, paresthesias in the affected extremity, and discrete-point tenderness in the lateral aspect of the quadrilateral space. MRI is useful for assessing the structural abnormalities within the quadrilateral space and other abnormalities in the shoulder joint that may be responsible for some of the symptoms and teres minor atrophy. MRA and catheter angiography show compression or occlusion of the circumflex humeral artery with abduction and external rotation of the arm. Often considered diagnostic, this finding may be seen in a significant portion of asymptomatic individuals.

Crutch Injury
Chronic use of axillary crutches may cause repetitive trauma to the axillary artery, leading to intimal injury, stenosis, poststenotic dilatation, aneurysm formation, thrombosis, and distal embolization (Fig. 47-25). Such compression is often encountered in patients with muscle wasting and loss of body fat around the axilla.

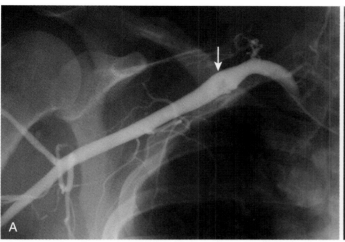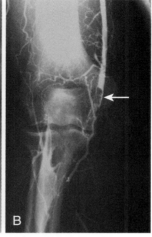

Figure 47-24 Thoracic outlet syndrome. Right subclavian angiogram shows focal dilatation (*arrow* in **A**) of the distal subclavian artery with distal embolus (*arrow* in **B**) to the brachial artery. Note the cervical rib in **A**.

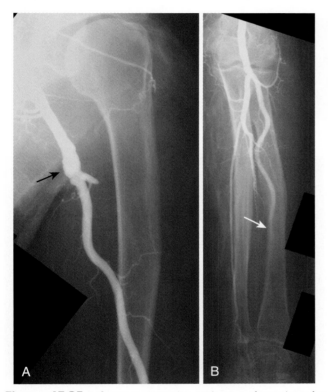

Figure 47-25 Left upper extremity angiogram shows irregular beaded appearance (*arrow* in **A**) of the axillary-brachial artery junction following repetitive injury from chronic use of crutches. Also note distal embolization (*arrow* in **B**) to the radial artery.

Patients may have distal embolization or acute upper extremity ischemia secondary to arterial thrombosis. The radial nerve is often compressed along with the axillary artery, and patients may have a flexed, limp wrist from paralysis of the extensor group of arm and forearm muscles. Color Doppler ultrasonography, CTA, and MRA demonstrate the characteristic stenosis, poststenotic dilatation, thrombus, and distal embolism. Catheter angiography is more accurate in depicting the distal emboli. Treatment involves thrombolysis and angioplasty if there are no aneurysms, and surgical thrombectomy and axillary-brachial bypass graft in patients with aneurysms.

Hypothenar Hammer Syndrome

Hypothenar hammer syndrome results from repetitive injury to the ulnar artery against the hook of hamate when the hypothenar eminence is used as a hammer. Such injury is common in carpenters, postal workers (stamping), and mechanics. Repetitive injury results in intimal and medial disruption of the ulnar artery with stenosis, aneurysm, thrombosis, artery occlusion, and distal embolization. Patients usually present with symptoms of distal embolization. Catheter angiography is the most useful imaging modality for assessing the ulnar artery abnormalities: occlusion, vessel irregularity, pseudoaneurysm, and distal emboli (Fig. 47-26). Recent advances in high-resolution MRI may also allow accurate delineation of arterial abnormalities. Treatment involves surgical resection and bypass graft.

Hand-Arm Vibration Syndrome

Hand-arm vibration syndrome results from many years' use of vibrating tools, such as a pneumatic drill, hammer drill, or chainsaw, that are used at frequencies of 2 Hz to 1500 Hz. Patients present with vascular symptoms of Raynaud phenomenon—blanching of the fingers, especially after exposure to cold, with delayed or poor recovery. Other symptoms result from neurologic or musculoskeletal damage—numbness, tingling, pain, sensory and motor deficits, Dupuytren contractures, and carpal tunnel syndrome. Vascular imaging of the fingers after exposure to cold shows findings similar to those seen with Raynaud syndrome.

■ IMAGING OF PALMAR COLLATERAL CIRCULATION BEFORE RADIAL ARTERY HARVESTING

Radial artery harvesting before coronary artery bypass graft requires assessment of palmar collateral circulation to prevent hand ischemia. Clinical assessment through the Allen test is often useful but has substantial false-positive and false-negative results. In this test the hand is elevated and the patient is asked to clench a fist. Then the radial and ulnar arteries are compressed

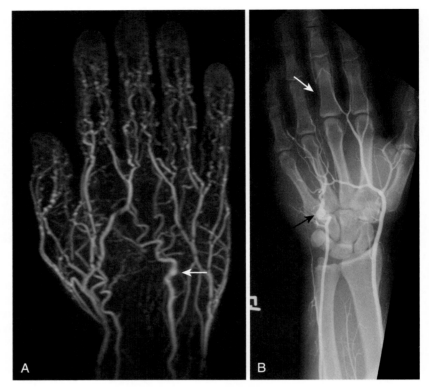

Figure 47-26 Hypothenar hammer syndrome. A, Magnetic resonance angiography of the hand shows focal aneurysm *(arrow)* of the ulnar artery at the expected location. **B,** Catheter angiography in a different patient shows ulnar artery aneurysm *(black arrow)* and distal emboli *(white arrow)* to the digital arteries.

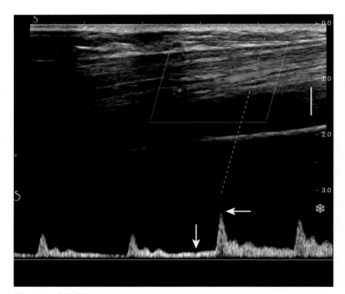

Figure 47-27 Doppler imaging of palmer collateral circulation. Note augmentation of flow *(horizontal arrow)* in the ulnar artery following manual compression *(vertical arrow)* of the radial artery.

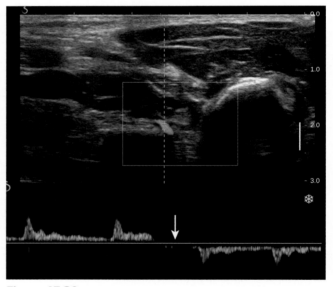

Figure 47-28 Evaluating patency of the palmer arch. Note flow reversal within the proximal segment of the deep palmar arch (in the thenar eminence) following manual compression *(arrow)* of the radial artery.

at the wrist till the hand blanches. Then the hand is observed for return of perfusion after releasing the compression over the ulnar artery. A successful reperfusion of the hand suggests an intact palmar collateral circulation through the deep (formed by the radial artery) and superficial (formed by the ulnar artery) palmar arches. Similar to the Allen test, a Doppler demonstration of arterial flow augmentation in the ulnar artery following compression of the radial artery suggests an intact

palmar arch (Fig. 47-27). Though direct visualization of the palmar arch is often not possible with color Doppler ultrasonography, demonstration of flow reversal within the proximal segment of the deep palmar arch (in the thenar eminence) on radial artery occlusion suggests an intact arch and sufficient collateral flow within the hand (Fig. 47-28). This method may also be used before radial artery catheterization and creation of a radial artery to cephalic vein fistula for hemodialysis.

■ VASCULAR MALFORMATIONS

Τηε hand is commonly affected in various vascular malformations. A detailed description of vascular malformations can be found in Chapter 51.

Bibliography

Capers 4th Q, Phillips J. Advances in percutaneous therapy for upper extremity arterial disease. *Cardiol Clin*. 2011;29:351-361.

Demondion X, Herbinet P, Van Sint Jan S, Boutry N, Chantelot C, Cotten A. Imaging assessment of thoracic outlet syndrome. *Radiographics*. 2006;26:1735-1750.

Feldman DR, Vujic I, McKay D, Callcott F, Uflacker R. Crutch-induced axillary artery injury. *Cardiovasc Intervent Radiol*. 1995;18:296-299.

Patterson BO, Holt PJ, Cleanthis M, Tai N, Carrell T, Loosemore TM, et al. Imaging vascular trauma. *Br J Surg*. 2012;99:494-505. doi:http://dx.doi.org/10.1002/bjs.7763.

Weir E, Lander L. Hand-arm vibration syndrome. *CMAJ*. 2005;172:1001-1002.

Zimmerman P, Chin E, Laifer-Narin S, Ragavendra N, Grant EG. Radial artery mapping for coronary artery bypass graft placement. *Radiology*. 2001;220:299-302.

CHAPTER 48

Lower Extremity Arteries

Meghna Chadha, Chaitanya Ahuja, and Sanjeeva P. Kalva

The arteries of the lower extremities are commonly affected by atherosclerosis, trauma, and thromboembolism. Advanced vascular disease frequently results in limb loss and decreased life expectancy. In this chapter, key collateral pathways, noninvasive physiologic evaluation techniques, and imaging techniques, and imaging of various vascular disorders of the lower extremity arteries are discussed.

■ COLLATERAL PATHWAYS OF THE LOWER EXTREMITY ARTERIES

Extensive collateral pathways exist between the pelvic arteries and the profunda femoris artery. In the presence of common femoral artery occlusion, the profunda femoris artery receives blood flow from the branches of the internal iliac artery through the pudendal arteries, from the lumbar arteries through the lateral circumflex iliac artery and the lateral circumflex femoral artery, and from the contralateral profunda femoris artery through the external pudendal arteries. The muscular branches of the profunda femoris artery supply the distal superficial femoral artery in the presence of proximal superficial femoral artery occlusion (Fig. 48-1). Similarly, in the presence of distal superficial femoral artery occlusion, the profunda femoris artery reconstitutes the popliteal artery through the geniculate arteries. The geniculate branches of the superficial femoral artery and the muscular branches of the profunda femoris artery reconstitute the distal popliteal artery in the presence of proximal popliteal artery occlusion, whereas the sural and geniculate branches reconstitute the tibial arteries in the presence of distal popliteal artery occlusion. Similarly, the sural and geniculate arteries collateralize the tibial arteries in the presence of proximal tibial artery occlusion. Multiple cross-tibial collateral vessels exist among the anterior tibial, posterior tibial, and peroneal arteries. The plantar arch provides an excellent collateral pathway in the foot in the event of occlusion of either the dorsalis pedis artery or the posterior tibial artery.

Pearls and Pitfalls

1. The profunda femoris and peroneal arteries are the key pathways in maintaining leg perfusion in the event of occlusion of the major arteries in the leg.
2. Often, flow through the collateral vessels can be robust, resulting in normal pedal pulses despite occlusion of the superficial femoral artery.

3. When occlusive disease affects the common femoral artery, imaging of the abdominal and pelvic vessels is important, to assess the collateral supply to the leg.

■ NONINVASIVE PHYSIOLOGIC EVALUATION

Noninvasive evaluation of lower extremity arterial disease is important in assessing the physiologic impact of the occlusive disease because the severity of the occlusive process does not often correlate with the symptoms. For example, good collateral supply in the presence of superficial femoral artery occlusion may result in normal distal pulses, and the patient may remain asymptomatic. Noninvasive physiologic evaluation provides objective means to assess the severity of the disease and helps monitor disease progression and outcomes of various therapies. Commonly used physiologic tests include the ankle-brachial index (ABI), segmental limb pressures, and pulse volume recordings (PVR) (Fig. 48-2). These tests can be performed at rest and after standardized exercise. Occlusive disease that is well compensated at rest may be unmasked on exercise testing. Physical examination is part of noninvasive evaluation; skin integrity, temperature, capillary refill, and palpable pulses can be assessed.

Ankle-Brachial Index

The ABI refers to the ratio of the highest upper arm pressure on either side to the highest ankle pressure obtained through Doppler evaluation of the dorsalis pedis and posterior tibial arteries at the ankle by using appropriately sized blood pressure cuffs and continuous wave Doppler imaging. The ABI provides information about the presence and severity of peripheral arterial disease, but it does not contain information about the level of the occlusive process. An ABI of 1 or more indicates the absence of peripheral arterial disease, and a lower ABI usually correlates with the severity of occlusive disease (Table 48-1). The ABI may be falsely elevated in the presence of noncompressible arteries, as often seen in diabetes as a result of calcific medial sclerosis. In such cases, the toe-brachial index (normal >0.6) is a useful measure to assess disease severity because the digital arteries are rarely affected by calcific medial sclerosis. During exercise, the ABI remains normal or elevated in the absence of peripheral arterial disease.

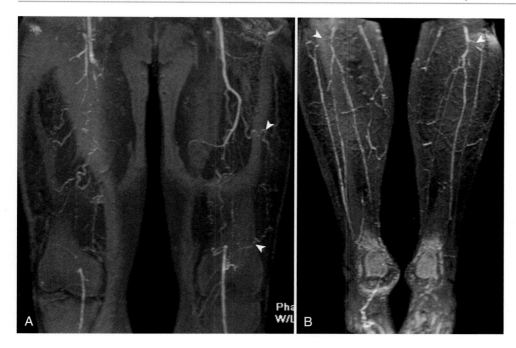

Figure 48-1 Gadolinium-enhanced magnetic resonance angiography of lower extremities. Long segment occlusion of bilateral superficial femoral arteries is visible. **A,** The proximal popliteal artery is reconstituted through muscular branches *(arrowheads)* of the profunda femoris artery. **B,** Distal runoff vessels show multifocal disease *(arrowheads).* Atherosclerosis is a multifocal disease with involvement of multiple vessels.

Segmental Limb Pressures

The segmental limb pressure test consists of obtaining blood pressure measurements at the thigh, calf, and ankles with appropriately sized blood pressure cuffs. A drop of 20 to 30 mm Hg pressure at any level or a difference of more than 20 mm Hg compared with the opposite side indicates hemodynamically significant occlusive disease in that vascular segment. The test is usually combined with Doppler evaluation of arterial flow at each level. Doppler analysis of the arterial waveform provides information about the presence and severity of occlusive disease. The normal Doppler pattern of peripheral arteries is triphasic. In the presence of occlusive disease, the arterial waveform becomes monophasic, with decreased amplitude.

Pulse Volume Recordings

PVRs are obtained by applying appropriately sized blood pressure cuffs at various levels in the thigh, calf, and ankle, inflating the cuffs to 60 to 65 mm Hg pressure, and recording the changes in the pressure in the cuff. The pressure changes within the cuff represent changes in the blood volume during systole and diastole. These recordings are in a waveform. The waveforms are assessed for changes in amplitude and contour. Loss of the normal dicrotic notch and flattening of waveforms indicate the presence of peripheral arterial disease at that vascular segment.

Pearls and Pitfalls

- Physiologic evaluation of limb arteries through the ABI, segmental limb pressures, and PVRs provides information about the presence, severity, and location of disease.

- In the presence of a normal ABI at rest, exercise testing provides information about occult or subclinical disease.
- The ABI may be falsely elevated in the presence of noncompressible arteries; in such cases, toe pressures should be obtained.
- Physiologic testing can be performed to assess cold-induced digital ischemia. The test should be repeated after cold exposure to the hand, to assess changes in leg perfusion.

■ IMAGING TECHNIQUES

Imaging evaluation of the peripheral arteries is indicated to assess the presence and location of occlusive or aneurysmal disease that is suspected on physiologic evaluation or when arteriovenous shunting (fistulas or malformation or tumor) is suggested, as well as to localize a bleeding vessel. Imaging studies should be interpreted with concurrent knowledge of the patient's symptoms, earlier surgical procedures, and results of physiologic tests. Various imaging modalities are used to assess lower extremity arteries.

Color Doppler Ultrasound

Color Doppler ultrasound allows evaluation of the superficial arteries and bypass grafts. Every arterial segment is evaluated with grayscale, color flow, and spectral Doppler imaging, with special emphasis on peak systolic velocity and Doppler waveforms. Stenosis of 50% or more is suspected when the peak systolic velocity is twice or more than that of the proximal arterial segment. A peak systolic velocity four times or more than that of the proximal arterial segment suggests 75% or more luminal narrowing. Occlusion is seen as absence of flow on color flow imaging and spectral Doppler.

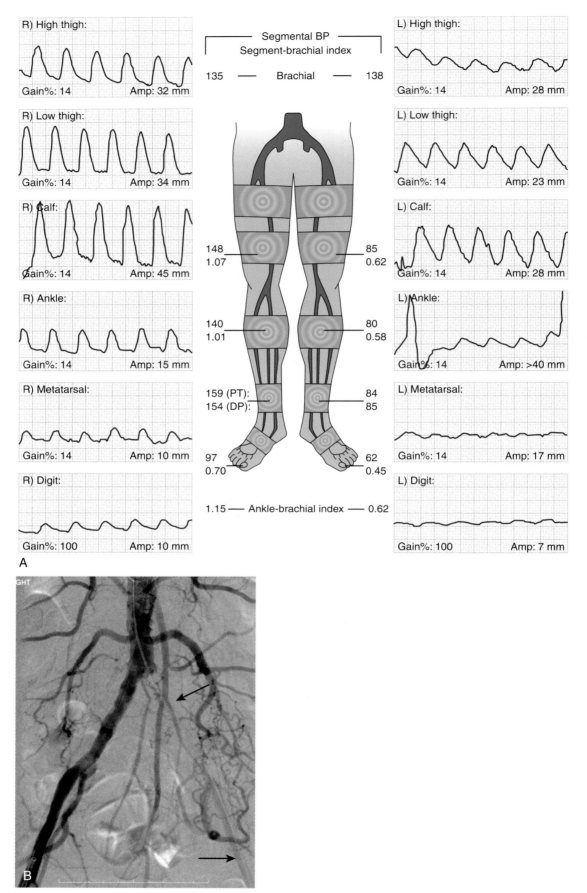

Figure 48-2 A 50-year-old female patient with left hip pain. Physical examination revealed diminished pulses in the left leg. **A,** Physiologic testing demonstrates an ankle-brachial index of 0.62 on the left that suggests moderate peripheral vascular disease. Segmental limb pressures demonstrate a decrease in the left thigh blood pressure (BP) compared with the opposite thigh, a finding suggesting left iliac artery disease. Corresponding pulse volume recordings show decreased amplitude and flattening of waveforms. **B,** Pelvic angiography shows an occluded left common iliac artery *(top arrow)* with a reconstituted left external iliac artery *(bottom arrow).*

On spectral Doppler imaging, peripheral arteries demonstrate a triphasic flow pattern. At the site of stenosis, the waveforms become monophasic or biphasic with increased peak systolic velocity, whereas distal to a hemodynamically significant stenosis, the waveforms become monophasic with a tardus parvus pattern (Fig. 48-3). The presence of a distal arteriovenous communication results in a monophasic flow pattern with increased diastolic flow but preserved systolic upstroke. In addition, arterialized waveforms are seen in the draining veins. Color Doppler flow settings must be adjusted to evaluate arteries with slow flow distal to an occlusion and to assess the digital arteries.

Computed Tomography Angiography

Computed tomography (CT) angiography (CTA) with multidetector CT technology provides excellent soft tissue resolution. Advances in dual energy CT allow accurate identification of calcium and contrast material and thus allow less blooming artifact from dense calcium.

Table 48-1   Ankle-Brachial Index and Severity of Peripheral Arterial Disease

Ankle-Brachial Index	Disease Severity
>0.95	None
0.75-0.95	Mild peripheral arterial disease
0.5-0.75	Moderate peripheral arterial disease
0.3-0.5	Severe peripheral arterial disease
<0.3	Critical

Dual energy CTA permits excellent subtraction of calcium from contrast-enhanced arteries and therefore provides calcium-free three-dimensional (3-D) maximum intensity projections.

Current 64-slice scanners allow scanning of the entire abdomen and lower extremities in a few seconds, with extended scanning within a single breath hold even in sick patients. However, such fast scanning can be a problem when assessing asymmetric aortoiliac and peripheral arterial occlusive disease. The scanner may run faster than the contrast material in the diseased leg, with resulting poor contrast opacification of the distal arteries. In such cases, a delayed scan of the diseased territory is helpful, to limit false interpretation of occluded arteries. In addition, the scanner parameters must be adjusted to improve intravascular contrast and reduce the radiation dose. Such adjustments include applying lower peak kilovoltage (80 to 100 kVp instead of 120 to 140 kVp), automated current adjustment, autotriggered timing of the scan, adequate contrast material (4 to 6 mL/second, to a total volume of 90 to 120 mL), and submillimeter slice thickness. The axial scan data are reconstructed in coronal and sagittal planes, 3-D maximum intensity projections (Fig. 48-4), 3-D surface shaded display, and 3-D volume rendered images. These images provide a catheter angiography–like picture of the arterial tree and allow assessment of the longitudinal extent of the occlusive disease. Reconstructed true axial scans provide accurate assessment of luminal narrowing.

Magnetic Resonance Angiography

Both noncontrast and contrast-enhanced magnetic resonance angiography (MRA) techniques provide means for assessing the lower extremity arteries. The sensitivity and

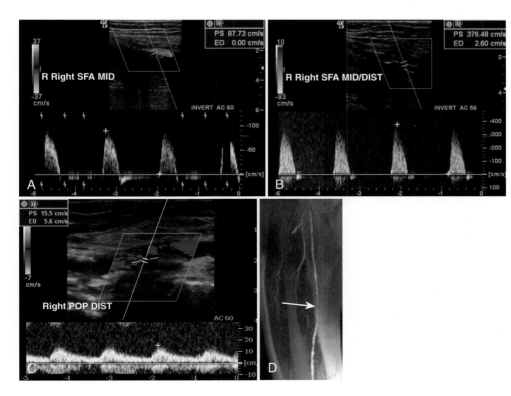

Figure 48-3 A 60-year-old male patient with right leg claudication. A, Color Doppler interrogation of the midsuperficial femoral artery (SFA MID) demonstrates a biphasic flow pattern with a peak systolic velocity of 87 cm/second. **B,** Just distal (DIST) to this location, a fourfold increase in peak systolic velocity suggests a hemodynamically significant stenosis. **C,** Distal to the stenosis, the popliteal artery (POP DIST) demonstrates a tardus parvus pattern. **D,** Magnetic resonance angiography confirms stenosis of the distal superficial femoral artery *(arrow)*.

specificity of contrast-enhanced MRA exceed 95% for detecting 50% or greater luminal stenosis. Noncontrast steady-state free precision MRA provides accurate assessment of large arterial steno-occlusive disease, whereas two-dimensional time of flight imaging provides reasonable assessment of distal arteries with slow flow.

Gadolinium-enhanced 3-D gradient recalled echo techniques allow rapid evaluation of the extremity arteries with a multistation technique (see Figs. 48-1 and 48-3). In addition, lower leg arterial evaluation can be supplemented by using time-resolved techniques such as time-resolved imaging with contrast kinetics (TRICKS). This approach provides highly accurate assessment of small vessel arteries. Moreover, it shows temporal changes in blood flow and thus allows detection of dominant collateral pathways in the presence of an occlusion and assessment of venous drainage pathways during evaluation of arteriovenous communications. MRA with protein-bound gadolinium allows high-resolution imaging of the arteries and veins for an accurate assessment of small vessel disease. In addition to vascular evaluation, MRA allows soft tissue and bone imaging to differentiate ischemic foot from soft tissue or bone infection, commonly encountered in diabetic patients.

Catheter Angiography

Catheter angiography remains the gold standard for evaluation of lower extremity arteries. Current angiography systems allow multistation overlapping imaging of both lower extremities with a catheter positioned in the lower abdominal aorta. Imaging through the delayed phase until all the collateral pathways are filled is important, to assess distal reconstitution in the presence of occlusion (see Fig. 48-2). As in CT, adequate contrast material injection and temporal acquisition are necessary. Distal abdominal aorta and pelvic arteries must be evaluated during assessments of the extremities for peripheral arterial disease. Selective catheter angiogra-

phy provides high-resolution imaging of arteries of the foot and distal leg.

Pearls and Pitfalls

- Noninvasive physiologic tests should precede imaging evaluation of lower extremity arteries. Imaging tests provide morphologic assessment of steno-occlusive disease but little information about the physiologic impact of the disease.
- Color Doppler evaluation is sufficient in most cases, especially for assessing superficial native arteries and bypass grafts. Assessment of distal vessels in the presence of proximal occlusion can be misleading unless the technical parameters of color Doppler imaging are adjusted for slow flow.
- CTA provides accurate assessment of the longitudinal extent of disease; the blooming effects of calcium can be minimized by using dual energy scanners. Care must be used when studying asymmetric peripheral arterial disease with current scanners; delayed scanning is often required.
- Noncontrast MRA is a boon for patients with kidney disease. The technique allows accurate assessment of large and medium-sized arteries. However, small leg and foot arteries are best evaluated with high-resolution contrast-enhanced MRA.
- Catheter angiography should be limited to interventional procedures. Assessment of reconstituted distal arteries requires administration of contrast material above the origin of collateral pathways and delayed imaging of the territory in question.

■ CHRONIC STENO-OCCLUSIVE DISEASE

Chronic steno-occlusive disease is most commonly the result of atherosclerosis. Other less common causes include thromboangiitis obliterans, popliteal artery

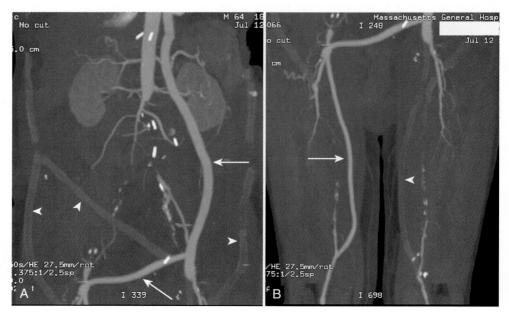

Figure 48-4 Three-dimensional maximum intensity projection of bypass grafts on computed tomography angiography. A and **B,** This study was performed to assess patency of left aortofemoral (*top arrow* in **A**), cross femoral (*bottom arrow* in **A**), and right femoropopliteal grafts (*horizontal arrow* in **B**). This patient had distal abdominal aortic resection for an infected aneurysm with subsequent multiple bypass grafts for lower extremity revascularization. Also seen are occluded axillary-femoral bypass grafts (*arrowheads* in **A**) and a left femoropopliteal bypass graft (*arrowhead* in **B**).

entrapment syndrome, cystic adventitial disease, vasculitis, chronic embolism, and trauma.

Atherosclerosis

Atherosclerosis affects middle-aged and older patients, with a higher prevalence in old patients; 20% of the population more than 70 years old has atherosclerosis. Risk factors include smoking, diabetes, hyperlipidemia, homocystinemia, and hypertension. Symptomatic disease is less common. More than half of the patients with atherosclerosis have no symptoms of leg ischemia. Symptoms may include claudication (often described as muscular cramping and tightening that occurs with exercise but resolves with rest), rest pain, skin ulcers, and gangrene. Critical limb ischemia is manifested by rest pain, tissue necrosis, and ulceration. The Fontaine and Rutherford classifications help grade the clinical severity of peripheral arterial disease. The distribution of disease is symmetric in more than three fourths of patients, but the severity of disease may differ. In addition, the disease tends to affect adjacent vascular segments. Common locations of steno-occlusive disease are the superficial femoral artery at the Hunter canal, common iliac artery, midpopliteal artery, tibioperoneal trunk, and origins of the tibial arteries. These sites reflect the areas of maximum shear stress on the arterial wall.

Physiologic tests provide information on the severity and location of the disease (see Fig. 48-2). Color Doppler ultrasound provides information on hemodynamically significant stenosis (see Fig. 48-3). The longitudinal extent, multifocal disease, and distal runoff are best assessed on CTA and MRA (see Figs. 48-1 and 48-3). Stenosis is seen as luminal narrowing secondary to calcified or noncalcified plaque. Luminal narrowing of 50% or more is considered physiologically significant. Similarly, the presence of collateral pathways suggests hemodynamically significant stenosis or occlusion. CTA is more accurate in assessing the true extent of luminal narrowing compared with MRA because MRA generally overestimates the percentage of stenosis. However, asymptomatic disease rarely requires revascularization despite the presence of arterial stenosis or occlusion. Imaging should provide the following information: location and extent of steno-occlusive disease, patency of distal runoff, major collateral vessels, presence of dissection, suitability for endovascular intervention based on Trans-Atlantic Society Consensus (TASC) guidelines, suitability of distal vessels for bypass graft, and presence of any arteriovenous communications.

In general, endovascular recanalization is highly successful in short, solitary, concentric, noncalcified, nonocclusive disease with patent distal runoff. Occlusions that are not amenable to endovascular revascularization are treated with bypass grafts using either autologous veins or synthetic polytetrafluoroethylene grafts. Similar to native arteries, grafts are evaluated with physiologic tests and color Doppler ultrasound for any focal stenosis. A fall in ABI of 0.2 or presence of a 50% or greater luminal narrowing either within the graft or at the anastomotic site on color Doppler imaging requires further evaluation. Color Doppler criteria to detect 50% or greater stenosis in bypass grafts are similar to those in native arteries.

Isolated common femoral artery stenosis and occlusion are uncommon in the absence of arterial trauma. These conditions are treated with endarterectomy. Similarly, isolated profunda femoris artery disease is uncommon. It is usually concurrent with proximal superficial femoral arterial disease. It is usually treated with endarterectomy, although the results of angioplasty are similar to those of surgery. Superficial femoral artery occlusion is three times more common than is stenosis. These occlusions are usually treated with balloon angioplasty. Bare metallic stents or stent grafts are used when the results of balloon angioplasty are suboptimal or when angioplasty is complicated by flow-limiting dissection (Fig. 48-5).

Chronic long segment occlusions may be difficult to treat by endovascular means because crossing such occlusions may be nearly impossible. Various techniques are helpful, including subintimal angioplasty, retrograde access through a distal runoff vessel, and procedures using various newer instruments including radiofrequency probes and forceps-like devices. Long segment chronic occlusions are best treated with bypass grafts. Popliteal artery disease is usually treated with angioplasty; stents are not used because of the risk of stent fracture across the knee joint. Treatment of tibioperoneal and tibial vessel disease is indicated for limb salvage and to treat nonhealing ischemic ulcer (Fig. 48-6). Despite angioplasty and stenting, 1-year patency rates remain dismal in these vessels.

Popliteal Artery Entrapment Syndrome

Normally, the popliteal artery runs between the heads of the gastrocnemius muscle and superficial to the popliteus muscle. An abnormal course of the artery or an abnormal insertion of the medial head of the gastrocnemius results in muscular compression of the artery during exercise. Repeated compression leads to intimal injury, fibrosis, aneurysm formation, thrombosis, and distal embolization. Five types of anatomic popliteal artery entrapment have been described (see Table 49-2 in Chapter 49). Another type, often referred to as a functional type of popliteal entrapment, occurs in patients with hypertrophy of calf muscles that compresses a normal popliteal artery.

Popliteal entrapment syndrome is common in young patients, affects men more often than women, and is bilateral in 25% of patients. The incidence of symptomatic popliteal entrapment syndrome appears to be less than 2 per 1000. Patients may present with exercise-induced calf claudication. Acute limb ischemia may develop from thrombosis of popliteal artery aneurysm. Distal embolization may result in tissue loss.

Physiologic tests including the ABI may be normal at rest, but the exercise ABI is always abnormal. Segmental limb pressures and PVRs following exercise point to popliteal artery disease. Color Doppler ultrasound

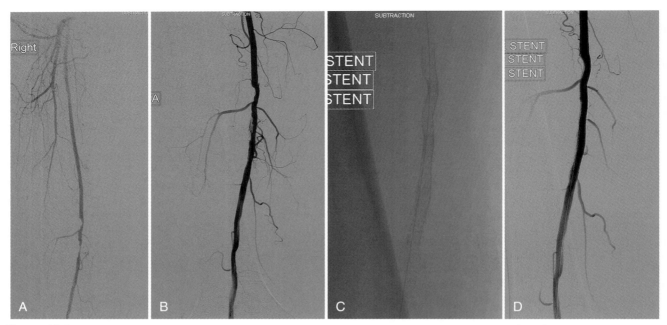

Figure 48-5 Angioplasty and stenting of superficial femoral artery for claudication. A, Right superficial femoral arteriogram shows eccentric, short segment, high-grade stenosis affecting the distal superficial femoral artery. **B,** Angioplasty (A) with a 5-mm balloon resulted in a suboptimal result with a small dissection. **C** and **D,** Subsequently, the patient was treated with a metallic stent, with excellent angiographic results.

may be helpful to identify the abnormal medial course of the artery and the presence of a muscle between the popliteal artery and vein (normally, the artery and vein run close to each other without any intervening muscle). It may also identify aneurysm and thrombus. Arterial stenosis may become apparent following active plantar flexion or passive dorsiflexion at the ankle. CTA and MRA with axial imaging help identify the abnormal relationship of the artery with the gastrocnemius or popliteus muscle. Again, a muscle may be identified between the artery and the vein, and the artery may course medial to the medial head of the gastrocnemius (Fig. 48-7, A). Dynamic MRA and catheter angiography during active plantar flexion or passive dorsiflexion of the ankle may demonstrate narrowing of the popliteal artery. Aneurysm or thrombosis may be identified in patients with chronic cases (see Fig. 48-7, B). The contralateral limb should always be examined to assess for bilateral disease even if the patient is asymptomatic on the other side. Treatment usually involves surgical resection of the medial head of gastrocnemius or the popliteus muscle. Acute thrombosis may be treated with thrombolysis.

Cystic Adventitial Disease

Cystic adventitial disease is rare and results from compression of the arterial lumen from focal accumulation of mucinous fluid within the arterial wall. The popliteal artery is commonly affected. The disease affects young men during the fourth or fifth decade. Patients may present with calf claudication or popliteal artery occlusion. Ultrasound, CTA, and MRA demonstrate extrinsic compression of the midpopliteal artery by a cystic mass (Fig. 48-8). The mass exhibits

low signal on T1-weighted images and bright signal on T2-weighted images. Treatment consists of surgical excision with bypass.

Thromboangiitis Obliterans (Buerger Disease)

Buerger disease affects young male smokers. Patients present with intermittent claudication, rest pain, or ischemic ulcers. In this disease, panvasculitis occurs, with preferential involvement of medium-sized and small vessels. The inflammatory debris occludes the vessel lumen. Proximal thigh vessels are preserved, with occlusion of below-knee arteries. The upper extremities may be involved in half of the patients. The vasa vasorum within the occluded vessels enlarge and give an appearance of corkscrew collateral vessels on angiography. Associated migratory thrombophlebitis affecting the superficial veins has been reported. Treatment involves cessation of smoking and medical therapy. Endovascular procedures and open surgical repairs are not usually successful because of early loss of distal runoff vessels.

Pearls and Pitfalls

- Dense calcified plaques may result in blooming artifact that limits the evaluation of the lumen with CTA imaging. In such cases, calcium removal using dual energy CT may be helpful.
- Dynamic imaging plays a significant role in assessing arterial compression in patients with suspected popliteal entrapment syndrome. This imaging can be achieved during active plantar flexion or passive dorsiflexion of the ankle.

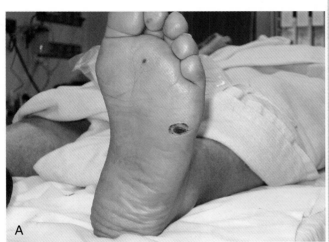

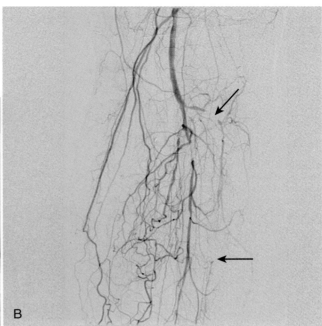

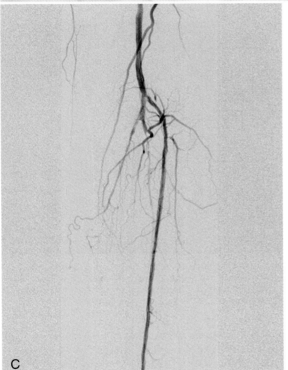

Figure 48-6 *Tibial artery angioplasty for nonhealing ulcer.* **A,** This patient presented with a nonhealing ulcer in the foot. **B,** Angiography shows multifocal occlusions in the anterior tibial artery *(arrows)*, tibioperoneal trunk, and posterior tibial artery. Note the extensive collateral vessels in the leg. **C,** Angioplasty of the anterior tibial artery was performed, with excellent angiographic results noting disappearance of collateral vessels.

■ Axial T1- and T2-weighted images of the popliteal fossa are essential when cystic adventitial disease is suspected.

■ The diagnosis of Buerger disease is based on recognition of characteristic corkscrew collateral vessels along the expected course of normal distal arteries that are otherwise occluded.

■ ACUTE LOWER EXTREMITY ISCHEMIA

An acutely ischemic leg is a surgical emergency, given the risk of irreversible loss of limb after 6 hours of ischemia. Causes include embolization from cardiac disorders (left atrial or ventricular aneurysms, valvular

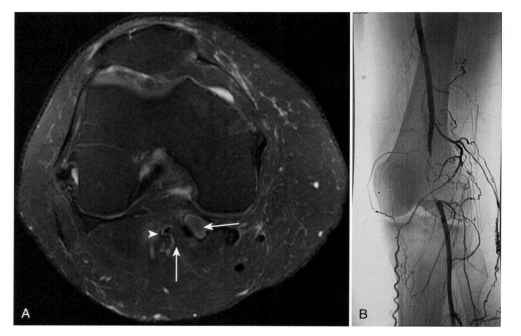

Figure 48-7 Popliteal entrapment syndrome. A, Axial fat-suppressed T2-weighted magnetic resonance imaging demonstrates muscle (the medial head of gastrocnemius; *vertical arrow*) between the popliteal artery *(horizontal arrow)* and the popliteal vein *(arrowhead)*. **B,** Angiography in another patient demonstrates occlusion of the popliteal artery secondary to thrombosis from popliteal entrapment. Note the multiple collateral vessels reconstituting the distal arteries.

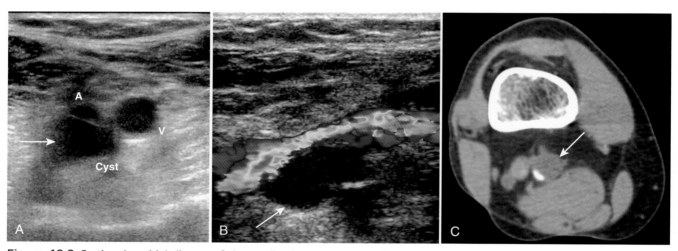

Figure 48-8 Cystic adventitial disease of the popliteal artery. A, Grayscale ultrasound demonstrates a mural cyst *(arrow)* compressing the arterial lumen. *A,* Artery; *V,* vein. **B,** Color flow imaging confirms the avascular nature of the cyst *(arrow),* with extrinsic compression over the popliteal artery resulting in flow turbulence (note aliasing). **C,** Contrast-enhanced computed tomography angiography demonstrates a mural cyst *(arrow)* with severe narrowing of the popliteal artery. Treatment consists of surgical resection.

vegetations) (Fig. 48-9) or proximal vessel disease (thromboembolism from a proximal diseased artery), as well as in situ thrombosis of diseased native arteries (Fig. 48-10) and bypass grafts. Symptoms differ based on the presence of collateral vessels in the leg. Given the development of collateral pathways in chronic peripheral arterial disease, in situ thrombosis is usually better tolerated compared with embolic occlusion, in which collateral vessels are absent. Patients may present with pain, sensory loss, skin discoloration, and loss of motor function depending on the severity and time from the onset of arterial occlusion.

The diagnosis of acute lower extremity ischemia is based on clinical findings, and imaging is rarely sought, to prevent delay in revascularization. Color Doppler ultrasound may demonstrate intraluminal thrombus, the extent of thrombus, and the presence of collateral flow. It is a useful bedside test to assess the proximal extent of the disease. CTA and MRA are rarely performed, but they may show occluded arteries with collateral vessels, if any are present. The presence of diffuse plaques in addition to thrombus usually suggests acute on chronic limb ischemia. Echocardiography helps identify the cardiac source of the emboli. Treatment involves systemic heparinization and revascularization through locoregional pharmacomechanical thrombolysis or surgical thrombectomy. Intraoperative angiography may be performed to rule out underlying steno-occlusive lesions; if found, such lesions are treated to prevent recurrence of thrombosis. Bypass grafts are often occluded by anastomotic stenosis and require prompt therapy.

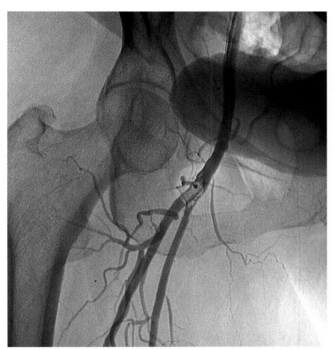

Figure 48-9 Nonocclusive embolus to the common femoral artery from a left atrial thrombus. The filling defect at the bifurcation of the right common femoral artery is consistent with an embolus. Emboli usually lodge at vessel bifurcation points.

Pearls and Pitfalls

- Acute limb ischemia is a clinical diagnosis. Imaging is rarely obtained. However, differentiating embolic occlusion from in situ thrombosis is important.
- Intraoperative angiography plays a significant role in diagnosis of underlying steno-occlusive disease that caused in situ thrombosis.

■ BLUE TOE SYNDROME

Blue toe syndrome results from microembolization of cholesterol crystals, atheromatous debris, and platelet aggregates from a ruptured plaque to the toe arteries. Clinically, this condition manifests as localized painful purple discoloration of toes; the distal pulses are often preserved. Plaque rupture may be spontaneous or secondary to endovascular or open arterial interventions. Imaging is required to identify the location of the source of such emboli. CTA and MRA are highly helpful to identify ulcerated plaques in the aorta and iliofemoral arteries. Catheter angiography, which is rarely performed unless CTA and MRA findings are inconclusive, may demonstrate stenosis with irregular margins, ulcerated plaques, or an aneurysm. Treatment involves heparinization and exclusion of the embolic source either through stent graft or surgery.

Pearls and Pitfalls

- Identification and exclusion of the embolic source are important in preventing recurrence of blue toe syndrome. The recurrence rate in untreated cases is as high as 90% within 5 years.

- A normal angiogram does not rule out atheroembolism, given the limitation of catheter angiography in identifying microemboli in the digital arteries.

■ ANEURYSMAL DISEASE

Aneurysms of lower extremity arteries may result from iatrogenic or noniatrogenic trauma, infection, inflammatory vasculitis, and degenerative disease. Degenerative aneurysms are often associated with abdominal aortic aneurysm. Connective tissue disorders such as Ehlers-Danlos syndrome and Marfan syndrome may result in aneurysms in young persons.

Common Femoral Artery Aneurysm

Aneurysms of the common femoral artery may be degenerative or pseudoaneurysms. Degenerative aneurysms are true aneurysms, often bilateral, and found in older patients. A diameter of 2 cm is considered aneurysmal, and aneurysms are treated if they are symptomatic (thromboembolism, rupture) or if the aneurysm is larger than 2.5 cm in diameter. Ultrasound, CTA, and MRA may demonstrate a dilated common femoral artery with a diameter of 2 cm or more, mural thrombus, and perianeurysmal fluid in cases of rupture. Evaluation of the thoracoabdominal aorta is recommended when degenerative common femoral artery aneurysm is detected on imaging.

Pseudoaneurysms result from iatrogenic trauma, following femoral artery catheterization and surgical interventions. The incidence of femoral artery pseudoaneurysm following cardiac catheterization is up to 5% and may be affected by the use of closure devices and concurrent anticoagulation. The aneurysm may arise from the common femoral, superficial femoral, or profunda femoris artery. Imaging plays a significant role in identifying the aneurysms that can be treated with local thrombin injection. Pseudoaneurysms with a wide or short neck, large aneurysm size resulting in compression of adjacent veins, and the presence of an arteriovenous fistula require surgical therapy. Ultrasound is sufficient in identifying the characteristics of the pseudoaneurysm (Fig. 48-11); however, CTA and MRA could be helpful when the neck of the lesion is not well visualized. When thrombin injection is contemplated, it is performed under ultrasound guidance, with the utmost precaution taken to prevent distal embolization of thrombin.

Anastomotic pseudoaneurysms occur in 2% to 5% of all femoral surgical anastomoses and may be a result of graft degeneration or infection. These pseudoaneurysms require surgical therapy.

Popliteal Artery Aneurysm

Most of the popliteal artery aneurysms are degenerative, secondary to atherosclerosis. These aneurysms are bilateral in 60% to 70% of cases and are often associated with common femoral artery aneurysms. These aneurysms may affect the entire popliteal artery, or they may be focal, involving the above-knee popliteal artery. Popliteal artery aneurysms may manifest with swelling, but patients often present with thrombosis, distal embolization, and compression of adjacent veins that results in deep venous thrombosis.

Because degenerative aneurysms are often systemic, imaging should always include the aorta and femoropopliteal arteries. Ultrasound demonstrates a dilated popliteal artery, an associated mural thrombus, and patency of the distal vessels (Fig. 48-12). CTA and MRA are helpful when endovascular therapy is planned. These imaging techniques depict the extent of the aneurysm, the size of the proximal and distal vessels, distal runoff, and suitability for treatment with a stent graft. Catheter angiography is an integral part of endovascular interventions such as thrombolysis or endovascular stent graft placement (see Fig. 48-12). Surgical therapy involves excision of the aneurysm and bypass graft.

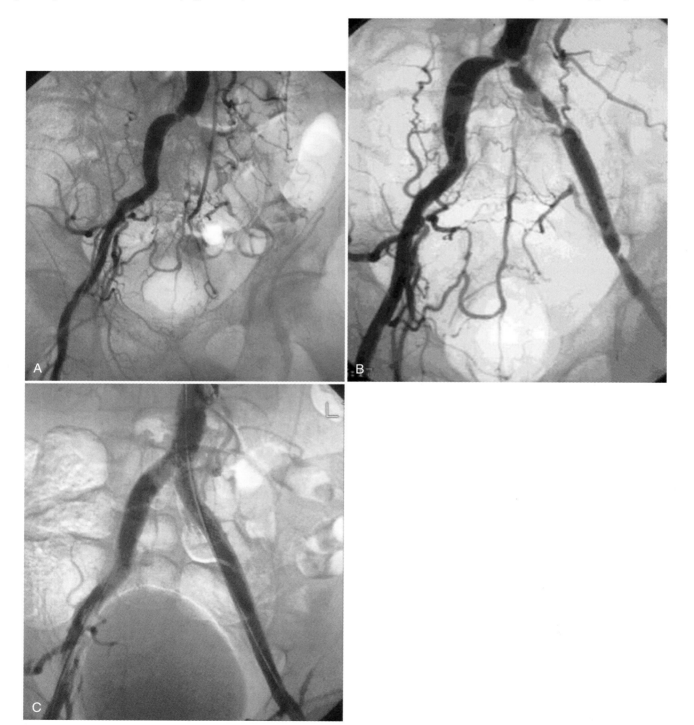

Figure 48-10 *Acute limb ischemia secondary to in situ thrombosis of the left iliofemoral arteries.* **A,** Pelvic angiogram shows occlusion of the left iliofemoral arteries. **B,** Following thrombolysis, flow is restored. Underlying chronic atherosclerotic stenoses are apparent. **C,** This patient was treated with angioplasty and stent placement.

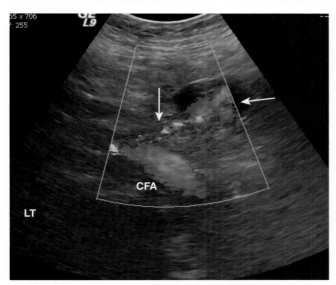

Figure 48-11 *Right common femoral artery (CFA) pseudoan-eurysm following catheterization.* Color Doppler imaging shows a long, narrow neck *(vertical arrow)* connecting the pseudoaneurysm *(horizontal arrow)* with the common femoral artery. Pseudoaneurysms with a long, narrow neck are well suited for thrombin injection. *LT,* Left.

Pseudoaneurysms of the popliteal artery are rare and occur secondary to catheterization and at the anastomotic sites of femoropopliteal bypass grafts. Treatment is surgical.

Persistent Sciatic Artery Aneurysm

Aneurysms of the persistent sciatic artery occur secondary to repetitive trauma to the superficial vessel against the greater trochanter of the femur. Patients may present with buttock swelling or distal thromboembolism. Rupture of these aneurysms is rare. Ultrasound, CTA, and MRA demonstrate the location, extent, and size of the aneurysm with associated mural thrombus (Fig. 48-13). The course of the distal runoff vessel can also be assessed. Treatment is usually surgical.

Pearls and Pitfalls

■ Degenerative aneurysms tend to affect multiple arteries. Assessing the aorta and femoropopliteal arteries is important when a degenerative aneurysm is found in any one of the arteries.

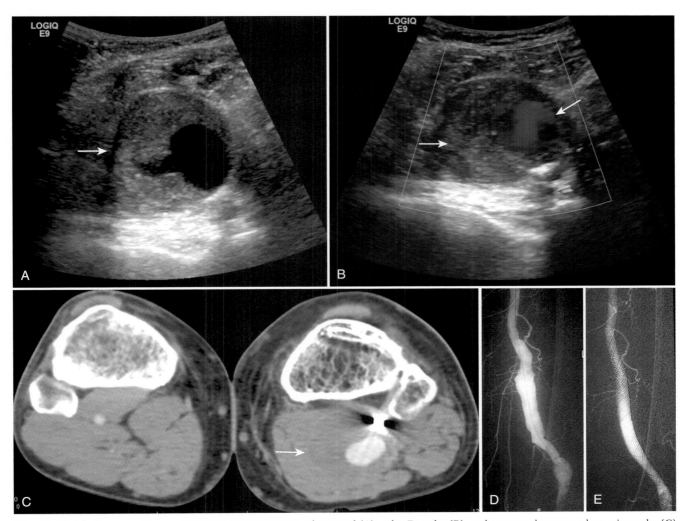

Figure 48-12 *Degenerative popliteal artery aneurysm.* Ultrasound (A), color Doppler (B), and computed tomography angiography (C) demonstrate a large left popliteal artery aneurysm with mural thrombus *(horizontal arrows)*. The patent lumen is marked with an *oblique arrow* in **B**. **D** and **E**, The aneurysm was treated with a stent graft.

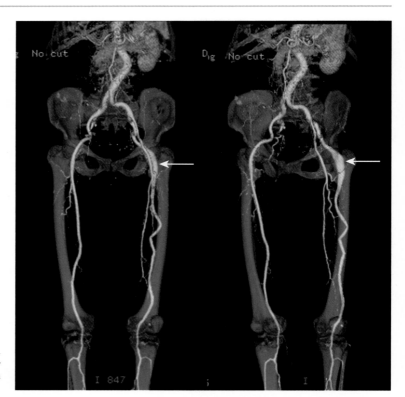

Figure 48-13 Persistent sciatic artery aneurysm. Volume rendered three-dimensional computed tomography angiography demonstrates an aneurysm *(arrow)* affecting a persistent sciatic artery.

- Before thrombin injection for a common femoral artery pseudoaneurysm is contemplated, the presence of an arteriovenous fistula must be excluded.
- Surgical bypass graft aneurysms can be degenerative or infective.

■ TRAUMA

Injury to the arteries of the lower extremities can occur during penetrating or blunt trauma to the leg, following surgical or endovascular procedures, or during orthopedic trauma. Trauma can result in various forms of arterial injury including rupture, dissection, intimal injury, thrombosis, arteriovenous fistula, and pseudoaneurysm. Color Doppler imaging is usually the first noninvasive method to assess arterial and venous injuries. It may demonstrate periarterial hematoma, thrombosis, pseudoaneurysm, and arteriovenous fistula. Identifying dissection and intimal injury is often difficult with ultrasound. CTA may demonstrate the same findings, but dissection and intimal irregularity, intraluminal debris, and contour abnormalities including vessel transection may also be seen. Catheter angiography is reserved for when clinical suspicion of arterial injury is high and surgical or endovascular therapy is planned. Angiography may demonstrate intimal injury, abrupt vessel cutoff, active bleeding, dissection, pseudoaneurysm (Fig. 48-14), or arteriovenous fistula (Fig. 48-15). Treatment consists of endovascular embolization or exclusion with a stent graft or surgical reconstruction.

Pearls and Pitfalls

- Signs of arterial injury can be subtle. In such cases, CTA with thin slices or angiography may be helpful.
- Arterial transection may be missed on axial CTA. Coronal or sagittal reformations are useful to detect arterial transection.

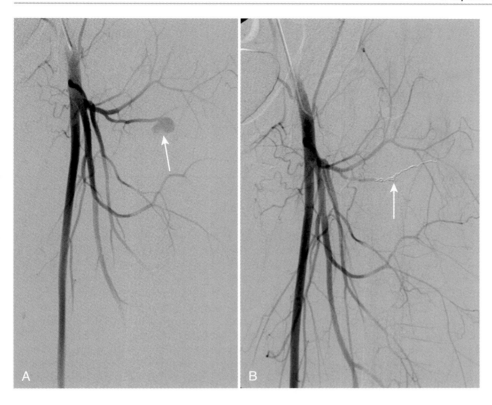

Figure 48-14 Traumatic pseudoaneurysm. A, Traumatic pseudoaneurysm *(arrow)* of the profunda femoris artery following penetrating injury with a knife. **B,** The pseudoaneurysm was successfully treated with coil embolization *(arrow).*

Bibliography

Abou-Sayed H, Berger DL. Blunt lower extremity trauma and popliteal artery injuries: revisiting the case for selective arteriography. *Arch Surg.* 2002;137:585-589.

Andrews RT. Diagnostic angiography of the pelvis and lower extremities. *Semin Interv Radiol.* 2000;17:71-111.

Comerota AJ, Throm RC, Mathias SD, et al. Catheter directed thrombolysis for ilio-femoral deep venous thrombosis improves health related quality of life. *J Vasc Surg.* 2000;32:130-137.

Dorros G, Jaff MR, Dorros AM, et al. Tibioperoneal (outflow lesion) angioplasty can be used as primary treatment in 235 patients with critical limb ischemia: five year follow-up. *Circulation.* 2001;104:2057-2062.

Fraser JD, Anderson DR. Deep venous thrombosis: recent advances and optimal investigation with US. *Radiology.* 1999;211:9-24.

Hafez HM, Woolgar J, Robbs JV. Lower extremity arterial injury: results of 550 cases and review of risk factors associated with limb loss. *J Vasc Surg.* 2001;33:1212-1219.

Kandarpa K, Becker GJ, Hunink MG, et al. Transcatheter interventions for the treatment of peripheral atherosclerotic lesions. *J Vasc Interv Radiol.* 2001;12:413-421.

Kaufman JA, Lee MJ. *The Requisites: Vascular and Interventional Radiology.* St. Louis: Mosby; 2004.

Lofberg AM, Karacagil S, Ljingman C, et al. Percutaneous transluminal angioplasty of femoropopliteal arteries in limbs with chronic critical limb ischemia. *J Vasc Surg.* 2001;34:114-121.

Matxhett WJ, McFarland DR, Eidt JF, et al. Blue toe syndrome: treatment with intraarterial stents and review of therapies. *J Vasc Interv Radiol.* 2000;11:585-592.

Ouriel K. Peripheral arterial disease. *Lancet.* 2001;358:1257-1264.

Valji K. *Vascular and Interventional Radiology.* 2nd ed. Philadelphia: Saunders; 2006.

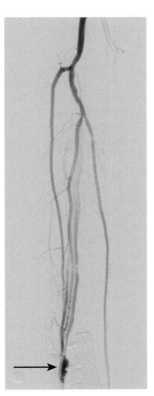

Figure 48-15 Traumatic arteriovenous fistula. Traumatic arteriovenous fistula *(arrow)* following surgical repair of a tibial fracture with early draining peroneal veins.

CHAPTER 49

Deep Venous Thrombosis

Sanjeeva P. Kalva

Venous thromboembolism (VTE) is an important worldwide clinical entity. It includes asymptomatic deep venous thrombosis (DVT), symptomatic DVT, and pulmonary embolism (PE). Each year, DVT and PE affect 1 to 2 per 1000 people in the United States. In persons more than 80 years old, the incidence of DVT increases to 1 in 100. One third of the people who had DVT may go on to develop long-term complications (e.g., post-thrombotic syndrome) with symptoms of swelling, pain, and discoloration of the affected limb. Recurrent DVT occurs in one third of patients within 10 years of the initial diagnosis. Approximately 60,000 to 100,000 people die of DVT or PE each year in the United States.

■ DIAGNOSTIC METHODS

Clinical and ancillary findings are useful for the diagnosis of DVT. Clinical scoring systems such as the Wells score can be used to select patients for an appropriate diagnostic test. Noninvasive tests, such as the D-dimer test, and plethysmography may be used for diagnosis of DVT. However, sensitivity varies, and specificity is poor (Table 49-1). The definitive diagnosis depends on identifying the presence, location, and extent of the thrombus on imaging studies. Ultrasonography and color Doppler imaging are commonly used; computed tomography venography (CTV) and magnetic resonance venography (MRV) play significant roles in identifying pelvic, abdominal, and chest DVT. Ascending venography has little role in the diagnosis of DVT, although it is used in therapeutic interventions (see Table 49-1).

Ultrasonography

Ultrasonography is the imaging test of choice for assessment of DVT in the extremities. This technique is recommended for symptomatic patients in whom the suspicion of acute DVT is high. Grayscale ultrasound is coupled with Doppler (duplex ultrasound) imaging for an accurate assessment of the venous system. This approach has greater than 95% sensitivity and specificity for detecting above-knee DVT.

Technique

The deep and superficial veins of the extremities are usually examined from proximal to distal locations (i.e., from the common femoral vein to the tibial veins or from the subclavian vein to the forearm veins). At each location, the vein is compressed directly with the ultrasound probe to assess compressibility. In addition, Doppler evaluation of the vein is performed (either with or without color flow imaging) to assess presence of flow changes to respiration and cardiac motion and the response to distal compression. Normal veins are compressible and demonstrate an anechoic lumen (Fig. 49-1). The venous flow is phasic with respiration and shows an augmentation response to distal compression (Fig. 49-2). Upper extremity veins often demonstrate flow variations secondary to cardiac pulsations. This phenomenon is often observed in the jugular, subclavian, and axillary veins. Deep inspiration may collapse a normal subclavian or jugular vein.

Findings

An enlarged vein that is noncompressible and demonstrates low-level echoes within the lumen is diagnostic of acute DVT (Fig. 49-3, *A*). Color flow and Doppler imaging techniques demonstrate no flow within the lumen (see Fig. 49-3, *B*). The response to distal compression is blunted. Partial thrombosis of the vein manifests as a partially compressible vein with partial flow noted on color flow imaging (Fig. 49-4). Subacute thrombosis is depicted as a normal-caliber vein that is noncompressible or partially compressible with a moderately echogenic lumen and an absence of color flow or Doppler signal. Partial recanalization of the thrombus results in the appearance of flow channels within the thrombus; these channels are best observed on color flow or power Doppler imaging (Fig. 49-5). As the thrombosis becomes chronic, the caliber of the vein becomes small, with little or no flow. Calcification of the venous wall indicates chronic DVT and may be seen as a highly echogenic focus with or without distal acoustic shadowing.

Upper extremity DVT has similar imaging characteristics. The absence of normal cardiac pulsations and of a response to deep inspiration may suggest the presence of DVT in the proximal veins.

Pearls and Pitfalls
■ Ultrasound may identify other causes of leg pain, such as a ruptured or unruptured Baker cyst, hematoma, and tendon injury.
■ Visualizing the intrathoracic and abdominopelvic veins is often difficult. Proximal (or central) venous

Table 49-1   Diagnostic Tests for Deep Venous Thrombosis

Test	Advantages	Disadvantages
D-dimer test	Rapid Inexpensive	Variable sensitivity Poor specificity in certain patient populations
Ultrasound	Relatively inexpensive Can be performed at bedside Highly sensitive for above-knee symptomatic DVT	Operator dependent Poor specificity for calf vein and pelvic vein DVT
CT venography	Highly sensitive and specific for central and pelvic vein DVT Can be used in patients with inherent contraindications for MRI	Expensive Radiation exposure Adverse reactions to contrast material
MRV	Highly sensitive and specific for central and pelvic vein DVT Can be used in patients allergic to iodinated contrast material Both noncontrast and gadolinium-enhanced studies possible	Expensive Poor availability Cannot be used in patients with pacemakers or aneurysm clips and in those who are claustrophobic Gadolinium contraindicated in patients with renal failure
Ascending venography	Highly sensitive and specific for DVT, including calf vein DVT	Invasive Poor availability Radiation exposure Adverse reactions to contrast material Risk of thrombophlebitis and contrast material extravasation

CT, Computed tomography; *DVT,* deep venous thrombosis; *MRI,* magnetic resonance imaging; *MRV,* magnetic resonance venography.

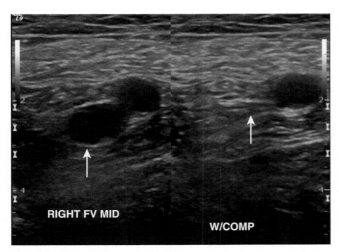

Figure 49-1 Compression ultrasound study. Grayscale ultrasound examination shows anechoic lumen with thin walls of right femoral vein (FV MID; *left arrow*). The vein is compressible (W/COMP; *right arrow*), a finding suggesting that the vein is patent.

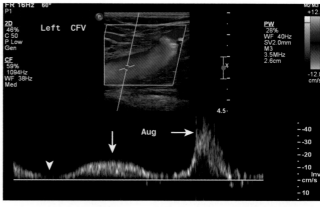

Figure 49-2 Spectral Doppler evaluation of the left common femoral vein (CFV). Imaging shows respiratory flow variations (*arrowhead,* flow during expiration; *vertical arrow,* flow during inspiration) and augmentation response (Aug; *horizontal arrow*) to distal compression.

compression or thrombosis may be suspected when respiratory phasic variations in the distal veins are absent (see the later section on May-Thurner syndrome).
- When DVT is detected, the examiner must assess its proximal extent because pelvic DVT is more often associated with PE.
- The sensitivity of duplex ultrasound in detecting symptomatic DVT is greater than 95%; however, it falls to 50% for detection of asymptomatic DVT. When the ultrasound study result is negative in patients with a high clinical suspicion of DVT, a repeat ultrasound study 1 week later is recommended.

Computed Tomography Venography

CTV allows visualization of central thoracic and abdominopelvic veins that are often obscured on ultrasound. One of the main advantages of CTV is that the study can be combined with computed tomography pulmonary angiography (CTPA) without the requirement of additional intravenous contrast material. These protocols allow 20% higher detection of VTE compared with CTPA alone. The extent of the computed tomography (CT) scan ranges from the popliteal fossa to the groin or the pelvis. The scan may be extended to the upper abdomen if thrombosis of the inferior vena cava (IVC) or gonadal or renal veins is suspected.

Technique

CTV may be performed following intravenous injection of diluted (10%) iodinated contrast material in the foot veins or upper extremity veins to assess regional venous thrombosis. This technique is referred to as direct CTV and is rarely practiced now, but it can be useful when other studies are indeterminate. Indirect CTV refers to CT assessment of the regional and nonregional veins following intravenous administration of regular-strength contrast material. The veins are imaged during equilibrium phase (approximately 3 minutes following the injection of contrast material). Images

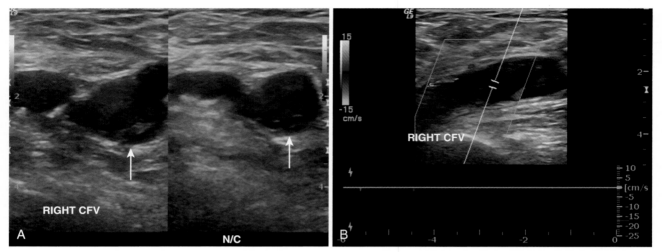

Figure 49-3 Acute deep venous thrombosis on ultrasound. A, Grayscale ultrasound examination of the right common femoral vein (CFV) demonstrates an enlarged vein *(arrows)* with low-level intraluminal echoes. The vein is noncompressible (N/C). **B,** Corresponding color flow and spectral Doppler image shows an absence of color flow and spectral tracing that suggests no flow within the vein.

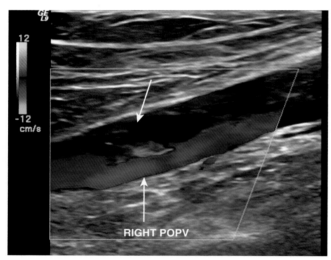

Figure 49-4 Partial thrombosis of right popliteal vein (POPV) on color flow imaging. Wall-adherent mixed echogenic thrombus *(top arrow)* with minimal peripheral flow *(bottom arrow)* is visible.

are reconstructed at 5- to 7.5-mm slice thickness with no interslice gap. Venous enhancement is considered adequate when the attenuation in the vein is higher than in the adjacent muscles; the enhanced veins rarely achieve an attenuation of more than 150 HU.

Findings

CTV allows direct visualization of thrombus in the vein as a filling defect within the contrast-filled lumen (Fig. 49-6). When thrombus fills the entire lumen and extends for a few CT slices, that segment of the vein fails to enhance with contrast material. Additional findings of acute thrombosis include an enlarged vein, rim enhancement of the vein (see Fig. 49-6), and perivenous edema or stranding. The sensitivity and specificity of CTV in detecting above-knee DVT are 90% to 95% compared with those of venous ultrasonography. Chronic thrombosis may be seen as nonenhancing small-caliber vein or intraluminal webs with

enhancement of recanalized channels; the presence of calcification within the venous wall is diagnostic of chronic DVT (Fig. 49-7).

Pearls and Pitfalls

- Excellent visualization of the central and peripheral veins makes CTV an optimal test for the diagnosis of DVT.
- CTV allows detection of other leg disorders such as popliteal cysts, iliopectineal bursitis, joint effusions, and intramuscular hemorrhage.
- Radiation exposure can be minimized by limiting the study to the thighs and scanning at lower peak kilovoltage.
- Inadequate enhancement of the veins can be minimized by using autotriggered scanning while keeping a region of interest in the femoral vein with a threshold of 60 HU. Larger volume of contrast material, low peak kilovoltage (80 kVp), and reconstruction at 50 keV on a dual energy scanner allow better visualization of the veins on indirect CTV.
- Image visualization at narrow window length and coronal reformations are also helpful to delineate the thrombus and its longitudinal extent.

Magnetic Resonance Venography

MRV is less commonly used for detection of lower extremity DVT. It is often used to assess the central veins of the thorax and body. It is equally sensitive and specific for detection of DVT in both the central and peripheral veins. MRV can be performed either with or without the use of gadolinium. Noncontrast MRV methods include bright-blood techniques such as time of flight (TOF) imaging, true fast imaging with steady-state precession (true FISP), and electrocardiogram-gated three-dimensional fast spin echo (FSE) imaging and black-blood techniques such as FSE T2-weighted and double inversion recovery FSE imaging. Contrast-enhanced MRV techniques use three-dimensional gradient echo techniques

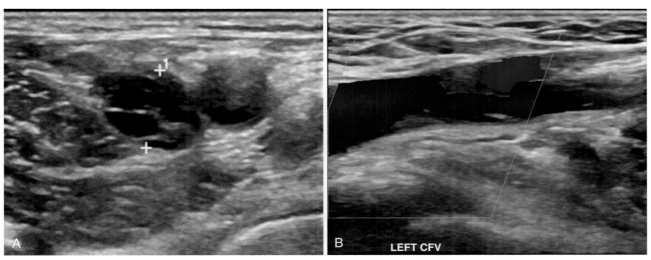

Figure 49-5 Partial recanalization of thrombus. A, Grayscale ultrasound examination shows multiple intraluminal septa resulting from recanalized thrombus. **B,** Corresponding color flow image shows partial flow within the thrombus. *CFV,* Common femoral vein.

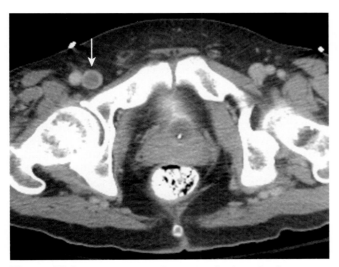

Figure 49-6 Right common femoral vein thrombosis on computed tomography venography. The vein *(arrow)* is enlarged, with an intraluminal filling defect and rim enhancement.

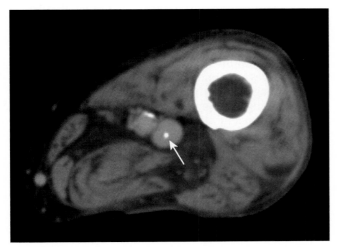

Figure 49-7 Chronic deep venous thrombosis of the left popliteal vein on computed tomography venography. Calcification of the vein *(arrow)* with faint intraluminal webs is visible.

similar to magnetic resonance angiography (MRA) for venous phase imaging. Rarely, direct MRV (similar to direct CTV) is performed with diluted (2%) gadolinium. Blood pool contrast materials (e.g., gadofosveset trisodium) are best suited for venous imaging.

Technique
The axial two-dimensional TOF technique is employed for abdominopelvic and lower extremity veins, with a saturation band applied superiorly to prevent artifacts from the arterial inflow. True FISP imaging is usually performed in the coronal plane for the body and in the axial plane for extremities. Images are acquired in 3- to 5-mm slice thickness. Contrast-enhanced MRV is usually performed in the coronal plane.

Findings
On bright-blood techniques and contrast-enhanced MRV, thrombus is seen as a filling defect within the vein (Fig. 49-8). Long segment thrombosis is best appreciated on coronal or sagittal images and is visualized as discontinuity of the vessel. However, the venous wall may enhance on contrast-enhanced MRV, thus giving a tram-track appearance (Fig. 49-9). Perivenous edema is rarely appreciated, but it can be seen on T2-weighted FSE sequences. On black-blood techniques, thrombus is seen as a mass of low signal intensity within the lumen of the vein. Chronic thrombus is seen as a small-caliber, nonenhancing vein with or without venous stenosis. Collateral veins are often seen bypassing the obstructed vein.

Pearls and Pitfalls
■ Flow directional abnormalities may result in signal void on TOF sequences. Additional imaging either with true FISP or contrast-enhanced MRV may be required to limit false positive diagnosis of DVT. On the other hand, the flow directional nature of TOF sequence can be utilized for advantage while assessing the hemodynamic significance of venous stenoses as collateral veins may show flow directional abnormalities (see the later section on May-Thurner Syndrome).

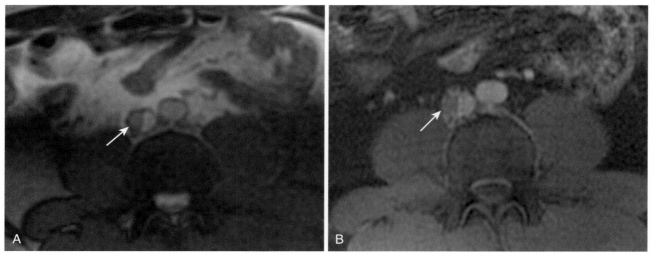

Figure 49-8 Partial thrombosis of the inferior vena cava (IVC) on magnetic resonance venography (MRV). Bright-blood technique (true fast imaging with steady-stage precession) (**A**) shows low signal intensity on the right half (*arrow*) of the IVC that does not enhance on contrast-enhanced MRV (**B**), a finding suggesting partial thrombosis of the IVC.

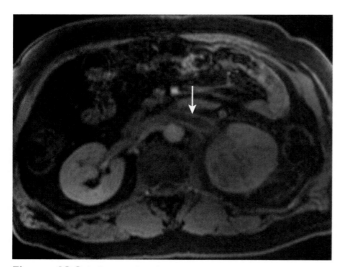

Figure 49-9 Left renal vein thrombosis on magnetic resonance venography (MRV). Contrast-enhanced MRV shows the tram-track appearance of the left renal vein (*arrow*) with an intraluminal filling defect secondary to tumor thrombus from left renal cell carcinoma.

- True FISP imaging can be combined with background suppression to provide better contrast resolution of the veins. During contrast-enhanced MRV, delayed (2 minutes), axial fat-saturated gradient echo, high-resolution T1-weighted images allow assessment of partial and wall-adherent thrombus.
- Similar to CTPA, MRV can be combined with pulmonary MRA, especially with the use of blood pool contrast materials.

Ascending Venography

Although ascending venography remains the gold standard, it is rarely performed for the diagnosis of DVT because it has been replaced by ultrasonography for extremity DVT. Ascending venography has 95% specificity and 100% sensitivity for thrombi measuring 0.5 cm

or more, and it is still the test of choice for detection of below-knee DVT. It is used in interventional procedures such as thrombolysis, placement of an IVC filter, and revascularization of venous occlusion.

Technique

Upper extremity venography is performed with the patient supine, with hands abducted and supinated. A superficial vein in the dorsum of the hand is accessed with an 18-gauge needle. A blood pressure cuff that is inflated to nearly systolic pressure or a tourniquet is applied in the upper arm, and diluted (240 mg iodine/mL) contrast material is injected. Multiple overlapping fluoroscopic images are obtained for the forearm and arm. The central veins are imaged while the contrast material is injected and the blood pressure cuff is deflated. Proximal venous access is often helpful for visualizing the central veins.

Lower extremity venography is best performed with the patient in the reverse Trendelenburg position at 30 to 60 degrees. The limb examined is kept nonweight bearing, and a dorsal foot vein is cannulated with an 18-gauge needle. A tourniquet applied at the ankle helps direct contrast material in to the deep venous system. Diluted contrast material (240 mg iodine/mL) is injected to a volume of 50 to 100 mL, and serial fluoroscopic images are obtained of the extremity. Pelvic veins are best imaged with the patient in the supine position.

Descending venography is performed for assessing venous insufficiency. In this procedure, a short sheath is placed in the common femoral vein, the patient is positioned at 60 degrees in the reverse Trendelenburg position, and 20 mL of contrast material is injected. Retrograde flow into the femoral and saphenous veins indicates the presence of venous reflux.

Findings

As with CT, acute thrombus is seen as a filling defect within the contrast-filled lumen (Fig. 49-10). The vein may be enlarged, and collateral veins may be visualized. Chronic thrombosis results in nonvisualization

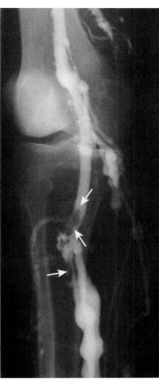

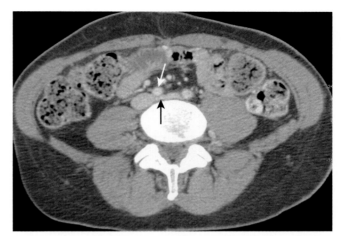

Figure 49-11 Anatomy of May-Thurner syndrome on computed tomography venography. The right common iliac artery *(white arrow)* compresses the left common iliac vein *(black arrow)* against the spine.

Figure 49-10 Ascending venography showing tibial and tibioperoneal trunk deep venous thrombosis *(arrows)*.

of the vein, with multiple collateral veins bypassing the occluded vein. Recanalized veins may appear as linear channels within the expected course of a vein.

Pearls and Pitfalls

- When the study is performed to assess subclavian vein compression at the thoracic inlet, the examiner must perform venography in abduction and neutral position of the upper extremity.
- Higher-density contrast material may obscure DVT.
- The venous system must be flushed with saline solution following contrast material injection to limit contrast-induced venous thrombosis.

■ VENOUS COMPRESSION SYNDROMES

Extrinsic venous compression results from an acquired or congenital abnormality in the course of the vein or adjacent arterial, muscular, ligamentous, or osseous structures. Such compression may lead to repetitive trauma to venous endothelium. The trauma may cause internal "spur" and "web" formation and subsequent symptomatic acute thrombosis or chronic thrombosis with venous hypertension and varicose veins. Four common venous compression syndromes are discussed here.

May-Thurner Syndrome

May-Thurner syndrome or iliac vein compression syndrome results from compression of the left common iliac vein between the right common iliac artery and the

spine, with subsequent development of DVT and chronic venous insufficiency in the left lower extremity. This entity was first described by Virchow in 1851, but detailed anatomic description was given by May and Thurner in 1957. The prevalence of symptomatic May-Thurner syndrome ranges from 18% to 49% among patients with left lower extremity DVT. Young and middle-aged women are commonly affected.

Anatomy and Pathophysiology

In contrast to the right common iliac vein, which runs almost vertically to the IVC, the left common iliac vein takes a more transverse course. Along its course, the left common iliac vein crosses under the right common iliac artery and may be compressed against the lumbar spine (Fig. 49-11). A combination of chronic compression between the spine and right common iliac artery and vibratory pressure of the artery leads to rubbing of the two walls of the left common iliac vein, with resultant chronic trauma to the endothelium. This damage further leads to irregular proliferation of the endothelium and deposition of elastin and collagen, thus forming irregular intraluminal spurs and webs that predispose to DVT. Patients may present with swelling, pain, varicose veins, and symptoms of postthrombotic syndrome (swelling, skin discoloration, and ulceration affecting the left lower extremity). Clinically, three stages are recognized: stage 1, asymptomatic stage; stage 2, development of a venous spur; and stage 3, thrombosis of the left common iliac vein.

Imaging

Exercise plethysmography is highly sensitive in identifying venous obstruction. Compression ultrasound and color Doppler imaging can accurately detect DVT. Iliac vein compression is difficult to visualize on ultrasound, but lack of respiratory variations and the absence of response to the Valsalva maneuver during Duplex evaluation of the common femoral vein suggest a proximal obstruction (Fig. 49-12). Intravascular ultrasound allows direct visualization of iliac vein compression,

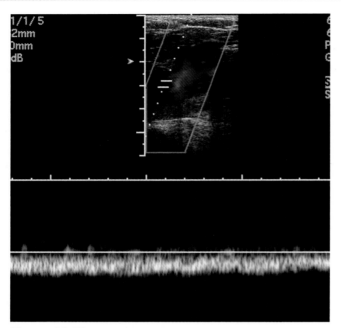

Figure 49-12 Spectral Doppler imaging of the left common femoral vein in a patient with May-Thurner syndrome. The left common femoral vein is patent, but the lack of respiratory variation in the flow suggests proximal obstruction.

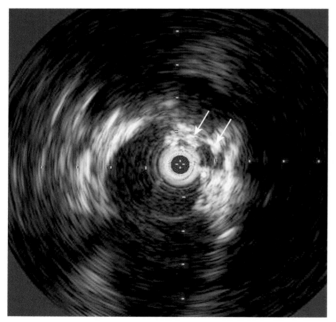

Figure 49-13 Intravascular ultrasound of the left common iliac vein in a patient with May-Thurner syndrome. Imaging demonstrates multiple mural echogenic foci (arrows) indicating the presence of spurs.

mural abnormalities such as spurs and webs, and multiple intraluminal channels (Fig. 49-13). It also allows accurate placement of a guidewire across the stenosed segments during endovascular intervention.

CTV and MRV allow direct visualization of DVT, compression of the left common iliac vein by the right common iliac artery, and pelvic venous collateral vessels. Morphologically, iliac venous compression has three grades on CTV: grade I, focal compression of the left common iliac vein at the crossing point of the right common iliac artery; grade II, diffuse atrophy of the left common iliac vein between the compression site and the confluence of the internal and external iliac arteries; and grade III, cordlike obliteration of the left common iliac vein. The presence of retrograde flow in the ipsilateral internal iliac vein (seen as flow void) and the ascending lumbar vein (seen as bright signal to the left of the lumbar spine) on TOF MRV and of pelvic collateral vessels on contrast-enhanced MRV suggests a hemodynamically significant venous compression (Fig. 49-14).

Left common femoral and iliac venography studies confirm the presence of venous obstruction. They may also demonstrate multiple venous channels secondary to intraluminal webs. An oblique, smooth filling defect with widening of the lumen of the left common iliac vein may be seen. As in MRV, the presence of flow reversal in the ipsilateral internal iliac vein and the ascending lumbar vein and of pelvic collateral vessels on left common femoral or external iliac venography suggests hemodynamically significant venous compression (Fig. 49-15). A pressure gradient of more than 2 mm Hg across the stenosis also suggests hemodynamically significant venous compression.

Variants of May-Thurner Anatomy

Morphologic variations in the course of the iliac arteries and veins may result in compression of the iliac veins and the IVC. The left common iliac vein may be compressed by a tortuous or aneurysmal left common iliac artery. Occasionally, the left common iliac vein may course between the iliopsoas muscle and the spine and cause venous compression (Fig. 49-16). The right common iliac vein may be compressed by the right common iliac artery (Fig. 49-17) because of a high aortic bifurcation or tortuosity and ectasia of the right common iliac artery. A high aortic bifurcation may also result in compression of the IVC or iliac venous confluence by the right common iliac artery. In addition, the right common iliac vein may be compressed by the left common iliac artery in patients with a left-sided IVC.

Treatment and Imaging Follow-up

Standard therapy for acute DVT consists of anticoagulation and compression stockings. Currently, endovascular pharmacomechanical thrombolysis is advocated for DVT to prevent postthrombotic syndrome. In addition, iliac venous compression is treated with self-expanding metallic stents (see Fig. 49-15). Long-term anticoagulation and compression stockings are required to prevent recurrent DVT and stent occlusion. The reported primary and secondary patency rates of iliac venous stents are 79% and 93%, respectively, at 1 year. Stent occlusion or stenosis may be suspected when symptoms recur or ultrasound imaging shows an absence of respiratory flow variations within the left common femoral vein. Thin-section CTV and intravascular ultrasound are highly useful to assess stent occlusion or stenosis. CT may show wall-adherent soft tissue resulting from either thrombus or intimal hyperplasia within the stent with

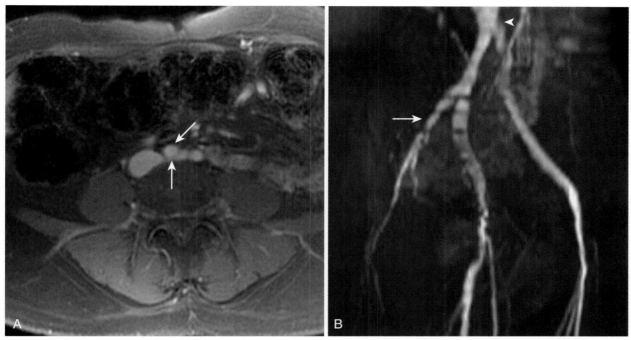

Figure 49-14 **Assessing the hemodynamic significance of iliac vein compression on time of flight (TOF) magnetic resonance venography (MRV).** **A,** Contrast-enhanced MRV shows compression of the left common iliac vein *(bottom arrow)* by the right common iliac artery *(top arrow)*. **B,** The hemodynamic significance of such venous compression can be assessed on TOF MRV. The right internal iliac vein *(arrow)* is well visualized; however, the left internal iliac vein is not seen secondary to retrograde flow. Contrast-enhanced MRV (not shown here) demonstrated a patent left internal iliac vein.

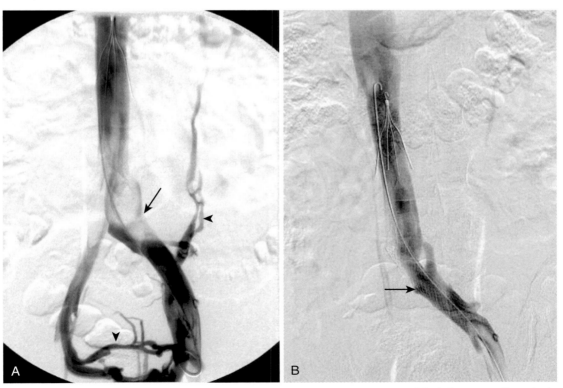

Figure 49-15 **A,** Left external iliac venography shows hemodynamically significant compression of the left common iliac vein *(arrow)*. Pelvic collateral vessels *(vertical arrowhead)* and an enlarged ascending lumbar vein *(horizontal arrowhead)* are visible. **B,** The patient subsequently underwent iliac venous stent placement *(arrow)*.

the appearance of new pelvic collateral veins. Treatment involves angioplasty with or without thrombolysis and stent placement.

Pearls and Pitfalls

- Asymptomatic iliac venous compression of 50% or greater may be seen in 25% of physiologically normal individuals. Two thirds of normal individuals have 25% or greater iliac vein compression.
- Intravascular ultrasound is key in diagnosing stage 2 disease, to identify mural spurs and webs.

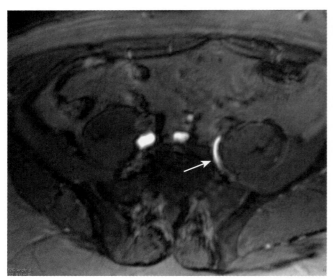

Figure 49-16 Variant of May-Thurner syndrome. Magnetic resonance venography (axial two-dimensional time of flight) shows compression of the left common iliac vein *(arrow)* between the spine and the left iliopsoas muscle.

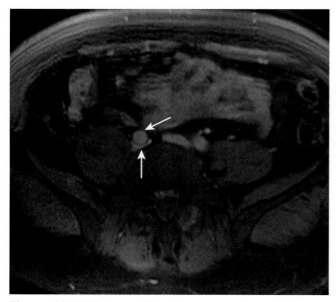

Figure 49-17 Variant of May-Thurner syndrome. Right common iliac venous compression *(bottom arrow)* by the right common iliac artery *(top arrow)* as a result of high aortic bifurcation.

- In patients with equivocal pressure gradient across the stenosis, repeat pressure measurements during the Valsalva maneuver may be helpful.
- Rarely, patients with iliac venous compression may present with pelvic congestion syndrome secondary to enlarged pelvic collateral vessels.

Paget-Schroetter Syndrome

Also known as effort thrombosis, idiopathic thrombosis, spontaneous thrombosis, and primary upper extremity DVT, Paget-Schroetter syndrome refers to DVT of the axillary and subclavian veins caused by excessive upper limb activity. It results from chronic compression of the subclavian vein at the level of the thoracic outlet and constitutes approximately 25% of cases of upper extremity DVT. This syndrome was first described by Paget in 1875 and then by Von Schroetter in 1884. Hughes named it the Paget-Schroetter syndrome in 1948. Its etiology appears to be complex and multifactorial. This syndrome develops more frequently in the dominant arm, usually after sports activities, including long-distance swimming, body building exercises, wrestling, hand ball, and baseball throwing, in which the shoulder is often depressed repetitively for prolonged periods. Men are affected twice as often as are women.

Anatomy and Pathophysiology

Anatomically, subclavian venous compression occurs in the costoclavicular space (Fig. 49-18) as a result of muscular, ligamentous, or osseous abnormalities that impinge on the vein and lead to decreased mobility, stasis of blood flow, and subsequent thrombosis. Such abnormalities include cervical rib, congenital bands, hypertrophy of scalenus tendons, abnormal insertion of the costoclavicular ligament, tumors, and excessive callus formation subsequent to clavicular fracture. Repeated venous compression from shoulder activities leads to endothelial trauma, inflammation, fibrosis, thrombus, and subsequent development of collateral

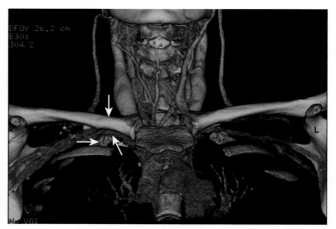

Figure 49-18 Anatomy of thoracic outlet. The subclavian vein *(oblique arrow)* passes through the costoclavicular space, in which it is compressed between the clavicle *(vertical arrow)* and the first rib *(horizontal arrow)*.

veins. Many patients also have hypercoagulable status secondary to factor V Leiden deficiency and thrombophilia. Patients present with upper extremity swelling, pain, and enlarged collateral vessels in the shoulder and chest.

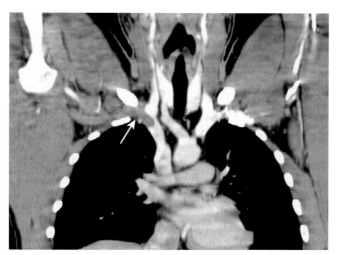

Figure 49-19 Computed tomography (CT) venography in Paget-Schroetter syndrome. CT venography is accurate in identifying thrombus *(arrow)* in the subclavian vein. It can also rule out the presence of anatomic abnormalities such as the cervical rib.

Imaging Findings

Ultrasound is highly accurate in identifying DVT affecting the axillary and distal subclavian veins; however, the proximal subclavian vein is often not well visualized. CTV and MRV are useful in accurately identifying the extent of thrombosis, the presence of collateral vessels, and anatomic abnormalities (Fig. 49-19). Contrast venography is the gold standard and accurately identifies the extent of thrombosis, the presence of collateral vessels, and intraluminal channels at the site of compression (Fig. 49-20). It is also used in endovascular therapy. Dynamic studies with abduction of the arm are performed during CTV, MRV, and conventional venography to assess venous compression at the thoracic outlet (Fig. 49-21).

Treatment and Imaging Follow-up

Acute axillary-subclavian vein thrombosis of less than 2 weeks' duration is best treated with catheter-directed pharmacomechanical thrombolysis, followed by surgical decompression of the vein through resection of the first rib or subclavius tendon, anterior and middle scalenectomy, and circumferential external venolysis. If symptoms recur following surgical treatment, angioplasty and stenting of the vein may be performed. Patients usually require long-term anticoagulation.

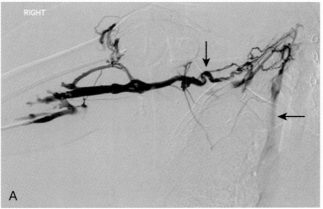
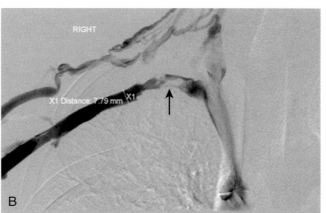
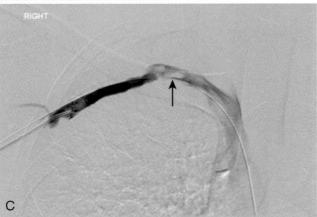

Figure 49-20 Paget-Schroetter syndrome. This patient presented with right upper extremity pain and swelling. **A,** Venography demonstrates occlusion of the right axillary and subclavian veins with opacification of the collateral veins *(vertical arrow)* that drain into the superior vena cava *(horizontal arrow)*. The patient underwent thrombolysis and balloon thrombectomy. **B,** Flow is restored in the axillary and subclavian veins with persistent thrombus *(arrow)* and collateral vessels at 12 hours following thrombolysis. **C,** Continued thrombolysis for 24 hours resulted in restoration of flow with minimal thrombus *(arrow)* in the subclavian vein. The collateral vessels disappeared. The patient subsequently underwent first rib resection.

Pearls and Pitfalls

- Dynamic imaging is key for detection of venous compression. The patient's arm is abducted and externally rotated to demonstrate venous compression at the costoclavicular space most clearly.
- Angioplasty and stenting should be avoided before surgical decompression.

Popliteal Venous Compression Syndrome

Unlike popliteal artery compression, popliteal venous compression is frequently interpreted as a benign radiologic finding without functional or pathologic significance. Morphologic venous entrapment can be seen in 27% of healthy population. The pathophysiology of this disease is same as that of popliteal arterial entrapment; however, large popliteal aneurysms may also impinge on the popliteal vein.

Anatomy and Pathophysiology

The popliteal artery and vein normally assume a straight course in the midline and posterior to the knee within the popliteal fossa. In patients with an entrapment, the medial head of the gastrocnemius muscle has an aberrant course and origin (a more lateral insertion, double head, fibrous band) separating the vein and the artery (Table 49-2). This configuration leads to compression of the vessels during active contraction of the gastrocnemius muscle, with hyperextension of the knee or with plantar flexion of the ankle with an extended knee. Less common causes include compression from an adjoining popliteal artery aneurysm, fibrous band across the vessels, popliteal cysts, and osteochondroma of the femur or tibia. Rarely, hypertrophied gastrocnemius and soleal muscles may compress the popliteal vein in the caudal aspect of the popliteal fossa; this condition is often referred to as functional entrapment. It may be asymptomatic or may result in venous insufficiency, venous thrombosis, and varicose veins. Chronic compression of the vein may result in sclerosis of the vein or poststenotic or prestenotic dilatation and chronic thrombosis.

Patients may present with signs and symptoms of popliteal arterial compression caused by concomitant arterial and venous compression (type 1), with leg edema and pain with no venous insufficiency (type 2), or with varicose veins, venous stasis dermatitis, and other symptoms of chronic venous insufficiency (type 3). Men are more often affected than are women. The disorder is bilateral in 20% to 35% of patients.

Imaging Findings

Ascending venography with dynamic maneuvers (active plantar flexion) remains the crucial test for diagnosis (Fig. 49-22). Venography may demonstrate an hourglass appearance or diffuse narrowing of the vein. Venous compression is either diffuse or at the midpopliteal level (across the joint line) and is rarely at a high or low popliteal level. Popliteal venous pressure measurements during dynamic maneuvers also provide information about the venous pressure changes. An increase in popliteal venous pressure or a decrease of less than 15% with exercise suggests outflow obstruction.

Ultrasound with color Doppler imaging allows accurate assessment of venous compression during dynamic maneuvers. It also detects the presence of

Table 49-2 Classification of Popliteal Venous Entrapment Syndromes

Type 1	Normal medial gastrocnemius, but aberrant course of the popliteal artery that courses medially around the head
Type 2	Abnormal medial head of the gastrocnemius that inserts lateral to the popliteal artery
Type 3	Abnormal slip of the medial head of the gastrocnemius surrounding the popliteal artery
Type 4	Popliteal artery located deeply within the popliteal fossa and entrapped by a fibrous band or the popliteus muscle
Type 5	Popliteal vein entrapped with any type 1 to 4
Type 6	Functional entrapment of the popliteal artery and vein caused by hypertrophy of the muscles

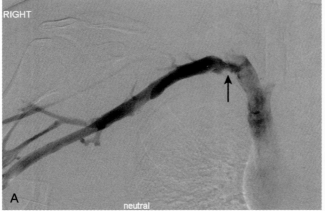
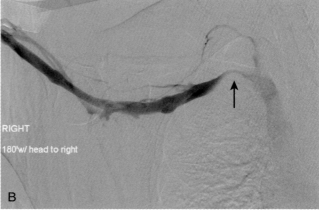

Figure 49-21 Dynamic venography for assessing venous compression *(arrows)* in a patient with suspected Paget-Schroetter syndrome. A, The subclavian vein is widely patent when the arm is adducted (neutral position). **B,** However, when the arm is abducted and externally rotated, significant stenosis of the subclavian vein is present.

venous insufficiency in the small saphenous vein and popliteal vein and DVT.

CT and magnetic resonance imaging (MRI) allow detection of abnormal muscle insertions and fibrous bands. The presence of a muscular or soft tissue density between the popliteal artery and vein on axial CT or MRI suggests popliteal entrapment. Dynamic MRV can also demonstrate the dynamic nature of the venous compression that increases with active plantar flexion of the foot. In patients with the functional variety of popliteal venous entrapment, CT and MRI demonstrate hypertrophy of the medial and lateral heads of the gastrocnemius muscles.

Treatment

Patients with minimal symptoms (type 2) benefit from compression stockings. Patients with severe symptoms require surgical decompression of the vessels through resection of the abnormal muscle or fibrous bands.

Pearls and Pitfalls

■ Dynamic imaging (through active plantar flexion) with ultrasound, MRV, or ascending venography is key for the diagnosis of popliteal venous compression. Associated arterial compression can also be diagnosed with ultrasound, MRI, and arteriography.

■ Isolated popliteal venous insufficiency noted on ultrasound imaging should raise the suspicion of popliteal venous entrapment, and further workup may be warranted.

■ Popliteal venous pressure measurements are useful in identifying patients who may benefit from surgery.

Nutcracker Syndrome

Nutcracker syndrome results from compression of the left renal vein between the superior mesenteric artery and the aorta. Rarely, it can also result from compression of the left renal vein between the aorta and the vertebral bodies in patients with a retroaortic left renal vein. This syndrome is commonly seen in young, healthy women in their third and fourth decades.

Anatomy and Pathophysiology

Compression of the left renal vein between the aorta and the superior mesenteric artery leads to localized left renal venous hypertension. This results in redistribution of venous flow through the ureteric and gonadal veins and leads to formation of varicosities around the ureter and pelvis. Rarely, the thin-walled intrarenal veins may rupture into the calyceal fornices and cause hematuria. Patients may present with left flank pain, abdominal pain with or without hematuria, and orthostatic proteinuria. Men may develop testicular pain with varicocele. Women may complain of chronic pelvic pain with dysmenorrhea, dysuria, and vulvar or pelvic varices. Long-standing pelvic venous hypertension may also lead to lower extremity varicose veins.

Imaging Findings

The definitive diagnosis is established through direct visualization of the venous compression, measuring the renal vein to IVC pressure gradient, and observing varices in the gonadal vein.

Doppler sonography has a sensitivity of 78% and a specificity of 100% in the diagnosis of the nutcracker

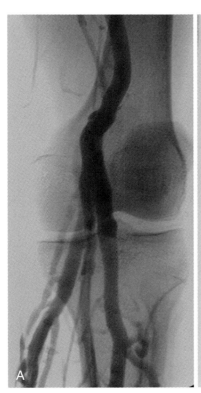
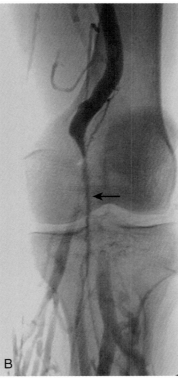

A   B

Figure 49-22 Dynamic venography for assessing popliteal venous compression. A, Ascending venography during neutral position of the ankle shows a patent popliteal vein. **B,** However, with active plantar flexion, the popliteal vein is diffusely narrowed *(arrow),* thus suggesting the presence of popliteal venous entrapment.

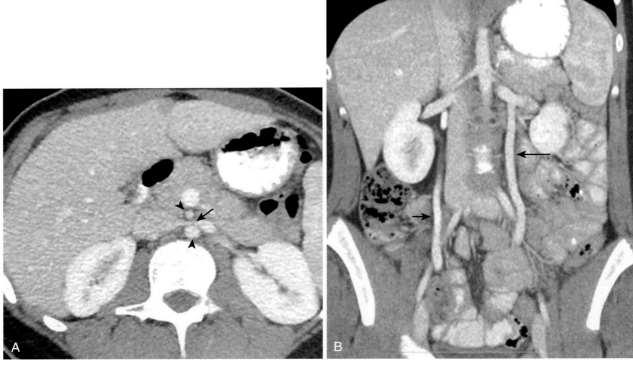

Figure 49-23 Computed tomography (CT) venography to assess nutcracker syndrome. A, Axial contrast-enhanced CT shows severe compression of the left renal vein *(arrow)* between the superior mesenteric artery *(top arrowhead)* and the aorta *(bottom arrowhead)*. **B,** Reconstructed coronal CT shows enlarged gonadal veins *(arrows)*. Large pelvic varices (not shown) were also present.

syndrome. The diagnostic criteria on ultrasound are as follows:

1. Peak systolic velocity of more than 100 cm/second at the site of renal vein compression while the patient is standing for at least 15 minutes
2. A diameter ratio of more than 3 between the narrowest portion of the renal vein and the renal vein at the hilum while the patient is supine, or a ratio of more than 5 while the patient is standing for 15 minutes

Contrast-enhanced CT and MRI can directly visualize compression of the left renal vein between the aorta and the superior mesenteric artery (Fig. 49-23). The enlarged left renal vein near the renal hilum and gonadal and pelvic varices may also be observed.

Left renal venography demonstrates the site of compression and retrograde flow through the gonadal varices (Fig. 49-24). The pressure gradient across the renal vein and IVC is elevated (normal gradient, 0 to 1; abnormal, 1 to 3).

Treatment and Imaging Follow-up

Patients with minor and tolerable symptoms can be managed conservatively with elastic compression stockings, whereas patients with significant hematuria, severe flank pain, renal functional impairment, pelvic pain, and failure of conservative therapy may benefit from surgery or endovascular therapy. Surgical options include medial nephropexy, gonadocaval bypass, transposition of the left renal vein or the superior mesenteric artery, and renal autotransplantation.

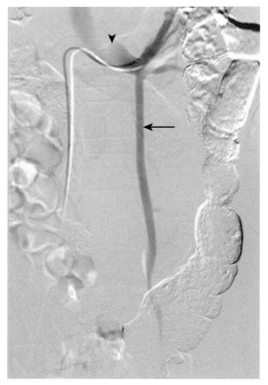

Figure 49-24 Left renal venography of the same patient as in Figure 49-23. Selective left renal venography shows reflux of contrast material into the left gonadal vein *(arrow)*. Extrinsic compression *(arrowhead)* over the left renal vein is also seen.

Laparoscopic extravascular scaffolding using polytetrafluoroethylene grafts around the compressed vein is another option. Endovascular therapy with stenting of the compressed left renal vein either with bare metallic stents or with stent grafts is becoming more popular because of excellent short-term results. Complications of stenting include stent occlusion, venous thrombosis, and thromboembolism. These complications are best assessed on ultrasound and contrast-enhanced CT. Symptomatic pelvic or gonadal varices can be embolized with a combination of chemical sclerosant agents and coils for symptom relief.

Pearls and Pitfalls

- Clinically significant venous compression is best diagnosed when symptoms are associated with the presence of anatomic compression and venous collateral vessels.
- When symptoms of pelvic congestion syndrome predominate, occlusion of the gonadal veins alone may provide symptomatic relief.
- Gonadal vein reflux may not be observed on supine studies. In such cases, repeat studies with the patient in the vertical position (standing MRI) or semierect venography during the Valsalva maneuver may demonstrate gonadal vein reflux.

Bibliography

Beitzke D, Wolf F, Juelg G, Lammer J, Loewe C. Diagnosis of popliteal venous entrapment syndrome by magnetic resonance imaging using blood-pool contrast agents. *Cardiovasc Intervent Radiol*. 2011;34(suppl 2):S12-S16.

di Marzo L, Cavallaro A. Popliteal vascular entrapment. *World J Surg*. 2005;29(suppl 1):S43-S45.

Forauer AR, Gemmete JJ, Dasika NL, Cho KJ, Williams DM. Intravascular ultrasound in the diagnosis and treatment of iliac vein compression (May-Thurner) syndrome. *J Vasc Interv Radiol*. 2002;13:523-527.

Gurel K, Gurel S, Karavas E, Buharalıoglu Y, Daglar B. Direct contrast-enhanced MR venography in the diagnosis of May-Thurner syndrome. *Eur J Radiol*. 2011;80:533-536.

Illig KA, Doyle AJ. A comprehensive review of Paget-Schroetter syndrome. *J Vasc Surg*. 2010;51:1538-1547.

Kibbe MR, Ujiki M, Goodwin AL, Eskandari M, Yao J, Matsumura J. Iliac vein compression in an asymptomatic patient population. *J Vasc Surg*. 2004;39:937-943.

Kim JY, Choi D, Guk Ko Y, Park S, Jang Y, Lee do Y. Percutaneous treatment of deep vein thrombosis in May-Thurner syndrome. *Cardiovasc Intervent Radiol*. 2006;29:571-575.

Kim KW, Cho JY, Kim SH, et al. Diagnostic value of computed tomographic findings of nutcracker syndrome: correlation with renal venography and renocaval pressure gradients. *Eur J Radiol*. 2011;80:648-654.

Oguzkurt L, Tercan F, Pourbagher MA, Kizilkilic O, Turkoz R, Boyvat F. Computed tomography findings in 10 cases of iliac vein compression (May-Thurner) syndrome. *Eur J Radiol*. 2005;55:421-425.

Raju S, Neglen P. Popliteal vein entrapment: a benign venographic feature or a pathologic entity? *J Vasc Surg*. 2000;31:631-641.

Sabharwal R, Boshell D, Vladica P. Multidetector spiral CT venography in the diagnosis of upper extremity deep venous thrombosis. *Australas Radiol*. 2007;51(suppl):B253-B256.

Thompson JF, Winterborn RJ, Bays S, White H, Kinsella DC, Watkinson AF. Venous thoracic outlet compression and the Paget-Schroetter syndrome: a review and recommendations for management. *Cardiovasc Intervent Radiol*. 2011;34:903-910.

Utsunomiya D, Sawamura T. Popliteal artery entrapment syndrome: non-invasive diagnosis by MDCT and MRI. *Australas Radiol*. 2007;51(spec no):B101-B103.

van Langevelde K, Tan M, Srámek A, Huisman MV, de Roos A. Magnetic resonance imaging and computed tomography developments in imaging of venous thromboembolism. *J Magn Reson Imaging*. 2010;32:1302-1312.

Venkatachalam S, Bumpus K, Kapadia SR, Gray B, Lyden S, Shishehbor MH. The nutcracker syndrome. *Ann Vasc Surg*. 2011;25:1154-1164.

Wang L, Yi L, Yang L, Liu Z, Rao J, Liu L, Yang J. Diagnosis and surgical treatment of nutcracker syndrome: a single-center experience. *Urology*. 2009;73:871-876.

Wolpert LM, Rahmani O, Stein B, Gallagher JJ, Drezner AD. Magnetic resonance venography in the diagnosis and management of May-Thurner syndrome. *Vasc Endovascular Surg*. 2002;36:51-57.

CHAPTER 50

Venous Insufficiency

Chieh-Min Fan

Venous insufficiency is defined as retrograde blood flow in the venous system resulting from incompetence of the venous valves. It is the most common pathologic process affecting the venous system. After the age of 50 years, more than half the human population will have some form of venous insufficiency, which spans a broad spectrum of clinical manifestations ranging from asymptomatic spider veins to symptomatic varicose veins to severe edema with skin inflammation and ulceration (Figure 50-1). Since 2000, the development and refinement of endovenous techniques have revolutionized the treatment of venous insufficiency and have relegated the once gold standard surgical vein stripping to an increasingly historical role.

As is the case with many minimally invasive therapies, achieving durable satisfactory outcomes with modern endovenous treatments depends on accurate diagnostic imaging for preprocedural planning, intraprocedural guidance, and postoperative assessment. Imaging the patient with venous insufficiency is straightforward provided one understands venous anatomy and is familiar with the spectrum of venous disease states and with the appropriate use of available venous imaging modalities. Avoiding the pitfalls of treating these patients requires awareness of the two forces at work in the development of venous insufficiency: valvular incompetence and venous obstruction. Because of the innate variability of the venous anatomy and disease patterns among individuals, errors of diagnosis or management typically arise when the operator fails to assess the patient fully clinically, uses poor technique, or fails to consider possible involvement of more remote venous structures.

This chapter reviews venous anatomy, basic physiology and pathophysiology of venous insufficiency, and the current role of imaging in the evaluation and treatment of the patient with venous insufficiency.

■ VENOUS ANATOMY

The two venous systems in the lower extremity work concordantly to conduct venous return to the central circulation. The deep venous system consists of a set of large-capacitance veins in the core of the limb. Deep venous components include the following: the paired peroneal, anterior tibial, and posterior tibial veins of the calf; the medial, lateral, and intergemellar (gastrocnemius) and soleal veins; the popliteal, femoral, and deep femoral veins; and the common femoral, external iliac, internal iliac, and common iliac veins of the pelvis. Venous drainage pathways out of the pelvis include the inferior vena cava, retroperitoneal ascending lumbar venous plexus, and gonadal veins.

The superficial venous system is a smaller dermal and subcutaneous network whose components include the great saphenous vein (GSV) and small saphenous vein (SSV), anterior and posterior accessory GSVs, cranial extension of the SSV and intersaphenous vein (vein of Giacomini), and superior accessory GSV. The inferior epigastric veins and external pudendal veins are the most cephalad components of the superficial system. The deep and superficial veins of the lower extremity communicate through up to 150 valved perforator veins that normally conduct venous blood in a superficial to deep direction. Historically, lower extremity venous nomenclature was notably inconsistent and confusing. Therefore, in 2001, an international interdisciplinary consensus committee convened in Italy, and the result was the publication of a consensus document that defined the currently accepted nomenclature for lower extremity veins.

■ VENOUS PHYSIOLOGY

Both superficial and deep venous systems function to collect the venous blood from the leg to the central circulation. Normally, the deep venous system dominates this process, by carrying 90% of the venous drainage load, compared with the 10% transported by the superficial veins. In the setting of deep venous dysfunction, this ratio shifts, and the superficial veins become the primary collateral drainage pathway. In contrast to the arterial circulation that maintains forward blood flow through an arterial pressure head, venous blood flow is propelled through the veins in the antegrade direction by external compression of the veins by the surrounding musculature (the calf and thigh muscular pumps), as well as by cyclic variations in intraabdominal pressure from respiratory motion. Contraction of the muscular pumps results in forward flow of the blood column, whereas one-way valves prevent retrograde reflux. When the muscular pump relaxes and the veins expand again, intravascular pressure in the deep veins decreases, resulting in a pressure gradient across

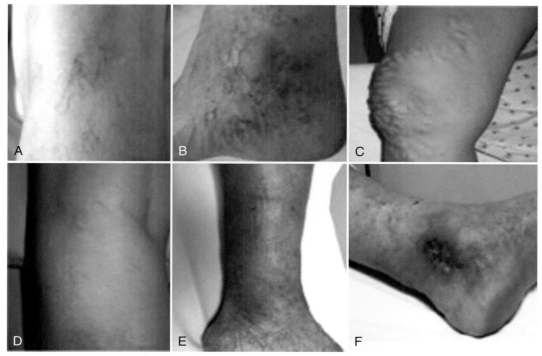

Figure 50-1 *Clinical manifestations of venous insufficiency.* **A,** Spider telangiectasia. **B,** Venulectasia in a corona phlebectatica distribution. **C,** Tributary varicose vein. **D,** Reticular varicose vein. **E,** Lipodermatosclerosis. **F,** Venous ulceration.

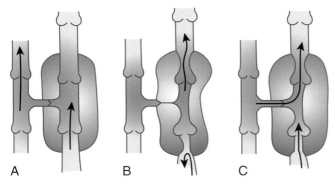

Figure 50-2 Schematic diagram of muscular pump function and venous flow dynamics. **A,** Neutral relaxation phase. **B,** Muscular contraction causing closure of perforator "gates" and deep vein compression with increased deep venous pressure resulting in antegrade flow. **C,** Muscular relaxation phase causing decreased venous pressure in empty deep vein, resulting in antegrade flow of blood from the surface through perforators and from distal segments.

the perforator vein system that promotes blood flowing from higher to lower pressure in the superficial to deep direction. Valves in the perforator veins prevent reflux of blood from the deep to superficial system during the contraction cycle of the pump. A schematic representation of venous flow dynamics is presented in Figure 50-2.

■ VENOUS PATHOPHYSIOLOGY

Development of venous valvular insufficiency is a multifactorial process likely involving genetic predisposition compounded by environmental and lifestyle factors.

Secondary venous insufficiency is generally presumed to result from postthrombotic valve destruction, compounded by postthrombotic obstruction to flow that promotes a state of chronic venous hypertension. In contrast, primary venous insufficiency likely results from an intrinsic structural derangement of the vein wall, rather than from valve leaflet damage. Compared with normal veins, primary varicose veins histologically demonstrate proportionally decreased muscle components secondary to increased wall infiltration by collagenous tissue. The abnormal collagen deposits are distributed in a nonuniform pattern and act to separate and disrupt the muscular grid of the vein wall. This process, in turn, results in discontinuous segments of dilatation, wall thinning (blow outs), and secondary expansion of the valve annuli that lead to valvular incompetence.

The mechanism by which venous hypertension incites inflammation and ulceration is a complex process not fully understood, but it seems to involve extravasation of erythrocytes and macromolecules that incite an inflammatory cascade in the dermal perivascular tissues. One theory postulates that venous hypertension causes increase capillary pore size, with resulting extravasation of erythrocytes and fibrinogen and α_2-macroglobulin into the dermal pericapillary extracellular matrix. This extravasated fibrinogen organizes into fibrin cuff around the capillaries and impairs nutrient and oxygen exchange. White blood cells have also been shown to accumulate in the setting of venous hypertension, and another theory suggests that inflammatory cytokines from red blood cell degradation promote leukocyte accumulation in the capillaries. This process, in turn, results in increased perivascular resistance and upregulation of inflammatory

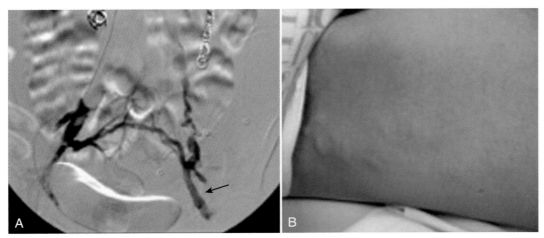

Figure 50-3 Pudendal collateral venous reflux with left thigh varicose vein. **A,** Balloon occlusion venography of the right internal iliac vein with cross-pelvic flow and retrograde reflux into the left pudendal vein *(arrow).* **B,** Typical appearance of a lower extremity varicose vein originating from a pelvic source of reflux.

cytokine and proteolytic enzyme release, with consequent tissue damage, inflammation, and ulceration. Reduction of the venous hypertension by leg elevation, compression therapy, and correction of the refluxing circuit reverses this process and promotes healing.

CLASSIFICATION OF CHRONIC VENOUS INSUFFICIENCY

Venous insufficiency may be classified by location as deep, superficial, or perforator reflux. The term axial reflux, applicable to either superficial (e.g., saphenous veins) or deep veins, refers to a continuous reflux column from the common femoral vein level to the knee, as opposed to segmental reflux, which is limited to a short section of vein. Venous insufficiency can also be classified broadly by presumed origin as either primary (developing de novo without an external inciting event) or secondary (from postthrombotic valve damage or venous obstruction). Because the deep and superficial venous structures work in a coordinated and compensatory fashion, prolonged reflux in one part of the system may, over time, overload and incite reflux in other venous structures.

The CEAP classification stratifies venous disorders on the zbasis of four parameters: clinical, etiology, anatomy, and pathophysiology. The clinical groupings range from no evidence of disease (C_0) through the spectrum of physical signs of venous insufficiency: telangiectasia or reticular veins (C_1), varicose veins (C_2), edema (C_3), skin changes such as lipodermatosclerosis (C_4), healed ulcer (C_5), and active ulcer (C_6). The etiology is classified as primary (E_p), congenital (E_c), or secondary (E_s). Anatomically, venous disease is divided into superficial (A_s), deep (A_d), and involving perforators (A_p). Pathophysiologically, venous disease is described as the result of reflux (P_r), obstruction (P_o), or both.

Pelvic congestion syndrome (PCS) is a distinct category of venous insufficiency involving the gonadal veins and internal iliac veins. It may occur either alone or in combination with lower extremity venous insufficiency resulting from transmission of venous reflux to the saphenofemoral junction through the external pudendal collateral veins. As is the case with varicose veins elsewhere, pelvic varicosities can result from primary valvular insufficiency or secondarily from more central outflow obstruction. The clinical presentation of PCS includes chronic pelvic pain (CPP) or pressure, which is typically worse when the patient is upright or sitting and relieved by recumbency, dyspareunia and postcoital discomfort, and the presence of vulvar, buttock, or proximal thigh varicosities. An example of thigh varicosities characteristic of PCS is presented in Figure 50-3.

IMAGING OF VENOUS INSUFFICIENCY

Duplex Ultrasound

Duplex ultrasound has emerged as the preferred initial imaging modality for evaluation of infrainguinal venous insufficiency, and it provides excellent anatomic detail, as well as localization and quantification of reflux. The study is best performed with a 7.5- to 13.5-MHz linear array transducer, with an ultrasound unit capable of grayscale imaging with both color and spectral Doppler interrogation.

Specific goals of the examination include the following:
1. Defining anatomy, position, and competence of saphenous junctions
2. Assessing the diameter and competence of superficial venous components including the GSV, accessory GSVs, SSV, major tributary branches, and perforators
3. Mapping all major varicosities to their originating source of reflux
4. Confirming status of the deep venous system including assessment for presence of reflux and exclusion of congenital absence, hypoplasia, or thrombotic occlusion of the deep veins

The duplex ultrasound venous reflux examination has two components: a supine examination using both grayscale scanning with dynamic compression and Doppler flow to rule out acute or chronic deep venous thrombus, followed by a reflux examination with pulse

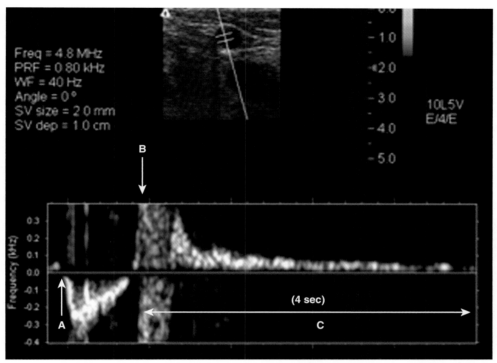

Figure 50-4 Spectral Doppler image of a great saphenous vein reflux waveform that demonstrates augmentation with calf compression (**A**), reversal of flow with release of compression (**B**), and duration of reflux (passive valve closure time) of 4 seconds (**C**).

wave or color Doppler interrogation of the superficial and deep veins with the patient in the upright position. For the reflux study, the patient is optimally standing with the leg of interest abducted slightly at the hip and with the foot resting fully on the ground but with the weight shifted to the contralateral leg. Calf perforator veins are most easily evaluated with the patient seated on the examining table with the lower leg in a relaxed dependent position. The ultrasound reflux examination includes diameter measurements serially along the length of the GSV and SSV and major accessory saphenous branches, with spectral Doppler assessment for reflux at each point of measurement. Reflux can be elicited by the Valsalva maneuver or by calf compression and release maneuvers.

Figure 50-4 illustrates the typical appearance of a spectral Doppler reflux waveform. The duration of retrograde flow is known as the passive valve closure time and is one quantitative parameter for assessing reflux. Abnormal reflux is defined as follows: greater than 1-second valve closure time at the common femoral, femoral, and popliteal veins; greater than 0.5 seconds for the deep femoral, saphenous, and deep calf veins; and greater than 0.35 seconds for perforator veins. However, the duration of reflux alone does not necessarily correlate with the severity of reflux. A patient with mild venous reflux may have a protracted valve closure time with low-amplitude spectral tracing, whereas a patient with severely incompetent valves may have a relative short duration of reflux of high amplitude as the bolus of blood refluxes across a severely incompetent valve.

The GSV and SSV travel in the saphenous space, which is demarcated by superficial and deep fascial layers that

are readily visible sonographically. In cross section, the saphenous veins in the saphenous space have an "Egyptian eye" appearance (Fig. 50-5). When a saphenous vein or a branch passes through the superficial fascia, it becomes a tributary vein.

Potential Pitfalls

1. Failure to stand the patient upright for the reflux examination. The duplex ultrasound examination for venous reflux must be performed with the patient in the upright position to maximize the gravitational effect on the blood column and the pressure gradient across the venous valves and too minimize the likelihood of a false-negative result. No pressure gradient exists in a horizontal vein in the supine position, so one cannot reliably assess the competence of the valves. Varicosities are also engorged in the upright position, thus facilitating visual assessment of disease distribution. To the experienced clinician, the pattern of varicose vein distribution often predicts the source of reflux, but it cannot be reliably assessed when the patient is supine and the veins are flat.

2. Failure to adjust the angle of insonation. Veins are typically branching and often serpiginous structures that change direction of flow as the course of the vessel changes. As the examiner interrogates for reflux along the course of a vein, it is technically important to adjust the angle of insonation constantly to 60 degrees or less to avoid loss of Doppler shift detection. Failure to do so will result in false-negative readings and underdetection of reflux.

3. Failure to trace the major varicosities to their source individually. Venous anatomy is highly variable, so

for accurate treatment planning, simply documenting reflux in the saphenous veins is inadequate. All major varicosities of clinical concern should be interrogated sonographically until the exact origin of the reflux is identified. For example, an incompetent midthigh hunterian perforator may give rise to a midthigh varicose vein pattern resembling one resulting from GSV reflux. Thorough duplex examination is especially useful in patients with varicose vein recurrence following earlier vein treatments because the pattern of neovein formation is unpredictable and variable from patient to patient.

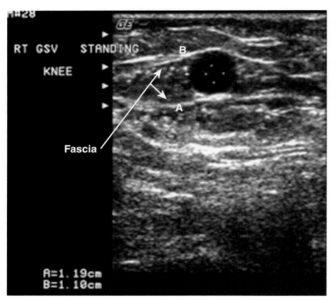

Figure 50-5 Cross-sectional appearance of the great saphenous vein (GSV) in the saphenous space that demonstrates a classic "Egyptian eye" appearance of the GSV between the superficial (B) and deep (A) fasciae *(arrows)*, which define the saphenous space.

Magnetic Resonance Venography and Computed Tomography Venography

Duplex ultrasound is technically limited for assessment of the calf veins and central pelvic veins, and, in certain situations, additional evaluation by computed tomography venography (CTV), magnetic resonance venography (MRV), or conventional contrast venography may be required. This is especially important in the setting of earlier deep venous thrombosis (DVT) because with obstruction of the deep venous system, the superficial veins become the primary drainage pathway of the lower limb. Removal or ablation of superficial veins is potentially contraindicated and clinically detrimental to these patients. Contrast-enhanced CTV and MRV provide excellent visual resolution of pelvic venous structures, as well as directional flow information, especially with time-resolved imaging of contrast kinetics (TRICKS) MRV sequencing. These imaging modalities are especially helpful in cases of suspected PCS. CTV and MRV also aid in the detection of venous obstruction resulting from extrinsic compression, which can be either benign or malignant.

Two examples of benign extrinsic compression resulting in venous hypertension and reflux include May-Thurner syndrome in which compression of the left common iliac vein by the right common iliac artery results in left lower extremity venous outflow obstruction (Fig. 50-6), and nutcracker syndrome in which compression of the left central renal vein occurs between the superior mesenteric artery and aorta resulting in left renal venous congestion and decompression through gonadal and collateral veins.

Contrast Venography

Conventional ascending contrast venography can easily be performed via an intravenous line in a foot vein, and therefore is in actuality no more invasive than CTV or

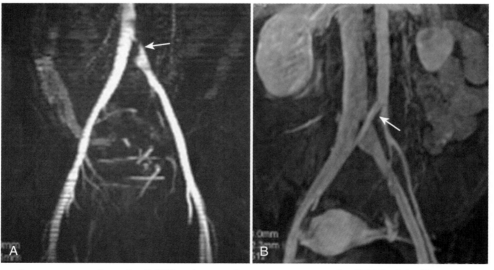

Figure 50-6 Magnetic resonance angiography (MRA) and magnetic resonance venography (MRV) of the iliac vein compression syndrome (May-Thurner syndrome). **A,** Time of flight MRV showing extrinsic compression of the left common iliac vein. **B,** With gadolinium-enhanced MRA and MRV, this condition is shown to result from compression by the crossing right common iliac artery.

MRV requiring an IV injection of contrast media. Contrast venography remains a useful modality for assessing lower extremity deep venous structures, especially in the calf where arterial contamination or bolus timing issues may erode diagnostic accuracy of CTV and MRV techniques. Venography is performed with the patient in reverse Trendelenburg position, with serial tourniquets on the ankle, calf, distal thigh, and midthigh to occlude the superficial venous system and preferentially drive the contrast into the deep venous structures. Spot images are obtained in multiple projections at each level. The location of incompetent perforators and presence of obstruction or scarring in the deep veins are noted. In the case of nonocclusive deep venous obstruction, the rapidity of contrast flow in the veins with release of the tourniquets can help clarify which system (deep or superficial) is the dominant drainage pathway for the limb. This point is illustrated in Figure 50-7.

Intravascular Ultrasound

Intravascular ultrasound (IVUS) has emerged as a uniquely useful tool for the assessment of central venous obstruction. IVUS has been shown to be more sensitive and specific than single plane venography for detection of iliac vein stenosis because many intraluminal synechiae and webs are poorly seen on venography and are beyond the imaging resolution of CTV and MRV. Luminal cross-sectional area reduction of more than 50% on IVUS is believed to be hemodynamically significant, and correction of the central venous obstruction alone by stenting has been shown to promote ulcer healing in 54% of patients with advanced C_6 venous disease.

■ TREATMENT OF VENOUS INSUFFICIENCY

Since 2000, the development of minimally invasive endovenous methods for correcting venous reflux and relieving chronic venous obstruction has revolutionized care of the patient with venous insufficiency. Compression therapy remains an integral adjunct to these newer treatment methods, and it is often the first intervention prescribed to control venous symptoms. Pressures of 30 to 40 mm Hg are required to compress superficial veins when patients are in a standing position. Systematic use of daily compression stockings for venous insufficiency can slow progression of disease, control symptoms, reduce ulceration, and promote ulcer healing. The use of compression stockings with anticoagulation has been shown to reduce the likelihood of post-thrombotic syndrome by 50% in patients with DVT. These benefits notwithstanding, compression stockings are perceived as difficult to wear, uncomfortable in warm weather, and cosmetically unsatisfactory.

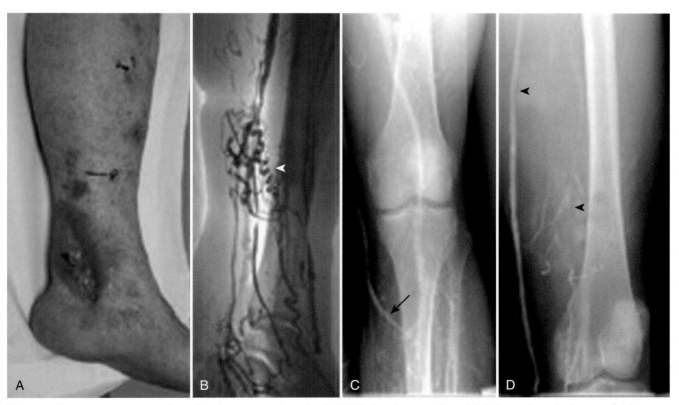

Figure 50-7 Venogram in a patient after deep venous thrombosis (DVT) that shows preferential drainage through the superficial venous system. **A,** Photograph of a nonhealing ulcer in a patient after DVT. **B,** Ascending venogram shows a large incompetent perforator at the level of the ulcer *(arrowhead)*. **C,** A second incompetent perforator *(arrow)* in the upper calf that drains into the great saphenous vein (GSV). Some filling of popliteal and lower femoral deep veins is noted. **D,** Venogram at the thigh level shows preferential drainage through the GSV *(top arrowhead)* that bypasses obstructing postthrombotic damage in the deep venous system *(bottom arrowhead)*.

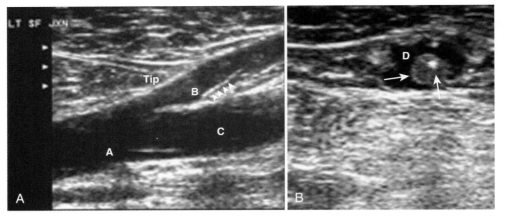

Figure 50-8 Intraprocedural ultrasound images of laser ablation of the great saphenous vein (GSV). **A,** Sagittal image of the saphenofemoral junction anatomy with the common femoral vein (A), GSV with laser tip (B and *arrowheads*), and femoral vein (C). **B,** Axial image of tumescent anesthesia injected circumferentially in the perivenous space (D), vein wall *(horizontal arrow)*, and laser fiber *(vertical arrow)*.

Endovenous treatments for venous insufficiency can be categorized as treatments for correction of axial reflux in the saphenous veins and treatments for more superficial varicosities. Saphenous vein ablation methods include chemical ablation with foamed sclerosant agents, surgical removal, and endovenous thermal ablation with radiofrequency (RF) or laser devices. Laser and RF ablation can also be used for straight segments of other tributary branches and for closure of incompetent perforator veins. Long-term data on endovenous thermal ablation demonstrate durable closure rates of 88% to 100% for laser and 87% to 89% for RF. Compared with RF ablation, laser ablation is associated with more postprocedural discomfort, but after 6 posttreatment weeks, both methods yield equivalent outcomes in terms of symptom resolution and improved quality of life. Surface varicosities, as well as perforator reflux, may be addressed with combined techniques of surgical phlebectomy, thermal ablation, and sclerotherapy.

The technique for endovenous thermal ablation of saphenous veins is essentially the same for both RF and laser techniques, and duplex ultrasound is the preferred image guidance modality. Under ultrasound guidance, the target vein is accessed at the lowest point of detectable reflux possible. The thermal heating device is positioned 0.5 cm below the saphenofemoral or saphenopopliteal junction. Under ultrasound observation, dilute 0.1% to 0.2% lidocaine tumescent anesthesia is injected around the entire length of vein targeted for thermal ablation. Sonographically, the goal is to encase the target segment in a column of tumescent fluid that has a threefold function: to isolate the vein and prevent thermal damage to surrounding tissue structures, to compress the vein onto the heating element, and provide local anesthesia. Once the tumescent anesthesia is in place, the heating element is activated and slowly withdrawn, thus delivering energy and causing thermal ablation of the vein. Intraprocedural images of endovenous laser ablation are presented in Figure 50-8.

After the ablation, the limb is placed into compression, and the patient is able to ambulate immediately. Follow-up at 1 to 2 weeks is standard postprocedural

care, and it usually includes a duplex ultrasound examination to confirm closure of the vein and to rule out thrombotic complications in adjacent deep venous structures. Postprocedural evaluation includes confirmation of patency of the common femoral or popliteal vein at the top of the ablated segment and documentation of occlusion of the ablated segment. The typical sonographic early appearance of an ablated saphenous vein is an occluded, noncompressible structure containing hyperechoic coagulum and surrounded by mild soft tissue inflammation (Fig. 50-9). After several months, the ablated vein segment involutes into a fine cord that can be difficult to visualize sonographically. DVT occurs rarely following saphenous vein thermal ablation, with a reported prevalence of 1% or less for both laser and RF methods.

Although conventional saphenous vein stripping has been largely replaced by endovenous thermal ablation, surgical treatments remain important therapeutic options for treatment of venous insufficiency. On the simplest level, phlebectomy removal of major branch varicosities is widely practiced as an adjunct to saphenous vein closure. In patients with combined lower extremity venous insufficiency and central pelvic vein occlusion, or extremely dilated saphenous veins, procedures combining endovenous techniques with surgical thrombectomy or ligation may be advantageous.

Pelvic Venous Congestion

Special discussion should be given to the topic of pelvic venous congestion, a form of venous insufficiency that has captured the interest and awareness of vein specialists. PCS is a condition of CPP resulting from venous insufficiency in the gonadal and parauterine deep pelvic veins. Characteristic features of the syndrome include CPP, pelvic and vulvar varicosities, and recurrent lower extremity varicosities. PCS is clinically significant because it may be the underlying disorder in 20% of women with CPP. CPP may be defined as nonmenstrual pelvic pain of more than 6 months' duration that is severe enough to cause functional disability or require medical or surgical treatment. As such, CPP is the primary indication for

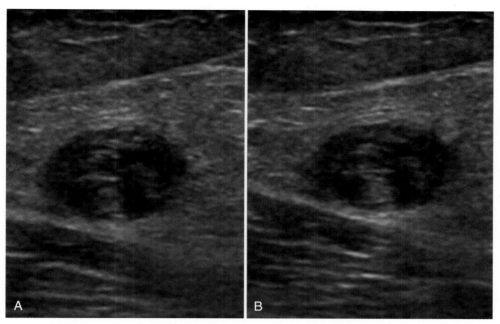

Figure 50-9 Transverse ultrasound images of the great saphenous vein without compression (**A**) and with compression (**B**) demonstrate hyperechoic coagulum in the lumen and noncompressibility.

10% of gynecologic referrals, 40% of diagnostic laparoscopies, and 12% of hysterectomies. As a major cause of CPP, PCS may be an underdiagnosed entity with significant socioeconomic relevance.

PCS has gained wider recognition for another reason. The syndrome has been implicated as a reason for early recurrence of superficial lower extremity venous insufficiency following saphenous closure and sclerotherapy. Reflux in the internal iliac veins may communicate with the saphenofemoral junction and lower extremity veins through pudendal, vulvar, and gluteal collateral vessels and varicosities. Pelvic venous reflux has been detected in 17% of 170 patients with recurrent varicose veins after surgery, a finding suggesting that the failure to recognize and address this potential "highest point of reflux" may compromise the efficacy of venous procedures lower down.

Pelvic varicosities are common incidental findings on imaging studies and laparoscopic examinations, and CPP is a frequent problem among premenopausal women. The two entities can coexist without a causal relationship, so identifying women with true PCS can be challenging. Clinical features that support the diagnosis include the following: positional pain that is worse when the patient is upright and improves with recumbency, multiparity, postcoital pelvic pain, premenopausal age, and the presence of perineal, gluteal, vulvar, and upper inner thigh varicose vein patterns. PCS is notably rare in nulliparous women. It is uncommon but not unheard of in postmenopausal women, in whom pelvic floor instability can often incite pain and symptoms mimicking those of PCS. A cyclic nature of the pain with menses suggests other disorders such as endometriosis.

Computed tomography (CT), magnetic resonance imaging (MRI), and laparoscopy can assist in the diagnosis of PCS. Characteristic imaging findings include dilated ovarian veins more than 10 mm in diameter and engorged pelvic varices in the parauterine and broad ligament regions (Figs. 50-10 and 50-11). Cross-sectional imaging can underdetect the problem because the gonadal venous congestion may not be fully apparent when the patient is supine. The defining diagnostic examination is gonadal venography demonstrating retrograde flow in the ovarian veins and cross-pelvic filling of pelvic varicosities. Internal iliac venography with balloon occlusion should also be routinely performed to assess for connections with parauterine varicosities that may benefit from sclerotherapy (Fig. 50-12). Although PCS can be bilateral, venous incompetence is often asymmetric, with left ovarian and right internal iliac veins the most commonly implicated vessels.

Treatment of PCS is a two-step process involving selective embolization of the ovarian vein or veins and balloon occlusion sclerotherapy of the internal iliac veins. The two components of treatment can be performed at one session or in a staged fashion. Many types of embolization agents have been used for gonadal vein occlusion including coils, vascular occluder devices, and foamed and liquid sclerosant agents. Because of the rich collateral venous network in the retroperitoneum, the entire length of the gonadal vein should be treated, to prevent collateralization and recurrent reflux in the gonadal vein. PCS treatment is typically performed on an outpatient basis and uses conscious sedation. The postprocedural course is usually uneventful. Transient mild paraspinal and pelvic discomfort may occur postprocedurally and is easily managed with nonsteroidal antiinflammatory medication. Following treatment, relief from CPP is usually significant and immediate, and embolotherapy of PCS is associated with a 75% to 100% success rate for combined complete resolution and partial relief of symptoms. Complications are rare

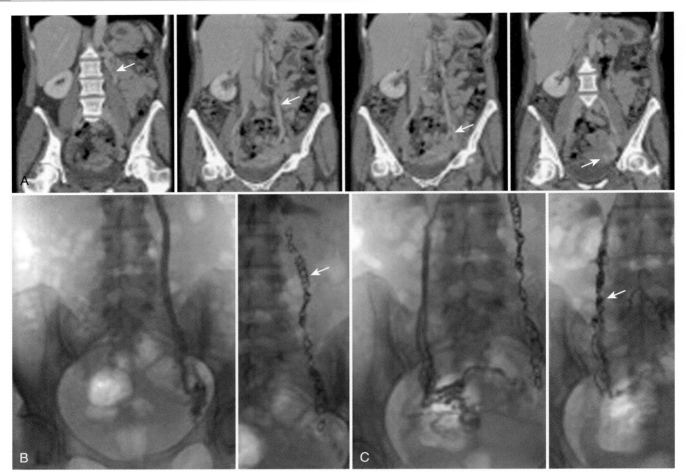

Figure 50-10 A, Coronal contrast-enhanced computed tomography angiography and computed tomography venography demonstrate a dilated gonadal vein extending from the left renal vein to pelvic varicosities *(arrows)*. **B,** Venographic correlation demonstrates left gonadal vein reflux and pelvic varicosities before and after *(arrow)* embolization. **C,** Venographic correlation demonstrates right gonadal vein reflux and pelvic varicosities before and after *(arrow)* embolization.

and include of migration of coils to the pulmonary bed and retroperitoneal pain.

As mentioned previously, pelvic venous compression syndromes cause regional venous obstruction and can contribute to pelvic venous insufficiency, especially on the left side. In May-Thurner syndrome, also known as iliac vein compression syndrome, the left common iliac vein is externally compressed by the crossing of the right common iliac artery. Over the long term, this chronic impingement can result in left iliac vein stenosis with left pelvic and lower extremity venous hypertension, reflux, and, most seriously, thrombotic occlusion. Nutcracker syndrome is a venous compression syndrome in which the central left renal vein is compressed and functionally obstructed between the aorta and the superior mesenteric artery. This entity results in a variant of pelvic venous congestion, manifesting with the constellation of flank pain, hematuria, and pelvic venous congestion as the left renal venous return is diverted through the left gonadal and retroperitoneal veins. Various surgical approaches to repair of nutcracker syndrome physiology have been tried, including left renal vein transposition, external renal vein stenting with ringed polytetrafluoroethylene, gonadal caval bypass, and nephrectomy. Most

recently, endovenous stenting of the compressed segment has been used.

Potential Pitfalls

1. Poor patient selection. Because pelvic pain and pelvic varicosities are both common findings but are not necessarily causally related in many women, a primary challenge of managing pelvic venous congestion is identifying patients in whom pelvic venous reflux is truly the cause of pelvic pain. A thorough clinical history of symptoms and a physical examination are essential for distinguishing patients with true pelvic venous insufficiency from those with other gynecologic issues such as pelvic floor relaxation or endometriosis, which can mimic PCS clinically.

2. Failure to address internal iliac venous reflux adequately. To obtain durable symptomatic relief, treatment of PCS must include evaluation and treatment of the parauterine deep pelvic veins, as well as the gonadal veins. When the gonadal veins alone are treated, recurrent symptoms develop in approximately 50% of cases. The deep pelvic veins form interconnecting plexuses with multiple points

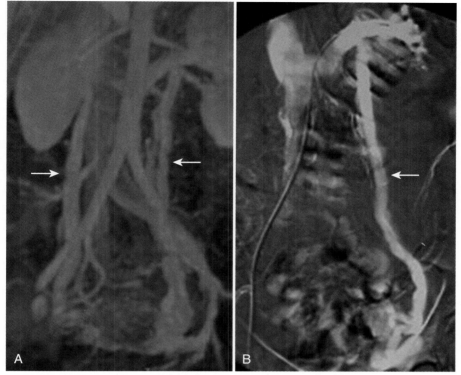

Figure 50-11 Magnetic resonance venography (**A**) and venography (**B**) in a patient with pelvic venous congestion *(arrows)* show correlation of the left gonadal vein anatomy.

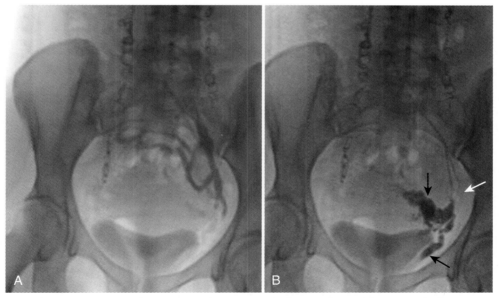

Figure 50-12 Selective venography of the left internal iliac vein without balloon occlusion (**A**) and with balloon occlusion (**B**, *arrow*) that demonstrates visualization of the connection with pelvic varicosities *(black arrows)* only with balloon occlusion technique.

of collateralization and central drainage pathways. Assessment and visualization of connections between iliac veins and pelvic varices require flow control with a balloon occlusion technique because simple injection without balloon occlusion fails to demonstrate the connections (see Fig. 50-12).

3. Failure to embolize the entire gonadal vein. Because the gonadal veins collateralize extensively with the ascending lumbar venous plexus, failure to close the entire course of the gonadal vein can result in recurrent reflux from collateral branches. This phenomenon is illustrated in Figure 50-13.

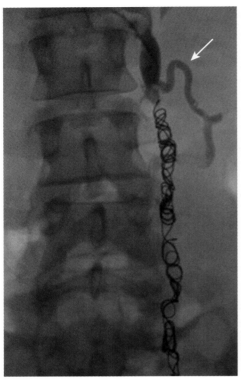

Figure 50-13 Venogram of the left gonadal vein after embolization shows filling of a large collateral branch *(arrow)* that could potentially be a conduit for recurrent reflux.

Varicocele

Varicocele, defined as venous incompetence of the testicular vein with retrograde venous congestion of the pampiniform plexus, is the most common correctable cause of male infertility. The prevalence of varicocele is 15% in the healthy male population and 40% in the subfertile male population. Most varicoceles are left unilateral lesions (~85%), and approximately 15% are bilateral lesions. Isolated right varicocele is a notably rare occurrence and a clinical red flag for other potential retroperitoneal disorders. The exact mechanism by which varicoceles adversely affect spermatogenesis is not fully understood; both hyperthermic effects of venous congestion and oxidative stress resulting from toxic metabolites have been implicated.

The clinical sequelae of varicocele include scrotal pain and swelling, testicular atrophy in adults and hypotrophy in pediatric population, oligozoospermia, and sperm dysmotility. The diagnosis of varicocele is made by clinical history and physical examination, correlated with duplex ultrasound demonstrating an engorged pampiniform plexus (Fig. 50-14) and reflux with the Valsalva maneuver on spectral or color Doppler imaging. Duplex ultrasound findings can be confirmed by retrograde venography, which is analogous to the venographic evaluation of pelvic venous congestion in women and demonstrates retrograde flow down the testicular vein into the varicocele (Fig. 50-15, *A*).

Many techniques are available for the treatment of varicoceles. Surgical ligation and varicocelectomy can be

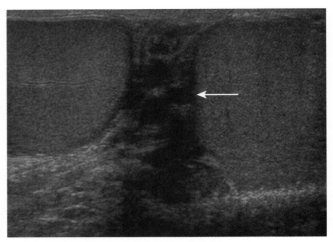

Figure 50-14 Grayscale ultrasound image of a left varicocele demonstrates dilated pampiniform veins *(arrow)*.

performed from a low inguinal or high retroperitoneal approach, and open, laparoscopic, robot-assisted, and microsurgical subinguinal methods have all been used. All methods of surgical varicocelectomy are effective in improving sperm count and sired pregnancy rates at 1 year, but the microsurgical infrainguinal approach has a significantly lower rate of postsurgical hydrocele and recurrent varicocele compared with other surgical techniques. Percutaneous methods of varicocele treatment include testicular vein occlusion with coil embolization or occluder devices and sclerotherapy from a retrograde testicular vein approach or antegrade injection through a pampiniform vein through cut-down exposure. Compared with surgical methods, these percutaneous approaches have similar rates of technical and clinical success with lower postprocedure complications. Figure 50-15, *B*, illustrates coil embolization of an incompetent left testicular vein associated with a varicocele.

Indications for treatment continue to a topic of debate, given that the prevalence of varicocele in men with infertility approaches 40%, but up to 15% of men with normal semen analysis have varicoceles. If one considers the surrogate end point of semen quality, treatment of varicocele improves sperm count and quality in up to 70% of patients, especially if pretreatment sperm count is greater than 10 million. However, available prospective randomized data are both lacking and conflicted on the impact of varicocele repair on rates of spontaneous conception. At present, the Best Practice Policy Committee of the American Urological Association (AUA) and the American Society for Reproductive Medicine (ASRM) recommend varicocele treatment for men with a palpable varicocele and abnormal semen parameters who have a female partner with normal fertility or a correctable cause of infertility.

■ CONCLUSION

Venous insufficiency remains one of the most common health issues of the adult aging population. Major growth in both interest and understanding of venous disease has occurred since 2000, and minimally invasive

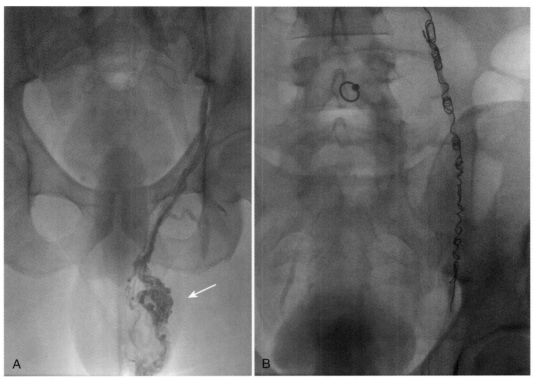

Figure 50-15 **Varicocele embolization.** **A,** Retrograde venography of the left testicular vein that demonstrates reflux into the left varicocele *(arrow).* **B,** Postcoiling image of the left testicular vein.

techniques to correct venous insufficiency and its deleterious effects have been developed. The high success rate and low complication rates of these treatments have shifted the risk-to-benefit ratio in favor of earlier treatment with image-guided endovenous methods over conventional surgical techniques.

Bibliography

Ahmed K, Sampath R, Khan M. Current trend in the diagnosis and management of renal nutcracker syndrome: a review. *Eur J Vasc Endovasc Surg.* 2006;31:410-416.

Al-Kandari A, Shabaan H, Elshebiny Y, Shokeir A. Comparison of outcomes of different varicocelectomy techniques: open inguinal, laparoscopic, and subinguinal microscopic varicocelectomy: a randomized clinical trial. *Urology.* 2007;69:417-420.

Antignani PL. Classification of chronic venous insufficiency: a review. *Angiology.* 2001;52(suppl 1):S17-S26.

Araki CT, Back TL, Padberg FT, et al. The significance of calf muscle pump function in venous ulceration. *J Vasc Surg.* 1994;20:872–877.

Asciutto G, Asciutto K, Mumme A, Geier B. Pelvic venous incompetence: reflux patterns and treatment results. *Eur J Vasc Endovasc Surg.* 2009;38:381-386.

Binkert C, Schoch E, Largiader J, Wigger P, Schoepke W, Zollikofer C. Treatment of pelvic venous spur (May-Thurner Syndrome) with self-expanding metallic endoprostheses. *Cardiovasc Intervent Radiol.* 1998;21:22-26.

Caggiati A, Bergan J, Gloviczki P, Eklof B, Allegra C, Partsch H. Nomenclature of the veins of the lower limb: extensions, refinements, and clinical application. *J Vasc Surg.* 2005;41:719-724.

Caggiati A, Bergan JJ, Gloviczki P, Janter G, Wendell-Smith CP, Partsch H. Nomenclature of the veins of the lower limb: an international interdisciplinary consensus statement. *J Vasc Surg.* 2002;36:416-422.

Chan P. Management of varicoceles. *Indian J Urol.* 2011;27:65-73.

Coleridge-Smith P, Labropoulos N, Partch H, Myers K, Nicolaides A, Cavezzi A. Duplex ultrasound investigation of the veins in chronic venous disease of the lower limbs: UIP consensus document. Part 1. Basic principles. *Eur J Vasc Endovasc Surg.* 2006;31:83-92.

Danielsson G, Eklof B, Grandinetti A, Lurie F, Kistner R. Deep axial reflux, an important contributor to skin changes or ulcer in chronic venous disease. *J Vasc Surg.* 2003;38:1336-1341.

Dick E, Burnett C, Anstee A, Hamady M, Black D, Gedroyc W. Time-resolved imaging of contrast kinetics three-dimensional (3D) magnetic resonance venography in patients with pelvic congestion syndrome. *Br J Radiol.* 2010;83:882-887.

Dubin L, Amelar R. Varicocelectomy: 986 cases in a twelve-year study. *Urology.* 1997;10:446-449.

Evers J, Collins J. Assessment of efficacy of varicocele repair for male subfertility: a systematic review. *Lancet.* 2003;361:1849-1852.

Flacke S, Schuster M, Kovacs A, et al. Embolization of varicoceles: pretreatment sperm motility predicts later pregnancy in partners of infertile men. *Radiology.* 2008;248:540-549.

Gale S, Lee J, Walsh E, Wojnarowski D, Comerota A. A randomized controlled trial of endovenous thermal ablation using 810 nm wavelength laser and the ClosurePLUS radiofrequency ablation methods for superficial venous insufficiency of the great saphenous vein. *J Vasc Surg.* 2010;52:645-650.

Gandini R, Konda D, Reale C, et al. Male varicocele: transcatheter foam sclerotherapy with sodium tetradecyl sulfate—outcome in 244 patients. *Radiology.* 2008;246:612-618.

Ganeshan A, Upponi S, Hon L, Uthappa M, Warajaulle D, Uberoi R. Chronic pelvic pain due to pelvic congestion syndrome: the role of diagnostic and interventional radiology. *Cardiovasc Intervent Radiol.* 2007;30:1105-1111.

Gloviczki P, Comerota A, Dalsing M, et al. The care of patients with varicose veins and associated diseases: clinical practice guidelines of the Society for Vascular Surgery and American Venous Forum. *J Vasc Surg.* 2011;53(suppl):2S-48S.

Herrick S, Sloan P, McGurk M, Freak L, McCollum C, Ferguson M. Sequential changes in histologic pattern and extracellular matrix deposition during the healing of chronic venous ulcers. *Am J Pathol.* 1992;141:1085–1095.

Hirai M, Iwata H, Hayakawa N. Effect of elastic compression stockings in patients with varicose veins and healthy controls measured by strain gauge plethysmography. *Skin Res Technol.* 2002;8:236-239.

Kahn S. The post-thrombotic syndrome: progress and pitfalls. *Br J Haematol.* 2006;134:357-365.

Kim H, Malhotra A, Rowe P, Lee J, Venbrux A. Embolotherapy for pelvic congestion syndrome: long-term results. *J Vasc Interv Radiol.* 2006;17:289-297.

Kistner RL, Eklof B, Masuda EM. Diagnosis of chronic venous disease of the lower extremities: the "CEAP" classification. *Mayo Clin Proc.* 1996;71:338-345.

Labropoulos N, Tiongson J, Kang S, Mansour A, Baker WH. The definition of venous reflux in the lower extremity veins. *J Vasc Surg.* 2003;38:793-798.

Ludbrook B. The musculovenous pump of the human lower limb. *Am Heart J.* 1966;7:635-641.

Maleux G, Stockx L, Wilms G, Marchal G. Ovarian vein embolization for the treatment of pelvic congestion syndrome: long-term technical and clinical results. *J Vasc Interv Radiol.* 2000;11:859-864.

Marsh P, Price B, Holdstock J, Harrison C, Whiteley M. Deep vein thrombosis (DVT) after venous thermoablation techniques: rates of endovenous heat-induced thrombosis (EHIT) and classical DVT after radiofrequency and endovenous laser ablation in a single centre. *Eur J Vasc Endovasc Surg.* 2010;40:521-527.

Meissner M, Glovickski P, Bergan J, et al. Primary chronic venous disorders. *J Vasc Surg.* 2007;46(suppl):54S-67S.

Min R, Khilnani N, Zimmet S. Endovenous laser treatment of saphenous vein reflux: long-term results. *J Vasc Interv Radiol.* 2003;14:991-996.

Mozes G, Gloviczki P. New discoveries in anatomy and new terminology of leg veins: clinical implications. *Vasc Endovasc Surg.* 2004;38:367-374.

Murthy G, Ballard R, Briet G, Watenpaugh D, Hargens R. Intramuscular pressures beneath elastic and inelastic leggings. *Ann Vasc Surg.* 1994;8:543-548.

Nabi G, Asterlings S, Greene D, Marsh R. Percutaneous embolization of varicoceles: outcomes and correlation of semen improvement with pregnancy. *Urology.* 2004;63:359-363.

Neglen P, Raju S. Intravascular ultrasound scan evaluation of the obstructed vein. *J Vasc Surg.* 2002;35:684-700.

Nicholson T, Basile A. Pelvic congestion syndrome, who should we treat and how? *Tech Vasc Interv Radiol.* 2006;9:19-23.

Pandley T, Shaikh R, Viswamitra S, Jambhekar K. Use of time resolved magnetic resonance imaging in the diagnosis of pelvic congestion syndrome. *J Magn Reson Imaging.* 2010;32:700-704.

Pappas P, Defouw D, Venezio L, et al. Morphometric assessment of the dermal microcirculation in patients with chronic venous insufficiency. *J Vasc Surg.* 1997;26:784-795.

Perrin M, Labropoulos N, Leon L. Presentation of the patient with recurrent varices after surgery (REVAS). *J Vasc Surg.* 2006;43:327-334.

Raju S, Neglen P. Unexpected major role for venous stenting in deep reflux disease. *J Vasc Surg.* 2010;51:401-408.

Scultetus A, Villavicencio L, Gillespie D. The nutcracker syndrome: its role in pelvic venous disorders. *J Vasc Surg.* 2001;34:812-819.

Sharlip I. Male Infertility Best Practice Policy Committee. *Infertility: report on varicocele and infertility.* American Urological Association, Inc. and American Society for Reproductive Medicine; Available at http://www.auanet.org/content/media/varicoceleinfertility.pdf. Accessed 01.10.12. 2001.

Sharma D, Dahiya K, Duhan N, Bansal R. Diagnostic laparoscopy in chronic pelvic pain. *Arch Gynecol Obstet.* 2011;283:295-297.

Thomas P, Nash G, Dormandy J. White cell accumulation in dependent legs of patients with venous hypertension: a possible mechanism for trophic changes. *Br Med J (Clin Res Ed).* 1988;296:1693-1695.

Travers J, Brookes C, Evans J, Baker D, Makin G, Mayhew T. Assessment of wall structure and composition of varicose veins with reference to collagen, elastin, and smooth muscle content. *Eur J Vasc Surg.* 1966;11:230-237.

Venbrux A, Chang A, Kim H, et al. Pelvic congestion syndrome (pelvic venous incompetence): impact of ovarian and internal iliac vein embolotherapy on menstrual cycle and chronic pelvic pain. *J Vasc Interv Radiol.* 2002;13:171-178.

CHAPTER 51

Vascular Anomalies

Philip R. John

The current classification of vascular anomalies into vascular tumors and vascular malformations and their subtypes has been used by the International Society for the Study of Vascular Anomalies (ISSVA) since 1996 (Table 51-1). This classification is based on the biologic and clinical behavior of these anomalies, including physical characteristics, natural history, and cellular features. Vascular tumors manifest in early infancy. Infantile hemangiomas are the most common type and during growth show increased endothelial cellularity and lumenized capillary-like structures. Vascular malformations are different and are congenital lesions, present at birth and resulting from errors in morphogenesis of vascular channels (capillaries, veins, arteries, and lymphatics) with normal endothelial cell turnover.

The nomenclature and biologic classification of vascular anomalies are shown in Table 51-1. This classification is extremely useful because it promotes a clear understanding of these disorders, allows radiologists to establish the correct diagnosis, and enables patients to be managed correctly with appropriate treatments undertaken and inappropriate treatments avoided. This classification, for example, allows radiologists to distinguish between infantile hemangiomas with a significant high-flow component from arteriovenous malformations (AVMs), which are also high-flow lesions without a parenchymal tumor component. A few patients, however, have exceptions to this classification. Some with vascular malformations are not evident until later in life because of either location or progressive expansion.

The interventional radiologist is pivotal to the success of any vascular anomalies program. That patients with these disorders are best treated by a multiprofessional team combining the skills and expertise in medicine, surgery, and radiology needed to diagnose and care effectively for these sometimes complex disorders is well recognized. Having a clear understanding of these conditions and their imaging features, an awareness of treatment options and when best to treat, skills in vascular interventions needed for these procedures, and a knowledge of potential complications and their management allows the interventional radiologist to become a clinical specialist in managing these patients.

Because misdiagnoses are not uncommon in some patients with these disorders, either clinically or on imaging, some patients receive inappropriate treatments. The radiologist is therefore well suited to ensuring the delivery of appropriate care for patients with vascular anomalies.

■ IMAGING

Not all patients with vascular anomalies require imaging to confirm the diagnosis because most (even up to 90%) of these anomalies can be diagnosed from clinical history and physical examination. For example, most babies with infantile hemangiomas do not need imaging, although close clinical follow-up is required. When imaging is undertaken to confirm the diagnosis and or to evaluate the anomaly fully, ultrasound and magnetic resonance imaging (MRI) are the most useful modalities because of their high tissue specificity. For most patients, magnetic resonance angiography (MRA) sequences are not needed to establish the diagnosis. In patients with high-flow lesions, however, MRA is useful for mapping the affected vascular anatomy. Ultrasound has limitations when lesions are extensive or deeply located, but it can be useful in selected patients to provide a rapid bedside diagnosis and to assess potential local complications that can sometimes be seen (e.g., superficial blood clots). Plain radiography and computed tomography (CT) are not required in most patients (these imaging techniques have low tissue specificity). However, they may be required when abnormalities of skeletal growth occur, such as in selected large facial malformations and extremity overgrowth in Klippel-Trenaunay syndrome (KTS).

Conventional venography and catheter angiography are not required in most patients. Venography is occasionally undertaken in KTS to assess anomalous veins and the deep venous system, for which magnetic resonance venography (MRV) may be inadequate. Catheter angiography is done in selected patients with high-flow vascular anomalies when catheter-directed treatments are undertaken. Direct percutaneous puncture venography of venous malformations (VMs) is required only during injection sclerotherapy. Nuclear medicine has no role in imaging of these disorders.

■ VASCULAR TUMORS

Infantile Hemangiomas

Hemangiomas are the most common tumors of infancy. They occur in the skin approximately 2 weeks after birth and are often found in the head and neck area. Twenty percent of babies have multiple lesions. When these tumors are internal, they can be present in the liver, gastrointestinal (GI) tract, and brain. Infantile

Table 51-1 Classification of Vascular Anomalies

Vascular Tumors	Vascular Malformations

Infantile Hemangioma
Superficial
Deep
	Low Flow
	Single channel
	  Capillary malformation (CM)
	  Venous malformation (VM)
	  Lymphatic malformation (LM)
	Combined channel
	  Capillary-lymphatic malformation (CLM)
	  Capillary-venous malformation (CVM)
	  Venous-lymphatic malformation (VLM)

Congenital Hemangioma Noninvolutionary congenital hemangioma (NICH) Rapid involutionary congenital hemangioma (RICH)	**High Flow** Arteriovenous malformation (AVM) Arteriovenous fistula (AVF)
Kaposiform Hemangioendothelioma (KHE)	**Complex Combined (Syndromic Low Flow)** Klippel-Trenaunay syndrome Maffucci syndrome Proteus syndrome
Tufted Angioma (TA)	**Complex Combined (Syndromic High Flow)** Parkes Weber syndrome PTEN gene mutation–related
Pyogenic Granuloma	

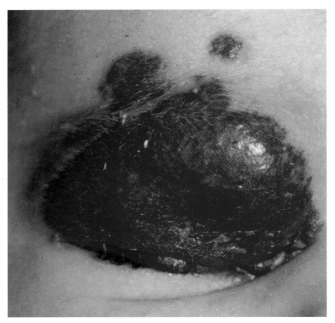

Figure 51-1 Proliferative infantile hemangioma. The *dense red* color is the result of dermal involvement by this vascular tumor affecting the upper eyelid of this 3-month-old baby.

hemangiomas have a characteristic three-phase life cycle, with tumors showing progression through three distinct phases. The first phase, the proliferative phase, occurs within the first 12 months of life with rapid tumor growth and tumor angiogenesis. During this phase, tumors are hypervascular, have prominent feeding arteries and veins, show high vascular flow, and can have intralesional vascular shunting. The second phase, the involuting phase, occurs between the ages of 1 and 5 to 7 years and is characterized by slow tumor involution, reduced angiogenesis, and reduction in overall size. During this phase, tumors show reduction in vascular flow and some fibrofatty replacement. Finally, the third phase, the involuted phase, occurs after 5 to 7 years, with resultant fibrofatty residue, small capillaries, and draining veins. After involution, lesions do not recur, and approximately half of all patients have nearly normal looking skin at the site of the lesion.

Clinically, tumors involving the superficial dermis manifest as red, raised lesions (Fig. 51-1). Ulceration and bleeding can be seen in large superficial tumors with rapid growth. Tumors in the lower dermis and subcutaneous tissue appear bluish or cause no alteration in color of the overlying skin. During involution, the color of the tumor fades, and a central pale area may be seen.

Congenital hemangiomas are rare and are distinct from infantile hemangiomas. They occur antenatally, are fully developed at birth, and do not usually exhibit postnatal tumor growth, in contrast to the more common infantile hemangiomas. The two types are the rapidly involuting congenital hemangioma (RICH) and the noninvoluting congenital hemangioma (NICH). Clinically, these lesions are quite different. RICHs are often impressive protuberant masses (Fig. 51-2), whereas a NICH tends to be a flat to slightly raised, rounded skin lesion, with telangiectasias and a pale surrounding halo (Fig. 51-3). RICHs regress spontaneously usually by 12 to 14 months of postnatal life, whereas NICHs persist throughout life. Both are hypervascular tumors. Significant arteriovenous (AV) shunting can occur in the RICH before tumor regression and can potentially lead to cardiac failure. An accurate history and physical examination can establish the diagnosis in 90% of patients.

Infantile hemangiomas can be mistaken for capillary malformations (CMs), and deeper (i.e., subcutaneous) hemangiomas can be mistaken for venous or lymphatic malformations because of the bluish discoloration through the skin. Hemangiomas showing high flow may be mistaken for AVMs, but the age at onset, growth pattern, and presence of tumor parenchyma in hemangiomas distinguishes these two lesions. Congenital hemangiomas can potentially be confused with vascular malformations, although their clinical features provide clues to the diagnosis.

The location of the infantile hemangioma may be associated with specific problems during the proliferative phase when the tumor is rapidly increasing in size. Airway obstruction, visual impairment, GI bleeding, high-output congestive heart failure from vascular shunting within large or multiple hemangiomas, (particularly in the liver), and tissue necrosis can potentially occur.

Hepatic Hemangiomas

Infantile hepatic hemangiomas (IHHs) have a pattern of involution similar to that of cutaneous hemangiomas. The classic presentation with heart failure, anemia,

SECTION V

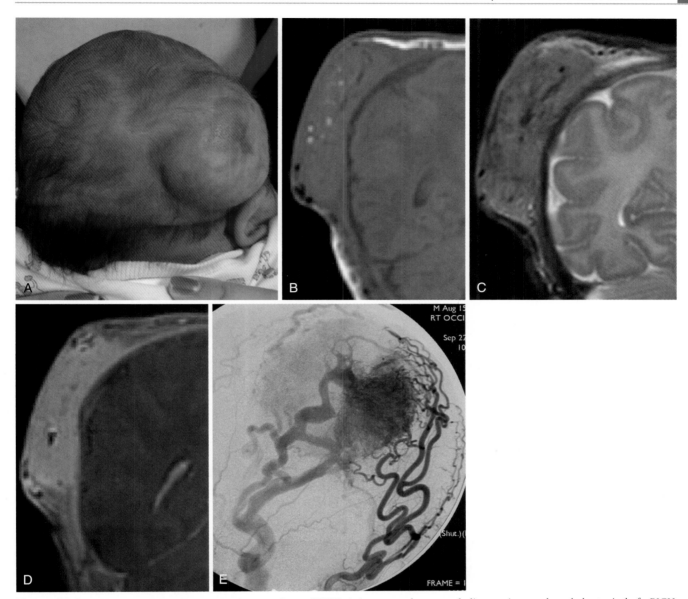

Figure 51-2 Rapidly involuting congenital hemangioma (RICH). A, Large protuberant cephalic mass in a newborn baby, typical of a RICH. **B to D,** Typical magnetic resonance imaging findings with hypointense tumor on a T1-weighted image (**B**), hyperintense tumor on a T2-weighted image (**C**), and tumor parenchymal enhancement after contrast administration (**D**). **E,** External carotid angiogram shows the hypervascular tumor, with prominent tortuous arterial inflow channels, parenchymal staining, and early venous outflow into enlarged tortuous channels. This angiogram was obtained immediately before transcatheter embolization using "PVA particles" through a microcatheter to promote tumor involution. Most infants with a RICH do not need catheter angiography and embolization because these lesions spontaneously regress by 12 months of age.

and hepatomegaly is rare, and certainly not all hepatic hemangiomas are life-threatening. Three predominant IHH forms exist: focal, multifocal, or diffuse (Fig. 51-4). Focal lesions are single, often large, and manifest antenatally. They do not grow after birth and are thought to represent RICH-type lesions, with regression in the first 12 to 14 months of life. Like RICH lesions, macrovascular shunts can result in high-output cardiac failure. Multifocal hepatic hemangiomas are similar to typical cutaneous infantile hemangiomas with similar three-phase life cycles. Small lesions, even if multiple, can be asymptomatic. Some IHHs with macrovascular shunts can lead to cardiac failure. In the diffuse type, most of the liver parenchyma is replaced by tumor, which typically causes massive hepatomegaly, abdominal compartment syndrome, and respiratory compromise. The diffuse type of IHH can lead to severe hypothyroidism until tumor involution occurs because the tumor produces type 3-iodothyronine deiodinase, which inactivates circulating thyroid hormones.

Imaging of Hemangiomas

In infantile hemangiomas, the imaging features depend on the phase of the life cycle of the tumor at the time of imaging (Fig. 51-5). During the proliferative phase, ultrasonography demonstrates a solid parenchymal mass with high vessel density and fast flow. MRI shows

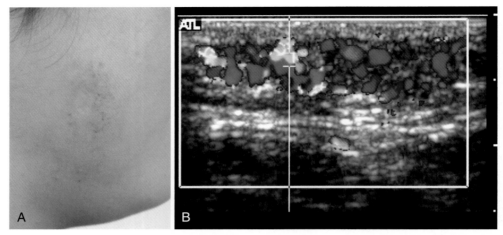

Figure 51-3 Noninvoluting congenital hemangioma (NICH). A, Flat facial lesion in a teenage patient that is typical of a NICH with telangiectasias surrounded by a *blue and pale "halo."* **B,** Ultrasound shows hypervascularity in the subcutaneous tissue immediately deep to the skin changes. The NICH is much less impressive than a rapidly involuting congenital hemangioma.

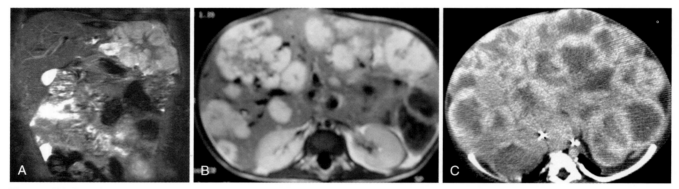

Figure 51-4 Types of infantile hepatic hemangiomas (IHH). The three variations are shown (**A** and **B,** magnetic resonance imaging; **C,** computed tomography scan). The difference between the multifocal and diffuse types is that the diffuse types have no or little normal intervening hepatic parenchyma between the tumor nodules.

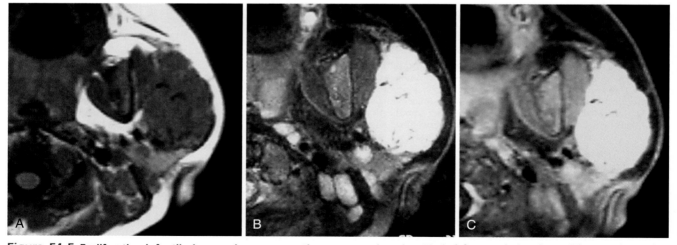

Figure 51-5 Proliferative infantile hemangioma: magnetic resonance imaging. Typical features during the proliferative phase of an infantile parenchymal hemangioma: T1 isodensity or hypointensity (**A**), T2 hyperintensity (**B**), and avid contrast enhancement (**C**).

a lobulated solid mass of intermediate signal intensity on T1-weighted sequences and hyperintense signal on T2-weighted sequences. Enlarged inflow arteries and draining veins can be seen. Flow voids are present. During the involuting phase, the vascularity is reduced, and

the tumor becomes smaller. MRI shows decreased flow voids, and the mass becomes more lobular, with evidence of fatty changes and less parenchymal enhancement.

During imaging, RICH can be confused with AVM because of AV shunting. However, a parenchymal tumor

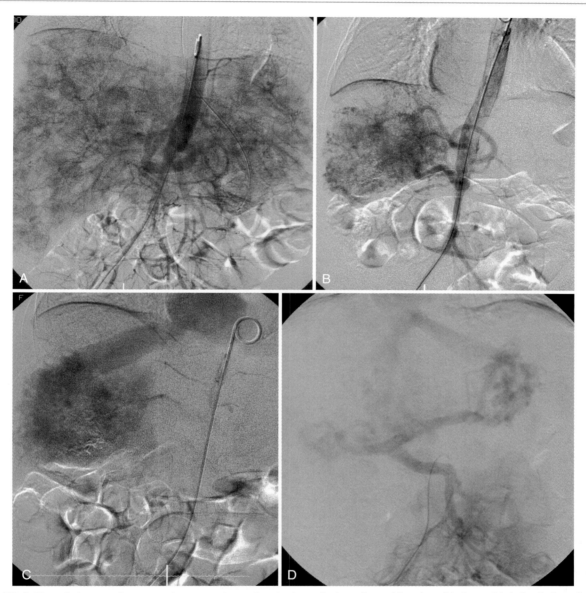

Figure 51-6 Hepatic hemangiomas: catheter angiography. Angiography is performed in selected infants with infantile hepatic hemangioma (IHH) who are in cardiac failure, to close vascular shunts and reduce the cardiac failure. **A,** Aortography in an infant with multifocal proliferative IHH shows widespread hypervascularity throughout the liver secondary to multiple IHH nodules with no vascular shunting. The aorta below celiac trunk is smaller than that above (secondary to increased hepatic arterial flow), with an enlarged hepatic artery. **B** and **C,** Aortography in another infant with a large right focal hepatic IHH shows arteriovenous shunts (hepatic artery to hepatic vein) through the vascular tumor with very large draining right hepatic vein. **D,** Superior mesenteric artery arterioportogram in another infant with multifocal IHH shows portovenous shunts (portal to hepatic veins) in the tumor nodules.

mass present in RICH is not present in AVM (see Fig. 51-2). Ultrasound studies of NICHs show subcutaneous hypervascularity in these relatively flat lesions (see Fig. 51-3). Because RICHs and NICHs are vascular tumors, the tumor parenchyma on MRI is hypointense on T1-weighted sequences and hyperintense on T2-weighted sequences and shows contrast enhancement. Calcification can be present in congenital hemangiomas. Catheter angiography is done in only a minority of infants with hemangiomas, such as at the same time as embolization, to close shunts to improve cardiac failure as in hepatic hemangiomas (Fig. 51-6), to devascularize challenging lesions in patients with kaposiform hemangioendothelioma (KHE) and

Kasabach-Merritt phenomenon (KMP) if medical therapy is ineffective, and in selected patients preoperatively.

Treatment of Hemangiomas

Most infantile hemangiomas do not require specific treatment other than observation and reassurance to the family. Previously, approximately only 10% of infantile hemangiomas were treated because they were "endangering" by virtue of their location or functional risks (e.g., airway compromise or heart failure). With current treatments readily available, more infants with hemangiomas are treated. Regular follow-up by a dermatologist is essential.

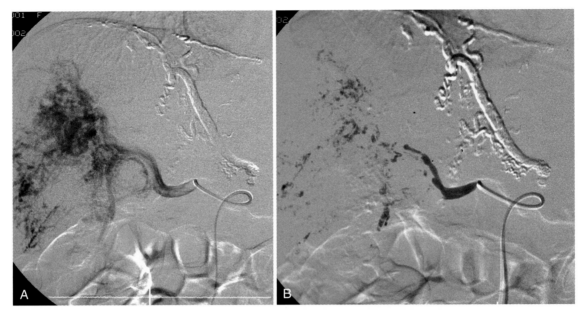

Figure 51-7 Catheter embolization of hepatic hemangiomas. Catheter angiography in an infant with a large focal right intrahepatic hemangioma and cardiac failure (same patient as in Fig. 51-6, **B** and **C**) shows the arterial supply of the hemangioma from enlarged right hepatic (**A**) and right phrenic arteries (not shown). Glue embolization of both arteries was performed to devascularize the arteriovenous shunts. Glue cast is shown in **A** (into the phrenic artery) and **B** (into the right hepatic artery).

Patients with infantile hemangiomas are treated usually with angiogenesis inhibitors, mainly corticosteroids (oral prednisone), often up until 10 to 12 months of age; the response rate is between 80% and 90%. Intralesional corticosteroid injection can be administered and is indicated for hemangiomas that cause local deformity or ulceration. Ultrasound guidance can sometimes be helpful to target the injection into the solid tumor component. Oral medication with the beta-blocker propranolol is gaining popularity as an alternative or as an adjunctive drug to prednisone. Systemic low-dose, high-frequency vincristine may be considered in challenging cases.

In selected patients, other options such as surgery with excision and debulking can be offered. Surgical resection is considered during the involuting phase in early childhood for large infantile hemangiomas and for NICHs. Laser therapy remains controversial in the treatment of infantile hemangiomas. Flash-lamp pulse dye laser must not be used because most cutaneous hemangiomas are deeper and are not affected by this laser. The neodymium:yttrium-aluminum-garnet (Nd:YAG) laser, however, can be useful for lesions in certain locations. Life-threatening large hemangiomas, especially in the liver with significant vascular shunting, require angiographic embolization (sometimes performed as staged procedures) to manage high-output cardiac failure by closing vascular shunts (Fig. 51-7). These often extremely sick infants require intensive care support throughout this life-threatening period.

Tufted Angioma and Kaposiform Hemangioendothelioma

These sometimes aggressive and invasive vascular tumors are often present at birth, although they can manifest later. KHE is usually more extensive than tufted angioma (TA). The tumors are often located on the trunk, shoulder, thigh, or retroperitoneum. TA appears as a red skin plaque and KHE as violaceous skin lesion (Fig. 51-8).

Tissue biopsy is not always required; however, percutaneous image-guided needle biopsy can be helpful. Histologic examination reveals infiltrating sheets of slender endothelial cells with positive staining for lymphatic elements.

Kasabach-Merritt Phenomenon

KMP is associated with KHE and TA. Typically, profound thrombocytopenia (platelet count usually $<10 \times 10^9/L$), coagulopathy (with reduced fibrinogen levels and elevated prothrombin and partial thromboplastic times), and bleeding are evident. Treatment is medical because the tumor is large and extensive. Low-dose intravenous vincristine and oral corticosteroids are usually given. In KMP, the mortality rate is between 20% and 30%. These tumors show proliferation into early childhood, with eventual incomplete regression, even though patients are otherwise asymptomatic.

■ VASCULAR MALFORMATIONS

Vascular malformations are classified according to the type of vascular channel affected (capillaries, lymphatics, veins, and arteries) or combinations of such channels. Clinical phenotypes include focal and diffuse forms, and although most of these malformations occur sporadically, inheritance is observed in familial cases. Complex forms can be associated with soft tissue and skeletal abnormalities.

Investigators have proposed that vascular malformations result from genetic mutations leading to dysfunction in the regulation of endothelial proliferation. Mutations in the following causative genes have been

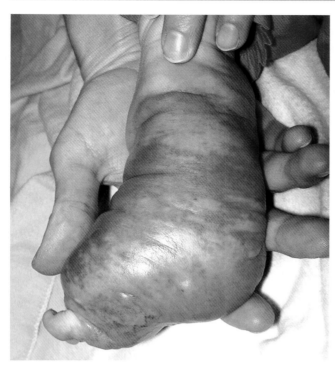

Figure 51-8 Kaposiform hemangioendothelioma (KHE). KHE affecting the lower extremity in this infant shows typical intense violaceous discoloration of the skin with swelling of the affected area.

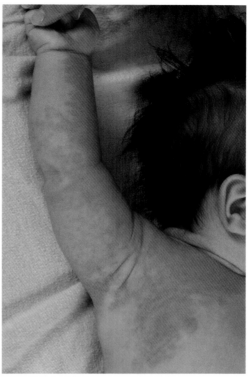

Figure 51-9 Capillary malformation (CM). Typical pink and red skin discoloration of a CM, otherwise known as a port-wine stain.

identified in patients with inherited phenotypes; the *RASA-1* gene (in CM-AVM and Parkes Weber syndrome), the glomulin gene (in glomovenous malformation), and the angiopoietin/*TIE2* receptor gene (in mucocutaneous VMs). Autosomal dominant inheritance patterns have been identified in hereditary hemorrhagic telangiectasia (HHT) and in the *PTEN* hamartoma tumor syndrome, in which AVMs are seen.

Lymphatic vessels are thought to develop from preexisting veins and express a unique receptor for vascular endothelial growth factor (e.g., VEGF-3). Posterior cervical lymphatic malformations are seen in several sporadic chromosomal syndromes including trisomy 13, 18, and 21, as well as in Turner and Noonan syndromes.

Occasionally, vascular malformations exhibit enlargement and sometimes endothelial hyperplasia, triggered by clotting, ischemia, or partial resection. These features account for their propensity for recurrence after certain treatments.

Capillary Malformations

CMs are commonly called port-wine stains. CM is the most common vascular malformation and is present at birth as a flat, pink-red cutaneous lesion (Fig. 51-9). The skin stains are commonly located as focal lesions in the head and neck area. They can be localized or extensive. On histologic examination, cutaneous CMs have dilated capillary to venule-size vessels located in the dermis that slowly dilate over time, thus resulting in a darker color and nodular appearance. CMs do not fade and are permanent throughout life.

Syndromic CMs occur more rarely, such as in Sturge-Weber syndrome (in which the CM affects the first and second trigeminal dermatomes and is associated with ipsilateral leptomeningeal vascular malformations and cerebral atrophy) and in complex combined vascular malformations such as KTS.

The diagnosis of CM is clinical, and no imaging is required. In patients with syndromic CMs, imaging with MRI is done to evaluate the associated underlying anomalies (e.g., in patients with Sturge-Weber syndrome, MRI reveals intracranial pial vascular enhancement and gyriform calcifications).

Treatment of CMs is for cosmesis, and flash-lamp pulse dye laser therapy is the treatment of choice. Multiple treatments are needed. Up to 70% of patients will show lightening of the skin stain.

■ LYMPHATIC MALFORMATIONS

Lymphatic malformations (LMs) are defined as macrocystic LMs (maximum cyst diameter, >1 cm), microcystic LMs (maximum cyst diameter, <1 cm), or mixed macrocystic and microcystic LMs. This classification better describes these lesions, and older terminology such as cystic hygromas and lymphangiomas should no longer be used because they do not describe the components of the LM.

Clinical Features

LMs often manifest as localized masses, sometimes infiltrative (Fig. 51-10), although they can also manifest with fluid leakage such as chylous fluid in body cavities or weeping from skin vesicles. LMs are usually noted at birth; however, they can be seen at any age, including prenatally on imaging. Although skin and soft tissues are most commonly affected, LMs can involve subcutaneous tissues, muscle (along the fascial planes), bone, and, more rarely, viscera such as the GI tract and lungs. The axilla, thorax, cervicofacial region. mediastinum, retroperitoneum, buttock, and anogenital regions are commonly affected. Soft tissue and skeletal hypertrophy can occur in patients with LMs. Macrocystic LMs appear as soft, compressible masses. Slight blue skin discoloration result from intralesional bleeding. Lymphedema can occur with diffuse infiltration of subcutaneous tissues. Infection and intralesional bleeding can occur in LMs and sometimes lead to alarming expansion of the lesion.

The problems associated with LMs can often be related to their location (e.g., proptosis from periorbital LMs, airway obstruction in cervicofacial LMs, protein-losing enteropathy in GI tract disease). LMs of the extremities can be associated with overgrowth and limb length discrepancy. In Gorham syndrome (soft tissue and skeletal LMs leading to progressive osteolysis), pathologic fractures and vertebral instability can occur.

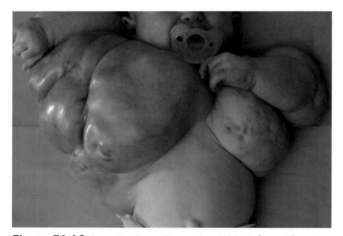

Figure 51-10 Lymphatic malformation (LM). Infant with a giant mixed LM with expansion of the chest wall and upper extremities as a result of disease involvement.

Imaging

LMs are best characterized by ultrasonography and MRI (Figs. 51-11 and 51-12). MRI better documents the full extent of deeper, larger, and more complex LMs. Cystic components on ultrasound and MRI are easily seen when cysts are larger than 1 cm in diameter. Microcystic LMs have cysts ranging in size up to 1 cm in diameter and often appear as predominantly solid lesions with no identifiable cysts on imaging. On MRI, LMs are hypointense on T1-weighted imaging and hyperintense on T2-weighted imaging (because of high water content). Macrocystic LMs show septal contrast enhancement. Microcystic LMs may show either no contrast enhancement or ill-defined enhancement of the entire lesion. Fluid-fluid levels in cysts result from layering of protein or blood. Enlarged or anomalous venous channels can sometimes be seen in close proximity to LMs. Contrast lymphangiography can identify abnormal lymphatic channels and leaks in those lymphatic anomalies of the thoracic duct and chylous effusions.

Treatment

The indications for treatment of LMs include recurrent infections, cosmesis, deformity, dysfunction, and leakage of fluid from the LM into body cavities or skin. Treatment options include injection sclerotherapy, surgery, and occasionally laser (interstitial and bare fiber surface laser treatment). Various treatment modalities may be needed. Focal and macrocystic lesions can be treated by both sclerotherapy and resection (Fig. 51-13). The advantage of sclerotherapy for macrocystic LMs is that the patient has no surgical scar, and surgical treatment may have a risk of neurovascular injury and other potential complications, depending on the location of the lesion. Diffuse and predominantly microcystic LMs are difficult to eradicate, although sclerotherapy can offer some reduction in lesion size, depending on the number of cysts that can be injected.

Surgical resection of complex and microcystic LM can be beneficial and usually must be well planned and staged. The recurrence rate after surgery for this type of LM is approximately 40% and is the result of regrowth and reexpansion of residual disease that

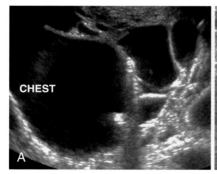
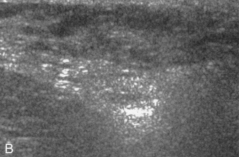
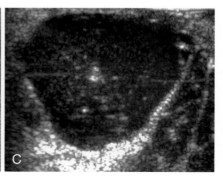

Figure 51-11 Lymphatic malformation (LM): ultrasound (same patient as in Fig. 51-10). **A,** Cysts of varying size (macrocysts and microcysts). **B,** "Solid" echogenic tissue in a different location in LM secondary to microcystic disease with no ultrasonically visible cysts. **C,** Echogenic fluid in LM cyst from intralesional hemorrhage.

remains at surgery. Scars from multiple surgical procedures are not uncommon and can themselves lead to disfigurement, pain, and functional impairment. New disease can develop in the skin along the edges of surgical scars. Investigators have suggested that sclerotherapy of the resection cavity may help reduce disease recurrence.

Intralesional bleeding causing sudden enlargement of LMs and pain can be treated conservatively with analgesics. LM enlargement occurring with systemic viral or bacterial infections usually resolves without specific treatment. Bacterial infections in the LM and resulting in a cellulitis-like presentation with reddening, enlargement, hardening, and pain require appropriate antibiotics, often intravenous.

When sclerotherapy for LMs is performed in children, most procedures are carried out using general anesthesia (as when treating most other vascular anomalies in childhood). This approach provides a safe, controlled, pain-free environment enabling procedures to be done efficiently and effectively. Cysts to be treated are evaluated with ultrasound, the patient is placed into an optimum position to access the cysts, and the skin is prepared. Dexamethasone (0.1 mg/kg body weight; maximum, 8 mg) and cefazolin (30 mg/kg body weight; maximum, 1 g) are given intravenously. Cysts are then punctured with a 21- or 22-gauge needle (sheathed or nonsheathed) with ultrasound guidance. Fluid is aspirated, and sclerosant is injected. Small drains (5 French) can be placed into one or more of the larger macrocysts, again with ultrasound

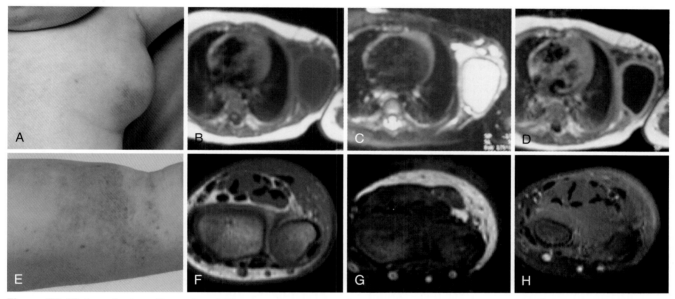

Figure 51-12 Lymphatic malformation (LM): magnetic resonance imaging (MRI) appearance. MRI can differentiate microcystic LM (A to D) from macrocystic LM (E to H). Both types appear hypointense on T1-weighted images (B and F) and hyperintense on T2-weighted images (C and G). Contrast enhancement patterns are different, with cyst wall enhancement in macrocystic LMs (D) and none to minimal overall lesion enhancement in microcystic LMs (H). Blood and protein contents in larger cysts alter the appearance.

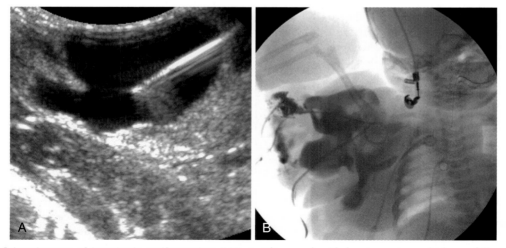

Figure 51-13 Sclerotherapy of lymphatic malformation (LM). A, Ultrasound-guided cyst puncture, which was followed by cyst aspiration and sclerosant injection for LM. For patients with large macrocysts, percutaneous drains (B) can be placed, and sclerosant injection can be repeated in 24 hours through the existing drains.

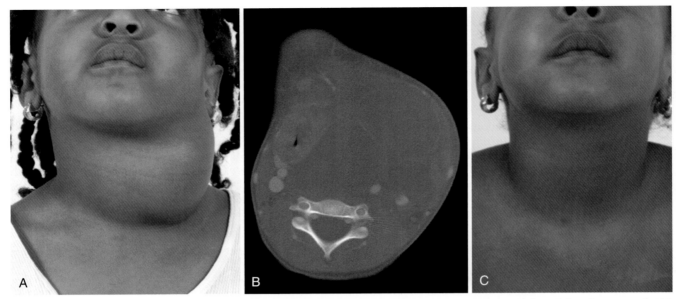

Figure 51-14 Macrocystic lymphatic malformation (LM): sclerotherapy results. A, A young patient with large left neck macrocystic LM. **B,** Computed tomography scan shows several large macrocysts causing displacement of the airway to the left side. **C,** Significant improvement and normal neck appearance are noted following doxycycline sclerotherapy with cyst drainage.

guidance, and cyst fluid is aspirated before the sclerosant is injected. Sclerosant agents used for intralesional sclerotherapy of LMs include doxycycline, sodium tetradecyl sulphate, ethanol, and bleomycin.

Doxycycline is commonly used as a solution with sterile water, at a concentration of 10 mg/mL in doses up to 300 mg for babies and 1200 mg for children 12 years old and older. When doxycycline is used, half the volume of the aspirated fluid is replaced with the doxycycline solution. Some cysts visible on ultrasound are too small to be aspirated, and therefore, a small volume of sclerosant is injected into these cysts. When drains have been placed into the larger macrocysts, these should be closed for 4 to 6 hours after sclerosant injection and then opened. If needed, repeat sclerosant can be injected the following day before drain removal. LM sclerotherapy results in scarring and cyst collapse and may need to be repeated at a 6-week interval between injection treatments. For well-localized macrocystic LMs, sclerotherapy can be curative (Fig. 51-14). For more diffuse and complex LMs, sclerotherapy can lead to much improvement, and treatments usually must be staged. Weeping or bleeding from cutaneous vesicles can be controlled with local injection sclerotherapy, although leakage generally resumes within 24 months.

Additional therapies such as tracheostomy are sometimes required to support vital functions. This need depends on the location of the LM and the consequences either of the disease or the treatments needed.

■ VENOUS MALFORMATIONS

Clinical Features

VMs, like LMs, are slow-flow lesions. However, VMs consist of venous channels that can arise anywhere in the body, although they are more commonly seen in the skin and soft tissues. VMs may be evident at birth or, more commonly, later in childhood. Their appearance is variable and includes varicosities, vein ectasias, discrete spongy masses, and complex channels permeating tissues and organs. VMs are the most common type of vascular malformation seen in specialized clinics. These lesions may be focal, multifocal, or diffuse in their involvement, and they generally enlarge slowly, with normal growth during childhood and increased growth during puberty. However, VMs can become symptomatic at any age. On physical examination, they appear as soft, bluish, compressible lesions that increase in size with dependency or during the Valsalva maneuver (Fig. 51-15). Localized intralesional coagulopathy is seen, particularly in VMs with diffuse intramuscular involvement (in which elevated D-dimer and low fibrinogen levels can be detected in peripheral blood). Intralesional clotting occurs, sometimes associated with acute pain.

Associated muscle wasting can be evident in patients with diffuse disease. Involvement of bones and joints may lead to pathologic fractures, recurrent hemarthroses, and arthritis. The arthritis resembles hemophiliac arthropathy. In patients with a diffuse type of VM, pulmonary hypertension has been recognized. Whether this is caused by recurrent silent pulmonary emboli is unclear, and screening is recommended.

VMs can affect any part of the GI tract and are often multiple. When associated with VMs of the pelvis and perineum, these malformations are more commonly located in the descending colon and rectum. GI bleeding, which is typically chronic, can result in anemia. In the blue rubber bleb nevus syndrome (or Bean syndrome), multifocal VMs are seen in the skin (typically on the palms of the hands and soles of the feet) and soft tissues in addition to the GI tract. Polypoid GI VMs can cause intussusception. The diagnosis of the GI involvement is best made by endoscopy, including wireless

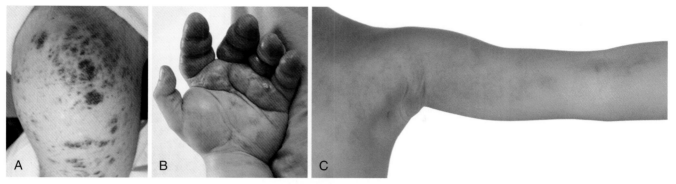

Figure 51-15 *Venous malformations (VMs): variable clinical appearance.* **A,** Typical blue skin lesions of VM. **B,** In a different patient, compressible swelling of the palm and fingers in extremity VM. **C,** In a different patient, a "varicose" type of extremity VM.

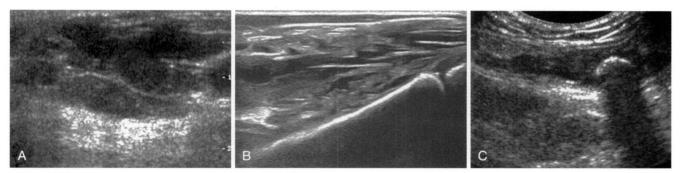

Figure 51-16 *Venous malformations (VMs): ultrasound appearance.* **A,** Typical "lakelike" hyporeflective soft tissue VM. Echogenic fibrin stranding is often noted, and intralesional thrombi are sometimes seen. **B,** Intramuscular VM. **C,** Echogenic phlebolith within the VM.

capsule endoscopy. Surgical and endoscopic treatment options should be considered for patients with GI VMs if bleeding is problematic. The VMs outside the GI tract in the blue rubber bleb nevus syndrome generally respond well to injection sclerotherapy.

Hepatic VMs of the liver, which are often incidental findings, are commonly diagnosed in adults as hepatic hemangiomas. Spontaneous or traumatic rupture, often with devastating consequences, is extremely rare. The most common indications for treatment of these lesions are persistent abdominal discomfort and when malignant disease cannot be excluded; in these cases, surgical excision is required.

Histologically, VMs most often consist of sinusoidal vascular spaces with thin walls, abnormal smooth muscle cells, and variable communications with adjacent veins. Intralesional thrombi can occur and calcify, thus forming phleboliths. In glomovenous malformations, a VM variant, the vascular channels are lined by glomus cells.

Imaging

Ultrasound and MRI are the imaging modalities of choice to identify the lesion, evaluate local involvement (including potential osseous and articular disease), and confirm the diagnosis when required (Figs. 51-16 to 51-18). Ultrasound is helpful to assess more superficial and focal lesions. Ultrasound typically shows a hyporeflective lesion, sometimes compressible and showing refilling when the transducer pressure is reduced, with variable solid elements within the lesion and occasionally hyperreflective phleboliths. MRI is highly tissue specific, with lesions hypointense on T1-weighted sequences, hyperintense on T2-weighted sequences, and showing lesion enhancement after contrast. Intralesional high signal on T1-weighted sequences results from intralesional thrombi. Contrast enhancement is seen and may be nonuniform throughout the lesion. Pathognomonic phleboliths (calcified thrombi) can be seen within the lesion as signal voids on T2-weighted sequences. Phleboliths do not occur in vascular tumors or other vascular malformations, and their presence, together with the contrast enhancement pattern, distinguishes VMs from other vascular anomalies.

Direct puncture venography and conventional venography may be required and are undertaken at the time of injection sclerotherapy. No reason exists to perform direct puncture venography before sclerotherapy.

Treatment

The indications for treatment of VMs are appearance, pain, loss of function, and bleeding (i.e., symptoms). A cure for VMs is difficult to achieve, apart from the most localized and therefore less problematic lesions. For extensive VMs of the extremities, conservative management with the use or graded compression stockings can achieve significant improvement in symptoms. The effectiveness of these stockings depends on their correct size, shape, and pressure (using commonly either a 20 to 30 mm Hg or a 30 to 40 mm Hg pressure garment).

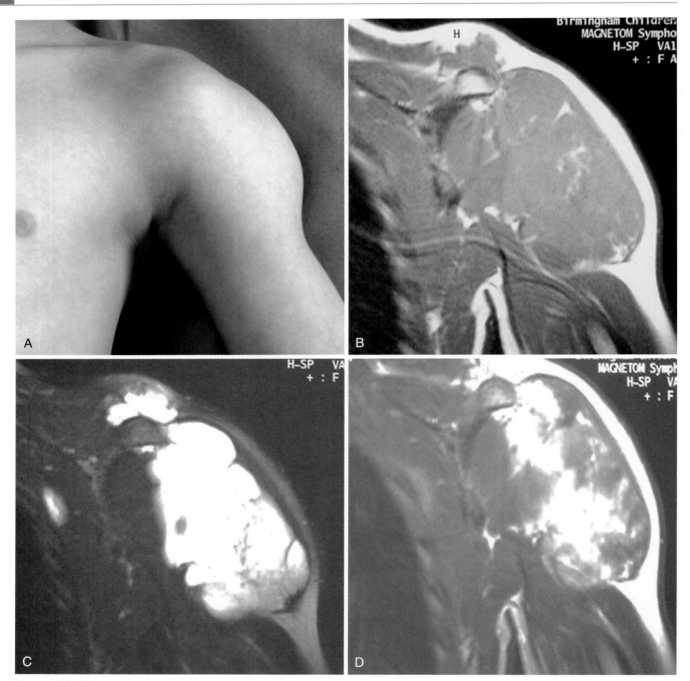

Figure 51-17 *Venous malformation (VM): magnetic resonance imaging (MRI) appearance.* **A,** A young patient with intramuscular upper extremity VM. The swelling was compressible, with an increase in size after release of the compression. The overlying skin was normal in color because of the absence of skin or subcutaneous involvement. Typical MRI findings are present with T1 isointensity (**B**), T2 hyperintensity from slowly flowing blood (**C**), and lesional contrast enhancement (**D**) with gadolinium. Hyperintense intralesional foci are the result of thrombi in the VM. Rounded focal hypointense lesions on T2-weighted imaging represent intralesional phleboliths as in **C**. Heterogenous and nonuniform contrast enhancement may be seen in VMs.

Regular stocking renewal (three to four times each year) is required because the elasticity diminishes over time, and the garment becomes less effective. Patient compliance is important to achieve the best results. In patients with troublesome pain from intralesional thrombosis (in which D-Dimer levels are elevated), low molecular weight heparin (LMWH) can be considered and must be given for several weeks, often resulting in excellent symptom relief. In patients with diffuse VMs, compression stockings should still be worn at during LMWH treatment.

Intralesional sclerotherapy is the mainstay of treatment for most VMs. The sclerosing agents most commonly used are 3% sodium tetradecyl sulfate (STS) foam and absolute alcohol, which cause direct endothelial damage, thrombosis, scarring, and reduction in size of the VM. The use of 3% STS has gained popularity

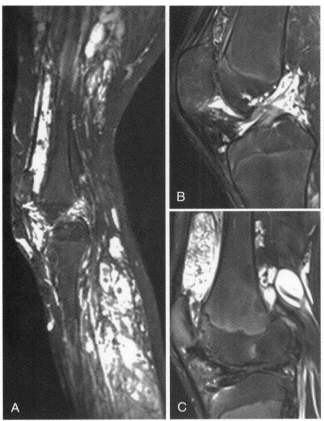

Figure 51-18 Diffuse extremity venous malformation (VM): magnetic resonance imaging (MRI). A and **B**, T2-weighted MRI (in two different patients) shows typical diffuse intramuscular VM affecting the entire lower extremity, with involvement of the suprapatellar bursa, knee joint, and cruciate ligament. **C**, Gradient T2-weighted imaging in a different patient shows intraarticular hemosiderin artifact from intraarticular VM bleeding. Recurrent intraarticular hemorrhage can lead to end-stage knee joint degenerative disease.

because of fatalities and major systemic complications associated with alcohol in adult patients with vascular malformations. Bleomycin can also be used; however, a small amount of conventional sclerosant is initially injected to promote thrombosis and blood stasis in the VM before bleomycin administration. Otherwise, the bleomycin will rapidly exit the VM at the time of injection. For 3% STS and alcohol, the maximum doses used at any one treatment should not exceed 0.5 mL 3% STS or 1 mL alcohol/kg body weight. STS can be easily made into a foam by agitating an equal volume of air with the STS liquid immediately before injecting. The injected sclerosant may be opacified for injection; however, the STS foam does not need opacification.

General anesthesia is often used for sclerotherapy. The VM is initially punctured, often at several locations with ultrasound guidance. The size (20 to 23 gauge), type (sheathed or not), and length of access needles used depend on the size and depth of the VM. Although a tourniquet can be used during treatment of an extremity VM to reduce venous outflow, tourniquets should be used with caution because they can lead to serious complications as a result of diverting sclerosant to nontarget

channels (venous and arterial) during sclerosant injection. Extremity tourniquets can aid initial direct puncture of the VM by causing distention of the VM. Once punctures are completed, venography is performed through access needles using digital substraction angiography to estimate the volume needed to fill the VM and assess possible communication of the VM with functional veins. This technique provides an estimate of the volume of sclerosant needed, which can then be injected through the puncture needles using "road mapping" (Fig. 51-19). For small very superficial VMs only, sclerosant can be injected without image guidance (office sclerotherapy). Occasional closure of large venous channels, including draining veins, is needed and this can be done using coils, glue, and endovenous laser.

In patients with a diffuse VM who have localized pain despite being compliant with garments and treated with LMWH, the site of the pain from the VM can be treated by injection sclerotherapy.

At the treated site, tissue swelling occurs following the injection of sclerosant. This swelling may be less appreciated when deeply located lesions are treated. Skin staining can also be seen when superficial lesions are treated. Swelling increases over the initial few hours after sclerotherapy and lasts for several days. Blistering of skin and mucosa may occur immediately after sclerotherapy. This blistering represents minor tissue injury and heals within 1 week, with no specific treatment needed. Complications (Box 51-1) require appropriate management and close observation and follow-up.

VMs have a propensity for recanalization and recurrent enlargement. Therefore, repeat injection sclerotherapy treatments are needed in many patients. Staged sclerotherapy is often required, and this can be done, for example, every 6 weeks. The aim of sclerotherapy is to relieve symptoms, and not necessarily significant reduction of the VM as shown on imaging, although a reduction in size can be seen (Fig. 51-20).

Laser therapy can be used in a few patients either as endovenous laser ablation (EVLA) or for interstitial treatment. EVLA may provide a useful adjunct to sclerotherapy and can be undertaken to reduce venous outflow from VMs, thus making sclerotherapy more effective. Interstitial laser (e.g., using Nd:YAG) can be used directly through percutaneous access into the VM.

When surgical resection is considered, it typically is reserved for well-localized lesions. Surgical treatment can be associated with procedural morbidity from intraprocedural bleeding in large lesions associated with intralesional coagulopathy and recurrence. Preoperative sclerotherapy should be considered to reduce the size of the VM and to decrease bleeding during resection. Other surgical techniques can be done, such as compartmentalizing of large lesions. Sometimes at the time of sclerotherapy, placing sutures throughout the lesion can reduce the size of the venous spaces in large lesions and can therefore render sclerotherapy potentially more effective. Surgical excision is often needed for patients with GI VMs that cause troublesome bleeding.

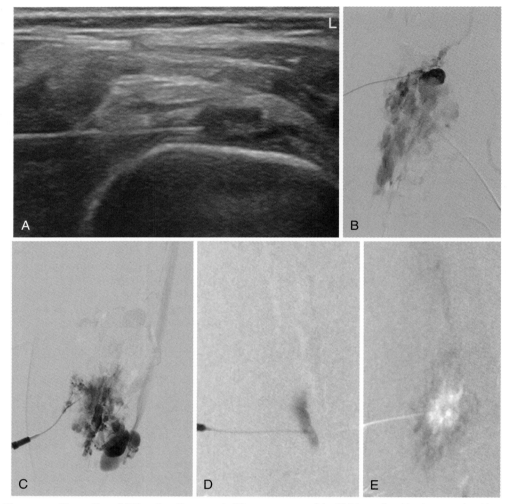

Figure 51-19 *Venous malformation (VM): sclerotherapy.* **A,** Direct puncture of the VM is made with ultrasound guidance. Often, multiple punctures are made using 20- to 22-gauge needles and sheaths, and blood is aspirated to confirm the position. Direct puncture venography is then done through puncture sites by using digital subtraction angiography with a slow frame rate. **B** and **C,** Filling of the VM during contrast injection with minor escape into the exiting veins. Sclerosant is then injected through the puncture sites by using road mapping. The volume injected is partly determined by the contrast volume needed to fill the VM. **D** and **E,** Injection of nonopacified foam sclerosant on road mapping.

BOX 51-1   Potential Complications of Alcohol and Sodium Tetradecyl Sulphate Sclerotherapy

Sclerosant effects
  Local tissue injury (blisters, tissue necrosis, nerve palsy, compartment syndrome)
  Hemoglobinuria
  Venous thromboembolic events
  Metabolic complications (e.g., acidosis, hypoglycemia)*
  Cardiorespiratory events (respiratory depression, cardiopulmonary collapse, arrhythmias)*
  Seizures*
  Perilesional fibrosis
Coagulation derangement
Procedure and device risk from catheters and implantable devices (e.g., embolic and occlusion devices)
Inadvertent embolization of blood clots and embolic agents (e.g., glue)
Age-related risk (e.g., avoidance of alcohol in neonates because of central nervous system susceptibility)

*Sclerosant effects observed with alcohol, whereas all other effects possible using both sclerosant agents.

■ ARTERIOVENOUS MALFORMATIONS

Clinical Features

AVMs are fast-flow vascular malformations characterized by an abnormal AV precapillary shunt, the so-called nidus. The presence of a nidus differentiates AVMs from congenital AV fistulas (AVFs). Often, multiple nidi are present. These shunts can be localized or extensive, and common locations include the extremities, trunk, and viscera. AVMs usually undergo slow progression in stages over many years. During childhood, the AVM grows in proportion to the child (Table 51-2). At birth, an AVM appears as a pink cutaneous skin stain and can be mistaken for a CM or the premonitory sign of an infantile hemangioma. However, high flow from AV shunting is present beneath the vascular skin stain, and this can easily be detected with Doppler ultrasound. The high flow is characterized clinically by increased growth and warmth of the affected body part, bruits, thrills, arterial aneurysms, and enlargement of draining veins. These features become progressively evident throughout childhood (Fig. 51-21). Tissue ischemia from AV shunting results in

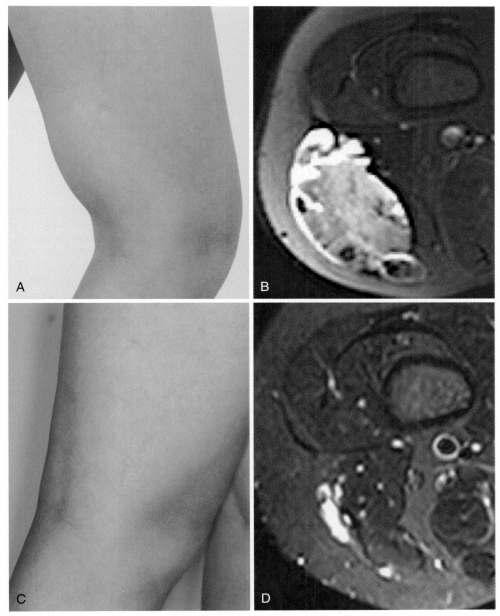

Figure 51-20 Venous malformation (VM) after sclerotherapy. A, Swelling of the lower posterior thigh from soft tissue VM. **B,** VM before sclerotherapy on T2-weighted magnetic resonance imaging (MRI). **C,** Nearly complete resolution of the swelling in the posterior thigh following sclerotherapy. **D,** Significant reduction in size of the VM with little residue on T2-weighted MRI.

Table 51-2   Schobinger Clinical Severity Classification of Arteriovenous Malformations

Stage 1	Quiescent stage (warm skin vascular stain present, mimicking a capillary malformation)
Stage 2	Expansion stage (lesion becoming warmer, bruits and thrills present, lesion enlarging)
Stage 3	Destructive stage (ulcers, hemorrhage, bone lysis, and pain)
Stage 4	Cardiac decompensation (cardiac failure from overload)

tissue pain, ulceration, and bleeding. Puberty, pregnancy, and local trauma are known to trigger rapid expansion in these lesions and increase shunting. High-output cardiac failure can be seen in patients with large, extensive AVMs.

Imaging

The diagnosis can usually be established clinically, based on history and physical examination. Ultrasound with Doppler is an excellent bedside imaging modality when lesions can be visualized. Ultrasound can easily differentiate AVMs from other lesions mentioned previously and also from other vascular malformations such as VMs. MRI and MRA are the most useful noninvasive imaging techniques to demonstrate

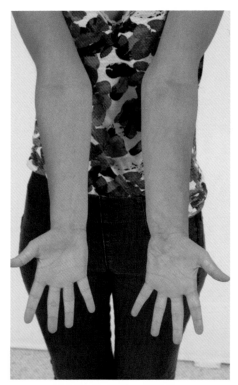

Figure 51-21 Arteriovenous malformation (AVM): upper extremity. A young teenage girl with left arm AVM affecting the forearm and hand. On physical examination, the distal extremity is larger than the opposite arm, it is warm on palpation, thrills are present at the elbow and wrist, an arterial aneurysm is palpable below the elbow, and prominent veins are visible in the forearm. These clinical signs indicate a high-flow vascular malformation.

the extent of involvement. An important imaging feature is that unlike hemangiomas, which are vascular tumors, AVMs show no evidence of parenchymal tumor, although soft tissue edema can be seen surrounding the abnormal shunts. High flow with a high density of vessels is seen on ultrasound, and on MRI, numerous characteristic flow voids are present. These lesions do not respect tissue boundaries. Catheter angiography is not needed for diagnosis and is reserved for patients when treatment is planned and undertaken (Fig. 51-22).

Treatment

Most AVMs eventually require treatment because of continued lesion expansion, which can be associated with troublesome symptoms including tissue ischemia and pain. Angiographic embolization has been the mainstay of treatment, either alone or in combination with surgical excision. Investigators have suggested that well-localized stage 1 AVMs may be amenable to surgical excision, and the outcome is better even without preoperative embolization. However, given that the full extent of the AVM may be underrecognized during early disease, embolization and surgery during infancy and early childhood are rarely undertaken because of the high risk of disease progression. An accepted practice is to observe AVMs in the early stages, monitor carefully on a yearly basis, and commence treatment when symptoms develop that indicate stage 3 disease (see Table 51-2).

Cures of AVM are rare and are reported infrequently when either embolization combined with surgery or surgery alone is undertaken. Well-localized, early-stage lesions have the best surgical results when complete resection is performed. Embolization does not cure these lesions and at best can provide control. Variance

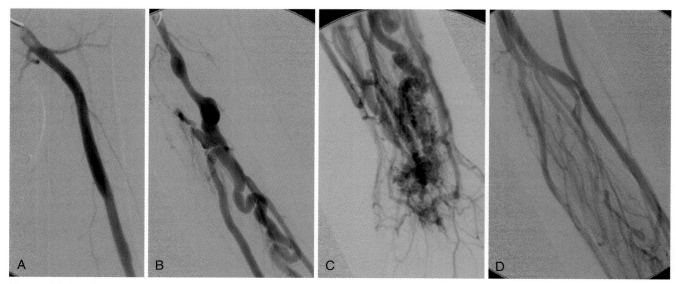

Figure 51-22 Catheter angiogram of upper extremity arteriovenous malformation (AVM). Catheter angiography is done when AVM treatment is undertaken. Global angiography is recommended so the entire arterial anatomy, shunts, and venous drainage can be studied from a proximal arterial injection. This catheter angiogram is from the patient in Figure 51-21. **A** to **D,** Arterial injection for the entire study done with a catheter in the distal axillary artery; features are consistent with an AVM. **A,** Enlargement of the brachial artery. **B,** Arterial aneurysms of the distal brachial artery with enlargement of the radial, ulnar, and interosseous arteries; the interosseous artery is tortuous. **C,** Multiple nidi in the distal forearm and palm. **D,** Early drainage into enlarged forearm veins.

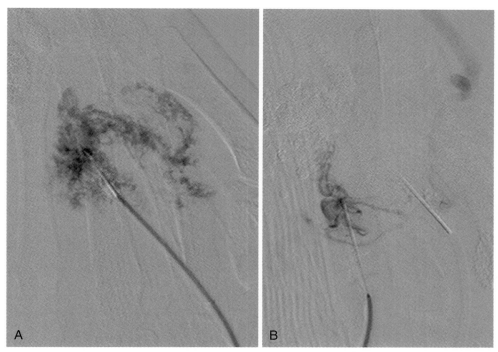

Figure 51-23 Direct puncture embolization of an arteriovenous malformation (AVM) nidus. Embolization (using alcohol or glue) of the AVM nidi can be done through an arterial microcatheter placed as close to the nidus as possible or by direct percutaneous puncture of the nidus. **A,** Direct puncture of a nidus with a 23-gauge needle and contrast injection into the nidus. Absolute alcohol was then injected. **B,** Significant closure of the nidus during repeat contrast injection after alcohol injection.

in practice is seen regarding when to commence treatment including embolization. Treatments, including embolization, are not without risk. Risk from embolization can result from the local and systemic problems related to the injected embolic agent or sclerosant, the catheter technique and devices used, and the risks from inadvertent embolization (see Box 51-1). Arterial embolizations frequently are multistage procedures targeting closure of the AV shunts through the nidi (Figs. 51-23 and 51-24). If nidal closure is not undertaken and closure, for example, is done to the proximal feeding arteries, the nidus will subsequently recruit adjacent arteries, thus leading to disease progression. Such proximal closure will compromise further embolizations because the inflow arteries have been occluded. For similar reasons, surgical ligation or closure of proximal arteries should not be performed. Direct percutaneous puncture of the AVM nidus can be an alternative technique or used in combination with arterial embolization. This procedure is not easy given that the nidi, identified on catheter angiography, can be difficult to puncture because of the small size of the channels. Closure of the venous drainage of the nidus can also be effective in achieving nidal closure, either by a transvenous retrograde approach or by direct percutaneous puncture.

Direct percutaneous nidal closure and closure of the venous drainage are techniques to consider when a transarterial approach cannot be performed, for example, when the proximal feeding arteries are too tortuous or have been previously ligated or embolized. Repeated and staged embolization procedures are typically needed, although overall they usually provide only temporary

improvement. The reason is that the large number of often small shunts makes it difficult to achieve complete occlusion. Despite this limitation, patients often have significant symptom improvement after embolization, and some cures with embolization alone have been reported.

In selected patients, surgical resection can be undertaken 2 to 3 days after preoperative embolization of the nidus. Although angiographic embolization decreases intraoperative bleeding, it does not reduce the amount or extent of tissue resected. Given that cures are rarely seen, all patients after treatment should have long-term follow-up. In patients with extensive AVMs, surgical options are not possible, and embolization is therefore the only option for symptom control. Surgical amputation is an option when extremity AVMs are located distally, the patient is severely affected, and the limb is nonfunctional.

■ COMBINED VASCULAR MALFORMATIONS

Combined vascular malformations are classified as either low flow or high flow (see Table 51-1). These more complex disorders, as a rule, are associated with soft tissue and skeletal overgrowth. The eponyms applied to several of the complex malformations can cause confusion, and it is better to describe the vascular channels affected, in addition to other tissue abnormalities.

Klippel-Trenaunay Syndrome

KTS is a low-flow combined vascular malformation involving abnormal capillary, lymphatic, and venous

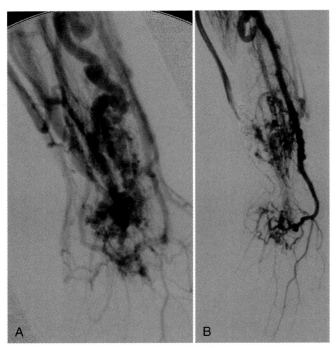

Figure 51-24 Angiography after embolization of arteriovenous malformation. The same patient as in Figures 51-21, 51-22, and 51-23, after multiple embolization procedures (transcatheter and direct percutaneous techniques). Preembolization (**A**) and postembolization (**B**) nonselective angiograms. After embolization, closure of nidal shunts in the distal forearm and palm is significant, with good preservation of digital flow, although the distal ulnar artery has been occluded during embolization procedures. The patient underwent embolization because of extremity pain, which was abolished by embolization.

channels (CLVM) associated with prominent soft tissue and bony hypertrophy. Commonly, the malformation affects a single lower extremity, although more than one extremity can be affected, in addition to truncal involvement (Fig. 51-25). The diagnosis is established clinically when the patient has at least two of the following three features: a cutaneous CM, a VM or varicosities, and hypertrophy of soft tissue and bone in the affected body part. This syndrome is sporadic, evident at birth, and varying in severity. The CM component is present in the skin often as a "geographic" stain. The venous component consists of anomalous superficial embryonic veins (especially the so-called lateral marginal vein of Serville). Deep venous anomalies can occur, such as hypoplasia and segmental atresias. A lymphatic component (LM) is variable and includes lymph channel hypoplasia, lymphedema, and cystic LMs. Often, small LMs are embedded in the surface of the cutaneous CM and can bleed intermittently.

Extremity overgrowth is obvious at birth, and although it is progressive, major changes after birth are unusual. Overgrowth can affect the length and girth of a limb, including the hand and foot. Yearly monitoring of leg length (done when the malformation affects the lower extremity) is important to assess for a potential leg length discrepancy (LLD). Radiographic monitoring of leg length is done in those children with an LLD who are older than the toddler age group, to decide whether surgical correction of an LLD is needed. Infrequently, the affected limb may be smaller and not larger than the contralateral limb.

Extremity pain is not uncommon and can have a variety of causes such as venous hypertension and chronic venous insufficiency, cellulitis, deep venous thrombosis, thrombophlebitis, osseous VMs, arthropathy, neuropathy, and growing pain.

Thrombophlebitis of the anomalous veins occurs in up to 45% of patients, and pulmonary emboli are reported in 4% to 25% of patients. Pulmonary hypertension has been recognized in patients with KTS. Whether this is the result of recurrent silent pulmonary emboli is unclear, and screening is recommended.

Bleeding can be problematic from the skin and the genitourinary and GI tracts. Patients can also be troubled with recurrent LM infections, cellulitis, and lymphedema.

Imaging has an important role in evaluating patients with KTS. Radiographs (often a CT scanogram) are needed to document LLDs. MRI can assess the type and extent of VMs and LMs and hypertrophic fatty tissue in areas of overgrowth (Fig. 51-26). MRV can help define the anatomy of the deep venous system and venous anomalies. Occasionally, this may require further invasive assessment with conventional venography performed by various techniques, including conventional pedal venography, percutaneous injection of tibial veins, retrograde catheter venography, and diversion venography (Fig. 51-27).

In general, treatment for KTS is conservative. When lower extremities are affected, leg lengths should be measured, and an LLD should be managed appropriately. Specific problems must be addressed when they arise, such as infections, bleeding, venothromboembolic events, and extremity pain. Graded compression stockings can be extremely helpful in patients with leg enlargement, venous anomalies, venous hypertension, chronic venous insufficiency, and lymphedema. Various topical treatments can be effective for skin bleeding. Although sclerotherapy can treat certain components such as focal VMs, macrocystic LMs, and bleeding capillary lymphatic vesicles, recurrence after sclerotherapy is recognized.

EVLA or surgical removal of anomalous veins producing pain or potential sources of pulmonary emboli is an option. Symptom recurrence after surgical excision of these channels is not uncommon. To reduce the size of the affected extremity (particularly the leg), surgical debulking of hypertrophic fatty tissue can be helpful. More recently, radical debulking of the subcutaneous tissues of affected extremities has been undertaken. Prophylactic anticoagulation and inferior vena cava filter placement should be considered in patients with KTS when they are undergoing long and complex interventions and surgical procedures because of the known increased venous thromboembolic risk.

Parkes Weber Syndrome

The Parkes Weber syndrome is a sporadic complex combined fast-flow vascular malformation affecting the extremities and trunk and associated with a *RASA-1* gene

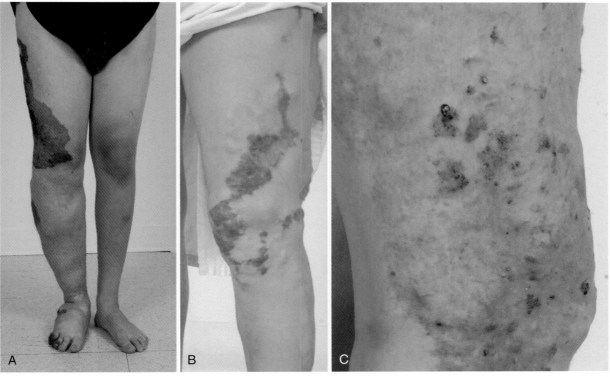

Figure 51-25 Lower extremity Klippel-Trenaunay syndrome (KTS). Three different patients with lower extremity KTS. **A,** Typical overgrowth of the affected right leg and foot with a "geographic" port-wine stain in the skin. **B,** A teenager with a typical port-wine stain and lateral varicosities. **C,** Port-wine stain that is thicker, nodular, and has blood-filled lymphatic vesicle blebs embedded on the surface of the stain.

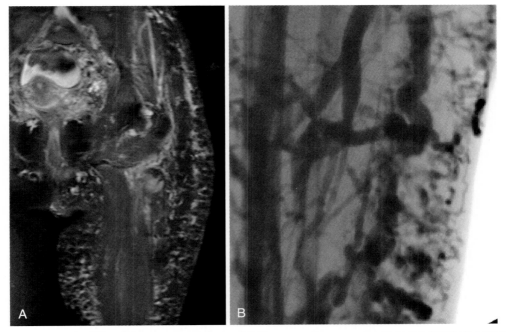

Figure 51-26 Lower extremity Klippel-Trenaunay syndrome (KTS): magnetic resonance imaging (MRI) and venography. In KTS, overgrowth of all affected tissues occurs, including the subcutaneous fat. **A** and **B,** In a single patient, numerous horizontal subcutaneous channels on T2-weighted imaging on MRI (**A**) correspond to multiple small venous channels seen on venography (**B**).

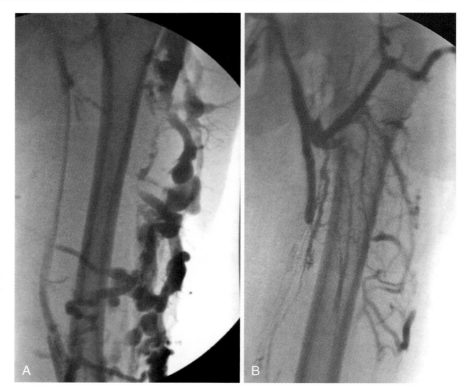

Figure 51-27 Klippel-Trenaunay syndrome (KTS): lower extremity venography. Anomalies of the deep and superficial venous system are seen in KTS. **A,** Typical embryonic vein, known as the lateral marginal vein of Serville, with multiple channels on the lateral aspect of the leg. The femoral vein is slightly hypoplastic but patent. **B,** In a different patient, partial atresia of the femoral vein.

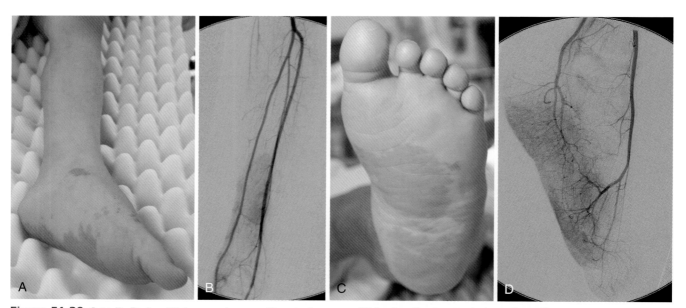

Figure 51-28 A to D, Parkes Weber syndrome with arteriovenous (AV) microfistulas. Typical pseudocapillary stain on the skin of the foot and ankle (**A** and **C**). The foot is enlarged, and several prominent veins in the foot and lower leg are present. Catheter angiography (**B** and **D**) shows multiple AV microfistulas in soft tissues of the foot and calf musculature. No macroshunts are seen. Not all patients with Parkes Weber syndrome require catheter angiography.

mutation. The lower extremity is most frequently affected. This condition can be confused with KTS because of the presence of a skin vascular stain, overgrowth of the affected body part, and prominent veins. Unlike KTS, however, the Parkes Weber syndrome is a high-flow vascular malformation because of AV shunting through multiple AV fistulas. The skin stain is not a true CM and has been described as a pseudo-CM (Fig. 51-28). The stain is warm because of the high flow, unlike the stain seen in KTS. The condition is obvious at birth, and it appears as overgrowth with a "geographic" macular pink skin stain. The clinical findings of high flow are characteristic, with increased warmth of affected area, bruits, or thrills.

MRI demonstrates enlargement of the main inflow arteries and outflow veins in the affected extremity and the region of the AVFs. MRI also depicts other associated channel anomalies.

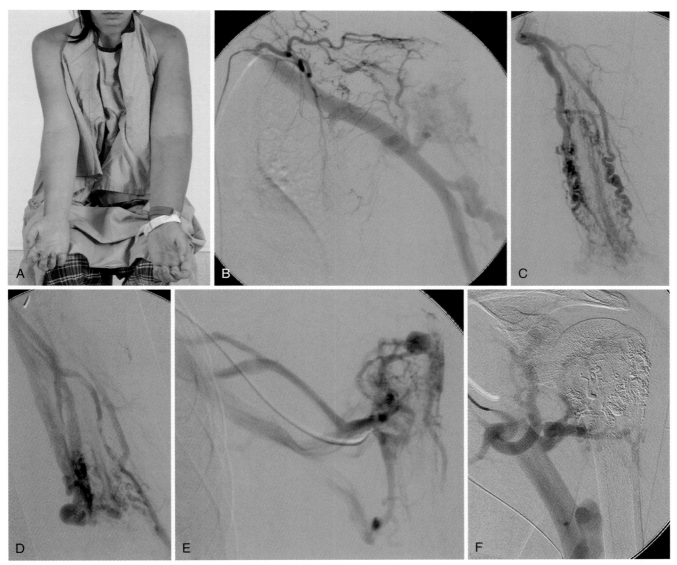

Figure 51-29 *Parkes Weber syndrome with arteriovenous (AV) macrofistulass.* A teenage girl (**A**) with cardiac overload from AV macrofistulas and shunts (**B** to **E**) in the left upper extremity at the shoulder and in the upper arm. Transcatheter glue embolization was performed to close the macroshunts at the shoulder AV fistulas. Angiography before (**E**) and after embolization (**F**) at the shoulder shows good closure of the fistulas.

Catheter angiography is not usually undertaken unless the patient has problems related to local pain or cardiac failure from volume overload. The catheter angiogram depicts enlargement of inflow arteries and draining veins and the AVFs. The fistulas are usually microfistulas, although macrofistulas can be seen (see Fig. 51-28; Fig. 51-29). AV microfistulas are unsuitable for catheter embolization. In patients with AV macrofistulas, shunt closure by superselective embolization can improve pain and high-output cardiac failure (see Fig. 51-29).

Maffucci Syndrome

The vascular malformations in Maffucci syndrome are VMs, which typically are exophytic and involve soft tissues and bones. Exostoses and enchondromas appear and manifest earlier than the VMs. Spindle cell hemangioendotheliomas are recognized as reactive vascular proliferations within preexisting VMs. Malignant transformation of endochondromas into chondrosarcomas has been reported to occur in up to 30% of cases.

Bannayan Riley-Ruvalcaba Syndrome

Bannayan Riley-Ruvalcaba syndrome is an autosomal dominant syndrome caused by mutation of the tumor suppressor gene *PTEN*. In this overgrowth syndrome, the dominant features include macrocephaly, multiple lipomas, and hamartomatous polyps of the ileum and colon. Vascular malformations occur and include cutaneous CMs, VMs, or AVMs. Typically, AVMs are located in areas of increased fatty tissue and are extremely difficult to control. Patients require long-term surveillance because of the risk of developing malignant disease, including thyroid carcinoma.

Proteus Syndrome

This rare overgrowth disorder is sporadic. Variable asymmetric features are seen in proteus syndrome, including vascular, skeletal, and soft tissue anomalies. Lipomas or lipomatosis, macrocephaly, and acral gigantism of the hands or feet may occur.

Bibliography

Alomari AI. Diversion venography—a modified technique in Klippel-Trenaunay syndrome: initial experience. *J Vasc Interv Radiol.* 2010;21:685-689.

Al-Saleh S, John PR, Letarte M, et al. Symptomatic liver involvement in neonatal hereditary hemorrhagic telangiectasia. *Pediatrics.* 2011;127:e1615-e1620.

Boon LM, Burrows PE, Paltiel H, et al. Hepatic vascular anomalies in infancy: a twenty-seven-year experience. *J Pediatr.* 1996;129:346-354.

Boon LM, MacDonald DM, Mulliken JB. Complications of systemic corticosteroid therapy for problematic haemangiomas. *Plast Reconstr Surg.* 1999;104:1616-1623.

Boyd JB, Mulliken JB, Kaban LB, et al. Skeletal changes associated with vascular malformations. *Plast Reconstr Surg.* 1984;74:789-795.

Brouillard P, Vikkula M. Genetic causes of vascular malformations. *Hum Mol Genet.* 2007;16:R140-R149.

Brouillard P, Vikkula M. Vascular malformations: localized defects in vascular morphogenesis. *Clin Genet.* 2003;63:340-351.

Burrows PE, Laor T, Paltiel H, Robertson RL. Diagnostic imaging in the evaluation of vascular birthmarks. *Pediatr Dermatol.* 1998;16:455-488.

Burrows PE, Mason KP. Percutaneous treatment of low flow vascular malformations. *J Vasc Interv Radiol.* 2004;15:431-445.

Cahill AM, Nijs E, Ballah D, et al. Percutaneous sclerotherapy in neonatal and infant head and neck lymphatic malformations: a single center experience. *J Pediatr Surg.* 2011;46:2083-2095.

Chaft J, Steckman DA, Blei F, et al. Genetics of vascular anomalies: an update. *Lymphat Res Biol.* 2003;1:283-289.

Christison-Legay ER, Burrows PE, Alomari A, et al. Hepatic haemangiomas: subtype classification and development of a clinical practice algorithm and registry. *J Pediatr Surg.* 2007;42:62-68.

De la Torre L, Carrasco D, Mora MA, et al. Vascular malformations of the colon in children. *J Pediatr Surg.* 2002;37:1754-1757.

Dubois J, Garel L, Grignon A, et al. Imaging of haemangiomas and vascular malformations in children. *Acad Radiol.* 1998;5:390-400.

Dubois J, Patriquin HB, Garel L, et al. Soft tissue haemangiomas in infants and children: diagnosis using Doppler sonography. *AJR Am J Roentgenol.* 1998;171:247-252.

Enjolras O, Chapot R, Merland JJ. Vascular anomalies and the growth of limbs: a review. *J Pediatr Orthop B.* 2004;13:349-357.

Enjolras O, Mulliken JB. Vascular tumors and vascular malformations (new issues). *Adv Dermatol.* 1997;13:375-423.

Enjolras O, Mulliken JB, Wassef M, et al. Residual lesions after Kasabach-Merritt phenomenon in 41 patients. *J Am Acad Dermatol.* 2000;42:225-235.

Enjolras O, Riche MC, Merland JJ, et al. Management of alarming haemangiomas in infancy: a review of 25 cases. *Pediatrics.* 1990;85:491-498.

Enjolras O, Wassef M, Mazoyer E, et al. Infants with Kasabach-Merritt syndrome do not have "true" haemangiomas. *J Pediatr.* 1997;130:631-640.

Fishman SJ, Burrows PE, Leichtner AM, et al. Gastrointestinal manifestations of vascular anomalies in childhood: varied etiologies require multiple therapeutic modalities. *J Pediatr Surg.* 1998;33:1163-1167.

Frieden I, Enjolras O, Esterly N. Vascular birthmarks and other abnormalities of blood vessels and lymphatics. In: Schachner LA, Hansen RC, eds. 3rd ed. *Pediatric Dermatology.* St. Louis: Mosby; 2003:833-862.

Gloviczki P, Noel AA, Hollier LH, Strandness Jr DE, et al. Arteriovenous fistulas and vascular malformations. In: Ascher E, Hollier LA, eds. *Haimovici's Vascular Surgery.* 5th ed. Oxford: Blackwell Science; 2004:991-1014.

Gloviczki P, Driscoll DJ. Klippel-Trenaunay syndrome: current management. *Phlebology.* 2007;22:291-298.

Gorincour G, Kokta V, Rypens F, et al. Imaging characteristics of two subtypes of congenital haemangiomas: rapidly involuting congenital haemangiomas and non-involuting congenital haemangiomas. *Pediatr Radiol.* 2005;35:1178-1185.

Greene AK, Perlyn CA, Alomari AI. Management of lymphatic malformations. *Clin Plastic Surg.* 2011;38:75-82.

Hassanein AH, Mulliken JB, Fishman SJ, et al. Venous malformation: risk of progression during childhood adolescence. *Ann Plast Surg.* 2012;68:198-201.

Jacob AG, Driscoll DJ, Shaughnessy WJ, et al. Klippel-Trenaunay syndrome: spectrum and management. *Mayo Clin Proc.* 1998;73:28-36.

Kassarjian A, Zurakowski D, Dubois J, et al. Infantile hepatic haemangiomas: clinical and imaging findings and their correlation with therapy. *AJR Am J Roentgenol.* 2004;182:785-795.

Leaute-Labreze C, Dumas de la Roque E, Hubiche T, et al. Propranolol for severe haemangiomas of infancy. *N Engl J Med.* 2008;358:2649-2651.

Lee A, Driscoll D, Gloviczki P, Clay R, Shaughnessy W, Stans A. Evaluation and management of pain in patients with Klippel-Trenaunay syndrome: a review. *Pediatrics.* 2005;115:744-749.

Liu AS, Mulliken JB, Zurakowski D, Fishman SJ, Greene AK. Extracranial arteriovenous malformations: natural progression and recurrence after treatment. *Plast Reconstr Surg.* 2010;125:1185-1194.

Lobo-Mueller E, Amaral JG, Babyn PS, et al. Complex combined vascular malformations and vascular malformation syndromes affecting the extremities in children. *Semin Musculoskelet Radiol.* 2009;13:255-276.

Lobo-Mueller E, Amaral JG, Babyn PS, et al. Extremity vascular anomalies in children: introduction, classification, and imaging. *Semin Musculoskelet Radiol.* 2009;13:210-235.

Marler JJ, Fishman SJ, Upton J, et al. Prenatal diagnosis of vascular anomalies. *J Pediatr Surg.* 2002;37:318-326.

Marler JJ, Mulliken JB. Current management of haemangiomas and vascular malformations. *Clin Plastic Surg.* 2005;32:99-116.

Mazoyer E, Enjolras O, Laurian C, et al. Coagulation abnormalities associated with extensive venous malformations of the limbs: differentiation from Kasabach-Merritt syndrome. *Clin Lab Haematol.* 2002;24:243-251.

Meyer JS, Hoffer FA, Barnes P, et al. Biological classification of soft-tissue vascular anomalies: MR correlation. *AJR Am J Roentgenol.* 1991;157:559-564.

Mulliken JB, Boon LM, Takahashi K, et al. Pharmacologic therapy for endangering haemangiomas. *Curr Opin Dermatol.* 1995;2:109-113.

Mulliken JB, Enjolras O. Congenital haemangiomas and infantile haemangiomas: missing links. *J Am Acad Dermatol.* 2004;50:875-882.

Mulliken JB, Glowacki J. Hemangiomas and vascular malformations in infants and children: a classification based on endothelial characteristics. *Plast Reconstr Surg.* 1982;69:412-420.

Revencu N, Boon L, Mulliken J, et al. Parkes Weber syndrome, vein Galen aneurysmal malformations, and other fast-flow vascular anomalies are caused by RASA1 mutations. *Hum Mutat.* 2008;29:959-965.

Rodriguez-Manero M, Aguado L, Redondo P. Pulmonary arterial hypertension in patients with slow-flow vascular malformations. *Arch Dermatol.* 2010;146:1347-1352.

Ryan C, Price V, John P, et al. Kasabach-Merritt phenomenon: a single centre experience. *Eur J Haematol.* 2010;84:97-104.

Sloan GM, Reinisch JF, Nichter LS, et al. Intralesional corticosteroid therapy for infantile haemangiomas. *Plast Reconstr Surg.* 1989;83:459-467.

Tan WH, Baris HN, Burrows PE, et al. The spectrum of vascular anomalies in patients with PTEN mutations: implications for diagnosis and management. *J Med Genet.* 2007;44:594-602.

Tan OT, Sherwood K, Gilchrest BA. Treatment of children with port-wine stains using the flashlamp pumped tunable dye laser. *N Engl J Med.* 1989;320:416-421.

Yakes WF, Rossi P, Odink H. Arteriovenous malformations management. *Cardiovasc Invent Radiol.* 1996;19:65-71.

Zuckerberg LR, Nikoloff BJ, Weiss SW. Kaposiform hemangioendothelioma of infancy and childhood: an aggressive neoplasm associated with Kasabach-Merritt syndrome and lymphangiomatosis. *Am J Surg Pathol.* 1993;17:321-328.

Index

A

Abscess
  aortic root, 564, 565f
  in endocarditis, 603f, 604
Absolute stent, 316b, 322, 325f
Accessory hemiazygos vein, 255–256
Acute aortic syndrome
  abdominal, 735–741
    dissection in, 740, 744f
    hematoma in, 740–741, 745f
    penetrating ulcers in, 740, 744f
  thoracic, 711–717
    aneurysm in, 715–716, 715f–716f
    dissection in, 712–713, 713f
    hematoma in, 711–712, 714f
    penetrating ulcers in, 714–715, 714f
    traumatic transection in, 713–714
Acute coronary syndrome, 382–393, 620–621. See
    also Coronary artery disease (CAD);
    Myocardial infarction (MI)
  angiography in, 620, 620f
  biomarkers in, 383
  calcium score in, 385–388, 386f–387f. See also
    Coronary artery calcium
  CT in, 389, 390f
  CTA in, 388–391, 620–621, 621t, 622f
  diagnosis of, 382–383
  echocardiography in, 384–385
  electrocardiography in, 382–383
  exercise tolerance testing in, 384
  mortality with, 621–622
  MRI in, 388, 388f, 446–447
  noninvasive imaging in, 383–385
  PET in, 465–466
  radiography in, 383–384, 384f
  risk stratification in, 383
  SPECT in, 384–385, 385f, 465–466
  symptoms of, 382–383
  troponin in, 383, 446–447
Agitated saline contrast, in echocardiography,
    18–19, 19f
Air
  mediastinal, 396
  pericardial, 209, 214f
  perigraft, 396
Air embolism, in cardiac catheterization, 47–49
ALCAPA (anomalous origin of the left coronary
    artery from the pulmonary artery), 240, 241f,
    610–611
Allen test, 769–770
Allergy, contrast-related, 20
ALN filter, 316b, 330, 330f
Amplatzer septal occluder, 304, 306f
Amplatzer vascular plug, 330–331, 331f
Amyloidosis, 514
  echocardiography of, 11f, 31f, 514
  MRI of, 462f, 462t, 514, 514f, 654, 655f
  vs. retroperitoneal fibrosis, 747, 747f
Anaconda stent graft, 313–315, 316b, 317f
Ancure endograft, 316–317, 316b, 319f
Anesthesia, in transesophageal echocardiography,
    21
AneuRx stent graft, 313, 316b, 316f
Aneurysm
  aberrant right subclavian artery, 187, 188f
  anterior communicating artery, 160–161, 161f
  aortic. See Aortic aneurysm
  aortic arch, in tuberculous aortitis, 421, 421f
  brachial artery, 761–763, 763f
  bronchial artery, 721–722, 723f–724f
  coronary artery, 243, 243f, 535, 611–612,
    612f–613f
  coronary artery bypass graft, 638–639, 640f
  femoral artery, 781, 783f
  interatrial septum, 28, 28f, 648–649, 649f
  interventricular septum, 662–663, 663f
  left ventricular apex, 8f
  in Loeys-Dietz syndrome, 717
  mitral valve, 565f
  persistent sciatic artery, 783, 784f
  popliteal artery, 781–783, 783f

Aneurysm (*Continued*)
  pulmonary artery, 678–679, 679f, 681
  Rasmussen, 679–680
  saphenous vein graft, 638–639, 640f
  sinus of Valsalva, 716–717, 717f
  splenic artery, 751, 753f–754f
  ulnar artery, 769, 770f
  ultrasound of, 117–118
  upper extremity artery, 761–763, 763f–764f,
    769, 770f
  ventricular, 202–203, 205f, 458, 459f–460f
  visceral artery, 751, 753f–754f
Angiography. See also Catheter angiography;
    Computed tomography angiography (CTA);
    Coronary angiography; Magnetic resonance
    angiography (MRA)
  left internal mammary artery, 51–52, 53f–54f
  pulmonary artery, 57, 57b, 669
Angioma, tufted, 818
Angiosarcoma, 531–533
  CT of, 532–533, 533f, 653–654, 654f
  echocardiography of, 34, 34f
  MRI of, 532–533, 533f
  right atrium, 202f
Ankle-brachial index, 772, 774f, 775t
Annuloaortic ectasia (annular dilatation), 23f
Antebrachial vein, 264f
Antecubital vein, 264f
Anterior communicating artery, aneurysm of,
    160–161, 161f
Aorta
  abdominal, 726–757
    atherosclerosis of, 726, 727f
    coarctation of, 726–728
    coral reef, 726, 728f
    CTA of, 124, 129, 256, 256f, 264f, 726,
      727f–729f
    digital subtraction angiography of, 159f
    dissection of. See Aortic dissection
    endovascular therapy of, 732–735. See also
      Stent graft
      aorto-uni-iliac stent graft in, 733–734,
        740f
      chimney/snorkel stent in, 734, 742f
      endoleak with, 124, 732–733, 739f
      in juxtarenal aneurysm, 734–735, 742f
      stent migration with, 732, 739f
      in thoracoabdominal aneurysm, 734–735,
        743f
      vascular graft conduit in, 734, 741f
      visceral artery bypass grafts in, 734–735,
        743f
    fistula of, 742, 745f–746f
    hypoplastic, 726–728, 729f
    inflammation of, 743–747, 746f
    MRA of, 726, 727f
    occlusive disease of, 726–729
    postoperative, 732–735
    pseudoaneurysm of, 730, 737f
    in retroperitoneal fibrosis, 745–747,
      747f–748f
    rupture of, 741–742
    syphilitic infection of, 421
    trauma to, 741–743
    tuberculous infection of, 421
  dissection of. See Aortic dissection
  thoracic, 394–411, 701–718. See also Aortic arch
    aneurysm of. See Aortic aneurysm
    ascending, 230–231, 253
      anatomy of, 705–711, 705f
      aneurysm of, 8f, 715–716, 715f–716f. See
        also Aortic aneurysm
      aortic valve–sparing procedure of, 400–401,
        401f
      biologic graft of, 399–400, 400f
      calcification of, 191, 421
      composite artificial graft of, 397–399,
        398f–400f
      digital subtraction angiography of, 160f
      dimensions of, 15t
      echocardiography of, 23f, 24–28

Aorta (*Continued*)
  left main coronary artery from, 240, 241f,
    607–608
  MRA of, 134f, 135–137, 153f
  radiography of, 185–187
  size of, 716, 716t
  supracoronary graft of, 394–397, 395f–398f
  thrombus of, 24–28, 27f
  transection of, 713–714
  descending, 231, 253
    anatomy of, 705–711, 705f
    aneurysm of, 419, 419f, 715–716. See also
      Aortic aneurysm
    atheroma of, 24–28, 27f
    calcification of, 191, 421, 422f
    catheter malposition in, 179, 182f
    coarctation of, 708
      CT of, 193f, 708, 710f
      Doppler echocardiography of, 10, 14f
      echocardiography of, 14f
      MRI of, 573f
      vs. pseudocoarctation, 709–710
      radiography of, 189–191, 193f
    digital subtraction angiography of, 160f
    dilatation of, 205, 206f
    diverticulum of, 714, 714f
    echocardiography of, 4f, 24–28
    hematoma of, 139f, 153, 703f, 711–712
    interrupted, 707–708, 709f
    MRA of, 137, 139f, 153f
    MRI of, 226f–227f
    penetrating atherosclerotic ulcers of,
      714–715, 714f
    pseudoaneurysm of, 189, 192f
    pseudocoarctation of, 191, 194f, 706, 707f,
      709–710
    radiography of, 185–191
    syphilitic infection of, 421, 422f
    transection of, 713–714
    treatment of, 403. See also Aorta, thoracic,
      endovascular therapy of
    tuberculous infection of, 421, 421f
  dissection of. See Aortic dissection
  endovascular therapy of, 403–409. See also
    Stent graft
    CT of, 124, 125f, 127f, 129, 129f
    dissection after, 407, 408f
    endograft collapse after, 406, 407f–408f
    endoleaks after, 124, 125f, 404–406,
      404f–406f, 404t
    fistula formation after, 407–409, 409f
    infection after, 407–409, 419, 421f
    stent migration after, 407
    transient postimplantation syndrome after,
      409
  imaging of
    CT in, 701–704
      noncontrast, 701–702, 703f
      CTA in, 702–704, 702f
    digital subtraction angiography in, 160f
    echocardiography in, 4f, 8f, 13f–14f, 23f,
      24–28, 27f
    MRI in, 87, 230–231, 704–705
      black-blood, 705
      contrast-enhanced, 704
      gradient echo, 705
      noncontrast, 704–705
    radiography in, 179, 180f, 185–191, 701,
      702f–703f
  postoperative, 394–411. See also Aorta,
    thoracic, endovascular therapy of
    anastomoses imaging in, 394–395, 395f–
      396f
    fluid collections in, 395, 396f
    graft imaging in, 394–395, 395f
    perigraft gas collections in, 396
    sternal osteomyelitis and, 396, 397f
  variants of, 705–706, 705f–707f
Aortic aneurysm
  abdominal, 729–732
    aortobifemoral bypass graft for, 732, 738f

Page numbers followed by *f* refer to figures, by *t* to tables, and by *b* to boxes.

835

Aortic aneurysm (Continued)
in connective tissue disorders, 730–732
CTA of, 729–730, 731f–732f
degenerative, 729–730, 731f–734f
diameter of, 729–730
endovascular therapy of, 732–735. See also
Stent graft
aorto-uni-iliac stent graft in, 733–734,
740f
chimney/snorkel stent in, 734, 742f
endoleak with, 124, 732–733, 739f
in juxtarenal aneurysm, 734–735, 742f
stent migration with, 732, 739f
in thoracoabdominal aneurysm, 734–735,
743f
vascular graft conduit in, 734, 741f
visceral artery bypass grafts in, 734–735,
743f
in IgG4-mediated disease, 730, 737f
inflammatory, 730, 737f
multiplanar CT of, 730, 734f
mycotic, 418–419, 730, 735f–736f
radiography of, 729–730
rupture of, 729–730, 732f
stent graft for. See Stent graft
treatment of, 730, 734f
ultrasound of, 729–730, 733f
thoracic, 715–716, 715f–716f
endovascular therapy of, 403–409. See also
Stent graft
dissection after, 407, 408f
endograft collapse after, 406, 407f–408f
endoleaks after, 124, 125f, 404–406,
404f–406f, 404t
fistula formation after, 407–409, 409f
infection after, 407–409, 419, 421f
stent migration after, 407
transient postimplantation syndrome after,
409
fusiform, 189
location of, 715
mycotic, 418–419
CTA of, 419, 420f
digital subtraction angiography of, 419,
419f
MRA of, 419, 420f
PET of, 419, 421f
radiography of, 189, 191f–192f
rupture of, 715–716
saccular, 189, 191f, 419, 419f, 422f
syphilis-related, 421, 422f
Aortic annulus, 11, 15t
Aortic arch
arch-first procedure on, 402
bovine, 187, 231, 253–254, 254f, 271f,
705–706, 705f
cervical, 705–706, 706f
CT of, 253, 254f, 271f
double, 254, 707, 708f
MRI of, 190f
radiography of, 189, 190f
vs. right arch with mirror image branching,
710–711, 711f
echocardiography of, 10, 13f, 271f
elephant trunk procedure on, 401–402, 402f
hemiarch procedure on, 401
MRA of, 253, 254f
MRI of, 230–231, 271f
penetrating atherosclerotic ulcers of, 714–715,
714f
pseudoaneurysm of, 189, 192f
radiography of, 179, 180f, 185–187
right, 253–254, 254f, 706–707, 707f
with mirror-branching morphology, 187–189,
253–254, 710–711
radiography of, 187–189, 189f
tuberculous aneurysm of, 421, 421f
variants of, 187
Aortic dissection, 712–713
abdominal, 738f, 740, 744f
in connective tissue disorders, 730–732
thoracic, 712–713
beak sign in, 713, 713f
catheter-based imaging of, 712–713
classification of, 712
cobweb sign in, 713, 713f
CT of, 382, 390f, 701–704, 703f, 712, 713f
echocardiography of, 24–28, 27f, 712–713
after endovascular therapy, 397, 397f, 407,
408f

Aortic dissection (Continued)
intimointimal intussusception in, 713
location of, 712
MRA of, 153, 153f
MRI of, 712
radiography of, 701, 703f, 712–713
after supracoronary graft placement, 397, 397f
type A, 712, 713f
hemopericardium with, 542, 543f
type B, 712
Aortic knob, 185–187, 192f–194f
Aortic nipple, 183
Aortic regurgitation
aortic stenosis and, 551
CTA of, 592–595, 593f, 594t
Doppler imaging of, 9, 553–554, 555f
echocardiography of, 9, 553–554, 554f–555f,
554t
ejection fraction in, 577
etiology of, 553
LVOT in, 553
MRI of, 88–89, 89f, 573–575, 574t, 575f–576f,
576t, 578b
planimetry in, 592–594, 593f–595f
quantification of, 575–577, 576f, 576t
vena contracta in, 554
Aortic root
abscess of, 564, 565f
aortic valve–sparing procedures for, 400–401,
401f
Bentall procedure for, 397–399, 399f
Cabrol procedure for, 397–399, 400f
calcium of, 372, 372f
CTA of, 589–590, 590f
Aortic stenosis
aortic enlargement with, 579f
calcium scores for, 591
CTA of, 590–592, 591f, 591t
Doppler imaging of, 16, 551, 554f
echocardiography of, 23f, 25f, 551–553,
552f–554f, 553t
etiology of, 577–578, 578b
in hypertrophic cardiomyopathy, 582f
low-gradient, 551–553, 592, 593f
MRI of, 577–578, 578t, 579f–580f, 581b
planimetry in, 580, 581f, 591–592, 591f, 591t
quantification of, 579–580, 580f
radiography of, 205, 206f, 268f, 702f
transcatheter valve implantation in, 308, 309f
treatment of, 308, 309f, 552f–553f, 578
Aortic valve, 23f
area of, 14–15, 551, 592, 593f
bicuspid, 336–337
classification of, 595–596, 596f
CT of, 336, 337f
CTA of, 594f, 595–596, 596f
echocardiography of, 336, 551, 552f, 555f
fish-mouth appearance of, 337f
MRI of, 336, 337f, 573f, 576f, 578f, 580f
treatment of, 337
congenital disease of, 595–596, 596f
CT of, 218, 218f, 269f
CTA of, 589–596, 589f–590f, 594f, 596f
Doppler imaging of, 6, 16t, 551, 554f
echocardiography of, 5–6, 9, 23f, 25f, 269f,
551–554, 552f
Lambl excrescence of, 551, 552f
MRI of, 229–230, 269f, 571, 571b, 571t,
572f–573f
systematic approach to, 571–573
papillary fibroelastoma of, 565–566, 566f–567f,
605f
prosthetic
CT of, 568f
CTA of, 594–595, 595f
echocardiography of, 565f, 566–569, 568f–569f
quadricuspid, 596
radiography of, 204–205, 206f
transcatheter implantation of, 308, 309f
unicuspid, 551, 552f, 596f
vegetations on, 8f, 564, 564f, 603–604, 603f
Aortitis
syphilitic, 421, 422f
Takayasu. See Takayasu arteritis/aortitis
tuberculous, 421, 421f
Aortobifemoral bypass graft, 732, 738f
Aortocaval fistula, 742, 745f
Aortoenteric fistula, 742, 746f
Aortography, 158, 159f–160f
catheters for, 158–159

Aortopulmonary collateral vessels, 346, 347f
Aortopulmonary window, 179, 180f
Apadenoson, 102
Apical ballooning syndrome. See Cardiomyopathy,
stress (takotsubo)
Apical thin point, 228, 229f
ARCAPA (anomalous origin of the right coronary
artery from the pulmonary artery), 240, 610,
610f
Arch-first procedure, 402
Arrhythmias
in coronary artery disease, 621–622
in single ventricle disorders, 355
Arrhythmogenic right ventricular cardiomyopathy/
dysplasia (ARVC/D), 362–364, 508–510
criteria for, 509–510, 509t, 510f
echocardiography of, 31, 509
MRI of, 88, 173, 363, 462t, 509–510, 510f
overdiagnosis of, 363
Arterial switch procedure, 349–350, 349f, 351f
Arteriovenous fistula
lower extremity, 784, 785f
in Parkes Weber syndrome, 832–833, 832f–833f
upper extremity, 758, 759f
Arteriovenous malformation, 826–829
catheter angiography of, 827–828, 828f
clinical manifestations of, 826–827, 827t, 828f
vs. congenital hemangioma, 816–817
embolization of, 828–829, 829f–830f
pulmonary, 676–678, 678f
treatment of, 828–829, 829f–830f
visceral artery, 752–753, 756f
Arteriovenous shunt, ultrasound of, 118
Arteritis. See Giant cell arteritis; Takayasu arteritis/
aortitis
Artery. See specific arteries
Artifacts
cardiac CT, 72, 72f
carotid artery duplex ultrasound, 687
CTA, 625–626, 627f
Doppler, 114, 115t
echocardiography, 21–24
MDCT, 371–372, 372f
MRA, 148, 149f, 152–153, 152f
SPECT, 167
Ascending venography
in deep venous thrombosis, 787t, 790–791, 791f
in venous insufficiency, 804–805, 805f
Atelectasis, in pulmonary embolism, 670–671
Atheroma, aortic, 24–28, 27f
Atherosclerosis
abdominal aorta, 726, 727f
coronary. See Coronary artery disease (CAD)
lower extremity artery, 777
catheter angiography of, 774f, 776
CTA of, 128f, 775, 776f, 777
MRA of, 773f, 775–777, 775f
treatment of, 777, 778f–779f
ultrasound of, 117, 118f–119f, 773–775, 775f
upper extremity artery, 758–760
arteriovenous fistula and, 758, 759f
catheter angiography of, 759, 760f
CTA of, 758–759, 759f
duplex ultrasound of, 758
MRA of, 759, 759f
visceral artery, 747–750, 748f
Atherosclerotic plaque, 370, 371f
vs. atherosclerotic ulcer, 714–715
Atherosclerotic ulcers
abdominal aorta, 740, 744f
vs. plaque, 714–715
thoracic aorta, 714–715, 714f
Atrial fibrillation
CT in, 68–69
Doppler echocardiography in, 28–29, 30f
radiofrequency ablation of, 643–645, 655–656
thrombus formation and, 535
Atrial septal aneurysm, 338
Atrial septal defect (ASD), 338–340, 647,
657–662, 658f
closure of, 29f, 35, 340
CT of, 340, 660f–661f, 661
echocardiography of, 9, 21, 28, 29f, 338–339,
661
flow quantification in, 340
inferior sinus venosus, 660, 662f
MRI of, 339–340, 339f, 660f–662f, 661–662
occluder repair in, 303–307, 306f, 340
ostium primum, 338, 339f, 647, 660
CT of, 648f, 658f, 660f

Atrial septal defect (ASD) (Continued)
MRI of, 339f, 660f
treatment of, 662
ostium secundum, 338, 647, 658f, 660
CT of, 196f, 648f, 661f
Doppler echocardiography of, 29f
echocardiography of, 24f, 29f
MRI of, 339f
treatment of, 662
pulmonary circulation in, 194, 196f
radiography of, 194, 196f
sinus venosus, 338, 339f, 647, 658f, 660, 661f–662f
CT of, 339f
MRI of, 648f
treatment of, 662
unroofed coronary sinus, 647, 648f, 660–661
Atrial switch procedure, 347–348, 348f, 350, 351f, 655, 656f
Atrioventricular nodal artery, 221
Atrioventricular septal defect (AVSD), 340–341
echocardiography of, 340
flow quantification in, 340
MRI of, 339f, 340
Axillary artery, 262, 263f
crutch-related injury to, 768–769, 769f
narrowing of, 760f
Axillary nerve, compression of, 768
Axillary vein, 264f
thrombosis of, 794–796, 795f
Azygos fissure, 182–183, 185f
Azygos vein, 255
catheter malposition in, 182–183, 185f
dilatation of
CT of, 183f–184f, 260f
radiography of, 182–183, 183f–184f
incidental, 185f
MRI of, 227f
radiography of, 182–183, 183f–185f

B
Bachmann bundle, 215
Bahnson fabric cusp valve, 280
Bannayan-Riley-Ruvalcaba syndrome, 833–834
Barlow syndrome, 558, 597, 599f
Basilar arteries
CTA of, 248–250, 251f, 695, 695f–696f
MRA of, 248–250, 251f
Basilic vein, 262–263, 264f
Beam hardening artifact, 72, 72f
coronary artery calcium score and, 371–372, 372f
Behçet disease, 679, 679f
Bentall procedure, 397–399, 399f
Bernoulli equation, 14, 16
Binoadenoson, 102
Bird beaking, vs. type IA endoleak, 404, 405f
Bird's Nest filter, 316b, 326, 327f
Björk-Shiley valve, 282–283, 282f
Blalock-Taussig shunt, 344f
Bland-White-Garland syndrome, 240, 241f, 610–611
Blood flow
arterial, 114–116, 116f
laminar, 114–115, 116f
peripheral resistance in, 115
pulsatile, 115–116, 116f
venous, 117
Blue toe syndrome, 781
Bovine arch, 187, 231f, 271f, 705–706, 705f
Bovine pericardial valves, 288–289, 288f–289f
Brachial artery, 262
aneurysm of, 761–763, 763f
for cardiac catheterization, 44–45
catheter angiography of, 263f
dissection of, 760, 761f
embolism of, 763, 765f
fibromuscular dysplasia of, 760–761, 762f
radiation arteritis of, 766f
thrombosis of, 766–767, 768f
Brachial plexus, compression of, 767–768, 768f–769f
Brachial vein, 264f
Brachiocephalic artery, Takayasu arteritis of, 765f
Brachiocephalic vein, 226f, 255, 264f
Braunwald-Cutter valve, 280
Breathing artifact, in MRA, 153
Broken heart syndrome. See Cardiomyopathy, stress (takotsubo)

Bronchial artery (arteries), 719–725
anastomoses of, 723–724, 723f
anatomy of, 719, 720f
aneurysm of, 721–722, 723f–724f
angiography of, 721f–724f, 724
CT of, 720–721, 720f–721f
anastomoses on, 723–724, 723f
nonbronchial collateral arteries on, 722, 722f, 724b
dilation of, 721–722
embolization of, 724–725
systemic artery communications with, 723–724, 723f
Bubble study, in echocardiography, 18–19, 19f
Buerger disease, 764–765, 766f, 778

C
C-Pulse, 303, 304f
C-reactive protein, vs. coronary calcium score, 377
Cabrol procedure, 397–399, 398f, 400f
Calcification
aortic valve, 204–205, 206f
carotid artery, 688
left atrium, 201–202, 647
left ventricle, 202–203, 205f
mitral annulus. See Mitral annular calcification
mitral leaflet, 206
myocardial, 383–384, 384f
pericardial, 209, 213f, 547, 548f
prosthetic cardiac valve, 291, 292f–293f
pulmonary artery, 197f, 673, 674f
pulmonic valve, 210f
thoracic aorta, 191, 421, 422f
Calcium
in cardiac CT, 62, 71–73, 72b
coronary artery. See Coronary artery calcium
Capillary malformation, 819, 819f
vs. infantile hemangioma, 814
Carbomedics valve, 286–287
Carbon dioxide (CO_2) contrast, in catheter angiography, 157
Carcinoid syndrome
pulmonic stenosis in, 207, 209f
tricuspid regurgitation in, 560–561, 561f
Cardiac catheterization, 39–55. See also Coronary angiography
brachial artery for, 44–45
complications of, 39–40, 40b, 40t, 44t, 54–55
equipment for, 40, 45f
femoral artery for, 40–45, 40t, 41f, 42b
fractional flow reserve pressure wire placement with, 55–56, 56f
intravascular ultrasound with, 56, 56f
optical coherence tomography with, 56–57, 56f
pressure waveform ventricularization with, 47
radial artery for, 42–44, 43f, 44t
right heart, 57, 57b, 57f
risk assessment for, 40, 40b
Cardiac computed tomography, 60–78, 490–504. See also Computed tomography angiography (CTA), coronary
acquisition time in, 64
artifacts with, 71–73, 72f
atrial fibrillation in, 68–69
bradycardia in, 66
calcium in, 62, 71–73, 72b
delayed phase, 495–497, 496f
dual energy, 500–503, 501f–503f
dynamic perfusion, 498–500, 499f
ECG-gated, 60–63, 61f, 432, 432f
ectopy in, 67–68, 68f–69f
end-systolic window in, 64, 67, 67f
high heart rate in, 63–67, 66b, 66f–67f
left ventricular function analysis on, 493–495
low cardiac output in, 73–74, 74f
low heart rate in, 66
metal in, 62, 71–73, 72b, 73f
motion artifact in, 67–68, 67f, 69f
multicycle reconstruction in, 64–66, 65f–66f
noise in, 61–62
non–ECG-gated, 490–491, 491f
obesity in, 69–71, 70b, 71f–72f
physiologic considerations in, 62
radiation exposure in, 74–77, 75f
dose reduction strategies for, 75b, 76f
scan timing in, 73–74, 74f
slice thickness in, 61, 62f
stressed arterial phase, 493, 494f
technical considerations in, 62–63, 63b, 63f
x-ray tube settings in, 70–71, 71f

Cardiac magnetic resonance (CMR) imaging, 79–90, 167–169
anatomy on, 225–231, 273See also at specific structures
angiographic, 81f, 85, 452–453, 453f
black-blood, 80, 81f–82f
bright-blood, 80–81, 82f
in cardiomyopathy, 357–369, 362f, 365f–366f
cine, 81
contraindications to, 163
contrast enhancement for, 81f, 83–85
first-pass perfusion with, 83
late gadolinium enhancement with, 83–85, 84f
ECG gating in, 79
vs. echocardiography, 174
edema imaging with, 80, 82f
gradient echo, 80
imaging planes in, 85–86
limitations of, 168–169
morphologic imaging with, 80, 81f
in myocardial infarction. See Myocardial infarction (MI), MRI of
in myocardial ischemia. See Myocardial ischemia, MRI of
in myocarditis. See Myocarditis, MRI of
oblique planes in, 82f, 85–86
phase contrast, 82–83, 84f
protocols for, 86–90, 442–445, 442f
steady-state free precession, 80–81, 89f
stress perfusion, 453–456, 454f–456f, 454t
adenosine for, 86–87, 453, 455f
dipyridamole for, 86–87
dobutamine for, 82f, 87, 453
indications for, 455–456
sensitivity and specificity of, 455–456, 456f
vs. SPECT perfusion, 454–455
T1-weighted, 79–80
T2*-weighted, 79–80, 82
Cardiac tamponade, 543
CT of, 543
echocardiography of, 32f, 33, 543, 543f
MRI of, 543
Cardiac valves. See also Valvular heart disease and at specific heart valves and valvular diseases
CT of, 217–219, 218f
CTA of, 589–590, 590f, 594f, 596–597, 597f–598f, 600–602
echocardiography of, 551–555, 552f, 560, 562
MRI of, 571–573, 572f
prosthetic. See Prosthetic cardiac valves
radiography of, 179, 203–209
Cardiac veins
CT of, 221, 223f
MRI of, 230
Cardiomegaly, 200–201
CardioMEMS heart failure pressure measurement system, 302–303, 303f
Cardiomyopathy, 505–521
amyloid, 514
echocardiography of, 11f, 31f, 514
MRI of, 462f, 462t, 514, 514f
classification of, 506t
dilated, 511–512
CT of, 511–512
echocardiography of, 10f, 15f, 29, 31f
etiology of, 511, 511b
mitral regurgitation in, 558
MRI of, 88, 512, 512f
radiography of, 511
SPECT of, 512
echocardiography of, 29–33, 505
hypertrophic, 361–362, 506–508
criteria for, 507
CT of, 508, 509f
Doppler echocardiography of, 32f
echocardiography of, 10f, 31, 32f, 173, 507
vs. mass, 537
MRI of, 88, 173, 361–362, 362f, 462f, 462t, 507–508, 507f–508f
stress echocardiography in, 20
sudden cardiac death in, 361
valve assessment in, 581–582, 581f–582f
inflammatory. See Myocarditis
ischemic. See also Myocardial ischemia
echocardiography of, 22f, 25f, 29
mitral regurgitation in, 558
MRI in, 358, 360
revascularization for, 357–358, 358f
scar detection in, 360

Cardiomyopathy *(Continued)*
  sudden cardiac death in, 358–361
  viable myocardium in, 357–358, 358f
  MRI of, 460, 461f–462f, 462t, 505–506, 506t
    black-blood, 505
    contrast-enhanced, 506, 506t
    functional, 506
    T2*-weighted, 506
  peripartum, 513–514
    CT of, 513–514, 513f
    differential diagnosis of, 513
    echocardiography of, 513–514
    MRI of, 513–514, 513f
    radiography of, 505
  restrictive
    vs. constrictive pericarditis, 549–550
    echocardiography of, 11f, 29–31, 31f
  sarcoid. *See* Sarcoidosis
  siderotic, 519, 519f
  stress (takotsubo), 514–516, 515b
    angiography of, 515
    CT of, 516
    echocardiography of, 515
    MRI of, 515–516, 515f
Carotid artery
  common
    CTA of, 693–695, 695f
    dissection of, 691, 691f
    duplex ultrasound of, 689, 689f
    echocardiography of, 13f, 271f
    intima-media thickness of, 692, 693f–694f
    intimal hyperplasia of, 692, 694f
    MRA of, 248, 249f, 696–698
    MRI of, 226f, 271f
    Takayasu arteritis of, 765f
  external
    catheter angiography of, 248, 249f
    Doppler ultrasound of, 115–116, 117f
    vs. internal carotid artery, 689
    internalized, 690
    MRA of, 249f
  internal
    calcification in, 688
    CTA of, 686, 693–695, 694f
      accuracy of, 694–695
      limitations of, 695
      postprocessing algorithms for, 695
      safety of, 693–694
    dissection of, 690–691, 691f
    Doppler ultrasound of, 120f, 695
    duplex ultrasound of, 685–693
      anatomic limitations in, 689, 689f
      B-mode, 688
      color flow, 688, 688f
      contralateral occlusions on, 690, 690f
      delayed systolic upstrokes on, 689
      dissection on, 690–691, 691f
      distal lesion limitation of, 689, 689f
      excessive color gain in, 687, 687f–688f
      vs. external carotid artery, 689–690
      hairline lumina on, 689–690, 690f
      heavily calcified plaque and, 688
      indications for, 686
      insonation angle for, 686–687
      interpretation of, 689–693
      intima-media thickness on, 692
      intimal hyperplasia on, 692
      limitations of, 687–689
      luminal echo in, 687
      mirror image artifact in, 687
      normal waveform characteristics of,
        685–686, 686t
      postoperative, 686
      protocol for, 685
      pseudo-occlusion on, 689–690
      pseudoaneurysm on, 693
      pseudonormalization on, 690
      pulse repetition frequency in, 687, 688f
      rationale for, 685
      sharp systolic upstrokes on, 689, 689f
      tandem lesions and, 688–689, 689f
      technical pitfalls in, 686–687
      transducer for, 686
      velocities falling off on, 690
      vs. external carotid artery, 689
    intima-media thickness of, 692
    intimal hyperplasia of, 692
    MRA of, 150–151, 248, 249f–250f, 686,
      696–698, 697f
    contrast-enhanced, 696

Carotid artery *(Continued)*
    metal effects in, 698
    safety of, 698
    stenosis overestimation on, 698
    stents on, 698
    subclavian steal on, 698
    pseudo-occlusion of, 689–690
    pseudoaneurysm of, 693
    tandem stenosis of, 688–689, 689f
    thrombus of, 688f
Carotid body, tumor of, 691, 692f
Carpentier-Edwards perimount valve, 288,
    288f–289f
Carpentier-Edwards supra-annular valve, 289–290
Catheter angiography, 155–162. *See also*
    Computed tomography angiography (CTA),
      vascular; Magnetic resonance angiography
      (MRA), vascular
    access sheath removal in, 161
    access site for, 158, 159t
    aortic, 158, 159f–160f
    axillary artery access for, 159t
    brachial artery access for, 159t
    catheters for, 158
    color-coded display in, 160–161, 162f
    complications of, 162
    contraindications to, 156
    contrast for, 157, 160, 160t
    dilators for, 158
    equipment for, 157–158
    femoral artery access for, 159f, 159t
    guidewires for, 157–158
    historical perspective on, 155
    image acquisition/display in, 160–161, 160f–
      162f
    indications for, 155–156
    limitations of, 162
    needles for, 157
    patient assessment before, 155, 156t
    premedication for, 156–157
    pressure measurements with, 159
    radial artery access for, 159t
    sheath for, 158, 161
    subclavian artery access for, 159t
    technique of, 156–161, 157f
Catheterization
    cardiac. *See* Cardiac catheterization
    pulmonary artery, 57, 57b, 57f
    vascular. *See* Catheter angiography
Cavernous sinuses, MRV of, 253
Celect filter, 316b, 329, 329f
Celiac artery
    catheter angiography of, 256, 257f
    CTA of, 256, 258f
Central venous catheter
    complications of, 185
    fracture of, 179
    malposition of, 179–185
      in azygos vein, 182–183, 185f
      in descending aorta, 179, 182f
      extravascular, 185
      in extravascular location, 187f
      in internal jugular vein, 181f
      in left innominate vein, 181f
      in left internal mammary vein, 183–185, 186f
      in pericardiophrenic vein, 183–185, 187f
Cephalic vein, 262–263, 264f
Cerebellar veins, 251–252
Cerebral arteries
    CTA of, 248, 250f–251f, 695, 696f
    MRA of, 248, 250f, 696–698, 697f
Cerebral veins, 251
Cerebrovascular accident (CVA), cardiac
    catheterization and, 54–55
Cervical aortic arch, 705–706, 706f
Charcot joint, 422f
Chest pain
    acute, 620–621. *See also* Acute coronary
      syndrome
    stable, 618–620, 618t
Chest radiography
    in acute coronary syndrome, 383–384, 384f
    aorta on, 179, 180f, 185–191, 701, 702f–703f
    cardiovascular anatomy on, 179, 180f, 267–272,
      267f–268f
    central venous catheter malposition on. *See*
      Central venous catheter, malposition of
    heart on, 179, 180f, 200–209, 267–272,
      267f–268f. *See also at specific structures*
    pericardium on, 209–211, 212f–214f

Chest radiography *(Continued)*
    pulmonary vasculature on, 191–200, 195b
    venous anatomy on, 179–185. *See also at specific*
      veins
Chiari network, 3–5
Chordae tendineae
    CT of, 218
    MRI of, 228
Circle of Willis
    CTA of, 250–251, 252f
    MRA of, 250–251, 252f
Circumflex humeral artery
    catheter angiography of, 263f
    compression of, 768
    pseudoaneurysm of, 767f
Coarctation of aorta, 708
    CT of, 193f, 708, 710f
    Doppler echocardiography of, 10, 14f
    echocardiography of, 14f
    MRI of, 573f
    vs. pseudocoarctation, 709–710
    radiography of, 189–191, 193f
Color gain, in carotid artery duplex ultrasound,
    687, 687f–688f
Combined vascular malformations, 814t, 829–834
Computed tomography (CT). *See* Cardiac com-
    puted tomography; Computed tomography
    angiography (CTA), coronary
Computed tomography angiography (CTA)
    carotid artery, 693–695, 694f–695f
    coronary, 166, 617. *See also* Cardiac computed
      tomography
      in acute chest pain, 388–391
      arterial phase, 491–493, 492f
      artifacts on, 625–626, 627f
      in atrial fibrillation, 68–69
      bolus tracking method in, 74
      delayed phase scan with, 495–497, 496f
      dynamic perfusion imaging with, 498–500,
        499f
      indications for, 166, 618–621, 618t–619t,
        620f, 621t, 622f
      late diastolic window in, 64
      left ventricular function analysis in, 493–495
      obesity and, 69–71, 71f–72f
      in percutaneous coronary interventions, 625,
        626f
      prospective triggering in, 391
      radiation in, 74–77, 75b, 75f, 431–438
        body weight and, 435
        dose estimation for, 431
        dose for, 389, 431–432
        dose-reduction training and, 435
        heart rate and, 435
        iterative image reconstruction and, 435
        vs. noninvasive imaging radiation doses,
          436
        patient-related factors and, 435
        prospective ECG-triggered axial scan
          technique and, 433, 433f
        prospective ECG-triggered helical high-
          pitch scan technique and, 434, 434f
        protocol-related factors and, 435–436
        retrospective ECG-gated technique and,
          432, 432f–433f
        scan length and, 434, 434f
        x-ray tube current and, 76–77, 76f,
          434–435
        x-ray tube potential and, 435
        x-ray tube voltage and, 76
      risk stratification with, 621–624, 622f–624f,
        624t
      scan timing in, 73–74
      SPECT with, 482–483, 484f
      stenosis overestimation on, 626–627, 628f
      stent on, 627–628, 629f
      stressed arterial phase, 493
      timing bolus method in, 74
      triple rule-out protocol with, 389, 390f
    valvular, 587–605, 589f. *See also at specific*
      valvular diseases
      optimization of, 587–589
      postprocessing in, 588–589, 589f–591f,
        593f–594f
    vascular, 121–130
      advances in, 127–129
      automated bolus triggering in, 126, 126f
      body habitus in, 122
      cardiac output in, 122
      vs. catheter-based angiography, 121

Computed tomography angiography (CTA) (Continued)
  contrast-related factors in, 122–124
  contrast volume in, 123–124
  dual energy, 127–129
  injection duration in, 123
  injection rate in, 123
  intravenous access in, 122
  iodine concentration in, 123
  patient-related factors in, 122
  postprocessing in, 126–127, 127f–128f
  principles of, 121–126
  renal function in, 122
  saline flush in, 124
  scan coverage in, 124
  scan delay in, 124–125
  scanning parameters in, 124
  technical parameters in, 73, 124–125, 127–129
  test bolus technique in, 125, 125f
  unenhanced CT before, 124, 125f
Computed tomography venography (CTV), 129, 787–788, 787t, 789f
Congenital heart disease, 333–356. See also specific congenital diseases
  imaging techniques in, 335–336
  MRI of, 88
Congenital hemangioma, 814, 815f–816f, 816–817
Congenital pulmonary venolobar syndrome, 200, 201f, 644, 676, 677f
Continuity equation, 14–15, 551
Contrast
  agitated saline, in echocardiography, 18–19, 19f
  in catheter angiography, 157, 160, 160t
  gadolinium-based, in MRA, 138–140, 143, 148–150
  microbubble, 19–20, 19f–20f
Cor triatriatum, 647, 648f
Coral reef aorta, 726, 728f
CoreValve device, 308, 309f
Coronary angiography, 37–59, 616–617, 618f. See also Computed tomography angiography (CTA), coronary
  air embolism with, 47–49
  anatomy on, 232–247, 233f–234f, 273. See also at Coronary artery (arteries)
  anomalous artery, 239–246, 239b, 240f–242f. See also Coronary artery (arteries)
  arterial sheath removal in, 55
  blood flow on, 234, 235t
  cardiac catheterization for, 39–55
    brachial artery, 44–45
    complications of, 54–55
    femoral artery, 40–45, 41f, 42b
    radial artery, 42–44, 43f, 44t, 52–54
  contraindications to, 39b
  evaluation before, 37–39
  false-negative, 628, 630f
  false-positive, 628, 630f
  graft, 51, 53b, 53f–54f
  indications for, 37, 38b–39b, 164–166, 619–620, 619f–620f. See also Coronary artery disease (CAD), angiography of
  left coronary artery, 45–46, 45f–47f
    anterior descending, 46f–47f, 50, 235, 237f–238f, 273f–274f
    complications of, 47–49
    left circumflex, 46f–47f, 50, 235–238, 238f, 274f
    left main, 45–46, 46f–47f, 235, 237f, 237t
    views for, 46f–47f, 49–50
  limitations of, 55
  in percutaneous coronary interventions, 624–625, 625f–626f
  planes for, 232, 233f, 234t
  pressure waveform ventricularization with, 47
  renal dysfunction with, 55
  right coronary artery, 48f–49f, 50, 53f–54f, 238, 239f, 275f–276f
  risk stratification with, 621–624, 623f
  segmental flow models and, 234–235, 236f
  segmental nomenclature for, 234, 234f
  single artery, 242–243, 243f
  stent on, 627–628, 629f
  stroke with, 54–55
  SYNTAX score in, 234
  TIMI grading system in, 234, 235t
  views for, 46f–47f, 49–50, 232, 233f, 234t

Coronary artery (arteries), 606–615
  aneurysm of, 243, 243f, 535, 611–612, 612f–613f
  angiography of. See Computed tomography angiography (CTA), coronary; Coronary angiography
  anomalous, 606–608
    angiography of, 239–246, 239b. See also specific anomalies
    in athletes, 607
    classification of, 607
    CT of, 239
    echocardiography of, 239
    MRI of, 87
    sudden death and, 607
    symptoms of, 607
  atherosclerosis of, 464–465, 464b, 465f. See also Acute coronary syndrome; Coronary artery disease (CAD); Myocardial infarction (MI)
  communications between, 244–245, 244f
  CT of, 219–221, 219f–220f
  dominance of, 221
  ectasia of, 243, 243f, 611, 612f
  fistula of, 245, 245f, 612–615, 613f–614f
  high-takeoff, 240, 241f, 607–608
  hypoplasia of, 243–244, 244f
  intramural, 244, 244f
  left anterior descending, 221, 222f, 222t, 273f, 606
    aneurysm of, 243, 243f
    angiography of, 46f–47f, 50, 235, 237f–238f, 273f–274f
    CT of, 219, 219f–220f, 273f–274f
    diameter of, 237t
    ectasia of, 243, 243f
    hypoplasia of, 243–244, 244f
    right coronary sinus origin of, 242
  left circumflex, 221, 222f, 222t, 273f, 606
    absence of, 608
    aneurysm of, 243, 243f
    angiography of, 46f–47f, 50, 235–238, 238f, 274f
    CT of, 219–220, 219f–220f, 274f
    diameter of, 237t
    ectasia of, 243, 243f
    fistula of, 245, 245f, 614f
    nondominant, 238
    right coronary artery origin of, 608
    right sinus of Valsalva origin of, 242, 242f, 608
    separate left sinus of Valsalva origin of, 240, 240f, 608
  left main, 221, 222f, 222t, 273f, 606
    absence of, 219, 219f, 240, 240f
    angiography of, 45–46, 46f–49f, 49–50, 235, 237f
    ascending aorta origin of, 240, 241f, 607–608
    CT of, 219–220
    diameter of, 235, 237t
    noncoronary sinus origin of, 242, 242f
    opposite-sinus origin of, 240–242, 242f
    ostial stenosis of, 243, 243f
    posterior sinus of Valsalva origin of, 608
    pulmonary artery origin of, 240, 241f, 610–611
    right sinus of Valsalva origin of, 242, 607–609, 609f
    rudimentary, 242–243, 243f
    separate left sinus of Valsalva origin of, 608
  myocardial bridging of, 244, 244f, 611, 611f
  ostial stenosis of, 243, 243f
  radionuclide imaging of. See Positron emission tomography (PET); Single-photon emission computed tomography (SPECT)
  right, 221, 275f, 606
    acute marginal branch of, 220, 220f
    aneurysm of, 613f
    angiography of, 48f–49f, 50, 238, 239f, 275f–276f
    anomalous opposite-sinus origin of, 240–242, 242f
    CT of, 220–221, 220f, 275f–276f
    diameter of, 237t
    left circumflex artery origin from, 608
    left sinus of Valsalva origin of, 242, 242f, 609–610, 610f
    noncoronary sinus origin of, 242, 242f
    posterior sinus of Valsalva origin of, 608
    pulmonary artery origin of, 610–611, 610f

Coronary artery (arteries) (Continued)
  segmentation classification of, 221, 222f, 222t, 234, 234f
  single, 242–243, 243f, 608, 609f
  spasm of, 628, 630f
  stress testing of. See Stress testing
Coronary artery bypass graft (CABG), 632–642
  aneurysm of, 638–639, 640f
  angiography of, 51, 53b, 53f–54f
  CT perfusion imaging of, 498–500, 499f
  kinking of, 637
  left internal mammary artery graft in, 473, 474f, 634–635, 636f
  malposition of, 637
  multidetector CT of, 632
    limitations of, 641
    radiation dose with, 641
    for reoperation, 640, 641f
    technique of, 633
  occlusion of, 638, 638f–639f
  patency of, 638, 638f–639f
  PET of, 473
  radial artery graft in, 635–636, 769–770, 770f
  reoperation for, 640, 641f
  right gastroepiploic artery graft in, 636
  right internal mammary artery graft in, 635, 637f
  rubidium-82 perfusion imaging of, 473, 474f
  saphenous vein graft in, 633–634, 634f–635f
    occlusion of, 638, 638f–639f
  SPECT of, 473
  thrombosis of, 637
  vasospasm of, 637
Coronary artery calcium, 370–381
  in asymptomatic patients, 379
  EDTA effects on, 378
  electron beam tomography for, 370
  in end-stage renal disease, 378–379
  estrogen effects on, 378
  garlic effects on, 378
  lipid effects on, 377–378
  multidetector CT for, 370, 371f–372f
  nanobacteria effects on, 378
  pathophysiology of, 370
  plaque area and, 370, 371f
  progression of, 377–379
  scoring for, 370–371
    in acute coronary syndrome, 385–388, 386f–387f
    aortic root calcium and, 372, 372f
    beam hardening artifact and, 372f
    vs. C-reactive protein, 377
    in CAD risk stratification, 621–622, 624t
    vs. carotid IMT, 377
    in diabetes, 376
    epidemiology of, 372–373, 374f
    guidelines for, 373–375
    in heart failure, 376
    vs. lipoprotein levels, 376–377
    mitral annular calcification and, 371, 372f
    nomogram for, 372–373, 373f
    prognostic value of, 375–376
    with radionuclide imaging, 481–483, 483f
    sensitivity of, 376
    specificity of, 376
    in symptomatic patients, 376
    treatment recommendations and, 376
    very high scores with, 375
    very low scores with, 375–376
  sevelamer effects on, 378–379
  statin effects on, 377–378
Coronary artery disease (CAD), 616–631. See also Acute coronary syndrome; Myocardial infarction (MI); Myocardial ischemia
  angiography of, 616–617, 618f–620f, 628. See also Coronary angiography
    false-negative, 628, 630f
    false-positive, 628, 630f
    indications for, 619–620, 619f–620f
    risk stratification with, 621–622, 623f
    spasm on, 628, 630f
  asymptomatic, 171
  calcium scoring in. See Coronary artery calcium
  CTA of, 616–617, 618f, 618t, 620f. See also Computed tomography angiography (CTA), coronary
    artifacts on, 625–626, 627f
    indications for, 618–621, 618t–619t, 621t
    risk stratification with, 621–624, 623f–624f, 624t

Coronary artery disease (CAD) *(Continued)*
  stenosis overestimation on, 626–627, 628f
  stent on, 627–628, 629f
  definition of, 616, 617f
  ECG in, 473
  fractional flow reserve in, 164–165
  heart failure and, 473–481, 621
  imaging of, 163–176, 165f
    anatomic methods for, 164–166, 166t.
      See also Computed tomography
        angiography (CTA), coronary;
        Coronary angiography
    in asymptomatic individuals, 171
    indications for, 163–164, 164b
    physiologic methods for, 166t, 167–169. *See
      also* Echocardiography, stress;
      Positron emission tomography (PET);
      Single-photon emission computed
      tomography (SPECT)
    pretest disease probability in, 164, 166t
    radiation dose in, 171, 171t
    test selection in, 164–171, 165f
  molecular imaging in, 485
  MRA of, 452–453
  multivessel
    PET of, 473, 476f–477f
    SPECT of, 473
  pathophysiology of, 370, 464–465, 464b, 465f
  perfusion MRI of, 453–456, 454f–456f, 454t
  PET of, 466–473
    calcium scoring with, 481–483, 483f
    cold pressor, 470
    coronary flow reserve on, 469–470
    cost effectiveness of, 472–473
    multivessel disease on, 473, 476f–477f
    patient management with, 471
    risk stratification with, 469–470, 472t
    sensitivity and specificity of, 466–467
  plaque area in, 370, 371f
  preclinical, 464–465, 464b, 465f
  risk stratification in
    coronary angiography in, 621–622, 623f
    CTA in, 621–624, 623f–624f, 624t
    PET in, 469–470, 472t
    SPECT in, 467–469, 469b, 470f–471f, 471t
  SPECT of, 466–473
    attenuation artifacts in, 467
    attenuation correction in, 467, 468f–469f
    cost effectiveness of, 472–473
    CT-based attenuation correction in, 467
    multivessel disease on, 473
    patient management with, 471, 472f
    risk stratification with, 467–469, 469b,
      470f–471f, 471t
    sensitivity and specificity of, 466–467
  stable chest pain and, 618–620, 618t–619t
  stent for, CTA of, 627–628, 629f
Coronary sinus
  CT of, 215–216, 216f, 221, 223f, 271f
  echocardiography of, 271f
  MRI of, 225–226, 227f, 228, 230, 271f
Coronary vein, 261–262
Coumadin ridge, 227f, 649–650
Crista terminalis, 534
  CT of, 215, 216f
  echocardiography of, 3–5
  MRI of, 226f, 649–650, 650f
Crutch injury, 768–769, 769f
Cryoglobulinemic vasculitis, hepatitis C
  virus–associated, 419–420
CTA. *See* Computed tomography angiography
  (CTA)
CTV. *See* Computed tomography venography
  (CTV)
Cyst(s)
  hydatid, 9f, 33–34
  lymphatic. *See* Lymphatic malformations
  pericardial, 33–34, 546, 546f

D
D-dimer, 668, 787t
Damus-Kaye-Stansel procedure, 344f
DeBakey-Surgitool valve, 280
Deceleration time, in mitral inflow velocity profile,
  17
Deep venous thrombosis (DVT), 786–799
  ascending venography of, 787t, 790–791,
    804–805, 805f
  clinical manifestations of, 668
  CTV of, 787–788, 787t, 789f

Deep venous thrombosis (DVT) *(Continued)*
  D-dimer in, 787t
  MRV of, 787t, 788–790, 790f
  treatment of, 792–794
  ultrasound of, 786–787, 787f–789f, 787t
  upper extremity, 786, 790
    in Paget-Schroetter syndrome, 794–796,
      794f–796f
Dextrocardia, 245–246, 246f, 647, 647f
Diabetes mellitus, coronary artery calcium in, 376
Digital arteries
  in Buerger disease, 764–765, 766f
  in frostbite, 761, 763f
Digital subtraction angiography, 159f–161f,
  160–161
Digital vein, 262–263
Dilated cardiomyopathy. *See* Cardiomyopathy,
  dilated
Dissection
  aortic. *See* Aortic dissection
  brachial artery, 760, 761f
  common carotid artery, 691, 691f
  internal carotid artery, 690–691, 691f
  pulmonary artery, 673–674
  upper extremity artery, 760, 761f
Diverticulum
  ductus, 714, 714f
  Kommerell, 189f, 254f, 761–763, 764f
  left atrium, 646
  pericardial, 546
Doppler echocardiography. *See* Echocardiography,
  Doppler *and at specific diseases and structures*
Dorsalis pedis artery, 265f
Ductus diverticulum, 714, 714f
Dural sinuses, MRV of, 252–253, 252f

E
E/A ratio, 16t, 17, 18f
Ebstein anomaly
  CTA of, 602–603, 602f
  echocardiography of, 561, 562f
ECG. *See* Electrocardiography (ECG)
Echocardiography, 1–36, 272–273. *See also at
  specific structures and disorders*
  agitated saline contrast for, 18–19, 19f
  artifacts with, 21–24
  Doppler, 13–18, 16t
    color flow, 14
    continuous wave, 14
    left ventricular diastolic function on, 17–18,
      18f
    modalities of, 13–18
    pulsed wave, 13
  interventional, 34–35, 36f
  left ventricular opacification for, 19–20, 19f
  M-mode, 10–12, 15t
  microbubble contrast for, 19–20, 19f
  vs. MRI, 174
  stress, 20, 167
    indications for, 167
  transesophageal, 17t, 20–21, 26f
    anesthesia in, 21
    of aorta, 24–28, 27f
    bicaval view for, 21, 24f
    blind spot on, 24–28
    complications of, 21
    four-chamber view for, 21, 22f
    indications for, 21
    long-axis aortic and mitral valve view for,
      21, 23f
    long-axis aortic valve view for, 21, 23f
    short-axis view for, 21, 25f
    three-dimensional, 21
    transgastric view for, 21, 25f–26f
    two-chamber view for, 21, 22f
  transthoracic, 3–10, 17t
    apical five-chamber view for, 6, 8f, 270f
    apical four-chamber view for, 6, 8f, 270f, 272f
    apical long-axis view for, 9, 10f
    apical two-chamber view for, 9, 9f, 271f
    left ventricular function on, 12, 15f–16f
    measurements on, 10–12, 15t
    parasternal long-axis view for, 3, 4f, 268f,
      272f
    parasternal short-axis view for, 5–6, 5f–7f,
      269f
    right parasternal view for, 10
    right ventricular inflow view for, 3–5, 4f, 268f
    right ventricular outflow view for, 5, 270f
    subcostal view for, 9–10, 11f–12f, 271f–272f

Echocardiography *(Continued)*
  suprasternal view for, 10, 13f–14f, 271f–272f
  views for, 3–10, 272
Eclipse filter, 316b, 329–330
Ectasia
  annuloaortic, 23f
  coronary artery, 243, 243f, 611, 612f
Ectopy, CT and, 67–68, 68f–69f
Edema
  myocardial, 423–424, 424f–425f, 427–428
  pulmonary, 195–197
EDTA (ethylenediaminetetraacetic acid), coronary
  artery calcium and, 378
Edwards MIRA valve, 287
Edwards SAPIEN valve, 308, 309f
Effective regurgitant orifice area, in mitral regurgitation, 15
Effort thrombosis. *See* Paget-Schroetter syndrome
Egyptian eye sign, 803, 804f
Ehlers-Danlos syndrome, 679, 730–732, 750–751,
  753f
Eisenmenger syndrome, 195, 197f, 340
Ejection fraction, 12
  in aortic regurgitation, 577, 577f
  in mitral regurgitation, 577
  in tetralogy of Fallot, 582, 583f
Electrocardiography (ECG)
  in acute coronary syndrome, 382–383
  in coronary artery disease, 473
  in left ventricular noncompaction, 365, 366f
  in myocardial infarction, 445
  in sarcoidosis, 364, 365f
Elephant trunk procedure, 401–402, 402f
Embolism
  in catheter angiography, 162
  pulmonary. *See* Pulmonary embolism
  tumor, 681–682, 683f
  upper extremity artery, 763, 765f
Embolization coils, 331, 331f
Embolization device, 330–331
  Amplatzer vascular plug, 330–331, 331f
  coil, 331, 331f
Emergency department, chest pain in. *See* Acute
  coronary syndrome
Empty pericardial sign, 546
Endocarditis
  abscess in, 603f, 604
  complications of, 584
  CT of, 292–295
  CTA of, 603–604, 603f
  Doppler imaging of, 565f–566f
  echocardiography of, 564, 604
    aneurysm on, 565f
    aortic root abscess on, 564, 565f
    calcification on, 566f
    regurgitation on, 564, 566f
    vegetations on, 564, 564f–566f
  MRI of, 584–585, 584f
  paravalvular leak in, 603f, 604
Endograft. *See* Stent graft
Endoleak, 404–406, 404t
  after dissection repair, 406
  type I, 404, 404f, 404t, 732–733
    type IA, 404, 404f–405f, 404t, 407f
      vs. bird beaking, 404, 405f
  type II, 404, 404t, 405f–406f, 733, 739f
  type III, 404–405, 404t, 408f, 732–733
  type IV, 732–733
Endologix endograft, 315, 316b, 318f
Endomyocardial fibrosis, 518–519
Endurant endograft, 313, 315f, 316b
Epicardial fat, 423, 424f
Erdheim-Chester disease, 747, 747f
Esophageal-endograft fistula, 408–409, 409f
Estrogen, coronary artery calcium and, 378
Eustachian valve, 535
  CT of, 215–216
  echocardiography of, 3–5, 4f
  MRI of, 225–226, 649–650, 650f
Excluder endograft, 313, 316b, 316f
Express stent, 316b, 325–326, 326f

F
Fabry disease, 519–520
  echocardiography of, 520
  MRI of, 462f, 520
  radiography of, 520
False chordae, 228
Femoral artery, 772, 773f
  aneurysm of, 781, 783f

Femoral artery (Continued)
  atherosclerosis of, 117, 119f, 772, 773f, 775f, 777, 778f
  for cardiac catheterization, 40–45, 40t, 41f, 42b
  for catheter angiography, 159f, 159t
  CTA of, 263–264, 264f
  Doppler ultrasound of, 115–118, 117f, 120f
  embolus of, 779–780, 781f
  pseudoaneurysm of, 117–118, 120f
Femoral vein
  thrombosis of, 786, 788f–789f. See also Deep venous thrombosis (DVT)
  ultrasound of, 786–787, 787f–788f
Fenfluramine, valvular heart disease with, 569
Fibroelastoma, papillary, 525–526, 652–653
  CT of, 526, 527f
  CTA of, 604, 605f
  echocardiography of, 25f, 526, 527f, 561f, 565–566, 566f–567f
  MRI of, 526, 527f, 584–585, 584f
Fibroma, 526
  CT of, 526, 528f
  echocardiography of, 35f
Fibromuscular dysplasia
  of renal artery, 750, 751f
  of upper extremity arteries, 760–761, 762f
Fibromyxosarcoma, 565–566, 567f
Fibrosis, in myocarditis, 425–426, 426f, 428, 428f
Figure 3 sign, 189–190, 193f
Fistula
  aortocaval, 742, 745f
  aortoenteric, 742, 746f
  arteriovenous
    lower extremity, 784, 785f
      in Parkes Weber syndrome, 832–833, 832f–833f
    upper extremity, 758, 759f
  coronary artery, 245, 245f, 612–615
  coronary-cameral, 612–614
  left atrium, 654
  right atrium, 654, 655f
  after thoracic endovascular therapy, 407–409, 409f
Flair stent graft, 316b, 318, 321f
Fleischner sign, 197
Fluency stent graft, 316b, 317–318, 321f
Fluorine-18, 94–95, 97t, 107t
Fluorine-18 flurpiridaz, 94
Fontan procedure, 352–354, 353f–354f
Fractional flow reserve (FFR) pressure wire, 55–56, 56f
Frostbite, 761, 763f

G
G2 Express filter, 316b, 329–330
G2 X filter, 316b, 329–330, 330f
Garlic, coronary artery calcium and, 378
Genicular artery, 264f
Giant cell arteritis, 412–415, 743–745
  catheter angiography of, 764, 766f
  color-coded duplex sonography of, 413, 413f, 415
  CTA of, 764, 766f
  MRA of, 764, 766f
  MRI of, 413–415, 414f–415f, 743–745
  PET of, 413, 414f
  ultrasound of, 743–745
Glenn anastomosis, 352–354, 353f–354f
Gore HELEX occluder, 304, 306f
Gore TAG thoracic endoprosthesis, 316b, 317, 320f
Gorham syndrome, 820
Gorlin syndrome, 526, 528f
Graft. See Coronary artery bypass graft (CABG); Stent graft
Granulomatosis, with polyangiitis, 417–418
Great arteries, transposition of. See Transposition of the great arteries
Great cardiac vein, 221, 274f
Great saphenous vein, 265, 800
  duplex ultrasound of, 802–804, 803f–804f
  insufficiency of. See Venous insufficiency
  laser ablation of, 806, 806f
  venography of, 804–805, 805f
Greenfield filter, 316b, 326, 327f
Gunther Tulip filter, 316b, 328–329, 329f

H
Hamartoma, 529, 530f
Hampton hump, 197, 669, 670f
Hancock valve, 289, 290f

Hand-arm vibration syndrome, 769
Harken-Soroff ball valve, 279
Heart
  anatomy of. See also Cardiac valves; Coronary artery (arteries); Left atrium; Left ventricle; Right atrium; Right ventricle
  angiography of, 232–247, 273. See also Coronary angiography
    CT of, 215–224, 267, 267f–268f, 273. See also Computed tomography angiography (CTA), coronary
    MRI of, 225–231. See also Cardiac magnetic resonance (CMR) imaging and at specific structures
    radiography of, 179, 180f, 200–209, 267–272, 267f–268f
    ultrasound of, 272–273. See also Echocardiography
  angiography of. See Computed tomography angiography (CTA); Coronary angiography
  carcinoid disease of, 207, 209f, 560–561, 561f
  dextrocardia of, 245–246, 246f
  enlargement of, 200–201
  herniation of, 546
  imaging of, 163–176, 165f. See also at Coronary artery disease (CAD) and specific imaging modalities
    in noncoronary disease, 171–174, 172t
  innervation of, 484–485
  left-dominant, 221
  masses of, 522–538
    vs. anatomic variants, 534–535
    aneurysmal, 535
    benign, 524–529. See also specific tumors
    CT of, 523–524
    echocardiography of, 33–34, 174, 523
    imaging of, 172t, 522–524
    malignant, 529–533. See also specific tumors
    MRI of, 90, 174, 524
    radiography of, 522–523
    thrombotic, 535
    metastatic disease of, 529–531, 531f–532f
  MRI of. See Cardiac magnetic resonance (CMR) imaging
  radionuclide imaging of, 91–110. see also Positron emission tomography (PET); Single-photon emission computed tomography (SPECT)
  right-dominant, 221
  size of, 200–201
  ultrasound of. See Echocardiography
Heart disease
  atherosclerotic. See Acute coronary syndrome; Coronary artery disease (CAD); Myocardial infarction (MI); Myocardial ischemia
  valvular. See Valvular heart disease and specific valvular diseases
Heart failure
  CardioMEMS in, 302–303, 303f
  coronary artery calcium in, 376
  coronary artery disease and, 473–481, 621
  I-123 MIBG imaging in, 484–485
  imaging in, 172–173, 172t
  myocardial viability testing in, 473–481
    carbon-11 PET for, 478
    F-18 FDG PET for, 475–481, 481t
    metabolism imaging for, 475–481
    perfusion imaging for, 475, 477f
    rationale for, 473–475
    thallium-201 redistribution imaging for, 475
HeartNet, 302, 302f
Hemangioendothelioma, kaposiform, 818, 819f
Hemangioma
  cardiac, 527–529, 586f, 652
  congenital, 814, 814t, 815f–816f, 816–817
  hepatic, 823
    infantile, 814–815, 817f–818f, 818
  infantile, 813–814, 814t
    CT of, 816f
    MRI of, 815–816, 816f
    proliferative, 814f, 816f
    treatment of, 817–818, 818f
Hematoma, intramural
  abdominal, 740–741, 745f
  thoracic, 139f, 153, 703f, 712
    vs. aortitis, 712
Hemiarch procedure, 401
Hemiazygos vein, 255–256
Hemochromatosis, 519, 519f
Hemopericardium, 542, 543f

Hemopneumopericardium, 546f
Hemoptysis, 724–725
  bronchial artery angiography in, 721f–722f, 724, 724f
  bronchial artery CT in, 719–722, 721f, 724, 724f
  bronchial artery embolization in, 724–725
  massive, 724
Hemorrhage, with pulmonary artery catheter, 311
Hemorrhoidal veins, 260
Hepatic artery, 256
  angiography of, 160, 161f
  variants of, 256
Hepatic infantile hemangioma, 814–815, 817f–818f
Hepatic veins
  CT of, 260, 261f
  Doppler imaging of, 561–562, 563f
  variants of, 260
Hepatitis C virus–associated cryoglobulinemic vasculitis, 419–420
Hereditary hemorrhagic telangiectasis, 676–678
HeRO graft, 316b, 322, 324f
Hiatal hernia, 654, 655f
Hibernating myocardium, 473–475, 478, 479f
Hip, Charcot joint of, 422f
Hufnagel aortic ball valve, 279
Hughes-Stovin syndrome, 679
Human immunodeficiency virus (HIV) infection, 420
Humeral artery, circumflex
  catheter angiography of, 263f
  compression of, 768
  pseudoaneurysm of, 767f
Hydatid cyst, 9f, 33–34
Hyperemia, in myocarditis, 424–425, 425f, 428
Hypereosinophilic syndrome, 518–519
  CT of, 519
  echocardiography of, 518
  MRI of, 518–519, 518f
  radiography of, 518
Hypertrophic cardiomyopathy. See Cardiomyopathy, hypertrophic
Hypogenetic lung syndrome, 198, 200, 201f, 676, 677f
  pulmonary venous drainage in, 644
Hypoplastic aortic syndrome, 726–728, 729f
Hypoplastic left heart syndrome, 350–352, 353f–354f, 647
Hypoplastic lung syndrome, 198
Hypothenar hammer syndrome, 769, 770f
Hypoxia, single ventricle and, 354–355

I
I-123 metaiodobenzylguanidine (I-123 MIBG) imaging, 484–485
iCAST stent graft, 316b, 322, 323f
IgG4-mediated disease, abdominal aorta aneurysm in, 730, 737f
Iliac artery, 264f
  catheter angiography of, 256–258, 259f
  CTA of, 263, 264f
  MRA of, 132, 132f
Iliac vein, 259–260
  compression of. See May-Thurner syndrome
Iliofemoral artery, thrombus of, 779–780, 782f
Impella Circulatory Support system, 298, 300f
Implantable cardioverter-defibrillator, 310–311
  complications of, 310–311
  lead-related complications of, 310–311
Implantable loop recorders, 307–308, 308f
Infantile hemangioma, 813–814, 814f, 814t
  vs. arteriovenous malformation, 816–817
  CT of, 816f
  MRI of, 815–816, 816f
  proliferative, 816f
  treatment of, 817–818, 818f
Infection. See also Endocarditis
  aneurysmal. See Aortic aneurysm, thoracic, mycotic
  of cardiac device, 311
  after thoracic endovascular therapy, 407–409, 419, 421f
Inferior sagittal sinus, MRV of, 252, 252f
Inferior vena cava, 259
  CT of, 259, 260f, 271f
  diameter of, 9–10
  duplicated, 259, 260f
  echocardiography of, 9–10
  interrupted, 182–183, 184f
  measurement of, 11–12, 15t

Inferior vena cava *(Continued)*
  MRI of, 227f, 271f
  radiography of, 179, 180f, 182
  renal cell cancer to, 136f, 653, 653f
  thrombus of, 789, 790f
    CT of, 182–183, 183f
    echocardiography of, 12f
  variants of, 259, 260f
Inferior vena cava filter, 326–330
  ALN, 316b, 330, 330f
  Bird's Nest, 316b, 326, 327f
  Celect, 316b, 329, 329f
  Eclipse, 316b, 329–330
  G2 Express, 316b, 329–330
  G2 X, 316b, 329–330, 330f
  Greenfield, 316b, 326, 327f
  Gunther Tulip, 316b, 328–329, 329f
  OptEase, 316b, 328
  Option, 316b, 330, 330f
  Simon nitinol, 316b, 327, 328f
  TrapEase, 316b, 328, 328f
  Vena Tech, 316b, 327, 327f
Innominate artery, 226f
Innominate vein
  left
    accessory, anomalous, 181–182, 182f
    catheter malposition in, 179, 181f
    radiography of, 179, 181f
  right, radiography of, 179, 180f–181f
Interatrial septum
  amyloidosis of, 654, 655f
  aneurysm of, 28, 28f, 648–649, 649f
    CT of, 271f
  defect of. *See* Atrial septal defect (ASD)
  definition of, 657–658, 658f
  development of, 658, 659f
  echocardiography of, 9, 11f, 24f, 28, 28f, 271f
  lipomatous hypertrophy of, 535, 650
    CT of, 650, 650f, 658f
    echocardiography of, 11f, 24f
    F-18 FDG PET of, 535, 536f
    MRI of, 226f, 650f
  MRI of, 226–227, 226f, 229f, 271f
Intercoronary communications, 244–245, 244f
Intercostal vein, 183
Interventional echocardiography, 34–35
Interventricular septum
  aneurysm of, 662–663, 663f
  defect of. *See* Ventricular septal defect (VSD)
  development of, 662, 663f
  flattening of, 7f
  measurement of, 15t
Interventricular veins, 221
Intraaortic balloon pump, 298, 299f
Intravascular ultrasound (IVUS)
  central venous, 805
  coronary, 56, 56f, 165
  in May-Thurner syndrome, 791–792, 792f
Iodine-123, 94
Iron, myocardial accumulation of, 519, 519f
Isovolumetric relaxation time, in mitral inflow
    velocity profile, 17

J
Jantene procedure, 349–350, 349f, 351f
Jugular vein, internal
  catheter malposition in, 179, 181f
  radiography of, 179, 181f

K
k-space, in MRA, 140
Kaposi sarcoma, 748f
Kaposiform hemangioendothelioma, 818, 819f
Kasabach-Merritt phenomenon, 818
Kawasaki disease, 417
Kerley A lines, 195
Kerley B lines, 195, 198f
Kidneys
  cardiac catheterization effects on, 55
  disease of, coronary artery calcium and,
    378–379
  transplantation of, 128f
Klippel-Trenaunay syndrome, 829–830, 831f–832f
Kommerell diverticulum, 189f, 254f, 761–763, 764f

L
Lambl excrescence, 551, 552f
Laser ablation
  of saphenous vein, 806, 806f
  of vascular malformation, 825

Left atrial appendage, 645–646, 654
  closure of, 35, 36f, 656
  CT of, 215, 216f–217f, 217
  Doppler echocardiography of, 30f
  echocardiography of, 28–29, 30f
  emptying velocity of, 30f
  enlargement of, 204f
  MRI of, 228, 229f
  occluder device for, 307, 307f
  radiography of, 201, 204f
  thrombus of, 30f, 650–651, 651f, 654
Left atrium, 645–646
  amyloidosis of, 654, 655f
  benign tumors of, 651–653
  calcification of, 201–202, 647
  CT of, 217, 217f, 268f–271f
  dilatation of, 8f
  dimensions of, 646
  diverticulum of, 646
  echocardiography of, 8f, 28–29, 30f, 268f–271f
  emptying velocity of, 30f
  enlargement of, 201, 203b, 204f, 646, 646f
  fibroelastoma of, 652–653
  fistula of, 654
  hemangioma of, 652
  hypoplasia of, 647
  leiomyosarcoma of, 585f
  lipoma of, 651
  lung cancer extension to, 653, 653f
  malignant tumors of, 653–654
  masses of, 649–654
  measurement of, 11, 15t, 17–18, 228
  mediastinal compression of, 654, 655f
  MRI of, 226f–227f, 228, 268f–271f
  myxoma of, 22f, 651
  paraganglioma of, 652
  postoperative, 655–656
  radiography of, 201–202
  sarcoma of, 653–654, 654f
  size of, 646–647
  thrombus of, 30f, 650–651, 651f
  volume of, 11
Left internal mammary artery graft, 473, 474f,
    634–635, 636f
Left ventricle
  aneurysm of, 202–203, 205f
  apical thin point of, 228, 229f
  CT of, 217, 268f–271f
  echocardiography of, 9, 25f–26f, 174, 268f–271f
    contrast for, 19–20, 19f–20f
  enlargement of, 202, 204b
  measurement of, 11, 15t, 217, 228, 230f
  MRI of, 86, 226f–227f, 228–230, 229f–230f,
    268f–271f
  radiography of, 179, 180f, 202–203
  vs. right ventricle, 217
  thrombus of, 7f, 9f, 28f
Left ventricular apex
  aneurysm of, 8f
  echocardiography of, 6, 7f–9f, 28f
  hypertrophy of, 20, 20f
  thrombus of, 7f, 9f, 28f
Left ventricular apicoaortic conduit, 303, 305f
Left ventricular diastolic function
  Doppler echocardiography of, 17, 18f
  echocardiography of, 17–18, 18f
Left ventricular ejection fraction (LVEF)
  in aortic regurgitation, 577, 577f
  PET of, 97, 475, 477f
  SPECT of, 106
Left ventricular function
  CT of, 493–495
  echocardiography of, 12, 15f–16f
  myocardial viability testing for. *See* Myocardial
    viability
Left ventricular noncompaction (LVNC), 365–367,
    510–511
  CTA of, 511, 511f
  differential diagnosis of, 510
  echocardiography of, 7f, 31f, 33, 510
  electrocardiography of, 365, 366f
  MRI of, 365–367, 366f, 510–511
  pathogenesis of, 510
Left ventricular outflow tract (LVOT)
  in aortic regurgitation, 553
  in aortic stenosis, 579f, 592, 593f
  congenital obstruction of, 553, 554f
  CT of, 268f, 270f
  diameter of, 11, 592, 593f
  Doppler measurement of, 16t

Left ventricular outflow tract (LVOT) *(Continued)*
  echocardiography of, 268f, 270f
  measurement of, 551
  MRI of, 268f, 270f
  narrowing of, 581
  obstruction of, in hypertrophic cardiomyopathy,
    581, 581f
Left ventriculography, 50–51, 52f
Leiomyosarcoma
  cardiac, 532, 585f
  pelvic, 532f
Levocardia, 544–546
LifeStent, 316b, 322–324, 325f
Ligament of Marshall, 221
Lillehei-Kaster valve, 283–284
Linear artifact, echocardiography-related, 23
Lipids, coronary artery calcium and, 377–378
Lipoma, 526
  CT of, 526, 528f, 651, 652f
  echocardiography of, 526, 528f
  MRI of, 528f, 651
Lipomatous hypertrophy, interatrial septum, 535,
    650
  CT of, 650, 650f
  echocardiography of, 11f, 24f
  F-18 FDG PET of, 535, 536f
  MRI of, 226f, 650f
Lipoproteins, vs. coronary calcium score, 376–377
Liver
  hemangioma of, 823
  infantile hemangioma of, 814–815, 817f–818f,
    818
  vascular malformation of, 823
Loeys-Dietz syndrome, 717
Lower extremity arteries, 772–785
  anatomy of, 263–264, 264f–265f
  aneurysm of, 781–784, 783f–784f
  ankle-brachial index for, 772, 775t
  arteriovenous fistula of, 784, 785f
  atherosclerosis of, 777
    catheter angiography of, 774f, 776
    CTA of, 128f, 775, 776f, 777
    MRA of, 773f, 775–777, 775f
    treatment of, 777, 778f–779f
    ultrasound of, 117, 118f–119f, 773–775, 775f
  Buerger disease of, 778
  catheter angiography of, 774f, 776
  chronic steno-occlusive disease of, 773f–775f,
    776–779, 778f–780f
  collateral pathways of, 772, 773f
  color Doppler ultrasound of, 773–775, 775f
  CTA of, 128f, 775, 776f, 777
  cystic adventitial disease of, 778, 780f
  ischemic disease of, 779–781, 781f–782f
  MRA of, 773f, 775–777, 775f
  noninvasive evaluation of, 772–773, 774f
  pseudoaneurysm of, 784, 785f
  pulse volume recordings of, 773
  segmental limb pressures of, 773
  thromboangiitis obliterans of, 778
  ultrasound of, 117, 118f–119f, 773–775, 774f
Lung cancer
  left atrium invasion by, 653, 653f
  pulmonary artery invasion by, 680–682, 683f
LVOT. *See* Left ventricular outflow tract (LVOT)
Lymphangioma, 529
Lymphatic malformations, 819–822
  clinical manifestations of, 819–820, 820f
  MRI of, 820, 821f
  treatment of, 820–822, 821f–822f
  ultrasound of, 820, 820f
Lymphoma, 533
  CT of, 533, 534f, 748f
  radiography of, 533

M
Maffucci syndrome, 833
Magnetic resonance angiography (MRA)
  coronary. *See* Cardiac magnetic resonance
    (CMR) imaging
  vascular, 131–154
    balanced steady-state free precession,
      133–137, 136f, 153, 153f
    breathing artifact with, 153
    bright-blood, 131–137, 132f, 134f
      balanced steady-state free precession,
        133–137, 136f, 153, 153f
      ECG-gated fast spin echo, 133, 135f
      phase contrast, 132–133, 134f
      quiescent interval single shot, 137, 138f

Magnetic resonance angiography (MRA)
  (Continued)
    time-of-flight, 131–132, 132f
  bypass graft on, 132f, 138f
  contrast-enhanced, 138–154
    agent injection for, 143
    agent timing for, 143, 148–150, 149f
    asymmetric flow in, 150
    automated agent detection for, 143–144
    blood pool materials for, 139–140,
      141f
    breathing artifact on, 153
    extracellular materials for, 138–139
    extraluminal abnormalities and, 153
    field of view in, 152–154, 152f
    fluoroscopic triggering for, 144
    gadolinium for, 138–140
    k-space in, 140
    parallel imaging techniques in, 142
    partial Fourier techniques in, 142
    phase ghosting in, 153, 153f
    pseudostenosis in, 150–152
    ringing artifact in, 148, 149f
    sequences for, 140–143
    slow flow in, 150
    stenosis on, 154
    three-dimensional spoiled gradient recalled
      echo sequences for, 141–143
    time-resolved, 144, 145f–146f
    venous contamination in, 148–150
    venous enhancement in, 150, 151f
    vs. CTA, 131
  dark-blood, 137, 139f, 142f
  double inversion recovery in, 137
  ECG-gated fast spin echo, 133, 135f
  extraluminal abnormalities on, 153
  fast spin echo, 133, 135f
  field of view in, 152–154, 152f
  flow void phenomenon in, 137
  noncontrast, 131–137
    bright-blood, 131–137, 132f, 134f–136f,
      138f
    dark-blood, 137, 139f, 142f
  phase contrast, 132–133, 134f
  phase ghosting with, 153, 153f
  postprocessing for, 147–148
    maximum intensity projection in, 147,
      151–152
    multiplanar reconstruction in, 147
    pseudostenosis in, 151–152f
    shaded surface display in, 147–148, 148f
    subtraction images in, 147
    volume rendering in, 148, 149f
  pseudostenosis on, 150–152
  quiescent interval single shot, 137, 138f
  stenosis on, 154
  time-of-flight, 131–132, 132f
  venous contamination with, 148–150
Magnetic resonance imaging (MRI). See also
    Cardiac magnetic resonance (CMR) imaging;
    Magnetic resonance angiography (MRA)
  cardiac device and, 311
  stent compatibility with, 316b
Magnetic resonance venography (MRV), 787t,
    788–790, 790f
Magovern-Cromie ball valve, 280
Maki artifact, 148, 149f
Mammary artery, internal
  angiography of, 51–52, 53f–54f
  MRI of, 226f
Mammary vein, internal
  catheter malposition in, 183–185, 186f
  MRI of, 226f
Marfan syndrome, 679
  aneurysm in, 716–717, 730–732, 738f
  aortic dissection in, 738f
Marshall, vein of, 221
May-Thurner syndrome, 791–794, 804, 808
  anatomy of, 791–792, 791f, 794f
  CTV of, 791f, 792
  MRV of, 792, 793f–794f, 804, 804f
  ultrasound of, 791–792, 792f
  venography of, 792, 793f
Median arcuate ligament syndrome, 749–750,
    749f
Median vein, 262–263
Mediastinum, hiatal hernia of, 654, 655f
Medtronic Freestyle valve, 290
Medtronic Hall valve, 283, 284f–285f
Mercedes Benz sign, 229–230

Mesenteric artery
  inferior, catheter angiography of, 256, 257f
  occlusive disease of, 747–750, 748f–749f
  superior
    catheter angiography of, 256, 257f
    occlusive disease of, 747–749, 748f
    stents in, 753, 756f
Mesenteric vein, 261–262
Mesothelioma, 550, 550f
Metacarpal vein, 262–263
Metaiodobenzylguanidine (MIBG) imaging,
    484–485
Metal
  in cardiac CT, 62, 71–73, 72b, 73f
  in carotid MRA, 698
Metastatic disease
  cardiac, 34, 35f, 529–531
    CT of, 530–531, 531f–532f, 653
    MRI of, 530–531, 653
    PET-CT of, 531f
  retroperitoneal, 747, 748f
Microbubble study, 19–20, 19f–20f
Middle aortic syndrome, 726–728, 729f
Mirror-image artifact, 23, 687
Mitral annular calcification
  caseous, 535, 537f, 556–557, 557f
  coronary artery calcium score and, 371, 372f
  CT of, 207f, 535, 537f
  echocardiography of, 535, 556–557, 557f
  MRI of, 537f
  radiography of, 206, 207f
Mitral inflow velocity profile, 17, 18f
Mitral regurgitation
  in cardiomyopathy, 558
  CTA of, 597, 599f
  Doppler imaging of, 557f, 558–559, 559f
  echocardiography of, 15–16, 557–560,
    557f–558f, 558t, 560t
  effective regurgitant orifice area in, 15
  ejection fraction in, 577
  in endocarditis, 566f
  etiology of, 573
  flow convergence in, 559, 559f
  functional, 558
  in hypertrophic cardiomyopathy, 581, 582f
  mitral valve prolapse in, 557–558, 557f–558f
  MRI of, 573–575, 574f–576f, 577t, 578b
  planimetry in, 597
  proximal isovelocity surface area (PISA) in, 559,
    559f
  pulmonary vein flow in, 559–560, 559f
  quantification of, 576–577, 577t
  regurgitant jet area in, 557f, 558
  vena contracta in, 558–559
Mitral ring, 599–600, 600f
Mitral stenosis
  congenital, 599–600, 600f
  CTA of, 597–598, 599f, 599t
  Doppler echocardiography of, 556, 556f–557f
  echocardiography of, 6, 6f, 8f, 555–557, 556t,
    557f
    hockey-stick appearance on, 555, 556f
    mitral annular calcification on, 556–557,
      557f
    valve area on, 555–556, 556f, 556t
  etiology of, 555
  hockey-stick appearance of, 597–598, 599f
  left atrial enlargement in, 201, 204f, 646, 646f
  mitral annular calcification in, 556–557, 557f
  MRI of, 578–579, 578t, 579f
  planimetry in, 597–598, 599f
  quantification of, 579–580
  severity of, 555–557, 556f–557f, 556t
  treatment of, 557, 557f
Mitral valve, 23f
  aneurysm of, 565f
  area of, 554–556, 556f, 556t
    pressure half-time for, 15–16, 555–556, 556f
  congenital disease of, 599–600, 600f
  CT of, 218, 218f
  CTA of, 596–600, 597f–598f, 600f
  Doppler echocardiography of, 16t, 18f, 32f
  echocardiography of, 6, 6f, 554–560
  fibromyxosarcoma of, 565–566, 567f
  fish-mouth appearance of, 6f
  leiomyosarcoma of, 585f
  metastatic sarcoma of, 586f
  MRI of, 228, 571, 571b, 571t, 572f
    systematic approach to, 571–573
  myxoma of, 584, 585f

Mitral valve (Continued)
  parachute, 599–600, 600f
  prosthetic, echocardiography of, 566–569, 568f
  radiography of, 206, 207f
  replacement of, 211f
  thrombus of, 584, 584f
  vegetations on, 564, 565f–566f
Mitral valve prolapse
  CTA of, 597, 599f
  Doppler echocardiography of, 3
  echocardiography of, 3, 557–558, 557f–558f
  MRI of, 574f
  treatment of, 558
Moderator band, 3–5, 216–217, 216f, 227, 227f
Moderator band artery, 216–217
Monostrut valve, 284
MRA. See Magnetic resonance angiography (MRA)
Myocardial bridging, 244, 244f, 611, 611f
Myocardial infarction (MI). See also Acute coro-
    nary syndrome; Myocardial ischemia
  acuity of, 447–448, 450f
  complications of, 456–459
    aneurysmal, 458, 459f–460f
    thrombotic, 457, 457f, 460f
  CTA of, 495–497, 496f
  dual energy CT of, 500–503, 501f
  ECG of, 445
  mortality with, 621–622
  MRI of, 86, 86f, 444f, 445–446, 447f
    acute vs. chronic disease on, 447–448, 450f
    cine, 443
    clinical reporting of, 444–445, 445f
    vs. CT, 495, 496f, 497
    delayed enhancement, 443, 443f, 445–446,
      491f
    vs. CT, 495, 496f
    no-reflow zone on, 447–448, 450f, 458
    non–ST-segment MI on, 446, 448f
    pathophysiologic correlation with, 444–
      445, 445f–446f, 459–463, 461f
    vs. SPECT, 445–446, 447f
    ST-segment elevation MI on, 446–447,
      449f
    no-reflow zone on, 447–448, 450f, 458
    vs. SPECT, 445–446, 447f
    T2-weighted, 443–444, 443f
    thrombus on, 457, 457f–458f, 460f
    ventricular aneurysm on, 458, 459f–460f
  non–ECG-gated CT of, 490–491, 491f
  vs. nonischemic disease, 459–463, 461f–462f
  non–ST-segment, 446, 448f
  SPECT of, 445–446, 447f
  ST-segment elevation, 446–447, 449f
  subendocardial, 445–446, 447f
  ventricular aneurysm after, 458, 459f–460f
  viability study in. See Myocardial viability
Myocardial ischemia. See also Coronary artery
    disease (CAD); Myocardial infarction (MI)
  balanced, 473
  complications of, 456–459
    aneurysmal, 458, 459f–460f
    thrombotic, 457, 457f, 460f
  CT of, 490–504
    delayed phase, 495–497, 496f
    dual energy, 500–503, 501f–503f
    dynamic perfusion, 498–500, 499f
    left ventricular function analysis on,
      493–495
    non–ECG-gated, 490–491, 491f
    stressed arterial phase, 493, 494f
  CTA of, 491–503
    arterial phase, 491–493, 492f
    stressed arterial phase, 493, 494f
  MRI of, 86–87, 86f, 439–463, 442f. See also
    Cardiac magnetic resonance (CMR)
    imaging
    angiographic, 442
    cine, 442–444, 442f–444f
    clinical reporting of, 444–445, 445f
    delayed enhancement, 442f, 443–445,
      444f–445f, 455, 456f
    pathophysiologic correlation with,
      459–463, 461f–462f
    vs. SPECT, 454–455
    stress perfusion, 442, 442f, 453–456, 454f,
      454t, 456f
      adenosine, 453, 455f
      dobutamine, 453
    T2-weighted, 442–444, 443f
    vs. nonischemic disease, 459–463, 461f–462f

Myocardial ischemia *(Continued)*
  pathophysiology of, 370, 441–442, 442t,
    459–460, 461f
  PET of, 466–473
    after coronary artery bypass graft, 473
    cost effectiveness of, 472–473
    CT-based attenuation correction with, 467
    F-18 FDG, 483–484
    in patient management, 471
    risk stratification with, 469–470, 472t, 473
    sensitivity and specificity of, 466–467
  SPECT of, 466–473, 483–484
    attenuation artifacts with, 467, 473
    after coronary artery bypass graft, 473
    cost effectiveness of, 472–473
    CT-based attenuation correction with, 467
    in patient management, 471, 472f
    radionuclide attenuation correction with,
      467, 468f–469f
    risk stratification with, 467–469, 469b, 471t,
      473
    sensitivity and specificity of, 466–467
    vs. stress ECG, 473
  viability study in. *See* Myocardial viability
Myocardial perfusion imaging. *See* Cardiac
    computed tomography, dynamic perfusion;
    Cardiac magnetic resonance (CMR) imaging,
    stress perfusion; Positron emission tomogra-
    phy (PET), cardiac; Single-photon emission
    tomography (SPECT), cardiac
Myocardial stunning, 441, 473–475
Myocardial viability, 357–358, 358f, 473–481
  carbon-11 PET for, 478
  delayed enhanced MRI for, 448–452, 450f–452f,
    496, 496f
  delayed phase CT for, 495–497, 496f
  dual-energy CT for, 502f–503f, 503
  F-18 FDG PET for, 475–481, 479f–480f, 481t
  radionuclide perfusion imaging for, 475, 477f
  rationale for, 473–475
  SPECT for, 451, 475
  thallium-201 redistribution imaging for, 475
Myocarditis, 517–518
  chest radiography of, 517
  CT of, 518
  echocardiography of, 517
  etiology of, 517, 517b
  MRI of, 88, 423–430, 427t, 462f, 462t, 517–518,
    517f
    early gadolinium enhancement on, 424–425,
      425f, 428
    edema on, 423–424, 424f–425f, 427–428
    fibrosis on, 425–426, 426f, 428, 428f
    follow-up, 428–429, 429f
    hyperemia on, 424–425, 425f
    Lake Louise criteria in, 426, 427t
    late gadolinium enhancement on, 425–426,
      426f, 428–429, 428f–429f
    protocol for, 426–428
    ventricular abnormalities on, 423, 424f
Myocardium
  hibernating, 473–475, 478, 479f
  stunned, 441, 473–475
  viability of. *See* Myocardial viability
Myxoma, 524–525
  CTA of, 525, 525f
  echocardiography of, 22f, 34, 34f
  MRI of, 525, 585f, 651, 652f

N
Nanobacteria, coronary artery calcium and, 378
Nitrogen-13 ammonia, 94–95, 107t
Noninvoluting congenital hemangioma, 814,
    816–817, 816f
Nutcracker syndrome, 797–799
  anatomy of, 797
  CT of, 798, 798f
  Doppler ultrasound of, 797–798
  MRI of, 798
  treatment of, 798–799
  venography of, 798, 798f

O
Obesity, CT and, 69–71, 70b
Oblique sinus, 224
Occipital sinus, MRV of, 252–253
Occluder devices, 303–307
  left atrial appendage, 307, 307f
  septal, 303–307, 306f
Omicarbon valve, 283–284

Omniscience valve, 283–284
Ophthalmic veins, 253
OptEase filter, 316b, 328
Optical coherence tomography (OCT), 56–57,
    56f, 165
Option filter, 316b, 330, 330f
Oreo cookie sign, 212f, 541, 541f
Osler-Weber-Rendu syndrome, 676–678
Osteomyelitis, sternal, 396, 397f
Osteosarcoma, CT of, 653–654, 654f
Oxygen-15, 94–95, 107t

P
Pacemaker, 308–310
  biventricular, 310
  cardiac CT and, 72–73
  complications of, 310–311
  dual-chamber, 309–310
  lead-related complications of, 310–311
  single-chamber, 309–310
  single pass, 310
Paget-Schroetter syndrome, 794–796
  anatomy of, 794–795, 794f
  CTV of, 795, 795f
  treatment of, 795
  venography of, 795, 795f–796f
Palmar collaterals, imaging of, 769–770, 770f
Palmaz stent, 316b, 326, 326f
Pannus, with prosthetic cardiac valves, 291
Papillary fibroelastoma, 652–653
  CT of, 526, 527f
  CTA of, 604, 605f
  echocardiography of, 25f, 526, 527f, 561f,
    565–566, 566f–567f
  MRI of, 526, 527f, 584–585, 584f
Papillary muscles
  CT of, 217, 217f
  echocardiography of, 6, 7f
  MRI of, 228, 229f
Parachute mitral valve, CTA of, 599–600, 600f
Paraganglioma, 529
  CT of, 529, 529f, 652
  echocardiography of, 5f, 34, 35f
  MRI of, 652, 653f
Parkes Weber syndrome, 830–833, 832f–833f
Partial anomalous pulmonary venous return
    (PAPVR), 644, 645f, 656
Patent ductus arteriosus (PDA), 665
  CT of, 665, 666f
  CTA of, 665, 666f
  Doppler echocardiography of, 14f, 24
  echocardiography of, 5f, 13f, 24
  radiography of, 665
  treatment of, 665
Patent foramen ovale (PFO), 338, 648–649, 658
  CT of, 339f, 649f, 659f
  echocardiography of, 9, 18–19, 19f, 28
  occluder repair in, 303–307
Pectinate muscles
  CT of, 217, 217f
  echocardiography of, 28–29, 30f
Pelvic congestion syndrome, 802, 802f,
    806–809
  CT of, 807, 808f
  MRV of, 807, 809f
  treatment of, 807–808, 809f–810f
  venography of, 809f
Pelvic pain, 802, 806–808
Penetrating atherosclerotic ulcers
  of abdominal aorta, 740, 744f
  of thoracic aorta, 714–715, 714f
Percutaneous coronary intervention (PCI)
  angiography-guided, 624–625, 625f–626f
  CTA-guided, 625, 626f
  imaging for, 624–625, 625f–626f
  PET after, 473
  SPECT after, 473
Perforating arteries, 264f
Perforating veins, 265
Pericardial constriction, 547–550
  CT of, 173–174, 549–550
  echocardiography of, 33, 548–549
  MRI of, 173–174, 548–550, 549f
Pericardial cyst, 546
  CT of, 546
  echocardiography of, 33–34
  MRI of, 546, 546f
Pericardial disease, 539–550. *See also specific*
    diseases
  imaging in, 172t, 173–174

Pericardial effusion, 539–543
  CT of, 212f, 224f, 542, 543f, 547f
  echocardiography of, 4f, 7f, 32f, 33, 34f, 173,
    541–542, 542f–543f
  MRI of, 541
  in myocarditis, 423, 424f
  Oreo cookie sign in, 212f, 541, 541f
  vs. pericardial thickening, 542–543
  vs. pleural effusion, 3, 4f
  radiography of, 209, 212f, 541, 541f
Pericardial recesses, 539
  CT of, 223–224, 224f
  MRI of, 225, 226f
Pericardial sinuses, 539
Pericardial space, 539
Pericardial thickening, 89–90, 89f
  vs. pericardial effusion, 542–543, 542f
Pericardiophrenic vein, catheter malposition in,
    183–185, 187f
Pericarditis, 547
  constrictive
    effusive, 549
    vs. restrictive cardiomyopathy, 549–550
  CT of, 547, 547f
Pericardium
  absence of
    congenital, 209–211, 544–546, 545f
    differential diagnosis of, 544–546
    postsurgical, 211
  anatomy of, 539, 539f–540f
  calcification of, 209, 547
    CT of, 548f
    radiography of, 209, 213f, 548f
  constriction of, 547–550
    CT of, 173–174, 549–550
    echocardiography of, 33, 548–549
    MRI of, 173–174, 548–550, 549f
  CT of, 223–224, 542, 542f
  development of, 544, 544f
  diverticulum of, 546
  echocardiography of, 33
  fat layers of, 539, 539f, 541f
  fibrous, 539, 539f
  imaging of, 173–174
  metastatic tumor of, 34
  MRI of, 89–90, 89f, 225, 226f
  parietal layer of, 223, 539, 539f
  radiography of, 209–211
  rupture of, 546–547
    CT of, 547, 547f
    radiography of, 546
  serous, 223, 539, 539f
  thickening of, 89–90, 89f
    vs. effusion, 542–543, 542f
  trauma to, 542, 546–547
    CT of, 547, 547f
    radiography of, 546, 546f
  tumors of, 550, 550f
  visceral, 223, 539, 539f
Perigraft fluid, 395, 396f
Perigraft gas, 396
Peripherally inserted central catheter. *See* Central
    venous catheter
Peroneal artery, 264f
PET. *See* Positron emission tomography (PET)
Petrosal sinuses, 253
Phase ghosting, in MRA, 153, 153f
Phentermine, 569
Phosphate-binding therapy, coronary artery
    calcium and, 378–379
Pleural effusion
  vs. pericardial effusion, 3, 4f
  in pulmonary embolism, 670–671
Pneumopericardium, 209, 214f
Pneumothorax, cardiac device and, 311
Polyarteritis nodosa, 417, 418f, 419
Popliteal artery, 263–264, 264f, 772, 773f
  aneurysm of, 781–783, 783f
  cystic adventitial disease of, 778, 780f
  entrapment syndrome of, 777–778,
    780f
Popliteal vein
  compression of, 796–797
    anatomy of, 796, 796t
    CT of, 797
    MRI of, 797
    ultrasound of, 796–797
    venography of, 796–797, 797f
  thrombosis of, 786, 788, 788f–789f
Porcine valves, 289–290, 290f

Port-wine stain, 819, 819f
  vs. infantile hemangioma, 814
Portal vein, 261–262, 262f
Portosystemic collateral vessels, 262
Positron emission tomography (PET), cardiac,
    91–110. *See also* Coronary artery disease
    (CAD); Myocardial infarction (MI);
    Myocardial ischemia
  F-18 FDG, 475–478, 479f–480f
  image display in, 106
  indications for, 97, 167, 169f
  interpretation of, 104–106, 106t
  patient-related factors in, 104
  protocols for, 96f, 97–99, 97t, 98f
  quantification of, 106
  radiation exposure with, 436
  radiation risk reduction in, 107–108
  radiotracers in, 94–95, 97t, 107–108, 107t
  scanners for, 91–93, 92f, 92t
  software for, 93–94
  vs. SPECT, 98b
  stress test, 100–101, 104b, 104t
  troubleshooting for, 104, 105t
Posterior sinus of Valsalva, 606
Potts shunt, in tetralogy of Fallot, 344f
Pressure waveform ventricularization, in cardiac
    catheterization, 47
Prosthetic cardiac valves, 277–297
  Bahnson fabric cusp valve, 280
  bileaflet, 284–287, 286f–287f
  bioprosthetic, 287–291, 288f–289f
    calcification with, 291, 292f–293f
    stented, 288–289, 288f–290f
    stentless, 290–291
  Björk-Shiley valve, 282–283, 282f
  Braunwald-Cutter valve, 280
  caged ball, 279–280, 281f
  calcification with, 291, 292f–293f
  Carbomedics valve, 286–287
  Carpentier-Edwards perimount valve, 288,
    288f–289f, 292f
  Carpentier-Edwards supra-annular valve,
    289–290
  complications of, 291–295
  CT of, 211f
  DeBakey-Surgitool valve, 280
  dehiscence with, 294–295, 294f
  echocardiography of, 565f, 566–569, 568f–569f
    problems with, 566–567, 567t
  Edwards MIRA valve, 287
  functional assessment of, 291–295
  Hancock valve, 289, 290f
  Harken-Soroff ball valve, 279
  historical perspective on, 279
  Hufnagel aortic ball valve, 279
  infective endocarditis with, 292–295
  Lillehei-Kaster valve, 283–284
  Magovern-Cromie ball valve, 280
  Medtronic Hall valve, 283, 284f–285f
  Monostrut valve, 284
  Omicarbon valve, 283–284
  Omniscience valve, 283–284
  pannus with, 291
  patient-prosthesis mismatch and, 295
  pseudoaneurysm with, 292–295, 292f–293f
  radiography of, 209, 211f
  St. Jude valve, 284–286, 286f–287f
  Smelloff-Cutter ball valve, 280
  Sorin Bicarbon valve, 287
  Sorin Mitroflow valve, 288–289, 289f
  Starr-Edwards valve, 280, 281f
  thrombus with, 291
  tilting disk, 282–284, 282f, 284f–285f
  vegetations with, 292–295
Protegé stent, 316b, 322, 324f
Proteus syndrome, 834
Pseudoaneurysm
  abdominal aorta, 730, 737f
  aortic arch, 189, 192f
  after Bentall procedure, 399, 399f
  carotid artery, 693
  femoral artery, 120f, 785f
  prosthetic cardiac valve, 292–295, 292f–293f
  pulmonary artery, 311, 679–681, 680f
  renal artery, 751, 755f
  subclavian artery, 141f
  thoracic aorta, 189, 192f
  ultrasound of, 117–118
  upper extremity artery, 766–767, 767f
  visceral artery, 751, 755f

Pseudocoarctation of aorta, 191, 194f, 706, 707f,
    709–710
Pseudostenosis, in MRA, 150–152
Pulmonary arterial hypertension, 672–673
  calcifications in, 673, 674f
  chronic pulmonary embolism and, 671–672,
    672f
  CT of, 673, 674f
  definition of, 672–673
  MRI of, 673
  pathogenesis of, 672–673
  postcapillary, 673, 674f
  precapillary, 673
  radiography of, 195, 197b, 197f, 673, 674f
Pulmonary arteriovenous malformation, 676–678,
    678f
Pulmonary artery (arteries), 191–200, 254,
    668–684
  anatomy of, 668
  aneurysm of, 678–679, 679f, 681
  anomalies of, 674–676, 675f, 677f
  catheter-related infarction of, 311–312
  CT of, 270f
  decreased vascularity of, 193, 195b
  diameter of, 230, 668
  dilation of
    embolism-related, 671–672, 672f
    idiopathic, 675
  dimensions of, 15t
  dissection of, 673–674
  echocardiography of, 270f
  embolism of. *See* Pulmonary embolism
  hilar, 192
  idiopathic dilation of, 675
  increased pressure of, 195, 197f
  increased vascularity of, 193–194, 196b, 196f
  left, 668
    aberrant course (sling) of, 198–200, 200f,
      676, 677f
    proximal interruption of, 676
    radiography of, 179, 180f
    left coronary artery origin from, 240, 241f,
      610–611
    lung cancer invasion of, 682, 683f
  main, 191–192, 668
    dimensions of, 15t
    idiopathic dilation of, 675
    radiography of, 179, 180f
  MRI of, 226f, 230, 270f
  parenchymal, 192
  poststenotic dilatation of, 207, 210f
  proximal interruption of, 198, 199f, 676
  pseudoaneurysm of, 311, 679–681, 680f
  radiography of, 192–197, 195b
  right, 179, 180f, 668
    left pulmonary artery from, 198–200, 200f,
      676, 677f
    proximal interruption of, 676
    right coronary artery origin from, 240, 610, 610f
  sarcoma of, 681, 682f
  Takayasu arteritis of, 708–709, 711f
  tumor emboli of, 681–682, 683f
Pulmonary artery catheter, 57, 57b, 57f, 311–312
  complications of, 311–312
  hemorrhage with, 311
  indications for, 311
  malposition of, 311, 680–681, 680f
  pseudoaneurysm with, 311
  pulmonary infarction with, 311–312
Pulmonary artery sling, 198–200, 200f, 676, 677f
Pulmonary capillary wedge pressure (pulmonary
    venous pressure), 195–197
Pulmonary edema, 195–197
Pulmonary embolism, 197, 668–671
  angiography of, 669
  atelectasis in, 670–671
  chronic, 671–672, 672f
  CT of, 382, 389, 390f, 669–671, 669f–671f
  Hampton hump in, 669, 670f
  massive, 671
  mortality with, 669
  MRA of, 149f, 671
  MRI of, 671
  pathogenesis of, 668–669
  pleural effusion in, 670–671
  radiography of, 669, 669f–670f
  right-sided cardiac strain in, 671, 671f
  ventilation-perfusion scintigraphy of, 669
  Westermark sign in, 669, 669f
Pulmonary/systemic flow (Qp/Qs), 16

Pulmonary valve. *See* Pulmonic valve
Pulmonary vein(s), 191–200, 643–645
  anatomy of, 643–645, 644f–645f
  anomalous drainage of, 644, 644f–645f, 656
    ipsilateral (scimitar vein), 198, 200, 201f,
      644, 676, 677f
  CT of, 221–223, 223f, 643–644, 644f
  Doppler imaging of, 6, 17–18, 559–560, 559f
  left, 221–223, 223f
  MRI of, 87–88, 226f–227f, 228, 643
  parenchymal, 192
  radiography of, 192–197
  right, 221–223, 223f
  stenosis of, 645, 645f
  velocity profile of, 17–18
Pulmonary venous hypertension, 195–197, 197b,
    198f, 673
Pulmonary venous pressure (pulmonary capillary
    wedge pressure), 195–197
Pulmonic regurgitation
  Doppler echocardiography of, 6
  echocardiography of, 564
  MRI of, 208f, 573, 582f–583f
  quantification of, 575–577
  radiography of, 208f
  after tetralogy of Fallot repair, 207, 208f, 343,
    345f, 573, 582, 582f–583f
Pulmonic stenosis, 674–675
  in carcinoid syndrome, 207, 209f
  CT of, 267f, 674–675, 675f
  Doppler imaging of, 562–563, 563f, 563t
  echocardiography of, 562–563, 563f, 563t
  MRI of, 578, 580f, 674–675
  quantification of, 579–580, 580f
  radiography of, 207, 210f, 267f, 674–675, 675f
  in tetralogy of Fallot, 562–563, 563f
Pulmonic valve
  bicuspid, 601, 601f
  CT of, 218–219
  CTA of, 600–601, 601f
  Doppler measurement of, 16t
  echocardiography of, 562–564
  MRI of, 228, 571, 571b, 571t, 572f
    systematic approach to, 571–573
  papillary fibroelastoma of, 584f
  quadricuspid, 601, 601f
  radiography of, 207, 208f–210f
  tricuspid, 601, 601f
Pulse repetition frequency, in carotid artery duplex
    ultrasound, 687, 688f
Pulse volume recording, 773
  in Raynaud syndrome, 761, 762f
Pulseless disease. *See* Takayasu arteritis/aortitis

Q
Q waves, in myocardial infarction, 445
Quadrilateral space syndrome, 768

R
Radial artery, 262
  for cardiac catheterization, 42–44, 43f, 44t,
    52–54
  catheter angiography of, 263f
  crutch-related injury to, 768–769, 769f
Radial artery graft, 635–636
  palmar collateral imaging for, 769–770, 770f
Radial strain, in left ventricular function assess-
    ment, 12, 16f
Radiation
  arterial effects of, 765, 766f
  CTA-related. *See* Computed tomography angiog-
    raphy (CTA), radiation in
  valvular effects of, 569
Radiofrequency ablation, in atrial fibrillation,
    643–645, 655–656
Radionuclide imaging. *See* Positron emission
    tomography (PET); Single-photon emission
    computed tomography (SPECT)
Radiotracers, in cardiac radionuclide imaging,
    94–95, 107–108, 107t
Rapidly involuting congenital hemangioma, 814,
    814t, 815f, 816–817
Rasmussen aneurysm, 679–680
Rastelli operation, 344f, 349
Raynaud syndrome, 761
Regadenoson, 102, 104
Renal artery
  accessory, 256, 259f
  catheter angiography of, 256, 258f, 750
  CTA of, 256, 258f, 750

Renal artery (Continued)
  Doppler ultrasound of, 115–116, 116f
  in Ehlers-Danlos syndrome, 750–751, 753f
  fibromuscular dysplasia of, 750, 751f
  MRA of, 750
  neurofibromatosis of, 750–751, 753f
  pseudoaneurysm of, 751, 755f
  segmental arterial mediolysis of, 750–751, 752f
  stenosis of, 750, 750f
Renal cell carcinoma
  metastases from, 34, 35f, 653, 653f
  MRA in, 136f
Renal vein(s), 260
  CT of, 261f
  left, compression of. See Nutcracker syndrome
  renal cell cancer of, 136f
  thrombosis of, 789, 790f
  variants of, 261, 261f
Retroperitoneal fibrosis, 745–747, 747f–748f
Reverberation artifact, 23, 687
Rhabdomyoma, 526–527, 529f
Rheumatic disease
  left atrial enlargement in, 201, 204f
  mitral leaflet calcification in, 206
  mitral stenosis in, 597–598
  tricuspid stenosis in, 207–209
Rib notching, in coarctation of aorta, 190–191, 193f
Right atrial appendage, 645–646, 654
  CT of, 215, 216f
  MRI of, 225–226
  radiography of, 179, 180f
  thrombus of, 654
Right atrium, 645–646
  amyloidosis of, 654, 655f
  angiosarcoma of, 202f
  benign tumors of, 651–653, 652f
  CT of, 202f–203f, 215, 268f–270f
  dilatation of, 11–12
  dimensions of, 11–12, 227, 646–647, 646f
  echocardiography of, 28–29, 268f–270f
  enlargement of, 201, 202b, 203f, 646–647, 646f
  fibroelastoma of, 652–653
  fistula of, 654, 655f
  hemangioma of, 652
  lipoma of, 651, 652f
  malignant tumors of, 35f, 653–654
  masses of, 649–654, 650f
  MRI of, 225–227, 226f–227f, 268f–270f
  myxoma of, 651, 652f
  paraganglioma of, 652, 653f
  postoperative, 655–656
  radiography of, 179, 180f, 201, 202f–203f
  renal cancer extension to, 653, 653f
  sarcoma of, 653–654
  size of, 646–647
  thrombus of, 650–651
    echocardiography of, 12f, 33f
    MRI of, 174, 175f, 650–651, 651f
Right gastroepiploic artery graft, 636
Right heart catheterization, 57f
Right internal mammary artery graft, 635, 637f
Right ventricle
  CT of, 216–217, 216f, 268f–270f
  device perforation of, 311
  dilatation of, 7f
  echocardiography of, 6, 7f, 25f, 174, 268f–270f
  vs. left ventricle, 217
  measurement of, 11–12, 15t
  MRI of, 86, 226f–227f, 227–228, 268f–270f
  radiography of, 180f
Right ventricular ejection fraction, in tetralogy of Fallot, 582, 583f
Right ventricular inflow tract (RVIT), echocardiography of, 3–5, 4f, 25f
Right ventricular outflow tract (RVOT), 217
  CT of, 268f–270f
  dimensions of, 11, 15t
  echocardiography of, 5, 25f, 268f–270f
  MRI of, 226f–227f, 227, 268f–270f
  tumor of, 5f
Right ventricular wall thickness, 15t
Ringing artifact, 148, 149f
Ross procedure, 399–400, 400f
  CTA evaluation for, 601, 601f
Rubidium-82, 94–95, 107t

S
St. Jude valve, 284–286, 286f–287f
Saphenous vein, 265, 800
  duplex ultrasound of, 802–804, 803f–804f

Saphenous vein (Continued)
  insufficiency of. See Venous insufficiency
  laser ablation of, 806, 806f
  venography of, 804–805, 805f
Saphenous vein graft, 633–634, 634f–635f
  aneurysm of, 638–639, 640f
  occlusion of, 638, 638f–639f
Sarcoidosis, 364–365, 516–517
  chest radiography of, 516
  CT of, 517
  echocardiography of, 516
  electrocardiography of, 364, 365f
  F-18 FDG PET of, 481, 482f
  MRI of, 364–365, 365f, 462f, 462t, 516, 516f
Sarcoma, 531–533
  CT of, 526, 533, 533f–534f, 653–654, 654f
  echocardiography of, 34, 34f–35f
  metastatic, 586f
  MRI of, 526, 533, 533f
  pulmonary artery, 681, 682f
Sciatic artery, persistent, 263–264, 265f
  aneurysm of, 783, 784f
Scimitar syndrome, 198, 200, 201f, 644, 676, 677f
Sclerotherapy
  in lymphatic malformation, 820–822, 821f–822f
  in vascular malformation, 824–825, 826b, 826f–827f
Segmental arterial mediolysis, 750–751, 752f
Segmental limb pressure test, 773
Seminoma, 748f
Sevelamer, coronary artery calcium and, 378–379
Shone complex, 599–600, 600f
Side lobe artifact, 23
Sigmoid sinus, MRV of, 252f
Simon nitinol filter, 316b, 327, 328f
Single-photon emission computed tomography (SPECT), cardiac, 91–110, 92t, 167. See also Coronary artery disease (CAD); Myocardial infarction (MI); Myocardial ischemia
  ECG-gated, 98, 101f, 106
  false-negative, 167, 168f
  first-pass, 99
  image display in, 106
  interpretation of, 104–106, 106t
  multigated, 99–100, 102f, 106–107
  patient-related factors in, 104
  vs. PET, 98b
  protocols for, 96f, 97–99, 98f, 99t–100t
  quantification of, 106
  radiation exposure with, 436
  radiation risk reduction in, 107–108
  radiotracers in, 94–97, 107t
  scanners for, 91–93, 92f
  software for, 93–94
  stress test, 100–101, 104b, 104t
  troubleshooting in, 104, 105t
Sinoatrial nodal artery, 215, 220f
Sinoatrial node, 215
Sinotubular junction, 11
Sinus venosus, 215
Sinuses of Valsalva, 606
  aneurysm of, 716–717, 717f
  dilation of, 4f
  dimensions of, 15t
  MRI of, 229–230
S.M.A.R.T. stent, 316b, 324, 325f
Smelloff-Cutter ball valve, 280
Sorin Bicarbon valve, 287
Sorin Mitroflow valve, 288–289, 289f
Spasm
  coronary artery, 628, 630f
  coronary artery bypass graft, 637
SPECT. See Single-photon emission computed tomography (SPECT)
Spermatic veins, 260
Spindle cell sarcoma, 653–654, 654f
Splenic artery, 256
  aneurysm of, 751, 753f–754f
Splenic vein, 261–262
Starr-Edwards valve, 280, 281f
Statins, coronary artery calcium and, 377–378
Steal phenomenon. See Subclavian steal phenomenon
Stent, 322–326
  Absolute, 316b, 322, 325f
  carotid Wallstent, 316b, 324–325, 326f
  Express, 316b, 325–326, 326f
  LifeStent, 316b, 322–324, 325f

Stent (Continued)
  migration of, 407
  Palmaz, 316b, 326, 326f
  Protegé, 316b, 322, 324f
  S.M.A.R.T., 316b, 324, 325f
  visceral artery, 753
  Wallstent, 316b, 324, 325f
  Zilver, 316b, 322, 324f
Stent graft, 313–322. See also Thoracic endovascular aortic repair (TEVAR)
  Anaconda, 313–315, 316b, 317f
  Ancure, 316–317, 316b, 319f
  AneuRx, 313, 316b, 316f
  Endologix, 315, 316b, 318f
  Endurant, 313, 315f, 316b
  Excluder, 313, 316b, 316f
  Flair, 316b, 318, 321f
  Fluency, 316b, 317–318, 321f
  Gore TAG thoracic, 316b, 317, 320f
  HeRO, 316b, 322, 324f
  iCAST, 316b, 322, 323f
  Talent abdominal, 313, 315f, 316b
  Talent thoracic, 316b, 317, 320f
  Vanguard, 316, 316b, 319f
  Viabahn, 316b, 318, 321f
  Viabil, 316b, 318, 322f
  Viatorr, 316b, 318, 322f
  WallFlex, 316b, 318–322, 323f
  Zenith abdominal, 313, 314f, 316b
  Zenith thoracic, 316b, 317, 320f
Straight sinus, MRV of, 252, 252f
Strain imaging, in left ventricular function assessment, 12, 16f
Streak artifact, 72, 72f
Stress testing, 169
  CT, 493, 494f
  echocardiographic, 20, 167
    indications for, 167
    exercise vs. pharmacologic, 169–171, 170t
  MRI, 453–456, 454f–456f, 454t
    adenosine for, 453, 455f
    dobutamine for, 82f, 87, 453
    indications for, 455–456
    interpretation of, 455–456, 456f
    vs. SPECT perfusion, 454–455
    vasodilator for, 86–87
  pharmacologic vs. exercise, 169–171, 170t
  radionuclide, 100–101, 103f
    adenosine for, 102, 104
    defect interpretation in, 106, 106t
    dipyridamole for, 102–103
    dobutamine for, 104
    exercise for, 101–104, 104t
    interpretation of, 106
    pharmacologic, 101–104, 104t
    protocols for, 102–104
    regadenoson for, 102, 104
    termination of, 104b
    vasodilator for, 101–102
Stroke, cardiac catheterization and, 54–55
Stroke volume, 14–15
Sturge-Weber syndrome, 819
Subaortic membrane, 553, 554f
Subaortic stenosis, in hypertrophic cardiomyopathy, 581f
Subclavian artery, 262
  left
    aberrant, 706–707, 707f
    CT of, 253–254, 254f
    radiography of, 189f
    compression of, 767–768, 768f
    echocardiography of, 13f
    MRA of, 140, 141f
    MRI of, 226f
    pseudoaneurysm of, 141f
    radiography of, 179, 180f, 182f
    stenosis of, 117–118, 120f, 692, 758–760, 759f
    Takayasu arteritis of, 765f
    transection of, 766–767, 767f
  right
    aberrant, 706
      aneurysm of, 187, 188f, 761–763, 764f
      CT of, 253–254, 255f
      MRA of, 706f
      radiography of, 187, 188f, 706f
    compression of, 767–768, 769f
    stenosis of, 692, 758–760, 760f
    transection of, 766–767

Subclavian steal phenomenon, 118, 120f, 692, 693f, 698, 758, 759f–760f
Subclavian vein, 262–263, 264f
  radiography of, 179, 181f–182f
  thrombosis of, 794–796, 794f–796f
Subscapular artery, catheter angiography of, 263f
Sudden cardiac death
  anomalous coronary arteries and, 239
  coronary artery anomalies and, 607
  coronary artery hypoplasia and, 243–244
  in hypertrophic cardiomyopathy, 361
  I-123 MIBG imaging and, 484–485
  in ischemic cardiomyopathy, 358–361
Sulcus terminalis, 215
Superior sagittal sinus, MRV of, 252, 252f
Superior vena cava, 264f
  CT of, 255, 255f
  left-sided, 181–182, 182f, 230, 255, 255f
    vs. anomalous accessory left innominate vein, 181–182, 182f
  MRI of, 226f, 231
  radiography of, 179, 180f–182f, 181–182
Supracoronary graft, 394–397, 395f, 397f
  dissection with, 397, 397f
  fluid collection with, 395, 396f–397f
  pseudoaneurysm with, 397, 398f
Supraventricular crest, 227, 227f
Swan-Ganz catheter. See Pulmonary artery catheter
Swyer-James syndrome, 198
Syphilitic aortitis, 421, 422f

T
Takayasu arteritis/aortitis, 415–417
  abdominal aorta, 416–417f, 743–745, 746f
  carotid artery, 765f
  CT of, 764, 765f
  CTA of, 415–416, 416f, 710f–711f
  digital subtraction angiography of, 417f
  vs. intramural hematoma, 712
  MRA of, 142f, 415–416, 416f–417f, 764, 765f
  MRI of, 415–416, 418f
  ostial stenosis in, 243, 243f
  PET of, 416–417
  pulmonary artery, 708–709, 711f
  subclavian artery, 765f
  thoracic aorta, 142f, 418f, 708–709, 710f
Takotsubo cardiomyopathy. See Cardiomyopathy, stress (takotsubo)
Talent endograft
  abdominal, 313, 315f, 316b
  thoracic, 316b, 317, 320f
Tamponade. See Cardiac tamponade
TandemHeart, 298–299, 301f
Technetium-99m, 94–95, 107t
Temporal arteritis. See Giant cell arteritis
Tendon of Todaro, 215–216
Teratoma, 527
Terminal groove, 215
Testicular vein, varicocele of, 810, 810f–811f
Tetralogy of Fallot, 341–345
  MRI of, 343–345, 345f, 582, 582f–583f
  pulmonic regurgitation in, 207, 208f, 343, 345f, 582, 582f–583f
  pulmonic stenosis in, 207, 562–563, 563f
  right ventricular function in, 582, 583f
  treatment of, 343, 344f
Thallium-201, 94, 107t
Thebesian valve
  CT of, 215–216, 216f
  MRI of, 225–226, 227f
Thoracic endovascular aortic repair (TEVAR)
  dissection after, 407, 408f
  endograft collapse after, 406, 407f–408f
  endoleaks after, 404–406, 404t
    after dissection repair, 406
    type I, 404, 404f, 404t
    type IA, 404, 404f–405f, 404t, 407f
    type II, 404, 404t, 405f–406f, 408f
    type III, 404–405, 404t
  fistula after, 407–409, 409f
  infection after, 407–409, 419, 421f
  stent migration after, 407
  transient postimplantation syndrome after, 409
Thoracic outlet syndrome, 141f, 767–768, 768f–769f
Thromboangiitis obliterans (Buerger disease), 764–765, 766f, 778
Thrombus
  brachial artery, 766–767, 768f
  carotid artery, 688f

Thrombus (Continued)
  coronary artery bypass graft, 637
  iliofemoral artery, 779–780, 781f
  inferior vena cava, 12f, 182–183, 183f
  intracavitary, 535
    postinfarction, 457, 457f–458f
  left atrial appendage, 30f, 650–651, 651f, 654
  left atrium, 30f, 650–651, 651f
  left ventricle, 7f, 9f, 28f, 535
  left ventricular apex, 7f, 9f, 28f
  mitral valve, 584, 584f
  postinfarction, 457, 457f–458f, 460f
  prosthetic cardiac valve, 291
  right atrial appendage, 654
  right atrium, 535, 650–651
    echocardiography of, 4f, 12f, 33f
    MRI of, 174, 175f, 650–651, 651f
  in single ventricle disorders, 355
  superior mesenteric artery, 747–749, 748f
  thoracic aorta, 24–28, 27f
  tricuspid valve, 4f, 584, 584f
  vs. tumor, 33
  upper extremity artery, 766–767, 767f
  venous, 118. See also Deep venous thrombosis (DVT)
Tibial artery, 263–264, 264f–265f
  angioplasty of, 777, 779f
Tibial vein, thrombosis of, 791f
Toes, microembolization of, 781
Toronto Stentless valve, 290
Total anomalous pulmonary venous return (TAPVR), 644
Transcatheter aortic valve implantation, 308, 309f
Transesophageal echocardiography. See Echocardiography, transesophageal
Transient postimplantation syndrome, 409
Transposition of the great arteries, 345–350
  aortic interruption and, 707–708, 709f
  arch analysis in, 346
  blood flow analysis in, 346
  chamber analysis in, 346
  CT of, 348f, 349–350
  dextro-, 346–350, 348f–349f, 647, 655, 656f
  levo-, 350, 351f, 647
  mediastinal collateral vessels in, 346, 347f
  MRI of, 350
  pulmonary venous analysis in, 346
  septal analysis in, 346
  surgical repair of, 346–349, 348f–349f, 655, 656f
  venous analysis in, 346
Transthoracic echocardiography. See Echocardiography, transthoracic
Transverse sinus, 223
  MRV of, 252–253, 252f
TrapEase filter, 316b, 328, 328f
Tricuspid regurgitation
  annuloplasty for, 209, 211f
  carcinoid-related, 560–561, 561f
  causes of, 209
  Doppler imaging of, 6, 561–562, 562f–563f
  echocardiography of, 3–5, 560–562, 561f–563f, 562f
  etiology of, 560
  giant right atrium in, 646–647, 646f
  MRI of, 573–575
  quantification of, 576–577
Tricuspid stenosis, 207–209
  echocardiography of, 560, 560t
Tricuspid valve
  carcinoid tumor of, 560–561, 561f
  CT of, 218, 268f
  CTA of, 601–603, 602f
  Doppler measurement of, 16t
  Ebstein anomaly of
    CTA of, 602–603, 602f
    echocardiography of, 561, 562f
  echocardiography of, 268f, 560–562
  hemangioma of, 586f
  MRI of, 227, 268f, 571, 571b, 571t, 572f, 584f
    systematic approach to, 571–573
  papillary fibroelastoma of, 561f
  prolapse of, 561
  radiography of, 207–209
  thrombus of, 4f, 584f
  vegetations on, 535, 536f, 564, 565f, 584, 584f
Troponin, in acute coronary syndrome, 383, 446–447
Tuberculous aortitis, 421, 421f
Tufted angioma, 818

Tumor
  cardiac. See also specific tumors
    echocardiography of, 33–34, 174
    metastatic. See Metastatic disease
    MRI of, 90, 174
  carotid body, 691, 692f
  pulmonary artery, 681–682, 682f–683f
  retroperitoneal, 747, 748f
  right ventricular outflow tract, 5f
  vascular, 813–818. See also Hemangioma
Twiddler syndrome, 310

U
Ulcers, atherosclerotic
  of abdominal aorta, 740, 744f
  of thoracic aorta, 714–715, 714f
Ulnar artery, 262
  aneurysm of, 769, 770f
  catheter angiography of, 263f
Ultrasound. See also Echocardiography; Vascular ultrasound
  fetal, rhabdomyoma on, 529f
  intravascular
    coronary, 56, 56f, 165
    iliac vein, 791–792, 792f, 805
Univentricular AV connection, 352
Upper extremity arteries, 758–771
  anatomy of, 262, 263f
  aneurysm of, 761–763, 763f–764f
  atherosclerosis of, 758–760
    arteriovenous fistula and, 758, 759f
    catheter angiography of, 759, 760f
    CTA of, 758–759, 759f
    duplex ultrasound of, 758
    MRA of, 759, 759f
  Buerger disease of, 764–765, 766f
  contrast extravasation injury to, 766–767, 767f
  crutch injury of, 768–769, 769f
  dissection of, 760, 761f
  embolism of, 763, 765f
  fibromuscular dysplasia of, 760–761, 762f
  frostbite of, 761, 763f
  giant cell arteritis of, 764, 766f
  hand-arm vibration syndrome of, 769
  hypothenar hammer syndrome of, 769, 770f
  pseudoaneurysm of, 766–767, 767f
  quadrilateral space syndrome of, 768
  radiation arteritis of, 765, 766f
  Raynaud syndrome of, 761, 762f
  repetitive trauma of, 767–769, 768f–770f
  small vessel arteritis of, 765–766
  Takayasu arteritis of, 764, 765f
  thoracic outlet syndrome of, 767–768, 768f–769f
  trauma to, 766–769, 767f–768f
  vasculitis of, 763–766
    large vessel, 764, 765f–766f
    medium vessel, 764–765, 766f
    small vessel, 765–766
Uterine fibroids, 148f

V
Valvular heart disease. See also at specific heart valves and valvular diseases
  CTA of, 587–605. See also at specific valvular diseases
    optimization of, 587–589
    postprocessing in, 588–589, 589f–591f, 593f–594f
  echocardiography of, 551–570. See also at specific valvular diseases
  imaging in, 172t, 173
  MRI of, 88–89, 89f, 571–586
    in hypertrophic cardiomyopathy, 581–582, 581f–582f
    in masses, 584–585, 584f–586f
    systematic approach to, 571–573, 571b, 571t
    after tetralogy of Fallot repair, 582–584, 582f–583f
  prosthetic valves for. See Prosthetic cardiac valves
  radiation-induced, 569
Vanguard stent graft, 316, 316b, 319f
Varicocele, 810, 810f–811f
Varicose veins. See Venous insufficiency
Vascular malformations, 813, 814t, 818–819. See also Arteriovenous malformation
  in Bannayan Riley-Ruvalcaba syndrome, 833–834
  combined, 814t, 829–834

Vascular malformations (*Continued*)
  in Klippel-Trenaunay syndrome, 829–830, 831f–832f
  in Maffucci syndrome, 833
  in Parkes Weber syndrome, 830–833, 832f–833f
  in proteus syndrome, 834
Vascular system
  anatomy of. *See specific structures*
  angiography of. *See* Catheter angiography; Computed tomography angiography (CTA), vascular; Magnetic resonance angiography (MRA), vascular
  ultrasound of. *See* Vascular ultrasound
Vascular ultrasound, 111–120
  artifacts in, 114, 115t
  B-flow, 113
  Doppler, 111–113, 112f, 118f, 773–775
    artifacts in, 115t
    color, 113, 116f–117f
    continuous wave, 112
    power, 113
    pulsed wave, 112–113
    spectral, 113, 116f–117f, 117
  image optimization in, 113–114
  principles of, 111–113
Vasculitides
  infectious, 419–420
  large vessel, 412–417. *See also* Giant cell arteritis; Takayasu arteritis/aortitis
  medium vessel, 417, 418f
  small vessel, 417–418, 765–766
Vasospasm
  coronary artery, 628, 630f
  coronary artery bypass graft, 637
Vegetations
  aortic valve, 8f, 564, 564f, 603–604, 603f
  CTA of, 603–604
  echocardiography of, 564, 564f–566f
  mitral valve, 564, 565f–566f
  prosthetic valve, 292–295
  tricuspid valve, 535, 536f, 564, 565f, 584, 584f
Vein(s). *See also specific veins*
  lower extremity, 265
  upper extremity, 262–263, 264f
Vein of Marshall, 221
Vena contracta
  in aortic regurgitation, 554
  in mitral regurgitation, 558–559, 558t
Vena Tech filter, 316b, 327, 327f
Venography
  ascending, 787t, 790–791, 791f, 796, 797f, 804–805, 805f
  CT, 129, 787–788, 787t, 789f
  MR, 787t, 788–790, 790f

Venous compression syndromes, 791–799. *See also* May-Thurner syndrome; Nutcracker syndrome; Paget-Schroetter syndrome; Popliteal vein, compression of
Venous contamination, in MRA, 148–150
Venous enhancement, in MRA, 150, 151f
Venous insufficiency, 800–812
  ascending venography of, 804–805, 805f
  classification of, 802, 802f
  CTV of, 804
  definition of, 800, 801f
  duplex ultrasound of, 802–804, 803f–804f
  intravascular ultrasound of, 805
  MRV of, 804, 804f
  pathophysiology of, 801–802
  pelvic, 806–809, 808f–810f
  treatment of, 800, 805–810, 806f–807f
Venous malformations, 822–825
  clinical manifestations of, 822–823, 823f
  hepatic, 823
  MRI of, 823, 824f–825f
  treatment of, 823–825, 826b, 826f–827f
  ultrasound of, 823, 823f
Venous system
  anatomy of, 800
  insufficiency of. *See* Venous insufficiency
  physiology of, 800–801, 801f
  thrombosis of, 118. *See also* Deep venous thrombosis (DVT)
Ventilation-perfusion scintigraphy, in pulmonary embolism, 669
Ventricle. *See also* Left ventricle; Right ventricle
  double inlet, 352
  single, 350–355
    aortopulmonary collateral vessels with, 347f, 355
    arrhythmias with, 355
    hypoxia with, 354–355
    thrombus with, 354f, 355
    treatment of, 352–355, 353f
    venovenous collateral vessels with, 354f, 355
  single inlet, 352
Ventricular assist devices, 299–302
  complications of, 300–302
  imaging of, 300, 301f
Ventricular septal defect (VSD), 341, 657, 658f, 662–665
  acquired, 664–665, 665f
  closure of, 341
  CT of, 341, 342f, 664f–665f
  in dextro-transposition of the great arteries, 347
  Doppler echocardiography of, 22f
  echocardiography of, 22f, 25f, 341
  inflow, 664

Ventricular septal defect (VSD) (*Continued*)
  in levo-transposition of the great arteries, 350
  membranous, 662–663, 664f
  MRI of, 341, 342f, 664f
  muscular, 341, 342f, 663, 664f
  nonrestrictive, 341
  occluder repair in, 303–307, 341
  outlet, 341, 342f
  restrictive, 341
  supracristal, 658f, 663–664, 664f
  traumatic, 664–665, 665f
  treatment of, 665
Ventricular tachycardia, 359–360, 359f
Ventriculography
  left, 50–51, 52f
  radionuclide, 99–100, 102f, 106–107
Vertebral arteries
  CTA of, 248–250, 251f
  Doppler ultrasound of, 118, 120f
  duplex ultrasound of, 685, 686t, 692, 693f
  MRA of, 248–250, 251f
Vertebral veins, 253
Viabahn stent graft, 316b, 318, 321f
Viabil stent graft, 316b, 318, 322f
Viatorr stent graft, 316b, 318, 322f
Visceral artery (arteries)
  aneurysm of, 751, 753f–754f
  arteriovenous malformation of, 752–753, 756f
  fibromuscular dysplasia of, 750, 751f
  neurofibromatosis of, 750–751, 753f
  occlusive disease of, 747–750, 748f
  pseudoaneurysm of, 751, 755f
  segmental mediolysis of, 750–751, 752f
  stents in, 753, 756f

W
Wall motion score, 12
WallFlex stent, 316b, 318–322, 323f
Wallstent, 316b, 324, 325f
  carotid, 316b, 324–325, 326f
Warfarin ridge, MRI of, 227f, 649–650
Warping artifact, in MRA, 152–153, 152f
Watchman device, 307, 307f
Westermark sign, 197, 669, 669f
Wheat procedure. *See* Supracoronary graft
Williams syndrome, 553

Z
Zenith endograft
  abdominal, 313, 314f, 316b
  thoracic, 316b, 317, 320f
Zilver stent, 316b, 322, 324f